mTOR in Human Diseases

Special Issue Editor

Olivier Dormond

MDPI • Basel • Beijing • Wuhan • Barcelona • Belgrade

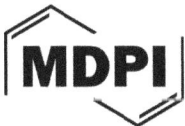

MDPI

Special Issue Editor
Olivier Dormond
Lausanne University Hospital
Switzerland

Editorial Office
MDPI
St. Alban-Anlage 66
4052 Basel, Switzerland

This is a reprint of articles from the Special Issue published online in the open access journal *International Journal of Molecular Sciences* (ISSN 1422-0067) from 2018 to 2019 (available at: https: //www.mdpi.com/journal/ijms/special_issues/mTOR_human)

For citation purposes, cite each article independently as indicated on the article page online and as indicated below:

LastName, A.A.; LastName, B.B.; LastName, C.C. Article Title. *Journal Name* **Year**, *Article Number, Page Range.*

ISBN 978-3-03921-060-2 (Pbk)
ISBN 978-3-03921-061-9 (PDF)

mTOR in Human Diseases

Contents

About the Special Issue Editor

Olivier Dormond, born in Basel, Switzerland, received his medical diploma from the University of Lausanne in 1997. He did his MD-PhD at the CePO in Lausanne from 1998 to 2001. Between 2001 and 2004, he specialized in internal medicine at Lausanne University Hospital. He did a post-doctoral fellowship at Children's Hospital in Boston from 2004 to 2007. Since 2008, he has served as group leader of the research laboratory of the Department of Visceral Surgery at Lausanne University Hospital.

International Journal of
Molecular Sciences

MDPI

Editorial

mTOR in Human Diseases

Olivier Dormond

Department of Visceral Surgery Lausanne University Hospital and University of Lausanne, Pavillon 4, Av de Beaumont, 1011 Lausanne, Switzerland; Olivier.Dormond@chuv.ch

Received: 5 May 2019; Accepted: 9 May 2019; Published: 11 May 2019

The human body regenerates constantly in part under the control of signaling pathways that regulate cell growth. Among these pathways, the mechanistic target of rapamycin (mTOR) has emerged as a major cellular crossroad that links favorable environmental conditions with cell growth. Accordingly, mTOR is implicated in different physiological and pathological conditions, and inhibition of mTOR has been approved for various clinical situations. This special issue "mTOR in human diseases" covers different aspects of the implication of mTOR in physiological processes as well as in various diseases.

The role of mTOR and the consequences of mTOR inhibition has been extensively explored in cancer. Tian et al. review mTOR signaling in solid malignancies and discuss results of clinical trials that have tested mTOR inhibitors in eight different tumors, including lung, colorectal, gastric, renal, bladder, prostate and breast cancers as well as head and neck squamous cell carcinoma [1]. The rationale to target mTOR in advanced biliary tract cancers and in medulloblastoma is also presented by Wu et al. and Aldaregia et al., respectively [2,3]. Besides solid tumors, two reviews highlight the role of mTOR signaling in leukemia and particularly in T-cell acute lymphoblastic leukemia and provide future perspective regarding mTOR-targeting agents [4,5]. All together, these reviews acknowledge the participation of mTOR signaling pathway in tumorigenesis but also highlight the lack of major anti-tumor efficacy of mTOR inhibitors in patients. Limitations include activation of alternate proliferative signaling pathways following mTOR inhibition, tumor heterogeneity and treatment-resistant mTOR mutations. Hence, additional studies are needed to further understand the role of mTOR signaling pathway in cancer and to characterize resistance mechanisms developed by cancer cells to bypass mTOR inhibition. In this context, Tavares et al. present the contribution of mTORC1 and mTORC2 in papillary thyroid carcinoma [6]. Hsu et al. provide results on mTOR in oral cavity squamous cell carcinoma and show the anti-cancer efficacy of the dual PI3K/mTOR inhibitor NVP-BEZ235 [7]. Harachi et al. describe the importance of mTORC1 and mTORC2 in cancer cell metabolism [8]. Identification of biomarkers that predict response to mTOR inhibitors will further help improve the anti-cancer efficacy of these inhibitors. Nepstad et al. found metabolic differences in human acute myeloid leukemia cells between responders and non-responders to mTOR inhibition [9]. Whereas next-generation sequencing is a valuable tool to identify biomarkers, Seeboeck et al. demonstrate, however, that commercially available ready-made gene panels show limited applicability for mTOR pathway-related genes [10]. Besides cancer cells, mTOR signaling pathway regulates cellular processes of non-tumorous cells present in the tumor microenvironment, such as endothelial cells, lymphocytes and macrophages. Conciatori et al. review the role of mTOR in these cells and highlight the anti-cancer benefits that result from mTOR inhibition in the microenvironment [11]. Finally, tumor cachexia is associated with poor prognosis in cancer patients. Emerging evidence suggests that mTOR influences cachexia, as discussed by Duval et al. [12].

Besides cancer, the implication of mTOR signaling pathway in neurological and neuropsychiatric disorders has been demonstrated. Ryskalin et al. present evidence that autophagy impairment is involved in synaptic dysfunction found in some psychiatric disorders, such as schizophrenia. Accordingly, mTOR inhibitors that induce autophagy might represent a therapeutic intervention [13].

Similarly, accelerating autophagic flux appears to be an effective treatment strategy in Parkinson's and Alzheimer's diseases and two reviews present the role of mTOR and the therapeutic opportunities for mTOR inhibitors in these diseases [14,15]. Neurodegenerative diseases are also part of age-related pathologies. Interestingly, recent studies have highlighted mTOR inhibitors as promising treatment for various age-related disorders and are discussed by Walters and Cox [16]. mTOR is further involved in Hutchinson–Gilford progeria syndrome, a rare premature ageing syndrome. Chiarini et al. provide a complete review on the role of mTOR in this disease as well as in other laminopathies and discuss therapeutic opportunities for mTOR inhibitors [17].

Several side effects have been observed in patients treated with mTOR inhibitors. In particular, lung toxicity such as lung fibrosis results in frequent therapy discontinuation. Granata et al. performed mRNA and microRNA profiling on primary bronchial epithelial cells treated or not treated with mTOR inhibitors, which led to the identification of novel potential targets [18]. mTOR inhibitors also reduce male fertility, and the mechanisms controlled by mTOR in the male reproductive tract are presented by Moreira et al. [19]. Toxicities mediated by drugs might also involve mTOR activation. For instance, general anesthetic agents harm brain development. Xu et al. suggest that anesthetic agents-mediated neuron disruption involves upregulation of mTOR activity [20].

Over the last decade, multiple studies have unveiled the complex role played by mTOR signaling pathway in cellular metabolism. Mao and Zhang discuss recent findings on the role of mTOR signaling pathway in metabolic tissues and organs including liver, adipose tissue, muscle and pancreas [21]. Sangüesa et al. highlight the consequences of mTOR activation by excessive consumption of sugar [22]. In addition to cellular metabolism, mTOR regulates autophagy. Wang et al. show that mTOR participates in dopamine receptor D3-mediated autophagy regulation [23]. Finally, Kim et al. found mTOR pathway activation by fluid shear stress and melatonin in preosteoblast cells [24].

In summary, this special issue highlights the fascinating role played by mTOR in cellular processes. It further addresses a non-exhaustive panel of human diseases in which mTOR is implicated, from rare disorders to cancer.

Conflicts of Interest: The author declares no conflict of interest.

References

1. Tian, T.; Li, X.; Zhang, J. Mtor signaling in cancer and mtor inhibitors in solid tumor targeting therapy. *Int. J. Mol. Sci.* **2019**, *20*, 755. [CrossRef]
2. Wu, C.E.; Chen, M.H.; Yeh, C.N. Mtor inhibitors in advanced biliary tract cancers. *Int. J. Mol. Sci.* **2019**, *20*, 500. [CrossRef] [PubMed]
3. Aldaregia, J.; Odriozola, A.; Matheu, A.; Garcia, I. Targeting mtor as a therapeutic approach in medulloblastoma. *Int. J. Mol. Sci.* **2018**, *19*, 1838. [CrossRef] [PubMed]
4. Mirabilii, S.; Ricciardi, M.R.; Piedimonte, M.; Gianfelici, V.; Bianchi, M.P.; Tafuri, A. Biological aspects of mtor in leukemia. *Int. J. Mol. Sci.* **2018**, *19*, 2396. [CrossRef] [PubMed]
5. Evangelisti, C.; Chiarini, F.; McCubrey, J.A.; Martelli, A.M. Therapeutic targeting of mtor in t-cell acute lymphoblastic leukemia: An update. *Int. J. Mol. Sci.* **2018**, *19*, 1878. [CrossRef]
6. Tavares, C.; Eloy, C.; Melo, M.; Gaspar da Rocha, A.; Pestana, A.; Batista, R.; Bueno Ferreira, L.; Rios, E.; Sobrinho Simoes, M.; Soares, P. Mtor pathway in papillary thyroid carcinoma: Different contributions of mtorc1 and mtorc2 complexes for tumor behavior and slc5a5 mrna expression. *Int. J. Mol. Sci.* **2018**, *19*, 1448. [CrossRef] [PubMed]
7. Hsu, C.M.; Lin, P.M.; Lin, H.C.; Tsai, Y.T.; Tsai, M.S.; Li, S.H.; Wu, C.Y.; Yang, Y.H.; Lin, S.F.; Yang, M.Y. Nvp-bez235 attenuated cell proliferation and migration in the squamous cell carcinoma of oral cavities and p70s6k inhibition mimics its effect. *Int. J. Mol. Sci.* **2018**, *19*, 3546. [CrossRef] [PubMed]
8. Harachi, M.; Masui, K.; Okamura, Y.; Tsukui, R.; Mischel, P.S.; Shibata, N. Mtor complexes as a nutrient sensor for driving cancer progression. *Int. J. Mol. Sci.* **2018**, *19*, 3267. [CrossRef]

9. Nepstad, I.; Reikvam, H.; Brenner, A.K.; Bruserud, O.; Hatfield, K.J. Resistance to the antiproliferative in vitro effect of pi3k-akt-mtor inhibition in primary human acute myeloid leukemia cells is associated with altered cell metabolism. *Int. J. Mol. Sci.* **2018**, *19*, 382. [CrossRef]
10. Seeboeck, R.; Sarne, V.; Haybaeck, J. Current coverage of the mtor pathway by next-generation sequencing oncology panels. *Int. J. Mol. Sci.* **2019**, *20*, 690. [CrossRef] [PubMed]
11. Conciatori, F.; Bazzichetto, C.; Falcone, I.; Pilotto, S.; Bria, E.; Cognetti, F.; Milella, M.; Ciuffreda, L. Role of mtor signaling in tumor microenvironment: An overview. *Int. J. Mol. Sci.* **2018**, *19*, 2453. [CrossRef]
12. Duval, A.P.; Jeanneret, C.; Santoro, T.; Dormond, O. Mtor and tumor cachexia. *Int. J. Mol. Sci.* **2018**, *19*, 2225. [CrossRef]
13. Ryskalin, L.; Limanaqi, F.; Frati, A.; Busceti, C.L.; Fornai, F. Mtor-related brain dysfunctions in neuropsychiatric disorders. *Int. J. Mol. Sci.* **2018**, *19*, 2226. [CrossRef]
14. Zhu, Z.; Yang, C.; Iyaswamy, A.; Krishnamoorthi, S.; Sreenivasmurthy, S.G.; Liu, J.; Wang, Z.; Tong, B.C.; Song, J.; Lu, J.; et al. Balancing mtor signaling and autophagy in the treatment of parkinson's disease. *Int. J. Mol. Sci.* **2019**, *20*, 728. [CrossRef]
15. Kou, X.; Chen, D.; Chen, N. Physical activity alleviates cognitive dysfunction of alzheimer's disease through regulating the mtor signaling pathway. *Int. J. Mol. Sci.* **2019**, *20*, 1591. [CrossRef] [PubMed]
16. Walters, H.E.; Cox, L.S. Mtorc inhibitors as broad-spectrum therapeutics for age-related diseases. *Int. J. Mol. Sci.* **2018**, *19*, 2325. [CrossRef] [PubMed]
17. Chiarini, F.; Evangelisti, C.; Cenni, V.; Fazio, A.; Paganelli, F.; Martelli, A.M.; Lattanzi, G. The cutting edge: The role of mtor signaling in laminopathies. *Int. J. Mol. Sci.* **2019**, *20*, 847. [CrossRef]
18. Granata, S.; Santoro, G.; Masola, V.; Tomei, P.; Sallustio, F.; Pontrelli, P.; Accetturo, M.; Antonucci, N.; Carratu, P.; Lupo, A.; et al. In vitro identification of new transcriptomic and mirnomic profiles associated with pulmonary fibrosis induced by high doses everolimus: Looking for new pathogenetic markers and therapeutic targets. *Int. J. Mol. Sci.* **2018**, *19*, 1250. [CrossRef] [PubMed]
19. Moreira, B.P.; Oliveira, P.F.; Alves, M.G. Molecular mechanisms controlled by mtor in male reproductive system. *Int. J. Mol. Sci.* **2019**, *20*, 1633. [CrossRef] [PubMed]
20. Xu, J.; Mathena, R.P.; Xu, M.; Wang, Y.; Chang, C.; Fang, Y.; Zhang, P.; Mintz, C.D. Early developmental exposure to general anesthetic agents in primary neuron culture disrupts synapse formation via actions on the mtor pathway. *Int. J. Mol. Sci.* **2018**, *19*, 2183. [CrossRef]
21. Mao, Z.; Zhang, W. Role of mtor in glucose and lipid metabolism. *Int. J. Mol. Sci.* **2018**, *19*, 2043. [CrossRef] [PubMed]
22. Sanguesa, G.; Roglans, N.; Baena, M.; Velazquez, A.M.; Laguna, J.C.; Alegret, M. Mtor is a key protein involved in the metabolic effects of simple sugars. *Int. J. Mol. Sci.* **2019**, *20*, 1117. [CrossRef] [PubMed]
23. Wang, D.; Ji, X.; Liu, J.; Li, Z.; Zhang, X. Dopamine receptor subtypes differentially regulate autophagy. *Int. J. Mol. Sci.* **2018**, *19*, 1540. [CrossRef] [PubMed]
24. Kim, C.H.; Jeung, E.B.; Yoo, Y.M. Combined fluid shear stress and melatonin enhances the erk/akt/mtor signal in cilia-less mc3t3-e1 preosteoblast cells. *Int. J. Mol. Sci.* **2018**, *19*, 2929. [CrossRef]

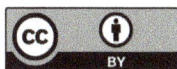

International Journal of
Molecular Sciences

MDPI

Review

mTOR Signaling in Cancer and mTOR Inhibitors in Solid Tumor Targeting Therapy

Tian Tian, Xiaoyi Li and Jinhua Zhang *

College of Life Science and Bioengineering, Beijing Jiaotong University, Beijing 100044, China;
ttian@bjtu.edu.cn (T.T.); 15271074@bjtu.edu.cn (X.L.)
* Correspondence: zhangjh@bjtu.edu.cn; Tel./Fax: +86-10-51684351

Received: 10 January 2019; Accepted: 1 February 2019; Published: 11 February 2019

Abstract: The mammalian or mechanistic target of rapamycin (mTOR) pathway plays a crucial role in regulation of cell survival, metabolism, growth and protein synthesis in response to upstream signals in both normal physiological and pathological conditions, especially in cancer. Aberrant mTOR signaling resulting from genetic alterations from different levels of the signal cascade is commonly observed in various types of cancers. Upon hyperactivation, mTOR signaling promotes cell proliferation and metabolism that contribute to tumor initiation and progression. In addition, mTOR also negatively regulates autophagy via different ways. We discuss mTOR signaling and its key upstream and downstream factors, the specific genetic changes in the mTOR pathway and the inhibitors of mTOR applied as therapeutic strategies in eight solid tumors. Although monotherapy and combination therapy with mTOR inhibitors have been extensively applied in preclinical and clinical trials in various cancer types, innovative therapies with better efficacy and less drug resistance are still in great need, and new biomarkers and deep sequencing technologies will facilitate these mTOR targeting drugs benefit the cancer patients in personalized therapy.

Keywords: mTOR; PI3K; cancer; inhibitor; therapy

---

1. Introduction

The mammalian or mechanistic target of rapamycin (mTOR) is a serine/threonine kinase that acts through two structurally and functionally distinct protein complexes, mTOR complex 1 (mTORC1) and mTOR complex 2 (mTORC2), to sense and integrate multiple intracellular and environmental signals [1,2]. mTOR signaling is generally involved in regulating cell survival, cell growth, cell metabolism, protein synthesis and autophagy, as well as homeostasis [3]. The pathological relevance of dysregulation of mTOR signal is illustrated in many human diseases, especially the multitude of different human cancers. As reported, mTOR is aberrantly overactivated in more than 70% of cancers [4]. Over the past few years, it has been extensively demonstrated in animal models and clinical patients of cancer that mTOR dysfunction contributes to tumorigenesis [5].

Since the mTOR pathway regulates many basic biological and physiological processes such as cell proliferation, survival and autophagy, it is logical that components in the mTOR pathway are among the most frequently mutated genes in cancers [6]. The regulation of mTOR pathway is also influenced by its positive and negative regulators that have cross talk with mTOR, such as the phosphoinositide 3-kinase (PI3K)/Akt, mitogen activated protein kinase (MAPK), vascular endothelial growth factor (VEGF), nuclear factor-κB (NF-κB), and p53 etc., which comprise a much more complicated signaling cascade [7].

Several types of mTOR inhibitors such as rapamycin, its rapalogs and mTORC1/2 kinase inhibitors have been examined in various cancer models, including breast cancer, lung cancer, gastric carcinoma, colorectal cancer, prostate cancer, head and neck cancer, gynecologic cancer, glioblastoma, lymphoma, urinary bladder cancer, renal cancer and medulloblastoma, etc. However, the effects of mTOR inhibitors utilized as monotherapy in cancer are sometimes dampened by several resistance mechanisms [8]. Combined therapies with mTOR inhibitors and other pathway inhibitors or conventional therapies are under investigation in preclinical and clinical trials in different tumor types. Hence, novel therapeutic strategies based on mTOR inhibition still need to be developed.

2. mTOR (The mammalian or mechanistic target of rapamycin) Signaling in Cancer

2.1. mTORC1 and mTORC2

mTOR is a serine/threonine kinase, which is attributed to the phosphoinositide 3-kinase related protein kinase (PIKK) super family, and was first discovered from a genetic screening for rapamycin-resistant mutations in yeast *Saccharomyces cerevisiase* [9,10]. In mammalian cells, mTOR mainly acts through its two evolutionarily conserved complexes, mTORC1 and mTORC2, which share some common subunits, such as the mTOR kinase, the mammalian lethal with SEC13 protein 8 (mLST8), dishevelled, EGL-10 and pleckstrin (DEP) domain-containing mTOR-interacting protein (DEPTOR), telomere maintenance 2 (Tel2) and Tel2-interacting protein 1(Tti1) complex as shown in Figure 1.

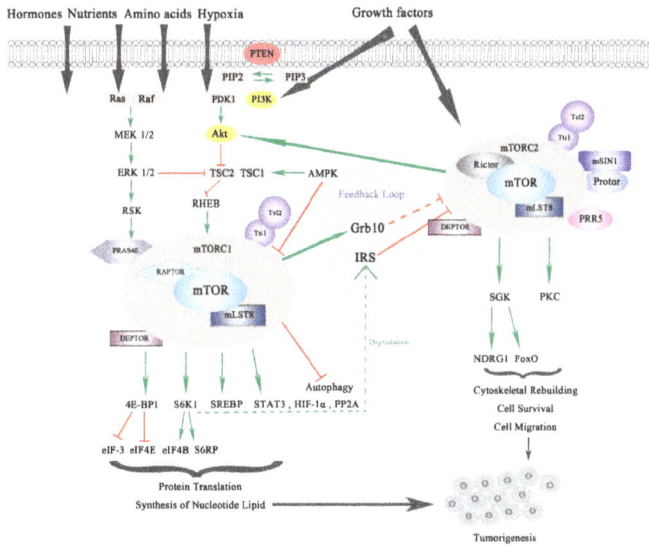

Figure 1. The mammalian or mechanistic target of rapamycin (mTOR) complexes and signaling pathway of mTORC1 and mTORC2. mTORC1 is responsive to nutrients, hormones, amino acids, hypoxia and growth factors, while mTORC2 responds to growth factors. mTORC1 and mTORC2 share common subunits of mTOR kinase, mLST8, DEPTOR (DEP domain-containing mTOR-interacting protein), Tel 2 and Tti 1. mTORC1 additionally binds with RAPTOR (Regulatory-associated protein of mTOR) and PRAS40 (Proline-rich substrate of 40 kDa), and mTORC2 combines with RICTOR and mSIN1 (Mammalian stress-activated protein kinase interacting protein 1) as well as Protor and PRR5 (Proline-rich protein 5). mTORC1 is regulated by PI3K/Akt (Phosphoinositide 3-kinase/serine-threonine protein kinase) and Ras-MAPK (Mitogen activated protein kinase) signaling pathways. mTORC1 regulates protein translation and synthesis of nucleotide lipid via 4E-BP1 and S6K1 and downstream effectors. mTORC1 also activates STAT3 (Signal transducer and activator of transcription), HIF-1α (Hypoxia-inducible factor 1α) and PP2A (Protein phosphatase 2A) in tumorigenesis. mTORC2 regulates SGK (Serum glucose kinase) and PKC (Protein kinase C) to promote cell survival, cytoskeleton reorganization and cell migration. mTORC2 is negatively modulated by mTORC1 via different feedback loops mediated by IRS (insulin receptor substrate) or Grb10. mTORC1 and mTORC2 can both contribute to turmorigenesis through different mechanisms [7,11].

mTORC1 and mTORC2 are different in the aspects of rapamycin sensitivity, specific binding components, subcellular localization, downstream substrates, and regulation [12]. mTORC1 is sensitive to rapamycin whereas mTORC2 is comparatively resistant to rapamycin [13]. In addition to the common binding subunits, mTORC1 and mTORC2 respectively harbor distinct components that contribute to the specificity of substrates, different subcellular localization, and specific regulation. mTORC1 also contains the regulatory-associated protein of mTOR (RAPTOR), which is a significant scaffolding protein in the mTORC1 assembly and its stability and regulation, and proline-rich substrate of 40 kDa (PRAS40) is a negative regulator of mTORC1 by releasing mTORC1 inhibition upon the activation of growth factors [14,15]. mTORC2 uniquely contains rapamycin-insensitive companion of mTOR (RICTOR) and the mammalian stress-activated protein kinase interacting protein 1 (mSIN1), both of which can mutually affect their protein levels and stabilize each other. Previous research has demonstrated that RICTOR is a scaffolding protein essential for the assembly, stability, substrate recognition, and subcellular localization activation of mTORC2. In addition, mSIN1, which is essential for plasma membrane localization of mTORC2, negatively regulates mTORC2 kinase activity [16,17]. Newly discovered interactors include Protein observed with RICTOR 1/2 (Protor-1/2), which are required for mTORC2 assembly and catalytic process, and Proline-Rich Protein (PRR) 5, which is necessary for mTOR activity and mTOR–RICTOR binding [18,19].

mTORC1 and mTORC2 have differing subcellular localization binding with their own respective, specific subunits, which also determine their distinct functions and independent regulations. mTORC1 is associated with endosomal and lysosomal membranes, where it interacts with its effectors. mTORC2 is affiliated with the plasma membrane, as well as ribosomal membranes, where it binds with its key substrasts, AGC family kinases (subgroup of Ser/Thr protein kinases named after 3 representative families, the cAMP-dependent protein kinase (PKA), the cGMP-dependent protein kinase (PKG) and the protein kinase C (PKC) families), such as serum glucose kinase (SGK) isoforms and protein kinase C (PKC), which are essential for mTORC2 activation [20]. Both mTORC1 and mTORC2 play significant and differing roles in a variety of intracellular processes. They are regulated by various endogenous and exogenous stimuli, such as nutrients, growth factors, energy, hormones and hypoxia, and they can also affect glucose metabolism through different physiological mechanisms [1,21–23]. Generally, mTORC1 can phosphorylate its downstream effectors, such as eukaryotic translation initiation factor 4E binding protein 1 (4EBP1), S6 kinase (S6K), and sterol regulatory element-binding protein (SREBP), to motivate protein translation, synthesis of nucleotides and lipids, biogenesis of lysosomes, and to suppress the process of autophagy [24]. On the other hand, mTORC2 is more sensitive to extracellular growth factors though the molecular mechanism remains to be elucidated [25]. Upon activation, mTORC2 phosphorylates its downstream targets SGK and PKC, as mentioned previously, to intensify the signaling cascade [26]. mTORC2 mainly increases cytoskeletal rebuilding and cell migration, inhibits apoptosis and affects metabolism [27] (as shown in Figure 1).

2.2. Signaling of mTORC1

The mTOR signaling pathway is crucial in cell growth, proliferation and metabolism. mTORC1 is regulated by several signaling pathways including the PI3K/Akt pathway, the Ras-MAPK pathway, and some other intracellular factors (see Figure 1).

Activation of mTORC1 is primarily dependent on the PI3K/AKT pathway to respond to oncogenic growth factors or insulin [28]. Even though the second messenger phosphatidylinositol (3,4,5)-triphosphate (PIP3) binds and activates mTORC2 directly, mTORC1 can also be indirectly activated by PI3K through Akt. Akt is activated by phosphorylation at Ser473 by mTORC2 and at Thr308 by another serine-threonie kinase PDK1 (Phosphoinositide-dependent Kinase 1). Then, phosphorylation of tuberous sclerosis complex 2 (TSC2) by active Akt results in blockage of TSC2 and TSC1 combination [29–31]. The activator of mTORC1, Ras homolog enriched in brain (RHEB), which is negatively regulated by TSC1/2, is released by TSC to allow the activation of mTORC1 in lysosomes [32]. In addition, AKT can activate mTORC1 by phosphorylating and dissociating the inhibitor PRAS40 from RAPTOR independent of TSC1/2 [33].

Moreover, TSC2 can also be phosphorylated by extracellular signal-regulated kinases (ERKs) and ribosomal protein S6 kinase (RSK) from the Ras-MAPK signaling pathway, which results in inhibiting TSC1/2 and promoting RHEB-mediated mTORC1 activation. In addition, similar to AKT, PRAS40 can also be phosphorylated by RSK to release RAPTOR and activate mTORC1 [34–36].

mTORC1 is also responsive to fluctuations of cellular factors such as DNA damage, intracellular adenosine triphosphate (ATP), glucose, amino acids, and oxygen. Several signaling pathways that are responsive to DNA damage suppress mTORC1 via p53 target genes, leading to TSC2 activation: for example, $5'$-AMP activated protein kinase β (AMPKβ) and phosphatase and tensin homolog on chromosome 10 (PTEN) [37]. Upon energy exhaustion, AMP kinase (AMPK), which is activated by low ATP/high AMP levels, promotes TSC1/2 complex formation and phosphorylates RAPTOR, leading to indirect inhibition of mTORC1 [38]. This outcome also implies that in a situation of energy shortage, AMP accumulation will cover the growth factor signals and suppress cellular replication. Through a sensing signal cascade of amino acids, mTORC1 can be positively regulated by amino acids, activation of which motivates the Rag complex to combine with RAPTOR. Along with this process, mTORC1 is recruited to the lysosomal surface [39,40]. Rag-GTPase, which is associated with RAPTOR and localizes mTORC1 to lysosomal membranes, is especially activated by arginine in lysosomes or by leucine in the cytoplasm [41–44].

Once activated, mTORC1 will transfer the signal to downstream effectors, such as 4EBP1 and S6K1, both of which are essential modulators of cap-dependent and cap-independent translation. After phosphorylation of 4EBP1 and S6K1 by mTORC1, the binding partners, eukaryotic initiation factor (eIF)-4E and eukaryotic initiation factor-3 (eIF-3), will be respectively liberated, facilitating initiating complex formation for translation and intensifying ribosome genesis [45]. In the following signal cascade, eIF-4E will form the eIF-4F complex and increase protein translation, which is significant for the G1-S phase transition. Upon low mTORC1 activity, 4E-BP1 is dephosphorylated, and protein translation is inhibited [46]. On the other side, eIF-4B and S6 ribosomal protein (S6RP) are phosphorylated by S6K1, which initiates protein translation and continues translation elongation [47,48]. Actually, mTORC1-related signals seem to prefer to affect the translation of oncogenic proteins involved in protein synthesis, invasion and metastasis [49]. Moreover, mTORC1 also regulates some other proteins such as hypoxia-inducible factor 1α (HIF-1α), protein phosphatase 2A (PP2A), glycogen synthase, and signal transducer and activator of transcription (STAT) 3, through which mTORC1 promotes biosynthesis of proteins, lipids and nucleotides in aberrant cells, tissue and organism growth in cancer [2,50–54].

In brief, mTORC1 activation induces cap-dependent translation that leads to increases in cell size and proliferation, which are two typical characteristics of cancer [55,56].

2.3. Signaling of mTORC2

Although the regulatory mechanism of mTORC1 is well depicted, the regulators of mTORC2 are much less characterized. This is partly due to the difficulties in teasing apart the functional differences between mTORC1 and mTORC2 [13]. As we mentioned previously, through mSIN1, mTORC2 localizes at the plasma membrane where it binds with its substrates Akt, SGK and PKC. Notably, the localization of mTORC2 is significant for its regulation [16] (see Figure 1).

First, mSIN1 regulates mTORC2 depending on different mechanisms. mTORC2-Akt signaling can be sustained by a positive feedback loop from mSIN1 phosphorylation of Akt, whereas mSIN 1 phosphorylation by S6K1 at the same site suppresses mTORC2 activity [57–59]. On the other hand, recent research found that mSIN1 can also combine with Rb in the cytoplasm, which results in the inhibition of mTORC2 complex formation and Akt signaling [60].

Likewise, mTORC2 is regulated by PI3K/Akt, as well as by mTORC1 itself. PI3K activates mTORC2 to bind to ribosomes both in normal physiological and pathological conditions, such as cancer [61]. Akt, which is commonly found to be hyperactive in cancers, is an important substrate of mTORC2. Akt aggregates signals from PI3K/mTORC2 and PI3K/PDK1 to accelerate cell proliferation. Localization of Akt to the plasma membrane is regulated by PIP3, which is similar to mTORC2. Akt also activates mTORC1 signaling in addition to mTORC2, leading to a more complicated signal network [29]. In addition, mTORC2 is negatively modulated by mTORC1 via feedback loops. For example, the S6K1 promotes insulin receptor substrate (IRS) 1/2 degradation resulting in inhibition of mTORC2 and the PI3K/Akt pathway. Another feedback mechanism is through growth factor receptor-bound protein 10 (Grb10), which is positively modulated by mTORC1 [62–64].

For downstream effectors, serum and glucocorticoid kinase (SGK) and protein kinase C (PKC) are two key phosphorylation substrates of mTORC2. SGK substrates include N-myc downstream-regulated gene 1 protein (NDRG1) and Forkhead box family transcription factors (FoxO), which promote cell survival under oxygen or nutrient depletion conditions or in response to PI3K inhibition [65,66]. Through phosphorylation of different PKC family members, mTORC2 is reported to regulate cytoskeleton reorganization and cell movements involved in tumorigenesis [17,25,67,68] (See Figure 1).

2.4. mTOR Signaling in Cancer

Since mTOR signaling regulates fundamental activities including cell cycle, proliferation, growth, and survival, as well as protein synthesis and glucose metabolism, there is no doubt that mTOR has a close association with cancer. As reported, mTOR signaling is enhanced in various types of cancers. Data in solid tumors demonstrated that the mTOR signal is dysregulated in almost 30% of cancers and is one of the most frequently affected cascades in human cancers [69].

Activation of mTOR signaling in cancer mainly depends on three different levels of mechanisms: first, mutations in the mTOR gene lead to a constitutively hyperactive mTOR signaling cascade; second, mutations in the components of mTORC1 and mTORC2 result in activation of mTOR signaling; and lastly but most importantly, aberrant mTOR signaling can also result from mutations in upstream genes, that is, loss-of- function mutations in suppressor genes and gain-of-function mutations in oncogenes [7]. We discuss these mechanisms in the following text.

Mutation of mTOR, which is the core gene of the mTOR signaling and encodes the kinase, will directly lead to hyperactivation of mTOR signaling. A study utilizing public tumor genome sequencing data in 2014 reported that 33 mTOR mutations were found to contribute to the hyperactivation of mTOR signaling in various cancer types. Most of these mutations assemble in six different regions of the c-terminal region of mTOR in several cancer types, and one is specifically abundant in kidney cancer, all of which maintain the sensitivity to mTOR inhibition by pharmacological therapies [70].

Moreover, genetic aberrations in components of mTOR complexes are reported to have a close relationship with cancer. RICTOR, a component of mTORC2, was found to be amplified in beast cancer, non-small cell lung cancer (NSCLC), and particularly in squamous cell lung carcinoma (SQCLC), in which RICTOR amplification is significantly related to poor prognosis and short survival [71–73]. Overexpression of RICTOR was also observed in gliomas with high Akt activity in nearly 70% of patients and HER2 (human epidermal growth factor receptor-2)-positive breast cancers, leading to Akt hyperactivity and tumor aggravation [72,74].

Except for the above, mTOR signaling hyper-activation can commonly result from mutations of upstream genes including oncogenes and tumor suppressor genes [75]. The PI3K signaling pathway, which is upstream of both mTOR complexes, often has various kinds of mutations of its components in cancer, such as mutation and amplification of Akt and of PIK3CA and amplification of growth factor receptors, Epidermal Growth Factor Receptor (EGFR) and insulin growth factor receptor (IGFR) [76–78]. Since PI3K and RAS are two parallel pathways, amplification of growth factor receptors that are upstream of either signal can also result in abnormal signal transduction on both mTOR complexes [6]. Furthermore, loss of functions in tumor suppressor genes, such as PTEN, p53, TSC1/TSC2 and Serine Threonine Kinase 11 (STK11), all contribute to mTOR activation in the pathological state of cancer [79]. PTEN, which is the second most frequently mutated gene after p53 in human cancer, can be downregulated through mutation, methylation, protein instability and intracellular localization [80]. Aberrations in the PTEN genes also influence cancer cells in myeloma, breast cancer and endometrium cancer, which are sensitive to mTOR inhibitors [81–84]. Inactivation of TSC1 or TSC2, which are negative regulators of mTORC1, is responsible for Tuberous Sclerosis and leads to benign tumor genesis. This also demonstrates that mTORC1 serves as a potent driver of cell proliferation. Mutations of TSC1 and TSC2 are reported in bladder cancer, urothelial carcinoma, clear cell renal carcinoma and well-differentiated pancreatic neuroendocrine tumors [85–87]. Actually, mutations in TSC1, TSC2 and mTOR are much less frequent than those in components that are higher upstream in the signaling pathway.

mTOR signaling mainly regulates cell proliferation and metabolism involved in tumor initiation and progression. As reported, at the level of 4E-BP1/eIF-4E, dysregulation of protein synthesis downstream of mTORC1 play a central role in tumorigenesis. eIF-4E promotes the translation of specific pro-oncogenic proteins that regulate cell survival, cell cycle progression, angiogenesis, energy metabolism, and metastasis. Besides, mTOR activation also leads to increased ribosome biogenesis, providing machinery to maintain high levels of cell growth [1]. In cancer cells, metabolism seems to reprogram to sustain the demands of rapid cell growth. mTOR complex is recently depicted as a nutrient sensor in metabolism of cancer, especially on glucose and amino acid, nucleotide, fatty acid and lipid, growth factors and other stresses. Nutrient sensing mainly activates mTORC1 and the metabolic changes in cancer cells sustain mTOC1 activation in turn [2,22,23,88]. In glucose metabolism, mTORC1 can enhance the translation of two key transcription factors, hypoxia inducible factor (HIF)-1α and Myc, which drive expression of a variety of glycolytic enzymes to regulate glycolysis [89–91]. mTORC2 can also increase glucose metabolism through its downstream effector AKT [92]. For lipid synthesis, mTORC1 activates the critical transcription factor sterol regulatory element-binding protein 1 (SRE-BP1) driving gene transcription in lipid synthesis via Akt activation and phosphorylation of Lipin1 and S6K1 [93,94]. The increased levels of SRE-BP mRNA and protein are associated with mTORC1 upregulation in human breast cancer tissues [95]. In addition, purine and pyrimidine synthesis, which is significant for cancer cell DNA replication, can also be promoted by mTORC1 via S6K1 phosphorylation [96,97].

Moreover, mTOR is involved in the regulation of autophagy, a process that degrades and recycles cytosolic components in response to a shortage of nutrients and energy. Autophagy is commonly regarded as an inhibition process against tumorigenesis, and blockage of autophagy contributes to cancer initiation [98]. However, some conflicting research results have demonstrated that autophagy may play a dual role in cancer development under specific conditions: for example, it is dependent on different P53 status in pancreatic cancer [99–101]. mTORC1 is reported to inactivate UNC-5-like autophagy-activating kinase 1 (ULK1) by phosphorylation resulting in failure to form ULK1-ATG13-FIP200 complex, which is required for autophagy initiation [102–104], while mTORC2 can inhibit autophagy indirectly by activating mTORC1. mTORC1 also regulates autophagy at the transcription level by modulating a key transcription factor, Transcription Factor EB (TFEB), for genes in lysosomes and autophagy [105]. Moreover, mTORC1 is likely to affect autophagy through some other ways such as the death-associated protein 1 (DAP1) which suppresses autophagy, WD repeat domain phophoinositide-interacting protein 2 (WIPI2) and a mammalian ortholog of Atg18 [23].

3. mTOR Inhibitors in Therapies of Different Types of Cancer

As stated above, the mTOR signaling pathway plays a central role in cancer initiation and progression, and is the second most frequently altered pathway after the p53 pathway in human cancers [106]. Therapies utilizing mTOR inhibitors have been developed to reduce the high mTOR signaling levels in various cancer types.

Rapamycin, which lead to mTOR discovery of mTOR in the target screening, is the original inhibitor of mTOR. Rapamycin binds to FK506 Binding Protein 12 (FKBP12), resulting in the unbinding

RAPTOR from mTORC1. In addition, the downstream effect is inactivation of S6K1 and 4E-BP1 by inhibiting phosphorylation, which leads to a decrease in protein synthesis and cell cycle arrest in the G1 phase [107]. Rapamycin also negatively regulates VEGF, platelet-derived growth factor (PDGF), basic fibroblast growth factor (bFGF) and so on, which are transcriptional targets of hypoxia-inducible factor 1α (HIF-1α) and contribute to vascular development and cancer progression [108]. Moreover, rapamycin can act indirectly on mTORC2 also by binding FKBP12, leading to dissociation of RICTOR from mTOR, thus decreasing the levels of mTORC2 and possibly in a specific cell type [13,109]. Due to poor solubility and undeterminate kinetic and pharmacological properties of rapamycin, a series of allosteric mTOR inhibitors (named rapalogs) have been developed to achieve better efficacy in patients [110]. Four rapalogs of rapamycin: temsirolimus (by intravenous administration), everolimus and ridaforolimus (by oral administration) and ABI-009 (nanoparticle albumin-bound-rapamycin) have been applied in monotherapy or combination therapies in a variety of cancer types in different phases of clinical trials [111]. Apart from rapalogs, ATP competitive inhibitors, such as vistusertib (AZD2014), AZD8055, CC-223 and OSI027 that suppress mTORC1 and mTOR2 kinase simultaneously, and PI3K/mTOR dual inhibitors might result in improved anticancer effect in preclinical and clinical studies [112]. Several potential biomarkers, including PIK3CA and PTEN mutation status, AKT activity, and other members of the mTOR pathway, have also been explored according to preclinical results and clinical data.

In the following parts of our review, we focus on the alterations of mTOR signaling in eight different types of solid tumors and applications of various mTOR inhibitors in therapeutic strategies in these specific tumors.

3.1. Lung Cancer

In non-small cell carcinomas (NSCLC), PI3K pathway activation is found in 50–70% of patients with AKT phosphorylation [113]. Mutations in EGFR, Kirsten rat sarcoma viral oncogene (KRAS), PI3K, amplification of PIK3CA and loss of PTEN can lead to PI3K pathway activation [114]. As reported by The Cancer Genome Atlas (TCGA) Research Group, alterations in the PI3K/Akt pathway, which is upstream of mTOR signaling, were detected in 47% of squamous cancers (including *PIK3CA* alterations in 16%, *PTEN* alterations in 15%, *AKT3* alterations in 16%, *AKT2* alterations in 4% and *AKT1* alterations < 1% of the total samples) [114]. Actually, genomic amplification is much more frequent than somatic mutations in *PI3KCA* in lung cancers. In addition, *PI3KCA* was found to have copy number amplifications in 33% of squamous cell lung carcinomas, which occurred independently of the *PI3KCA* gene mutation, demonstrating that each event is probably sufficient to initiate tumorigenesis. Besides, in a report of 51 Japanese small cell lung cancinoma (SCLC) patients, 36% of the tumors had genetic mutations related with mTOR pathway [115]. Phophorylated mTOR is demonstrated to contribute to SCLC progression [116].

Although some reports indicated that expression of mTOR/phosphorylated-mTOR (p-mTOR) has no significant association with prognosis in NSCLC patients [117], mTOR inhibitors including everolimus, temsirolimus, and ridaforolimus have been extensively applied in NSCLC patients in clinical trials. Although both everolimus and ridaforolimus demonstrated promise in phase I studies, neither of them achieved such promising results in phase II studies in NSCLC patients due to toxicity of these traditional mTOR inhibitors [118–120]. Everolimus either combined with chemotherapy (CT) or radiotherapy also showed non-significant results in NSCLC patients [121,122]. A phase II study in advanced NSCLC patients treated with chemotherapy (CT) or CT and EGFR inhibitors demonstrated that everolimus at a dose of 10 mg/day achieved a response rate of 4.7% and a disease control rate of 47.1% [123]. Another phase II clinical trial of everolimus (5 mg/day) combined with the EGFR inhibitor gefitinib (250 mg/day) in 62 advanced NSCLC patients did not indicate a definite result because the partial response rate did not meet the threshold to continue further investigation [124]. Temsirolimus is reported to suppress cell proliferation in NSCLC cell lines relying on different doses [125]. A phase I clinical trial of temsirolimus confirmed a partial response rate in one patient with NSCLC out of 63 patients of various types of advanced cancer [126]. In a phase II study, 35% of NSCLC patients (*n* = 52) benefited from temsirolimus, among which 8% patients had confirmed PR and 27% had a stable disease [127]. On the other hand, both everolimus and temsirolimus have some adverse events (AEs), such as fatigue, dyspnea, stomatitis, mucositis, asthenia, nausea and mucositis, and combination therapies with other inhibitors, radiotherapy or chemotherapy are still under investigation. Sirolimus, which is an allosteric inhibitor of mTORC1, was demonstrated to possibly inhibit the NSCLC cell proliferation in a preclinical study [128]. Clinical trials are still under way in phase I or II of sirolimus combined with other therapies in patients with NSCLC harboring specific gene mutations [121]. Reports on mTOR inhibitors in SCLC are relatively rare, and temsirolimus was shown to fail to benefit SCLC patients [129].

3.2. Gastric Cancer (GC)

Researches demonstrated that PIK3CA, PIK3CB, AKT1 and mTOR are overexpressed in GC cell lines, and mTOR pathway is active in almost 60% of gastric cancer patients [130]. *PIK3CA* is reported to be commonly mutated and amplified at frequencies of around 18% and 5%, respectively [131]. Three mutation hotspots that exist in almost 80% of *PIK3CA* mutations are E545K (exon 9), E542K (exon 9) and H1047R (exon 20) [132]. As reported, *PIK3CA* mutation frequency in gastric cancer is associated with cancer stage and Epstein–Barr virus (EBV) infection [131,133]. *PTEN*, which is a key inhibitor of the PI3K pathway, is a significant tumor suppressor gene. According to the TCGA database of gastric cancer, deletion, mutation and amplification of *PTEN* each occur in 0.3%, 3.1% and 4% of cases, respectively. The alteration frequency of *PIK3CA* and *PTEN* varies significantly in different populations: for example, between Asian and Caucasian GC patients, the rate is 7% compared to 15% for *PIK3CA* mutations, 21% compared to 4% for *PTEN* deletion, and 47% compared to 78% for *PTEN* loss, respectively [134]. Another research found 19% *PTEN* mutations in GC patients in a Chinese population, including missense, nonsense, deletion, and mutations in intron 6 [135]. PTEN tends to be mutated more frequently in advanced stage or less differentiated GC [136]. Despite AKT overexpression in 74% of GC patients examined by immunochemistry, the genetic alterations in AKT are very few at approximately 1% to 3% in GC [137,138]. Although the exact genomic changes that occur in mTOR signaling downstream of PI3K/Akt are not well clarified, it is reported that phosphorylated-mTOR overexpression is related to some clinicopathological features and poor prognosis in GC patients alone or combined with TSC1 downregulation [139,140]. In an Eastern Chinese population, mTORC1 polymorphisms contribute to the risk of GC [141]. Moreover, an immunohistochemical study via GC tissue microarray demonstrated that aberrant S6K1 expression may lead to cancer initiation, invasion and metastasis of GC [142].

The mTOR inhibitors have also been utilized in preclinical studies and clinical trials of GC. Everolimus and sirolimus showed obvious G1 cell cycle arrest effects and suppressed proliferation in gastric cancer cell lines [143,144]. Rapamycin was responded well in cancer cells harboring PIK3CA and/or PTEN mutations (*P* = 0.0123) in a preclinical study, and inhibited tumor volume and microvasculature growth when was applied in a mouse xenograft model [145,146]. Temsirolimus demonstrated a favorable toxicity profile, pharmacokinetics features, and cancer resistant efficacy in a phase I trial in advanced cancer including GC and is continuing to a phase II trial [126]. Everolimus showed a good disease control rate (DCR) (56%), median progression-free survival (PFS; 2.7 months) and overall survival (OS; 10.1 months) in advanced GC patients (*n* = 53) in phase II trails [147]. And biomarkers exploration has also been executed in a phase II study of everolimus in advanced gastric cancer patients, and pS6 (Ser240/4) was found to be a potential predictive marker [148]. Although some side effects of everolimus (stomatitis, anorexia, fatigue, rash, nausea, peripheral edema, diarrhea and pruritus) existed and improvements of the overall survival and primary endpoint were not obvious, the PFS for six months and safety were significant in previously treated GC patients in phase III trials, which also made everolimus the only drug to progress to phase III tirals for advanced GC treatments [149,150]. Ridaforolimus, also an analog of rapamycin, demonstrated good antitumor effects during preclinical and phase Ib clinical trials combined with capecitabine [151].

mTORC1/2 kinase inhibitors other than rapalogs, such as PP242, AZD 2014, AZD8055, and OSI-027 have also attracted interests due to their competition with ATP in mTOR kinase activity. PP242 showed outstanding antiproliferative and antiangiogenesis capabilities in GC cell lines, while there are no future reports of other inhibitors on GC therapies so far and most of these inhibitors are still in phase I trials [138,152].

3.3. Colorectal Cancer (CRC)

The PI3K/Akt pathway is genetically altered in many CRC cell lines [153]. Mutations of PI3K and PTEN are dominant among those alterations in CRC patients. As reported, approximately 15% of metastatic CRC patients carried *PI3K3CA* mutations, and loss of PTEN was found in 20% to 40% of CRC patients [154,155]. In addition, PI3K subunit p85α and AKT1/2 were overexpressed, particularly in advanced tumor stages, and the phosphorylation level of mTOR and S6K1 was increased in CRC [156]. Mutation of the p53 gene or deletion of the 17p chromosome is significant for tumor initiation, especially from adenoma to carcinoma in CRC [157,158]. p53 inhibits mTOR activity via AMPK-β1 and TSC2 in CRC cell lines. p53 also regulates the mTOR pathway by a target gene, DNA damage and development 1 (REDD1), which is essential for hypoxia activation of TSC1/2 and modulated by oxidative stress [159,160]. Previous immunohistochemical studies demonstrated that mTORC1 signaling was involved in tumorigenesis at an early stage and contributed to progression from normal cells to a neoplastic state in human colorectal adenoma and cancers [161]. mTORC1 and mTORC2 both overexpress and play significant roles in CRC.

As for clinical trials of mTOR inhibitors, neither everolimus nor temsirolimus showed satisfactory effects as monotherapies in treating metastatic CRC in several clinical trials. The effects of temsirolimus were limited, especially in metastatic CRC patients with KRAS mutations [162,163]. Partial suppression of the mTOR signaling pathway by rapamycin and rapalogs was found to be attributed to 4E-BP1 kinase, which led to resistance in CRC [164]. Combination treatments of rapalogs and other drugs have exhibited potential in CRC therapies. For example, combination of the VEGF inhibitor bevacizumab and an mTOR inhibitor achieved fewer adverse effects and prolonged stable disease in metastatic CRC patients [165]. Sorafenib was reported to improve the efficacy of rapamycin in CRC patients harboring *K-RAS* and *PIK3CA* mutations [166]. Everolimus together with octreotide LAR (long-acting release) achieved an obviously prolonged PFS in advanced colorectal neuroendocrine cancers in a phase III study, while the combination of everlimus and irinotecan was well tolerated in a phase I study in mCRC patients [167,168]. And everolimus and tivozanib, which inhibits angiogenesis, demonstrated a 50% disease control in a phase II trial [165]. The combined therapies with mitogen-activated protein kinase kinase (MEK) inhibitors and mTOR inhibitors also attracted more attention because these treatments can overcome the resistance to MEK suppression in CRC [169]. Moreover, dual PI3K/mTOR inhibitors have a reduced possibility to induce drug resistance than rapalogs, and mTOR kinase inhibitors can suppress mTORC1 and mTORC2 simultaneously; thus, these drugs are introduced as the second generation of mTOR inhibitor drugs in preclinical and clinical trials [170]. For instance, NVP-BEZ235, a dual inhibitor of PI3K and mTOR signaling, inhibited tumor growth in a genetically engineered mouse model of sporadic CRC [171]. mTORC1/2 inhibitors OSI-027 showed obvious antitumor activity in several human xenograft models with various histologies [172,173]. In another study of human colon cancer cell line xenograft, both the ATP competitive mTOR inhibitor PP242 and dual inhibitor of PI3K and mTOR NVP-BEZ235 significantly suppressed the xenograft growth, and they achieved better efficacy combined with a MEK inhibitor, implying a prosperous future for second generation mTOR inhibitors in combination therapies for CRC [174].

3.4. Renal Cancer (RCC)

RCC is regarded as one of the most lethal cancers because of the rare available therapies and lack of proper diagnosis biomarkers at early stages. RCC is mainly classified as clear cell renal cell carcinoma (ccRCC, 85%), papillary renal cell carcinoma (PRCC, 0–15%), chromophobe renal cell carcinoma (chRCC, 5%) and collecting duct carcinoma and medullary carcinoma (1%).

Generally, mTOR signaling regulates cell metabolism, and RCC is also a cancer of metabolism dysregulation [175]. Data from TCGA on a ccRCC study in 2013 demonstrated genetic alterations in components of each level of the PI3K/Akt signaling pathway cascade (PIK3CA, PIK3R1, PIK3R2, PTEN, PDPK1, AKT1, AKT2, AKT3, FOXO1, FOXO3, MTOR, RICTOR, TSC1, TSC2, RHEB, AKT1S1, and PRTOR), mainly including *GNB2L1* amplification (6%), *PI3KCA* amplifications or mutations (5%), *PTEN* deletions or mutations (5%) or *MTOR* mutations (6%). Clustered *MTOR* mutations, as well as mutations in *AKT1*, *AKT3* and *RHEB*, contributed to PI3K/Akt and mTOR hyperactivation in ccRCC [70,176,177]. In addition, the cross talk between VHL/HIF and the PI3K/Akt pathway via a positive feedback mechanism contributes to the sustaining activation of PI3K/Akt signaling in ccRCC [178,179]. The rate of genetic alterations in PI3K/Akt pathway components in pRCC is 28% according to the TCGA database, including mutations of *PTEN* and PI3K subunits and amplifications of *GNB2L1*, *PDK1* and *RPTOR* amplifications. In chRCC, *PTEN* was mutated most frequently which occurred in 11% of patients, and mutations of *AKT1*, *TSC1/TSC2* and *mTOR* in the mTOR signaling pathway have also been shown [180].

For targeted therapy towards the mTOR signal pathway in ccRCC, the treatment strategies are at the leading edge, and many drugs have been authorized by the US Food and Drug Administration (FDA). Among these approved drugs, temsirolimus and everolimus are rapalogs that partially inhibit mTORC1 activation, leading to modest survival benefits in advanced ccRCC patients according to the results of the phase III Global ARCC trial [69,181,182]. For metastatic renal cell carcinoma (mRCC), temsirolimus and everolimus are the only mTOR inhibitors authoried by the US FDA. The clinical data demonstrated that mTOR inhibitors can treat mRCC effectively as long as the adverse events were appropriately handled [183]. As reported, ccRCC patients harboring *TSC1* mutation tended to respond to mTOR inhibitors [184]. In a study of 79 patients with mRCC, when treated by mTOR inhibitors, those with mTOR, TSC1, or TSC2 mutations were found to benefit more than others who progressed [185]. Some studies found that resistance to temsirolimus was related to low levels of phosphorylated protein kinase B (p-Akt) and p70 ribosomal S6 Kinase (p-S6K1) in RCC, suggesting that patients with these features should be eliminated from temsirolimus treatments in the future [108]. These data also imply that predicative biomarkers are especially in great need for selecting therapies in future personalized management of RCC [186]. Besides, combination therapy of everolimus together with lenvatinib was regarded to be the first strategy for mRCC, and cabozantinib and nibolumab are subsequent choices, all of which achieved a better efficacy than everolimus alone [187]. mTORC1/2 inhibitors including AZD8055, LN0128 and OSI-027, seem to have potential for greater efficacy than rapalogs in clinical trials of ccRCC [188]. A combination of MAPK- and mTOR-targeted therapies was reported to utilize temsirolimus and tivozanib, which achieved better efficacy in RCC patients [189].

3.5. Urinary Bladder Cancer (UBC)

Urinary bladder cancer (UBC), the malignancy that occurs in the urinary system, ranks as the ninth most common cancer [190]. UBC is classified into non-muscle-invasive UBC (NMIUBC) and muscle-invasive UBC (MIUBC) according to the invasion status into the urinary bladder wall and nearby structures. Genetic alterations of the mTOR pathway occur in over 40% of UBC patients, including deletion or mutations of *PTEN*, *TSC1* or *TSC2* and mutations or amplifications of *PI3KCA* or *AKT1* according to the TCGA database [191–194]. These alterations in the mTOR pathway are reported to be associated with progression and mortality in bladder cancers ($n = 887$) and are valuable for prognosis [195]. UBC patients with a higher grade often harbor mutations that hyperactivate the mTOR pathway or KRAS genes and decrease expression of tumor suppressor genes compared to lower grade UBC patients in whom the FGFR3 mutation dominates [195,196]. Loss of PTEN is common in MIUBC, while is hardly found in NMIUBC [197,198]. In a research composed of both NMIUBC and MIUBC patients, mTOR was expressed in NMIUBC and had a poor prognosis in

MIUBC [199]. Another case study (*n* = 208) indicated that mTOR activation evaluated by 4E-BP1 or S6K1 phosphorylation contributed to tumorigenesis and was an indicator of recurrence and poor survival of UBC patients [200].

Research on UBC cell lines 5637, T24, and HT1376 indicated that everolimus and temsirolimus applied as single agent only showed limited efficacy in these experimental trials [201,202]. In ICR mice induced by *N*-butyl-*N*-(4-hydroxybutyl) nitrosamine (BBN), sirolimus decreased tumor incidence and proliferation, as implied by histopathological and immunohistochemical results, while everolimus demonstrated little effects on bladder tumors [203,204]. In addition, sirolimus also showed benefits in a genetically engineered mouse model of invasive UBC [205]. As reported from a phase II study, everolimus demonstrated mild antitumor effects in metastatic UBC patients resistant to chemotherapy [206]. In another phase II study, only a small portion of patients with advanced UBC responded to everolimus [207]. It seems that rapalogs utilized as monotherapy are not as effctive as expected in the treatment of UBC. For combination therapies, the results from 5637 and T24 cell lines were much more exciting because either everolimus or temsirolimus combined with gemcitabine showed a better response, and cisplatin together with everolimus or temsirolimus also achieved a promising results in 5637 and HT1376 cell lines [208]. A synergistic combination of mTOR inhibitors and EGFR/HER2 inhibitors in UBC cell lines implied a potential efficacy in NMIUBC and MIUBC treatments [209]. A study in patient-derived xenograft models with dual inhibition of mTOR and MEK suggested potential clinical efficacy in UBC [210]. Application of mTOR inhibitors in UBC treatments should depend on careful selection of the tumor type: NMIUBC seems to respond to combination of rapalogs and other drugs, while only those MIUBC patients with phosphorylated mTOR are suitable to accept mTOR inhibitors treatments.

3.6. Prostate Cancer (PCa)

The mTOR pathway is reported to be significantly active in prostate cancer [211,212]. The PI3K/Akt pathway is found aberrant in PCa cell lines, xenograft models, and 30–50% primary PCa tissue samples [213]. Genetic alterations of the mTOR pathway were detected in 42% of primary prostate tumors and all metastatic tumors [211]. Aberrant PTEN/Akt expression was found in 42% of PCa tissues [214]. As PTEN loss was demonstrated to be associated with a high Gleason score, PCa pathological stages and promoted the progression of lymph node metastasis, PTEN may serve as a potential early prognostic marker in prostate cancers [215–219]. High levels of phosphorylated-4EBP1 and eIF-4E are significantly related to increased mortality in PCa patients, implying that downstream effectors of the mTOR pathway may be a potential prognostic indicator for PCa progression [220]. Studies in PCa cell lines indicated that the PI3K/Akt/mTOR pathway contributed to PCa radioresistance (RR) through mechanisms of intrinsic radioresistance, cancer cell proliferation and hypoxia, and in those PCa RR cell lines, the PI3K/Akt/mTOR pathway was the most active [221,222]. Moreover, activation of the PI3K/Akt/mTOR pathway was also reported to be involved in epithelial mesenchymal transition (EMT) and cancer stem cells (CSCs) in prostate cancer radioresistance [223].

Despite the antitumor efficacy demonstrated by the mTOR inhibitors (rapalogs) rapamycin and everolimus in murine models of Pca [90,224,225], the performances of rapalogs in phase I and II clinical trials were not so satisfactory, leading to application of second generation mTOR inhibitors or further combination therapies in Pca [226–229]. As reported, the ATP competitive mTOR inhibitor MLN0128 showed better efficacy in reducing tumor size and invasion in cell lines and Pca mouse models [49]. These ATP competitive mTOR inhibitors, such as MLN0128, AZD2014, ZAD8055, CC-223, DS-378a and OSI-027, are in early clinical trials. In preclinical studies, the dual PI3K/mTOR inhibitors BEZ235 and GDC-0980 demonstrated effective inhibition of cell proliferation in prostate cancer cells [230,231]. BEZ235 was also reported to reduce tumor volume in a mouse model harboring PTEN loss, and the effects were enhanced when combined with AR antagonist enzalutamide, implying a potential prospect in synergy treatments cotargeting the AR, PI3K and mTOR signaling pathways in PCa [232]. BEZ235 and GDC-0980 are currently being tested as single agents or combination therapies with abiraterone acetate in the process of phase I/II clinical trials in castration-resistance prostate cancer (CRPC).

3.7. Breast Cancer

In breast cancer, most genetic alterations and mutations lie upstream of mTOR resulting in hyperactivation of mTOR signaling. *PIK3CA* is frequently mutated in breast cancer in three "hotspots": E545K, E542K in exon 9 (helical domain) and H1047R in exon 20 (kinase domain) [233]. As reported, *PIK3CA* mutations occurred in 20–50% of breast cancers, especially including 35% of hormone receptor (HR)-positive breast cancers, 23% of human epidermal growth factor receptor 2 (HER2)-positive breast cancers and less than 10% in triple-negative breast cancer (TNBC) [234]. PTEN mutations occur in less than 3% of breast cancers, while PTEN loss occurs in approximately 30% of breast cancers [234,235]. Although Akt mutations in the catalytic domains have not been detected, E17K substitution occurred in the pleckstrin homology domain of AKT1 resulting in constitutive activation in 3% of HR-positive breast cancers [236]. Studies also found mutations in mTOR itself in various cancer types with FAT and FATC domains frequently mutated [237,238]. Moreover, mTOR expression is correlated with poor prognosis in breast cancer, and phosphor-mTOR was more common in TNBC [239–241].

Everolimus has been proved by the FDA in treating hormone receptor-positive, HER2-negative breast cancer. And the mTOR inhibitors have been utilized in many clinical trials in beast cancer treatments, such as HORIZON, BOLERO-1, BOLERO-2, BOLERO-3 and TAMRAD, which are all Phase III or II randomized clinical practices evaluating the combination therapies with different mTOR inhibitors in different settings. The HORIZON trial was executed in first-line patients of Hormone Receptor (HR) positive advanced breast cancer to compare the combined therapy of temsiroliumus with letrozole to therapy of placebo with letrozole. Analysis of the HORIZON trial demonstrated the combination therapy failed to improve PFS and may be account for more grade 3 or 4 adverse effects (37% vs. 24%) [242]. The BOLERO-1 trial was another randomized phase III evaluating everolimus (10 mg) with paclitaxel and trastuzumab in patients of HER2 positive advance breast cancer. PFS was not obviously increased in the group of everolimus (14.9 months) compared to the group of placebo (*P* = 0.1167), while in the HR-negative subgroup, the PFS was prolonged 7.2 months with everolimus administration (*P* = 0.049) [243]. A high rate of adverse events correlated with deaths in everolimus treatments of BOLERO-1 was also reported indicating the necessity to monitor the adverse events in early stage. The object of BOLERO-2 trial is to evaluating combination of mTOR inhibitor everolimus with aromatase inhibitor (AI) in HR positive advanced breast cancers. Application of everolimus increased the PFS to 10.6 months compared to 4.1 months originally with single exemestane administration (*P* < 0.0001) [244], which directly led to the permission of FDA for everolimus with exemestane in advanced breast cancer patients with HR positive and HER2 negative following unsuccessful therapy with letrozole or anastrozole. A recently reported study of BOLERO-2 demonstrated an improvement in overall survival in combination therapy group (31.0 months) compared to the control group with exemestane and placebo (26.6 months) [245]. The TAMRAD trial compared the combination of everolimus with tamoxifen to single tamosifen application in 111 HR positive/HER2 negative, AI resistant metastatic breast cancer patients, implying a significant increase of clinical benefit rate (CBR), time to progression (TTP) and OS by everolimus addition [246]. Analysis of results from HORIZON and BOLERO-2 illuminated that endocrine-resistant patients may gain more benefits from temsirolimus administration. So far, researches have mainly focused on clinical efficacy in HR positive and HER2 negative breast cancer patients, in which everolimus has been approved for combined application with exemestane. Ridaforolimus was reported to benefit HER2 positive metastatic breast cancer patients when applied with trastuzumab in a phase II trial, indicating ridaforolimus may improve the efficacy of trastuzumab [247].

Aside from the rapalogs, other mTOR inhibitors, such as ATP competitive inhibitors and PI3K /mTOR dual inhibitors, have also been studied in breast cancer. ATP competitive inhibitors, AZD2014, which showed better anti-proliferative capabilities in breast cancer cell lines, xenograft and primary explant models, is now in process of phase II clinical trials designed to be combined with other compounds or therapies [112,248,249]. MLN0128 inhibited cell viability in five breast cell lines (HR−/+, HER2−/+) and acted synergistically with TSA [250]. In a phase I trial, CC223 was reported to be tolerated well and achieved partial response in breast cancer patients, implying its promising potential in the future [251]. Dual inhibitors of PI3K and mTOR, BEZ235 and PF-04691502, both demonstrated antitumor efficacy in breast cancer cells and xenograft models [252,253], but were also inclined to cause serious side effects in clinical practices. More combination therapies with mTOR inhibitors are still underway in different settings [254].

3.8. Head and Neck Squamous Cell Carcinoma (HNSCC)

Head and neck squamous cell carcinoma (HNSCC) accounts for almost 90% of human head and neck cancers, including cancers in the oral cavity, oropharynx, nasopharynx, hypopharynx, and larynx.

A whole-exome sequencing research in 151 HNSCC patients demonstrated that PI3K pathway was frequently mutated in 30.5% of HNSCC [255]. The genes with genetic alterations in HNSCC mainly include *PIK3CA, PIK3CD, PTEN, PDK1, Akt, RICTOR, RAPTOR, TSC1, TSC2* and *mTOR* [256–260]. Especially, *PI3KCA* amplifications and *PTEN* mutation are prevalent in human papilloma virus (HPV) infected HNSCC [261]. Another separate study indicated that HPV positive HNSCC had a different mutated gene cluster from HPV negative HNSCC [262]. PI3KCA amplification was observed in early stage in the carcinogenesis as well as in the malignancies, implying PI3K pathway contributes to the oncogenic process of HNSCC [263]. In addition, advanced HNSCC patients often harbor multiple aberrations including mutations in *PIK3CA* and *mTOR* or *PIK3CA* and *PTEN*, suggesting these simultaneously existing mutations are also associated with HNSCC progression [264]. A phase II clinical trial showed that the single-nucleotide polymorphisms (SNP) in PTEN (rs12569998) and AKT2 (rs8100018) are related with the progression risk and PFS in metastatic HNSCC treated with combination of docetaxel and cetuximab [265]. mTOR is reported to be activated in 80–90% HNSCC, particularly those with HPV infection [266,267]. As reported, mTOR and its downstream effectors, eIF-4E, 4EBP1, S6K1, and S6 are all biomarkers for diagnosis and prognosis in head and neck cancer, demonstrating the promising prospect for mTOR inhibitors in HNSCC treatments [268].

In preclinical studies of mTOR inhibitors, rapamycin and its rapalog temsirolimus, everolimus all showed efficacy in xenograft HNSCC models [268,269]. An in vivo retroinhibition approach applied in HNSCC cells demonstrated that rapamycin and its rapalogs can prevent angiogenesis, and another study in xenograft model implied that rapamycin and rapalog everolimus also inhibit lymphangiogenesis and lymph node metastasis in HNSCC [270,271]. Besides, mTOR inhibition can also act synergistically with radiation therapy to reinforce the anti-angiogenic effects and suppress HNSCC tumor growth in xenograft models [272,273]. Besides, several reports demonstrated the promising results of mTOR inhibitors in HNSCC patient-derived tumorgraft (PDX) models [274–276].

Rapamycin, originally regarded as a specific inhibitor of mTORC1, was found to supress both mTORC1 and mTORC2 in HNSCC cells [267]. And in a study of newly diagnosed HNSCC patients, rapamycin (NCT01995922) achieved improved effectiveness, as most patients responded and one patient got complete response [260]. Everolimus has been utilized in combination with cisplatin and radiation therapy or with erlotinib or with cisplatin and docetaxel in HNSCC treatment, and was tolerated well in these phase I or II clinical trials [277–279]. Another combination therapy in a phase I study with temsirolimus, carboplatin and paclitaxel in HNSCC achieved a partial response rate of 22%, while temsirolimus combined with erlotinib was poorly tolerated with common adverse effects including fatigue, hyperglycemia, diarrhea and peritonitis in recurrent or metastatic HNSCC patients in a phase II strudy [280,281]. Actually, most clinical practices of mTOR inhibitors as single agent in HNSCC have been applied in those patients that failed in other therapies or general patients without selection. Clinical trails focusing on mTOR inhibitors in HPV+ HNSCC patients have seldom been conducted yet, although previous researches confirmed the potential of this strategy. Dual PI3K/mTOR inhibitors like BEZ235 showed anti-tumor effects in HNSCC cell lines and tumorgrafts with PIK3CA mutations, its efficacy in HNSCC patients remained unknown [255]. Besides, combination therapies of mTOR inhibitors with other molecular-targeted therapies (EGFR, VEGFR, MEK, MAPK and MET) or conventional therapies may shed lights in HNSCC clinical success.

4. Discussions and Future Prospects

Among these eight solid tumor types we discussed, it seems that mTOR inhibitors achieved better efficacy and relatively more attentions in treatments of renal cancer and breast cancer. Although these tumors originate from different primary organs, they share similar genetic alterations in PI3K or mTOR signal pathway (as summarized in Table 1), which imply that genetical and molecular biological methods should be applied to classify cancer subtypes in addition to those organs affected especially before targeted therapy application. Then we can get some related clues from clinical trials about which specific mTOR inhibitors or combinations may benefit cancer patients with what kind of genetic alterations in mTOR signaling [112]. We also summarize mTOR inhibitors that are under preclinical and clinical trials in these eight solid cancer types (as shown in Table 2). Apart from those eight types of solid tumors we mentioned, mTOR inhibitors have also been utilized in the therapies of gynecologic cancer, osteosarcoma, leukemia, lymphoma, thyroid carcinoma, glioblastoma, neuroendocrine tumors and medulloblastoma, and we won't go into details here [282–289].

To summarize, mTOR inhibitors can be classified into three generations: the first generation inhibitors, mainly include rapamycin and its rapalogs temsirolimus (CCI-779), everolimus (RAD001) and ridaforolimus; second generation inhibitors refer to ATP-competitive inhibitor of mTOR kinase which inhibit both mTORC1 and mTORC2 simutaneously (MLN0128, AZD2014, AZD8055, CC223, etc.) as well as some dual PI3K/mTOR inhibitors (PP242, MLN0128, KU-0063794, BEZ235, etc.); Third generation inhibitor, which has been seldom reported in clinical trials yet, has a bivalent structure to take advantage of the two docking sites and avoid resistance against the original compounds. Better efficacy with less toxicity in large individual variability is always the ultimate aim for designing targeting drugs. Rapalogs, as the first generation mTOR inhibitors, have been tested in many clinical trials, but they achieved only modest efficacy applied as monotherapies in cancer treatments due to multiple mechanisms: First, rapalogs partially inhibit mTORC1 activity, and a negative feed back loop will arouse the PI3K and Akt signal via PI3K/mTORC2/Akt cascade, leading to increased cell growth and enhanced cell survival [290,291]. mTOR signal pathway is a complicated system which has various cross-talks with other signaling pathways that can counteract rapalogs' functions [292]. Second, although phosphorylation of S6K1 is totally blocked by rapalogs, 4EBP1 phosphorylation is modestly suppressed. Thus, proteins translation regulated by 4EBP1 in tumorigenesis can still be translated to promote cancer progression. Also, rapalogs decrease the inhibition of IRS-1 by S6K1 phosphorylation, inducing Akt signaling and downstream pathways [291]. Besides, mTORC1 inhibition can also promote cell proliferation by catabolism of extracellular proteins in nutrient deprived conditions, and enhance cell survival via autophagy [293,294]. Therefore, new focuses are turned to the second generation mTOR inhibitors with dual inhibition on PI3K and mTOR signaling or mTOR kinase inhibitors, which are less possible to induce drug resistance than rapalogs alone and already have been introduced in preclinical study or entered the clinical practices [170]. Combination therapies with rapalogs and other signal pathway inhibitors as well as conventional therapies are more prosperous, and many clinical trials have already confirmed the benefits of this treating strategy in various cancer types as we discussed above. However, whether these therapy strategies will offer improved benefits need to be verified in further clinical trials.

For future directions of mTOR targeting therapy, we should clarify the following issues: first, we need to establish appropriate dose schedules of mTOR inhibitors that ensure the efficacy and better toleration in patients; second, all the mTOR inhibitors related treatments no matter monotherapies or combination therapies should continue to be carefully optimized and evaluated to achieve the best effectiveness in clinical trials; third, we should improve the ability to predict who will respond to a certain targeted therapy of mTOR according to the analysis of genetic variations from the patients; fourth, molecular biomarkers for the prognosis and prediction need to be explored to help selecting suitable therapy plans and monitoring the treatment response to mTOR inhibitors in patients.

Table 1. The incidence of genetic variations in mTOR (The mammalian or mechanistic target of rapamycin) signal pathway components in 8 types of solid human cancers summarized in this review.

Cancer Type	Refs	Type of Genetic Variation	Gene (Incidence)
Lung cancer			
Squamous cancer	[114]	genetic alterations	PI3CA (16%), PTEN (15%), AKT3 (16%), AKT2 (4%), AKT1(<1%)
		amplifications	PI3CA (33%)
SCLC	[115]	genetic alterations	PI3CA (6%), PTEN (4%), AKT3 (4%), AKT2 (9%), RICTOR (9%), mTOR (4%)
Gastric cancer			
	[131,132]	mutations	PI3CA (18%) (E545K, E542K-exon9, H1047R-exon20)
		amplifications	PI3CA (5%)
	TCGA	deletions, mutations, amplifications	PTEN (0.3%, 3.1%, 4%)
	[135]	deletions and mutations	PTEN (19%, Chinese population
	[137,138]	genetic alterations	AKT (1–3%)
Colorectal cancer			
	[154,155]	mutations	PI3CA (15%)
		deletions	PTEN (20–40%)
Renal cancer			
ccRcc	[70,176,177]	amplifications	GNB2L1 (6%)
		amplifications or mutations	PI3KCA (5%)
		deletions or mutations	PTEN (5%)
		mutations	mTOR (6%)
pRcc	TCGA	mutations	PTEN, PI3K
		amplifications	GNB2L1, PDK1, RPTOR (total: 28%)
chRCC	[180]	mutations	PTEN (11%)
Urinary bladder cancer			
	[192]	activating point mutations	PI3KCA (17%)
		mutations or deletions	TSC1 or TSC2 (9%)
		mutations	AKT3 (10%)
Prostate cancer			
	[211]	genetic alterations	mTOR pathway (42% primary PCa, 100% metastatic PCa)
		mutations	PTEN (4% primary PCa, 42% metastatic PCa); PIK3CA (6% primary PCa, 16% metastatic PCa)
Breast cancer			
	[233–235]	mutations	PIK3CA (20–50%) (E545K, E542K-exon9, H1047R-exon20)
		mutations, loss	PTEN (<3%, 30%)
HR-positive	[234]	mutations	PIK3CA (35%)
	[236]	E17K substitution	AKT1 (3%)
HER2-positive	[234]	mutations	PIK3CA (23%)
TNBC	[234]	mutations	PIK3CA (<10%)
Head and neck squamous cell carcinoma			
	[255,257,258,260]	mutations	PIK3CA (12.6%, 11–40%) (E545K, E542K-exon9, H1047R-exon20) TSC1 (11%), TSC2 (13%)
		amplifications	PIK3CA (24.4%)
		loss	PTEN (8.16%, 10–15%)

Table 2. mTOR inhibitors that are under preclinical and clinical trials in eight solid cancer types summerized in this review.

Cancer Type	Drug Class	Drugs	Refs
Lung cancer			
NSCLC	mTORC1 inhibitors	everolimus	[118–124]
		temsirolimus	[125–127]
		sirolimus	[128]
Gastric cancer			
	mTORC1 inhibitors	rapamycin	[145,146]
		temsirolimus	[126]
		everolimus	[143,144,148–150]
		ridaforolimus	[151]
	mTORC1 and mTORC2 inhibitors	PP242	[138,152]
Colorectal cancer			
	mTORC1 inhibitor	temsirolimus	[162,163]
		rapamycin	[164,166]
		everolimus	[165,167,168]
	PI3K and mTOR inhibitors	NVP-BEZ235	[171,174]
	mTORC1 and mTORC2 inhibitors	OSI-027	[172,173]
		PP242	[174]
Renal cancer			
ccRCC	mTORC1 inhibitor	temsirolimus	[108,181,189]
		everolimus	[182,187]
	mTORC1 and mTORC2 inhibitors	AZD8055, IN-0128, OSI-027	[188]
mRCC		rapamycin	[184,185]
Urinary bladder cancer			
	mTORC1 inhibitor	rapamycin	[201,205]
		everolimus	[202,204,206–208]
		sirolimus	[203,205]
		temsirolimus	[208]
	mTORC1 and mTORC2 inhibitors	PP242 or OSI-027	[209]
Prostate cancer			
	mTORC1 inhibitor	rapamycin	[225,227]
		everolimus	[226,228,229]
	mTORC1 and mTORC2 inhibitors	MLN0128	[49]
	PI3K and mTOR inhibitors	NVP-BEZ235, GDC-0980	[230,231]
Breast cancer			
	mTORC1 inhibitor	rapamycin	[242]
		everolimus	[243–246]
		ridaforolimus	[247]
	mTORC1 and mTORC2 inhibitors	AZD2014	[112,248,249]
		MLN0128	[250]
		CC-223	[251]
	PI3K and mTOR inhibitors	PF-04691502	[252]
		NVP-BEZ235	[253]
Head and neck squamous cell carcinoma			
	mTORC1 inhibitor	rapamycin	[267–271]
		temsirolimus	[268,273,280,281]
		everolimus	[268,270,274,277–279]
	PI3K and mTOR inhibitors	PF-05212384	[272]

In the present review, we discuss the mTOR components of mTORC1 and mTORC2 and the upstream and downstream effectors of mTOR signaling pathway in physiological and pathological status.

Genetic alterations occurred in eight solid tumors and preclinical as well as clinical trials targeting mTOR in these tumor types. As we know, most tumors are heterogeneous and caused by multiple genetic and environmental factors, so it is difficult to have one single drug to fit all patients with the same tumor type. More thorough realization of genetic profile and molecular characterization of different cancer subtypes will surely help us select the most appropriate drugs in targeting mTOR signaling in cancer therapy. With the rapid development of biomarkers and deep sequencing technology, personalized therapy utilizing more specific mTOR targeting drugs that have better efficacy and more safety, will be translated into clinical cancer treatments in the near future.

Funding: This research was funded by the Ministry of Science and Technology of China (grant number 2015CB553705), the National Natural Science Foundation of China (grant number 31301022 and 81772497) and the Natural Science Foundation of Beijing (grant number 7162116).

Conflicts of Interest: The authors declare no conflicts of interest.

Abbreviations

4EBP1	Eukaryotic translation initiation factor 4E binding protein 1
AEs	Adverse events
AMPK	AMP kinase
AMPKβ	AMP activated protein kinaseβ
ATP	Adenosine Tri-Phosphate
BBN	N-butyl-N-(4-hydroxybutyl) nitrosamine
Bgff	Basic fibroblast growth factor
CBR	Clinical benefit rate
ccRCC	Clear cell renal cell carcinoma
chRCC	Chromophobe renal cell carcinoma
CRC	Colorectal cancer
CRPC	Castration-resistance prostate cancer
CSC	Cancer stem cells
CT	Chemotherapy
DAP1	Death-associated protein 1
DCR	Disease control rate
DEP	EGL-10 and Pleckstrin
DEPTOR	DEP domain-containing mTOR-interacting protein
EBV	Epstein-Barr virus
EGFR	Epidermal Growth Factor Receptor
eIF-3	Eukaryotic initiation factor-3
eIF-4E	Eukaryotic translation Initiation Factor
EMT	Epithelial mesenchymal transition
ERKs	Extracellular signal-regulated kinases
FDA	Food and Drug Administration
FKBP12	FK506 Binding Protein 12
FoxO	Forkhead box family transcription factors
GC	Gastric cancer
Grb10	Growth factor receptor-bound protein 10
HER2	Human epidermal growth factor receptor 2
HIF-1α	Hypoxia-inducible factor 1α
HNSCC	Head and neck squamous cell carcinoma
HPV	Papilloma virus
HR	Hormone Receptor
IGFR	Insulin growth factor receptor
IRS	Insulin receptor substrate
LAR	Long-acting release
MAPK	Mitogen activated protein kinase
MEK	Mitogen-activated protein kinase kinase

MIUBCs	Muscle-invasive UBCs
mLST8	Mammalian lethal with SEC13 protein 8
mRCC	Metastatic renal cell carcinoma
mSIN1	Mammalian stress-activated protein kinase interacting protein 1
mTOR	The mammalian or mechanistic target of rapamycin
mTORC	mTOR complex
NDRG1	N-myc Downstream-Regulated Gene 1 protein
NF-κB	Nuclear factor-κB
NMIUBCs	Non-muscle-invasive UBCs
NSCLC	Non-small cell lung cancer
OS	Overall survival
p-Akt	Phosphor-protein kinase B
PCa	Prostate cancer
PDGF	Platelet-derived growth factor
PDK1	Phosphoinositide-dependent Kinase 1
PFS	Progression free survival
PI3K	Phosphoinositide 3-kinase
PIKK	Phosphoinositide 3-kinase related protein kinase
PIP3	Phosphatidylinositol (3, 4, 5)-triphosphate
PKA	cAMP-dependent protein kinase
PKC	Protein kinase C
PKG	cGMP-dependent protein kinase
p-mTOR	Phosphorylated-mTOR
PP2A	Protein phosphatase 2A
PRAS40	Proline-rich substrate of 40 kDa
PRCC	Papillary renal cell carcinoma
Protor-1/2	Protein observed with RICTOR 1/2
PRR 5	Proline-rich protein 5
p-S6K1	p70 ribosomal S6 Kinase
PTEN	Phosphatase and tensin homolog on chromosome 10
RAPTOR	Regulatory-associated protein of mTOR
RCC	Renal cancer
REDD1	DNA damage and development 1
RHEB	Ras homolog enriched in brain
RICTOR	Rapamycin-insensitive companion of mTOR
RR	Radioresistance
RSK	Ribosomal protein S6 kinase
S6K	S6 kinase
S6RP	S6 ribosomal protein
SCLC	Small cell lung cancinoma
SGK	Serum glucose kinase
SNP	Single-nucleotide polymorphisms
SQCLC	Squamous cell lung carcinoma
SREBP	Sterol regulatory element-binding protein
SRE-BP1	Sterol regulatory element-binding protein 1
STAT	Signal transducer and activator of transcription
STK11	Serine threonine kinase 11
TCGA	The cancer genome atlas
Tel2	Telomere maintenance 2
TFEB	Transcription factor transcription factor EB
TNBC	Triple-negative breast cancer
TSC	Tuberous sclerosis complex
Tti1	Tel2-interacting protein 1
TTP	Time to progression

UBC	Urinary bladder cancer
ULK1	UNC-5 Like autophagy activating Kinase 1
VEGF	Vascular endothelial growth factor
WIPI2	WD repeat domain phophoinositide-interacting protein 2

References

1. Laplante, M.; Sabatini, D.M. mTOR signaling in growth control and disease. *Cell* **2012**, *149*, 274–293. [CrossRef] [PubMed]
2. Saxton, R.A.; Sabatini, D.M. mTOR Signaling in Growth, Metabolism, and Disease. *Cell* **2017**, *169*, 361–371. [CrossRef] [PubMed]
3. Watanabe, R.; Wei, L.; Huang, J. mTOR signaling, function, novel inhibitors, and therapeutic targets. *J. Nucl. Med.* **2011**, *52*, 497–500. [CrossRef] [PubMed]
4. Forbes, S.A.; Bindal, N.; Bamford, S.; Cole, C.; Kok, C.Y.; Beare, D.; Jia, M.; Shepherd, R.; Leung, K.; Menzies, A.; et al. COSMIC: Mining complete cancer genomes in the Catalogue of Somatic Mutations in Cancer. *Nucleic Acids Res.* **2011**, *39*, D945–D950. [CrossRef] [PubMed]
5. Ciuffreda, L.; Di Sanza, C.; Incani, U.C.; Milella, M. The mTOR pathway: A new target in cancer therapy. *Curr. Cancer Drug Targets* **2010**, *10*, 484–495. [CrossRef] [PubMed]
6. Mayer, I.A.; Arteaga, C.L. The PI3K/AKT Pathway as a Target for Cancer Treatment. *Annu. Rev. Med.* **2016**, *67*, 11–28. [CrossRef] [PubMed]
7. Conciatori, F.; Ciuffreda, L.; Bazzichetto, C.; Falcone, I.; Pilotto, S.; Bria, E.; Cognetti, F.; Milella, M. mTOR Cross-Talk in Cancer and Potential for Combination Therapy. *Cancers* **2018**, *10*, 23. [CrossRef] [PubMed]
8. Faes, S.; Demartines, N.; Dormond, O. Resistance to mTORC1 Inhibitors in Cancer Therapy: From Kinase Mutations to Intratumoral Heterogeneity of Kinase Activity. *Oxid. Med. Cell. Longev.* **2017**, *2017*, 1726078. [CrossRef]
9. Bakkenist, C.J.; Kastan, M.B. Initiating cellular stress responses. *Cell* **2004**, *118*, 9–17. [CrossRef]
10. Heitman, J.; Movva, N.R.; Hall, M.N. Targets for cell cycle arrest by the immunosuppressant rapamycin in yeast. *Science* **1991**, *253*, 905–909. [CrossRef]
11. Rad, E.; Murray, J.T.; Tee, A.R. Oncogenic Signalling through Mechanistic Target of Rapamycin (mTOR): A Driver of Metabolic Transformation and Cancer Progression. *Cancers* **2018**, *10*, 5. [CrossRef] [PubMed]
12. Shimobayashi, M.; Hall, M.N. Making new contacts: The mTOR network in metabolism and signalling crosstalk. *Nat. Rev. Mol. Cell Biol.* **2014**, *15*, 155–162. [CrossRef] [PubMed]
13. Sarbassov, D.D.; Ali, S.M.; Sengupta, S.; Sheen, J.H.; Hsu, P.P.; Bagley, A.F.; Markhard, A.L.; Sabatini, D.M. Prolonged rapamycin treatment inhibits mTORC2 assembly and Akt/PKB. *Mol. Cell* **2006**, *22*, 159–168. [CrossRef] [PubMed]
14. Fonseca, B.D.; Smith, E.M.; Lee, V.H.; MacKintosh, C.; Proud, C.G. PRAS40 is a target for mammalian target of rapamycin complex 1 and is required for signaling downstream of this complex. *J. Biol. Chem.* **2007**, *282*, 24514–24524. [CrossRef] [PubMed]
15. Peterson, T.R.; Laplante, M.; Thoreen, C.C.; Sancak, Y.; Kang, S.A.; Kuehl, W.M.; Gray, N.S.; Sabatini, D.M. DEPTOR is an mTOR inhibitor frequently overexpressed in multiple myeloma cells and required for their survival. *Cell* **2009**, *137*, 873–886. [CrossRef] [PubMed]
16. Liu, P.; Gan, W.; Chin, Y.R.; Ogura, K.; Guo, J.; Zhang, J.; Wang, B.; Blenis, J.; Cantley, L.C.; Toker, A.; et al. PtdIns(3,4,5)P3-Dependent Activation of the mTORC2 Kinase Complex. *Cancer Discov.* **2015**, *5*, 1194–1209. [CrossRef]
17. Sarbassov, D.D.; Ali, S.M.; Kim, D.H.; Guertin, D.A.; Latek, R.R.; Erdjument-Bromage, H.; Tempst, P.; Sabatini, D.M. Rictor, a novel binding partner of mTOR, defines a rapamycin-insensitive and raptor-independent pathway that regulates the cytoskeleton. *Curr. Biol.* **2004**, *14*, 1296–1302. [CrossRef]
18. Pearce, L.R.; Huang, X.; Boudeau, J.; Pawlowski, R.; Wullschleger, S.; Deak, M.; Ibrahim, A.F.; Gourlay, R.; Magnuson, M.A.; Alessi, D.R. Identification of Protor as a novel Rictor-binding component of mTOR complex-2. *Biochem. J.* **2007**, *405*, 513–522. [CrossRef]
19. Woo, S.Y.; Kim, D.H.; Jun, C.B.; Kim, Y.M.; Haar, E.V.; Lee, S.I.; Hegg, J.W.; Bandhakavi, S.; Griffin, T.J.; Kim, D.H. PRR5, a novel component of mTOR complex 2, regulates platelet-derived growth factor receptor beta expression and signaling. *J. Biol. Chem.* **2007**, *282*, 25604–25612. [CrossRef]

20. Kim, L.C.; Cook, R.S.; Chen, J. mTORC1 and mTORC2 in cancer and the tumor microenvironment. *Oncogene* **2017**, *36*, 2191–2201. [CrossRef]

21. Wullschleger, S.; Loewith, R.; Hall, M.N. TOR signaling in growth and metabolism. *Cell* **2006**, *124*, 471–484. [CrossRef]

22. Harachi, M.; Masui, K.; Okamura, Y.; Tsukui, R.; Mischel, P.S.; Shibata, N. mTOR Complexes as a Nutrient Sensor for Driving Cancer Progression. *Int. J. Mol. Sci.* **2018**, *19*, 3267. [CrossRef] [PubMed]

23. Paquette, M.; El-Houjeiri, L.; Pause, A. mTOR Pathways in Cancer and Autophagy. *Cancers* **2018**, *10*, 18. [CrossRef] [PubMed]

24. Ben-Sahra, I.; Manning, B.D. mTORC1 signaling and the metabolic control of cell growth. *Curr. Opin. Cell Biol.* **2017**, *45*, 72–82. [CrossRef]

25. Jacinto, E.; Loewith, R.; Schmidt, A.; Lin, S.; Ruegg, M.A.; Hall, A.; Hall, M.N. Mammalian TOR complex 2 controls the actin cytoskeleton and is rapamycin insensitive. *Nat. Cell Biol.* **2004**, *6*, 1122–1128. [CrossRef] [PubMed]

26. Pearce, L.R.; Komander, D.; Alessi, D.R. The nuts and bolts of AGC protein kinases. *Nat. Rev. Mol. Cell Biol.* **2010**, *11*, 9–22. [CrossRef] [PubMed]

27. Nobes, C.D.; Hall, A. Rho GTPases control polarity, protrusion, and adhesion during cell movement. *J. Cell Biol.* **1999**, *144*, 1235–1244. [CrossRef] [PubMed]

28. Zhang, H.; Bajraszewski, N.; Wu, E.; Wang, H.; Moseman, A.P.; Dabora, S.L.; Griffin, J.D.; Kwiatkowski, D.J. PDGFRs are critical for PI3K/Akt activation and negatively regulated by mTOR. *J. Clin. Investig.* **2007**, *117*, 730–738. [CrossRef] [PubMed]

29. Inoki, K.; Li, Y.; Zhu, T.; Wu, J.; Guan, K.L. TSC2 is phosphorylated and inhibited by Akt and suppresses mTOR signalling. *Nat. Cell Biol.* **2002**, *4*, 648–657. [CrossRef] [PubMed]

30. Manning, B.D.; Tee, A.R.; Logsdon, M.N.; Blenis, J.; Cantley, L.C. Identification of the tuberous sclerosis complex-2 tumor suppressor gene product tuberin as a target of the phosphoinositide 3-kinase/akt pathway. *Mol. Cell* **2002**, *10*, 151–162. [CrossRef]

31. Potter, C.J.; Pedraza, L.G.; Xu, T. Akt regulates growth by directly phosphorylating Tsc2. *Nat. Cell Biol.* **2002**, *4*, 658–665. [CrossRef] [PubMed]

32. Puertollano, R. mTOR and lysosome regulation. *F1000Prime Rep.* **2014**, *6*, 52. [CrossRef] [PubMed]

33. Sancak, Y.; Thoreen, C.C.; Peterson, T.R.; Lindquist, R.A.; Kang, S.A.; Spooner, E.; Carr, S.A.; Sabatini, D.M. PRAS40 is an insulin-regulated inhibitor of the mTORC1 protein kinase. *Mol. Cell* **2007**, *25*, 903–915. [CrossRef] [PubMed]

34. Ballif, B.A.; Roux, P.P.; Gerber, S.A.; MacKeigan, J.P.; Blenis, J.; Gygi, S.P. Quantitative phosphorylation profiling of the ERK/p90 ribosomal S6 kinase-signaling cassette and its targets, the tuberous sclerosis tumor suppressors. *Proc. Natl. Acad. Sci. USA* **2005**, *102*, 667–672. [CrossRef] [PubMed]

35. Carriere, A.; Cargnello, M.; Julien, L.A.; Gao, H.; Bonneil, E.; Thibault, P.; Roux, P.P. Oncogenic MAPK signaling stimulates mTORC1 activity by promoting RSK-mediated raptor phosphorylation. *Curr. Biol.* **2008**, *18*, 1269–1277. [CrossRef] [PubMed]

36. Ma, L.; Chen, Z.; Erdjument-Bromage, H.; Tempst, P.; Pandolfi, P.P. Phosphorylation and functional inactivation of TSC2 by Erk implications for tuberous sclerosis and cancer pathogenesis. *Cell* **2005**, *121*, 179–193. [CrossRef] [PubMed]

37. Feng, Z.; Zhang, H.; Levine, A.J.; Jin, S. The coordinate regulation of the p53 and mTOR pathways in cells. *Proc. Natl. Acad. Sci. USA* **2005**, *102*, 8204–8209. [CrossRef]

38. Gwinn, D.M.; Shackelford, D.B.; Egan, D.F.; Mihaylova, M.M.; Mery, A.; Vasquez, D.S.; Turk, B.E.; Shaw, R.J. AMPK phosphorylation of raptor mediates a metabolic checkpoint. *Mol. Cell* **2008**, *30*, 214–226. [CrossRef]

39. Sancak, Y.; Bar-Peled, L.; Zoncu, R.; Markhard, A.L.; Nada, S.; Sabatini, D.M. Ragulator-Rag complex targets mTORC1 to the lysosomal surface and is necessary for its activation by amino acids. *Cell* **2010**, *141*, 290–303. [CrossRef]

40. Sancak, Y.; Peterson, T.R.; Shaul, Y.D.; Lindquist, R.A.; Thoreen, C.C.; Bar-Peled, L.; Sabatini, D.M. The Rag GTPases bind raptor and mediate amino acid signaling to mTORC1. *Science* **2008**, *320*, 1496–1501. [CrossRef]

41. Bonfils, G.; Jaquenoud, M.; Bontron, S.; Ostrowicz, C.; Ungermann, C.; De Virgilio, C. Leucyl-tRNA synthetase controls TORC1 via the EGO complex. *Mol. Cell* **2012**, *46*, 105–110. [CrossRef] [PubMed]

42. Han, J.M.; Jeong, S.J.; Park, M.C.; Kim, G.; Kwon, N.H.; Kim, H.K.; Ha, S.H.; Ryu, S.H.; Kim, S. Leucyl-tRNA synthetase is an intracellular leucine sensor for the mTORC1-signaling pathway. *Cell* **2012**, *149*, 410–424. [CrossRef] [PubMed]

43. Wang, S.; Tsun, Z.Y.; Wolfson, R.L.; Shen, K.; Wyant, G.A.; Plovanich, M.E.; Yuan, E.D.; Jones, T.D.; Chantranupong, L.; Comb, W.; et al. Metabolism. Lysosomal amino acid transporter SLC38A9 signals arginine sufficiency to mTORC1. *Science* **2015**, *347*, 188–194. [CrossRef] [PubMed]

44. Wolfson, R.L.; Chantranupong, L.; Saxton, R.A.; Shen, K.; Scaria, S.M.; Cantor, J.R.; Sabatini, D.M. Sestrin2 is a leucine sensor for the mTORC1 pathway. *Science* **2016**, *351*, 43–48. [CrossRef] [PubMed]

45. Ma, X.M.; Blenis, J. Molecular mechanisms of mTOR-mediated translational control. *Nat. Rev. Mol. Cell Biol.* **2009**, *10*, 307–318. [CrossRef] [PubMed]

46. Gingras, A.C.; Kennedy, S.G.; O'Leary, M.A.; Sonenberg, N.; Hay, N. 4E-BP1, a repressor of mRNA translation, is phosphorylated and inactivated by the Akt(PKB) signaling pathway. *Genes Dev.* **1998**, *12*, 502–513. [CrossRef] [PubMed]

47. Browne, G.J.; Proud, C.G. A novel mTOR-regulated phosphorylation site in elongation factor 2 kinase modulates the activity of the kinase and its binding to calmodulin. *Mol. Cell Biol.* **2004**, *24*, 2986–2997. [CrossRef] [PubMed]

48. Holz, M.K.; Ballif, B.A.; Gygi, S.P.; Blenis, J. mTOR and S6K1 mediate assembly of the translation preinitiation complex through dynamic protein interchange and ordered phosphorylation events. *Cell* **2005**, *123*, 569–580. [CrossRef]

49. Hsieh, A.C.; Liu, Y.; Edlind, M.P.; Ingolia, N.T.; Janes, M.R.; Sher, A.; Shi, E.Y.; Stumpf, C.R.; Christensen, C.; Bonham, M.J.; et al. The translational landscape of mTOR signalling steers cancer initiation and metastasis. *Nature* **2012**, *485*, 55–61. [CrossRef]

50. Azpiazu, I.; Saltiel, A.R.; DePaoli-Roach, A.A.; Lawrence, J.C. Regulation of both glycogen synthase and PHAS-I by insulin in rat skeletal muscle involves mitogen-activated protein kinase-independent and rapamycin-sensitive pathways. *J. Biol. Chem.* **1996**, *271*, 5033–5039.

51. Hudson, C.C.; Liu, M.; Chiang, G.G.; Otterness, D.M.; Loomis, D.C.; Kaper, F.; Giaccia, A.J.; Abraham, R.T. Regulation of hypoxia-inducible factor 1alpha expression and function by the mammalian target of rapamycin. *Mol. Cell Biol.* **2002**, *22*, 7004–7014. [CrossRef] [PubMed]

52. Huffman, T.A.; Mothe-Satney, I.; Lawrence, J.C., Jr. Insulin-stimulated phosphorylation of lipin mediated by the mammalian target of rapamycin. *Proc. Natl. Acad. Sci. USA* **2002**, *99*, 1047–1052. [CrossRef] [PubMed]

53. Peterson, R.T.; Desai, B.N.; Hardwick, J.S.; Schreiber, S.L. Protein phosphatase 2A interacts with the 70-kDa S6 kinase and is activated by inhibition of FKBP12-rapamycinassociated protein. *Proc. Natl. Acad. Sci. USA* **1999**, *96*, 4438–4442. [CrossRef] [PubMed]

54. Yokogami, K.; Wakisaka, S.; Avruch, J.; Reeves, S.A. Serine phosphorylation and maximal activation of STAT3 during CNTF signaling is mediated by the rapamycin target mTOR. *Curr. Biol.* **2000**, *10*, 47–50. [CrossRef]

55. Dowling, R.J.; Topisirovic, I.; Alain, T.; Bidinosti, M.; Fonseca, B.D.; Petroulakis, E.; Wang, X.; Larsson, O.; Selvaraj, A.; Liu, Y.; et al. mTORC1-mediated cell proliferation, but not cell growth, controlled by the 4E-BPs. *Science* **2010**, *328*, 1172–1176. [CrossRef] [PubMed]

56. Fingar, D.C.; Salama, S.; Tsou, C.; Harlow, E.; Blenis, J. Mammalian cell size is controlled by mTOR and its downstream targets S6K1 and 4EBP1/eIF4E. *Genes Dev.* **2002**, *16*, 1472–1487. [CrossRef] [PubMed]

57. Humphrey, S.J.; Yang, G.; Yang, P.; Fazakerley, D.J.; Stockli, J.; Yang, J.Y.; James, D.E. Dynamic adipocyte phosphoproteome reveals that Akt directly regulates mTORC2. *Cell Metab.* **2013**, *17*, 1009–1020. [CrossRef]

58. Liu, P.; Gan, W.; Inuzuka, H.; Lazorchak, A.S.; Gao, D.; Arojo, O.; Liu, D.; Wan, L.; Zhai, B.; Yu, Y.; et al. Sin1 phosphorylation impairs mTORC2 complex integrity and inhibits downstream Akt signalling to suppress tumorigenesis. *Nat. Cell Biol.* **2013**, *15*, 1340–1350. [CrossRef]

59. Yang, G.; Murashige, D.S.; Humphrey, S.J.; James, D.E. A Positive Feedback Loop between Akt and mTORC2 via SIN1 Phosphorylation. *Cell Rep.* **2015**, *12*, 937–943. [CrossRef]

60. Zhang, J.; Xu, K.; Liu, P.; Geng, Y.; Wang, B.; Gan, W.; Guo, J.; Wu, F.; Chin, Y.R.; Berrios, C.; et al. Inhibition of Rb Phosphorylation Leads to mTORC2-Mediated Activation of Akt. *Mol. Cell* **2016**, *62*, 929–942. [CrossRef]

61. Willems, L.; Tamburini, J.; Chapuis, N.; Lacombe, C.; Mayeux, P.; Bouscary, D. PI3K and mTOR signaling pathways in cancer: New data on targeted therapies. *Curr. Oncol. Rep.* **2012**, *14*, 129–138. [CrossRef] [PubMed]

62. Hsu, P.P.; Kang, S.A.; Rameseder, J.; Zhang, Y.; Ottina, K.A.; Lim, D.; Peterson, T.R.; Choi, Y.; Gray, N.S.; Yaffe, M.B.; et al. The mTOR-regulated phosphoproteome reveals a mechanism of mTORC1-mediated inhibition of growth factor signaling. *Science* **2011**, *332*, 1317–1322. [CrossRef]

63. Um, S.H.; Frigerio, F.; Watanabe, M.; Picard, F.; Joaquin, M.; Sticker, M.; Fumagalli, S.; Allegrini, P.R.; Kozma, S.C.; Auwerx, J.; et al. Absence of S6K1 protects against age- and diet-induced obesity while enhancing insulin sensitivity. *Nature* **2004**, *431*, 200–205. [CrossRef] [PubMed]

64. Yu, Y.; Yoon, S.O.; Poulogiannis, G.; Yang, Q.; Ma, X.M.; Villen, J.; Kubica, N.; Hoffman, G.R.; Cantley, L.C.; Gygi, S.P.; et al. Phosphoproteomic analysis identifies Grb10 as an mTORC1 substrate that negatively regulates insulin signaling. *Science* **2011**, *332*, 1322–1326. [CrossRef] [PubMed]

65. Bakker, W.J.; Harris, I.S.; Mak, T.W. FOXO3a is activated in response to hypoxic stress and inhibits HIF1-induced apoptosis via regulation of CITED2. *Mol. Cell* **2007**, *28*, 941–953. [CrossRef] [PubMed]

66. Weiler, M.; Blaes, J.; Pusch, S.; Sahm, F.; Czabanka, M.; Luger, S.; Bunse, L.; Solecki, G.; Eichwald, V.; Jugold, M.; et al. mTOR target NDRG1 confers MGMT-dependent resistance to alkylating chemotherapy. *Proc. Natl. Acad. Sci. USA* **2014**, *111*, 409–414. [CrossRef]

67. Gan, X.; Wang, J.; Wang, C.; Sommer, E.; Kozasa, T.; Srinivasula, S.; Alessi, D.; Offermanns, S.; Simon, M.I.; Wu, D. PRR5L degradation promotes mTORC2-mediated PKC-delta phosphorylation and cell migration downstream of Galpha12. *Nat. Cell Biol.* **2012**, *14*, 686–696. [CrossRef]

68. Thomanetz, V.; Angliker, N.; Cloetta, D.; Lustenberger, R.M.; Schweighauser, M.; Oliveri, F.; Suzuki, N.; Ruegg, M.A. Ablation of the mTORC2 component rictor in brain or Purkinje cells affects size and neuron morphology. *J. Cell Biol.* **2013**, *201*, 293–308. [CrossRef]

69. Fruman, D.A.; Rommel, C. PI3K and cancer: Lessons, challenges and opportunities. *Nat. Rev. Drug Discov.* **2014**, *13*, 140–156. [CrossRef]

70. Grabiner, B.C.; Nardi, V.; Birsoy, K.; Possemato, R.; Shen, K.; Sinha, S.; Jordan, A.; Beck, A.H.; Sabatini, D.M. A diverse array of cancer-associated MTOR mutations are hyperactivating and can predict rapamycin sensitivity. *Cancer Discov.* **2014**, *4*, 554–563. [CrossRef]

71. Cheng, H.; Zou, Y.; Ross, J.S.; Wang, K.; Liu, X.; Halmos, B.; Ali, S.M.; Liu, H.; Verma, A.; Montagna, C.; et al. RICTOR Amplification Defines a Novel Subset of Patients with Lung Cancer Who May Benefit from Treatment with mTORC1/2 Inhibitors. *Cancer Discov.* **2015**, *5*, 1262–1270. [CrossRef] [PubMed]

72. Morrison Joly, M.; Hicks, D.J.; Jones, B.; Sanchez, V.; Estrada, M.V.; Young, C.; Williams, M.; Rexer, B.N.; Sarbassov dos, D.; Muller, W.J.; et al. Rictor/mTORC2 Drives Progression and Therapeutic Resistance of HER2-Amplified Breast Cancers. *Cancer Res.* **2016**, *76*, 4752–4764. [CrossRef] [PubMed]

73. Balko, J.M.; Giltnane, J.M.; Wang, K.; Schwarz, L.J.; Young, C.D.; Cook, R.S.; Owens, P.; Sanders, M.E.; Kuba, M.G.; Sanchez, V.; et al. Molecular profiling of the residual disease of triple-negative breast cancers after neoadjuvant chemotherapy identifies actionable therapeutic targets. *Cancer Discov.* **2014**, *4*, 232–245. [CrossRef] [PubMed]

74. Masri, J.; Bernath, A.; Martin, J.; Jo, O.D.; Vartanian, R.; Funk, A.; Gera, J. mTORC2 activity is elevated in gliomas and promotes growth and cell motility via overexpression of rictor. *Cancer Res.* **2007**, *67*, 11712–11720. [CrossRef] [PubMed]

75. Zhang, Y.; Kwok-Shing Ng, P.; Kucherlapati, M.; Chen, F.; Liu, Y.; Tsang, Y.H.; de Velasco, G.; Jeong, K.J.; Akbani, R.; Hadjipanayis, A.; et al. A Pan-Cancer Proteogenomic Atlas of PI3K/AKT/mTOR Pathway Alterations. *Cancer Cell* **2017**, *31*, 820–832 e823. [CrossRef] [PubMed]

76. Guertin, D.A.; Sabatini, D.M. Defining the role of mTOR in cancer. *Cancer Cell* **2007**, *12*, 9–22. [CrossRef] [PubMed]

77. Liu, P.; Cheng, H.; Roberts, T.M.; Zhao, J.J. Targeting the phosphoinositide 3-kinase pathway in cancer. *Nat. Rev. Drug Discov.* **2009**, *8*, 627–644. [CrossRef] [PubMed]

78. Guertin, D.A.; Stevens, D.M.; Saitoh, M.; Kinkel, S.; Crosby, K.; Sheen, J.H.; Mullholland, D.J.; Magnuson, M.A.; Wu, H.; Sabatini, D.M. mTOR complex 2 is required for the development of prostate cancer induced by Pten loss in mice. *Cancer Cell* **2009**, *15*, 148–159. [CrossRef] [PubMed]

79. Zoncu, R.; Efeyan, A.; Sabatini, D.M. mTOR: From growth signal integration to cancer, diabetes and ageing. *Nat. Rev. Mol. Cell Biol.* **2011**, *12*, 21–35. [CrossRef]

80. Milella, M.; Falcone, I.; Conciatori, F.; Cesta Incani, U.; Del Curatolo, A.; Inzerilli, N.; Nuzzo, C.M.; Vaccaro, V.; Vari, S.; Cognetti, F.; et al. PTEN: Multiple Functions in Human Malignant Tumors. *Front. Oncol.* **2015**, *5*, 24. [CrossRef]

81. Shi, Y.; Gera, J.; Hu, L.; Hsu, J.H.; Bookstein, R.; Li, W.; Lichtenstein, A. Enhanced sensitivity of multiple myeloma cells containing PTEN mutations to CCI-779. *Cancer Res.* **2002**, *62*, 5027–5034. [PubMed]

82. DeGraffenried, L.A.; Fulcher, L.; Friedrichs, W.E.; Grunwald, V.; Ray, R.B.; Hidalgo, M. Reduced PTEN expression in breast cancer cells confers susceptibility to inhibitors of the PI3 kinase/Akt pathway. *Ann. Oncol.* **2004**, *15*, 1510–1516. [CrossRef] [PubMed]

83. Milam, M.R.; Celestino, J.; Wu, W.; Broaddus, R.R.; Schmeler, K.M.; Slomovitz, B.M.; Soliman, P.T.; Gershenson, D.M.; Wang, H.; Ellenson, L.H.; et al. Reduced progression of endometrial hyperplasia with oral mTOR inhibition in the Pten heterozygote murine model. *Am. J. Obstet. Gynecol.* **2007**, *196*, 247-e1. [CrossRef] [PubMed]

84. Pulito, C.; Mori, F.; Sacconi, A.; Goeman, F.; Ferraiuolo, M.; Pasanisi, P.; Campagnoli, C.; Berrino, F.; Fanciulli, M.; Ford, R.J.; et al. Metformin-induced ablation of microRNA 21-5p releases Sestrin-1 and CAB39L antitumoral activities. *Cell Discov.* **2017**, *3*, 17022. [CrossRef] [PubMed]

85. Platt, F.M.; Hurst, C.D.; Taylor, C.F.; Gregory, W.M.; Harnden, P.; Knowles, M.A. Spectrum of phosphatidylinositol 3-kinase pathway gene alterations in bladder cancer. *Clin. Cancer Res.* **2009**, *15*, 6008–6017. [CrossRef] [PubMed]

86. Sjodahl, G.; Lauss, M.; Gudjonsson, S.; Liedberg, F.; Hallden, C.; Chebil, G.; Mansson, W.; Hoglund, M.; Lindgren, D. A systematic study of gene mutations in urothelial carcinoma; inactivating mutations in TSC2 and PIK3R1. *PLoS ONE* **2011**, *6*, e18583. [CrossRef]

87. Jiao, Y.; Shi, C.; Edil, B.H.; de Wilde, R.F.; Klimstra, D.S.; Maitra, A.; Schulick, R.D.; Tang, L.H.; Wolfgang, C.L.; Choti, M.A.; et al. DAXX/ATRX, MEN1, and mTOR pathway genes are frequently altered in pancreatic neuroendocrine tumors. *Science* **2011**, *331*, 1199–1203. [CrossRef]

88. Mossmann, D.; Park, S.; Hall, M.N. mTOR signalling and cellular metabolism are mutual determinants in cancer. *Nat. Rev. Cancer* **2018**, *18*, 744–757. [CrossRef]

89. Duvel, K.; Yecies, J.L.; Menon, S.; Raman, P.; Lipovsky, A.I.; Souza, A.L.; Triantafellow, E.; Ma, Q.; Gorski, R.; Cleaver, S.; et al. Activation of a metabolic gene regulatory network downstream of mTOR complex 1. *Mol. Cell* **2010**, *39*, 171–183. [CrossRef]

90. Majumder, P.K.; Febbo, P.G.; Bikoff, R.; Berger, R.; Xue, Q.; McMahon, L.M.; Manola, J.; Brugarolas, J.; McDonnell, T.J.; Golub, T.R.; et al. mTOR inhibition reverses Akt-dependent prostate intraepithelial neoplasia through regulation of apoptotic and HIF-1-dependent pathways. *Nat. Med.* **2004**, *10*, 594–601. [CrossRef]

91. Gordan, J.D.; Thompson, C.B.; Simon, M.C. HIF and c-Myc: Sibling rivals for control of cancer cell metabolism and proliferation. *Cancer Cell* **2007**, *12*, 108–113. [CrossRef] [PubMed]

92. Elstrom, R.L.; Bauer, D.E.; Buzzai, M.; Karnauskas, R.; Harris, M.H.; Plas, D.R.; Zhuang, H.; Cinalli, R.M.; Alavi, A.; Rudin, C.M.; et al. Akt stimulates aerobic glycolysis in cancer cells. *Cancer Res.* **2004**, *64*, 3892–3899. [CrossRef] [PubMed]

93. Peterson, T.R.; Sengupta, S.S.; Harris, T.E.; Carmack, A.E.; Kang, S.A.; Balderas, E.; Guertin, D.A.; Madden, K.L.; Carpenter, A.E.; Finck, B.N.; et al. mTOR complex 1 regulates lipin 1 localization to control the SREBP pathway. *Cell* **2011**, *146*, 408–420. [CrossRef] [PubMed]

94. Porstmann, T.; Santos, C.R.; Griffiths, B.; Cully, M.; Wu, M.; Leevers, S.; Griffiths, J.R.; Chung, Y.L.; Schulze, A. SREBP activity is regulated by mTORC1 and contributes to Akt-dependent cell growth. *Cell Metab.* **2008**, *8*, 224–236. [CrossRef]

95. Ricoult, S.J.; Yecies, J.L.; Ben-Sahra, I.; Manning, B.D. Oncogenic PI3K and K-Ras stimulate de novo lipid synthesis through mTORC1 and SREBP. *Oncogene* **2016**, *35*, 1250–1260. [CrossRef] [PubMed]

96. Ben-Sahra, I.; Howell, J.J.; Asara, J.M.; Manning, B.D. Stimulation of de novo pyrimidine synthesis by growth signaling through mTOR and S6K1. *Science* **2013**, *339*, 1323–1328. [CrossRef] [PubMed]

97. Ben-Sahra, I.; Hoxhaj, G.; Ricoult, S.J.H.; Asara, J.M.; Manning, B.D. mTORC1 induces purine synthesis through control of the mitochondrial tetrahydrofolate cycle. *Science* **2016**, *351*, 728–733. [CrossRef]

98. White, E. The role for autophagy in cancer. *J. Clin. Investig.* **2015**, *125*, 42–46. [CrossRef]

99. Rosenfeldt, M.T.; O'Prey, J.; Morton, J.P.; Nixon, C.; MacKay, G.; Mrowinska, A.; Au, A.; Rai, T.S.; Zheng, L.; Ridgway, R.; et al. p53 status determines the role of autophagy in pancreatic tumour development. *Nature* **2013**, *504*, 296–300. [CrossRef]

100. Iacobuzio-Donahue, C.A.; Herman, J.M. Autophagy, p53, and pancreatic cancer. *N. Engl. J. Med.* **2014**, *370*, 1352–1353. [CrossRef]

101. White, E.; DiPaola, R.S. The double-edged sword of autophagy modulation in cancer. *Clin. Cancer Res.* **2009**, *15*, 5308–5316. [CrossRef] [PubMed]
102. Kim, Y.C.; Guan, K.L. mTOR: A pharmacologic target for autophagy regulation. *J. Clin. Investig.* **2015**, *125*, 25–32. [CrossRef] [PubMed]
103. Hosokawa, N.; Hara, T.; Kaizuka, T.; Kishi, C.; Takamura, A.; Miura, Y.; Iemura, S.; Natsume, T.; Takehana, K.; Yamada, N.; et al. Nutrient-dependent mTORC1 association with the ULK1-Atg13-FIP200 complex required for autophagy. *Mol. Biol. Cell* **2009**, *20*, 1981–1991. [CrossRef] [PubMed]
104. Jung, C.H.; Jun, C.B.; Ro, S.H.; Kim, Y.M.; Otto, N.M.; Cao, J.; Kundu, M.; Kim, D.H. ULK-Atg13-FIP200 complexes mediate mTOR signaling to the autophagy machinery. *Mol. Biol. Cell* **2009**, *20*, 1992–2003. [CrossRef] [PubMed]
105. Settembre, C.; Fraldi, A.; Medina, D.L.; Ballabio, A. Signals from the lysosome: A control centre for cellular clearance and energy metabolism. *Nat. Rev. Mol. Cell Biol.* **2013**, *14*, 283–296. [CrossRef] [PubMed]
106. Klempner, S.J.; Myers, A.P.; Cantley, L.C. What a tangled web we weave: Emerging resistance mechanisms to inhibition of the phosphoinositide 3-kinase pathway. *Cancer Discov.* **2013**, *3*, 1345–1354. [CrossRef] [PubMed]
107. Gingras, A.C.; Raught, B.; Gygi, S.P.; Niedzwiecka, A.; Miron, M.; Burley, S.K.; Polakiewicz, R.D.; Wyslouch-Cieszynska, A.; Aebersold, R.; Sonenberg, N. Hierarchical phosphorylation of the translation inhibitor 4E-BP1. *Genes Dev.* **2001**, *15*, 2852–2864.
108. Faivre, S.; Kroemer, G.; Raymond, E. Current development of mTOR inhibitors as anticancer agents. *Nat. Rev. Drug Discov.* **2006**, *5*, 671–688. [CrossRef]
109. Huang, J.; Wu, S.; Wu, C.L.; Manning, B.D. Signaling events downstream of mammalian target of rapamycin complex 2 are attenuated in cells and tumors deficient for the tuberous sclerosis complex tumor suppressors. *Cancer Res.* **2009**, *69*, 6107–6114. [CrossRef]
110. Benjamin, D.; Colombi, M.; Moroni, C.; Hall, M.N. Rapamycin passes the torch: A new generation of mTOR inhibitors. *Nat. Rev. Drug Discov.* **2011**, *10*, 868–880. [CrossRef]
111. Gonzalez-Angulo, A.M.; Meric-Bernstam, F.; Chawla, S.; Falchook, G.; Hong, D.; Akcakanat, A.; Chen, H.; Naing, A.; Fu, S.; Wheler, J.; et al. Weekly nab-Rapamycin in patients with advanced nonhematologic malignancies: Final results of a phase I trial. *Clin. Cancer Res.* **2013**, *19*, 5474–5484. [CrossRef] [PubMed]
112. Janku, F.; Yap, T.A.; Meric-Bernstam, F. Targeting the PI3K pathway in cancer: Are we making headway? *Nat. Rev. Clin. Oncol.* **2018**, *15*, 273–291. [CrossRef] [PubMed]
113. Cooper, W.A.; Lam, D.C.; O'Toole, S.A.; Minna, J.D. Molecular biology of lung cancer. *J. Thorac. Dis.* **2013**, *5* (Suppl. 5), S479–S490. [PubMed]
114. Cancer Genome Atlas Research Network. Comprehensive genomic characterization of squamous cell lung cancers. *Nature* **2012**, *489*, 519–525. [CrossRef] [PubMed]
115. Umemura, S.; Mimaki, S.; Makinoshima, H.; Tada, S.; Ishii, G.; Ohmatsu, H.; Niho, S.; Yoh, K.; Matsumoto, S.; Takahashi, A.; et al. Therapeutic priority of the PI3K/AKT/mTOR pathway in small cell lung cancers as revealed by a comprehensive genomic analysis. *J. Thorac. Oncol.* **2014**, *9*, 1324–1331. [CrossRef] [PubMed]
116. Lee, J.H.; Kang, K.W.; Lee, H.W. Expression of phosphorylated mTOR and its clinical significances in small cell lung cancer. *Int. J. Clin. Exp. Pathol.* **2015**, *8*, 2987–2993. [PubMed]
117. Li, L.; Liu, D.; Qiu, Z.X.; Zhao, S.; Zhang, L.; Li, W.M. The prognostic role of mTOR and p-mTOR for survival in non-small cell lung cancer: A systematic review and meta-analysis. *PLoS ONE* **2015**, *10*, e0116771. [CrossRef]
118. O'Donnell, A.; Faivre, S.; Burris, H.A., 3rd; Rea, D.; Papadimitrakopoulou, V.; Shand, N.; Lane, H.A.; Hazell, K.; Zoellner, U.; Kovarik, J.M.; et al. Phase I pharmacokinetic and pharmacodynamic study of the oral mammalian target of rapamycin inhibitor everolimus in patients with advanced solid tumors. *J. Clin. Oncol.* **2008**, *26*, 1588–1595.
119. Besse, B.; Leighl, N.; Bennouna, J.; Papadimitrakopoulou, V.A.; Blais, N.; Traynor, A.M.; Soria, J.C.; Gogov, S.; Miller, N.; Jehl, V.; et al. Phase II study of everolimus-erlotinib in previously treated patients with advanced non-small-cell lung cancer. *Ann. Oncol.* **2014**, *25*, 409–415. [CrossRef]
120. Mellema, W.W.; Dingemans, A.M.; Thunnissen, E.; Snijders, P.J.; Derks, J.; Heideman, D.A.; Van Suylen, R.; Smit, E.F. KRAS mutations in advanced nonsquamous non-small-cell lung cancer patients treated with first-line platinum-based chemotherapy have no predictive value. *J. Thorac. Oncol.* **2013**, *8*, 1190–1195. [CrossRef]

121. Deutsch, E.; Le Pechoux, C.; Faivre, L.; Rivera, S.; Tao, Y.; Pignon, J.P.; Angokai, M.; Bahleda, R.; Deandreis, D.; Angevin, E.; et al. Phase I trial of everolimus in combination with thoracic radiotherapy in non-small-cell lung cancer. *Ann. Oncol.* **2015**, *26*, 1223–1229. [CrossRef] [PubMed]

122. Ramalingam, S.S.; Owonikoko, T.K.; Behera, M.; Subramanian, J.; Saba, N.F.; Kono, S.A.; Gal, A.A.; Sica, G.; Harvey, R.D.; Chen, Z.; et al. Phase II study of docetaxel in combination with everolimus for second- or third-line therapy of advanced non-small-cell lung cancer. *J. Thorac. Oncol.* **2013**, *8*, 369–372. [CrossRef] [PubMed]

123. Soria, J.C.; Shepherd, F.A.; Douillard, J.Y.; Wolf, J.; Giaccone, G.; Crino, L.; Cappuzzo, F.; Sharma, S.; Gross, S.H.; Dimitrijevic, S.; et al. Efficacy of everolimus (RAD001) in patients with advanced NSCLC previously treated with chemotherapy alone or with chemotherapy and EGFR inhibitors. *Ann. Oncol.* **2009**, *20*, 1674–1681. [CrossRef] [PubMed]

124. Price, K.A.; Azzoli, C.G.; Krug, L.M.; Pietanza, M.C.; Rizvi, N.A.; Pao, W.; Kris, M.G.; Riely, G.J.; Heelan, R.T.; Arcila, M.E.; et al. Phase II trial of gefitinib and everolimus in advanced non-small cell lung cancer. *J. Thorac. Oncol.* **2010**, *5*, 1623–1629. [CrossRef] [PubMed]

125. Ohara, T.; Takaoka, M.; Toyooka, S.; Tomono, Y.; Nishikawa, T.; Shirakawa, Y.; Yamatsuji, T.; Tanaka, N.; Fujiwara, T.; Naomoto, Y. Inhibition of mTOR by temsirolimus contributes to prolonged survival of mice with pleural dissemination of non-small-cell lung cancer cells. *Cancer Sci.* **2011**, *102*, 1344–1349. [CrossRef] [PubMed]

126. Hidalgo, M.; Buckner, J.C.; Erlichman, C.; Pollack, M.S.; Boni, J.P.; Dukart, G.; Marshall, B.; Speicher, L.; Moore, L.; Rowinsky, E.K. A phase I and pharmacokinetic study of temsirolimus (CCI-779) administered intravenously daily for 5 days every 2 weeks to patients with advanced cancer. *Clin. Cancer Res.* **2006**, *12*, 5755–5763. [CrossRef] [PubMed]

127. Reungwetwattana, T.; Molina, J.R.; Mandrekar, S.J.; Allen-Ziegler, K.; Rowland, K.M.; Reuter, N.F.; Luyun, R.F.; Dy, G.K.; Marks, R.S.; Schild, S.E.; et al. Brief report: A phase II "window-of-opportunity" frontline study of the MTOR inhibitor, temsirolimus given as a single agent in patients with advanced NSCLC, an NCCTG study. *J. Thorac. Oncol.* **2012**, *7*, 919–922. [CrossRef]

128. Wislez, M.; Spencer, M.L.; Izzo, J.G.; Juroske, D.M.; Balhara, K.; Cody, D.D.; Price, R.E.; Hittelman, W.N.; Wistuba, I.I.; Kurie, J.M. Inhibition of mammalian target of rapamycin reverses alveolar epithelial neoplasia induced by oncogenic K-ras. *Cancer Res.* **2005**, *65*, 3226–3235. [CrossRef]

129. Mamdani, H.; Induru, R.; Jalal, S.I. Novel therapies in small cell lung cancer. *Transl. Lung Cancer Res.* **2015**, *4*, 533–544.

130. Riquelme, I.; Tapia, O.; Espinoza, J.A.; Leal, P.; Buchegger, K.; Sandoval, A.; Bizama, C.; Araya, J.C.; Peek, R.M.; Roa, J.C. The Gene Expression Status of the PI3K/AKT/mTOR Pathway in Gastric Cancer Tissues and Cell Lines. *Pathol. Oncol. Res.* **2016**, *22*, 797–805. [CrossRef]

131. Sukawa, Y.; Yamamoto, H.; Nosho, K.; Ito, M.; Igarashi, H.; Naito, T.; Mitsuhashi, K.; Matsunaga, Y.; Takahashi, T.; Mikami, M.; et al. HER2 expression and PI3K-Akt pathway alterations in gastric cancer. *Digestion* **2014**, *89*, 12–17. [CrossRef] [PubMed]

132. Markman, B.; Atzori, F.; Perez-Garcia, J.; Tabernero, J.; Baselga, J. Status of PI3K inhibition and biomarker development in cancer therapeutics. *Ann. Oncol.* **2010**, *21*, 683–691. [CrossRef] [PubMed]

133. Cancer Genome Atlas Research Network. Comprehensive molecular characterization of gastric adenocarcinoma. *Nature* **2014**, *513*, 202–209.

134. Chong, M.L.; Loh, M.; Thakkar, B.; Pang, B.; Iacopetta, B.; Soong, R. Phosphatidylinositol-3-kinase pathway aberrations in gastric and colorectal cancer: Meta-analysis, co-occurrence and ethnic variation. *Int. J. Cancer* **2014**, *134*, 1232–1238. [CrossRef] [PubMed]

135. Wen, Y.G.; Wang, Q.; Zhou, C.Z.; Qiu, G.Q.; Peng, Z.H.; Tang, H.M. Mutation analysis of tumor suppressor gene PTEN in patients with gastric carcinomas and its impact on PI3K/AKT pathway. *Oncol. Rep.* **2010**, *24*, 89–95. [PubMed]

136. Carracedo, A.; Alimonti, A.; Pandolfi, P.P. PTEN level in tumor suppression: How much is too little? *Cancer Res.* **2011**, *71*, 629–633. [CrossRef] [PubMed]

137. Nam, S.Y.; Lee, H.S.; Jung, G.A.; Choi, J.; Cho, S.J.; Kim, M.K.; Kim, W.H.; Lee, B.L. Akt/PKB activation in gastric carcinomas correlates with clinicopathologic variables and prognosis. *APMIS* **2003**, *111*, 1105–1113. [CrossRef] [PubMed]

138. Tran, P.; Nguyen, C.; Klempner, S.J. Targeting the Phosphatidylinositol-3-kinase Pathway in Gastric Cancer: Can Omics Improve Outcomes? *Int. Neurourol. J.* **2016**, *20*, S131–S140. [CrossRef]

139. Byeon, S.J.; Han, N.; Choi, J.; Kim, M.A.; Kim, W.H. Prognostic implication of TSC1 and mTOR expression in gastric carcinoma. *J. Surg. Oncol.* **2014**, *109*, 812–817. [CrossRef]

140. Yu, G.; Wang, J.; Chen, Y.; Wang, X.; Pan, J.; Li, G.; Jia, Z.; Li, Q.; Yao, J.C.; Xie, K. Overexpression of phosphorylated mammalian target of rapamycin predicts lymph node metastasis and prognosis of Chinese patients with gastric cancer. *Clin. Cancer Res.* **2009**, *15*, 1821–1829. [CrossRef]

141. He, J.; Wang, M.Y.; Qiu, L.X.; Zhu, M.L.; Shi, T.Y.; Zhou, X.Y.; Sun, M.H.; Yang, Y.J.; Wang, J.C.; Jin, L.; et al. Genetic variations of mTORC1 genes and risk of gastric cancer in an Eastern Chinese population. *Mol. Carcinog.* **2013**, *52* (Suppl. 1), E70–E79. [CrossRef] [PubMed]

142. Xiao, L.; Wang, Y.C.; Li, W.S.; Du, Y. The role of mTOR and phospho-p70S6K in pathogenesis and progression of gastric carcinomas: An immunohistochemical study on tissue microarray. *J. Exp. Clin. Cancer Res.* **2009**, *28*, 152. [CrossRef] [PubMed]

143. Cejka, D.; Preusser, M.; Woehrer, A.; Sieghart, W.; Strommer, S.; Werzowa, J.; Fuereder, T.; Wacheck, V. Everolimus (RAD001) and anti-angiogenic cyclophosphamide show long-term control of gastric cancer growth in vivo. *Cancer Biol. Ther.* **2008**, *7*, 1377–1385. [CrossRef]

144. Fuereder, T.; Jaeger-Lansky, A.; Hoeflmayer, D.; Preusser, M.; Strommer, S.; Cejka, D.; Koehrer, S.; Crevenna, R.; Wacheck, V. mTOR inhibition by everolimus counteracts VEGF induction by sunitinib and improves anti-tumor activity against gastric cancer in vivo. *Cancer Lett.* **2010**, *296*, 249–256. [CrossRef] [PubMed]

145. Lang, S.A.; Gaumann, A.; Koehl, G.E.; Seidel, U.; Bataille, F.; Klein, D.; Ellis, L.M.; Bolder, U.; Hofstaedter, F.; Schlitt, H.J.; et al. Mammalian target of rapamycin is activated in human gastric cancer and serves as a target for therapy in an experimental model. *Int. J. Cancer* **2007**, *120*, 1803–1810. [CrossRef] [PubMed]

146. Meric-Bernstam, F.; Akcakanat, A.; Chen, H.; Do, K.A.; Sangai, T.; Adkins, F.; Gonzalez-Angulo, A.M.; Rashid, A.; Crosby, K.; Dong, M.; et al. PIK3CA/PTEN mutations and Akt activation as markers of sensitivity to allosteric mTOR inhibitors. *Clin. Cancer Res.* **2012**, *18*, 1777–1789. [CrossRef]

147. Doi, T.; Muro, K.; Boku, N.; Yamada, Y.; Nishina, T.; Takiuchi, H.; Komatsu, Y.; Hamamoto, Y.; Ohno, N.; Fujita, Y.; et al. Multicenter phase II study of everolimus in patients with previously treated metastatic gastric cancer. *J. Clin. Oncol.* **2010**, *28*, 1904–1910. [CrossRef]

148. Yoon, D.H.; Ryu, M.H.; Park, Y.S.; Lee, H.J.; Lee, C.; Ryoo, B.Y.; Lee, J.L.; Chang, H.M.; Kim, T.W.; Kang, Y.K. Phase II study of everolimus with biomarker exploration in patients with advanced gastric cancer refractory to chemotherapy including fluoropyrimidine and platinum. *Br. J. Cancer* **2012**, *106*, 1039–1044. [CrossRef]

149. Ohtsu, A.; Ajani, J.A.; Bai, Y.X.; Bang, Y.J.; Chung, H.C.; Pan, H.M.; Sahmoud, T.; Shen, L.; Yeh, K.H.; Chin, K.; et al. Everolimus for previously treated advanced gastric cancer: Results of the randomized, double-blind, phase III GRANITE-1 study. *J. Clin. Oncol.* **2013**, *31*, 3935–3943. [CrossRef]

150. Farran, B.; Muller, S.; Montenegro, R.C. Gastric cancer management: Kinases as a target therapy. *Clin. Exp. Pharmacol. Physiol.* **2017**, *44*, 613–622. [CrossRef]

151. Perotti, A.; Locatelli, A.; Sessa, C.; Hess, D.; Vigano, L.; Capri, G.; Maur, M.; Cerny, T.; Cresta, S.; Rojo, F.; et al. Phase IB study of the mTOR inhibitor ridaforolimus with capecitabine. *J. Clin. Oncol.* **2010**, *28*, 4554–4561. [CrossRef] [PubMed]

152. Xing, X.; Zhang, L.; Wen, X.; Wang, X.; Cheng, X.; Du, H.; Hu, Y.; Li, L.; Dong, B.; Li, Z.; et al. PP242 suppresses cell proliferation, metastasis, and angiogenesis of gastric cancer through inhibition of the PI3K/AKT/mTOR pathway. *Anticancer Drugs* **2014**, *25*, 1129–1140. [CrossRef] [PubMed]

153. Parsons, D.W.; Wang, T.L.; Samuels, Y.; Bardelli, A.; Cummins, J.M.; DeLong, L.; Silliman, N.; Ptak, J.; Szabo, S.; Willson, J.K.; et al. Colorectal cancer: Mutations in a signalling pathway. *Nature* **2005**, *436*, 792. [CrossRef] [PubMed]

154. De Roock, W.; De Vriendt, V.; Normanno, N.; Ciardiello, F.; Tejpar, S. KRAS, BRAF, PIK3CA, and PTEN mutations: Implications for targeted therapies in metastatic colorectal cancer. *Lancet Oncol.* **2011**, *12*, 594–603. [CrossRef]

155. Zhang, J.; Roberts, T.M.; Shivdasani, R.A. Targeting PI3K signaling as a therapeutic approach for colorectal cancer. *Gastroenterology* **2011**, *141*, 50–61. [CrossRef] [PubMed]

156. Johnson, S.M.; Gulhati, P.; Rampy, B.A.; Han, Y.; Rychahou, P.G.; Doan, H.Q.; Weiss, H.L.; Evers, B.M. Novel expression patterns of PI3K/Akt/mTOR signaling pathway components in colorectal cancer. *J. Am. Coll. Surg.* **2010**, *210*, 767–776. [CrossRef]

157. Markowitz, S.D.; Bertagnolli, M.M. Molecular origins of cancer: Molecular basis of colorectal cancer. *N. Engl. J. Med.* **2009**, *361*, 2449–2460. [CrossRef]

158. Baker, S.J.; Preisinger, A.C.; Jessup, J.M.; Paraskeva, C.; Markowitz, S.; Willson, J.K.; Hamilton, S.; Vogelstein, B. p53 gene mutations occur in combination with 17p allelic deletions as late events in colorectal tumorigenesis. *Cancer Res.* **1990**, *50*, 7717–7722.

159. Ellisen, L.W.; Ramsayer, K.D.; Johannessen, C.M.; Yang, A.; Beppu, H.; Minda, K.; Oliner, J.D.; McKeon, F.; Haber, D.A. REDD1, a developmentally regulated transcriptional target of p63 and p53, links p63 to regulation of reactive oxygen species. *Mol. Cell* **2002**, *10*, 995–1005. [CrossRef]

160. Brugarolas, J.; Lei, K.; Hurley, R.L.; Manning, B.D.; Reiling, J.H.; Hafen, E.; Witters, L.A.; Ellisen, L.W.; Kaelin, W.G., Jr. Regulation of mTOR function in response to hypoxia by REDD1 and the TSC1/TSC2 tumor suppressor complex. *Genes Dev.* **2004**, *18*, 2893–2904. [CrossRef]

161. Zhang, Y.J.; Dai, Q.; Sun, D.F.; Xiong, H.; Tian, X.Q.; Gao, F.H.; Xu, M.H.; Chen, G.Q.; Han, Z.G.; Fang, J.Y. mTOR signaling pathway is a target for the treatment of colorectal cancer. *Ann. Surg. Oncol.* **2009**, *16*, 2617–2628. [CrossRef] [PubMed]

162. Ng, K.; Tabernero, J.; Hwang, J.; Bajetta, E.; Sharma, S.; Del Prete, S.A.; Arrowsmith, E.R.; Ryan, D.P.; Sedova, M.; Jin, J.; et al. Phase II study of everolimus in patients with metastatic colorectal adenocarcinoma previously treated with bevacizumab-, fluoropyrimidine-, oxaliplatin-, and irinotecan-based regimens. *Clin. Cancer Res.* **2013**, *19*, 3987–3995. [CrossRef] [PubMed]

163. Spindler, K.L.; Sorensen, M.M.; Pallisgaard, N.; Andersen, R.F.; Havelund, B.M.; Ploen, J.; Lassen, U.; Jakobsen, A.K. Phase II trial of temsirolimus alone and in combination with irinotecan for KRAS mutant metastatic colorectal cancer: Outcome and results of KRAS mutational analysis in plasma. *Acta Oncol.* **2013**, *52*, 963–970. [CrossRef] [PubMed]

164. Zhang, Y.; Zheng, X.F. mTOR-independent 4E-BP1 phosphorylation is associated with cancer resistance to mTOR kinase inhibitors. *Cell Cycle* **2012**, *11*, 594–603. [CrossRef]

165. Wolpin, B.M.; Ng, K.; Zhu, A.X.; Abrams, T.; Enzinger, P.C.; McCleary, N.J.; Schrag, D.; Kwak, E.L.; Allen, J.N.; Bhargava, P.; et al. Multicenter phase II study of tivozanib (AV-951) and everolimus (RAD001) for patients with refractory, metastatic colorectal cancer. *Oncologist* **2013**, *18*, 377–378. [CrossRef] [PubMed]

166. Gulhati, P.; Zaytseva, Y.Y.; Valentino, J.D.; Stevens, P.D.; Kim, J.T.; Sasazuki, T.; Shirasawa, S.; Lee, E.Y.; Weiss, H.L.; Dong, J.; et al. Sorafenib enhances the therapeutic efficacy of rapamycin in colorectal cancers harboring oncogenic KRAS and PIK3CA. *Carcinogenesis* **2012**, *33*, 1782–1790. [CrossRef]

167. Castellano, D.; Bajetta, E.; Panneerselvam, A.; Saletan, S.; Kocha, W.; O'Dorisio, T.; Anthony, L.B.; Hobday, T. Group R-S: Everolimus plus octreotide long-acting repeatable in patients with colorectal neuroendocrine tumors: A subgroup analysis of the phase III RADIANT-2 study. *Oncologist* **2013**, *18*, 46–53. [CrossRef]

168. Bradshaw-Pierce, E.L.; Pitts, T.M.; Kulikowski, G.; Selby, H.; Merz, A.L.; Gustafson, D.L.; Serkova, N.J.; Eckhardt, S.G.; Weekes, C.D. Utilization of quantitative in vivo pharmacology approaches to assess combination effects of everolimus and irinotecan in mouse xenograft models of colorectal cancer. *PLoS ONE* **2013**, *8*, e58089. [CrossRef]

169. Temraz, S.; Mukherji, D.; Shamseddine, A. Dual Inhibition of MEK and PI3K Pathway in KRAS and BRAF Mutated Colorectal Cancers. *Int. J. Mol. Sci.* **2015**, *16*, 22976–22988. [CrossRef]

170. Zhang, Y.J.; Duan, Y.; Zheng, X.F. Targeting the mTOR kinase domain: The second generation of mTOR inhibitors. *Drug Discov. Today* **2011**, *16*, 325–331. [CrossRef]

171. Roper, J.; Richardson, M.P.; Wang, W.V.; Richard, L.G.; Chen, W.; Coffee, E.M.; Sinnamon, M.J.; Lee, L.; Chen, P.C.; Bronson, R.T.; et al. The dual PI3K/mTOR inhibitor NVP-BEZ235 induces tumor regression in a genetically engineered mouse model of PIK3CA wild-type colorectal cancer. *PLoS ONE* **2011**, *6*, e25132. [CrossRef] [PubMed]

172. Bhagwat, S.V.; Gokhale, P.C.; Crew, A.P.; Cooke, A.; Yao, Y.; Mantis, C.; Kahler, J.; Workman, J.; Bittner, M.; Dudkin, L.; et al. Preclinical characterization of OSI-027, a potent and selective inhibitor of mTORC1 and mTORC2: Distinct from rapamycin. *Mol. Cancer Ther.* **2011**, *10*, 1394–1406. [CrossRef] [PubMed]

173. Bahrami, A.; Khazaei, M.; Hasanzadeh, M.; ShahidSales, S.; Joudi Mashhad, M.; Farazestanian, M.; Sadeghnia, H.R.; Rezayi, M.; Maftouh, M.; Hassanian, S.M.; et al. Therapeutic Potential of Targeting

PI3K/AKT Pathway in Treatment of Colorectal Cancer: Rational and Progress. *J. Cell. Biochem.* **2018**, *119*, 2460–2469. [CrossRef] [PubMed]

174. Blaser, B.; Waselle, L.; Dormond-Meuwly, A.; Dufour, M.; Roulin, D.; Demartines, N.; Dormond, O. Antitumor activities of ATP-competitive inhibitors of mTOR in colon cancer cells. *BMC Cancer* **2012**, *12*, 86. [CrossRef] [PubMed]

175. Linehan, W.M.; Srinivasan, R.; Schmidt, L.S. The genetic basis of kidney cancer: A metabolic disease. *Nat. Rev. Urol.* **2010**, *7*, 277–285. [CrossRef] [PubMed]

176. Sun, M.; Wang, G.; Paciga, J.E.; Feldman, R.I.; Yuan, Z.Q.; Ma, X.L.; Shelley, S.A.; Jove, R.; Tsichlis, P.N.; Nicosia, S.V.; et al. AKT1/PKBalpha kinase is frequently elevated in human cancers and its constitutive activation is required for oncogenic transformation in NIH3T3 cells. *Am. J. Pathol.* **2001**, *159*, 431–437. [CrossRef]

177. Lawrence, M.S.; Stojanov, P.; Mermel, C.H.; Robinson, J.T.; Garraway, L.A.; Golub, T.R.; Meyerson, M.; Gabriel, S.B.; Lander, E.S.; Getz, G. Discovery and saturation analysis of cancer genes across 21 tumour types. *Nature* **2014**, *505*, 495–501. [CrossRef]

178. Bernardi, R.; Guernah, I.; Jin, D.; Grisendi, S.; Alimonti, A.; Teruya-Feldstein, J.; Cordon-Cardo, C.; Simon, M.C.; Rafii, S.; Pandolfi, P.P. PML inhibits HIF-1alpha translation and neoangiogenesis through repression of mTOR. *Nature* **2006**, *442*, 779–785. [CrossRef]

179. Toschi, A.; Lee, E.; Gadir, N.; Ohh, M.; Foster, D.A. Differential dependence of hypoxia-inducible factors 1 alpha and 2 alpha on mTORC1 and mTORC2. *J. Biol. Chem.* **2008**, *283*, 34495–34499. [CrossRef]

180. Davis, C.F.; Ricketts, C.J.; Wang, M.; Yang, L.; Cherniack, A.D.; Shen, H.; Buhay, C.; Kang, H.; Kim, S.C.; Fahey, C.C.; et al. The somatic genomic landscape of chromophobe renal cell carcinoma. *Cancer Cell.* **2014**, *26*, 319–330. [CrossRef]

181. Hudes, G.; Carducci, M.; Tomczak, P.; Dutcher, J.; Figlin, R.; Kapoor, A.; Staroslawska, E.; Sosman, J.; McDermott, D.; Bodrogi, I.; et al. Temsirolimus, interferon alfa, or both for advanced renal-cell carcinoma. *N. Engl. J. Med.* **2007**, *356*, 2271–2281. [CrossRef]

182. Amato, R.J.; Jac, J.; Giessinger, S.; Saxena, S.; Willis, J.P. A phase 2 study with a daily regimen of the oral mTOR inhibitor RAD001 (everolimus) in patients with metastatic clear cell renal cell cancer. *Cancer* **2009**, *115*, 2438–2446. [CrossRef] [PubMed]

183. Gonzalez-Larriba, J.L.; Maroto, P.; Duran, I.; Lambea, J.; Flores, L.; Castellano, D.; The Changing, G. The role of mTOR inhibition as second-line therapy in metastatic renal carcinoma: Clinical evidence and current challenges. *Expert Rev. Anticancer Ther.* **2017**, *17*, 217–226. [CrossRef] [PubMed]

184. Kucejova, B.; Pena-Llopis, S.; Yamasaki, T.; Sivanand, S.; Tran, T.A.; Alexander, S.; Wolff, N.C.; Lotan, Y.; Xie, X.J.; Kabbani, W.; et al. Interplay between pVHL and mTORC1 pathways in clear-cell renal cell carcinoma. *Mol. Cancer Res.* **2011**, *9*, 1255–1265. [CrossRef] [PubMed]

185. Kwiatkowski, D.J.; Choueiri, T.K.; Fay, A.P.; Rini, B.I.; Thorner, A.R.; de Velasco, G.; Tyburczy, M.E.; Hamieh, L.; Albiges, L.; Agarwal, N.; et al. Mutations in TSC1, TSC2, and MTOR Are Associated with Response to Rapalogs in Patients with Metastatic Renal Cell Carcinoma. *Clin. Cancer Res.* **2016**, *22*, 2445–2452. [CrossRef] [PubMed]

186. Graham, J.; Heng, D.Y.C.; Brugarolas, J.; Vaishampayan, U. Personalized Management of Advanced Kidney Cancer. *Am. Soc. Clin. Oncol. Educ. Book* **2018**, *38*, 330–341. [CrossRef] [PubMed]

187. Ghidini, M.; Petrelli, F.; Ghidini, A.; Tomasello, G.; Hahne, J.C.; Passalacqua, R.; Barni, S. Clinical development of mTor inhibitors for renal cancer. *Expert Opin. Investig. Drugs* **2017**, *26*, 1229–1237. [CrossRef]

188. Cho, D. Novel targeting of phosphatidylinositol 3-kinase and mammalian target of rapamycin in renal cell carcinoma. *Cancer J.* **2013**, *19*, 311–315. [CrossRef]

189. Fishman, M.N.; Srinivas, S.; Hauke, R.J.; Amato, R.J.; Esteves, B.; Cotreau, M.M.; Strahs, A.L.; Slichenmyer, W.J.; Bhargava, P.; Kabbinavar, F.F. Phase Ib study of tivozanib (AV-951) in combination with temsirolimus in patients with renal cell carcinoma. *Eur. J. Cancer* **2013**, *49*, 2841–2850. [CrossRef]

190. Babjuk, M.; Bohle, A.; Burger, M.; Capoun, O.; Cohen, D.; Comperat, E.M.; Hernandez, V.; Kaasinen, E.; Palou, J.; Roupret, M.; et al. EAU Guidelines on Non-Muscle-invasive Urothelial Carcinoma of the Bladder: Update 2016. *Eur. Urol.* **2017**, *71*, 447–461. [CrossRef]

191. Carneiro, B.A.; Meeks, J.J.; Kuzel, T.M.; Scaranti, M.; Abdulkadir, S.A.; Giles, F.J. Emerging therapeutic targets in bladder cancer. *Cancer Treat. Rev.* **2015**, *41*, 170–178. [CrossRef] [PubMed]

192. Cancer Genome Atlas Research Network. Comprehensive molecular characterization of urothelial bladder carcinoma. *Nature* **2014**, *507*, 315–322. [CrossRef] [PubMed]

193. Houede, N.; Pourquier, P. Targeting the genetic alterations of the PI3K-AKT-mTOR pathway: Its potential use in the treatment of bladder cancers. *Pharmacol. Ther.* **2015**, *145*, 1–18. [CrossRef] [PubMed]

194. Audenet, F.; Attalla, K.; Sfakianos, J.P. The evolution of bladder cancer genomics: What have we learned and how can we use it? *Urol. Oncol.* **2018**, *36*, 313–320. [CrossRef] [PubMed]

195. Sun, C.H.; Chang, Y.H.; Pan, C.C. Activation of the PI3K/Akt/mTOR pathway correlates with tumour progression and reduced survival in patients with urothelial carcinoma of the urinary bladder. *Histopathology* **2011**, *58*, 1054–1063. [CrossRef] [PubMed]

196. Abraham, R.; Pagano, F.; Gomella, L.G.; Baffa, R. Chromosomal deletions in bladder cancer: Shutting down pathways. *Front. Biosci.* **2007**, *12*, 826–838. [CrossRef] [PubMed]

197. Puzio-Kuter, A.M.; Castillo-Martin, M.; Kinkade, C.W.; Wang, X.; Shen, T.H.; Matos, T.; Shen, M.M.; Cordon-Cardo, C.; Abate-Shen, C. Inactivation of p53 and Pten promotes invasive bladder cancer. *Genes Dev.* **2009**, *23*, 675–680. [CrossRef] [PubMed]

198. Calderaro, J.; Rebouissou, S.; de Koning, L.; Masmoudi, A.; Herault, A.; Dubois, T.; Maille, P.; Soyeux, P.; Sibony, M.; de la Taille, A.; et al. PI3K/AKT pathway activation in bladder carcinogenesis. *Int. J. Cancer* **2014**, *134*, 1776–1784. [CrossRef] [PubMed]

199. Afonso, J.; Longatto-Filho, A.; Da Silva, V.M.; Amaro, T.; Santos, L.L. Phospho-mTOR in non-tumour and tumour bladder urothelium: Pattern of expression and impact on urothelial bladder cancer patients. *Oncol. Lett.* **2014**, *8*, 1447–1454. [CrossRef] [PubMed]

200. Park, S.J.; Lee, T.J.; Chang, I.H. Role of the mTOR Pathway in the Progression and Recurrence of Bladder Cancer: An Immunohistochemical Tissue Microarray Study. *Korean J. Urol.* **2011**, *52*, 466–473. [CrossRef] [PubMed]

201. Garcia, J.A.; Danielpour, D. Mammalian target of rapamycin inhibition as a therapeutic strategy in the management of urologic malignancies. *Mol. Cancer Ther.* **2008**, *7*, 1347–1354. [CrossRef] [PubMed]

202. Chiong, E.; Lee, I.L.; Dadbin, A.; Sabichi, A.L.; Harris, L.; Urbauer, D.; McConkey, D.J.; Dickstein, R.J.; Cheng, T.; Grossman, H.B. Effects of mTOR inhibitor everolimus (RAD001) on bladder cancer cells. *Clin. Cancer Res.* **2011**, *17*, 2863–2873. [CrossRef] [PubMed]

203. Oliveira, P.A.; Arantes-Rodrigues, R.; Sousa-Diniz, C.; Colaco, A.; Lourenco, L.; De La Cruz, L.F.; Da Silva, V.M.; Afonso, J.; Lopes, C.; Santos, L. The effects of sirolimus on urothelial lesions chemically induced in ICR mice by BBN. *Anticancer Res.* **2009**, *29*, 3221–3226. [PubMed]

204. Vasconcelos-Nobrega, C.; Pinto-Leite, R.; Arantes-Rodrigues, R.; Ferreira, R.; Brochado, P.; Cardoso, M.L.; Palmeira, C.; Salvador, A.; Guedes-Teixeira, C.I.; Colaco, A.; et al. In vivo and in vitro effects of RAD001 on bladder cancer. *Urol. Oncol.* **2013**, *31*, 1212–1221. [CrossRef] [PubMed]

205. Seager, C.M.; Puzio-Kuter, A.M.; Patel, T.; Jain, S.; Cordon-Cardo, C.; Mc Kiernan, J.; Abate-Shen, C. Intravesical delivery of rapamycin suppresses tumorigenesis in a mouse model of progressive bladder cancer. *Cancer Prev. Res.* **2009**, *2*, 1008–1014. [CrossRef] [PubMed]

206. Milowsky, M.I.; Iyer, G.; Regazzi, A.M.; Al-Ahmadie, H.; Gerst, S.R.; Ostrovnaya, I.; Gellert, L.L.; Kaplan, R.; Garcia-Grossman, I.R.; Pendse, D.; et al. Phase II study of everolimus in metastatic urothelial cancer. *BJU Int.* **2013**, *112*, 462–470. [CrossRef] [PubMed]

207. Seront, E.; Rottey, S.; Sautois, B.; Kerger, J.; D'Hondt, L.A.; Verschaeve, V.; Canon, J.L.; Dopchie, C.; Vandenbulcke, J.M.; Whenham, N.; et al. Phase II study of everolimus in patients with locally advanced or metastatic transitional cell carcinoma of the urothelial tract: Clinical activity, molecular response, and biomarkers. *Ann. Oncol.* **2012**, *23*, 2663–2670. [CrossRef]

208. Pinto-Leite, R.; Arantes-Rodrigues, R.; Sousa, N.; Oliveira, P.A.; Santos, L. mTOR inhibitors in urinary bladder cancer. *Tumour. Biol.* **2016**, *37*, 11541–11551. [CrossRef]

209. Becker, M.N.; Wu, K.J.; Marlow, L.A.; Kreinest, P.A.; Vonroemeling, C.A.; Copland, J.A.; Williams, C.R. The combination of an mTORc1/TORc2 inhibitor with lapatinib is synergistic in bladder cancer in vitro. *Urol. Oncol.* **2014**, *32*, 317–326. [CrossRef]

210. Cirone, P.; Andresen, C.J.; Eswaraka, J.R.; Lappin, P.B.; Bagi, C.M. Patient-derived xenografts reveal limits to PI3K/mTOR- and MEK-mediated inhibition of bladder cancer. *Cancer Chemother. Pharmacol.* **2014**, *73*, 525–538. [CrossRef]

211. Taylor, B.S.; Schultz, N.; Hieronymus, H.; Gopalan, A.; Xiao, Y.; Carver, B.S.; Arora, V.K.; Kaushik, P.; Cerami, E.; Reva, B.; et al. Integrative genomic profiling of human prostate cancer. *Cancer Cell* **2010**, *18*, 11–22. [CrossRef] [PubMed]

212. Reid, A.H.; Attard, G.; Ambroisine, L.; Fisher, G.; Kovacs, G.; Brewer, D.; Clark, J.; Flohr, P.; Edwards, S.; Berney, D.M.; et al. Molecular characterisation of ERG, ETV1 and PTEN gene loci identifies patients at low and high risk of death from prostate cancer. *Br. J. Cancer* **2010**, *102*, 678–684. [CrossRef] [PubMed]

213. Morgan, T.M.; Koreckij, T.D.; Corey, E. Targeted therapy for advanced prostate cancer: Inhibition of the PI3K/Akt/mTOR pathway. *Curr. Cancer Drug Targets* **2009**, *9*, 237–249. [CrossRef] [PubMed]

214. Teng, D.H.; Hu, R.; Lin, H.; Davis, T.; Iliev, D.; Frye, C.; Swedlund, B.; Hansen, K.L.; Vinson, V.L.; Gumpper, K.L.; et al. MMAC1/PTEN mutations in primary tumor specimens and tumor cell lines. *Cancer Res.* **1997**, *57*, 5221–5225.

215. McMenamin, M.E.; Soung, P.; Perera, S.; Kaplan, I.; Loda, M.; Sellers, W.R. Loss of PTEN expression in paraffin-embedded primary prostate cancer correlates with high Gleason score and advanced stage. *Cancer Res.* **1999**, *59*, 4291–4296. [PubMed]

216. Dreher, T.; Zentgraf, H.; Abel, U.; Kappeler, A.; Michel, M.S.; Bleyl, U.; Grobholz, R. Reduction of PTEN and p27kip1 expression correlates with tumor grade in prostate cancer. Analysis in radical prostatectomy specimens and needle biopsies. *Virchows Arch.* **2004**, *444*, 509–517. [CrossRef] [PubMed]

217. Schmitz, M.; Grignard, G.; Margue, C.; Dippel, W.; Capesius, C.; Mossong, J.; Nathan, M.; Giacchi, S.; Scheiden, R.; Kieffer, N. Complete loss of PTEN expression as a possible early prognostic marker for prostate cancer metastasis. *Int. J. Cancer* **2007**, *120*, 1284–1292. [CrossRef] [PubMed]

218. Jamaspishvili, T.; Berman, D.M.; Ross, A.E.; Scher, H.I.; De Marzo, A.M.; Squire, J.A.; Lotan, T.L. Clinical implications of PTEN loss in prostate cancer. *Nat. Rev. Urol.* **2018**, *15*, 222–234. [CrossRef]

219. Perdomo, H.A.G.; Zapata-Copete, J.A.; Sanchez, A. Molecular alterations associated with prostate cancer. *Cent. Eur. J. Urol.* **2018**, *71*, 168–176.

220. Graff, J.R.; Konicek, B.W.; Lynch, R.L.; Dumstorf, C.A.; Dowless, M.S.; McNulty, A.M.; Parsons, S.H.; Brail, L.H.; Colligan, B.M.; Koop, J.W.; et al. eIF4E activation is commonly elevated in advanced human prostate cancers and significantly related to reduced patient survival. *Cancer Res.* **2009**, *69*, 3866–3873. [CrossRef] [PubMed]

221. Skvortsova, I.; Skvortsov, S.; Stasyk, T.; Raju, U.; Popper, B.A.; Schiestl, B.; von Guggenberg, E.; Neher, A.; Bonn, G.K.; Huber, L.A.; et al. Intracellular signaling pathways regulating radioresistance of human prostate carcinoma cells. *Proteomics* **2008**, *8*, 4521–4533. [CrossRef]

222. Karar, J.; Maity, A. PI3K/AKT/mTOR Pathway in Angiogenesis. *Front. Mol. Neurosci.* **2011**, *4*, 51. [CrossRef] [PubMed]

223. Chang, L.; Graham, P.H.; Hao, J.; Ni, J.; Bucci, J.; Cozzi, P.J.; Kearsley, J.H.; Li, Y. Acquisition of epithelial-mesenchymal transition and cancer stem cell phenotypes is associated with activation of the PI3K/Akt/mTOR pathway in prostate cancer radioresistance. *Cell Death Dis.* **2013**, *4*, e875. [CrossRef] [PubMed]

224. Nardella, C.; Carracedo, A.; Alimonti, A.; Hobbs, R.M.; Clohessy, J.G.; Chen, Z.; Egia, A.; Fornari, A.; Fiorentino, M.; Loda, M.; et al. Differential requirement of mTOR in postmitotic tissues and tumorigenesis. *Sci. Signal* **2009**, *2*, ra2. [CrossRef]

225. Kinkade, C.W.; Castillo-Martin, M.; Puzio-Kuter, A.; Yan, J.; Foster, T.H.; Gao, H.; Sun, Y.; Ouyang, X.; Gerald, W.L.; Cordon-Cardo, C.; et al. Targeting AKT/mTOR and ERK MAPK signaling inhibits hormone-refractory prostate cancer in a preclinical mouse model. *J. Clin. Investig.* **2008**, *118*, 3051–3064. [CrossRef] [PubMed]

226. Nakabayashi, M.; Werner, L.; Courtney, K.D.; Buckle, G.; Oh, W.K.; Bubley, G.J.; Hayes, J.H.; Weckstein, D.; Elfiky, A.; Sims, D.M.; et al. Phase II trial of RAD001 and bicalutamide for castration-resistant prostate cancer. *BJU Int.* **2012**, *110*, 1729–1735. [CrossRef] [PubMed]

227. Armstrong, A.J.; Netto, G.J.; Rudek, M.A.; Halabi, S.; Wood, D.P.; Creel, P.A.; Mundy, K.; Davis, S.L.; Wang, T.; Albadine, R.; et al. A pharmacodynamic study of rapamycin in men with intermediate- to high-risk localized prostate cancer. *Clin. Cancer Res.* **2010**, *16*, 3057–3066. [CrossRef]

228. Templeton, A.J.; Dutoit, V.; Cathomas, R.; Rothermundt, C.; Bartschi, D.; Droge, C.; Gautschi, O.; Borner, M.; Fechter, E.; Stenner, F.; et al. Phase 2 trial of single-agent everolimus in chemotherapy-naive patients with castration-resistant prostate cancer (SAKK 08/08). *Eur. Urol.* **2013**, *64*, 150–158. [CrossRef]

229. Statz, C.M.; Patterson, S.E.; Mockus, S.M. mTOR Inhibitors in Castration-Resistant Prostate Cancer: A Systematic Review. *Target Oncol.* **2017**, *12*, 47–59. [CrossRef]

230. Maira, S.M.; Stauffer, F.; Brueggen, J.; Furet, P.; Schnell, C.; Fritsch, C.; Brachmann, S.; Chene, P.; De Pover, A.; Schoemaker, K.; et al. Identification and characterization of NVP-BEZ235, a new orally available dual phosphatidylinositol 3-kinase/mammalian target of rapamycin inhibitor with potent in vivo antitumor activity. *Mol. Cancer Ther.* **2008**, *7*, 1851–1863. [CrossRef]

231. Wallin, J.J.; Edgar, K.A.; Guan, J.; Berry, M.; Prior, W.W.; Lee, L.; Lesnick, J.D.; Lewis, C.; Nonomiya, J.; Pang, J.; et al. GDC-0980 is a novel class I PI3K/mTOR kinase inhibitor with robust activity in cancer models driven by the PI3K pathway. *Mol. Cancer Ther.* **2011**, *10*, 2426–2436. [CrossRef] [PubMed]

232. Carver, B.S.; Chapinski, C.; Wongvipat, J.; Hieronymus, H.; Chen, Y.; Chandarlapaty, S.; Arora, V.K.; Le, C.; Koutcher, J.; Scher, H.; et al. Reciprocal feedback regulation of PI3K and androgen receptor signaling in PTEN-deficient prostate cancer. *Cancer Cell* **2011**, *19*, 575–586. [CrossRef] [PubMed]

233. Baselga, J. Targeting the phosphoinositide-3 (PI3) kinase pathway in breast cancer. *Oncologist* **2011**, *16* (Suppl. 1), 12–19. [CrossRef] [PubMed]

234. Stemke-Hale, K.; Gonzalez-Angulo, A.M.; Lluch, A.; Neve, R.M.; Kuo, W.L.; Davies, M.; Carey, M.; Hu, Z.; Guan, Y.; Sahin, A.; et al. An integrative genomic and proteomic analysis of PIK3CA, PTEN, and AKT mutations in breast cancer. *Cancer Res.* **2008**, *68*, 6084–6091. [CrossRef] [PubMed]

235. Engelman, J.A.; Luo, J.; Cantley, L.C. The evolution of phosphatidylinositol 3-kinases as regulators of growth and metabolism. *Nat. Rev. Genet.* **2006**, *7*, 606–619. [CrossRef] [PubMed]

236. Carpten, J.D.; Faber, A.L.; Horn, C.; Donoho, G.P.; Briggs, S.L.; Robbins, C.M.; Hostetter, G.; Boguslawski, S.; Moses, T.Y.; Savage, S.; et al. A transforming mutation in the pleckstrin homology domain of AKT1 in cancer. *Nature* **2007**, *448*, 439–444. [CrossRef]

237. Sato, T.; Nakashima, A.; Guo, L.; Coffman, K.; Tamanoi, F. Single amino-acid changes that confer constitutive activation of mTOR are discovered in human cancer. *Oncogene* **2010**, *29*, 2746–2752. [CrossRef]

238. Hardt, M.; Chantaravisoot, N.; Tamanoi, F. Activating mutations of TOR (target of rapamycin). *Genes Cells* **2011**, *16*, 141–151. [CrossRef]

239. Ueng, S.H.; Chen, S.C.; Chang, Y.S.; Hsueh, S.; Lin, Y.C.; Chien, H.P.; Lo, Y.F.; Shen, S.C.; Hsueh, C. Phosphorylated mTOR expression correlates with poor outcome in early-stage triple negative breast carcinomas. *Int. J. Clin. Exp. Pathol.* **2012**, *5*, 806–813.

240. Wazir, U.; Newbold, R.F.; Jiang, W.G.; Sharma, A.K.; Mokbel, K. Prognostic and therapeutic implications of mTORC1 and Rictor expression in human breast cancer. *Oncol. Rep.* **2013**, *29*, 1969–1974. [CrossRef]

241. Walsh, S.; Flanagan, L.; Quinn, C.; Evoy, D.; McDermott, E.W.; Pierce, A.; Duffy, M.J. mTOR in breast cancer: Differential expression in triple-negative and non-triple-negative tumors. *Breast* **2012**, *21*, 178–182. [CrossRef] [PubMed]

242. Mondesire, W.H.; Jian, W.; Zhang, H.; Ensor, J.; Hung, M.C.; Mills, G.B.; Meric-Bernstam, F. Targeting mammalian target of rapamycin synergistically enhances chemotherapy-induced cytotoxicity in breast cancer cells. *Clin. Cancer Res.* **2004**, *10*, 7031–7042. [CrossRef]

243. Hurvitz, S.A.; Andre, F.; Jiang, Z.; Shao, Z.; Mano, M.S.; Neciosup, S.P.; Tseng, L.M.; Zhang, Q.; Shen, K.; Liu, D.; et al. Combination of everolimus with trastuzumab plus paclitaxel as first-line treatment for patients with HER2-positive advanced breast cancer (BOLERO-1): A phase 3, randomised, double-blind, multicentre trial. *Lancet Oncol.* **2015**, *16*, 816–829. [CrossRef]

244. Baselga, J.; Campone, M.; Piccart, M.; Burris, H.A., 3rd; Rugo, H.S.; Sahmoud, T.; Noguchi, S.; Gnant, M.; Pritchard, K.I.; Lebrun, F.; et al. Everolimus in postmenopausal hormone-receptor-positive advanced breast cancer. *N. Engl. J. Med.* **2012**, *366*, 520–529. [CrossRef]

245. Piccart, M.; Hortobagyi, G.N.; Campone, M.; Pritchard, K.I.; Lebrun, F.; Ito, Y.; Noguchi, S.; Perez, A.; Rugo, H.S.; Deleu, I.; et al. Everolimus plus exemestane for hormone-receptor-positive, human epidermal growth factor receptor-2-negative advanced breast cancer: Overall survival results from BOLERO-2dagger. *Ann. Oncol.* **2014**, *25*, 2357–2362. [CrossRef] [PubMed]

246. Bachelot, T.; Bourgier, C.; Cropet, C.; Ray-Coquard, I.; Ferrero, J.M.; Freyer, G.; Abadie-Lacourtoisie, S.; Eymard, J.C.; Debled, M.; Spaeth, D.; et al. Randomized phase II trial of everolimus in combination with tamoxifen in patients with hormone receptor-positive, human epidermal growth factor receptor 2-negative metastatic breast cancer with prior exposure to aromatase inhibitors: A GINECO study. *J. Clin. Oncol.* **2012**, *30*, 2718–2724. [CrossRef] [PubMed]

247. Seiler, M.; Ray-Coquard, I.; Melichar, B.; Yardley, D.A.; Wang, R.X.; Dodion, P.F.; Lee, M.A. Oral ridaforolimus plus trastuzumab for patients with HER2+ trastuzumab-refractory metastatic breast cancer. *Clin. Breast Cancer* **2015**, *15*, 60–65. [CrossRef]

248. Guichard, S.M.; Curwen, J.; Bihani, T.; D'Cruz, C.M.; Yates, J.W.; Grondine, M.; Howard, Z.; Davies, B.R.; Bigley, G.; Klinowska, T.; et al. AZD2014, an Inhibitor of mTORC1 and mTORC2, Is Highly Effective in ER+ Breast Cancer When Administered Using Intermittent or Continuous Schedules. *Mol. Cancer Ther.* **2015**, *14*, 2508–2518. [CrossRef]

249. Bahrami, A.; Khazaei, M.; Shahidsales, S.; Hassanian, S.M.; Hasanzadeh, M.; Maftouh, M.; Ferns, G.A.; Avan, A. The Therapeutic Potential of PI3K/Akt/mTOR Inhibitors in Breast Cancer: Rational and Progress. *J. Cell. Biochem.* **2018**, *119*, 213–222. [CrossRef]

250. Wilson-Edell, K.A.; Yevtushenko, M.A.; Rothschild, D.E.; Rogers, A.N.; Benz, C.C. mTORC1/C2 and pan-HDAC inhibitors synergistically impair breast cancer growth by convergent AKT and polysome inhibiting mechanisms. *Breast Cancer Res. Treat.* **2014**, *144*, 287–298. [CrossRef]

251. Bendell, J.C.; Kelley, R.K.; Shih, K.C.; Grabowsky, J.A.; Bergsland, E.; Jones, S.; Martin, T.; Infante, J.R.; Mischel, P.S.; Matsutani, T.; et al. A phase I dose-escalation study to assess safety, tolerability, pharmacokinetics, and preliminary efficacy of the dual mTORC1/mTORC2 kinase inhibitor CC-223 in patients with advanced solid tumors or multiple myeloma. *Cancer* **2015**, *121*, 3481–3490. [CrossRef]

252. Britten, C.D.; Adjei, A.A.; Millham, R.; Houk, B.E.; Borzillo, G.; Pierce, K.; Wainberg, Z.A.; LoRusso, P.M. Phase I study of PF-04691502, a small-molecule, oral, dual inhibitor of PI3K and mTOR, in patients with advanced cancer. *Investig. New Drugs* **2014**, *32*, 510–517. [CrossRef] [PubMed]

253. Dey, N.; Sun, Y.; Carlson, J.H.; Wu, H.; Lin, X.; Leyland-Jones, B.; De, P. Anti-tumor efficacy of BEZ235 is complemented by its anti-angiogenic effects via downregulation of PI3K-mTOR-HIF1alpha signaling in HER2-defined breast cancers. *Am. J. Cancer Res.* **2016**, *6*, 714–746. [PubMed]

254. Hare, S.H.; Harvey, A.J. mTOR function and therapeutic targeting in breast cancer. *Am. J. Cancer Res.* **2017**, *7*, 383–404. [PubMed]

255. Lui, V.W.; Hedberg, M.L.; Li, H.; Vangara, B.S.; Pendleton, K.; Zeng, Y.; Lu, Y.; Zhang, Q.; Du, Y.; Gilbert, B.R.; et al. Frequent mutation of the PI3K pathway in head and neck cancer defines predictive biomarkers. *Cancer Discov.* **2013**, *3*, 761–769. [CrossRef] [PubMed]

256. Squarize, C.H.; Castilho, R.M.; Abrahao, A.C.; Molinolo, A.; Lingen, M.W.; Gutkind, J.S. PTEN deficiency contributes to the development and progression of head and neck cancer. *Neoplasia* **2013**, *15*, 461–471. [CrossRef] [PubMed]

257. Du, L.; Shen, J.; Weems, A.; Lu, S.L. Role of phosphatidylinositol-3-kinase pathway in head and neck squamous cell carcinoma. *J. Oncol.* **2012**, *2012*, 450179. [CrossRef]

258. Freudlsperger, C.; Burnett, J.R.; Friedman, J.A.; Kannabiran, V.R.; Chen, Z.; Van Waes, C. EGFR-PI3K-AKT-mTOR signaling in head and neck squamous cell carcinomas: Attractive targets for molecular-oriented therapy. *Expert Opin. Ther. Targets* **2011**, *15*, 63–74. [CrossRef]

259. Morris, L.G.; Taylor, B.S.; Bivona, T.G.; Gong, Y.; Eng, S.; Brennan, C.W.; Kaufman, A.; Kastenhuber, E.R.; Banuchi, V.E.; Singh, B.; et al. Genomic dissection of the epidermal growth factor receptor (EGFR)/PI3K pathway reveals frequent deletion of the EGFR phosphatase PTPRS in head and neck cancers. *Proc. Natl. Acad. Sci. USA* **2011**, *108*, 19024–19029. [CrossRef]

260. Wang, Z.; Valera, J.C.; Zhao, X.; Chen, Q.; Silvio Gutkind, J. mTOR co-targeting strategies for head and neck cancer therapy. *Cancer Metast. Rev.* **2017**, *36*, 491–502. [CrossRef]

261. Lechner, M.; Frampton, G.M.; Fenton, T.; Feber, A.; Palmer, G.; Jay, A.; Pillay, N.; Forster, M.; Cronin, M.T.; Lipson, D.; et al. Targeted next-generation sequencing of head and neck squamous cell carcinoma identifies novel genetic alterations in HPV+ and HPV- tumors. *Genome Med.* **2013**, *5*, 49. [CrossRef] [PubMed]

262. Seiwert, T.Y.; Zuo, Z.; Keck, M.K.; Khattri, A.; Pedamallu, C.S.; Stricker, T.; Brown, C.; Pugh, T.J.; Stojanov, P.; Cho, J.; et al. Integrative and comparative genomic analysis of HPV-positive and HPV-negative head and neck squamous cell carcinomas. *Clin. Cancer Res.* **2015**, *21*, 632–641. [CrossRef] [PubMed]

263. Rogers, S.J.; Box, C.; Harrington, K.J.; Nutting, C.; Rhys-Evans, P.; Eccles, S.A. The phosphoinositide 3-kinase signalling pathway as a therapeutic target in squamous cell carcinoma of the head and neck. *Expert Opin. Ther. Targets* **2005**, *9*, 769–790. [CrossRef] [PubMed]

264. Giudice, F.S.; Squarize, C.H. The determinants of head and neck cancer: Unmasking the PI3K pathway mutations. *J. Carcinog. Mutagen.* **2013**. [CrossRef]

265. Pfisterer, K.; Fusi, A.; Klinghammer, K.; Knodler, M.; Nonnenmacher, A.; Keilholz, U. PI3K/PTEN/AKT/mTOR polymorphisms: Association with clinical outcome in patients with head and neck squamous cell carcinoma receiving cetuximab-docetaxel. *Head Neck* **2015**, *37*, 471–478. [CrossRef] [PubMed]

266. Molinolo, A.A.; Hewitt, S.M.; Amornphimoltham, P.; Keelawat, S.; Rangdaeng, S.; Meneses Garcia, A.; Raimondi, A.R.; Jufe, R.; Itoiz, M.; Gao, Y.; et al. Dissecting the Akt/mammalian target of rapamycin signaling network: Emerging results from the head and neck cancer tissue array initiative. *Clin. Cancer Res.* **2007**, *13*, 4964–4973. [CrossRef]

267. Molinolo, A.A.; Marsh, C.; El Dinali, M.; Gangane, N.; Jennison, K.; Hewitt, S.; Patel, V.; Seiwert, T.Y.; Gutkind, J.S. mTOR as a molecular target in HPV-associated oral and cervical squamous carcinomas. *Clin. Cancer Res.* **2012**, *18*, 2558–2568. [CrossRef]

268. Gao, W.; Li, J.Z.; Chan, J.Y.; Ho, W.K.; Wong, T.S. mTOR Pathway and mTOR Inhibitors in Head and Neck Cancer. *ISRN Otolaryngol.* **2012**, *2012*, 953089. [CrossRef]

269. Coppock, J.D.; Vermeer, P.D.; Vermeer, D.W.; Lee, K.M.; Miskimins, W.K.; Spanos, W.C.; Lee, J.H. mTOR inhibition as an adjuvant therapy in a metastatic model of HPV+ HNSCC. *Oncotarget* **2016**, *7*, 24228–24241. [CrossRef]

270. Patel, V.; Marsh, C.A.; Dorsam, R.T.; Mikelis, C.M.; Masedunskas, A.; Amornphimoltham, P.; Nathan, C.A.; Singh, B.; Weigert, R.; Molinolo, A.A.; et al. Decreased lymphangiogenesis and lymph node metastasis by mTOR inhibition in head and neck cancer. *Cancer Res.* **2011**, *71*, 7103–7112. [CrossRef]

271. Amornphimoltham, P.; Patel, V.; Leelahavanichkul, K.; Abraham, R.T.; Gutkind, J.S. A retroinhibition approach reveals a tumor cell-autonomous response to rapamycin in head and neck cancer. *Cancer Res.* **2008**, *68*, 1144–1153. [CrossRef] [PubMed]

272. Leiker, A.J.; DeGraff, W.; Choudhuri, R.; Sowers, A.L.; Thetford, A.; Cook, J.A.; Van Waes, C.; Mitchell, J.B. Radiation Enhancement of Head and Neck Squamous Cell Carcinoma by the Dual PI3K/mTOR Inhibitor PF-05212384. *Clin. Cancer Res.* **2015**, *21*, 2792–2801. [CrossRef] [PubMed]

273. Ekshyyan, O.; Rong, Y.; Rong, X.; Pattani, K.M.; Abreo, F.; Caldito, G.; Chang, J.K.; Ampil, F.; Glass, J.; Nathan, C.O. Comparison of radiosensitizing effects of the mammalian target of rapamycin inhibitor CCI-779 to cisplatin in experimental models of head and neck squamous cell carcinoma. *Mol. Cancer Ther.* **2009**, *8*, 2255–2265. [CrossRef] [PubMed]

274. Klinghammer, K.; Raguse, J.D.; Plath, T.; Albers, A.E.; Joehrens, K.; Zakarneh, A.; Brzezicha, B.; Wulf-Goldenberg, A.; Keilholz, U.; Hoffmann, J.; et al. A comprehensively characterized large panel of head and neck cancer patient-derived xenografts identifies the mTOR inhibitor everolimus as potential new treatment option. *Int. J. Cancer* **2015**, *136*, 2940–2948. [CrossRef] [PubMed]

275. Mazumdar, T.; Byers, L.A.; Ng, P.K.; Mills, G.B.; Peng, S.; Diao, L.; Fan, Y.H.; Stemke-Hale, K.; Heymach, J.V.; Myers, J.N.; et al. A comprehensive evaluation of biomarkers predictive of response to PI3K inhibitors and of resistance mechanisms in head and neck squamous cell carcinoma. *Mol. Cancer Ther.* **2014**, *13*, 2738–2750. [CrossRef]

276. Tentler, J.J.; Tan, A.C.; Weekes, C.D.; Jimeno, A.; Leong, S.; Pitts, T.M.; Arcaroli, J.J.; Messersmith, W.A.; Eckhardt, S.G. Patient-derived tumour xenografts as models for oncology drug development. *Nat. Rev. Clin. Oncol.* **2012**, *9*, 338–350. [CrossRef]

277. Fury, M.G.; Lee, N.Y.; Sherman, E.; Ho, A.L.; Rao, S.; Heguy, A.; Shen, R.; Korte, S.; Lisa, D.; Ganly, I.; et al. A phase 1 study of everolimus + weekly cisplatin + intensity modulated radiation therapy in head-and-neck cancer. *Int. J. Radiat. Oncol. Biol. Phys.* **2013**, *87*, 479–486. [CrossRef] [PubMed]

278. Massarelli, E.; Lin, H.; Ginsberg, L.E.; Tran, H.T.; Lee, J.J.; Canales, J.R.; Williams, M.D.; Blumenschein, G.R., Jr.; Lu, C.; Heymach, J.V.; et al. Phase II trial of everolimus and erlotinib in patients with platinum-resistant recurrent and/or metastatic head and neck squamous cell carcinoma. *Ann. Oncol.* **2015**, *26*, 1476–1480. [CrossRef]

279. Fury, M.G.; Sherman, E.; Ho, A.L.; Xiao, H.; Tsai, F.; Nwankwo, O.; Sima, C.; Heguy, A.; Katabi, N.; Haque, S.; et al. A phase 1 study of everolimus plus docetaxel plus cisplatin as induction chemotherapy for patients with locally and/or regionally advanced head and neck cancer. *Cancer* **2013**, *119*, 1823–1831. [CrossRef]

280. Fury, M.G.; Sherman, E.; Ho, A.; Katabi, N.; Sima, C.; Kelly, K.W.; Nwankwo, O.; Haque, S.; Pfister, D.G. A phase I study of temsirolimus plus carboplatin plus paclitaxel for patients with recurrent or metastatic (R/M) head and neck squamous cell cancer (HNSCC). *Cancer Chemother. Pharmacol.* **2012**, *70*, 121–128. [CrossRef]

281. Bauman, J.E.; Arias-Pulido, H.; Lee, S.J.; Fekrazad, M.H.; Ozawa, H.; Fertig, E.; Howard, J.; Bishop, J.; Wang, H.; Olson, G.T.; et al. A phase II study of temsirolimus and erlotinib in patients with recurrent and/or metastatic, platinum-refractory head and neck squamous cell carcinoma. *Oral Oncol.* **2013**, *49*, 461–467. [CrossRef] [PubMed]

282. de Melo, A.C.; Paulino, E.; Garces, A.H. A Review of mTOR Pathway Inhibitors in Gynecologic Cancer. *Oxid. Med. Cell. Longev.* **2017**, *2017*, 4809751. [CrossRef] [PubMed]

283. Hu, K.; Dai, H.B.; Qiu, Z.L. mTOR signaling in osteosarcoma: Oncogenesis and therapeutic aspects (Review). *Oncol. Rep.* **2016**, *36*, 1219–1225. [CrossRef] [PubMed]

284. Dinner, S.; Platanias, L.C. Targeting the mTOR Pathway in Leukemia. *J. Cell. Biochem.* **2016**, *117*, 1745–1752. [CrossRef] [PubMed]

285. Blachly, J.S.; Baiocchi, R.A. Targeting PI3-kinase (PI3K), AKT and mTOR axis in lymphoma. *Br. J. Haematol.* **2014**, *167*, 19–32. [CrossRef] [PubMed]

286. Manfredi, G.I.; Dicitore, A.; Gaudenzi, G.; Caraglia, M.; Persani, L.; Vitale, G. PI3K/Akt/mTOR signaling in medullary thyroid cancer: A promising molecular target for cancer therapy. *Endocrine* **2015**, *48*, 363–370. [CrossRef] [PubMed]

287. Li, X.; Wu, C.; Chen, N.; Gu, H.; Yen, A.; Cao, L.; Wang, E.; Wang, L. PI3K/Akt/mTOR signaling pathway and targeted therapy for glioblastoma. *Oncotarget* **2016**, *7*, 33440–33450. [CrossRef]

288. Chan, J.; Kulke, M. Targeting the mTOR signaling pathway in neuroendocrine tumors. *Curr. Treat. Opt. Oncol.* **2014**, *15*, 365–379. [CrossRef]

289. Dimitrova, V.; Arcaro, A. Targeting the PI3K/AKT/mTOR signaling pathway in medulloblastoma. *Curr. Mol. Med.* **2015**, *15*, 82–93.

290. Sun, S.Y.; Rosenberg, L.M.; Wang, X.; Zhou, Z.; Yue, P.; Fu, H.; Khuri, F.R. Activation of Akt and eIF4E survival pathways by rapamycin-mediated mammalian target of rapamycin inhibition. *Cancer Res.* **2005**, *65*, 7052–7058. [CrossRef]

291. O'Reilly, K.E.; Rojo, F.; She, Q.B.; Solit, D.; Mills, G.B.; Smith, D.; Lane, H.; Hofmann, F.; Hicklin, D.J.; Ludwig, D.L.; et al. mTOR inhibition induces upstream receptor tyrosine kinase signaling and activates Akt. *Cancer Res.* **2006**, *66*, 1500–1508. [CrossRef] [PubMed]

292. Mendoza, M.C.; Er, E.E.; Blenis, J. The Ras-ERK and PI3K-mTOR pathways: Cross-talk and compensation. *Trends Biochem. Sci.* **2011**, *36*, 320–328. [CrossRef] [PubMed]

293. Palm, W.; Park, Y.; Wright, K.; Pavlova, N.N.; Tuveson, D.A.; Thompson, C.B. The Utilization of Extracellular Proteins as Nutrients Is Suppressed by mTORC1. *Cell* **2015**, *162*, 259–270. [CrossRef] [PubMed]

294. Degenhardt, K.; Mathew, R.; Beaudoin, B.; Bray, K.; Anderson, D.; Chen, G.; Mukherjee, C.; Shi, Y.; Gelinas, C.; Fan, Y.; et al. Autophagy promotes tumor cell survival and restricts necrosis, inflammation, and tumorigenesis. *Cancer Cell* **2006**, *10*, 51–64. [CrossRef] [PubMed]

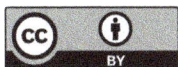

International Journal of
Molecular Sciences

MDPI

Review

mTOR Inhibitors in Advanced Biliary Tract Cancers

Chao-En Wu [1], Ming-Huang Chen [2,3] and Chun-Nan Yeh [4,*]

[1]   Division of Hematology-Oncology, Department of Internal Medicine, Chang Gung Memorial Hospital, Linkou branch, Chang Gung University, Taoyuan 333, Taiwan; jiaoen@gmail.com
[2]   School of Medicine, National Yang-Ming University, Taipei 112, Taiwan; mhchen9@gmail.com
[3]   Department of Oncology, Taipei Veterans General Hospital, Taipei 112, Taiwan
[4]   Department of General Surgery and Liver Research Center, Chang Gung Memorial Hospital, Linkou branch, Chang Gung University, Taoyuan 333, Taiwan
*   Correspondence: yehchunnan@gmail.com; Tel.: +886-3-3281200 (ext. 3219); Fax: +886-3-3285818

Received: 6 January 2019; Accepted: 22 January 2019; Published: 24 January 2019

Abstract: Patients with advanced biliary tract cancers (BTCs), including cholangiocarcinoma (CCA), have poor prognosis so novel treatment is warranted for advanced BTC. In current review, we discuss the limitations of current treatment in BTC, the importance of mTOR signalling in BTC, and the possible role of mTOR inhibitors as a future treatment in BTC. Chemotherapy with gemcitabine-based chemotherapy is still the standard of care and no targeted therapy has been established in advanced BTC. PI3K/AKT/mTOR signaling pathway linking to several other pathways and networks regulates cancer proliferation and progression. Emerging evidences reveal mTOR activation is associated with tumorigenesis and drug-resistance in BTC. Rapalogs, such as sirolimus and everolimus, partially inhibit mTOR complex 1 (mTORC1) and exhibit anti-cancer activity in vitro and in vivo in BTC. Rapalogs in clinical trials demonstrate some activity in patients with advanced BTC. New-generation mTOR inhibitors against ATP-binding pocket inhibit both TORC1 and TORC2 and demonstrate more potent anti-tumor effects in vitro and in vivo, however, prospective clinical trials are warranted to prove its efficacy in patients with advanced BTC.

Keywords: mTOR; advanced biliary tract cancers

1. Introduction of Bile Duct Cancers

Bile duct cancers (BTCs) including intrahepatic/extrahepatic cholangiocarcinoma (CCA), gallbladder cancer (GBC), and Ampullar Vater cancer, are the malignant neoplasms arising from epithelial cells of bile ducts [1]. CCA was considered as primary liver cancer and, currently, the term CCA has been used for bile duct cancers arising from intrahepatic and extrahepatic bile system, excluding the malignancies of gallbladder and Ampulla of Vater.

The estimated annual cases of primary liver cancers including intrahepatic CAA is 42,220 in the United States [2] and around 15% of them are intrahepatic CCA according to Surveillance, Epidemiology, and End Results (SEER) program [3,4]. Estimated 12,190 cases of gallbladder and other biliary cancers are diagnosed annually in the United States [2]. Although they are uncommon and relatively rare, the patients with BTC have a poor prognosis because most of them are locally advanced at presentation and high recurrence rate for the early stage after curative surgery [5,6]. The efficacy of systemic treatment is limited, therefore, novel agents are warranted for the patients with biliary tract cancers.

Int. J. Mol. Sci. **2019**, *20*, 500

2. Current Evidences of Systemic Treatment for Advanced Bile Duct Cancers

2.1. In the Era of Chemotherapy

Systemic chemotherapy is the standard treatment in biliary duct cancers based on a randomized study which showed fluorouracil (FU)-based systemic chemotherapy provided longer overall survival (6 versus 2.5 months) than best supportive care alone in 90 eligible patients with pancreatic (n = 53) or biliary cancer (n = 37) [7]. Therefore, chemotherapy with FU-based regimens proved the efficacy of chemotherapy and became the standard of care for patients with advanced BTC in 1996. A later study in patients with advanced pancreatic cancer showed gemcitabine-treated patients experienced better clinical benefit response compositing of measurements of pain, Karnofsky performance status, and body weight (23.8% vs. 4.8%, p = 0.0022) and longer overall survival (OS, 5.65 and 4.41 months, p = 0.0025) than 5-FU-treated patients [8], gemcitabine was also wildly used in patients with advanced BTC. Subsequently, chemotherapy with FU, and gemcitabine, with or without platinum has been studied, but the optimal chemotherapy regimen has been debated for more than a decade.

In 2007, pooled phase II studies by Eckel et al. showed superior response rates (RRs) and tumor control rates (TCRs) of gemcitabine- or platinum-based regimens and highest RRs and TCRs was found in the gemcitabine/platinum combination subgroup so this study concluded that gemcitabine/platinum combination represented the provisional standard for chemotherapy [9] even lack of direct comparison of gemcitabine and 5-FU in these patients. In 2010, ABC-02 trial, the first randomized phase III study in advanced BTC, reported that gemcitabine plus cisplatin has better TCRs (81.4% versus 71.8%, p = 0.049), median progression-free survival (PFS, 8.0 months versus 5.0 months, p < 0.001) and median OS (11.7 months versus 8.1 months, p < 0.001) than gemcitabine alone [10] so the combination of gemcitabine and cisplatin has been considered the standard of care as the first-line treatment in patients with advanced BTC and widely used in clinical practice [11]. This regimen has not been compared head to head with other gemcitabine-based combinations except gemcitabine plus TS-1 which demonstrated non-inferiority in the Japanese phase III FUGA-BT study [12]. This study enrolled a total of 354 patients with chemotherapy-naïve advanced BTC and a preliminary report presented at the 2018 American Society of Clinical Oncology (ASCO) Gastrointestinal Cancers Symposium showed the combination of gemcitabine/TS-1 was non-inferior in terms of median OS (15.1 versus 13.4 months), median PFS (6.8 versus 5.8 months), and objective RRs (30% versus 32%) so that this combination can be considered as another standard treatment in patients with advanced BTC.

2.2. Development of Targeted Therapy in Advanced BTC

Few prospective trials have been undertaken of first-line chemotherapy and targeted therapy in advanced BTC. Molecularly targeted agents targeting vascular endothelial growth factor (VEGF) or epidermal growth factor receptor (EGFR) were investigated in advanced BTC. Although the addition of bevacizumab [13] or cetuximab [14] to chemotherapy showed promising clinical results in phase II trials, randomized study [15,16] failed to demonstrate additional activity of cetuximab when it combined with chemotherapy. In a study of pooled trials published during January 2000 to January 2014, the authors concluded that triplet combinations of gemcitabine/FU/platinum and gemcitabine-based chemotherapy plus targeted therapy (predominantly targeting EGFR) are most effective concerning TCRs and survivals [17]. However, gemcitabine-based chemotherapy is still the standard of care in advanced BTC and the use of additional targeted therapy is questionable.

2.3. Immune Checkpoints Inhibitors

The immune checkpoints inhibitors against cytotoxic T-lymphocyte-associated protein 4 (CTLA-4), programmed cee death protein-1(PD-1), or programmed death-ligand 1 (PD-Ll) have been developed to show efficacy in a variety of cancers. Nakamura et al. found that the poorest prognosis for BTC patients was in those with significant enrichment of hypermutated tumors and elevated expression of immune checkpoint molecules such as CTLA-4 and IDO but which are associated with favourable clinical response to anti-PD-L1 treatment [18]. In this study, 45.2% of patients showed an increase in the expression of immune checkpoint molecules. In Keynote-026 (NCT02054806), a phase 1b trial to evaluate the safety and efficacy of pembrolizumab in advanced pre-treated BTC patients, Bang et al. [19] reported interim results that 8 out of 23 PD-L1-positive patients (35%) had PD and SD and some of them had disease control lasting for 40+ weeks. A number of immunotherapy studies are currently recruiting and ongoing [20].

In addition, based on data from the patients with microsatellite instability-high (MSI-H) or deficient mismatch repair (dMMR) cancers enrolled across uncontrolled, multi-cohort, multi-center, single-arm clinical trials, in May 2017, the US FDA approved pembrolizumab for treatment of a variety of advanced MSI-H or dMMR solid tumors (including BTC) [21] so the patients with advanced BTC harboring MSI-H or dMMR are candidates for immune checkpoint inhibitors.

3. Molecular Alterations in Cholangiocarcinoma

A variety of molecular alterations involving both oncogenes (e.g., *RAS* [22–24], *BRAF* [25], *ERBB2/HER2*, *EGFR* [26], and *PIK3CA* (phosphoinositide 3-kinase, catalytic, α-polypeptide) [27]) and tumor suppressor genes (e.g., *p53* [23], *SMAD4* [28], and *CDKN2A* [29]) have been described in invasive BTC [30]. Most of the genetic alterations involve phosphoinositide 3-kinase (PI3K)/AKT/mammalian target of rapamycin (mTOR) through MAPKinase activation or p53 suppression resulting in activation of mTOR. p53 negatively regulates the PI3K/AKT/mTOR pathway via its upregulation of phosphatase and tensin homolog (PTEN), TSC2, AMP-activated protein kinase (AMPK), and other proteins [31].

In addition, gene expression profiling of BTC compared with normal biliary epithelium has identified upregulated *ribosomal protein S6 kinase, 70kD* (*RPS6K* encoding p70-S6K) and *eukaryotic translation initiation factor 4E* (*EIF4E*), which are two important downstream mediators of AKT/mTOR signaling pathway, as well as the potential drug target insulin-like growth factor 1 receptor (IGF1-R) [32]. The collective evidences of genetic studies in BTC detailed above suggest mTOR plays a central and critical role in invasive BTC, therefore, targeting mTOR pathway by mTOR inhibitors could be envisioned as a novel treatment in advanced BTC (Figure 1).

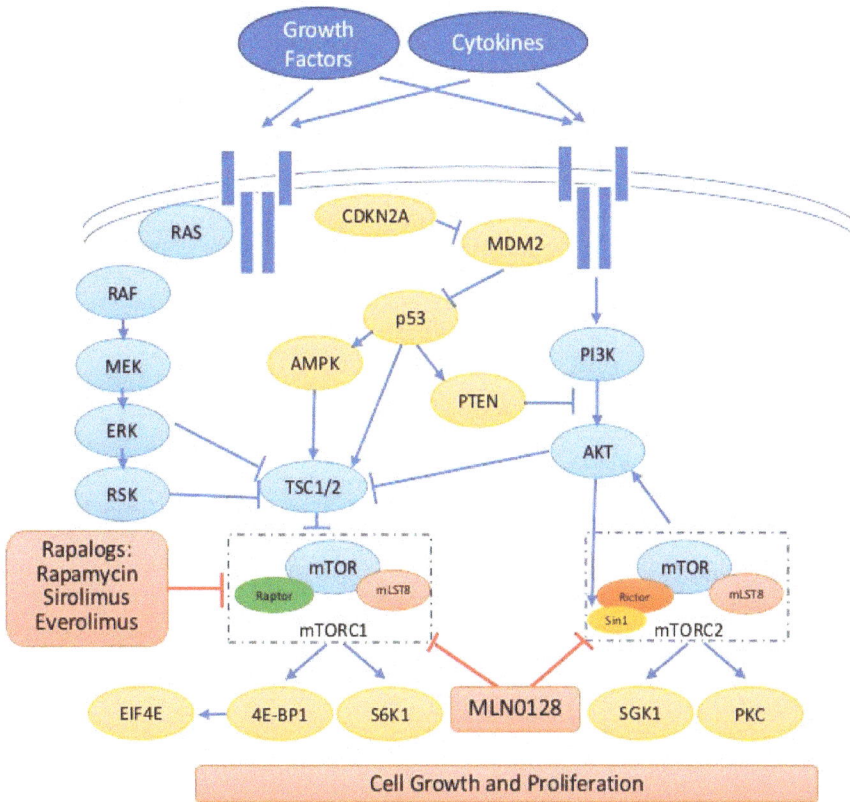

Figure 1. The signaling transduction of mTOR pathway. Extracellular signals such as growth factors and cytokines binding to the receptors stimulate RAS/RAF/MEK/ERK and PI3K/AKT/mTOR caspases. mTOR exists in two functionally and structurally distinct complexes, mTORC1 and mTORC2. Both mTORC1/2 contain different core components so they phosphorylate a distinct set of substrates and exhibit distinct function. PTEN is a negative regulator for PI3K/AKT. In addition, ERK/RSK, AMPK, and p53 regulate mTORC1 through TSC2 regulation. Rapalogs mainly inhibit mTORC1 and new-generation mTOR inhibitors such as MLN0128 inhibitor both mTORC1/2. Blue t-bar indicates inhibition, blue arrow indicates stimulation/activation, red t-bar indicates inhibition by drugs, and dashed square indicates mTOR1/2 complexes.

4. mTOR Pathway in Cancers

4.1. mTOR, Its Complexes and Downstream Regulations in Cancers

The serine/threonine kinase mTOR, a member in a family of protein kinase called *PI3K*-related kinases, integrates intracellular and extracellular signal transduction leading to regulation of in a variety of cellular functions such as cell cycle progression, cell metabolism, cell proliferation, survival [33–36]. The mTOR pathway is dysregulated in various cancers including cholangiocarcinoma [37,38], making mTOR an important target for the development of new anticancer drugs [39,40].

The mTOR exists in two structurally and functionally distinct complexes, mTOR complex 1 (mTORC1) and mTOR complex 2 (mTORC2), which regulated by and regulate distinct signaling pathways resulting from different complex co-factors. Both complexes contain mTOR and a protein, called mLST8, that associates with its kinase domain. It is considered that the functional differences between mTORC1 and mTORC2 result from the other core components such as Raptor in mTORC1 and a complex of Rictor and mSIN1 in mTORC2.

mTORC1 is the downstream of the two proto-oncogenes kinase pathways, PI3K/AKT as well as RAS/RAF/MEK/ERK, through inhibition of TSC2 and PRAS40, both are negative regulators of mTORC1 [41–46]. mTORC1 is the upstream of two distinct pathways which control translation of specific subsets of mRNA. One involves p70-S6K, and another pathway is related with eukaryotic initiation factor 4E binding protein-1 (4E-BP1) [47]. The PI3K/AKT/mTOR signaling cascade is central to cell survival, apoptosis, metabolism, motility, and angiogenesis [48].

In response to PI3K/AKT signaling activation, mTOR rapidly phosphorylates both downstream substrates, p70-S6K and 4E-BP1, the latter leading to release of EIF4E, resulting in initiation of translation. This pathway was also found to be up-regulated using tissue microarrays in CCA [27] and is a key pathway for CCA drug development [30]. mTOR can be inhibited by using the macrolide rapamycin. However, a subset of biliary cancers will be possibly resistant to mTOR inhibitors as the downstream activation bypass mTOR regulation. Therefore, in a study of gene expression comparing BTC and normal biliary epithelium identified two genes involving mTOR pathway, p70-S6K and EIF4E, which are differentially up-regulated in BTC so this study provides alternative downstream targets for inhibition [47].

In contrast, mTORC2 contains Rictor in place of Raptor so it phosphorylates a distinct set of substrates [49]. AKT/mTORC2 forms a positive feedback loop that AKT phosphorylates SIN1 at Tyrosine 86 which enhances mTORC2 kinase activity to phosphorylate and catalyse AKT(Serine 473) leading to AKT activation to control various cellular processes [50,51]. mTORC2 is tumorigenic and is reported to promote cancer via formation of lipids essential for growth and energy production in hepatocellular carcinoma model [52–54].

4.2. Upstream Regulation of mTOR in Cancers

4.2.1. The Physiological Regulation of mTOR Pathway

PI3Ks are a family of intracellular signal transducers and regulate a crucial signal transduction system linking multiple receptors and oncogenes to many essential cellular functions including cell survival, proliferation, and differentiation [55]. Upon signals from various growth factors and cytokines stimulating receptor tyrosine kinases (RTKs) and G protein-coupled receptors (GPCRs), PI3Ks transduce the signals into intracellular messages via activating the serine/threonine kinase AKT followed by downstream effector pathways.

Several classes of PI3K kinases have been identified in mammalian cells, and only class I PI3K can function as second-messenger being implicated in oncogenesis. The class I PI3K kinase consists of two main subunits, p85 and p110, which mediate regulatory and catalytic activity of kinase respectively [56]. Three different genes, *PIK3CA*, *PIK3CB*, and *PIK3CD*, encode three specific p110 isoforms, p110α, β, and δ, respectively [57], and activating missense mutations of *PIK3CA* have been found as oncogenic in a variety of cancers [58]. *PIK3CB* mutation is rare but has been reported to be activating and oncogenic [59].

The PI3K kinases activated by RTKs phosphorylate the 3′-hydroxyl group of phosphatidylinositol (4,5)-bisphosphate (PIP2) to generate phosphatidylinositol (3,4,5)-trisphosphate (PIP3) [60], which is an important second messenger that transduces signals through AKT to downstream activators of cellular growth and survival [61]. PTEN is a phosphatase which negatively regulates PIP3 activity by dephosphorylation [62].

AMPK activity can be regulated by the cellular energy level through the balance in ATP/AMP ratio, so low ratio under nutrient deprivation can activate AMPK followed by mTOR inhibition via TSC1/2 activation [63]. p53 was reported as a substrate of AMPK which activates p53 phosphorylation on serine 15 required to initiate AMPK-dependent cell cycle arrest [64]. In addition, AMPK, TSC2, and PTEN were also regulated by p53 [65]. Furthermore, MAPKinase pathway activates ERK/RSK which regulate mTOR via TSC-2 suppression [66]. Therefore, those pathways are tightly regulated to affect mTOR activities leading to the balance of cell survival and death (Figure 1).

4.2.2. Alterations of mTOR Pathway in Cancers

IGF1-R is a receptor on the cell surface and stimulated through the binding with IGF1 resulting in activation of PI3K/AKT/mTOR pathway. IGF1-R overexpression was reported to be associated with more aggressive phenotypes of cancer [67]. PTEN is a negative regulator of PI3K so is considered as a tumor suppressor in tumorigenesis [62]. Dysregulation of the above genes or proteins leads to mTOR activation resulting in tumor progression and survival in BTC.

PIK3CA mutations are commonly found in cancers such colon, breast, gastric, and brain cancers, but such mutations are rarely found in BTC [18,27] and are associated with poor prognosis [68]. Although not high rate of *PIK3CA* activating mutations, immunohistochemical evaluation of downstream *PIK3CA* targets EIF4E and 4E-BP1 suggests that additional mechanisms may play positively regulation in mTOR pathway in cancers. In addition, *PTEN* downregulation was reported to be associated with mTOR activation in BTC [69]. Expression profiling of BTC compared with normal biliary epithelium has identified upregulated AKT/mTOR signaling components, including the potential drug target IGF1-R [47]. Expression of IGF1-R and its ligands are seen in the majority of GBCs and metastases providing a targeted candidate for therapeutic strategies to interfering with IGF pathway [70]. Therefore, treating BTC cell lines with a small-molecule inhibitor of the IGF1-R was suggested and showed the efficacy of targeting this pathway [71].

5. mTOR Inhibitors

5.1. Rapalogs, First-Generation of mTOR Inhibitors

Rapalogs include rapamycin, also known as sirolimus, and its analogues such as everolimus, temsirolimus are all highly specific allosteric inhibitors of mTOR with the same mechanism of action [72,73]. Rapalogs binding to the intracellular protein FKBP12 forms a drug-protein complex. This FKBP12–rapalog complex binds to the FKBP12–rapamycin binding (FRB) domain of mTOR, which is located at just N-terminal next to the kinase domain [74,75]. Binding of FKBP12–rapalog complex to the FRB domain interferes the association of mTOR and Raptor in mTORC1 so that inhibits mTORC1 signaling within minutes at low doses of rapalogs. In contrast, higher doses or prolonged use of rapalogs can sequester mTOR from mTORC2 to block mTORC2 signaling [27]. Although rapalogs are highly specific to mTOR, it is well known that rapalogs can only partially inhibit the functions of mTORC1 [76,77]. For example, rapamycin highly inhibits S6K activity in all settings but does not inhibit 4E-BP1 which is also a direct substrate of mTORC1 [76]. Therefore, the sensitivity to rapalogs cannot determine whether the cellular processes are mTORC1-dependent or mTORC1-independent.

5.2. Second-Generation mTOR Inhibitors

For the limitations of rapalogs in mTOR inhibition, a number of second-generation mTOR inhibitors have been developed. Like most kinase inhibitors, second-generation mTOR inhibitors were designed to directly target the ATP-binding pocket of the mTOR kinase domain so these new generation mTOR inhibitors can inhibit both mTORC1 and mTORC2. The next important question is whether these compounds display superior anti-cancer activity via inhibition of both mTORC1 and mTORC2 and whether such treatments can be tolerated at the effective doses because of off-target effects on the evolutionarily related protein kinases [78]. Currently, several compounds such as AZD-2014, MLN0128 (INK128, TAK228), OSI-027, and GDC-0349 have been investigated in clinical trials to prove the clinical significance in cancer treatments. Furthermore, NVP-BEZ235, LY3023414, and PF-04691502 are dual PI3K/mTOR inhibitors and have been investigated in clinical trials.

AZD-2014, a dual mTORC1/2 inhibitor, showed superior activity than everolimus in vitro and in vivo in renal cell carcinoma [79] but demonstrate inferior efficacy in patients with renal cell carcinoma [80]. Therefore, although preliminary studies showed promising efficacy of dual mTOR inhibitors in various of cancers [81,82], the clinical significance should still be investigated in clinical trials to prove their activities in cancer treatment [83].

6. Sustained mTORC1/2 Signaling Activation as a Driver of Resistance to Anti-Cancer Treatment

Several studies in different cancer types have already shown that sustained mTORC1 signaling under certain targeted therapy is strongly associated with primary and acquired resistance to such treatment so mTORC1 inhibition seems to be an effective therapeutic strategy in combination with other targeted agents even the efficacy is limited as single-use [84,85]. mTORC1 activation has been also reported to be resistant to various anti-cancer treatments including chemotherapy, targeted therapy, and hormonal treatment. On the contrary, mTOR inhibition by rapalogs was shown sensitization to anti-cancer treatments [86].

mTORC2 activation and AKT phosphorylation have also been found to escape MAPKinase inhibition by sorafenib in CCA cells. Therefore, prevention of escape by suppressing mTORC2 activity may lead to promising new approaches in CCA therapy [87].

7. Preclinical Studies of mTOR Inhibitors in BTC

7.1. The Rationale of mTOR Inhibitors Alone or in Combination with Chemotherapeutic Agents in Cholangiocarcinoma

As discussed above, a number of genetic alterations directly or indirectly involving PI3K/AKT/mTOR activation were reported in advanced BTC [30]. In addition, gene expression profiling of invasive BTC has showed upregulation of downstream mediators in mTOR pathway, *RPS6K* and *EIF4E* as well as IGF1-R [32]. These genetic studies in BTC suggest mTOR plays an important role in invasive BTC, therefore, mTOR inhibitors targeting mTOR pathway could be considered as a reasonable therapeutic strategy.

Furthermore, in a preclinical study to investigate the functional role and mechanism of miR-199a-3p in the regulation of cisplatin sensitivities in CCA, Li et al. demonstrated that miR-199a-3p enhances cisplatin activity in CCA cell lines (GBC-SD and RBE) via both inhibiting the mTOR signaling pathway and decreasing the expression of MDR1. In this study, mTOR suppression by siRNA or miR-199a-3p potentiates cisplatin sensitivity of CCA cell lines indicating mTOR pathway regulates cisplatin activity in CCA although the exact mechanism is unclear [88].

Ling et al. found metformin increases AMPK phosphorylation and inhibits the activation of mTORC1 complex and can sensitize sorafenib, 5-FU, and As2O3 but not gemcitabine in cholangiocarcinoma cell lines (RBE and HCCC-9810) [89]. Wandee et al. found metformin sensitizes cisplatin in CCA cell lines (KKU-100 and KKU-452) via AMPK activation and AKT/mTOR/p70-S6K suppression [90]. Lyu et al. demonstrated Fyn was associated with AMPK/mTOR regulation [91] and was overexpressed in CCA cell lines. Furthermore, Fyn knockdown in CCA cell lines induces AMPK phosphorylation, followed by inhibiting downstream mTOR phosphorylation leading to inhibition of migration and invasion [92].

Above studies have shown mTOR pathway is crucial for regulation of tumor growth and sensitivities to anti-cancer drugs in CCA.

7.2. Preclinical Studies of Rapalogs in BTC

Everolimus exhibits in vitro multiple effects in a CCA cell line (RMCCA-1). Everolimus at low concentrations reduced in vitro invasion and migration and high concentrations exhibited cytotoxic effects such as suppression of cell proliferation and induction of apoptosis [93]. Everolimus was also found to inhibit the secretion of proinflammatory cytokines by cancer-associated myofibroblasts (CAFs) and inhibits proliferation of CCA cells (HuCCT1 and TFK1) at low concentrations [94]. Both studies confirmed the previous hypothesis that mTOR plays important role in CCA and mTOR inhibitors exert anticancer effects via mTOR inhibition. In addition, rapamycin was found to initiate AKT activation in CCA and inhibition of AKT by salubrinal potentiates the in vitro and in vivo efficacy of rapamycin in CCA both [95]. In terms of combination of rapalogs and cytotoxic agents, our group reported gemcitabine plus everolimus combination showed synergistic effect in the CCA cells in vitro and in vivo [96].

7.3. New Generation mTOR Inhibitors in BTC

Zhang et al. established a novel mouse model of intrahepatic CCA exhibiting activated AKT/mTOR cascade and found both mTORC1 and mTORC2 signalings are required for AKT/YapS127A-induced cholangiocarcinogenesis [97]. MLN0128, a second generation, ATP-competitive mTOR inhibitor, suppress cell growth and induce apoptosis in vitro and in vivo via suppression of both mTORC1 and mTORC2 signaling. An important finding in this study was that MLN0128 had better therapeutic efficacy than gemcitabine/oxaliplatin combination (one of the standard chemotherapy regimen) as well as everolimus in the treatment of AKT/YapS127A intrahepatic CCA model. In addition, the same group reported that the combination of palbociclib, a CDK4/6 inhibitor, and MLN0128 demonstrated a pronounced, synergistic growth inhibition in intrahepatic CCA cell lines and in AKT/YapS127A mice [98].

7.4. Dual PI3K/mTOR Inhibitors in BTC

New dual inhibitors targeted to PI3K/mTOR such as NVP-BEZ235, which exerts strong antiproliferative properties against primary cultures of intrahepatic CCA subtypes with differential drug sensitivity, have been developed [99]. In addition, our group identified both HSP90 overexpression and loss of PTEN were poor prognostic factors in patients with intrahepatic CCA. Thus, the combination of the HSP90 inhibitor (NVP-AUY922) and the PI3K/mTOR inhibitor (NVP-BEZ235) in CCA were evaluated and showed synergistic effects in vitro and in vivo. This combination not only inhibited the PI3K/AKT/mTOR pathway but also induced reactive oxygen species (ROS), which may enhance the vicious cycle of endoplasmic reticulum (ER) stress. Our data suggest the simultaneous targeting of the PI3K/mTOR and HSP pathways could be a novel and active therapeutic strategy for advanced CCA [100].

7.5. Other Indirect Inhibition of mTOR Pathway

VEGF can induce phosphorylation of both VEGFR1 and VEGFR2 but only VEGFR2 played a role in the promoting anti-apoptotic cell growth through activating a PI3K/AKT/mTOR signaling pathway. Apatinib, a VEGFR2-specific inhibitor, was reported to inhibit the anti-apoptosis induced by VEGF signaling, and promoted cell death in vitro and delayed tumor growth in vivo [101].

Besides direct inhibitors targeting mTOR, suppression of MAPKinase [102,103] or reactivation p53 [104,105] alone or in combination with mTOR inhibitors could be reasonably therapeutic strategies in advanced BTC.

8. mTOR Inhibitors in Clinical Setting

There are two settings for mTOR inhibitors used in the patients with advanced cholangiocarcinoma. Firstly, mTOR inhibitors could be used alone or in combination with other agents in the patients with advanced cholangiocarcinoma refractory to standard treatments. Secondly, mTOR inhibitors could be used in combination with standard treatment in patients with treatment-naïve advanced cholangiocarcinoma to investigate the possibly better response, progression-free survival and overall survival than conventional standard treatment. The combination of mTOR inhibitors with standard treatment aims to overcome resistance and potentiate the cytotoxicity of chemotherapy. Published clinical studies of mTOR inhibitors in advanced BTC were summarized in Table 1.

Table 1. Summary of published data regarding mTOR inhibitors in advanced BTC.

Compound(s)	Phase	Patients	Response	Survival
Everolimus, 1 L [106]	Case report	iCCA (*n* = 1) with PIK3CA mutation	PR	PFS > 6 m
Everolimus [107]	Phase I	Advanced BTC (*n* = 22)	DCR: 50% (11/22)	NA
Everolimus (>2 L) [108]	Phase II	Advanced BTC (*n* = 39)	DCR: 44.7% RR: 5.1% (including 1 CR)	mPFS: 3.2 m (1.8–4.0) mOS: 7.7 m (5.5–13.2)
Everolimus [109]	Phase II	CCA (*n* = 1), PTEN loss	SD	NA
Everolimus (1 L) [110]	Phase II	Advanced BTC (*n* = 27)	DCR at 12 weeks: 48% PR: 12% (3/25) SD: 60% (15/25)	mPFS: 5.5 m (2.2–10.0) mOS: 9.5 m (5.5–16.6)
Sirolimus [111]	Phase II	iCCA (*n* = 9)	SD: 33% (3/9) PD: 67% (6/9)	mOS:7 (2.6–35)
Sirolimus [112]	Phase II	hilar CCA (*n* = 1) with PIK3CA mutation	PD	PFS: 0.9 m
Everolimus, gemcitabine, cisplatin (1 L) [113]	Phase I	Cohort III, CCA and GBC (*n* = 10)	SD: 60% (6/10) PD: 40% (4/10)	NA

1 L, first line; 2 L, second line; iCCA, intrahepatic cholangiocarcinoma; GBC, gallbladder cancer; BTC, biliary tract cancer; CR, complete response; PR, partial response; SD, stable disease; PD, progressive disease; DCR, disease control rate; mPFS, median progression-free survival; mOS, median overall survival.

8.1. Clinical Studies of Everolimus in Advanced BTC

Bian et al. reported a 31-year-old male patient was diagnosed as stage IV intrahepatic CCA with *PIK3CA* mutation (E545G), which may result in activating mTOR pathway so patient received everolimus and achieved partial response (PR) after 2-month everolimus and at least 6-month PFS [106]. Larger series of everolimus in advanced BTC were studied. A phase I study reported that everolimus achieved 50% disease-control-rate (DCR) in a subgroup of 22 advanced BTC patients [107]. A phase II ITMO study in Italy enrolled 39 patients with previously chemotherapy-treated advanced BTC and the DCR was 44.7%, and the RR was 5.1%. Among two patients who experienced response, one patient showed a PR at 2 months and another patient showed a complete response (CR) sustained up to 8 months. The median PFS and OS were 3.2 (CI: 1.8–4.0) and 7.7 (CI: 5.5–13.2) months respectively [108]. In another phase II study to evaluate the activity of everolimus in 10 patients with *PIK3CA* amplification/mutation or *PTEN* loss refractory solid cancer, one patient with CCA with *PTEN* loss experienced disease control [109]. Recently, another phase II the RADiChol study published to evaluate the efficacy of everolimus as first-line treatment in treatment naïve advanced BTC, 27 patients enrolled showed DCR at 12 weeks was 48% and PFS and OS were 5.5 (2.2–10.0) and 9.5 (5.5–16.6) months, respectively [110]. Three (12%) of 25 patients evaluable for response experienced PR and 15 patients had stable diseases (SD). In addition, the authors performed immunohistochemistry (IHC) staining of PI3K/AKT/mTOR and found no association between IHC and clinical outcomes [110].

8.2. Clinical Studies of Sirolimus in Advanced BTC

In terms of other mTOR inhibitors, sirolimus, Rizell reported a cohort of sirolimus used in patients with hepatocellular carcinoma (*n* = 21) and iCCA (*n* = 9). Three (33%) of nine patients with intrahepatic CCA achieved SD after sirolimus treatment and others experienced progressive disease [111]. In a pilot study enrolling patients with PIK3CA mutant/amplified refractory solid cancer, sirolimus failed to demonstrate the clinical benefit in a patient with hilar cholangiocarcinoma (PIK3CA E545K mutation) who experienced disease progression following the second cycle of sirolimus with PFS of 0.9 months [112].

mTOR inhibitors alone, either sirolimus or everolimus showed some activity in advanced BTC with acceptable toxicities in treatment-naïve or pre-treated advanced BTC. The DCR (~50%) and survivals are compatible with the current standard of care. The use of mTOR inhibitors should be validated by larger randomized controlled trial (RCT) studies particularly in treatment naïve patients.

For refractory BTC patients, mTOR inhibitors provide limited disease control which might benefit some patients whose BTCs are refractory to standard treatment.

The only published study investigating the combination of everolimus and chemotherapy was performed to determine the maximally tolerated dose (MTD) of different combinations [113]. The MTD for Cohort I of the two-drug combination was everolimus 5 mg on Monday/Wednesday/Friday and gemcitabine 800 mg/m^2. Cohort II was to determine the MTC when cisplatin was added in everolimus/gemcitabine as a three-drug combination and cohort III was evaluation the activity of everolimus 5 mg on Monday/Wednesday/Friday, gemcitabine 600 mg/m^2, cisplatin 12.5 mg/m^2, 60% of 10 CCA and GBC carcinoma in cohort 3 experienced SD. The hematological DLT (mainly thrombocytopenia) limited the dosage used in three-drug combination and resulted in limited response rate. However, everolimus/gemcitabine could be an interesting regimen which demonstrated 2 CRs in this two-drug combination.

8.3. Clinical Studies of New Generation mTOR Inhibitors in Advanced BTC

Although new generation mTOR inhibitors and dual PI3K/mTOR inhibitors targeting both mTORC1 and mTORC2 showed anticancer activities in BTC (discussed in Sections 8.2 and 8.3), no clinical trials of these agents in advanced BTC were reported. All of these compounds are being investigated under early clinical trials to evaluate the efficacy in various refractory solid or hematologic cancers. Therefore, more and more results of new generation mTOR inhibitors will be released and published in the near future.

9. Summary of mTOR Inhibitors in BTC

In conclusion, mTOR signaling pathway connecting with several other pathways and networks regulates cancer proliferation and progression. Activation of mTOR is associated with drug-resistance in BTC. Rapalogs partially inhibit mTORC1 and exhibit anti-cancer activity. Rapalogs in clinical trials demonstrate some activity in patients with advanced BTC. New-generation mTOR inhibitors against ATP-binding pocket inhibit both TORC1 and TORC2 and demonstrate more potent anti-tumor effects in vitro and in vivo. Prospective clinical trials are warranted to prove its efficacy in patients with advanced BTC.

Funding: This research was supported by CMRPG310231, CMRPG310241, MOST107-2314-B-182A-134-MY3, NMRPG3H6211, CRRPG3F0031-3, and MOST105-2314-B-182A-MY2, NMRPG3F6021-2 to C.-N.Y.

Conflicts of Interest: The authors declare no conflicts of interest.

References

1. Patel, T. Cholangiocarcinoma. *Nat. Clin. Pract. Gastroenterol. Hepatol.* **2006**, *3*, 33–42. [CrossRef]
2. Siegel, R.L.; Miller, K.D.; Jemal, A. Cancer statistics, 2018. *CA Cancer J. Clin.* **2018**, *68*, 7–30. [CrossRef]
3. Patel, T. Increasing incidence and mortality of primary intrahepatic cholangiocarcinoma in the United States. *Hepatology* **2001**, *33*, 1353–1357. [CrossRef]
4. Shaib, Y.H.; Davila, J.A.; McGlynn, K.; El-Serag, H.B. Rising incidence of intrahepatic cholangiocarcinoma in the United States: A true increase? *J. Hepatol.* **2004**, *40*, 472–477. [CrossRef] [PubMed]
5. Jarnagin, W.R.; Fong, Y.; DeMatteo, R.P.; Gonen, M.; Burke, E.C.; Bodniewicz, B.J.; Youssef, B.M.; Klimstra, D.; Blumgart, L.H. Staging, resectability, and outcome in 225 patients with hilar cholangiocarcinoma. *Ann. Surg.* **2001**, *234*, 507–517. [CrossRef] [PubMed]
6. Valle, J.W.; Wasan, H.; Johnson, P.; Jones, E.; Dixon, L.; Swindell, R.; Baka, S.; Maraveyas, A.; Corrie, P.; Falk, S.; et al. Gemcitabine alone or in combination with cisplatin in patients with advanced or metastatic cholangiocarcinomas or other biliary tract tumours: A multicentre randomised phase II study—The UK ABC-01 Study. *Br. J. Cancer* **2009**, *101*, 621–627. [CrossRef] [PubMed]
7. Glimelius, B.; Hoffman, K.; Sjoden, P.O.; Jacobsson, G.; Sellstrom, H.; Enander, L.K.; Linne, T.; Svensson, C. Chemotherapy improves survival and quality of life in advanced pancreatic and biliary cancer. *Ann. Oncol.* **1996**, *7*, 593–600. [CrossRef] [PubMed]

8.   Burris, H.A., 3rd; Moore, M.J.; Andersen, J.; Green, M.R.; Rothenberg, M.L.; Modiano, M.R.; Cripps, M.C.; Portenoy, R.K.; Storniolo, A.M.; Tarassoff, P.; et al. Improvements in survival and clinical benefit with gemcitabine as first-line therapy for patients with advanced pancreas cancer: A randomized trial. *J. Clin. Oncol.* **1997**, *15*, 2403–2413. [CrossRef]

9.   Eckel, F.; Schmid, R.M. Chemotherapy in advanced biliary tract carcinoma: A pooled analysis of clinical trials. *Br. J. Cancer* **2007**, *96*, 896–902. [CrossRef]

10. Valle, J.; Wasan, H.; Palmer, D.H.; Cunningham, D.; Anthoney, A.; Maraveyas, A.; Madhusudan, S.; Iveson, T.; Hughes, S.; Pereira, S.P.; et al. Cisplatin plus gemcitabine versus gemcitabine for biliary tract cancer. *N. Engl. J. Med.* **2010**, *362*, 1273–1281. [CrossRef]

11. Wu, C.E.; Hsu, H.C.; Shen, W.C.; Lin, Y.C.; Wang, H.M.; Chang, J.W.; Chen, J.S. Chemotherapy with gemcitabine plus cisplatin in patients with advanced biliary tract carcinoma at Chang Gung Memorial Hospital: A retrospective analysis. *Chang Gung Med. J.* **2012**, *35*, 420–427. [PubMed]

12. Ueno, M.; Morizane, C.; Okusaka, T.; Mizusawa, J.; Katayama, H.; Ikeda, M. Randomized phase III study of gemcitabine plus S-1 combination therapy versus gemcitabine plus cisplatin combination therapy in advanced biliary tract cancer: A Japan Clinical Oncology Group study (JCOG1113, FUGA-BT). *J. Clin. Oncol.* **2018**, *36*, 205. [CrossRef]

13. Zhu, A.X.; Meyerhardt, J.A.; Blaszkowsky, L.S.; Kambadakone, A.; Muzikansky, A.; Zheng, H.; Clark, J.W.; Abrams, T.A.; Chan, J.A.; Enzinger, P.C.; et al. Efficacy and safety of gemcitabine, oxaliplatin, and bevacizumab in advanced biliary-tract cancers and correlation of changes in 18-fluorodeoxyglucose PET with clinical outcome: A phase 2 study. *Lancet Oncol.* **2010**, *11*, 48–54. [CrossRef]

14. Rubovszky, G.; Lang, I.; Ganofszky, E.; Horvath, Z.; Juhos, E.; Nagy, T.; Szabo, E.; Szentirmay, Z.; Budai, B.; Hitre, E. Cetuximab, gemcitabine and capecitabine in patients with inoperable biliary tract cancer: A phase 2 study. *Eur. J. Cancer* **2013**, *49*, 3806–3812. [CrossRef] [PubMed]

15. Malka, D.; Cervera, P.; Foulon, S.; Trarbach, T.; de la Fouchardiere, C.; Boucher, E.; Fartoux, L.; Faivre, S.; Blanc, J.F.; Viret, F.; et al. Gemcitabine and oxaliplatin with or without cetuximab in advanced biliary-tract cancer (BINGO): A randomised, open-label, non-comparative phase 2 trial. *Lancet Oncol.* **2014**, *15*, 819–828. [CrossRef]

16. Chen, J.S.; Hsu, C.; Chiang, N.J.; Tsai, C.S.; Tsou, H.H.; Huang, S.F.; Bai, L.Y.; Chang, I.C.; Shiah, H.S.; Ho, C.L.; et al. A KRAS mutation status-stratified randomized phase II trial of gemcitabine and oxaliplatin alone or in combination with cetuximab in advanced biliary tract cancer. *Ann. Oncol.* **2015**, *26*, 943–949. [CrossRef]

17. Eckel, F.; Schmid, R.M. Chemotherapy and targeted therapy in advanced biliary tract carcinoma: A pooled analysis of clinical trials. *Chemotherapy* **2014**, *60*, 13–23. [CrossRef]

18. Nakamura, H.; Arai, Y.; Totoki, Y.; Shirota, T.; Elzawahry, A.; Kato, M.; Hama, N.; Hosoda, F.; Urushidate, T.; Ohashi, S.; et al. Genomic spectra of biliary tract cancer. *Nat. Genet.* **2015**, *47*, 1003–1010. [CrossRef]

19. Bang, Y.J.; Doi, T.; De Braud, F.; Piha-Paul, S.; Hollebecque, A.; Razak, A.R.A.; Lin, C.C.; Ott, P.A.; He, A.R.; Yuan, S.S.; et al. Safety and efficacy of pembrolizumab (MK-3475) in patients (pts) with advanced biliary tract cancer: Interim results of KEYNOTE-028. *Eur. J. Cancer* **2015**, *51*, S112. [CrossRef]

20. Goldstein, D.; Lemech, C.; Valle, J. New molecular and immunotherapeutic approaches in biliary cancer. *ESMO Open* **2017**, *2*, e000152. [CrossRef]

21. Le, D.T.; Durham, J.N.; Smith, K.N.; Wang, H.; Bartlett, B.R.; Aulakh, L.K.; Lu, S.; Kemberling, H.; Wilt, C.; Luber, B.S.; et al. Mismatch repair deficiency predicts response of solid tumors to PD-1 blockade. *Science* **2017**, *357*, 409–413. [CrossRef] [PubMed]

22. Hanada, K.; Tsuchida, A.; Iwao, T.; Eguchi, N.; Sasaki, T.; Morinaka, K.; Matsubara, K.; Kawasaki, Y.; Yamamoto, S.; Kajiyama, G. Gene mutations of K-ras in gallbladder mucosae and gallbladder carcinoma with an anomalous junction of the pancreaticobiliary duct. *Am. J. Gastroenterol.* **1999**, *94*, 1638–1642. [CrossRef] [PubMed]

23. Kim, Y.T.; Kim, J.; Jang, Y.H.; Lee, W.J.; Ryu, J.K.; Park, Y.K.; Kim, S.W.; Kim, W.H.; Yoon, Y.B.; Kim, C.Y. Genetic alterations in gallbladder adenoma, dysplasia and carcinoma. *Cancer Lett.* **2001**, *169*, 59–68. [CrossRef]

24. Tannapfel, A.; Benicke, M.; Katalinic, A.; Uhlmann, D.; Kockerling, F.; Hauss, J.; Wittekind, C. Frequency of p16(INK4A) alterations and k-ras mutations in intrahepatic cholangiocarcinoma of the liver. *Gut* **2000**, *47*, 721–727. [CrossRef] [PubMed]

25. Tannapfel, A.; Sommerer, F.; Benicke, M.; Katalinic, A.; Uhlmann, D.; Witzigmann, H.; Hauss, J.; Wittekind, C. Mutations of the BRAF gene in cholangiocarcinoma but not in hepatocellular carcinoma. *Gut* **2003**, *52*, 706–712. [CrossRef] [PubMed]

26. Leone, F.; Cavalloni, G.; Pignochino, Y.; Sarotto, I.; Ferraris, R.; Piacibello, W.; Venesio, T.; Capussotti, L.; Risio, M.; Aglietta, M. Somatic mutations of epidermal growth factor receptor in bile duct and gallbladder carcinoma. *Clin. Cancer Res.* **2006**, *12*, 1680–1685. [CrossRef] [PubMed]

27. Riener, M.O.; Bawohl, M.; Clavien, P.A.; Jochum, W. Rare PIK3CA hotspot mutations in carcinomas of the biliary tract. *Genes Chromosomes Cancer* **2008**, *47*, 363–367. [CrossRef]

28. Argani, P.; Shaukat, A.; Kaushal, M.; Wilentz, R.E.; Su, G.H.; Sohn, T.A.; Yeo, G.J.; Cameron, J.L.; Kern, S.E.; Hruban, R.H. Differing rates of loss of Dpc4 expression and of p53 overexpression among carcinomas of the proximal and distal bile ducts—Evidence for biologic distinction. *Cancer* **2001**, *91*, 1332–1341. [CrossRef]

29. Ueki, T.; Hsing, A.W.; Gao, Y.T.; Wang, B.S.; Shen, M.C.; Cheng, J.; Deng, J.; Fraumeni, J.F., Jr.; Rashid, A. Alterations of p16 and prognosis in biliary tract cancers from a population-based study in China. *Clin. Cancer Res.* **2004**, *10*, 1717–1725. [CrossRef]

30. Hezel, A.F.; Deshpande, V.; Zhu, A.X. Genetics of biliary tract cancers and emerging targeted therapies. *J. Clin. Oncol.* **2010**, *28*, 3531–3540. [CrossRef]

31. Ekshyyan, O.; Anandharaj, A.; Nathan, C.A.O. Dual PI3K/mTOR Inhibitors: Does p53 Modulate Response? *Clin. Cancer Res.* **2013**, *19*, 3719–3721. [CrossRef] [PubMed]

32. Hansel, D.E.; Rahman, A.; Hidalgo, M.; Thuluvath, P.J.; Lillemoe, K.D.; Schulick, R.; Ku, J.L.; Park, J.G.; Miyazaki, K.; Ashfaq, R.; et al. Identification of novel cellular targets in biliary tract cancers using global gene expression technology. *Am. J. Pathol.* **2003**, *163*, 217–229. [CrossRef]

33. Zoncu, R.; Efeyan, A.; Sabatini, D.M. mTOR: From growth signal integration to cancer, diabetes and ageing. *Nat. Rev. Mol. Cell Biol.* **2011**, *12*, 21–35. [CrossRef] [PubMed]

34. Wullschleger, S.; Loewith, R.; Hall, M.N. TOR signaling in growth and metabolism. *Cell* **2006**, *124*, 471–484. [CrossRef] [PubMed]

35. Crino, P.B. The mTOR signalling cascade: Paving new roads to cure neurological disease. *Nat. Rev. Neurol.* **2016**, *12*, 379–392. [CrossRef] [PubMed]

36. Zhou, X.; Liu, W.; Hu, X.; Dorrance, A.; Garzon, R.; Houghton, P.J.; Shen, C. Regulation of CHK1 by mTOR contributes to the evasion of DNA damage barrier of cancer cells. *Sci. Rep.* **2017**, *7*, 1535. [CrossRef] [PubMed]

37. Chung, J.Y.; Hong, S.M.; Choi, B.Y.; Cho, H.; Yu, E.; Hewitt, S.M. The expression of phospho-AKT, phospho-mTOR, and PTEN in extrahepatic cholangiocarcinoma. *Clin. Cancer Res.* **2009**, *15*, 660–667. [CrossRef]

38. Ma, X.M.; Blenis, J. Molecular mechanisms of mTOR-mediated translational control. *Nat. Rev. Mol. Cell Biol.* **2009**, *10*, 307–318. [CrossRef]

39. Zhou, H.Y.; Huang, S.L. Current development of the second generation of mTOR inhibitors as anticancer agents. *Chin. J. Cancer* **2012**, *31*, 8–18. [CrossRef]

40. Faivre, S.; Kroemer, G.; Raymond, E. Current development of mTOR inhibitors as anticancer agents. *Nat. Rev. Drug Discov.* **2006**, *5*, 671–688. [CrossRef]

41. Mendoza, M.C.; Er, E.E.; Blenis, J. The Ras-ERK and PI3K-mTOR pathways: Cross-talk and compensation. *Trends Biochem. Sci.* **2011**, *36*, 320–328. [CrossRef]

42. Kim, L.C.; Cook, R.S.; Chen, J. mTORC1 and mTORC2 in cancer and the tumor microenvironment. *Oncogene* **2017**, *36*, 2191–2201. [CrossRef] [PubMed]

43. Sancak, Y.; Thoreen, C.C.; Peterson, T.R.; Lindquist, R.A.; Kang, S.A.; Spooner, E.; Carr, S.A.; Sabatini, D.M. PRAS40 is an insulin-regulated inhibitor of the mTORC1 protein kinase. *Mol. Cell* **2007**, *25*, 903–915. [CrossRef] [PubMed]

44. Wang, L.F.; Harris, T.E.; Roth, R.A.; Lawrence, J.C. PRAS40 regulates mTORC1 kinase activity by functioning as a direct inhibitor of substrate binding. *J. Biol. Chem.* **2007**, *282*, 20036–20044. [CrossRef] [PubMed]

45. Inoki, K.; Li, Y.; Xu, T.; Guan, K.L. Rheb GTPase is a direct target of TSC2 GAP activity and regulates mTOR signaling. *Gene Dev.* **2003**, *17*, 1829–1834. [CrossRef] [PubMed]

46. Huang, J.X.; Manning, B.D. A complex interplay between Akt, TSC2 and the two mTOR complexes. *Biochem. Soc. T* **2009**, *37*, 217–222. [CrossRef] [PubMed]

47. Schulick, R. Identification of Novel Cellular Targets in Biliary Tract Cancers Using Global Gene Expression Technology (vol 163, pg 217, 2003). *Am. J. Pathol.* **2017**, *187*, 936.
48. Markman, B.; Dienstmann, R.; Tabernero, J. Targeting the PI3K/Akt/mTOR pathway–beyond rapalogs. *Oncotarget* **2010**, *1*, 530–543.
49. Wang, X.M.; Proud, C.G. mTORC2 is a tyrosine kinase. *Cell Res.* **2016**, *26*, 1–2. [CrossRef]
50. Yang, G.; Murashige, D.S.; Humphrey, S.J.; James, D.E. A Positive Feedback Loop between Akt and mTORC2 via SIN1 Phosphorylation. *Cell Rep.* **2015**, *12*, 937–943. [CrossRef]
51. Sarbassov, D.D.; Ali, S.M.; Sengupta, S.; Sheen, J.H.; Hsu, P.P.; Bagley, A.F.; Markhard, A.L.; Sabatini, D.M. Prolonged rapamycin treatment inhibits mTORC2 assembly and Akt/PKB. *Mol. Cell* **2006**, *22*, 159–168. [CrossRef] [PubMed]
52. Guri, Y.; Colombi, M.; Dazert, E.; Hindupur, S.K.; Roszik, J.; Moes, S.; Jenoe, P.; Heim, M.H.; Riezman, I.; Riezman, H.; et al. mTORC2 Promotes Tumorigenesis via Lipid Synthesis. *Cancer Cell* **2017**, *32*, 807–823. [CrossRef] [PubMed]
53. Guertin, D.A.; Stevens, D.M.; Saitoh, M.; Kinkel, S.; Crosby, K.; Sheen, J.H.; Mullholland, D.J.; Magnuson, M.A.; Wu, H.; Sabatini, D.M. mTOR Complex 2 Is Required for the Development of Prostate Cancer Induced by Pten Loss in Mice. *Cancer Cell* **2009**, *15*, 148–159. [CrossRef] [PubMed]
54. Guri, Y.; Hall, M.N. mTOR Signaling Confers Resistance to Targeted Cancer Drugs. *Trends Cancer* **2016**, *2*, 688–697. [CrossRef]
55. Liu, P.; Cheng, H.; Roberts, T.M.; Zhao, J.J. Targeting the phosphoinositide 3-kinase pathway in cancer. *Nat. Rev. Drug Discov.* **2009**, *8*, 627–644. [CrossRef] [PubMed]
56. Whitman, M.; Downes, C.P.; Keeler, M.; Keller, T.; Cantley, L. Type I phosphatidylinositol kinase makes a novel inositol phospholipid, phosphatidylinositol-3-phosphate. *Nature* **1988**, *332*, 644–646. [CrossRef] [PubMed]
57. Owonikoko, T.K.; Khuri, F.R. Targeting the PI3K/AKT/mTOR pathway: Biomarkers of success and tribulation. *Am. Soc. Clin. Oncol. Educ. Book* **2013**. [CrossRef] [PubMed]
58. Samuels, Y.; Waldman, T. Oncogenic mutations of PIK3CA in human cancers. *Curr. Top. Microbiol. Immunol.* **2010**, *347*, 21–41. [PubMed]
59. Whale, A.D.; Colman, L.; Lensun, L.; Rogers, H.L.; Shuttleworth, S.J. Functional characterization of a novel somatic oncogenic mutation of PIK3CB. *Signal Transduct. Target. Ther.* **2017**, *2*, 17063. [CrossRef] [PubMed]
60. Czech, M.P. PIP2 and PIP3: Complex roles at the cell surface. *Cell* **2000**, *100*, 603–606. [CrossRef]
61. Cantley, L.C.; Neel, B.G. New insights into tumor suppression: PTEN suppresses tumor formation by restraining the phosphoinositide 3-kinase AKT pathway. *Proc. Natl. Acad. Sci. USA* **1999**, *96*, 4240–4245. [CrossRef] [PubMed]
62. Carracedo, A.; Pandolfi, P.P. The PTEN-PI3K pathway: Of feedbacks and cross-talks. *Oncogene* **2008**, *27*, 5527–5541. [CrossRef] [PubMed]
63. Mihaylova, M.M.; Shaw, R.J. The AMPK signalling pathway coordinates cell growth, autophagy and metabolism. *Nat. Cell Biol.* **2011**, *13*, 1016–1023. [CrossRef] [PubMed]
64. Jones, R.G.; Plas, D.R.; Kubek, S.; Buzzai, M.; Mu, J.; Xu, Y.; Birnbaum, M.J.; Thompson, C.B. AMP-activated protein kinase induces a p53-dependent metabolic checkpoint. *Mol. Cell* **2005**, *18*, 283–293. [CrossRef] [PubMed]
65. Feng, Z.; Hu, W.; de Stanchina, E.; Teresky, A.K.; Jin, S.; Lowe, S.; Levine, A.J. The regulation of AMPK beta1, TSC2, and PTEN expression by p53: Stress, cell and tissue specificity, and the role of these gene products in modulating the IGF-1-AKT-mTOR pathways. *Cancer Res.* **2007**, *67*, 3043–3053. [CrossRef] [PubMed]
66. Ma, L.; Chen, Z.; Erdjument-Bromage, H.; Tempst, P.; Pandolfi, P.P. Phosphorylation and functional inactivation of TSC2 by Erk implications for tuberous sclerosis and cancer pathogenesis. *Cell* **2005**, *121*, 179–193. [CrossRef] [PubMed]
67. Lopez, T.; Hanahan, D. Elevated levels of IGF-1 receptor convey invasive and metastatic capability in a mouse model of pancreatic islet tumorigenesis. *Cancer Cell* **2002**, *1*, 339–353. [CrossRef]
68. Roa, I.; Garcia, H.; Game, A.; de Toro, G.; de Aretxabala, X.; Javle, M. Somatic Mutations of PI3K in Early and Advanced Gallbladder Cancer Additional Options for an Orphan Cancer. *J. Mol. Diagn.* **2016**, *18*, 388–394. [CrossRef]

69. Petzold, J.; Lederer, E.; Reihs, R.; Ernst, C.; Bettermann, K.; Halbwedl, I.; Lax, S.; Park, Y.N.; Kim, K.S.; Kiesslich, T.; et al. Pten inactivation and alteration of the pi3k/AKT/MTOR pathway in biliary tract cancer. *Anticancer Res.* **2014**, *34*, 5942–5943.

70. Kornprat, P.; Rehak, P.; Ruschoff, J.; Langner, C. Expression of IGF-I, IGF-II, and IGF-IR in gallbladder carcinoma. A systematic analysis including primary and corresponding metastatic tumours. *J. Clin. Pathol.* **2006**, *59*, 202–206. [CrossRef]

71. Wolf, S.; Lorenz, J.; Mossner, J.; Wiedmann, M. Treatment of biliary tract cancer with NVP-AEW541: Mechanisms of action and resistance. *World J. Gastroenterol.* **2010**, *16*, 156–166. [CrossRef] [PubMed]

72. Guertin, D.A.; Sabatini, D.M. The Pharmacology of mTOR Inhibition. *Sci. Signal.* **2009**, *2*, pe24. [CrossRef] [PubMed]

73. Li, J.; Kim, S.G.; Blenis, J. Rapamycin: One Drug, Many Effects. *Cell Metab.* **2014**, *19*, 373–379. [CrossRef] [PubMed]

74. Vilella-Bach, M.; Nuzzi, P.; Fang, Y.; Chen, J. The FKBP12-rapamycin-binding domain is required for FKBP12-rapamycin-associated protein kinase activity and G1 progression. *J. Biol. Chem.* **1999**, *274*, 4266–4272. [CrossRef] [PubMed]

75. Choi, J.; Chen, J.; Schreiber, S.L.; Clardy, J. Structure of the FKBP12-rapamycin complex interacting with the binding domain of human FRAP. *Science* **1996**, *273*, 239–242. [CrossRef]

76. Choo, A.Y.; Yoon, S.O.; Kim, S.G.; Roux, P.P.; Blenis, J. Rapamycin differentially inhibits S6Ks and 4E-BP1 to mediate cell-type-specific repression of mRNA translation. *Proc. Natl. Acad. Sci. USA* **2008**, *105*, 17414–17419. [CrossRef]

77. Kang, S.A.; Pacold, M.E.; Cervantes, C.L.; Lim, D.; Lou, H.J.; Ottina, K.; Gray, N.S.; Turk, B.E.; Yaffe, M.B.; Sabatini, D.M. mTORC1 phosphorylation sites encode their sensitivity to starvation and rapamycin. *Science* **2013**, *341*, 1236566. [CrossRef] [PubMed]

78. Zheng, B.; Mao, J.H.; Qian, L.; Zhu, H.; Gu, D.H.; Pan, X.D.; Yi, F.; Ji, D.M. Pre-clinical evaluation of AZD-2014, a novel mTORC1/2 dual inhibitor, against renal cell carcinoma. *Cancer Lett.* **2015**, *357*, 468–475. [CrossRef]

79. Liu, Q.S.; Kirubakaran, S.; Hur, W.; Niepel, M.; Westover, K.; Thoreen, C.C.; Wang, J.H.; Ni, J.; Patricelli, M.P.; Vogel, K.; et al. Kinome-wide Selectivity Profiling of ATP-competitive Mammalian Target of Rapamycin (mTOR) Inhibitors and Characterization of Their Binding Kinetics. *J. Biol. Chem.* **2012**, *287*, 9742–9752. [CrossRef]

80. Powles, T.; Wheater, M.; Din, O.; Geldart, T.; Boleti, E.; Stockdale, A.; Sundar, S.; Robinson, A.; Ahmed, I.; Wimalasingham, A.; et al. A Randomised Phase 2 Study of AZD2014 Versus Everolimus in Patients with VEGF-Refractory Metastatic Clear Cell Renal Cancer. *Eur. Urol.* **2016**, *69*, 450–456. [CrossRef]

81. Petrossian, K.; Nguyen, D.; Lo, C.; Kanaya, N.; Somlo, G.; Cui, Y.X.; Huang, C.S.; Chen, S.A. Use of dual mTOR inhibitor MLN0128 against everolimus-resistant breast cancer. *Breast Cancer Res. Treat.* **2018**, *170*, 499–506. [CrossRef] [PubMed]

82. Vandamme, T.; Beyens, M.; de Beeck, K.O.; Dogan, F.; van Koetsveld, P.M.; Pauwels, P.; Mortier, G.; Vangestel, C.; de Herder, W.; Van Camp, G.; et al. Long-term acquired everolimus resistance in pancreatic neuroendocrine tumours can be overcome with novel PI3K-AKT-mTOR inhibitors. *Br. J. Cancer* **2016**, *114*, 650–658. [CrossRef] [PubMed]

83. Schmid, P.; Ferreira, M.; Dubey, S.; Zaiss, M.; Harper-Wynne, C.; Makris, A.; Brown, V.; Kristeleit, H.; Patel, G.; Perello, A.; et al. MANTA: A randomized phase II study of fulvestrant in combination with the dual mTOR inhibitor AZD2014 or everolimus or fulvestrant alone in estrogen receptor-positive advanced or metastatic breast cancer. *Cancer Res.* **2018**, *78*. Abstract GS2-07. [CrossRef]

84. Kelsey, I.; Manning, B.D. mTORC1 status dictates tumor response to targeted therapeutics. *Sci. Signal.* **2013**, *6*, pe31. [CrossRef] [PubMed]

85. Ilagan, E.; Manning, B.D. Emerging role of mTOR in the response to cancer therapeutics. *Trends Cancer* **2016**, *2*, 241–251. [CrossRef] [PubMed]

86. Jiang, B.H.; Liu, L.Z. Role of mTOR in anticancer drug resistance: Perspectives for improved drug treatment. *Drug Resist. Updates* **2008**, *11*, 63–76. [CrossRef] [PubMed]

87. Yokoi, K.; Kobayashi, A.; Motoyama, H.; Kitazawa, M.; Shimizu, A.; Notake, T.; Yokoyama, T.; Matsumura, T.; Takeoka, M.; Miyagawa, S.I. Survival pathway of cholangiocarcinoma via AKT/mTOR signaling to escape RAF/MEK/ERK pathway inhibition by sorafenib. *Oncol. Rep.* **2018**, *39*, 843–850. [CrossRef]

88. Li, Q.; Xia, X.; Ji, J.; Ma, J.; Tao, L.; Mo, L.; Chen, W. MiR-199a-3p enhances cisplatin sensitivity of cholangiocarcinoma cells by inhibiting mTOR signaling pathway and expression of MDR1. *Oncotarget* **2017**, *8*, 33621–33630. [CrossRef]

89. Ling, S.; Feng, T.; Ke, Q.; Fan, N.; Li, L.; Li, Z.; Dong, C.; Wang, C.; Xu, F.; Li, Y.; et al. Metformin inhibits proliferation and enhances chemosensitivity of intrahepatic cholangiocarcinoma cell lines. *Oncol. Rep.* **2014**, *31*, 2611–2618. [CrossRef]

90. Wandee, J.; Prawan, A.; Senggunprai, L.; Kongpetch, S.; Tusskorn, O.; Kukongviriyapan, V. Metformin enhances cisplatin induced inhibition of cholangiocarcinoma cells via AMPK-mTOR pathway. *Life Sci.* **2018**, *207*, 172–183. [CrossRef]

91. Ahn, C.S.; Han, J.A.; Lee, H.S.; Lee, S.; Pai, H.S. The PP2A regulatory subunit Tap46, a component of the TOR signaling pathway, modulates growth and metabolism in plants. *Plant Cell* **2011**, *23*, 185–209. [CrossRef] [PubMed]

92. Lyu, S.C.; Han, D.D.; Li, X.L.; Ma, J.; Wu, Q.; Dong, H.M.; Bai, C.; He, Q. Fyn knockdown inhibits migration and invasion in cholangiocarcinoma through the activated AMPK/mTOR signaling pathway. *Oncol. Lett.* **2018**, *15*, 2085–2090. [CrossRef] [PubMed]

93. Moolthiya, P.; Tohtong, R.; Keeratichamroen, S.; Leelawat, K. Role of mTOR inhibitor in cholangiocarcinoma cell progression. *Oncol. Lett.* **2014**, *7*, 854–860. [CrossRef] [PubMed]

94. Heits, N.; Heinze, T.; Bernsmeier, A.; Kerber, J.; Hauser, C.; Becker, T.; Kalthoff, H.; Egberts, J.H.; Braun, F. Influence of mTOR-inhibitors and mycophenolic acid on human cholangiocellular carcinoma and cancer associated fibroblasts. *BMC Cancer* **2016**, *16*, 322. [CrossRef] [PubMed]

95. Zhao, X.F.; Zhang, C.Y.; Zhou, H.; Xiao, B.; Cheng, Y.; Wang, J.J.; Yao, F.L.; Duan, C.Y.; Chen, R.; Liu, Y.P.; et al. Synergistic antitumor activity of the combination of salubrinal and rapamycin against human cholangiocarcinoma cells. *Oncotarget* **2016**, *7*, 85492–85501. [CrossRef] [PubMed]

96. Lin, G.G.; Lin, K.J.; Wang, F.; Chen, T.C.; Yen, T.C.; Yeh, T.S. Synergistic antiproliferative effects of an mTOR inhibitor (rad001) plus gemcitabine on cholangiocarcinoma by decreasing choline kinase activity. *Dis. Models Mech.* **2018**, *11*. [CrossRef] [PubMed]

97. Zhang, S.S.; Song, X.H.; Cao, D.; Xu, Z.; Fan, B.A.; Che, L.; Hu, J.J.; Chen, B.; Dong, M.J.; Pilo, M.G.; et al. Pan-mTOR inhibitor MLN0128 is effective against intrahepatic cholangiocarcinoma in mice. *J. Hepatol.* **2017**, *67*, 1194–1203. [CrossRef]

98. Song, X.; Liu, X.; Wang, H.; Wang, J.; Qiao, Y.; Cigliano, A.; Utpatel, K.; Ribback, S.; Pilo, M.G.; Serra, M.; et al. Combined CDK4/6 and Pan-mTOR Inhibition Is Synergistic Against Intrahepatic Cholangiocarcinoma. *Clin. Cancer Res.* **2018**. [CrossRef]

99. Fraveto, A.; Cardinale, V.; Bragazzi, M.C.; Giuliante, F.; De Rose, A.M.; Grazi, G.L.; Napoletano, C.; Semeraro, R.; Lustri, A.M.; Costantini, D.; et al. Sensitivity of Human Intrahepatic Cholangiocarcinoma Subtypes to Chemotherapeutics and Molecular Targeted Agents: A Study on Primary Cell Cultures. *PLoS ONE* **2015**, *10*, e0142124. [CrossRef]

100. Chen, M.H.; Chiang, K.C.; Cheng, C.T.; Huang, S.C.; Chen, Y.Y.; Chen, T.W.; Yeh, T.S.; Jan, Y.Y.; Wang, H.M.; Weng, J.J.; et al. Antitumor activity of the combination of an HSP90 inhibitor and a PI3K/mTOR dual inhibitor against cholangiocarcinoma. *Oncotarget* **2014**, *5*, 2372–2389. [CrossRef]

101. Peng, H.; Zhang, Q.Y.; Li, J.L.; Zhang, N.; Hua, Y.P.; Xu, L.X.; Deng, Y.B.; Lai, J.M.; Peng, Z.W.; Peng, B.G.; et al. Apatinib inhibits VEGF signaling and promotes apoptosis in intrahepatic cholangiocarcinoma. *Oncotarget* **2016**, *7*, 17220–17229. [CrossRef] [PubMed]

102. Wu, C.E.; Koay, T.S.; Esfandiari, A.; Ho, Y.H.; Lovat, P.; Lunec, J. ATM Dependent DUSP6 Modulation of p53 Involved in Synergistic Targeting of MAPK and p53 Pathways with Trametinib and MDM2 Inhibitors in Cutaneous Melanoma. *Cancers* **2018**, *11*, 3. [CrossRef]

103. Andersen, N.J.; Boguslawski, E.B.; Kuk, C.Y.; Chambers, C.M.; Duesbery, N.S. Combined inhibition of MEK and mTOR has a synergic effect on angiosarcoma tumorgrafts. *Int. J. Oncol.* **2015**, *47*, 71–80. [CrossRef]

104. Wu, C.E.; Esfandiari, A.; Ho, Y.H.; Wang, N.; Mahdi, A.K.; Aptullahoglu, E.; Lovat, P.; Lunec, J. Targeting negative regulation of p53 by MDM2 and WIP1 as a therapeutic strategy in cutaneous melanoma. *Br. J. Cancer* **2018**, *118*, 495–508. [CrossRef] [PubMed]

105. Laroche, A.; Chaire, V.; Algeo, M.P.; Karanian, M.; Fourneaux, B.; Italiano, A. MDM2 antagonists synergize with PI3K/mTOR inhibition in well-differentiated/dedifferentiated liposarcomas. *Oncotarget* **2017**, *8*, 53968–53977. [CrossRef] [PubMed]

106. Bian, J.L.; Wang, M.M.; Tong, E.J.; Sun, J.; Li, M.; Miao, Z.B.; Li, Y.L.; Zhu, B.H.; Xu, J.J. Benefit of everolimus in treatment of an intrahepatic cholangiocarcinoma patient with a PIK3CA mutation. *World J. Gastroenterol.* **2017**, *23*, 4311–4316. [CrossRef] [PubMed]

107. Verzoni, E.; Pusceddu, S.; Buzzoni, R.; Garanzini, E.; Damato, A.; Biondani, P.; Testa, I.; Grassi, P.; Bajetta, E.; DeBraud, F.; et al. Safety profile and treatment response of everolimus in different solid tumors: An observational study. *Future Oncol.* **2014**, *10*, 1611–1617. [CrossRef] [PubMed]

108. Buzzoni, R.; Pusceddu, S.; Bajetta, E.; De Braud, F.; Platania, M.; Iannacone, C.; Cantore, M.; Mambrini, A.; Bertolini, A.; Alabiso, O.; et al. Activity and safety of RAD001 (everolimus) in patients affected by biliary tract cancer progressing after prior chemotherapy: A phase II ITMO study. *Ann. Oncol.* **2014**, *25*, 1597–1603. [CrossRef]

109. Kim, S.T.; Lee, J.; Park, S.H.; Park, J.O.; Park, Y.S.; Kang, W.K.; Lim, H.Y. Prospective phase II trial of everolimus in PIK3CA amplification/mutation and/or PTEN loss patients with advanced solid tumors refractory to standard therapy. *BMC Cancer* **2017**, *17*, 211. [CrossRef]

110. Lau, D.K.; Tay, R.Y.; Yeung, Y.H.; Chionh, F.; Mooi, J.; Murone, C.; Skrinos, E.; Price, T.J.; Mariadason, J.M.; Tebbutt, N.C. Phase II study of everolimus (RAD001) monotherapy as first-line treatment in advanced biliary tract cancer with biomarker exploration: The RADiChol Study. *Br. J. Cancer* **2018**, *118*, 966–971. [CrossRef]

111. Rizell, M.; Andersson, M.; Cahlin, C.; Hafstrom, L.; Olausson, M.; Lindner, P. Effects of the mTOR inhibitor sirolimus in patients with hepatocellular and cholangiocellular cancer. *Int. J. Clin. Oncol.* **2008**, *13*, 66–70. [CrossRef] [PubMed]

112. Jung, K.S.; Lee, J.; Park, S.H.; Park, J.O.; Park, Y.S.; Lim, H.Y.; Kang, W.K.; Kim, S.T. Pilot study of sirolimus in patients with PIK3CA mutant/amplified refractory solid cancer. *Mol. Clin. Oncol.* **2017**, *7*, 27–31. [CrossRef] [PubMed]

113. Costello, B.A.; Borad, M.J.; Qi, Y.; Kim, G.P.; Northfelt, D.W.; Erlichman, C.; Alberts, S.R. Phase I trial of everolimus, gemcitabine and cisplatin in patients with solid tumors. *Investig. New Drugs* **2014**, *32*, 710–716. [CrossRef] [PubMed]

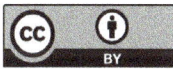

International Journal of
Molecular Sciences

MDPI

Review

Targeting mTOR as a Therapeutic Approach in Medulloblastoma

Juncal Aldaregia [1], Ainitze Odriozola [1], Ander Matheu [1,2,3] and Idoia Garcia [1,2,3,4,*]

1   Cellular Oncology Group, Biodonostia Research Institute, 20014 Donostia-San Sebastián, Spain;
     juncal.aldareguia@biodonostia.org (J.A.); ainitzeodri15@gmail.com (A.O.);
     ander.matheu@biodonostia.org (A.M.)
2   IKERBASQUE, Basque Foundation for Science, 48013 Bilbao, Spain
3   CIBER de fragilidad y envejecimiento saludable (CIBERfes), 28029 Madrid, Spain
4   Physiology Department, Faculty of Medicine and Nursing, University of the Basque Country (UPV/EHU),
     48940 Leioa, Spain
*   Correspondence: idoia.garcia@biodonostia.org; Tel.: +34-943-006-297

Received: 24 May 2018; Accepted: 20 June 2018; Published: 22 June 2018

Abstract: Mechanistic target of rapamycin (mTOR) is a master signaling pathway that regulates organismal growth and homeostasis, because of its implication in protein and lipid synthesis, and in the control of the cell cycle and the cellular metabolism. Moreover, it is necessary in cerebellar development and stem cell pluripotency maintenance. Its deregulation has been implicated in the medulloblastoma and in medulloblastoma stem cells (MBSCs). Medulloblastoma is the most common malignant solid tumor in childhood. The current therapies have improved the overall survival but they carry serious side effects, such as permanent neurological sequelae and disability. Recent studies have given rise to a new molecular classification of the subgroups of medulloblastoma, specifying 12 different subtypes containing novel potential therapeutic targets. In this review we propose the targeting of mTOR, in combination with current therapies, as a promising novel therapeutic approach.

Keywords: mTOR; Medulloblastoma; MBSCs

1. Mechanistic Target of Rapamycin (mTOR)

The mechanistic (formerly mammalian) target of rapamycin (mTOR) is a master signaling pathway that regulates organismal growth and homeostasis. This pathway is not only implicated in physiological conditions but it is also central in several pathological conditions [1]. mTOR is highly sensitive to rapamycin, a specific inhibitor of this serine/threonine kinase and an antiproliferative drug that is used clinically in antitumor and immunosuppressive therapy [2]. As represented in Figure 1, mTOR is activated by tyrosine kinase receptors via the phosphatidylinositol 3-kinase (PI3K)/AKT pathway. mTOR interacts with different proteins, forming two functionally distinct multiprotein complexes, mTOR complex 1 (mTORC1) and complex 2 (mTORC2) [3]. mTORC1 is composed of mTOR, Raptor, GβL, and DEP domain-containing mTOR-interacting protein (DEPTOR) [4]. It is a sensor of a wide variety of cellular signals, including growth factors, energy levels, oxygen, stress, or amino acids. These signals promote the regulation of cell growth and metabolism through a number of downstream effects, such as protein and lipid synthesis or autophagy inhibition [3]. Less is known about mTORC2, which is composed of mTOR, Rictor, GβL, Sin1, Proline rich protein 5 (PRR5)/Protor-1, and DEPTOR [5]. It responds to growth factors that control the cell proliferation, but it is insensitive to nutrients. mTORC2 can directly phosphorylate AKT, and it controls the cytoskeletal organization and cell survival [6] (Figure 1).

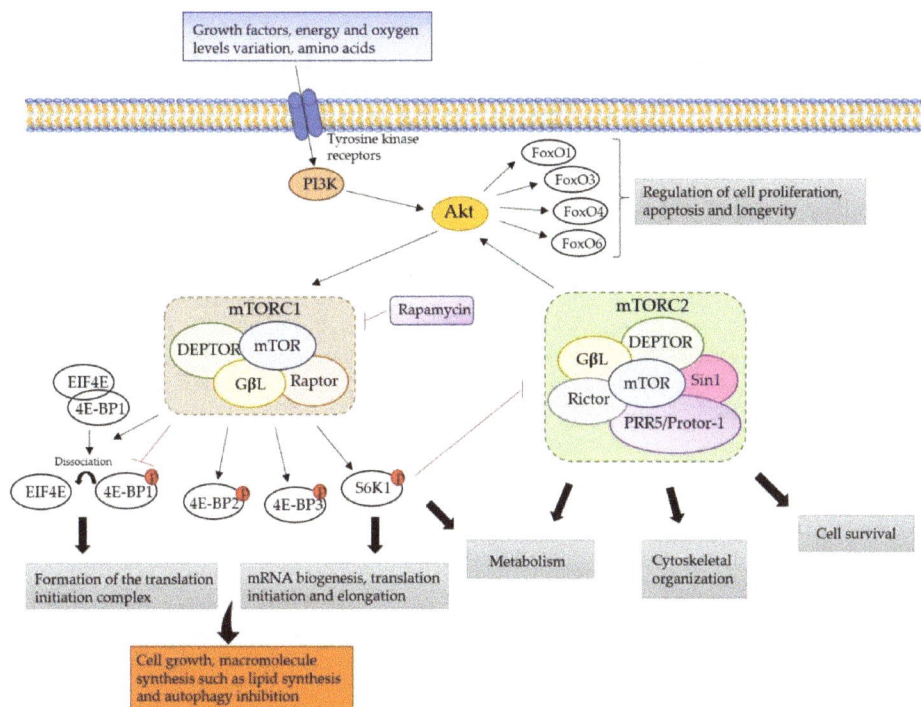

Figure 1. Mechanistic target of rapamycin (mTOR) signaling pathway. mTOR is part of two different complexes, mTOR complex 1 (mTORC1) and complex 2 (mTORC2). mTORC1 is activated by the phosphatidylinositol 3-kinase (PI3K)/AKT signaling pathway, and its downstream effectors activate cell growth, lipid synthesis, and metabolism, whereas it inhibits the autophagy. This complex can be inhibited by rapamycin. mTORC2 activates AKT, thus activating also mTORC1. Furthermore, mTORC2 activates the metabolism, cytoskeletal organization, and cell survival.

One of the most important downstream effects of mTORC1 is the upregulation of protein synthesis. It phosphorylates several translation regulators, including eukaryotic translation initiation factor 4E (eIF4E)-binding proteins (4E-BP1, 2, 3) [1] and the p70 ribosomal S6 kinase 1 and 2 (S6K1) [7]. The phosphorylation of 4EBP1 inactivates this protein and allows the dissociation of 4EBP1 from EIF4E, enabling the formation of the translation initiation complex. In the case of S6K1, when phosphorylated, it increases mRNA biogenesis, translational initiation, and elongation [1]. Furthermore, S6K1 establishes a negative-feedback mechanism between mTORC1 and mTORC2; when there is a strong activation of mTORC1, mTORC2 is inhibited [8,9]. Since mTORC2 activates AKT, the activation of mTORC1 indirectly inhibits AKT. AKT activation via mTORC2 is required for the phosphorylation of some AKT substrates, such as the members of the Forkhead boxO (FoxO) family (FoxO1, 3, 4, and 6), which are involved in the regulation of cellular processes such as cell proliferation, apoptosis, and longevity [9] (Figure 1).

It is more and more obvious that the mTOR signaling pathway has an important role in essential cellular functions. The key role of mTOR in controlling cell proliferation has raised the interest in rapamycin for cancer therapy. This drug disrupts mTORC1 protein complex formation, whereas mTORC2 is quite insensitive to the drug, and long-term treatments are required in order to inhibit its assembly [10] (Figure 1).

2. mTOR in Central Nervous System (CNS) Development

mTOR plays an important role in the development of an organism because of its implication in the growth, proliferation, and migration of every cell during normal brain development [11]. Accordingly, the first mTOR knockout (KO) mouse study demonstrated that mTOR is indispensable for normal development and viability [11,12]. Indeed, the importance of mTOR in the brain development was evidenced when Hentges and colleagues created a loss of function mutant of mTOR and it showed a defect in the telencephalon formation, and it died in mid-gestation [13].

Nowadays, it is known that the deregulation of mTOR signaling is associated with many brain diseases, including neurological diseases, psychiatric diseases, or pediatric brain tumors [9,14]. The activation of the PI3K/AKT/mTOR signaling pathway enhances the proliferation of progenitors, neuronal hypertrophy, and excessive dendritic branching, while the opposite consequences are presented when the pathway is suppressed [15].

When forming the cerebellum, cerebellar granule neuron precursors (CGNPs) undergo a rapid expansion in the external granule layer (EGL) on the dorsal surface of the cerebellum. Afterwards, they exit the cell cycle, migrate internally, and differentiate into interneurons [16]. In the expansion phase, the CGNPs require Sonic Hedgehog (SHH) signaling activation for cell proliferation and insulin-like growth factor (IGF), which positively regulates the mTOR pathway, for cell survival capacity [16]. Furthermore, Mainwaring and Kenney demonstrated that SHH signaling modulates the individual mTOR effectors separately, in order to maintain a proliferation-competent state. Unlike what has been observed in cell lines, the CGNPs positively regulate eIF4E and negatively regulate S6K, promoting cell proliferation and cell cycle progression [16].

3. Medulloblastoma

Medulloblastoma (MB) is the most frequent pediatric solid tumor, representing around 20% of the tumors of the CNS in childhood [17]. This tumor arises in the cerebellum and it is classified as a grade IV lesion by the World Health Organization (WHO) [18]. As mentioned above, cerebellum development needs a well-regulated rate of proliferation and differentiation of the CGNPs in order to form a correct cerebellum [19]. The SHH–Patched (PTCH1) [20], or WNT [21] signaling pathways are key regulators of this process. PTCH1 is the receptor of SHH. In the absence of SHH, PTCH1 inhibits the Smoothened (SMO)-GLI signaling pathway (Figure 2). When SHH is present, its binding to PTCH1 releases the negative regulation that PTCH1 is exerting to SMO and therefore the signaling pathway will be active, promoting cell proliferation [20]. The mechanism of action of the WNT signaling pathway is similar. As represented in Figure 2, in the absence of WNT, the multiprotein complex formed by Axin, and the Glycogen Synthase Kinase 3 Beta (GSK3β) and APC will phosphorylate cytoplasmic β-catenin that will then be degraded. When WNT is present, it will bind to its receptor Frizzled and this binding will inhibit the GSK3β inhibiting the function of the multiprotein complex. β-catenin will be accumulated and then it will translocate into the nucleus, promoting the cell cycle progression. If an excessive activation of these signaling pathways occurs, the MB progression may occur because of the incapacity of the cells to exit from a proliferative state and enter in a differentiation process [22]. Indeed, the patients with Gorlin's syndrome (PTCH1 mutation) and the patients with Turcot's syndrome (APC mutation) present increased incidence of MB [20]. Further evidence demonstrating that the hyperactivation of these signaling pathways are responsible for the loss of equilibrium in cerebellar growth are the WNT and SHH MB mice models [23–25].

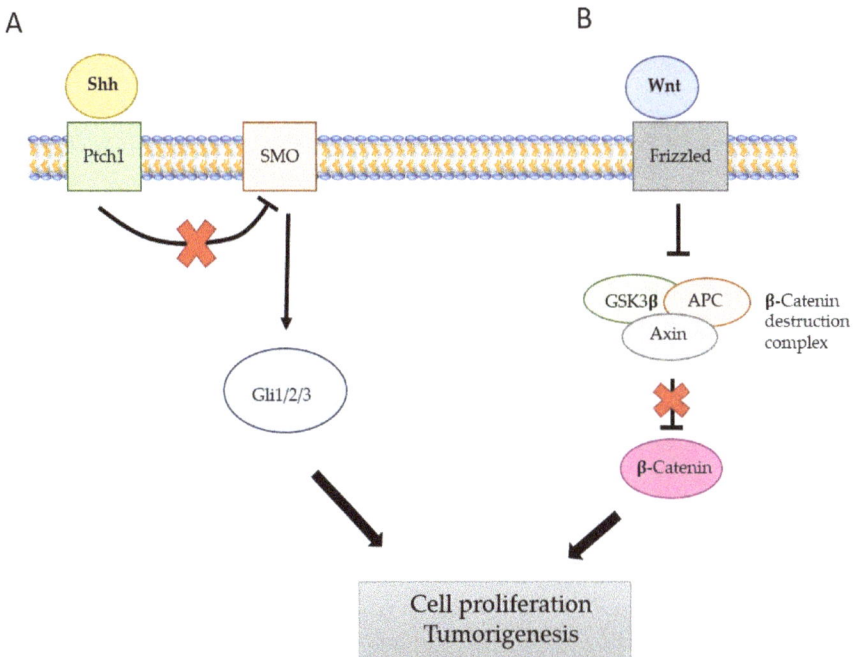

Figure 2. The Sonic Hedgehog (SHH)/Patched (PTCH1) and WNT signaling pathways. (**A**) The SHH ligand inactivates the PTCH1 receptor allowing Smoothened (SMO) to become active. Red cross represents the release of the inhibition exerted by PTCH1 on SMO when SHH is present. The SMO activates the GLI proteins, a family of transcription factors that turn on the expression of different target genes, giving raise to cell proliferation and tumorigenesis (activation of the pathway represented with black arrows). (**B**) The binding of WNT to the Frizzled receptor activates a cascade of downstream events, resulting in the inactivation of the β-catenin destruction complex. The red cross represent the release of the inhibition exerted by the β-catenin destruction complex on β-catenin. In consequence, β-catenin activates and promotes the transcription of genes that promote cell proliferation and tumorigenesis (represented with black arrows). Adapted from [21,23].

The progress in MB therapy has increased the survival rate of the patients, although it is very variable depending on the tumor subtype. The strategy that is used nowadays for MB patients is based on maximal tumor resection, followed by chemotherapy and craniospinal radiotherapy [17]. The prognostic of the patients is different depending on the type of resection (complete or not) and the age of the patient, since patients younger than 3 years old cannot receive craniospinal radiotherapy because of the risks that promote a second neoplasia [26]. Regarding to chemotherapy, the most used strategy is the combination of lomustine, vincristine, and cisplatin [17]. This therapy has improved the survival of patients, in some cases reaching a 70–90% of survival rate [27]. However, the high doses of chemotherapy and radiotherapy that need to be used in order to achieve a therapeutic response cause irreparable damage to the healthy tissue, causing permanent neurological sequelae and disability [28,29]. Furthermore, despite the improvement in the prognosis for children with MB, about 30% of the surviving patients relapse after the initial treatment [29,30].

Moreover, almost 30% of the patients present with disseminated tumor at the moment of diagnosis [31]. MBs spread from the cerebrospinal fluid (CFS), and the most common dissemination is leptomningeal. Metastases outside the CFS are very rare, but they can appear in the bone, lymph node, and lung, in decreasing order of occurrence [32].

4. Medulloblastoma Subgroups

The first classification of MBs was based on their histopathological features. Until 2007, three main subgroups were defined (classic, desmoplastic-nodular, and large cell anaplastic [LCA] MB), when the WHO classification defined four different histological subgroups, namely, desmoplastic-nodular, large cell, anaplastic, and MB with extensive nodularity (MBEN), the first one being the one with the best prognosis [33]. This classification was supplemented in 2011 with the studies of Northcott and colleagues. Using a bioinformatic analysis of transcriptional data from two cohorts from Toronto and Moscow, they discovered four distinct molecular variants of MB, which they denominated WNT, SHH, Group C, and Group D [34]. These and additional studies gave rise to a consensus conference in Boston in 2010, where the discussants came to a consensus of the existence of four MB subgroups, named WNT, SHH, Group 3, and Group 4 [35]. In a recent study that was carried out by Cavalli and colleagues, 763 MB samples were analyzed using the similarity network fusion approach [36]. The result of this work was the identification of new subtypes within the four MB subgroups, specifically, they identified a total of 12 subtypes, namely: two WNT, four SHH, three Group 3, and three Group 4 subtypes [36]. The main features and the relationship among these classifications are summarized in Table 1.

4.1. WNT subgroup

This subgroup is characterized by the aberrant activation of the WNT/β-catenin signaling pathway and the good prognosis of the patients [37]. In 2017, two subtypes were identified, WNT α and WNT β. The main molecular difference between the two subgroups is that the WNT α type tumors present monosomy 6, where β-catenin gene is located, whereas the WNT β type tumors are normally diploid for chromosome 6 (Table 1). The WNT α tumors are frequent in children and adolescents, whereas the WNT β tumors are more likely to appear in adolescents and adults [36] (Table 1).

Table representing key histological and clinical data of two different MB classifications, as well as genetic alterations, metastasis rates, age, and survival data of the Cavalli classification. The mTOR implication in some of the subgroups is also presented. The age groups are infant (0–3 years), children (>3–10 years), adolescent (>10–17 years), and adult (>17 years). Ado—adolescent; amp: amplification; child—children; dup—duplication; LCA—large cell/anaplastic; MBEN—medulloblastoma with extensive nodularity; mut—mutations; ↑—activation.

Int. J. Mol. Sci. **2018**, *19*, 1838

Table 1. Graphical summary of the different classification of medulloblastoma (MB) subgroups and their specifications.

Medulloblastoma Classification System	Clinical Features	WNT		SHH				Group 3			Group 4		
Taylor Classification	Histology	Classic, Rarely LCA		Desmoplastic/Nodular, Classic, LCA				Classic, LCA			Classic, LCA		
	Prognosis	Very good		Infants Good; Other Intermidiate				Poor			Intermidiate		
Cavalli classification		α	β	α	β	γ	δ	α	β	γ	α	β	γ
	Metastasis	9%	21%	20%	33%	9%	9%	43%	20%	40%	40%	41%	39%
	Genetic alterations	Monosomy 6		TP53 mutations	PTEN loss		TERT promoter mut	8q loss	GFI1 and GFI1B ↑, OTX2 amp, DDX31 loss	MYC amp	MYCN and CDK amp, 8p loss, 7q gain	SNCAIP dup, i17q	CDK amp, 8p loss, 7q gain
	Age	Child; Ado	Ado; Adult	Child; Ado	Infant	Infant	Adult	Infant; Child	Child; Ado	Infant; Children	Child; Ado	Child; Ado	Child; Ado
	Subtype histology			LCA, desmoplastic	Desmoplastic	MBEN, desmoplastic	Desmoplastic						
	Survival	97%	100%	70%	67%	88%	89%	66%	56%	42%	67%	75%	83%
mTOR				mTORC1 activation							PI3K/AKT/mTOR activation		

4.2. SHH Subgroup

This subgroup is characterized by the aberrant activation of the SHH signaling pathway that gives rise to the disease. Different genes belonging to this signaling pathway can be mutated, such as SHH, PTCH, SMO, SUFU, GLI1, or GLI2. The patients that are classified in the SHH subgroup have an intermediate prognosis, except the infants who have a good prognosis. This information has recently been complemented with the four subtypes that are defined within the SHH group: SHH α, SHH β, SHH γ, and SHH δ [36] (Table 1). The SHH α subtype mainly affects the children and adolescents, and, among other alterations, it is the only one presenting the TP53 mutations [36]. Furthermore, this subgroup is enriched with the expression of the genes that are involved in DNA repair and cell cycle progression [36]. Both SHH β and SHH γ tumors affect infants, but the survival rates are very different. As shown in Table 1, the SHH β tumors are characterized by phosphatase and tensin homolog (PTEN) loss and they present the lowest survival rate at 5 years within the SHH tumors. In addition to identifying specific mutations and genetic alterations, Cavalli and colleagues identified an enrichment on the developmental signaling pathways in the SHH β and SHH γ subgroups. In SHH δ, the main characteristic is the enrichment of mutations in TERT promoter [36] (Table 1).

4.3. Group 3

This subgroup presents the worst survival rate [38] and to date, a unique altered signaling pathway originating the disease has not been identified. Cavalli and colleagues have described three different subtypes within the Group 3 MB, namely: Group 3α, Group 3β, and Group 3γ. Group 3α is characterized by chromosome 8q loss (encoding v-myc avian myelocytomatosis viral oncogene homolog (MYC)). The Group 3β tumors are characterized by the activation of the GFI1 and GFI1B oncogenes, amplification of OTX2, and loss of DDX31 on chromosome 9. Finally, the Group 3γ tumors present the MYC amplification as a result of the gain of chromosome 8q [36] (Table 1).

Regarding to the implication of the signaling pathways, the Group 3α tumors are enriched in the expression of the photoreceptor, muscle contraction, and primary cilium-related genes, while Group 3β and 3γ present the enrichment of protein translation pathways. Furthermore, Group 3γ is also enriched in the expression of genes that are related to telomere maintenance [36].

4.4. Group 4

This is the most prevalent group; almost 40% of the MBs are included in this subgroup. As in Group 3, the deleterious signaling pathway that causes the disease has not been identified. There are three different subtypes that have been described within this subgroup: Group 4α, Group 4β, and Group 4γ. The main characteristics of the Group 4α tumors are the v-myc avian myelocytomatosis viral-related oncogene, neuroblastoma-derived (MYCN) and cyclin dependent kinase 6 (CDK6) amplifications, 8p loss and 7q gain. The Group 4β tumors are characterized with the synuclein alpha interacting protein (SNCAIP) duplications and ubiquitous i17q. Finally, the Group 4γ tumors present CDK6 amplifications, 8p loss, and 7q gain, as Group 4α tumors, but with the absence of MYCN amplifications [36] (Table 1).

The experiments that were performed by Cavalli and colleagues have identified differentially activated pathways for each subtype, supporting the existence of the three independent subtypes. The pathways that were identified were the activation of migration pathways in Group 4α, activation of mitogen activated kinase-like protein (MAPK) and fibroblast growth factor receptor 1 (FGFR1) signaling pathways in Group 4β, and activation of PI3K/AKT/mTOR and erb-b2 receptor tyrosine kinase 4 (ERBB4)-mediated nuclear signaling pathways in Group 4γ [36].

It is of relevance to underscore that in 2010, Gibson and colleagues demonstrated that the distinct subgroups of MB have different developmental origins, discovering that some WNT MBs were arisen from the cells in the dorsal brainstem [23]. Later, Grammel and colleagues discovered that some of the SHH MBs arise from the granule neuron precursors of the cochlear nuclei of the brainstem [39].

Two independent studies also reported two different cells of origin for Group 3 MB, with stem cell characteristics [40,41]. At last, several cell types were shown to be able to give rise the Group 4 tumors [26]. What all of these cells of origin have in common are the stem cell properties, and it is relevant to take into account that the majority of MB cells have a stem-like appearance [26].

5. Medulloblastoma Stem Cells (MBSCs)

The cancer stem cell (CSC) hypothesis explains the existence of a small fraction of tumor cells that have stem properties and the ability to proliferate and maintain the tumor growth [42]. These cells are characterized by two main properties, self-renewal and differentiation capacity, the self-renewal being the key property regulating the oncogenic potential, so that tumorigenesis is an effect that is derived by a deregulation of this process [43]. In the last years the presence of CSC has been described in different hematopoietic and solid-tumors, including MB [44]. These MBSCs are characterized by high levels of expression of CD133, Sox2, Musashi1, and Bmi1, which are all neural stem cell (NSC) genes [45]. As it occurs with CSCs, the MBSCs are considered responsible for therapeutic resistance and tumor recurrence [26], which is common in these tumors. Therefore, it would be necessary to develop targeted therapies against these MBSCs, in order to avoid tumor resistance and recurrence. Different studies have been focused on targeting different signaling pathways that are implicated in MBSCs, such as the SHH, PI3K/AKT/mTOR, Stat3, and Notch signaling pathways [26].

6. mTOR in Cancer

The activation of the mTOR pathway plays a key role in the development of several cancer types because of its importance in controlling cell growth and metabolism [1]. Aberrant mTOR activation can occur through oncogene stimulation or the loss of tumor suppressors [46]. Although the constitutive activation of the mTOR gene can occur, mutations in downstream and upstream components of both mTORC1 and mTORC2 [46] are more frequent, and these mutations are responsible for inducing cancer cell growth, survival, and proliferation [1].

The PI3K/AKT signaling pathway is found to be deregulated through a variety of mechanisms in many human cancers [1]. Mutations in different components produce constitutive activation of this signaling pathway, leading to a disturbance between the cell proliferation and apoptosis [47]. For instance, PIK3CA amplifications/mutations, AKT overexpression, and PTEN loss have been described in breast [48] or colorectal cancer [49].

Downstream of mTORC1, the overexpression of S6K1, 4EBP1, and eIF4E has been associated to cellular transformation [46]. eIF4E overexpression occurs in different human tumors, like breast, head and neck, colon, prostate, bladder, cervix, and lung cancer, enabling the selectable translation of some mRNAs that encode key proteins for cellular transformation [50]. Additionally, the loss of p53, a common event in cancer [1], negatively regulates some of the downstream targets of mTORC1, such as autophagy [51]. Thus, the function of the mTOR pathway in cancer development makes it interesting for targeted therapy in different tumors.

7. mTOR in Medulloblastoma

During brain development, the mTOR-mediated signaling pathway masters the differentiation of neurons and glia, as well as the maintenance of the stemness of NSCs [14]. In the expansion phase of CGNPs in the cerebellum, SHH and IGF are required [16], and it has been suggested that the activation of both pathways in CGNPs could interact and enhance tumor formation in the cerebellum [52–54]. Following this hypothesis, Rao and colleagues discovered that, in mice, the SHH induced tumor formation increases significantly when IGF-II is co-expresed, but no tumor formation was observed in the mice that were injected with IGF-II alone [53].

IGF positively regulates the mTOR pathway, which is frequently activated in malignant brain tumors, including MB [55]. Such an activation promotes the upregulation of protein translation by inhibition of 4E-BP1, through mTORC1 mediated phosphorylation [56]. Besides, a growing body of evidence points to the SHH signaling pathway as being the responsible for promoting the activity of mTORC1/4E-BP1-dependent translation and enhance tumor formation [6,57]. This evidence suggests that IGF-II, and therefore, the mTORC1/4E-BP1 pathway is a downstream transcriptional target of SHH, being critical in the SHH-mediated MB [58].

As a result of its role in the canonical SHH signaling pathway, mTORC1 seems to be a potentially important molecular target for treating SHH MBs [57]. However, the SHH signaling pathway also interacts with additional signaling pathways to promote MB growth and to induce treatment resistance. For instance, the Hippo pathway plays an important role in the control of organ development, and cross-talks with this pathway have been described [59].

Regarding the role of the PI3K/AKT/mTOR signaling pathway, its activation occurs in subgroup 4γ, the most prevalent subtype [36]. Moreover, Frasson et al. reported that the PI3K inhibition induces dramatic morphological changes and promotes apoptosis in DAOY human MB cells [60]. All of these data together suggest that targeting mTOR could be a potential therapeutic strategy for SHH-driven and Group 4 MBs. However, no relation between mTOR and the WNT or Group 3 MB subgroups has been described yet.

8. mTOR Signaling Pathway in MBSCs

Like all CSCs, the MBSCs possess the ability of self-renewal and differentiation, increasing the oncogenic potential of the heterogeneous tumor [61]. The transcription factors octamer-binding transcription factor 4 (OCT4), Nanog homeobox (NANOG), and SRY-box 2 (SOX2) are essential to maintain the pluripotency and self-renewal in embryonic stem cells and CSCs [14,62]. In addition to the expression of these transcription factors, one of the leading pathways that are involved in the regulation of embryonic stem cell differentiation and resistance of CSCs to therapy is the PI3K/AKT/mTOR signaling pathway [60]. This signaling pathway plays an essential role in the maintenance and survival of the CSCs by regulating multiple apoptosis-related proteins [61] and controlling the cell cycle progression [55]. Therefore, mTOR-mediated intracellular signaling is tightly regulated in the stem cells and it is considered one of the key modulators of the stemness in different stem cell populations [62]. Besides, it has been demonstrated that when inhibiting the mTOR signaling pathway, the CSC properties are reduced and the invasion potential is restrained in some of the cancer types [63].

The fact that PI3K inhibition has a heavy impact on the cell number of primary MB cells has already been demonstrated [60]. Following the hypothesis that stem cells could be the preferential target of PI3K/AKT inhibition, Frasson and colleagues showed that such inhibition indeed targets the CD133 positive cell fraction, reducing the number of the MBSC pool [60]. Furthermore, Hambardzumyan and colleagues discovered that the PI3K/AKT inhibitor, perifosine, increases the sensitivity to radiation-induced apoptosis in Nestin positive MBSCs [64]. Additionally, the PI3K/AKT axis is able to enhance the intracellular SHH signaling in CGNPs [65]. Different studies support the idea that the SHH signaling is also important in the regulation of CSC [66,67]. Ahlfeld and colleagues described that the constitutive activation of SHH signaling results in a significantly augmented expression of Sox2 that induces the cellular growth and proliferation of SHH MBs [68]. Therefore, targeting CSCs by the inhibition of mTOR or SHH may improve the outcome of patients with MB.

9. Targeted Therapy

As mentioned above, the current therapy is not enough to cure all of the MB patients, and the high doses of chemotherapy and radiotherapy that are needed induce severe side effects. This is the reason that recent investigations are directed toward improving targeted therapy in MB subgroups. There are two main objectives; on the one hand, to discover new drugs, and on the other hand, to optimize the doses of the drugs that are usually used. One consideration to be taken into account in MB treatment, as it occurs in all brain tumors, is that the drug must be able to cross the blood-brain barrier, which makes the development of new therapeutic agents difficult.

9.1. Targeting WNT Medulloblastomas

The WNT MBs present a good rate of cure compared with the other subgroups, since the WNT activation increases the tumor's radiosensitivity [69]. That is the reason that there are relatively few drugs that have been developed to target this signaling pathway. The current clinical trials are focused on the refinement of the standard treatment, with the objective of reducing the doses of chemotherapy and radiotherapy to decrease the neurotoxic side effects that are related to the treatment [27].

Two specific therapies have been developed to target the WNT MBs. The first one, norcantharidin, has been shown to block the WNT signaling pathway, impairing the growth of the MB [70]. The second one, lithium chloride, inhibits the GSK3β stabilizing β-catenin and reduces the MB growth [71].

9.2. Targeting SHH Medulloblastomas

Many specific treatments for SHH MB have been developed. Almost all of these treatments are focused on inhibiting SMO, a G protein type receptor that is implicated in the SHH signaling pathway. These treatments are based on the structure of cyclopamine, a naturally occurring plant alkaloid, the first SHH pathway inhibitor that was discovered with an anticancer effect. Cyclopamine inhibits the SMO protein, binding to its transmembrane domain and avoiding its change of conformation to the active form. However, cyclopamine has failed in clinical development, mainly because of its pharmacokinetic characteristics [26]. Therefore, research is focused on the development of new small molecules based on this compound, but with improved pharmacokinetic properties. Several small molecules have been developed, like vismodegib (GDC-0449), saridegib (IPI-926), erismodegib (LDE-225), TAK-441, XL-139 (BMS-833923), PF-04449913, and PF-5274857 [26].

The most studied of all of these analogs is vismodegib, the first food and drug administration (FDA)-approved drug as a SHH signaling inhibitor for advanced and metastatic basal cell carcinoma [72]. The patients with SHH-driven MB that were treated with vismodegib had a remarkable response and tumor size regression [73]. However, as vismodegib is a SMO inhibitor, it is not an effective treatment for the patients harboring genetic aberrations in genes downstream SMO, such as SUFU or GLI2 [74]. Furthermore, a number of patients that were treated with vismodegib acquired drug resistance because of a point mutation in SMO, the D473H mutation. This mutation would not prevent the activation of the SHH signaling pathway, but it would disrupt the ability of vismodegib to bind to the SMO [75]. Thus, a therapy targeting GLI using bromo- and extra-terminal BET domain inhibitors may be an alternative and efficient treatment for patients with genetic aberrations in SUFU or GLI, as well as for the patients who acquire resistance to SMO inhibitors, since they modulate GLI expression downstream of SMO and SUFU [76]. Another method to target GLI is the use of arsenic compounds. They have been tested in vitro and in vivo as a treatment for SHH-driven cancers and they have showed promising results [77].

9.3. Targeting Group 3 and 4 Medulloblastomas

The lack of an altered signaling pathway responsible for initiating the tumor makes it difficult to develop a targeted therapy for these subgroups of MBs. Among other alterations, some Group 3 MBs are characterized with MYC overexpression [36,74]. Two FDA-approved drugs targeting MYC, pemetrexed and gemcitabine, were used in combination to treat mouse allografts and xenografts. As a result of the treatment, the tumor growth was decreased [78]. Additionally, BET bromodomaim proteins have also been demonstrated to inhibit MYC-regulated signaling pathways in different cancers. Therefore, targeting these proteins could also be a promising strategy to target this subgroup of MBs. Nevertheless, MYC overexpression is only found in 10–20% of the patients in subgroup 3 [79].

9.4. Targeting the mTOR Pathway

As a result of the importance of the PI3K/AKT/mTOR pathway in cancer progression, targeting this signaling pathway has become one of the most studied strategies. Rapamycin is the first mTOR inhibitor that has been used in anti-cancer therapy. This compound is an antifungal agent that binds to FK506 Binding Protein 12 (FKBP12), forming a complex that allosterically inhibits the FKB12-Rapamycin Binding (FRB) domain of mTORC1, leading to the dissociation of Raptor from mTORC1 [80]. As rapamycin inhibits the mTORC1 complex, it also inhibits the protein translation and synthesis, and it induces cell cycle arrest in the G1 phase [10]. Even if rapamycin is not able to inhibit mTORC2, it can affect the mTORC2 complex indirectly [10,55]. However, poor solubility and unpredictable pharmacokinetic profiles of rapamycin have led to the development of rapamycin derivatives (rapalogs), new compounds based on the structure of rapamycin, but with improved pharmacological properties. These compounds have been tested and are approved for use in the treatment of different solid tumors [81–99] (Table 2).

Table 2. Mechanistic target of rapamycin (mTOR) inhibitors used in the clinic.

Types of mTOR Inhibitors	Name	Target	Disease	Trial Phase
Rapalogs	Temsirolimus	mTOR	RCC and MCL	Completed phase III
	Everolimus	mTOR	RCC, PNET, Lung, GEP, NET, Gastric, BC, mRCC	Completed phase III
	Ridaforolimus	mTOR	Sarcoma	Completed phase III
Second-generation mTOR inhibitors	BEZ235	PI3K/mTOR	BC, RCC, Endometrial, PNET	Discontinued
	GSK2126458	PI3K/mTOR	Colon/Rectum, RCC, BC, Endometrial, Melanoma, Ovary/Primary Peritoneal, Pancreas, Prostate	Phase I
	Gedatolisib (PF-04691502; PKI-587)	PI3K/mTOR	SCLC, Ovarian, Endometrial, Renal, Colorectal, Glioblastoma	Phase I
	Apitolisib (GDC-0980)	PI3K/mTOR	MPM, Colorectal, GIST, Sarcoma, BC	Phase I
Third-generation mTOR inhibitors	Rapalink-1	mTOR (mutant forms too)	Glioblastoma	No clinical data

mRRC—metastatic renal cell carcinoma; MCL—mantle cell lymphoma; PNET—pancreatic neuroendocrine tumor; GEP—gastro-entero-pancreatic; NET—neuroendocrine tumor; BC—breast cancer; SCLC—small cell lung cancer; MPM—malignant, pleural mesothelioma; GIST—gastrointestinal stromal tumor.

Some of these rapalogs have also been tested in MB, demonstrating promising results and leading to three clinical trials in phase I. These compounds are temsirolimus, sirolimus, and tesirolimus, in combination with perifpsine, an AKT inhibitor [55].

The PI3K/AKT/mTOR signaling pathway is primarily involved in SHH MBs. In these types of tumors, not only the mutations in the SMO receptor or the aberrant activation of the SHH pathway are the cause of MB initiation; an increased activation of the PI3K signaling or the alternative activation of the RAS-MAPK pathway could also eventually cause drug resistance [100]. Thus, combining SMO and PI3K/AKT/mTOR inhibitors may be a strategy to overcome resistance development.

Finally, it has been shown that the PI3K/AKT/mTOR signaling pathway is implicated in CSCs, and specifically in MBSCs, demonstrating that the inhibition of this signaling pathway reduces the MBSC population in the primary tumor culture [60]. Therefore, inhibiting mTOR may be a potential treatment to target the MBSCs, thus reducing the chances of tumor recurrence and therapy resistance (Figure 3).

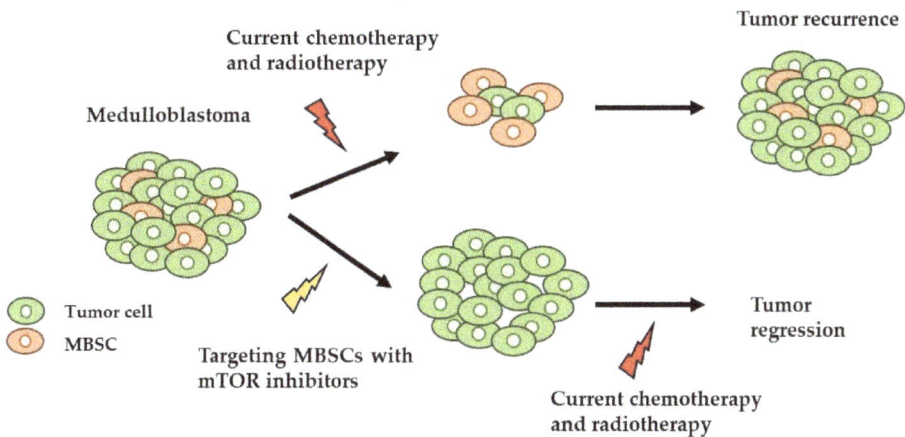

Figure 3. Schematic representation of a possible new approach to target medulloblastoma stem cells (MBSCs)s and MB. Medulloblastoma has an intracellular heterogeneity, having different cell types, such as normal tumor cells and MBSCs. With the classic treatment, the elimination of normal tumor cells is achieved, and the surviving MBSCs can form the tumor again. With the proposed new approach, the MBSCs are eliminated using mTOR inhibitors and the tumor cells are eliminated using the conventional therapy, achieving total tumor regression.

10. Concluding Remarks

MB is the most common malignant solid tumor in childhood, and even if the current therapies have improved the overall survival, the side effects that they generate are devastating for children. Improved knowledge of MB has given rise to a new and detailed classification of the subgroups of MB, which may lead, in the future, to a better stratification of the patients, based on the molecular characteristics of their tumor, moving towards a personalized therapy for each patient. To reach this goal, a deeper molecular profiling of each tumor is needed after the biopsy or surgery. Together with the new classification, new signaling pathways that are implicated in different subgroups of MB, have been identified. Signaling pathways such as the SHH or WNT signaling pathways, as well as PI3K/AKT/mTOR are therapeutic targets in MB.

mTOR is a master signaling pathway that regulates organismal growth and homeostasis, as a result of its implication in protein and lipid synthesis, and in the control of the cell cycle and the cellular metabolism. Different studies have shown that it is also necessary in cerebellar development and stem cell pluripotency maintenance. Being an essential protein in the homeostasis of the cells, when it is deregulated, it is implicated in different tumors, including MB. Furthermore, it has a decisive role in MBSCs, which is demonstrated by the fact that when the PI3K/AKT/mTOR signaling pathway is inhibited, the number of MBSCs decreases.

In this review we describe the targeting of mTOR as a promising therapeutic approach, mainly, but not only, for SHH-driven MB patients. Moreover, the combination of this approach with the current therapies could be a promising strategy, as the mTOR inhibition impairs the growth of MBSCs and increases the sensitivity to radiation-induced apoptosis in Nestin positive MBSCs, decreasing the possibility of tumor recurrence and therapy resistance (Figure 3).

Author Contributions: J.A., A.O., A.M. and I.G. contributed to the literature research of the topic, writing individual sections. J.A. and I.G. performed the proofreading of the final manuscript. I.G. and J.A. designed the figures. J.A. constructed all figures. J.A., A.O., A.M. and I.G. prepared the final manuscript.

Acknowledgments: J.A. is recipient of a predoctoral fellowship from the Department of Education of the Basque Government. This work was supported by grants from the Department of Industry of the Basque Government (SAIO13-PC13BN011), and the European Regional Developmental Fund, Institute of Health Carlos III (ISCIII) (PI16/01730) to I.G.

Conflicts of Interest: The authors declare no conflict of interest.

References

1. Laplante, M.; Sabatini, D.M. Mtor signaling in growth control and disease. *Cell* **2012**, *149*, 274–293. [CrossRef] [PubMed]
2. Chung, J.; Grammer, T.C.; Lemon, K.P.; Kazlauskas, A.; Blenis, J. Pdgf- and insulin-dependent pp70s6k activation mediated by phosphatidylinositol-3-OH kinase. *Nature* **1994**, *370*, 71–75. [CrossRef] [PubMed]
3. Chen, J.; Long, F. Mtor signaling in skeletal development and disease. *Bone Res.* **2018**, *6*, 1. [CrossRef] [PubMed]
4. Guertin, D.A.; Sabatini, D.M. Defining the role of mtor in cancer. *Cancer Cell* **2007**, *12*, 9–22. [CrossRef] [PubMed]
5. Oh, W.J.; Jacinto, E. Mtor complex 2 signaling and functions. *Cell Cycle* **2011**, *10*, 2305–2316. [CrossRef] [PubMed]
6. Pocza, T.; Sebestyen, A.; Turanyi, E.; Krenacs, T.; Mark, A.; Sticz, T.B.; Jakab, Z.; Hauser, P. Mtor pathway as a potential target in a subset of human medulloblastoma. *Pathol. Oncol. Res.* **2014**, *20*, 893–900. [CrossRef] [PubMed]
7. Ma, X.M.; Blenis, J. Molecular mechanisms of mtor-mediated translational control. *Nat. Rev. Mol. Cell Biol.* **2009**, *10*, 307–318. [CrossRef] [PubMed]
8. Julien, L.A.; Carriere, A.; Moreau, J.; Roux, P.P. Mtorc1-activated s6k1 phosphorylates rictor on threonine 1135 and regulates mtorc2 signaling. *Mol. Cell. Biol.* **2010**, *30*, 908–921. [CrossRef] [PubMed]
9. Bockaert, J.; Marin, P. Mtor in brain physiology and pathologies. *Physiol. Rev.* **2015**, *95*, 1157–1187. [CrossRef] [PubMed]
10. Sarbassov, D.D.; Ali, S.M.; Sengupta, S.; Sheen, J.H.; Hsu, P.P.; Bagley, A.F.; Markhard, A.L.; Sabatini, D.M. Prolonged rapamycin treatment inhibits mtorc2 assembly and akt/pkb. *Mol. Cell* **2006**, *22*, 159–168. [CrossRef] [PubMed]
11. Takei, N.; Nawa, H. Mtor signaling and its roles in normal and abnormal brain development. *Front. Mol. Neurosci.* **2014**, *7*, 28. [CrossRef] [PubMed]
12. Murakami, M.; Ichisaka, T.; Maeda, M.; Oshiro, N.; Hara, K.; Edenhofer, F.; Kiyama, H.; Yonezawa, K.; Yamanaka, S. Mtor is essential for growth and proliferation in early mouse embryos and embryonic stem cells. *Mol. Cell. Biol.* **2004**, *24*, 6710–6718. [CrossRef] [PubMed]
13. Hentges, K.E.; Sirry, B.; Gingeras, A.C.; Sarbassov, D.; Sonenberg, N.; Sabatini, D.; Peterson, A.S. Frap/mtor is required for proliferation and patterning during embryonic development in the mouse. *Proc. Natl. Acad. Sci. USA* **2001**, *98*, 13796–13801. [CrossRef] [PubMed]
14. Lee, D.Y. Roles of mtor signaling in brain development. *Exp. Neurobiol.* **2015**, *24*, 177–185. [CrossRef] [PubMed]
15. Wang, L.; Zhou, K.; Fu, Z.; Yu, D.; Huang, H.; Zang, X.; Mo, X. Brain development and akt signaling: The crossroads of signaling pathway and neurodevelopmental diseases. *J. Mol. Neurosci.* **2017**, *61*, 379–384. [CrossRef] [PubMed]
16. Mainwaring, L.A.; Kenney, A.M. Divergent functions for eif4e and s6 kinase by sonic hedgehog mitogenic signaling in the developing cerebellum. *Oncogene* **2011**, *30*, 1784–1797. [CrossRef] [PubMed]
17. Bartlett, F.; Kortmann, R.; Saran, F. Medulloblastoma. *Clin. Oncol.* **2013**, *25*, 36–45. [CrossRef] [PubMed]
18. Louis, D.N.; Perry, A.; Reifenberger, G.; von Deimling, A.; Figarella-Branger, D.; Cavenee, W.K.; Ohgaki, H.; Wiestler, O.D.; Kleihues, P.; Ellison, D.W. The 2016 world health organization classification of tumors of the central nervous system: A summary. *Acta Neuropathol.* **2016**, *131*, 803–820. [CrossRef] [PubMed]
19. Butts, T.; Green, M.J.; Wingate, R.J. Development of the cerebellum: Simple steps to make a 'little brain'. *Development* **2014**, *141*, 4031–4041. [CrossRef] [PubMed]
20. Wechsler-Reya, R.; Scott, M.P. The developmental biology of brain tumors. *Annu. Rev. Neurosci.* **2001**, *24*, 385–428. [CrossRef] [PubMed]

21. Haegele, L.; Ingold, B.; Naumann, H.; Tabatabai, G.; Ledermann, B.; Brandner, S. Wnt signalling inhibits neural differentiation of embryonic stem cells by controlling bone morphogenetic protein expression. *Mol. Cell. Neurosci.* **2003**, *24*, 696–708. [CrossRef]

22. Grimmer, M.R.; Weiss, W.A. Childhood tumors of the nervous system as disorders of normal development. *Curr. Opin. Pediatr.* **2006**, *18*, 634–638. [CrossRef] [PubMed]

23. Gibson, P.; Tong, Y.; Robinson, G.; Thompson, M.C.; Currle, D.S.; Eden, C.; Kranenburg, T.A.; Hogg, T.; Poppleton, H.; Martin, J.; et al. Subtypes of medulloblastoma have distinct developmental origins. *Nature* **2010**, *468*, 1095–1099. [CrossRef] [PubMed]

24. Goodrich, L.V.; Milenkovic, L.; Higgins, K.M.; Scott, M.P. Altered neural cell fates and medulloblastoma in mouse patched mutants. *Science* **1997**, *277*, 1109–1113. [CrossRef] [PubMed]

25. Dey, J.; Ditzler, S.; Knoblaugh, S.E.; Hatton, B.A.; Schelter, J.M.; Cleary, M.A.; Mecham, B.; Rorke-Adams, L.B.; Olson, J.M. A distinct smoothened mutation causes severe cerebellar developmental defects and medulloblastoma in a novel transgenic mouse model. *Mol. Cell. Biol.* **2012**, *32*, 4104–4115. [CrossRef] [PubMed]

26. Kumar, V.; Kumar, V.; McGuire, T.; Coulter, D.W.; Sharp, J.G.; Mahato, R.I. Challenges and recent advances in medulloblastoma therapy. *Trends Pharmacol. Sci.* **2017**, *38*, 1061–1084. [CrossRef] [PubMed]

27. Coluccia, D.; Figueiredo, C.; Isik, S.; Smith, C.; Rutka, J.T. Medulloblastoma: Tumor biology and relevance to treatment and prognosis paradigm. *Curr. Neurol. Neurosci. Rep.* **2016**, *16*, 43. [CrossRef] [PubMed]

28. Saury, J.M.; Emanuelson, I. Cognitive consequences of the treatment of medulloblastoma among children. *Pediatr. Neurol.* **2011**, *44*, 21–30. [CrossRef] [PubMed]

29. Musial-Bright, L.; Fengler, R.; Henze, G.; Hernaiz Driever, P. Carboplatin and ototoxicity: Hearing loss rates among survivors of childhood medulloblastoma. *Childs Nerv. Syst.* **2011**, *27*, 407–413. [CrossRef] [PubMed]

30. Kadota, R.P.; Mahoney, D.H.; Doyle, J.; Duerst, R.; Friedman, H.; Holmes, E.; Kun, L.; Zhou, T.; Pollack, I.F. Dose intensive melphalan and cyclophosphamide with autologous hematopoietic stem cells for recurrent medulloblastoma or germinoma. *Pediatr. Blood Cancer* **2008**, *51*, 675–678. [CrossRef] [PubMed]

31. Park, T.S.; Hoffman, H.J.; Hendrick, E.B.; Humphreys, R.P.; Becker, L.E. Medulloblastoma: Clinical presentation and management. Experience at the hospital for sick children, Toronto, 1950–1980. *J. Neurosurg.* **1983**, *58*, 543–552. [CrossRef] [PubMed]

32. Rochkind, S.; Blatt, I.; Sadeh, M.; Goldhammer, Y. Extracranial metastases of medulloblastoma in adults: Literature review. *J. Neurol. Neurosurg. Psychiatry* **1991**, *54*, 80–86. [CrossRef] [PubMed]

33. Louis, D.N.; Ohgaki, H.; Wiestler, O.D.; Cavenee, W.K.; Burger, P.C.; Jouvet, A.; Scheithauer, B.W.; Kleihues, P. The 2007 who classification of tumours of the central nervous system. *Acta Neuropathol.* **2007**, *114*, 97–109. [CrossRef] [PubMed]

34. Northcott, P.A.; Korshunov, A.; Witt, H.; Hielscher, T.; Eberhart, C.G.; Mack, S.; Bouffet, E.; Clifford, S.C.; Hawkins, C.E.; French, P.; et al. Medulloblastoma comprises four distinct molecular variants. *J. Clin. Oncol.* **2011**, *29*, 1408–1414. [CrossRef] [PubMed]

35. Taylor, M.D.; Northcott, P.A.; Korshunov, A.; Remke, M.; Cho, Y.J.; Clifford, S.C.; Eberhart, C.G.; Parsons, D.W.; Rutkowski, S.; Gajjar, A.; et al. Molecular subgroups of medulloblastoma: The current consensus. *Acta Neuropathol.* **2012**, *123*, 465–472. [CrossRef] [PubMed]

36. Cavalli, F.M.G.; Remke, M.; Rampasek, L.; Peacock, J.; Shih, D.J.H.; Luu, B.; Garzia, L.; Torchia, J.; Nor, C.; Morrissy, A.S.; et al. Intertumoral heterogeneity within medulloblastoma subgroups. *Cancer Cell* **2017**, *31*, 737–754.e6. [CrossRef] [PubMed]

37. Clifford, S.C.; Lusher, M.E.; Lindsey, J.C.; Langdon, J.A.; Gilbertson, R.J.; Straughton, D.; Ellison, D.W. Wnt/wingless pathway activation and chromosome 6 loss characterize a distinct molecular sub-group of medulloblastomas associated with a favorable prognosis. *Cell Cycle* **2006**, *5*, 2666–2670. [CrossRef] [PubMed]

38. Jiang, T.; Zhang, Y.; Wang, J.; Du, J.; Raynald; Qiu, X.; Wang, Y.; Li, C. A retrospective study of progression-free and overall survival in pediatric medulloblastoma based on molecular subgroup classification: A single-institution experience. *Front. Neurol.* **2017**, *8*, 198. [CrossRef] [PubMed]

39. Grammel, D.; Warmuth-Metz, M.; von Bueren, A.O.; Kool, M.; Pietsch, T.; Kretzschmar, H.A.; Rowitch, D.H.; Rutkowski, S.; Pfister, S.M.; Schuller, U. Sonic hedgehog-associated medulloblastoma arising from the cochlear nuclei of the brainstem. *Acta Neuropathol.* **2012**, *123*, 601–614. [CrossRef] [PubMed]

40. Pei, Y.; Moore, C.E.; Wang, J.; Tewari, A.K.; Eroshkin, A.; Cho, Y.J.; Witt, H.; Korshunov, A.; Read, T.A.; Sun, J.L.; et al. An animal model of myc-driven medulloblastoma. *Cancer Cell* **2012**, *21*, 155–167. [CrossRef] [PubMed]
41. Kawauchi, D.; Robinson, G.; Uziel, T.; Gibson, P.; Rehg, J.; Gao, C.; Finkelstein, D.; Qu, C.; Pounds, S.; Ellison, D.W.; et al. A mouse model of the most aggressive subgroup of human medulloblastoma. *Cancer Cell* **2012**, *21*, 168–180. [CrossRef] [PubMed]
42. Clarke, M.F.; Dick, J.E.; Dirks, P.B.; Eaves, C.J.; Jamieson, C.H.; Jones, D.L.; Visvader, J.; Weissman, I.L.; Wahl, G.M. Cancer stem cells—Perspectives on current status and future directions: Aacr workshop on cancer stem cells. *Cancer Res.* **2006**, *66*, 9339–9344. [CrossRef] [PubMed]
43. Manoranjan, B.; Venugopal, C.; McFarlane, N.; Doble, B.W.; Dunn, S.E.; Scheinemann, K.; Singh, S.K. Medulloblastoma stem cells: Where development and cancer cross pathways. *Pediatr. Res.* **2012**, *71*, 516–522. [CrossRef] [PubMed]
44. Singh, S.K.; Clarke, I.D.; Terasaki, M.; Bonn, V.E.; Hawkins, C.; Squire, J.; Dirks, P.B. Identification of a cancer stem cell in human brain tumors. *Cancer Res.* **2003**, *63*, 5821–5828. [PubMed]
45. Hemmati, H.D.; Nakano, I.; Lazareff, J.A.; Masterman-Smith, M.; Geschwind, D.H.; Bronner-Fraser, M.; Kornblum, H.I. Cancerous stem cells can arise from pediatric brain tumors. *Proc. Natl. Acad. Sci. USA* **2003**, *100*, 15178–15183. [CrossRef] [PubMed]
46. Populo, H.; Lopes, J.M.; Soares, P. The mtor signalling pathway in human cancer. *Int. J. Mol. Sci.* **2012**, *13*, 1886–1918. [CrossRef] [PubMed]
47. Osaki, M.; Oshimura, M.; Ito, H. Pi3k-akt pathway: Its functions and alterations in human cancer. *Apoptosis* **2004**, *9*, 667–676. [CrossRef] [PubMed]
48. Stemke-Hale, K.; Gonzalez-Angulo, A.M.; Lluch, A.; Neve, R.M.; Kuo, W.L.; Davies, M.; Carey, M.; Hu, Z.; Guan, Y.; Sahin, A.; et al. An integrative genomic and proteomic analysis of pik3ca, pten, and akt mutations in breast cancer. *Cancer Res.* **2008**, *68*, 6084–6091. [CrossRef] [PubMed]
49. Danielsen, S.A.; Eide, P.W.; Nesbakken, A.; Guren, T.; Leithe, E.; Lothe, R.A. Portrait of the pi3k/akt pathway in colorectal cancer. *Biochim. Biophys. Acta* **2015**, *1855*, 104–121. [CrossRef] [PubMed]
50. De Benedetti, A.; Graff, J.R. Eif-4e expression and its role in malignancies and metastases. *Oncogene* **2004**, *23*, 3189–3199. [CrossRef] [PubMed]
51. Feng, Z.; Zhang, H.; Levine, A.J.; Jin, S. The coordinate regulation of the p53 and mtor pathways in cells. *Proc. Natl. Acad. Sci. USA* **2005**, *102*, 8204–8209. [CrossRef] [PubMed]
52. Parathath, S.R.; Mainwaring, L.A.; Fernandez, L.A.; Campbell, D.O.; Kenney, A.M. Insulin receptor substrate 1 is an effector of sonic hedgehog mitogenic signaling in cerebellar neural precursors. *Development* **2008**, *135*, 3291–3300. [CrossRef] [PubMed]
53. Rao, G.; Pedone, C.A.; Del Valle, L.; Reiss, K.; Holland, E.C.; Fults, D.W. Sonic hedgehog and insulin-like growth factor signaling synergize to induce medulloblastoma formation from nestin-expressing neural progenitors in mice. *Oncogene* **2004**, *23*, 6156–6162. [CrossRef] [PubMed]
54. Malaguarnera, R.; Belfiore, A. The emerging role of insulin and insulin-like growth factor signaling in cancer stem cells. *Front. Endocrinol.* **2014**, *5*, 10. [CrossRef] [PubMed]
55. Dimitrova, V.; Arcaro, A. Targeting the pi3k/akt/mtor signaling pathway in medulloblastoma. *Curr. Mol. Med.* **2015**, *15*, 82–93. [CrossRef] [PubMed]
56. Truitt, M.L.; Ruggero, D. New frontiers in translational control of the cancer genome. *Nat. Rev. Cancer* **2016**, *16*, 288–304. [CrossRef] [PubMed]
57. Wu, C.C.; Hou, S.; Orr, B.A.; Kuo, B.R.; Youn, Y.H.; Ong, T.; Roth, F.; Eberhart, C.G.; Robinson, G.W.; Solecki, D.J.; et al. Mtorc1-mediated inhibition of 4ebp1 is essential for hedgehog signaling-driven translation and medulloblastoma. *Dev. Cell* **2017**, *43*, 673–688. [CrossRef] [PubMed]
58. Hahn, H.; Wojnowski, L.; Specht, K.; Kappler, R.; Calzada-Wack, J.; Potter, D.; Zimmer, A.; Muller, U.; Samson, E.; Quintanilla-Martinez, L.; et al. Patched target igf2 is indispensable for the formation of medulloblastoma and rhabdomyosarcoma. *J. Biol. Chem.* **2000**, *275*, 28341–28344. [CrossRef] [PubMed]
59. MacDonald, T.J.; Aguilera, D.; Castellino, R.C. The rationale for targeted therapies in medulloblastoma. *Neuro-Oncology* **2014**, *16*, 9–20. [CrossRef] [PubMed]
60. Frasson, C.; Rampazzo, E.; Accordi, B.; Beggio, G.; Pistollato, F.; Basso, G.; Persano, L. Inhibition of pi3k signalling selectively affects medulloblastoma cancer stem cells. *Biomed. Res. Int.* **2015**, *2015*, 973912. [CrossRef] [PubMed]

61. Huang, G.H.; Xu, Q.F.; Cui, Y.H.; Li, N.; Bian, X.W.; Lv, S.Q. Medulloblastoma stem cells: Promising targets in medulloblastoma therapy. *Cancer Sci.* **2016**, *107*, 583–589. [CrossRef] [PubMed]

62. Boyer, L.A.; Lee, T.I.; Cole, M.F.; Johnstone, S.E.; Levine, S.S.; Zucker, J.P.; Guenther, M.G.; Kumar, R.M.; Murray, H.L.; Jenner, R.G.; et al. Core transcriptional regulatory circuitry in human embryonic stem cells. *Cell* **2005**, *122*, 947–956. [CrossRef] [PubMed]

63. Yang, C.; Zhang, Y.; Zhang, Y.; Zhang, Z.; Peng, J.; Li, Z.; Han, L.; You, Q.; Chen, X.; Rao, X.; et al. Downregulation of cancer stem cell properties via mtor signaling pathway inhibition by rapamycin in nasopharyngeal carcinoma. *Int. J. Oncol.* **2015**, *47*, 909–917. [CrossRef] [PubMed]

64. Hambardzumyan, D.; Becher, O.J.; Rosenblum, M.K.; Pandolfi, P.P.; Manova-Todorova, K.; Holland, E.C. Pi3k pathway regulates survival of cancer stem cells residing in the perivascular niche following radiation in medulloblastoma in vivo. *Genes Dev.* **2008**, *22*, 436–448. [CrossRef] [PubMed]

65. Kenney, A.M.; Widlund, H.R.; Rowitch, D.H. Hedgehog and pi-3 kinase signaling converge on nmyc1 to promote cell cycle progression in cerebellar neuronal precursors. *Development* **2004**, *131*, 217–228. [CrossRef] [PubMed]

66. Merchant, A.A.; Matsui, W. Targeting hedgehog—A cancer stem cell pathway. *Clin. Cancer Res.* **2010**, *16*, 3130–3140. [CrossRef] [PubMed]

67. Liu, S.; Dontu, G.; Mantle, I.D.; Patel, S.; Ahn, N.S.; Jackson, K.W.; Suri, P.; Wicha, M.S. Hedgehog signaling and bmi-1 regulate self-renewal of normal and malignant human mammary stem cells. *Cancer Res.* **2006**, *66*, 6063–6071. [CrossRef] [PubMed]

68. Ahlfeld, J.; Favaro, R.; Pagella, P.; Kretzschmar, H.A.; Nicolis, S.; Schuller, U. Sox2 requirement in sonic hedgehog-associated medulloblastoma. *Cancer Res.* **2013**, *73*, 3796–3807. [CrossRef] [PubMed]

69. Salaroli, R.; Ronchi, A.; Buttarelli, F.R.; Cortesi, F.; Marchese, V.; Della Bella, E.; Renna, C.; Baldi, C.; Giangaspero, F.; Cenacchi, G. Wnt activation affects proliferation, invasiveness and radiosensitivity in medulloblastoma. *J. Neurooncol.* **2015**, *121*, 119–127. [CrossRef] [PubMed]

70. Cimmino, F.; Scoppettuolo, M.N.; Carotenuto, M.; De Antonellis, P.; Dato, V.D.; De Vita, G.; Zollo, M. Norcantharidin impairs medulloblastoma growth by inhibition of wnt/beta-catenin signaling. *J. Neurooncol.* **2012**, *106*, 59–70. [CrossRef] [PubMed]

71. Zinke, J.; Schneider, F.T.; Harter, P.N.; Thom, S.; Ziegler, N.; Toftgard, R.; Plate, K.H.; Liebner, S. Beta-catenin-gli1 interaction regulates proliferation and tumor growth in medulloblastoma. *Mol. Cancer* **2015**, *14*, 17. [CrossRef] [PubMed]

72. Chang, A.B.; Oppenheimer, J.J.; Weinberger, M.; Rubin, B.K.; Irwin, R.S. Children with chronic wet or productive cough—Treatment and investigations: A systematic review. *Chest* **2016**, *149*, 120–142. [CrossRef] [PubMed]

73. Robinson, G.W.; Orr, B.A.; Wu, G.; Gururangan, S.; Lin, T.; Qaddoumi, I.; Packer, R.J.; Goldman, S.; Prados, M.D.; Desjardins, A.; et al. Vismodegib exerts targeted efficacy against recurrent sonic hedgehog-subgroup medulloblastoma: Results from phase ii pediatric brain tumor consortium studies pbtc-025b and pbtc-032. *J. Clin. Oncol.* **2015**, *33*, 2646–2654. [CrossRef] [PubMed]

74. Kool, M.; Jones, D.T.; Jager, N.; Northcott, P.A.; Pugh, T.J.; Hovestadt, V.; Piro, R.M.; Esparza, L.A.; Markant, S.L.; Remke, M.; et al. Genome sequencing of shh medulloblastoma predicts genotype-related response to smoothened inhibition. *Cancer Cell* **2014**, *25*, 393–405. [CrossRef] [PubMed]

75. Yauch, R.L.; Dijkgraaf, G.J.; Alicke, B.; Januario, T.; Ahn, C.P.; Holcomb, T.; Pujara, K.; Stinson, J.; Callahan, C.A.; Tang, T.; et al. Smoothened mutation confers resistance to a hedgehog pathway inhibitor in medulloblastoma. *Science* **2009**, *326*, 572–574. [CrossRef] [PubMed]

76. Tang, Y.; Gholamin, S.; Schubert, S.; Willardson, M.I.; Lee, A.; Bandopadhayay, P.; Bergthold, G.; Masoud, S.; Nguyen, B.; Vue, N.; et al. Epigenetic targeting of hedgehog pathway transcriptional output through bet bromodomain inhibition. *Nat. Med.* **2014**, *20*, 732–740. [CrossRef] [PubMed]

77. Beauchamp, E.M.; Ringer, L.; Bulut, G.; Sajwan, K.P.; Hall, M.D.; Lee, Y.C.; Peaceman, D.; Ozdemirli, M.; Rodriguez, O.; Macdonald, T.J.; et al. Arsenic trioxide inhibits human cancer cell growth and tumor development in mice by blocking hedgehog/gli pathway. *J. Clin. Investig.* **2011**, *121*, 148–160. [CrossRef] [PubMed]

78. Morfouace, M.; Shelat, A.; Jacus, M.; Freeman, B.B., 3rd; Turner, D.; Robinson, S.; Zindy, F.; Wang, Y.D.; Finkelstein, D.; Ayrault, O.; et al. Pemetrexed and gemcitabine as combination therapy for the treatment of group3 medulloblastoma. *Cancer Cell* **2014**, *25*, 516–529. [CrossRef] [PubMed]

79. Northcott, P.A.; Jones, D.T.; Kool, M.; Robinson, G.W.; Gilbertson, R.J.; Cho, Y.J.; Pomeroy, S.L.; Korshunov, A.; Lichter, P.; Taylor, M.D.; et al. Medulloblastomics: The end of the beginning. *Nat. Rev. Cancer* **2012**, *12*, 818–834. [CrossRef] [PubMed]

80. Conciatori, F.; Ciuffreda, L.; Bazzichetto, C.; Falcone, I.; Pilotto, S.; Bria, E.; Cognetti, F.; Milella, M. Mtor cross-talk in cancer and potential for combination therapy. *Cancers* **2018**, *10*, 23. [CrossRef] [PubMed]

81. Hudes, G.; Carducci, M.; Tomczak, P.; Dutcher, J.; Figlin, R.; Kapoor, A.; Staroslawska, E.; Sosman, J.; McDermott, D.; Bodrogi, I.; et al. Temsirolimus, interferon alfa, or both for advanced renal-cell carcinoma. *N. Engl. J. Med.* **2007**, *356*, 2271–2281. [CrossRef] [PubMed]

82. Hutson, T.E.; Escudier, B.; Esteban, E.; Bjarnason, G.A.; Lim, H.Y.; Pittman, K.B.; Senico, P.; Niethammer, A.; Lu, D.R.; Hariharan, S.; et al. Randomized phase iii trial of temsirolimus versus sorafenib as second-line therapy after sunitinib in patients with metastatic renal cell carcinoma. *J. Clin. Oncol.* **2014**, *32*, 760–767. [CrossRef] [PubMed]

83. Rini, B.I.; Bellmunt, J.; Clancy, J.; Wang, K.; Niethammer, A.G.; Hariharan, S.; Escudier, B. Randomized phase iii trial of temsirolimus and bevacizumab versus interferon alfa and bevacizumab in metastatic renal cell carcinoma: Intoract trial. *J. Clin. Oncol.* **2014**, *32*, 752–759. [CrossRef] [PubMed]

84. Hess, G.; Barlev, A.; Chung, K.; Hill, J.W.; Fonseca, E. Cost of palliative radiation to the bone for patients with bone metastases secondary to breast or prostate cancer. *Radiat. Oncol.* **2012**, *7*, 168. [CrossRef] [PubMed]

85. Motzer, R.J.; Escudier, B.; Oudard, S.; Hutson, T.E.; Porta, C.; Bracarda, S.; Grunwald, V.; Thompson, J.A.; Figlin, R.A.; Hollaender, N.; et al. Efficacy of everolimus in advanced renal cell carcinoma: A double-blind, randomised, placebo-controlled phase iii trial. *Lancet* **2008**, *372*, 449–456. [CrossRef]

86. Yao, J.C.; Shah, M.H.; Ito, T.; Bohas, C.L.; Wolin, E.M.; Van Cutsem, E.; Hobday, T.J.; Okusaka, T.; Capdevila, J.; de Vries, E.G.; et al. Everolimus for advanced pancreatic neuroendocrine tumors. *N. Engl. J. Med.* **2011**, *364*, 514–523. [CrossRef] [PubMed]

87. Pavel, M.E.; Hainsworth, J.D.; Baudin, E.; Peeters, M.; Horsch, D.; Winkler, R.E.; Klimovsky, J.; Lebwohl, D.; Jehl, V.; Wolin, E.M.; et al. Everolimus plus octreotide long-acting repeatable for the treatment of advanced neuroendocrine tumours associated with carcinoid syndrome (radiant-2): A randomised, placebo-controlled, phase 3 study. *Lancet* **2011**, *378*, 2005–2012. [CrossRef]

88. Ohtsu, A.; Ajani, J.A.; Bai, Y.X.; Bang, Y.J.; Chung, H.C.; Pan, H.M.; Sahmoud, T.; Shen, L.; Yeh, K.H.; Chin, K.; et al. Everolimus for previously treated advanced gastric cancer: Results of the randomized, double-blind, phase iii granite-1 study. *J. Clin. Oncol.* **2013**, *31*, 3935–3943. [CrossRef] [PubMed]

89. Baselga, J.; Campone, M.; Piccart, M.; Burris, H.A., 3rd; Rugo, H.S.; Sahmoud, T.; Noguchi, S.; Gnant, M.; Pritchard, K.I.; Lebrun, F.; et al. Everolimus in postmenopausal hormone-receptor-positive advanced breast cancer. *N. Engl. J. Med.* **2012**, *366*, 520–529. [CrossRef] [PubMed]

90. Andre, F.; O'Regan, R.; Ozguroglu, M.; Toi, M.; Xu, B.; Jerusalem, G.; Masuda, N.; Wilks, S.; Arena, F.; Isaacs, C.; et al. Everolimus for women with trastuzumab-resistant, her2-positive, advanced breast cancer (bolero-3): A randomised, double-blind, placebo-controlled phase 3 trial. *Lancet Oncol.* **2014**, *15*, 580–591. [CrossRef]

91. Wolff, A.C.; Lazar, A.A.; Bondarenko, I.; Garin, A.M.; Brincat, S.; Chow, L.; Sun, Y.; Neskovic-Konstantinovic, Z.; Guimaraes, R.C.; Fumoleau, P.; et al. Randomized phase iii placebo-controlled trial of letrozole plus oral temsirolimus as first-line endocrine therapy in postmenopausal women with locally advanced or metastatic breast cancer. *J. Clin. Oncol.* **2013**, *31*, 195–202. [CrossRef] [PubMed]

92. Motzer, R.J.; Hutson, T.E.; Glen, H.; Michaelson, M.D.; Molina, A.; Eisen, T.; Jassem, J.; Zolnierek, J.; Maroto, J.P.; Mellado, B.; et al. Lenvatinib, everolimus, and the combination in patients with metastatic renal cell carcinoma: A randomised, phase 2, open-label, multicentre trial. *Lancet Oncol.* **2015**, *16*, 1473–1482. [CrossRef]

93. Demetri, G.D.; Chawla, S.P.; Ray-Coquard, I.; Le Cesne, A.; Staddon, A.P.; Milhem, M.M.; Penel, N.; Riedel, R.F.; Bui-Nguyen, B.; Cranmer, L.D.; et al. Results of an international randomized phase iii trial of the mammalian target of rapamycin inhibitor ridaforolimus versus placebo to control metastatic sarcomas in patients after benefit from prior chemotherapy. *J. Clin. Oncol.* **2013**, *31*, 2485–2492. [CrossRef] [PubMed]

94. Bendell, J.C.; Kurkjian, C.; Infante, J.R.; Bauer, T.M.; Burris, H.A., 3rd; Greco, F.A.; Shih, K.C.; Thompson, D.S.; Lane, C.M.; Finney, L.H.; et al. A phase 1 study of the sachet formulation of the oral dual pi3k/mtor inhibitor bez235 given twice daily (bid) in patients with advanced solid tumors. *Investig. New Drugs* **2015**, *33*, 463–471. [CrossRef] [PubMed]

95. Munster, P.; Aggarwal, R.; Hong, D.; Schellens, J.H.; van der Noll, R.; Specht, J.; Witteveen, P.O.; Werner, T.L.; Dees, E.C.; Bergsland, E.; et al. First-in-human phase i study of gsk2126458, an oral pan-class i phosphatidylinositol-3-kinase inhibitor, in patients with advanced solid tumor malignancies. *Clin. Cancer Res.* **2016**, *22*, 1932–1939. [CrossRef] [PubMed]

96. Shapiro, G.I.; Bell-McGuinn, K.M.; Molina, J.R.; Bendell, J.; Spicer, J.; Kwak, E.L.; Pandya, S.S.; Millham, R.; Borzillo, G.; Pierce, K.J.; et al. First-in-human study of pf-05212384 (pki-587), a small-molecule, intravenous, dual inhibitor of pi3k and mtor in patients with advanced cancer. *Clin. Cancer Res.* **2015**, *21*, 1888–1895. [CrossRef] [PubMed]

97. Fan, Q.; Aksoy, O.; Wong, R.A.; Ilkhanizadeh, S.; Novotny, C.J.; Gustafson, W.C.; Truong, A.Y.; Cayanan, G.; Simonds, E.F.; Haas-Kogan, D.; et al. A kinase inhibitor targeted to mtorc1 drives regression in glioblastoma. *Cancer Cell* **2017**, *31*, 424–435. [CrossRef] [PubMed]

98. Yao, J.C.; Fazio, N.; Singh, S.; Buzzoni, R.; Carnaghi, C.; Wolin, E.; Tomasek, J.; Raderer, M.; Lahner, H.; Voi, M.; et al. Everolimus for the treatment of advanced, non-functional neuroendocrine tumours of the lung or gastrointestinal tract (radiant-4): A randomised, placebo-controlled, phase 3 study. *Lancet* **2016**, *387*, 968–977. [CrossRef]

99. Dolly, S.O.; Wagner, A.J.; Bendell, J.C.; Kindler, H.L.; Krug, L.M.; Seiwert, T.Y.; Zauderer, M.G.; Lolkema, M.P.; Apt, D.; Yeh, R.F.; et al. Phase i study of apitolisib (gdc-0980), dual phosphatidylinositol-3-kinase and mammalian target of rapamycin kinase inhibitor, in patients with advanced solid tumors. *Clin. Cancer Res.* **2016**, *22*, 2874–2884. [CrossRef] [PubMed]

100. Buonamici, S.; Williams, J.; Morrissey, M.; Wang, A.; Guo, R.; Vattay, A.; Hsiao, K.; Yuan, J.; Green, J.; Ospina, B.; et al. Interfering with resistance to smoothened antagonists by inhibition of the pi3k pathway in medulloblastoma. *Sci. Transl. Med.* **2010**, *2*, 51ra70. [CrossRef] [PubMed]

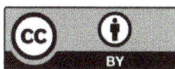

International Journal of
Molecular Sciences

MDPI

Review

Biological Aspects of mTOR in Leukemia

Simone Mirabilii [1], Maria Rosaria Ricciardi [1], Monica Piedimonte [1], Valentina Gianfelici [1], Maria Paola Bianchi [1] and Agostino Tafuri [1,2,*]

[1] Laboratory of Cell Kinetics and Applied Proteomics, Faculty of Medicine and Psychology, Department of Clinic and Molecular Medicine, Sapienza University of Rome, via Rovigo 1, 00161 Rome, Italy; simone.mirabilii@uniroma1.it (S.M.); mariarosaria.ricciardi@uniroma1.it (M.R.R.); monica.piedimonte@uniroma1.it (M.P.); gianfelici@bce.uniroma1.it (V.G.); mariapaolabianchi82@gmail.com (M.P.B.)

[2] Hematology, "Sant'Andrea" University Hospital, Sapienza University of Rome, via di Grottarossa 1035, 00189 Rome, Italy

* Correspondence: agostino.tafuri@uniroma1.it

Received: 17 July 2018; Accepted: 10 August 2018; Published: 14 August 2018

Abstract: The mammalian target of rapamycin (mTOR) is a central processor of intra- and extracellular signals, regulating many fundamental cellular processes such as metabolism, growth, proliferation, and survival. Strong evidences have indicated that mTOR dysregulation is deeply implicated in leukemogenesis. This has led to growing interest in the development of modulators of its activity for leukemia treatment. This review intends to provide an outline of the principal biological and molecular functions of mTOR. We summarize the current understanding of how mTOR interacts with microRNAs, with components of cell metabolism, and with controllers of apoptotic machinery. Lastly, from a clinical/translational perspective, we recapitulate the therapeutic results in leukemia, obtained by using mTOR inhibitors as single agents and in combination with other compounds.

Keywords: leukemia; cell signaling; metabolism; apoptosis; miRNA; mTOR inhibitors

1. mTOR Structure and Function

mTOR (also known as the mechanistic target of rapamycin) is a 289-kDa serine/threonine kinase belonging to the phosphatidylinositol kinase-related kinase (PIKK) family. Its COOH-terminal catalytic domain shows a very high homology to the phosphoinositide 3-kinase (PI3K) [1]. mTOR is structurally associated with other proteins forming two functionally distinct complexes, mTOR complex 1 (mTORC1) and mTOR complex 2 (mTORC2), characterized by a different response to rapamycin and its derivatives (rapalogs) [2,3]. mTORC1 includes mTOR, the regulatory-associated protein of mTOR (Raptor), the mammalian lethal with SEC13 protein 8 (mLST8), which stabilizes the kinase domain, and also the following inhibitory components: DEP domain-containing mTOR-interacting protein (Deptor), PRAS40 (proline-rich Akt substrate of 40 kDa), and FKBP38 (FK506-binding protein 38). mTORC1 is sensitive to rapamycin and its derivatives (Figure 1).

Similarly to mTORC1, mTORC2 also includes mTOR, mLST8, and Deptor, but contains the protein Rictor (Rapamycin-insensitive companion of mTOR) as a component, rather than Raptor. mTORC2 also associates with the mammalian stress-activated protein kinase interacting protein (mSIN1) and protein observed with Rictor-1 (Protor-1) (Figure 1).

Although rapamycin does not bind or directly inhibit mTORC2, it has been shown that prolonged treatment with rapamycin and its derivatives is able to abrogate mTORC2 signaling, probably due to the inability of mTOR linked to rapamycin to incorporate into new mTORC2 complexes [4,5]. mTORC1 and mTORC2 govern multiple cellular functions.

By integrating signals from the external environment with information on the metabolic status of the cell, mTORC1 controls the anabolic processes to promote protein synthesis and cell growth and inhibits autophagy [6]. Signal integration occurs at the level of the TSC1-TSC2 (tuberous sclerosis complex1-2) complex, the main inhibitor that is upstream of mTORC1. This complex acts as a molecular switch: during stress conditions, it suppresses mTOR activity thus limiting cell growth while it releases its inhibition under favorable conditions. TSC1 stabilizes TSC2, preventing its ubiquitin-mediated degradation.

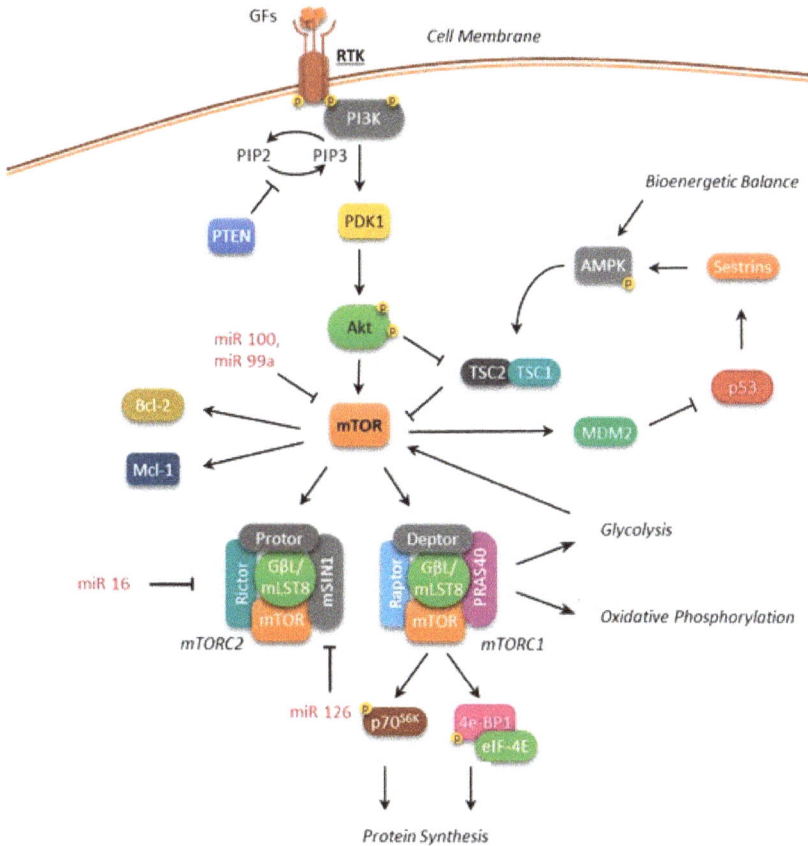

Figure 1. Overview of the mTOR regulation network. Arrows: positive interaction; T-bars: inhibition.

Activated mTORC1 phosphorylates "protein synthesis machine" components that include p70S6K (protein S6 kinase beta-1) and 4E-BP1 [eukaryotic translation initiation factor 4E (eIF4E)-binding protein 1]. Following activation, p70S6K enhances messenger RNA (mRNA) translation by phosphorylating the 40S ribosomal protein, S6. Conversely, phosphorylation of 4E-BP1 at multiple sites promotes its dissociation from eIF4E and allows the initiation of cap-dependent translation [7].

The mechanisms related to the regulation of mTORC2 activity remain poorly understood. It has been documented that mTORC2 controls the cell proliferation and survival, and the organization of the actin cytoskeleton [3,8]. In particular, it has been reported that one of the main functions of TORC2 is the rapamycin-insensitive cell cycle-dependent regulation of actin polymerization through the activation of Rho GTPase [9]. Moreover, the reported mTORC2-ribosome association suggests its role in protein synthesis [10] and in driving the oncogenic PI3K signaling in cancer [8]. In fact, compelling evidence has shown that aberrant activation of mTOR is associated with the development and progression of several types of cancers [11]. Recently, mTORC2 has emerged as an additional regulator of cellular and tumor metabolism, prompting further investigation.

2. mTOR Deregulation in Leukemias

There is increasing evidence that deregulation of the PI3K/Akt/mTORC1 signaling contributes to leukemogenesis. Increased mTORC1 and mTORC2 activity has been reported to play a critical role in leukemia initiation, propagation, and relapse [12–17]. Particularly, mTOR constitutive activation is frequently found in leukemia patients, contributing to chemoresistance, disease progression, and unfavorable outcomes.

In the view of mTOR functioning as a point of convergence between a nutrient-sensing pathway (via-mTORC1) and as a regulator of Akt itself (via-mTORC2), the definition of the role of mTOR in controlling cellular metabolism and energy homoeostasis in normal and cancer cells plays a fundamental role in developing effective therapies for leukemia treatment (Figure 1). Over the years, several small molecules that target the PI3K/Akt/mTOR signaling pathway have been investigated, showing potential therapeutic efficacy in hematologic malignancies, alone or in combination with chemotherapeutic drugs.

The efficacy of mTOR inhibition in the treatment of various types of cancer is still being evaluated, and there are many possibilities that have yet to be explored in identifying areas where rapamycin might prove to be an effective treatment for cancer.

3. mTOR Involvement in Leukemia Metabolism

From a metabolic perspective, mTOR has been traditionally considered as a central regulator that is involved in the promotion of anabolic processes. Signals from bioenergetics status, oxygen levels, DNA damage, and amino acids availability converge on mTOR, unleashing a series of metabolic responses [18]. In fact, it has been shown that mTOR, when incorporated in mTORC1, promotes the synthesis of proteins, lipids, and nucleotides, as well as the adoption of a glycolytic phenotype, and an increase of carbon flux in the pentose phosphate pathway [18,19]. Indeed, research efforts in the leukemia setting have been mainly focused on the glycolytic aspect, in an attempt to exploit this feature as a target for therapeutic intervention. Many studies are focused on the connection between mTOR and glycolysis, mainly using 2-deoxy-D-glucose (2DG) for the inhibition of the glycolytic process. 2DG is a long-known glucose analog, which cannot be metabolized by cells, thus competing with glucose and accumulating in the cytosol [20]. Adenosine monophosphate (AMP)-activated protein kinase (AMPK) acts as a key sensor of cellular energy status coordinating multiple metabolic pathways in order to maintain the balance between ATP production and consumption [21]. Once activated by metabolic stresses, AMPK promotes ATP production switching on catabolic pathways while inhibiting macromolecules biosynthesis. Moreover, AMPK affects cell growth and proliferation by inhibiting mTOR and stabilizing p53 and p27 [21,22]. Pradelli, et al. observed that the blockage of glycolysis, either through 2DG exposure or through glucose deprivation, induces AMPK-mediated inhibition of mTOR, with a subsequent reduction of myeloid cell leukemia-1 (Mcl-1) and a sensitization toward the action of death receptor ligands on Jurkat acute lymphoblastic leukemia (ALL) and U937 acute myeloid leukemia (AML) cell lines [23]. This finding has been confirmed by Coloff, et al. on lymphoid cells, this time assessing the synergy between glycolysis inhibition and exposure to the Bcl-2 (B-cell lymphoma 2) inhibitor ABT-737 [24]. Similarly, Liu, et al. observed mTOR inactivation following 2DG exposure on myeloid cell lines that were previously treated with aurora kinase inhibitors [25]. In addition, Rosilio, et al. corroborated the observation that AMPK activation inhibits mTOR in T-ALL cells via the use of metformin, phenformin, and AICAR (5-Aminoimidazole-4-carboxamide ribonucleotide) [26]. Conversely, Estañ, et al. reported an opposite mechanism, where 2DG action in acute leukemia cell lines provokes AMPK inhibition and subsequent mTOR activation, along with a reduction in the intracellular ATP pool [27]. Interestingly, they observed a difference in the sensitization of leukemia cells when they were treated with arsenic trioxide and either 2DG or glucose deprivation, the latter being weaker, suggesting that 2DG may act through additional undetermined mechanisms [27]. However, despite the differences in the reported mechanism of action, all authors agree that mTOR action is paramount in controlling glycolysis in leukemia cells, allowing the conclusion that the block of this metabolic process is an effective therapeutic strategy, which confers sensitization to various chemotherapeutic agents [23–27]. Moreover, the action of agents targeting mTOR, such as rapamycin, appears to be enhanced when combined with glycolytic inhibitors [28,29].

Since glycolysis is the only reliable source of ATP on the fluctuating oxygen pressure condition that characterizes bone marrow [30], it is not unexpected that mTOR interacts with HIF1α (hypoxia-inducible factor 1-alpha), the master regulator of hypoxic response. Indeed, Konopleva's group demonstrated that hypoxia conditions activate the Akt/mTOR pathway, while exposure to everolimus—one of the first mTOR inhibitors that were approved by the FDA for clinical use in the treatment of patients with cancer [31]—deactivates HIF1α, reverting the glycolytic phenotype of the ALL cell line [32]. Interestingly, Konopleva, et al. also reported that the Akt/mTOR pathway is strongly activated by co-culturing leukemia cells with mesenchymal stem cells in hypoxic conditions [32]; this observation is coherent with the idea that confers to mTOR the role of coordinating signals from microenvironment and subsequently adapting metabolism to these conditions. Accordingly, Brown, et al. confirmed the activation of mTOR, on AML cell lines and primary cells, caused by stromal co-culture, which gives rise to an upregulation of glycolysis; the authors identified the triggering signal in the chemokine CXCL12 (C-X-C motif chemokine 12), through a CXCR4 (C-X-C chemokine receptor type 4)/mTOR axis [33].

A recent work by Feng and Wu identified the enzyme phosphofructokinase-2/fructose-2, 6-bisphosphatase 3 (PFKFB3) among the downstream targets of mTOR [34]; it is directly involved in the glycolytic process, mediating the conversion of fructose 6-phosphate in fructose 2,6-bisphosphate (and vice versa). The latter in turn regulates phosphofructokinase-1, which controls the critical step of glycolysis, the conversion of fructose 6-phosphate in fructose 1,6-bisphosphate [35]. This interaction could explain the mechanism by which mTOR controls glycolysis.

Alternatively, it has been reported that mTOR has a deep impact on mitochondrial respiration, activating oxidative phosphorylation through a mechanism involving its association with Raptor in Jurkat cell lines, whereas exposure to rapamycin disrupted the association and caused a decrease in cellular oxygen consumption [36]. The exposure to agents that impaired mitochondrial membrane potential inactivated mTOR, thus suggesting the presence of a feedback-controlling mechanism [37]. Ramanathan and Schreiber confirmed this finding, showing a downregulation of mitochondrial metabolism coupled with an upregulation of glycolysis when the Jurkat cell line is exposed to rapamycin [38]. These two reports appear to be in contrast with the previously mentioned mTOR activation of glycolysis. However, the use of the same cell model may limit these studies, as these results have not been expanded to other cell lines and/or primary samples. On the other hand, it may be possible that other layers of regulation exist, thus prompting further studies to better clarify the different roles of mTOR in the choice between glycolytic and mitochondrial metabolism.

The mTOR control over the metabolic phenotype has been associated with the resistance of leukemia cells to various agents. Beesley, et al. characterized the transcriptional profile of a panel that was composed of glucocorticoid-resistant T-ALL cell lines, showing that these are characterized by exceptionally high expression of genes related to both glycolysis and oxidative phosphorylation [39]. Exposure to rapamycin restored cell sensitiveness to dexamethasone, indirectly linking metabolism upregulation and mTOR activity [39]. More compelling evidence has been presented by Sharma, et al. who detected mTOR hyperactivation in B-cell leukemia and lymphoma cell lines, and in primary cells that were resistant to fludarabine, which is associated with higher rates of glycolysis and oxidative phosphorylation [40]. The role of mTOR has been verified in the acquisition of this metabolic phenotype, since everolimus was able to revert this higher metabolism [40]. Similar data were generated by our group: exposure to NVP-BKM120, a pan class PI3K inhibitor, on AML cells brought to mTOR deactivation, followed by a decrease in both glycolysis and oxidative phosphorylation [41]. Interestingly, Nepstad, et al. characterized metabolic differences between primary AML cells sensitive and resistant to PI3K/Akt/mTOR inhibitors, including rapamycin, tracing them among glutamine and lipid metabolism [42]. Taken together, these results seem to suggest that (i) leukemic cells display a high degree of heterogeneity in their metabolism; (ii) those which turn out to be resistant to therapeutic agents are generally characterized by a highly active metabolism; (iii) mTOR is the master regulator of leukemic cell metabolism, but we are only beginning to understand the mechanisms by which it operates in the leukemia cell setting.

4. mTOR and Apoptosis Regulation in Leukemias

Among the many functions previously listed, mTOR indirectly inhibits apoptosis [43,44] through a mechanism that depends on the cellular context and on the control of target molecules such as p53, Bcl-2, BAD (Bcl-2-associated death promoter), p21, p27, and c-myc [45].

4.1. mTOR and p53

Recent studies suggest a multifaceted integration of p53 and mTORC1 pathways to drive successful cell growth and proliferation, while in the meantime preserving genome integrity (Figure 2) [46].

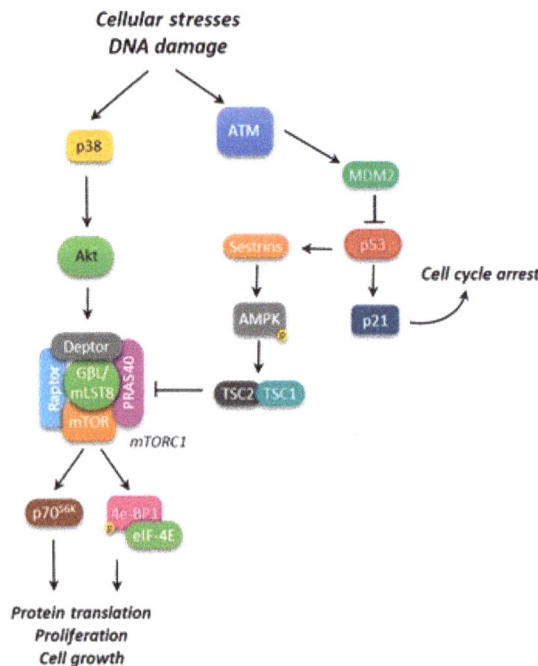

Figure 2. p53 and mTORC1 interaction. Arrows: positive interaction; T-bars: inhibition.

As a key point in such an intricate cooperation, p53 acts in balancing mTORC1 pro-growth activity. In response to cellular stresses and DNA damage, p53 inhibits mTORC1 activity through the upregulation of mTORC negative regulators, such as the activation of AMPK [47], the induction of PTEN (phosphatase and tensin homolog) and TSC2 transcription [47,48], and the decrease of S6K1 (ribosomal protein S6 kinase beta-1) activity or the dephosphorylation of 4E-BP1 [49]. In particular, glucose deprivation in normal cells causes AMPK to inhibit mTORC1 and stabilize p53, stalling cell growth and division [50].

Together, these observations highlighted that p53 inhibits mTOR by regulating a pathway that is used to detect nutrient/energy deprivation such as AMPK, and subsequently the TSC1/TSC2 complex [47].

More recently, it has been clarified that the products of two p53 target genes, Sestrin1 and Sestrin2, negatively regulate mTOR signaling by activating AMPK, which in turn phosphorylates TSC2 [51].

Nonetheless, it has been reported that lymphoma lesions, such as mutant EZH2 (enhancer of zeste homolog 2) in follicular lymphoma (FL), can override the p53-mediated induction of Sestrin1. Specifically, using a chimeric mouse model of lymphoma, Oricchio, et al. [52] demonstrated that Sestrin1 is epigenetically silenced by the lymphoma-specific mutant EZH2Y641X, resulting in mTORC1 activation. The reported EZH2-mediated epigenetic down-regulation of Sestrin1 increases the dependency of lymphomas on mTORC1 and induces sensitivity to mTORC1 inhibitors in EZH2 mutant lymphomas. On the other hand, it has also been reported that in cells that are exposed to genotoxic agents p38α/mTORC1/S6K1 down-regulate MDM2 (mouse double minute 2 homolog) levels, thereby inhibiting p53 ubiquitination and increasing p53 function [53]. This additional genotoxic stress-responsive pathway can contribute to regulate the p53-mediated cell response to DNA damage by sensing the cells' nutrient and energy status.

In a chronic myeloid leukemia (CML) model using the K562 cell line, which is resistant to imatinib, it was found that an increase of phospho-p70S6K and a decrease of phospho-p53Ser15, Bax (Bcl-2-associated X protein), and active caspase-3 compared to the wild-type K562 cell line occurred [54]. The authors also reported that dasatinib was able to induce p-p53Ser15 and active caspase-3 expression, thus promoting apoptosis by the downregulation of AktSer473 and the inhibition of mTOR/p70S6KThr389 activity [54].

Therefore, p53 and mTOR pathway activity could be integrated and combined to inhibit cell growth in response to DNA damage. Deciphering p53 and mTOR crosstalk could be the key to understanding their role in cancer suppression, and the potential clinical usefulness of mTORC1 inhibitors and modulators of the MDM2/p53 module.

Aberrant activation of the PI3K/Akt/mTOR pathway, as well as inactivation of wild-type p53 by MDM2 overexpression, are frequently observed in AML [55–57]. Kojima, et al. demonstrated that the simultaneous inhibition of PI3K/Akt/mTOR axis and of MDM2 induced the dephosphorylation of 4E-BP1, a decrease in MDM2, p21, Noxa, and Bcl-2 expression, and the conformational change of Bax, thus affecting mitochondrial stability and enhancing p53-mediated mitochondrial apoptosis in p53 wild-type AML [58]. Moreover, the use of a dual PI3K/mTOR inhibitor is more effective in blocking two separate inputs that promote mTOR activation: growth factors that stimulate mTOR through the class 1 PI3K, and the nutrients that activate mTOR through a class 3 PI3K.

Independent from a direct interaction between p53 and mTOR in cell death control, the effectiveness of their simultaneous modulation has been highlighted in leukemia. For example, Guo, et al. [59] reported that the reactivation of p53 by Nutlin-3, and Akt/mTOR inhibition by tanshinone IIA, exhibit a synergetic anti-leukemia effect with imatinib in Philadelphia positive (Ph +) ALL.

4.2. mTOR and Bcl-2 Family

Several research groups have shown that a high level mTOR expression is able to control apoptosis by modulating several molecules, including Bcl-2 family members, and thus promoting tumor cell survival (Figure 3) [44,45,60]. The activated PI3K/Akt/mTOR pathway has been shown to decrease the BH3 (Bcl-2 homology domain) mimetic effectiveness in cancer cells by upregulating anti-apoptotic Bcl-2 family members, such as Mcl-1 [61]. Consistently, rapamycin, an inhibitor of mTOR, has been shown to induce a decrease in Mcl-1 expression, and this mechanism is able to overcome drug resistance [62]. Moreover, it was reported that NVP-BEZ235, a PI3K/mTOR dual inhibitor, decreases Mcl-1 expression and sensitizes ovarian carcinoma cells to Bcl-xL (B-cell lymphoma-extra large)-targeting strategies.

Subsequently, simultaneous blockade of PI3K/mTOR and the Bcl-2 pathway was shown to have promising antileukemic activity in leukemia cell lines, primary samples, and xenograft models. Rahmani and colleagues [61] have demonstrated that co-exposure to the dual PI3K/mTOR inhibitor NVP-BEZ235 and the Bcl-2/Bcl-xL inhibitor ABT-737 strongly potentiated the cytotoxicity of single agents in AML. They found that antileukemic synergism involved multiple mechanisms, including Mcl-1 downregulation, the release of Bim (Bcl-2-like protein 11) from Bcl-2/Bcl-xL as well as Bak (Bcl-2 homologous antagonist/killer) and Bax from Mcl-1/Bcl-2/Bcl-xL, and GSK3α/β (glycogen synthase kinase 3 alpha/beta), culminating in a strong apoptosis induction [61].

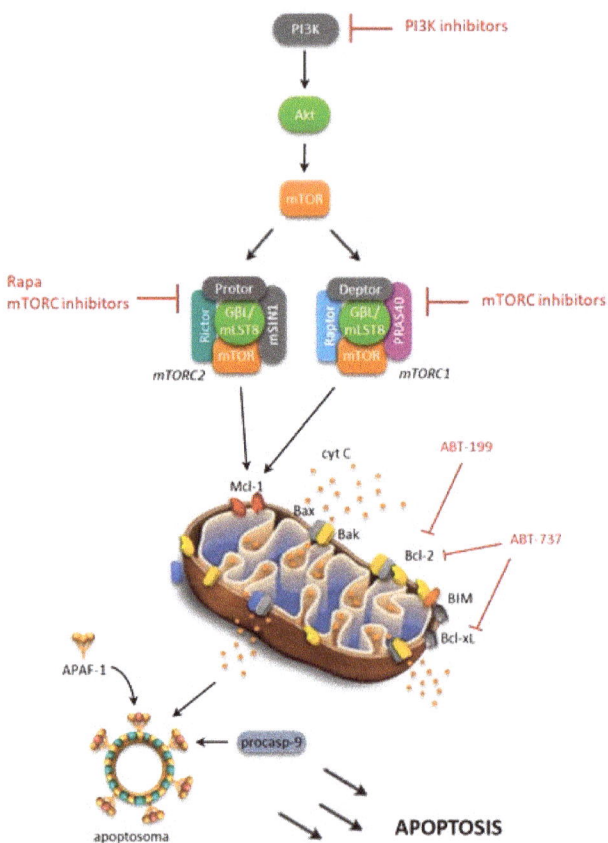

Figure 3. mTOR and Bcl-2 family member interactions. Arrows: positive interaction; T-bars: inhibition.

In a similar fashion, Spender, et al. suggested that the combined use of BH3 mimetics with mTORC1/2 inhibitors could be a novel and effective therapeutic approach for the management of Burkitt's lymphoma [63]. Authors demonstrated that exposure of Burkitt's lymphoma cells to dual PI3K/mTOR inhibitors, such as PI 103, was associated with an increase in Bim/Mcl-1 expression ratios and the loss of c-myc expression [63]. Remarkably, they also observed that dual PI3K/mTOR inhibitors or mTOR active site inhibitors were effective in overcoming resistance to ABT-737, thus indicating that inhibition of cap-dependent translation regulated by 4E-BP1/eIF4E represents a key point to overcome BH3 mimetics resistance.

Our group has previously explored a combined in vitro targeted approach to overcome ABT-737-acquired resistance in ALL with the simultaneous inhibition of the mTOR pathway by CCI-779 [64]. We observed that simultaneous inhibition strongly enhanced the cytotoxicity of single agents sensitizing ALL cells to apoptosis, and reverting the acquired ABT-737 resistance of cell models and primary samples, while sparing normal progenitors. Analysis of signaling modulations in newly sensitized ABT-737 resistant cells reveals that ABT-737 plus CCI-779 combination reduces 4E-BP1 phosphorylation and Mcl-1 expression. Since the involvement of proteasomal degradation was excluded, the inhibition of 4E-BP1-dependent protein translation may be responsible for the synergistic interaction between ABT-737 and CCI-779. However, in some ALL models, Mcl-1 may be not the unique determinant of ABT-737 resistance, since knockdown of protein expression by RNA interference does not result in significant changes of cytotoxicity [64].

A similar approach was used by Rahmani, et al. [65], which demonstrated the cooperation between the selective Bcl-2 inhibitor and PI3K inhibition (venetoclax/GDC-0980) in inducing Bax-dependent apoptosis, which exhibiting strong anti-AML activity both in vitro and in vivo, as well as against multiple forms of venetoclax resistance.

More recently, by the high-throughput profiling of signaling networks, Andreeff's group demonstrated that concomitant treatment with temsirolimus plus ABT-737 or the MDM2 inhibitor Nutlin-3a, is effective for eliminating microenvironmental resistance in AML, and it facilitated leukemic cell death [66].

Finally, it is interesting to mention the reported unsuspected role of mTOR as an apoptotic inducer. Indeed, Calastretti, et al. [67,68] stated that in human FL B-cell lines, characterized by high concentration of Bcl-2 protein, rapamycin increases the cellular concentration of p27kip1 and Bcl-2, leading to cell arrest in the G1 phase, and to the activation of an anti-apoptotic program. Moreover, prior treatment with rapamycin completely inhibited the taxol-induced apoptosis of human B-cell lines by phosphorylation/inactivation of Bcl-2.

This observation highlights the role of mTOR for a coordinated regulation of the cell cycle and apoptosis in normal and leukemia cells.

5. mTOR and MicroRNA Regulation in Leukemias

MicroRNAs (miRNAs) are ubiquitous regulators of biological processes that are involved in cellular differentiation, development, stress response, apoptosis, and cell growth. A number of studies have revealed differential expression of known miRNAs in different hematopoietic cell types, demonstrating that miRNAs play an important role in the decision by hematopoietic stem cells (HSC) and progenitor cells to self-renew or to differentiate into a specific cell type [69–71].

Most of these miRNAs have been reported to regulate the expression of key genes in the PI3K/Akt/mTOR pathway, and they are involved in the development and pathogenesis of hematological malignancies.

Among the miRNAs that directly target mTOR, miR-126 plays important functions in HSC, preserving quiescence and increasing self-renewal [70,72]. It is both highly expressed and functionally active within the murine and human HSC compartments, with progressive downregulation during the early steps of hematopoietic commitment. Lechman, et al. [70,72] reported interesting results that showed that miR-126 is involved in mTOR regulation by targeting mSIN1, together with several other members of the PI3K/Akt/mTOR axis. In particular, mSIN1 repression impairs the mTORC2 complex formation and full activation of Akt. They also showed that myeloid leukemia stem cells (LSC) express high endogenous levels of miR-126, compared with more differentiated AML populations [72]. Upregulation of miR-126 plays a critical role in promoting chemotherapy resistance of LSC.

Furthermore, mTOR and Rictor are direct targets of let-7 and miR-16. Marcais, et al. [73] showed that these miRNAs regulate the expression of mTOR components in CD4 T-cells and contribute to discriminate between T-cell activation and anergy.

MiR-100 and miR-99a are involved in mTOR regulation in ALL and contributed to the poor response to chemotherapy. Li, et al. [74] reported a downregulation of miR-100 and miR-99a in the cases of ALL, especially in T-ALL, and in ALL harboring mixed lineage leukemia (MLL) gene rearrangements and BCR-ABL1 fusion transcripts. Cases with lower levels of expression displayed shorter survival and a poorer outcome when compared to cases with higher expression. These miRNAs contribute to leukemia developments and progression by directly targeting the insulin-like growth factor 1 receptor (IGF1R) and mTOR. In fact, the protein levels of IGF1R and mTOR were reduced in Jurkat cells that were transfected with miR-100/99a mimics, while they were increased in cells that were transfected with the miR-100/99a inhibitors (antisense). Functional studies also showed that upregulation of mTOR induced the activation of Mcl-1 with consequent improvement of cell proliferation and inhibition of apoptosis.

Besides miRNAs which directly target mTOR components, several other miRNAs have been reported to targets that are upstream (mir-22, miR-26, miR-150, miR-193, miR-223, miR-3151) [75–79] or downstream (miR-29, miR-181) [80–82] of mTOR signaling, highlighting the importance of the PI3K/Akt/mTOR axis in leukemias.

6. mTOR Axis Inhibition in Leukemias

The role of the PI3K/Akt/mTOR pathway in leukemias has been widely studied, both for in vitro and in vivo models, in order to explore the therapeutic perspective of its inhibition. In fact, the use of the dual PI3K/mTOR inhibitor, dual Akt/tyrosine-kinase receptor (RTK) inhibitor, Akt inhibitor, selective inhibitor of PI3K, mTOR inhibitor, and the dual PI3K/phosphoinositide-dependent protein kinase-1 (PDK1) inhibitor in chronic and acute leukemias seem to have remarkable therapeutic effect as compared to conventional treatments [83].

6.1. Rapamycin and Rapalogs

Literature data have reported on first- and second-generation mTOR inhibitors. Among the first generation inhibitors, rapamycin and its analogs, called rapalogs, are the most well studied drugs, and they are now clinically used as cancer treatments. Rapamycin (sirolimus) is a macrolide antibiotic that is produced by the microorganism *Streptomyces hygroscopicus*, which has been discovered in 1975 as a potent antifungal agent [84]. In following studies, it was also associated with immunosuppression [85], which subsequently led to its development as a clinically useful drug in consideration of its anticancer activity [86]. Similarly to the immunosuppressant FK506, rapamycin binds to the intracellular receptor FKBP12 (FK506-binding protein 12), and they both share similar chemical structures. Nevertheless, the two macrolides have different mechanisms of action in cells, since FK506 inhibits T cell proliferation, whereas rapamycin interferes with cytokine signaling. However, the exact mechanism of how these interactions lead to inhibition of mTOR pathway remains to be understood.

In consideration of some pharmacological limitations of rapamycin, such as poor water solubility and chemical stability, rapalogs, including temsirolimus (CCI-779), everolimus (RAD001), and ridaforolimus (AP23573) have been developed, with minor immunosuppressive action [87]. Unfortunately, several studies have demonstrated that first generation inhibitors display limited anticancer activity, and that is partially due to the fact that the inhibition of mTORC1 by these drugs might lead to Akt upregulation and outgrowth of more aggressive lesions. Targeted strategies by combining rapamycin plus an inhibitor of Akt or PI3K, or the use of agents that target both PI3K and mTOR, or both mTORC1 and mTORC2, were then developed to circumvent this loop [88].

6.2. Dual Inhibitors

Selective dual mTORC1 and mTORC2 inhibitors are second-generation mTOR inhibitors. They are ATP-competitive inhibitors of mTOR that block the phosphorylation of all downstream targets of both mTORC complexes without inhibiting other kinases [89]. Among the second-generation mTOR inhibitors, AZD8055 is a compound that is able to prevent mTORC2-mediated Akt activation. This agent has been evaluated in a multicenter phase I study including patients with advanced solid tumors or lymphomas [90]. The most frequent adverse events (AEs) were elevated transaminases and fatigue, and not hypercholesterolemia or hypertriglyceridemia, as is often reported in patients who are treated with other mTOR inhibitors, including rapalogs. Another second-generation mTOR inhibitor is CC-223, which was evaluated in pre-treated patients with advanced solid tumors or multiple myeloma (MM) [91]. Common CC-223-related AEs were fatigue, nausea, diarrhea, and hyperglycemia. TAK-228, another dual mTORC1/mTORC2 kinase inhibitor, has been tested in patients with MM, non-Hodgkin lymphoma and Waldenström's macroglobulinemia (WM) [92]; reported toxicities included thrombocytopenia, fatigue, and neutropenia. Unfortunately, the best response achieved in a WM patient has been a partial remission (PR).

Dual PI3K/mTOR inhibitors are small molecules that are able to block the ATP binding sites of mTOR and PI3K, thus targeting all the three key enzymes, PI3K, Akt, and mTOR [93], although data from clinical trials are not entirely satisfying. In particular, NVP-BEZ235 has been tested in adult patients with relapse/refractory (R/R) acute leukemia, showing an anti-leukemic efficacy; this was more pronounced in an ALL setting, granting an encouraging overall response rate and a sustained molecular remission [94].

6.3. mTOR Inhibitors in AML

The activation of PI3K/Akt/mTOR has been observed in up to 80% of AML cases and has been associated with a poor prognosis [95].

Given the heterogeneity of leukemias, it is important to remark that there is variability within leukemias, in both in vitro and in vivo sensitivities to PI3K/Akt/mTOR inhibition. In this respect, Reikvam, et al. [96] investigated the functional effects on primary AML cells of two mTOR inhibitors (rapamycin, temsirolimus) and two PI3K inhibitors (GDC-0941, 3-methyladenine). They demonstrated that the antileukemic effect of PI3K/Akt/mTOR inhibition varies between patients. By unsupervised hierarchical clustering analysis, two main clusters were identified in this study: one included patients that exhibited remarkable antiproliferative effects to all inhibitors tested; the other patients proved to be resistant. Notably, resistant patients were characterized by a higher expression of *CDC25B*, a gene encoding a phosphatase involved in cell cycle progression [96,97]. In a recent study on AML patients, the same group identified two clusters that were characterized by high and low constitutive PI3K/Akt/mTOR activation [98]. Complex phenotypic differences, including genetic and molecular processes, cellular communication, and interactions with the microenvironment are reported to be involved in differences in pathway activation [98].

With regard to the heterogeneity of leukemias, additional crucial points that are related to the efficacy of targeted therapies are the leukemia-microenvironment crosstalk and subsequently the stem cell niche, a specialized microenvironment that helps to maintain stem cell characteristics [99,100]. Common pathways are potentially shared across multiple leukemias and are involved in microenvironment/leukemia interactions. Reikvam and colleagues [101] demonstrated that PI3K and mTOR inhibitors exerted direct and indirect antileukemic activity through the inhibition of angioregulatory mediators released by both AML and stromal cells. These effects are however mediated through the common targets represented by the PI3K/Akt/mTOR pathway.

The efficacy of several selective PI3K/Akt/mTOR inhibitors has been investigated on both AML cell lines and AML primary cells using mTOR inhibitors as single agents or in association with chemotherapy (Table 1). Recher, et al. [102] used rapamycin in monotherapy for patients with R/R de novo or secondary AML, showing partial responses in four out of nine patients. Perl, et al. [103] used rapamycin with the chemotherapy regimen MEC (mitoxantrone, etoposide, cytarabine) in patients with R/R or untreated secondary AML, reaching 22% of clinical responses (complete remission (CR) or PR), showing low synergy between rapamycin and chemotherapy. Furthermore, everolimus has been evaluated in association with low doses of cytarabine (LDAC) in naïve elderly AML patients who were not eligible for intensive chemotherapy [104]. Amadori, et al. [105] have combined temsirolimus with low dose of clofarabine as a salvage therapy. Temsirolimus has also been used for maintenance therapy in patients, achieving CR with or without full hematological recovery after induction (CRi). Despite these promising findings, the combination of rapalogs and chemotherapy failed to display the expected synergistic cytotoxicities in clinical trials.

In acute promyelocytic leukemia (APL), PI3K/Akt signaling is constitutively activated, and cells that are exposed to all-trans retinoic acid (ATRA) seem to be very sensitive to class I PI3K, p110beta, or p110delta inhibitors, and to rapamycin [83,106]. Therefore, PI3K and mTOR inhibitors in association with induction treatment regimens may provide therapeutic benefits [106]. In addition, the PI3K/Akt/mTOR pathway contributes to ATRA-induced granulocytic differentiation (Table 1) [107].

6.4. mTOR Inhibitors in ALL

The hyperactivation of the PI3K/Akt/mTOR pathway was reported also in B-ALL, where encouraging results have been obtained with the inhibitors of PI3K/mTOR and MEK1/2 [108]. In the study of Messina, et al. [108], ALL cells with mutated *NRAS* or *KRAS* showed sensitivity to rapamycin and to the dual PI3K/mTOR inhibitor NVP-BEZ235. Thus, the authors pointed out PI3K/mTOR inhibitors, among others, as alternative therapeutic approaches in frail patients (Table 2). Other selective mTORC1 inhibitors inducing apoptosis in ALL are RAD001, Torin-2, and CCI-779. RAD001 shows also a potent synergic effect with the Akt allosteric inhibitor MK2206 [83]. Instead, in the Ph + ALL setting, it has been shown that BCR-ABL is able to activate the survival pathway PI3K/ Akt/mTOR [109]. The use of the mTOR inhibitor and in combination with imatinib has also been proven to have a synergic effect even in imatinib-resistant cell lines [109].

The PI3K/Akt/mTOR pathway is also constitutively active in numerous T-ALL patients and this affects the patient outcome, indicating it as a potential therapeutic target for T-ALL. T-ALL, which represents 15% of pediatric ALL and 25% of adult ALL, is an aggressive disease where relapses are not infrequent, despite the good response to chemotherapy. The very poor prognosis suggests the need for new therapeutic strategies. The negative PI3K/mTOR pathway regulator, PTEN, is frequently mutated in T-ALL, leading to hyperactivation of the pathway [110]. The combination of rapamycin with the chemotherapeutic agent dexamethasone shows a synergic effect in T-ALL cells [111]. In addition, numerous pathway inhibitors, such as GDC-0941 (a pan class I PI3K inhibitor), MK-2206 (an allosteric Akt inhibitor), RAD001 (an mTORC1 inhibitor) and the dual PI3K/PDK1 inhibitors NVP-BAG956 and NVP-BEZ235, show a potent cytotoxic effect in T-ALL cell lines, as well as in patient-derived cells [112].

The NOTCH pathway, altered in about 50% of T-ALL patients [110], triggers the upregulation of the PI3K/Akt pathway through the transcription factor HES1 (hairy and enhancer of split-1), which negatively regulates the expression of PTEN [113]. Mutations of PTEN confer resistance to treatment with GSIs (gamma-secretase inhibitors) that blocks the NOTCH1 (Notch homolog 1, translocation-associated) pathway [113]. This interplay between NOTCH1 and PTEN suggests the possible efficacy of a combined inhibition of PI3K/Akt and the NOTCH1 pathway in T-ALL.

6.5. mTOR Inhibitors in Other Leukemias

The PI3k/Akt/mTOR pathway is one of the multiple signaling pathways that are activated by BCR-ABL in CML cells, so drugs targeting key molecules such as PI3K, Akt and mTOR have been reported to exert beneficial effects in CML progenitor and stem cell populations (Table 1). These drugs show synergic activity with tyrosine kinase inhibitors (TKis). In particular, the dual PI3K/PDK1 inhibitor NVP-BEZ235 is able to sensitize CML stem cells and progenitors to nilotinib, enhancing its cytotoxicity in TKi-resistant BCR-ABL mutant cells [114]. Moreover, a combination of dasatinib with rapamycin or LY294002 decreases FOXO1/3 (forkhead box proteins O1 and O3) phosphorylation and drives the apoptosis of CML cells [115]. Resveratrol, a phytoalexin, and a natural phenol produced by several plants, acts downstream of BCR-ABL, and inhibits Akt activity [116]. Conversely, in accelerated phase/blastic phase (AP/BP) CML patients, increased ABCG2 (drug pump, ATP-binding cassette sub-family G member 2) expression was associated with the lack of PTEN protein and subsequent Akt activation [117]. This suggests that PI3K/Akt could be an alternative therapeutic target in CML, since ABCG2 seems to be regulated by PTEN through the PI3K/Akt pathway [117]. TKi can also abrogate the activation of PI3K/Akt/mTOR, and therefore in the TKi-resistant cells, simultaneous inhibition of PI3K and Akt/mTOR is recommended to obtain a potent pro-apoptotic effect in CML cells.

Concerning chronic lymphocytic leukemia (CLL), one of the major prognostic factors is the specific characteristic of the B-cell receptor (BCR), upstream of a signal transduction pathway that is essential for survival and proliferation, with a major role in the context of prognosis and positive selection of the precursor tumoral cell. In fact, antigenic stimulation and therefore the constitutive activation of BCR signaling plays a fundamental role in the pathogenesis of CLL [118].

BCR stimulation triggers the activation of numerous intracellular pathways that regulate normal B cells or leukemia. In fact, BCR acts on kinases, such as spleen tyrosin kinase (SYK) and SRC kinase LYN, which phosphorylate immune receptors belonging to the complementary proteins of the BCR, CD79a, and CD79b complexes. This phosphorylation causes the recruitment of adaptive proteins and other kinases, such as Bruton tyrosine kinase (BTK) or PI3K to a complex formed by the accessory proteins of BCR and then it determines the downstream stimulation of Akt/mTOR, NF-kB (nuclear factor kappa-light-chain-enhancer of activated B cells), and/or ERK (extracellular-signal-regulated kinase) [119].

CC-115, a novel dual mTOR kinase and a DNA-dependent protein kinase (DNA-PK) inhibitor, was evaluated [120]. CC-115 showed encouraging preclinical data on the ability to overcome resistance to chemotherapy or venetoclax, as well as to idelalisib, proving to be an attractive compound for further combination studies in clinical settings (Table 2) [120].

In conclusion, the use of rapalogs, or of second-generation mTOR inhibitors—developed with the aim to overcome the weaknesses of rapalogs—showed a limited impact, despite the expected benefits in clinical trials. This could be due to several mechanisms, such as an incomplete blockage of the pathway, or the existence of feedback loops. Thus, these observations should prompt further studies that address the clarification of the mechanisms of drug resistance, and the design of a more precise and personalized treatment.

Table 1. mTOR inhibitors in myeloid leukemias.

Inhibitors	Disease	Response	Reference
Rapamycin monotherapy	R/R AML	PR	Recher, et al. [102]
Rapamycin + MEC	R/R or untreated secondary AML	CR/PR	Perl, et al. [103]
Everolimus + LDAC	Naïve elderly AML	CR/Cri/PR	Wei A.H., et al. [104]
Temsirolimus + LDClof	R/R AML	CR/Cri	Amadori, et al. [105]
ATRA + LY294002 and PD98059	APL	Increase granulocyte differentiation	Scholl S., et al. [106]
NVPBEZ235 + nilotinib	TKI-resistant BCR-ABL	Increase apoptosis	Airiau K., et al. [114]
Rapamycin + dasatinib	CML	Increase apoptosis	Pellicano F., et al. [115]
Resveratrol	CML	Inhibits Akt	Banerjee M. S., et al. [116]

Table 2. mTOR inhibitors in lymphoid leukemias.

Inhibitors	Disease	RESPONSE	Reference
CC-115	R/R CLL	PR	Thijssen, et al. [120]
Rapamycin + NVP-BEZ235	ALL	Increase apoptosis	Messina, et al. [108]
RAD001, Torin-2 and CCI-779	ALL	Increase apoptosis	Bertacchini et al. [83]
Imatinib + mTOR inhibitor	Imatinib-resistant Ph + ALL	Increase apoptosis	Xing H., et al. [109]

7. Summary

Over the last decade, it has been widely demonstrated that the mTOR pathway is physiologically activated during various cellular processes and that it is deregulated in human diseases such as cancer.

Int. J. Mol. Sci. **2018**, *19*, 2396

The critical role of mTOR in leukemia initiation, progression, and chemoresistance has also been proven by scientific and clinical studies evaluating its down-modulation. To date, several classes of pharmacological agents targeting the mTOR network have been developed. Each of them has their own pharmacokinetic properties, inhibitory activities, and toxicity profiles. Therefore, understanding which inhibitor is more clinically effective in each patient remains a constant challenge. The answer depends on the recognition of specific oncogenic addiction profile of leukemia cells, thus the need of new biomarkers for patient selection. The advances in the comprehension of the biological impact that mTOR has in the leukemia setting, described in this review, could contribute to the potential future development of effective mTOR-targeting based therapeutics.

Author Contributions: Writing-Original Draft Preparation, S.M., M.R.R., M.P., V.G.; Writing-Review & Editing, S.M., M.R.R., M.P., V.G., M.P.B., A.T.; Supervision, M.R.R., A.T.

Funding: This research was funded by Sapienza University (C26A14CPRB, C26A158NJR, RM116154EC670667, RP11715C7D08BDC2 and RM11715C7D01147A) grants, by Fondazione Internazionale D'AMATO Onlus and by Fondazione Frisiani-Santini.

Acknowledgments: We are grateful to RomAIL (Associazione Italiana contro le Leucemie-linfomi e mieloma) for providing laboratory space and to D. Calef for editing the manuscript.

Conflicts of Interest: The authors declare no conflict of interest.

References

1. Memmott, R.M.; Dennis, P.A. Akt-dependent and -independent mechanisms of mTOR regulation in cancer. *Cell Signal.* **2009**, *21*, 656–664. [CrossRef] [PubMed]
2. Laplante, M.; Sabatini, D.M. mTOR signaling at a glance. *J. Cell Sci.* **2009**, *122*, 3589–3594. [CrossRef] [PubMed]
3. Sarbassov, D.D.; Ali, S.M.; Kim, D.H.; Guertin, D.A.; Latek, R.R.; Erdjument-Bromage, H.; Tempst, P.; Sabatini, D.M. Rictor, a novel binding partner of mTOR, defines a rapamycin-insensitive and raptor-independent pathway that regulates the cytoskeleton. *Curr. Biol.* **2004**, *14*, 1296–1302. [CrossRef] [PubMed]
4. Lamming, D.W.; Ye, L.; Katajisto, P.; Goncalves, M.D.; Saitoh, M.; Stevens, D.M.; Davis, J.G.; Salmon, A.B.; Richardson, A.; Ahima, R.S.; et al. Rapamycin-induced insulin resistance is mediated by mTORC2 loss and uncoupled from longevity. *Science* **2012**, *335*, 1638–1643. [CrossRef] [PubMed]
5. Sarbassov, D.D.; Ali, S.M.; Sengupta, S.; Sheen, J.H.; Hsu, P.P.; Bagley, A.F.; Markhard, A.L.; Sabatini, D.M. Prolonged rapamycin treatment inhibits mTORC2 assembly and Akt/PKB. *Mol. Cell* **2006**, *22*, 159–168. [CrossRef] [PubMed]
6. Dibble, C.C.; Manning, B.D. Signal integration by mTORC1 coordinates nutrient input with biosynthetic output. *Nat. Cell Biol.* **2013**, *15*, 555–564. [CrossRef] [PubMed]
7. Jossé, L.; Xie, J.; Proud, C.G.; Smales, C.M. mTORC1 signalling and eIF4E/4E-BP1 translation initiation factor stoichiometry influence recombinant protein productivity from GS-CHOK1 cells. *Biochem. J.* **2016**, *473*, 4651–4664. [CrossRef] [PubMed]
8. Jacinto, E.; Loewith, R.; Schmidt, A.; Lin, S.; Rüegg, M.A.; Hall, A.; Hall, M.N. Mammalian TOR complex 2 controls the actin cytoskeleton and is rapamycin insensitive. *Nat. Cell Biol.* **2004**, *6*, 1122–1128. [CrossRef] [PubMed]
9. Goncharova, E.A.; Goncharov, D.A.; Li, H.; Pimtong, W.; Lu, S.; Khavin, I.; Krymskaya, V.P. mTORC2 is required for proliferation and survival of TSC2-null cells. *Mol. Cell Biol.* **2011**, *31*, 2484–2498. [CrossRef] [PubMed]
10. Zinzalla, V.; Stracka, D.; Oppliger, W.; Hall, M.N. Activation of mTORC2 by association with the ribosome. *Cell* **2011**, *144*, 757–768. [CrossRef] [PubMed]
11. McCubrey, J.A.; Abrams, S.L.; Fitzgerald, T.L.; Cocco, L.; Martelli, A.M.; Montalto, G.; Cervello, M.; Scalisi, A.; Candido, S.; Libra, M.; et al. Roles of signaling pathways in drug resistance, cancer initiating cells and cancer progression and metastasis. *Adv. Biol. Regul.* **2015**, *57*, 75–101. [CrossRef] [PubMed]
12. Lapidot, T.; Sirard, C.; Vormoor, J.; Murdoch, B.; Hoang, T.; Caceres-Cortes, J.; Minden, M.; Paterson, B.; Caligiuri, M.A.; Dick, J.E. A cell initiating human acute myeloid leukaemia after transplantation into SCID mice. *Nature* **1994**, *367*, 645–648. [CrossRef] [PubMed]

13. Hoshii, T.; Tadokoro, Y.; Naka, K.; Ooshio, T.; Muraguchi, T.; Sugiyama, N.; Soga, T.; Araki, K.; Yamamura, K.; Hirao, A. mTORC1 is essential for leukemia propagation but not stem cell self-renewal. *J. Clin. Investig.* **2012**, *122*, 2114–2129. [CrossRef] [PubMed]

14. Beauchamp, E.M.; Platanias, L.C. The evolution of the TOR pathway and its role in cancer. *Oncogene* **2013**, *32*, 3923–3932. [CrossRef] [PubMed]

15. Willems, L.; Tamburini, J.; Chapuis, N.; Lacombe, C.; Mayeux, P.; Bouscary, D. PI3K and mTOR signaling pathways in cancer: New data on targeted therapies. *Curr. Oncol. Rep.* **2012**, *14*, 129–138. [CrossRef] [PubMed]

16. Fang, Y.; Yang, Y.; Hua, C.; Xu, S.; Zhou, M.; Guo, H.; Wang, N.; Zhao, X.; Huang, L.; Yu, F.; et al. Rictor has a pivotal role in maintaining quiescence as well as stemness of leukemia stem cells in MLL-driven leukemia. *Leukemia* **2017**, *31*, 414–422. [CrossRef] [PubMed]

17. Evangelisti, C.; Chiarini, F.; McCubrey, J.A.; Martelli, A.M. Therapeutic targeting of mTOR in T-cell acute lymphoblastic leukemia: An update. *Int. J. Mol. Sci.* **2018**, *19*, 1878. [CrossRef] [PubMed]

18. Saxton, R.A.; Sabatini, D.M. mTOR signaling in growth, metabolism, and disease. *Cell* **2017**, *169*, 361–371. [CrossRef] [PubMed]

19. Ben-Sahra, I.; Manning, B.D. mTORC1 signaling and the metabolic control of cell growth. *Curr. Opin. Cell. Biol.* **2017**, *45*, 72–82. [CrossRef] [PubMed]

20. Mathupala, S.P.; Ko, Y.H.; Pedersen, P.L. Hexokinase II: Cancer's double-edged sword acting as both facilitator and gatekeeper of malignancy when bound to mitochondria. *Oncogene* **2006**, *25*, 4777–4786. [CrossRef] [PubMed]

21. Hardie, D.G. AMP-activated/SNF1 protein kinases: Conserved guardians of cellular energy. *Nat. Rev. Mol. Cell Biol.* **2007**, *8*, 774–785. [CrossRef] [PubMed]

22. Hardie, D.G.; Ross, F.A.; Hawley, S.A. AMP-activated protein kinase: A target for drugs both ancient and modern. *Chem. Biol.* **2012**, *19*, 1222–1236. [CrossRef] [PubMed]

23. Pradelli, L.A.; Bénéteau, M.; Chauvin, C.; Jacquin, M.A.; Marchetti, S.; Muñoz-Pinedo, C.; Auberger, P.; Pende, M.; Ricci, J.E. Glycolysis inhibition sensitizes tumor cells to death receptors-induced apoptosis by AMP kinase activation leading to Mcl-1 block in translation. *Oncogene* **2010**, *29*, 1641–1652. [CrossRef] [PubMed]

24. Coloff, J.L.; Macintyre, A.N.; Nichols, A.G.; Liu, T.; Gallo, C.A.; Plas, D.R.; Rathmell, J.C. Akt-dependent glucose metabolism promotes Mcl-1 synthesis to maintain cell survival and resistance to Bcl-2 inhibition. *Cancer Res.* **2011**, *71*, 5204–5213. [CrossRef] [PubMed]

25. Liu, L.L.; Long, Z.J.; Wang, L.X.; Zheng, F.M.; Fang, Z.G.; Yan, M.; Xu, D.F.; Chen, J.J.; Wang, S.W.; Lin, D.J.; et al. Inhibition of mTOR pathway sensitizes acute myeloid leukemia cells to aurora inhibitors by suppression of glycolytic metabolism. *Mol. Cancer Res.* **2013**, *11*, 1326–1336. [CrossRef] [PubMed]

26. Rosilio, C.; Lounnas, N.; Nebout, M.; Imbert, V.; Hagenbeek, T.; Spits, H.; Asnafi, V.; Pontier-Bres, R.; Reverso, J.; Michiels, J.F.; et al. The metabolic perturbators metformin, phenformin and AICAR interfere with the growth and survival of murine PTEN-deficient T cell lymphomas and human T-ALL/T-LL cancer cells. *Cancer Lett.* **2013**, *336*, 114–126. [CrossRef] [PubMed]

27. Estañ, M.C.; Calviño, E.; de Blas, E.; Boyano-Adánez Mdel, C.; Mena, M.L.; Gómez-Gómez, M.; Rial, E.; Aller, P. 2-Deoxy-D-glucose cooperates with arsenic trioxide to induce apoptosis in leukemia cells: Involvement of IGF-1R-regulated Akt/mTOR, MEK/ERK and LKB-1/AMPK signaling pathways. *Biochem. Pharmacol.* **2012**, *84*, 1604–1616. [CrossRef] [PubMed]

28. Xu, R.H.; Pelicano, H.; Zhang, H.; Giles, F.J.; Keating, M.J.; Huang, P. Synergistic effect of targeting mTOR by rapamycin and depleting ATP by inhibition of glycolysis in lymphoma and leukemia cells. *Leukemia* **2005**, *19*, 2153–2158. [CrossRef] [PubMed]

29. Akers, L.J.; Fang, W.; Levy, A.G.; Franklin, A.R.; Huang, P.; Zweidler-McKay, P.A. Targeting glycolysis in leukemia: A novel inhibitor 3-BrOP in combination with rapamycin. *Leuk. Res.* **2011**, *35*, 814–820. [CrossRef] [PubMed]

30. Schito, L.; Rey, S.; Konopleva, M. Integration of hypoxic HIF-α signaling in blood cancers. *Oncogene* **2017**, *36*, 5331–5340. [CrossRef] [PubMed]

31. Janku, F.; Yap, T.A.; Meric-Bernstam, F. Targeting the PI3K pathway in cancer: Are we making headway? *Nat. Rev. Clin. Oncol.* **2018**, *15*, 273–291. [CrossRef] [PubMed]

32. Frolova, O.; Samudio, I.; Benito, J.M.; Jacamo, R.; Kornblau, S.M.; Markovic, A.; Schober, W.; Lu, H.; Qiu, Y.H.; Buglio, D.; et al. Regulation of HIF-1α signaling and chemoresistance in acute lymphocytic leukemia under hypoxic conditions of the bone marrow microenvironment. *Cancer Biol. Ther.* **2012**, *13*, 858–870. [CrossRef] [PubMed]

33. Braun, M.; Qorraj, M.; Büttner, M.; Klein, F.A.; Saul, D.; Aigner, M.; Huber, W.; Mackensen, A.; Jitschin, R.; Mougiakakos, D. CXCL12 promotes glycolytic reprogramming in acute myeloid leukemia cells via the CXCR4/mTOR axis. *Leukemia* **2016**, *30*, 1788–1792. [CrossRef] [PubMed]

34. Feng, Y.; Wu, L. mTOR up-regulation of PFKFB3 is essential for acute myeloid leukemia cell survival. *Biochem. Biophys. Res. Commun.* **2017**, *483*, 897–903. [CrossRef] [PubMed]

35. Ros, S.; Schulze, A. Balancing glycolytic flux: The role of 6-phosphofructo-2-kinase/fructose 2,6-bisphosphatases in cancer metabolism. *Cancer Metab.* **2013**, *1*, 8. [CrossRef] [PubMed]

36. Hay, N.; Sonenberg, N. Upstream and downstream of mTOR. *Genes Dev.* **2004**, *18*, 1926–1945. [CrossRef] [PubMed]

37. Schieke, S.M.; Phillips, D.; McCoy, J.P., Jr.; Aponte, A.M.; Shen, R.F.; Balaban, R.S.; Finkel, T. The mammalian target of rapamycin (mTOR) pathway regulates mitochondrial oxygen consumption and oxidative capacity. *J. Biol. Chem.* **2006**, *281*, 27643–27652. [CrossRef] [PubMed]

38. Ramanathan, A.; Schreiber, S.L. Direct control of mitochondrial function by mTOR. *Proc. Natl. Acad. Sci. USA* **2009**, *106*, 22229–22232. [CrossRef] [PubMed]

39. Beesley, A.H.; Firth, M.J.; Ford, J.; Weller, R.E.; Freitas, J.R.; Perera, K.U.; Kees, U.R. Glucocorticoid resistance in T-lineage acute lymphoblastic leukaemia is associated with a proliferative metabolism. *Br. J. Cancer* **2009**, *100*, 1926–1936. [CrossRef] [PubMed]

40. Sharma, A.; Janocha, A.J.; Hill, B.T.; Smith, M.R.; Erzurum, S.C.; Almasan, A. Targeting mTORC1-mediated metabolic addiction overcomes fludarabine resistance in malignant B cells. *Mol. Cancer Res.* **2014**, *12*, 1205–1215. [CrossRef] [PubMed]

41. Allegretti, M.; Ricciardi, M.R.; Licchetta, R.; Mirabilii, S.; Orecchioni, S.; Reggiani, F.; Talarico, G.; Foà, R.; Bertolini, F.; Amadori, S.; et al. The pan-class I phosphatidyl-inositol-3 kinase inhibitor NVP-BKM120 demonstrates anti-leukemic activity in acute myeloid leukemia. *Sci. Rep.* **2015**, *5*, 18137. [CrossRef] [PubMed]

42. Nepstad, I.; Reikvam, H.; Brenner, A.K.; Bruserud, Ø.; Hatfield, K.J. Resistance to the antiproliferative in vitro effect of PI3K-Akt-mTOR inhibition in primary human acute myeloid leukemia cells is associated with altered cell metabolism. *Int. J. Mol. Sci.* **2018**, *19*, 382. [CrossRef] [PubMed]

43. Asnaghi, L.; Calastretti, A.; Bevilacqua, A.; D'Agnano, I.; Gatti, G.; Canti, G.; Delia, D.; Capaccioli, S.; Nicolin, A. Bcl-2 phosphorylation and apoptosis activated by damaged microtubules require mTOR and are regulated by Akt. *Oncogene* **2004**, *23*, 5781–5791. [CrossRef] [PubMed]

44. Zeng, X.; Kinsella, T.J. Mammalian target of rapamycin and S6 kinase 1 positively regulate 6-thioguanine-induced autophagy. *Cancer Res.* **2008**, *68*, 2384–2390. [CrossRef] [PubMed]

45. Castedo, M.; Ferri, K.F.; Kroemer, G. Mammalian target of rapamycin (mTOR): Pro- and anti-apoptotic. *Cell Death Differ.* **2002**, *9*, 99–100. [CrossRef] [PubMed]

46. Hasty, P.; Sharp, Z.D.; Curiel, T.J.; Campisi, J. mTORC1 and p53: Clash of the gods? *Cell Cycle* **2013**, *12*, 20–25. [CrossRef] [PubMed]

47. Feng, Z.; Zhang, H.; Levine, A.J.; Jin, S. The coordinate regulation of the p53 and mTOR pathways in cells. *Proc. Natl. Acad. Sci. USA* **2005**, *102*, 8204–8209. [CrossRef] [PubMed]

48. Stambolic, V.; MacPherson, D.; Sas, D.; Lin, Y.; Snow, B.; Jang, Y.; Benchimol, S.; Mak, T.W. Regulation of PTEN transcription by p53. *Mol. Cell* **2001**, *8*, 317–325. [CrossRef]

49. Horton, L.E.; Bushell, M.; Barth-Baus, D.; Tilleray, V.J.; Clemens, M.J.; Hensold, J.O. p53 activation results in rapid dephosphorylation of the eIF4E-binding protein 4E-BP1, inhibition of ribosomal protein S6 kinase and inhibition of translation initiation. *Oncogene* **2002**, *21*, 5325–5334. [CrossRef] [PubMed]

50. Feng, Z.; Hu, W.; de Stanchina, E.; Teresky, A.K.; Jin, S.; Lowe, S.; Levine, A.J. The regulation of AMPK beta1, TSC2, and PTEN expression by p53: Stress, cell and tissue specificity, and the role of these gene products in modulating the IGF-1-AKT-mTOR pathways. *Cancer Res.* **2007**, *67*, 3043–3053. [CrossRef] [PubMed]

51. Budanov, A.V.; Karin, M. p53 target genes sestrin1 and sestrin2 connect genotoxic stress and mTOR signaling. *Cell* **2008**, *134*, 451–460. [CrossRef] [PubMed]

52. Oricchio, E.; Katanayeva, N.; Donaldson, M.C.; Sungalee, S.; Pasion, J.P.; Béguelin, W.; Battistello, E.; Sanghvi, V.R.; Jiang, M.; Jiang, Y.; et al. Genetic and epigenetic inactivation of SESTRIN1 controls mTORC1 and response to EZH2 inhibition in follicular lymphoma. *Sci. Transl. Med.* **2017**, *9*, eaak9969. [CrossRef] [PubMed]

53. Lai, K.P.; Leong, W.F.; Chau, J.F.; Jia, D.; Zeng, L.; Liu, H.; He, L.; Hao, A.; Zhang, H.; Meek, D.; et al. S6K1 is a multifaceted regulator of Mdm2 that connects nutrient status and DNA damage response. *EMBO J.* **2010**, *29*, 2994–3006. [CrossRef] [PubMed]

54. Liu, J.; Zhang, Y.; Liu, A.; Wang, J.; Li, L.; Chen, X.; Gao, X.; Xue, Y.; Zhang, X.; Liu, Y. Distinct dasatinib-induced mechanisms of apoptotic response and exosome release in imatinib-resistant human chronic myeloid leukemia cells. *Int. J. Mol. Sci.* **2016**, *17*, 531. [CrossRef] [PubMed]

55. Xu, Q.; Simpson, S.E.; Scialla, T.J.; Bagg, A.; Carroll, M. Survival of acute myeloid leukemia cells requires PI3 kinase activation. *Blood* **2003**, *102*, 972–980. [CrossRef] [PubMed]

56. Kornblau, S.M.; Womble, M.; Qiu, Y.H.; Jackson, C.E.; Chen, W.; Konopleva, M.; Estey, E.H.; Andreeff, M. Simultaneous activation of multiple signal transduction pathways confers poor prognosis in acute myelogenous leukemia. *Blood* **2006**, *108*, 2358–2365. [CrossRef] [PubMed]

57. Tamburini, J.; Chapuis, N.; Bardet, V.; Park, S.; Sujobert, P.; Willems, L.; Ifrah, N.; Dreyfus, F.; Mayeux, P.; Lacombe, C.; et al. Mammalian target of rapamycin (mTOR) inhibition activates phosphatidylinositol 3-kinase/Akt by up-regulating insulin-like growth factor-1 receptor signaling in acute myeloid leukemia: Rationale for therapeutic inhibition of both pathways. *Blood* **2008**, *111*, 379–382. [CrossRef] [PubMed]

58. Kojima, K.; Shimanuki, M.; Shikami, M.; Samudio, I.J.; Ruvolo, V.; Corn, P.; Hanaoka, N.; Konopleva, M.; Andreeff, M.; Nakakuma, H. The dual PI3 kinase/mTOR inhibitor PI-103 prevents p53 induction by Mdm2 inhibition but enhances p53-mediated mitochondrial apoptosis in p53 wild-type AML. *Leukemia* **2008**, *22*, 1728–1736. [CrossRef] [PubMed]

59. Guo, Y.; Li, Y.; Xiang, B.; Huang, X.O.; Ma, H.B.; Wang, F.F.; Gong, Y.P. Nutlin-3 plus tanshinone IIA exhibits synergetic anti-leukemia effect with imatinib by reactivating p53 and inhibiting the AKT/mTOR pathway in Ph+ ALL. *Biochem. J.* **2017**, *474*, 4153–4170. [CrossRef] [PubMed]

60. Asnaghi, L.; Bruno, P.; Priulla, M.; Nicolin, A. mTOR: A protein kinase switching between life and death. *Pharmacol. Res.* **2004**, *50*, 545–549. [CrossRef] [PubMed]

61. Rahmani, M.; Aust, M.M.; Attkisson, E.; Williams, D.C., Jr.; Ferreira-Gonzalez, A.; Grant, S. Dual inhibition of Bcl-2 and Bcl-xL strikingly enhances PI3K inhibition-induced apoptosis in human myeloid leukemia cells through a GSK3- and Bim-dependent mechanism. *Cancer Res.* **2013**, *73*, 1340–1351. [CrossRef] [PubMed]

62. Wei, G.; Twomey, D.; Lamb, J.; Schlis, K.; Agarwal, J.; Stam, R.W.; Opferman, J.T.; Sallan, S.E.; den Boer, M.L.; Pieters, R.; et al. Gene expression-based chemical genomics identifies rapamycin as a modulator of MCL1 and glucocorticoid resistance. *Cancer Cell* **2006**, *10*, 331–342. [CrossRef] [PubMed]

63. Spender, L.C.; Inman, G.J. Phosphoinositide 3-kinase/AKT/mTORC1/2 signaling determines sensitivity of Burkitt's lymphoma cells to BH3 mimetics. *Mol. Cancer Res.* **2012**, *10*, 347–359. [CrossRef] [PubMed]

64. Iacovelli, S.; Ricciardi, M.R.; Allegretti, M.; Mirabilii, S.; Licchetta, R.; Bergamo, P.; Rinaldo, C.; Zeuner, A.; Foà, R.; Milella, M.; et al. Co-targeting of Bcl-2 and mTOR pathway triggers synergistic apoptosis in BH3 mimetics resistant acute lymphoblastic leukemia. *Oncotarget* **2015**, *6*, 32089–32103. [CrossRef] [PubMed]

65. Rahmani, M.; Nkwocha, J.; Hawkins, E.; Pei, X.; Parker, R.E.; Kmieciak, M.; Leverson, J.D.; Sampath, D.; Ferreira-Gonzalez, A.; Grant, S. Cotargeting BCL-2 and PI3K Induces BAX-Dependent Mitochondrial Apoptosis in AML Cells. *Cancer Res.* **2018**, *78*, 3075–3086. [CrossRef] [PubMed]

66. Zeng, Z.; Liu, W.; Tsao, T.; Qiu, Y.; Zhao, Y.; Samudio, I.; Sarbassov, D.D.; Kornblau, S.M.; Baggerly, K.A.; Kantarjian, H.M.; et al. High-throughput profiling of signaling networks identifies mechanism-based combination therapy to eliminate microenvironmental resistance in acute myeloid leukemia. *Haematologica* **2017**, *102*, 1537–1548. [CrossRef] [PubMed]

67. Calastretti, A.; Bevilacqua, A.; Ceriani, C.; Viganò, S.; Zancai, P.; Capaccioli, S.; Nicolin, A. Damaged microtubules can inactivate BCL-2 by means of the mTOR kinase. *Oncogene* **2001**, *20*, 6172–6180. [CrossRef] [PubMed]

68. Calastretti, A.; Rancati, F.; Ceriani, M.C.; Asnaghi, L.; Canti, G.; Nicolin, A. Rapamycin increases the cellular concentration of the BCL-2 protein and exerts an anti-apoptotic effect. *Eur. J. Cancer* **2001**, *37*, 2121–2128. [CrossRef]

69. Hu, W.; Dooley, J.; Chung, S.S.; Chandramohan, D.; Cimmino, L.; Mukherjee, S.; Mason, C.E.; de Strooper, B.; Liston, A.; Park, C.Y. mir29a maintains mouse hematopoietic stem cell self-renewal by regulating Dnmt3a. *Blood* **2015**, *125*, 2206–2216. [CrossRef] [PubMed]

70. Lechman, E.R.; Gentner, B.; van Galen, P.; Giustacchini, A.; Saini, M.; Boccalatte, F.E.; Hiramatsu, H.; Restuccia, U.; Bachi, A.; Voisin, V.; et al. Attenuation of miR-126 activity expands HSC in vivo without exhaustion. *Cell Stem Cell* **2012**, *11*, 799–811. [CrossRef] [PubMed]

71. Metzeler, K.H.; Maharry, K.; Kohlschmidt, J.; Volinia, S.; Mrozek, K.; Becker, H.; Nicolet, D.; Whitman, S.P.; Mendler, J.H.; Schwind, S.; et al. A stem cell-like gene expression signature associates with inferior outcomes and a distinct microRNA expression profile in adults with primary cytogenetically normal acute myeloid leukemia. *Leukemia* **2013**, *27*, 2023–2031. [CrossRef] [PubMed]

72. Lechman, E.R.; Gentner, B.; Ng, S.W.; Schoof, E.M.; van Galen, P.; Kennedy, J.A.; Nucera, S.; Ciceri, F.; Kaufmann, K.B.; Takayama, N.; et al. miR-126 Regulates Distinct Self-Renewal Outcomes in Normal and Malignant Hematopoietic Stem Cells. *Cancer Cell* **2016**, *29*, 214–228. [CrossRef] [PubMed]

73. Marcais, A.; Blevins, R.; Graumann, J.; Feytout, A.; Dharmalingam, G.; Carroll, T.; Amado, I.F.; Bruno, L.; Lee, K.; Walzer, T.; et al. microRNA-mediated regulation of mTOR complex components facilitates discrimination between activation and anergy in CD4 T cells. *J. Exp. Med.* **2014**, *211*, 2281–2295. [CrossRef] [PubMed]

74. Li, X.J.; Luo, X.Q.; Han, B.W.; Duan, F.T.; Wei, P.P.; Chen, Y.Q. MicroRNA-100/99a, deregulated in acute lymphoblastic leukaemia, suppress proliferation and promote apoptosis by regulating the FKBP51 and IGF1R/mTOR signalling pathways. *Br. J. Cancer* **2013**, *109*, 2189–2198. [CrossRef] [PubMed]

75. Palacios, F.; Abreu, C.; Prieto, D.; Morande, P.; Ruiz, S.; Fernández-Calero, T.; Naya, H.; Libisch, G.; Robello, C.; Landoni, A.I.; et al. Activation of the PI3K/AKT pathway by microRNA-22 results in CLL B-cell proliferation. *Leukemia* **2015**, *29*, 115–125. [CrossRef] [PubMed]

76. Yuan, T.; Yang, Y.; Chen, J.; Li, W.; Li, W.; Zhang, Q.; Mi, Y.; Goswami, R.S.; You, J.Q.; Lin, D.; et al. Regulation of PI3K signaling in T-cell acute lymphoblastic leukemia: A novel PTEN/Ikaros/miR-26b mechanism reveals a critical targetable role for PIK3CD. *Leukemia* **2017**, *31*, 2355–2364. [CrossRef] [PubMed]

77. Fang, Z.H.; Wang, S.L.; Zhao, J.T.; Lin, Z.J.; Chen, L.Y.; Su, R.; Xie, S.T.; Carter, B.Z.; Xu, B. miR-150 exerts antileukemia activity in vitro and in vivo through regulating genes in multiple pathways. *Cell Death Dis.* **2016**, *7*, e2371. [CrossRef] [PubMed]

78. Li, Y.; Gao, L.; Luo, X.; Wang, L.; Gao, X.; Wang, W.; Sun, J.; Dou, L.; Li, J.; Xu, C.; et al. Epigenetic silencing of microRNA-193a contributes to leukemogenesis in t(8;21) acute myeloid leukemia by activating the PTEN/PI3K signal pathway. *Blood* **2013**, *121*, 499–509. [CrossRef] [PubMed]

79. Jia, C.Y.; Li, H.H.; Zhu, X.C.; Dong, Y.W.; Fu, D.; Zhao, Q.L.; Wu, W.; Wu, X.Z. MiR-223 suppresses cell proliferation by targeting IGF-1R. *PLoS ONE* **2011**, *6*, e27008. [CrossRef] [PubMed]

80. Garzon, R.; Heaphy, C.E.; Havelange, V.; Fabbri, M.; Volinia, S.; Tsao, T.; Zanesi, N.; Kornblau, S.M.; Marcucci, G.; Calin, G.A.; et al. MicroRNA 29b functions in acute myeloid leukemia. *Blood* **2009**, *114*, 5331–5341. [CrossRef] [PubMed]

81. Pekarsky, Y.; Santanam, U.; Cimmino, A.; Palamarchuk, A.; Efanov, A.; Maximov, V.; Volinia, S.; Alder, H.; Liu, C.G.; Rassenti, L.; et al. Tcl1 expression in chronic lymphocytic leukemia is regulated by miR-29 and miR-181. *Cancer Res.* **2006**, *66*, 11590–11593. [CrossRef] [PubMed]

82. Zimmerman, E.I.; Dollins, C.M.; Crawford, M.; Grant, S.; Nana-Sinkam, S.P.; Richards, K.L.; Hammond, S.M.; Graves, L.M. Lyn kinase-dependent regulation of miR181 and myeloid cell leukemia-1 expression: Implications for drug resistance in myelogenous leukemia. *Mol. Pharmacol.* **2010**, *78*, 811–817. [CrossRef] [PubMed]

83. Bertacchini, J.; Heidari, N.; Mediani, L.; Capitani, S.; Shahjahani, M.; Ahmadzadeh, A.; Saki, N. Targeting PI3K/AKT/mTOR network for treatment of leukemia. *Cell Mol. Life Sci.* **2015**, *72*, 2337–2347. [CrossRef] [PubMed]

84. Vézina, C.; Kudelski, A.; Sehgal, S.N. Rapamycin (AY-22,989), a new antifungal antibiotic. I. Taxonomy of the producing streptomycete and isolation of the active principle. *J. Antibiot.* **1975**, *28*, 721–726. [CrossRef] [PubMed]

85. Yatscoff, R.W.; LeGatt, D.F.; Kneteman, N.M. Therapeutic monitoring of rapamycin: A new immunosuppressive drug. *Ther. Drug Monit.* **1993**, *15*, 478–482. [CrossRef] [PubMed]

86. Guertin, D.A.; Sabatini, D.M. Defining the role of mTOR in cancer. *Cancer Cell* **2007**, *12*, 9–22. [CrossRef] [PubMed]

87. Ballou, L.M.; Lin, R.Z. Rapamycin and mTOR kinase inhibitors. *J. Chem. Biol.* **2008**, *1*, 27–36. [CrossRef] [PubMed]

88. Feldman, M.E.; Apsel, B.; Uotila, A.; Loewith, R.; Knight, Z.A.; Ruggero, D.; Shokat, K.M. Active-site inhibitors of mTOR target rapamycin-resistant outputs of mTORC1 and mTORC2. *PLoS Biol.* **2009**, *7*, e1000038. [CrossRef] [PubMed]

89. Calimeri, T.; Ferreri, A.J.M. m-TOR inhibitors and their potential role in haematological malignancies. *Br. J. Haematol.* **2017**, *177*, 684–702. [CrossRef] [PubMed]

90. Naing, A.; Aghajanian, C.; Raymond, E.; Olmos, D.; Schwartz, G.; Oelmann, E.; Grinsted, L.; Burke, W.; Taylor, R.; Kaye, S.; et al. Safety, tolerability, pharmacokinetics and pharmacodynamics of AZD8055 in advanced solid tumours and lymphoma. *Br. J. Cancer* **2012**, *107*, 1093–1099. [CrossRef] [PubMed]

91. Bendell, J.C.; Kelley, R.K.; Shih, K.C.; Grabowsky, J.A.; Bergsland, E.; Jones, S.; Martin, T.; Infante, J.R.; Mischel, P.S.; Matsutani, T.; et al. A phase I dose-escalation study to assess safety, tolerability, pharmacokinetics, and preliminary efficacy of the dual mTORC1/mTORC2 kinase inhibitor CC-223 in patients with advanced solid tumors or multiple myeloma. *Cancer* **2015**, *121*, 3481–3490. [CrossRef] [PubMed]

92. Ghobrial, I.M.; Siegel, D.S.; Vij, R.; Berdeja, J.G.; Richardson, P.G.; Neuwirth, R.; Patel, C.G.; Zohren, F.; Wolf, J.L. TAK-228 (formerly MLN0128), an investigational oral dual TORC1/2 inhibitor: A phase I dose escalation study in patients with relapsed or refractory multiple myeloma, non-Hodgkin lymphoma, or Waldenström's macroglobulinemia. *Am. J. Hematol.* **2016**, *91*, 400–405. [CrossRef] [PubMed]

93. Wallin, J.J.; Edgar, K.A.; Guan, J.; Berry, M.; Prior, W.W.; Lee, L.; Lesnick, J.D.; Lewis, C.; Nonomiya, J.; Pang, J.; et al. GDC-0980 is a novel class I PI3K/mTOR kinase inhibitor with robust activity in cancer models driven by the PI3K pathway. *Mol. Cancer Ther.* **2011**, *10*, 2426–2436. [CrossRef] [PubMed]

94. Wunderle, L.; Badura, S.; Lang, F.; Wolf, A.; Schleyer, E.; Serve, H.; Goekbuget, N.; Pfeifer, H.; Bug, G. Safety and efficacy of BEZ235, a dual PI3-Kinase/mTOR inhibitor, in adult patients with relapsed or refractory acute leukemia: Results of a phase I study. *Blood* **2013**, *122*, 2675.

95. Min, Y.H.; Eom, J.I.; Cheong, J.W.; Maeng, H.O.; Kim, J.Y.; Jeung, H.K.; Lee, S.T.; Lee, M.H.; Hahn, J.S.; Ko, Y.W. Constitutive phosphorylation of Akt/PKB protein in acute myeloid leukemia: Its significance as a prognostic variable. *Leukemia* **2003**, *17*, 995–997. [CrossRef] [PubMed]

96. Reikvam, H.; Tamburini, J.; Skrede, S.; Holdhus, R.; Poulain, L.; Ersvaer, E.; Hatfield, K.J.; Bruserud, Ø. Antileukaemic effect of PI3K-mTOR inhibitors in acute myeloid leukaemia-gene expression profiles reveal CDC25B expression as determinate of pharmacological effect. *Br. J. Haematol.* **2014**, *164*, 200–211. [CrossRef] [PubMed]

97. Boutros, R.; Lobjois, V.; Ducommun, B. CDC25 phosphatases in cancer cells: Key players? Good targets? *Nat. Rev. Cancer* **2007**, *7*, 495–507. [CrossRef] [PubMed]

98. Nepstad, I.; Hatfield, K.J.; Aasebø, E.; Hernandez-Valladares, M.; Brenner, A.K.; Bartaula-Brevik, S.; Berven, F.; Selheim, F.; Skavland, J.; Gjertsen, B.T.; et al. Two acute myeloid leukemia patient subsets are identified based on the constitutive PI3K-Akt-mTOR signaling of their leukemic cells; a functional, proteomic, and transcriptomic comparison. *Expert Opin. Ther. Targets* **2018**, *22*, 639–653. [CrossRef] [PubMed]

99. Brenner, A.K.; Andersson Tvedt, T.H.; Bruserud, Ø. The Complexity of Targeting PI3K-Akt-mTOR Signalling in Human Acute Myeloid Leukaemia: The Importance of Leukemic Cell Heterogeneity, Neighbouring Mesenchymal Stem Cells and Immunocompetent Cells. *Molecules* **2016**, *21*, 1512. [CrossRef] [PubMed]

100. Duarte, D.; Hawkins, E.D.; Lo Celso, C. The interplay of leukemia cells and the bone marrow microenvironment. *Blood* **2018**, *131*, 1507–1511. [CrossRef] [PubMed]

101. Reikvam, H.; Nepstad, I.; Bruserud, Ø.; Hatfield, K.J. Pharmacological targeting of the PI3K/mTOR pathway alters the release of angioregulatory mediators both from primary human acute myeloid leukemia cells and their neighboring stromal cells. *Oncotarget* **2013**, *4*, 830–843. [CrossRef] [PubMed]

102. Récher, C.; Beyne-Rauzy, O.; Demur, C.; Chicanne, G.; Dos Santos, C.; Mas, V.M.; Benzaquen, D.; Laurent, G.; Huguet, F.; Payrastre, B. Antileukemic activity of rapamycin in acute myeloid leukemia. *Blood* **2005**, *105*, 2527–2534. [CrossRef] [PubMed]

103. Perl, A.E.; Kasner, M.T.; Tsai, D.E.; Vogl, D.T.; Loren, A.W.; Schuster, S.J.; Porter, D.L.; Stadtmauer, E.A.; Goldstein, S.C.; Frey, N.V.; et al. A phase I study of the mammalian target of rapamycin inhibitor sirolimus

and MEC chemotherapy in relapsed and refractory acute myelogenous leukemia. *Clin. Cancer Res.* **2009**, *15*, 6732–6739. [CrossRef] [PubMed]

104. Wei, A.H.; Sadawarte, S.; Catalano, J.; Hills, R.; Avery, S.; Patil, S.S.; Burnett, A.; Spencer, A. Phase Ib study combining the mTOR inhibitor everolimus (RAD001) with low-dose cytarabine in untreated elderly AML. *Blood* **2010**, *116*, 3299.

105. Amadori, S.; Stasi, R.; Martelli, A.M.; Venditti, A.; Meloni, G.; Pane, F.; Martinelli, G.; Lunghi, M.; Pagano, L.; Cilloni, D.; et al. Temsirolimus, an mTOR inhibitor, in combination with lower-dose clofarabine as salvage therapy for older patients with acute myeloid leukaemia: Results of a phase II GIMEMA study (AML-1107). *Br. J. Haematol.* **2012**, *156*, 205–212. [CrossRef] [PubMed]

106. Scholl, S.; Bondeva, T.; Liu, Y.; Clement, J.H.; Höffken, K.; Wetzker, R. Additive effects of PI3-kinase and MAPK activities on NB4 cell granulocyte differentiation: Potential role of phosphatidylinositol 3-kinase gamma. *J. Cancer Res. Clin. Oncol.* **2008**, *134*, 861–872. [CrossRef] [PubMed]

107. Ozpolat, B.; Akar, U.; Steiner, M.; Zorrilla-Calancha, I.; Tirado-Gomez, M.; Colburn, N.; Danilenko, M.; Kornblau, S.; Berestein, G.L. Programmed cell death-4 tumor suppressor protein contributes to retinoic acid-induced terminal granulocytic differentiation of human myeloid leukemia cells. *Mol. Cancer Res.* **2007**, *5*, 95–108. [CrossRef] [PubMed]

108. Messina, M.; Chiaretti, S.; Wang, J.; Fedullo, A.L.; Peragine, N.; Gianfelici, V.; Piciocchi, A.; Brugnoletti, F.; Di Giacomo, F.; Pauselli, S.; et al. Prognostic and therapeutic role of targetable lesions in B-lineage acute lymphoblastic leukemia without recurrent fusion genes. *Oncotarget* **2016**, *7*, 13886–13901. [CrossRef] [PubMed]

109. Xing, H.; Yang, X.; Liu, T.; Lin, J.; Chen, X.; Gong, Y. The study of resistant mechanisms and reversal in an imatinib resistant Ph+ acute lymphoblastic leukemia cell line. *Leuk. Res.* **2012**, *36*, 509–513. [CrossRef] [PubMed]

110. Gianfelici, V.; Chiaretti, S.; Demeyer, S.; Di Giacomo, F.; Messina, M.; La Starza, R.; Peragine, N.; Paoloni, F.; Geerdens, E.; Pierini, V.; et al. RNA sequencing unravels the genetics of refractory/relapsed T-cell acute lymphoblastic leukemia. Prognostic and therapeutic implications. *Haematologica* **2016**, *101*, 941–950. [CrossRef] [PubMed]

111. Zhang, C.; Ryu, Y.K.; Chen, T.Z.; Hall, C.P.; Webster, D.R.; Kang, M.H. Synergistic activity of rapamycin and dexamethasone in vitro and in vivo in acute lymphoblastic leukemia via cell-cycle arrest and apoptosis. *Leuk. Res.* **2012**, *36*, 342–349. [CrossRef] [PubMed]

112. Bressanin, D.; Evangelisti, C.; Ricci, F.; Tabellini, G.; Chiarini, F.; Tazzari, P.L.; Melchionda, F.; Buontempo, F.; Pagliaro, P.; Pession, A.; et al. Harnessing the PI3K/Akt/mTOR pathway in T-cell acute lymphoblastic leukemia: Eliminating activity by targeting at different levels. *Oncotarget* **2012**, *3*, 811–823. [CrossRef] [PubMed]

113. Palomero, T.; Sulis, M.L.; Cortina, M.; Real, P.J.; Barnes, K.; Ciofani, M.; Caparros, E.; Buteau, J.; Brown, K.; Perkins, S.L.; et al. Mutational loss of PTEN induces resistance to NOTCH1 inhibition in T-cell leukemia. *Nat. Med.* **2007**, *13*, 1203–1210. [CrossRef] [PubMed]

114. Airiau, K.; Mahon, F.X.; Josselin, M.; Jeanneteau, M.; Belloc, F. PI3K/mTOR pathway inhibitors sensitize chronic myeloid leukemia stem cells to nilotinib and restore the response of progenitors to nilotinib in the presence of stem cell factor. *Cell Death Dis.* **2013**, *4*, e827. [CrossRef] [PubMed]

115. Pellicano, F.; Scott, M.T.; Helgason, G.V.; Hopcroft, L.E.; Allan, E.K.; Aspinall-O'Dea, M.; Copland, M.; Pierce, A.; Huntly, B.J.; Whetton, A.D.; et al. The antiproliferative activity of kinase inhibitors in chronic myeloid leukemia cells is mediated by FOXO transcription factors. *Stem Cells* **2014**, *32*, 2324–2337. [CrossRef] [PubMed]

116. Banerjee Mustafi, S.; Chakraborty, P.K.; Raha, S. Modulation of Akt and ERK1/2 pathways by resveratrol in chronic myelogenous leukemia (CML) cells results in the downregulation of Hsp70. *PLoS ONE* **2010**, *5*, e8719. [CrossRef] [PubMed]

117. Huang, F.F.; Zhang, L.; Wu, D.S.; Yuan, X.Y.; Yu, Y.H.; Zhao, X.L.; Chen, F.P.; Zeng, H. PTEN regulates BCRP/ABCG2 and the side population through the PI3K/Akt pathway in chronic myeloid leukemia. *PLoS ONE* **2014**, *9*, e88298. [CrossRef] [PubMed]

118. Boddu, P.; Ferrajoli, A. Prognostic Factors in the Era of Targeted Therapies in CLL. *Curr. Hematol. Malig. Rep.* **2018**, *13*, 78–90. [CrossRef] [PubMed]

119. Kipps, T.J.; Stevenson, F.K.; Wu, C.J.; Croce, C.M.; Packham, G.; Wierda, W.G.; O'Brien, S.; Gribben, J.; Rai, K. Chronic lymphocytic leukaemia. *Nat. Rev. Dis. Primers* **2017**, *3*, 16096. [CrossRef] [PubMed]
120. Thijssen, R.; Ter Burg, J.; Garrick, B.; van Bochove, G.G.; Brown, J.R.; Fernandes, S.M.; Rodríguez, M.S.; Michot, J.M.; Hallek, M.; Eichhorst, B.; et al. Dual TORK/DNA-PK inhibition blocks critical signaling pathways in chronic lymphocytic leukemia. *Blood* **2016**, *128*, 574–583. [CrossRef] [PubMed]

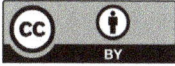

International Journal of
Molecular Sciences

MDPI

Review

Therapeutic Targeting of mTOR in T-Cell Acute Lymphoblastic Leukemia: An Update

Camilla Evangelisti [1,2], Francesca Chiarini [1,2], James A. McCubrey [3,*] and Alberto M. Martelli [4,*]

1   CNR Istituto di Genetica Molecolare, Unità di Bologna, 40136 Bologna, Italy; camilla.evangelisti@cnr.it (C.E.); francesca.chiarini@cnr.it (F.C.)
2   Istituto Ortopedico Rizzoli, 40136 Bologna, Italy
3   Department of Microbiology & Immunology, Brody School of Medicine, East Carolina University, Greenville, NC 27834, USA
4   Department of Biomedical and Neuromotor Sciences, University of Bologna, 40126 Bologna, Italy
*   Correspondence: mccubreyj@ecu.edu (J.A.M.); alberto.martelli@unibo.it (A.M.M.);
     Tel.: +39-051-209-1580 (A.M.M.)

Received: 13 June 2018; Accepted: 24 June 2018; Published: 26 June 2018

Abstract: T-cell acute lymphoblastic leukemia (T-ALL) is an aggressive blood malignancy that arises from the clonal expansion of transformed T-cell precursors. Although T-ALL prognosis has significantly improved due to the development of intensive chemotherapeutic protocols, primary drug-resistant and relapsed patients still display a dismal outcome. In addition, lifelong irreversible late effects from conventional therapy are a growing problem for leukemia survivors. Therefore, novel targeted therapies are required to improve the prognosis of high-risk patients. The mechanistic target of rapamycin (mTOR) is the kinase subunit of two structurally and functionally distinct multiprotein complexes, which are referred to as mTOR complex 1 (mTORC1) and mTORC2. These two complexes regulate a variety of physiological cellular processes including protein, lipid, and nucleotide synthesis, as well as autophagy in response to external cues. However, mTOR activity is frequently deregulated in cancer, where it plays a key oncogenetic role driving tumor cell proliferation, survival, metabolic transformation, and metastatic potential. Promising preclinical studies using mTOR inhibitors have demonstrated efficacy in many human cancer types, including T-ALL. Here, we highlight our current knowledge of mTOR signaling and inhibitors in T-ALL, with an emphasis on emerging evidence of the superior efficacy of combinations consisting of mTOR inhibitors and either traditional or targeted therapeutics.

Keywords: mTOR; T-cell acute lymphoblastic leukemia; targeted therapy; combination therapy

1. Introduction

T-cell acute lymphoblastic leukemia (T-ALL) is an aggressive disease that represents 10–15% of ALL cases in children and up to 25% in adults [1,2]. T-ALL is a genetically heterogeneous disorder caused by the accumulation of molecular alterations acting in a multistep pathogenic process [3]. While ≥80% of pediatric patients with T-ALL can expect to be cured [4], among adults younger than 60 years treated with conventional chemotherapy, the survival rates are in the range of 40–50%, and older patients have a much worse prognosis [5]. Although the use of high-dose multiagent chemotherapy results in a survival advantage, many patients still relapse and eventually experience refractory leukemia, which is associated with a poor likelihood of survival [5]. For example, only 20% of relapsed pediatric patients can be cured with current salvage protocols [6]. Moreover, especially childhood T-ALL survivors are at increased risk of developing long-term adverse health outcomes, including secondary malignancies due to the use of genotoxic drugs [7]. Therefore, novel, more effective and less toxic treatments are desired to improve the outcome of T-ALL patients, as well as their quality of life both during and after therapy.

Our increased knowledge of genetic alterations has significantly contributed to identify oncogenetic drivers and signaling cascades regulating T-ALL pathophysiology. This has opened the possibility of targeting pathways that are critical to prevent and/or treat relapse [8]. The mechanistic target of rapamycin (mTOR) is a key effector of signaling networks that are aberrantly regulated in T-ALL and negatively affect patient outcome [9]. In this context, it is also important to emphasize that very recent evidence has demonstrated that high mTOR expression is an independent negative prognosticator of clinical outcome to induction chemotherapy in T-ALL patients [10].

Here, we summarize and discuss recent advances in understanding and targeting mTOR in T-ALL settings with the aim of highlighting possible less toxic therapeutic strategies for improving the outcome of chemoresistant/refractory patients.

2. mTOR and Its Complexes: Structure, Activation, and Functions

mTOR is a 289-kDa protein encoded in humans by the *MTOR* gene mapping to chromosomal band 1p36.2 [11]. mTOR is an evolutionary conserved member of the phosphatidylinositol 3-kinase (PI3K)-related kinase (PIKK) family of protein kinases [12], and acts as the catalytic subunit of two large multiprotein complexes, which are referred to as mTOR complex 1 (mTORC1) and mTORC2. These complexes share some components, which include Tel2-interacting protein 1 (Tti1)/Tel2 complex, Dishevelled, Egl-10 and Pleckstrin (DEP) domain-containing mTOR-interacting protein (Deptor), and mammalian lethal with SEC13 protein 8 (mLST8) [13]. mTORC1 is defined by the association of mTOR with the regulatory-associated protein of mTOR (Raptor), which is a protein that is fundamental for mTORC1 assembly, stability, regulation, and substrate specificity [14]. Moreover, mTORC1 comprises proline-rich Akt substrate 1 40 kDa (PRAS40), which blocks mTORC1 activity until growth factor receptor signaling unlocks PRAS40-mediated mTORC1 inhibition [15]. The activation of mTORC1 is achieved by growth factors, cytokines, hormones, amino acids, high energy levels, and oxygen through multiple mechanisms. In contrast, intracellular and environmental stresses (low ATP levels, hypoxia, DNA damage) are powerful repressors of mTORC1 activity [13] (Figure 1). For the scope of this article, it is important to emphasize that growth factors, such as insulin-like growth factor-1 (IGF-1) or cytokines [interleukin (IL) 7, for example] activate PI3K. PI3K generates at the plasma membrane phosphatidylinositol 3,4,5 trisphosphate (PIP3) from phosphatidylinositol 4,5 bisphosphate (PIP2). PIP3 recruits to the plasma membrane phosphoinositide-dependent kinase 1 (PDK1) and Akt that is phosphorylated by PDK1 at Thr308 [16]. Akt phosphorylates tuberous sclerosis complex 2 (TSC2) at Thr1462 [17]. TSC2 is a GTPase activating protein (GAP) that functions in association with TSC1 to lock the small G-protein, RAS homolog enriched in brain (Rheb) in a GDP-bound, inactive state. Akt-mediated TSC1/TSC2 complex inhibition consequently allows Rheb to accumulate in a GTP-bound state, whereby Rheb-GTP binds and activates mTORC1 [18]. Moreover, Akt phosphorylates the mTORC1 inhibitor PRAS40 at Thr246. This phosphorylation causes PRAS40 dissociation from Raptor, allowing mTORC1 activation [19]. Also, the rat sarcoma (RAS)/rapidly accelerated fibrosarcoma (Raf)/mitogen-activated protein kinase (MEK)/extracellular signal-regulated kinase (ERK)/p90 ribosomal S6 kinase 1 (p90RSK1) cascade impinges on mTORC1, as both ERK and p90RSK1 phosphorylate TSC2 (at Ser664 and Ser1798, respectively), thereby inhibiting the TSC1/TSC2 complex and triggering Rheb-dependent mTORC1 activation [20]. Moreover, p90RSK1 can phosphorylate Raptor, causing mTORC1 activation [21]. As to the functions of mTORC1, they include the upregulation of cap-dependent and cap-independent translation, increased glycolysis, enhanced lipid and nucleotide synthesis, as well as positive regulation of ribosome biogenesis through the RNA polymerase (Pol) I-dependent and Pol III-dependent transcription of the different classes of ribosomal RNAs [13,22,23]. In contrast, mTORC1 is a repressor of autophagy [24] (Figure 1).

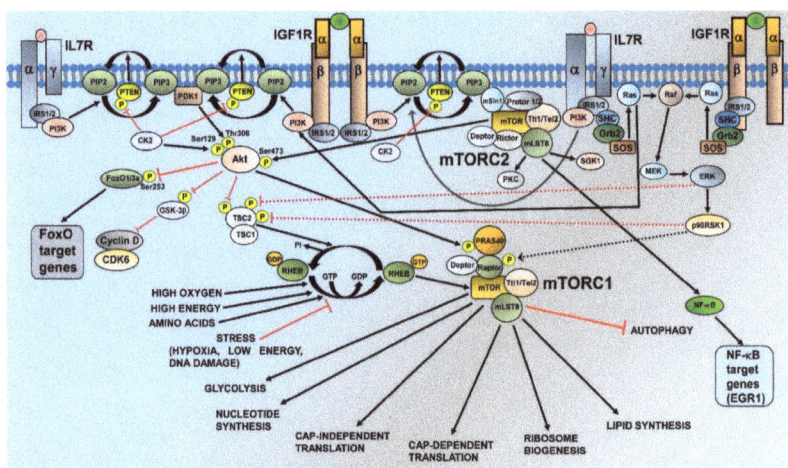

Figure 1. Regulation and functions of mechanistic target of rapamycin complex 1 (mTORC1) and mTORC2. For details, see the text. Black arrows indicate stimulatory events, while red lines indicate inhibitory events.

mTORC2 is characterized by the interactions of mTOR with the rapamycin independent companion of mTOR (Rictor), mammalian stress-activated protein kinase interacting protein 1 (mSin1), and protein observed with rictor (Protor) 1 or 2 [13]. Rictor is necessary for mTORC2 assembly, stability, and substrate interactions [25], while mSin1 is a repressor of mTORC2 kinase activity [26]. Nevertheless, it also drives mTORC2 localization to the plasma membrane, where Sin1-mediated mTORC2 inhibition is relieved in response to the growth factor receptor-dependent activation of PI3K [27]. Regarding Protor1, it may be involved in enabling mTORC2 to phosphorylate serum and glucocorticoid-activated kinase 1 (SGK1) [28]. In contrast to mTORC1, our knowledge of the control of mTORC2 activity is limited. However, recent evidence has highlighted that plasma membrane localization is a critical aspect of mTORC2 regulation. Indeed, the pleckstrin homology (PH) domain of mSin1 interacts with the mTOR kinase domain to restrain mTOR activity. PIP3, which is synthesized by PI3K at the cell membrane, binds mSin1-PH to release its inhibition on mTOR, thereby triggering mTORC2 activation [27].

As for the roles of mTORC2, this complex phosphorylates several members of the AGC family of protein kinases [29]. These include protein kinase C (PKC) isoforms $\alpha/\gamma/\delta/\epsilon/\zeta$ and SGK1 [13] (Figure 1). However, the most important and best known function of mTORC2 is the phosphorylation of Akt at Ser473, which fully activates the kinase activity of Akt [30]. Ser473 phosphorylation is required for Akt-mediated phosphorylation of Forkhead box O1/3a (FoxO1/3a) trascription factors, but not for that of other Akt targets, such as TSC2 and glycogen synthase kinase3β (GSK3β) [26]. In light of its substrates, mTORC2 is mainly involved in the control of cytoskeletal remodeling, cell migration, proliferation, and survival [13]. Nevertheless, it has been recently demonstrated that mTORC2 is a repressor of chaperone-mediated autophagy [31]. Furthermore, mTORC2 increases lipid synthesis, whereby promoting carcinogenesis [32].

3. Activation of mTORC1 and mTORC2 in T-ALL Cells

We will now review the multiple mechanisms that explain why the activities of both mTORC1 and mTORC2 are aberrantly regulated in T-ALL.

3.1. Phosphatase and Tensin Deleted on Chromsome 10

Compelling evidence indicates that phosphatase and tensin deleted on chromosome 10 (PTEN), which is the main negative regulator of the PI3K/Akt/mTOR cascade [33–35], plays a key role in the activation of this pathway in T-ALL cells [36]. PTEN dephosphorylates PIP3, thus yielding PIP2 and blunting PI3K activity (Figure 1). However, the gene encoding for PTEN is frequently either deleted or mutated in human T-ALL cell lines and primary samples [37], resulting in PI3K/Akt/mTOR upregulation. Interestingly, a very recent retrospective study has demonstrated that PTEN mutations, when combined with additional genetic anomalies (NOTCH1, FBXW7, and RAS mutations) and a high white blood cell count, were associated with a higher risk of relapse in childhood T-ALL [38].

Moreover, even when expressed in its wild-type form, PTEN is phosphorylated at a cluster of residues (Ser380/Thr382/Ser385) in the C-terminal, resulting in the downregulation of PTEN lipid phosphatase activity and high PIP3 levels [39]. Casein kinase 2 (CK2), which is overexpressed in T-ALL [40], has been identified as the kinase responsible for PTEN phosphorylation and inactivation in leukemic cells [41]. Furthermore, CK2 phosphorylates Akt at Ser129 (Figure 1). This phosphorylation positively contributes to Akt activity and increases Akt association with the chaperone protein heat shock protein 90 (HSP90), thus protecting Akt from protein phosphatase 2A (PP2A) activity at Thr308 [42]. However, PTEN is also a target of neurogenic locus notch homolog protein 1 (NOTCH1) signaling, as we will see later on in this article.

Apart from controlling PIP3 levels, PTEN induces miR-26b expression by regulating the differential expression of the Ikaros transcription factor isoforms that are upstream of miR-26b [43]. Accordingly, the levels of miR-26b were lower in PTEN-deficient mouse and human T-ALL cells. Intriguingly, it was shown that miR-26b negatively controls the expression of PI3K p110δ, which is a PI3K catalytic subunit important for PIP3 generation in T-ALL [43–45]. The overexpression of miR-26b decreased Ser473 p-Akt levels (which is indicative of mTORC2 inhibition), while either shRNA to PI3K p110δ or a PI3K p110δ-selective inhibitor (CAL-101) reduced the viability of T-ALL cell lines [43]. Overall, these findings highlighted a novel mechanism through which PTEN deficiency could result in a further increase in PI3K/Akt/mTOR signaling independently from PTEN lipid phosphatase activity.

3.2. NOTCH1 Signaling

NOTCH1 is a key oncogenetic driver of T-ALL, and NOTCH1 activating mutations occur in ≥50% of T-ALL patients [46]. Hairy and enhancer of split-1 (HES1) transcription factor, which is downstream of NOTCH1, represses PTEN expression and contributes to enhancing PI3K/AKT/mTOR signaling in NOTCH1-dependent T-ALL [47]. Furthermore, the NOTCH1/HES1 axis is somehow responsible for decreased PP2A activity on Thr308 and Ser473 p-Akt, resulting in the activation of downstream effectors, including mTORC1 [48].

Additional NOTCH1-dependent mechanisms that contribute to decreased PTEN levels have been identified. PTEN can be targeted and downregulated by miR-19 [49] or c-Myelocytomatosis oncogene protein (c-Myc) [50]. Moreover, NOTCH1 could control mTORC1 signaling through yet another mechanism, as documented by a study in which the treatment of T-ALL cell lines with a γ-secretase inhibitor (GSI) targeting NOTCH1 resulted in the dephosphorylation of mTORC1 downstream targets, including eukaryotic translation initiation factor 4E-binding protein 1 (4E-BP1), p70 S6 ribosomal protein kinase 1 (p70S6K1), and S6 ribosomal protein (S6RP), independently of PI3K/Akt activity. These effects on mTORC1 could be rescued by expression of the intracellular domain of NOTCH1 (ICN1) and mimicked by dominant negative mastermind-like transcriptional coactivator 1 (MAML1), which is a NOTCH1 regulator [51]. Furthermore, the expression of c-Myc opposed GSI-induced mTORC1 inhibition, thus implicating c-Myc as an intermediary between NOTCH1 and mTORC1 [51]. This observation could be related to c-Myc being a transcriptional repressor of TSC2; hence, high levels of c-Myc could result in upregulated mTORC1 activity, independently from PI3K/Akt [52].

Besides mTORC1, NOTCH1 has been proposed to somehow regulate mTORC2 activity as well, at least in a murine model of T-ALL, where hematopoietic bone marrow precursors were transduced to express ICN1 and transplanted into recipient mice [53]. Animals that received cells with Rictor conditional knockout showed at most a modest decrease in bone marrow and circulating leukemic cells. However, the median survival of these animals almost doubled when donor marrow was programmed to delete Rictor; moreover, the mice displayed decreased organ (lung, kidney, liver) invasion by ICN1-driven leukemic cells. Intriguingly, the expression of Nuclear factor κ-light-chain-enhancer of activated B cells (NF-κB) target genes (Bcl2a1, Nfkb2, and CCR7) was significantly decreased in the Rictor-depleted circulating T-ALL cells, whereas selected FoxO1/3 target genes (Il7ra, Sell, and S1p1) were not [53]. In this context, it is important to emphasize that C-C chemokine receptor type 7 (CCR7) has been shown to act as an important determinant of NOTCH1-driven T-ALL pathogenesis and death because of its critical role in regulating the trafficking of the leukemic cells into tissues [54]. Therefore, this study provided evidence that mTORC2 is an important determinant of the capacity of active NOTCH1 to induce NF-κB activity and CCR7 expression (most likely through Akt phosphorylation at Ser473 [55]), as well as accelerated tissue invasion and death in a murine T-ALL model. Nevertheless, a different group demonstrated that, in a NOTCH1-driven murine model of T-ALL, Rictor deletion—hence, mTORC2 inactivation—affected the activity of FoxO transcription factors as well. Indeed, in mice where Rictor expression was genetically suppressed, leukemia progression was hampered by a slower cell proliferation and decreased infiltration of organs such as the lung, liver, and kidney. This was accompanied by decreased phosphorylation of Ser473 p-Akt and Ser253 p-FoxO3a, as well as by increased expression of FoxO3a target genes (Figure 1), including those encoding for negative regulators of cell cycle progression, such as p21^{Cip1} and p27^{Kip1}. In contrast, the expression levels of positive regulators of cell cycle, cyclin-dependent kinase (CDK) 1 and 4, were decreased in Rictor-deleted T-ALL cells [56]. Moreover, this study documented that the absence of Rictor led to the overexpression of chemotaxis-related proteins, such as CCR2, CCR4, and C-X-C chemokine receptor (CXCR) 4, which most likely contributed to increased migration and the homing of Rictor-deficient T-ALL cells to the spleen, whereas migration to bone marrow was negatively affected. However, FoxO3a downregulation by shRNA did not affect the migration of T-ALL cells, suggesting a different type of control [56], although previous studies had documented that FoxO transcription factors are somehow involved in CXCR4 expression [57].

Overall, the results by Lee et al. [53] and Hua et al. [56] support the concept that in murine NOTCH1-mutated T-ALL models, mTORC2 is a critical regulator of leukemia progression that impacts a variety of genes targeted by both NFκB and FoxO3a.

Deptor has been identified as an mTORC1/mTORC2 component that is under the control of NOTCH1, as NOTCH1 directly binds to and activates Deptor promoter in T-ALL cells [58]. Deptor depletion by shRNA abolished cell proliferation, attenuated glycolytic metabolism, and enhanced cell death, whereas ectopically expressed Deptor significantly promoted cell growth and glycolysis. Furthermore, Deptor ablation delayed T-ALL onset in a xenograft model. These effects were mostly related to the control of Akt phosphorylation at both Thr308 and Ser473, as Deptor depletion inhibited Akt activation, while its overexpression enhanced it [56]. These findings may appear surprising at a first glance, as Deptor inhibits both mTORC1 and mTORC2 [59]. However, it was found that while Deptor depletion increased p70S6K1 phosphorylation, its overexpression inhibited p70S6K1 phosphorylation [56]. This suggested that Deptor activates Akt at least in part through the inhibition of mTORC1 activity, as reported in several studies (e.g., [60]).

3.3. RAS Signaling

RAS proteins include Harvey-RAS (H-RAS), neuroblastoma-RAS (N-RAS), and Kirsten-RAS (K-RAS) [61]. They are a family of small GTPases acting as molecular switches that oscillate between an inactive GDP-bound and an active GTP-bound status. RAS genes are the most frequently mutated genes in human cancer [62]. RAS proteins transduce signals from a variety of cell receptors, including receptor tyrosine kinases (RTKs) and cytokine receptors, to downstream effectors such as PI3K/Akt and MEK/ERK (Figure 1). By doing so, they regulate a plethora of functions that are fundamental for both healthy and tumor cells [63]. Activating RAS mutations have the potential for inducing T-ALL in murine models when combined with other genetic anomalies, including enhancer of Zeste 2 (EZH2) inactivation [64] as well as NOTCH1 [65,66] or IL7 receptor (IL7R) α chain mutations [67]. RAS signaling is overactive in about ≥50% of childhood T-ALL patients [68]. N-RAS and K-RAS activating mutations seem to occur more frequently in early T-cell progenitor (ETP)-ALL [69] than in other subtypes [70–72]. Of note, ETP-ALL is a T-ALL subtype characterized by a poor outcome [73]. In this context, it is important to highlight that in a murine model of T-ALL evoked by K-RAS activation, Raptor deficiency dramatically inhibited the cell cycle progression of T-cell progenitors and prevented leukemia development, thus emphasizing the key role played by mTORC1 in this setting [74].

However, RAS signaling cascade upregulation could also arise from mutations or alterations in the activity/expression of key regulatory components of the RAS pathway, including RAS guanine nucleotide-releasing protein 1 (RASGRP1, that is frequently overexpressed in human T-ALL cell lines and primary samples) [75,76], or RAS GTPase-activating proteins (RAS-GAPs), such as neurofibromin 1 or p120 RAS-GAP [77,78]. In murine T-ALL cells with increased RASGRP1 expression, RASGRP1 contributed to cytokine receptor-activated RAS pathway that stimulated the proliferation of T-ALL cells in vivo [75]. Remarkably, RASGRP1 overexpression in T-ALL cells seems to impinge primarily on PI3K/Akt rather than on MEK/ERK signaling [79,80].

3.4. RTK Signaling

Aberrant signals originating from RTKs have been implicated in PI3K/Akt/mTOR upregulation in T-ALL. A well-documented example is increased IGF1/IGF1 receptor (IGF1R) activity [81]. Indeed, IGF1R levels are increased both transcriptionally [82,83] and post-transcriptionally [84] by NOTCH1 in T-ALL cells [46]. As to the source of IGF1, a recent study has revealed how, in the thymic microenvironment of murine T-ALL models and T-ALL primary patient samples, leukemic cells overexpressed IGF1R while tumor-associated dendritic cells (DCs) synthesized and released IGF1, which drove T-ALL growth ex-vivo [85]. Importantly, it has been shown that IGF1/IGF1R signaling contributes to proliferation and survival not only of the bulk T-ALL cells, but also of cells endowed with leukemia-initiating activity [82].

Another RTK that is overexpressed and cooperates with PTEN deficiency to activate PI3K/Akt/mTOR in T-ALL cell lines and primary samples is neurotrophic tyrosine receptor kinase type 2 (NTRK2, also known as TrkB) [44]. Interestingly, the NTRK2 transcript levels were consistently higher in PTEN-deficient T-ALL cell lines and primary samples compared with PTEN wild-type cells. However, the significance of such an inverse correlation is still unclear.

3.5. IL7 Signaling

IL7/IL7R signaling has been documented to play a critical role in mTOR activation in T-ALL. IL7 and IL7R are essential for normal T-cell development and homeostasis, whereas disregulated IL7/IL7R activity promotes T-ALL [8]. In T-ALL, gain of function mutations of IL7Rα, which could be detected in about 10% of pediatric patients, resulted in the activation of PI3K/Akt/mTOR signaling [86,87]. Interestingly, both IGF1/IGF1R and IL7/IL7R activate not only PI3K/Akt but also the MEK/ERK module [81,88] (Figure 1). However, at least in human T-ALL cell lines, PI3K/Akt signaling was dominant over MEK/ERK in mediating cell proliferation and/or survival [81], although in the article by Triplett et al. [85], MEK/ERK activation by IGF1/IGF1R was detected in T-ALL cells co-cultured with thymic DCs. Moreover, IGF1/IGF1R and IL7/IL7R displayed non-overlapping roles in the control of T-ALL cell line growth [81]. However, further studies will be required to determine to which extent these findings apply to primary patient samples. In any case, it should be emphasized that NOTCH1 is a transcriptional activator also of the gene encoding IL7Rα [89].

3.6. Integrins and Chemokines

Integrin and chemokine signals are known for activating both PI3K/Akt and MEK/ERK [90,91]; hence, they have the potential for positively impacting mTORC1 and mTORC2. Accordingly, integrins and chemokines are important for regulating several aspects of T-ALL cell biology, including proliferation, survival, drug-resistance, migration, and infiltration of the central nervous system [2,8,92,93].

3.7. PI3K Activating Mutations

Although genetic anomalies of the PI3K p110α catalytic subunit are frequently detected in some types of solid cancers [94,95], they seem to be exceedingly rare in T-ALL [96].

3.8. mTOR Mutations

An emerging theme in mTOR biology is the identification of activating mutations that could confer increased sensitivity to mTOR inhibitors. Several such mutations have been identified in solid cancer cell lines and patients [97]. However, at present, the only activating mutation described in T-ALL cells is C1483Y, which has been identified in the MOLT-16 human cell line [98]. This mutation occurs in the FRAP, ATM, TRRAP (FAT) domain of mTOR, and leads to lower levels of Raptor bound to mTORC1/mTORC2 and higher levels of Rictor interacting with mTORC2. Therefore, the final effect is an increase in the activity of both mTORC1 and mTORC2 [99]. However, MOLT-16 cells are PTEN-deleted [100]. Therefore, their PTEN status also most likely contributes to mTORC1/mTORC2 activation.

4. Roles of mTORC1 and mTORC2 in T-ALL

The roles of the individual mTOR complexes were recently explored by shRNA knockdown strategy in a mouse model where T-ALL had been induced by ΔTrkA, which is a mutant of TrkA isolated from a patient with acute myeloid leukemia [101]. Some of the T-ALL clones also displayed PTEN mutations, abrogating the lipid phosphatase activity, and NOTCH1-activating mutations. While ΔTrkA was sufficient for upregulating mTORC1 (most likely through MEK/ERK signaling, as Akt was barely active in this model), increased mTORC2 activity required both inactivating PTEN and activating NOTCH1 mutations. Separate depletion of either Raptor (mTORC1) or Rictor (mTORC2) reduced the proliferation rate and the size of T-ALL cells, but was not sufficient to induce apoptosis [102]. In contrast, knockdown of eukaryotic translation initiation factor 4E (eIF4E, the rate limiting factor of mTORC1-dependent mRNA-translation [103]) had a dramatic impact, leading to significantly reduced cell size and proliferation, as well as remarkable apoptosis. Similar results were obtained using 4EGI-1, which is a small molecule that abrogates cap-dependent translation through direct binding to eIF4E [104]. As expected, either eIF4E knockdown or treatment with 4EGI-1 reduced the expression of key oncogenetic proteins and shifted the mitochondrial outer membrane toward an apoptosis-facilitating state [102]. At first glance, these findings are difficult to reconcile with Raptor knockdown by shRNA in T-ALL cells being ≥96%; therefore, cap-dependent translation should have been almost completely switched off. However, it should be considered that MEK/ERK/p90RSK1 signaling directly converges on eIF4E through mitogen-activated protein kinase interacting kinases (MNKs), partially bypassing mTORC1 [105]. Since MER/ERK was constitutively active in the murine T-ALL model used by Schwarzer et al. [102], it might be that Raptor knockdown did not attain a level of cap-dependent translation inhibition that was sufficient for inducing apoptosis, whereas eIF4E downregulation was more effective in this respect.

5. Therapeutic Targeting of mTORC1 and mTORC2 in T-ALL Cells: Preclinical Studies

mTOR was originally discovered as the target of rapamycin, which is a macrolide antibiotic isolated in 1972 from the bacterium Streptomyces hygroscopicus in the soil collected on Easter

Island (Rapa Nui in the local language) [97,106]. Three classes of mTOR inhibitors are at present available: allosteric inhibitors (rapamycin and its derivatives or rapalogs, i.e., RAD001/everolimus, CCI-779/temsirolimus) that mainly target mTORC1 [107]; ATP-competitive dual PI3K/mTOR inhibitors that target PI3K, mTORC1 and mTORC2 [108]; and ATP-competitive mTOR kinase inhibitors (TORKIs) that target mTORC1 and mTORC2, but not PI3K [109].

5.1. Allosteric mTOR Inhibitors

Allosteric mTOR inhibitors have proven their efficacy against T-ALL cells in several preclinical studies. This class of drugs mainly exerts cytostatic effects [109]. Accordingly, rapamycin or temsirolimus blocked IL7-dependent T-ALL proliferation and cell cycle progression. mTOR inhibition was accompanied by an increased expression of the CDK inhibitor, $p27^{Kip1}$ [110,111]. Rapamycin or temsirolimus also induced apoptosis of T-ALL cells cultured in the presence of IL7. Apoptotic cell death was characterized by the activation of p53, as documented by upregulated levels of Ser46 p-p53 [111], which is in agreement with previous findings [112]. Moreover, it has been demonstrated that rapamycin restored the expression of other cell cycle negative regulators, p14 and p15, in the MOLT-4 human T-ALL cell line [113]. Interestingly, these effects were related to the demethylation of the promoters of the genes encoding for p14 and p15, as rapamycin decreased total DNA methyltransferase (DNMT) activity in MOLT-4 cells. Although other groups have reported that mTORC1 controls the expression of DNMT1 [114], the molecular mechanism underlying this regulation remains unexplained.

The proapoptotic effects of rapamycin and rapalogs could be significantly increased by co-treatment with drugs that are currently employed in T-ALL patients, including doxorubicin [111,115], idarubicin [116], cyclophosphamide [117], and methotrexate [118]. Moreover, mTOR allosteric inhibitors synergize with glucocorticoids (GCs), that are widely used in current protocols for treating T-ALL [111,119,120]. It should be emphasized here that pediatric T-ALL patients often display GC resistance [121]. These patients, who are classified as prednisone poor responders (PPP), have worse outcome than other T-ALL patients receiving a high-risk adapted therapy [122]. Therefore, GC-resistance represents an important challenge for improving the prognosis of PPP.

In particular, it has been shown that rapamycin downregulated the expression of myeloid leukemia cell differentiation 1 (MCL-1), which is a critical regulator of GC-induced apoptosis, as it sequesters the BH3-only proapoptotic protein B-cell lymphoma-2 (Bcl-2) -like protein 11 (BIM) in GC-resistant CEM T-ALL cells [123]. Wei et al. [123] could not detect an increase in the expression levels of either BIM or p53-upregulated modulator of apoptosis (PUMA), which is another BH3-only proapoptotic protein. However, in a subsequent study that also took advantage of GC-resistant CEM cells, it was reported that rapamycin, when combined with GCs, upregulated GC receptor α isoform as well as BIM [124].

Allosteric mTOR inhibitors also have proven their efficacy in T-ALL cells when combined with other targeted therapeutics, which included inhibitors of NOTCH1 [125], MEK [111], Janus kinase 3 (Jak3) [111], Bcl-2 [126], and glycolysis [127].

More recently, it has been shown that a combination consisting of LEE011 (ribociclib), which is an investigator-grade CDK 4/6 inhibitor, and everolimus, was synergistic in vitro in reducing cell proliferation and increasing the apoptosis of human T-ALL cell lines [128]. The rationale for using this drug combination is that both CDK6 and its upstream regulator, cyclin D3, are frequently upregulated in T-ALL [129–132]. Cyclin D3 is a downstream target of NOTCH1 signaling in T-ALL [133]. However, CDK4/6 inhibition in cancer cells is usually cytostatic; therefore, monotherapy is unlikely to be optimal [134]. Moreover, CDK4/6 inhibitor could unleash adaptive responses that lead to an acquired resistance to this class of drugs. Some of these responses are orchestrated by mTORC1 or mTORC2 [135]. Indeed, previous studies that have been carried out in solid cancers have demonstrated the efficay of combining a CDK4/6 inhibitor with everolimus [136]. Pikman et al. [128] also investigated the effects of the LEE011 and everolimus combination in an orthotopic mouse model of T-ALL, where MOLT-16 cells were injected into NOD-SCID IL2Rγ^{null} (NSG) mice. They found that the drug combination resulted in a significantly prolonged mice survival compared with either drug alone.

5.2. Dual PI3K/mTOR Inhibitors

This class of drugs was originally developed to overcome some of the drawbacks of allosteric mTOR inhibitors, such as the only partial inhibition of mTORC1-dependent translation and the feedback activation of oncogenetic pathways, including PI3K/Akt [97,108,137]. When used in T-ALL cell models, some of these drugs (PI-103, NVP-BEZ235) displayed a more potent proapoptotic activity than rapamycin, and inhibited one of the rapamycin-resistant outputs of mTORC1, i.e., 4E-BP1 phosphorylation [138–140]. However, it has been demonstrated that PI-103 upregulated NOTCH1/c-Myc signaling in NOTCH1-mutated T-ALL cell lines, thus leading to an impaired cytotoxic response [141]. Drug combinations consisting of PI-103 and either a GSI or a small molecule c-Myc inhibitor (10058-F4) overcame resistance to the dual PI3K/mTOR targeting agent. Also, dual PI3K/mTOR inhibitors synergized with chemotherapeutic drugs used for T-ALL treatment [139,142]. In particular, NVP-BEZ235 enhanced GC-induced anti-leukemic activity in vitro (cell lines and primary samples) and systemic in vivo models of T-ALL, including a patient-derived xenograft [86,143]. Through the inhibition of Akt, NVP-BEZ235 alleviated the Akt-mediated suppression of GC-induced apoptotic pathways, thus leading to the increased expression of proapoptotic BIM. Furthermore, downregulation of MCL-1 protein by NVP-BEZ235 further contributed to the modulation of GC-resistance by increasing the amount of BIM available to induce apoptosis, especially in PTEN-null T-ALL cells, where the inhibition of Akt only partially overcame Akt-induced BIM suppression [143]. A recently described, highly synergistic drug combination comprises NVP-BEZ235 and calcineurin (Cn) inhibitors, and was effective both in vitro and in vivo in xenograft models [144]. Cn is a Ca^{2+}-activated protein phosphatase that plays several key roles in healthy T-cell physiology [145]. However, Cn is also somehow involved in some critical aspects of T-ALL pathophysiology, including GC resistance [121], migration [146], and adhesion [147].

5.3. TORKIs

This class of ATP-competitive molecules, which block only the mTOR catalytic domain, was developed to reduce toxicity due to the use of dual PI3K/mTOR inhibitors [97]. TORKIs, when compared with rapamycin, completely blocked in vitro and in vivo the phosphorylation of Ser473 p-Akt and Thr37/46 p-4E-BP1, markedly inhibited cell proliferation, and negatively affected cap-dependent translation under conditions where rapamycin had no effects [148,149]. We investigated the efficacy of two TORKIs, PP-242 and OSI-027, in T-ALL primary samples and cell lines. At variance with rapamycin, we found that the TORKIs induced a marked inhibition of mRNA translation, which led to lower levels of oncogenetic proteins, including MCL-1, survivin, and CDK-2. The inhibitors strongly synergized with both vincristine and the Bcl-2 inhibitor, ABT-263 [150]. Similar results were reported by another group that used the TORKI Torin-2 in human T-ALL cell lines and ICN1-transduced mouse T-ALL cells [151]. Interestingly, Torin-2 increased the expression levels of proapototic genes such as Bcl2l11 (which encodes for BIM) and Bbc3 (encoding for PUMA [152]) as well as of the p53 target gene, Cdkn1b (which encodes for the cell cycle progression, inhibitor p27^{Kip1} [153]). However, it should not be forgotten that p27^{Kip1} expression could be also under the control of FoxO3a [56], which is a target of mTORC2 through Akt (Figure 1). These mechanisms have been confirmed in human NOTCH1 mutated T-ALL Jurkat cells, where treatment with OSI-027, by inhibiting mTORC1-mediated 4E-BP1 phosphorylation, led to the decreased expression of c-Myc and subsequent upregulation of PUMA [154]. In contrast, the inhibition of mTORC2 activity resulted in NFκB–mediated expression of the early growth response 1 (EGR1) gene (Figure 1), which encodes a transcription factor that binds and transactivates the BCL2L11 locus, encoding BIM. Importantly, both of these pathways contributed to T-ALL cell death, which was observed in reponse to OSI-027 treatment [154].

6. Clinical Trials

At present, we know the results of three clinical trials where either everolimus or temsirolimus was combined with chemotherapy for treating relapsed/refractory T-ALL patients. The first trial was a Phase I/II study where everolimus was combined with Hyper-CVAD (cyclophosphamide, vincristine, adriamycin, dexamethasone) high-intensity chemotherapy [155] in adult patients with either B-lineage or T-lineage acute leukemia [156]. A partial or complete response was noted in five of 10 heavily pretreated T-ALL patients (median of four prior salvage regimens). Everolimus significantly inhibited the phosphorylation of S6RP, but this did not correlate with clinical response. However, no significant decrease in p-4E-BP1 and p-Akt levels was noted. Interestingly, the combined Hyper-CVAD and everolimus regimen did not result in significantly increased toxicity compared with Hyper-CVAD alone. Therefore, it was concluded that this drug combination was well tolerated and moderately effective in relapsed T-ALL patients [156].

The second study was a Phase I trial of temsirolimus in combination with UKALL R3 re-induction chemotherapy, which was conducted in children and adolescents with second or greater relapse of ALL [157]. Unfortunately, in this study, only one of 16 enrolled patients had T-ALL, while the others had B-ALL. Although the regimen induced remission in seven of 15 evaluable patients, the addition of temsirolimus to reinduction chemotherapy resulted in excessive toxicity and was not tolerable. In any case, the single T-ALL patient did not respond to treatment [157].

The third study was a Phase I trial of everolimus in combination with multiagent chemotherapy (vincristine, prednisone, pegylated asparaginase and doxorubicin) in pediatric ALL patients experiencing a first bone marrow relapse [158]. A total of 22 patients were enrolled, and 19 of them (86%) achieved a second complete remission. Remarkably, everolimus combined with four-drug reinduction chemotherapy was generally well tolerated. However, also in this study, there was only one T-ALL patient who did not respond at all to therapy.

Therefore, given the extremely limited number of T-ALL cases that were enrolled in the aforementioned studies, it is impossible to draw at present any firm conclusions, although it would seem that rapalogs have some potential in combination therapy in adult patients.

Further trials are being performed with rapalogs or the TORKI TAK-228 (Sapanisertib®) in combination with a variety of chemotherapeutics (see for example www.clinicaltrials.gov: NCT01614197, NCT03328104, NCT02484430). A very important aspect for development of the field will be the identification of chemotherapeutics that best combine with targeted inhibitors, and whether changes to the schedule and/or dose may alleviate adverse effects.

7. Conclusions

The evidence reviewed here demonstrates that mTORC1/mTORC2-generated signals play key roles in the control of T-ALL cell proliferation, survival, metabolism, and drug-resistance, making these complexes critical targets for novel anti-leukemic therapies. Although the use of mTOR inhibitors is continuously yielding a flood of promising preclinical data, initial clinical trials based on these drugs have not resulted in widespread and durable patient responses. As a consequence of these trials, only everolimus and temsirolimus have been approved as anticancer agents in the United States and Europe. They are used for treating advanced renal cell carcinoma, hormone receptor-positive/HER2-negative breast cancer in postmenopausal women, pancreatic and other selected neuroendocrine tumors, adult renal angiomyolipoma associated with TSC disease, pediatric or adult subependymal giant cell astrocytoma with TSC, and relapsed/refractory mantle cell lymphoma [97].

The limited effectiveness of mTOR targeting was initially explained on the basis of the activation of compensatory signaling pathways unleashed by mTOR inhibitors in cancer cells [97]. However, more recently, it became apparent that the low efficacy of these drugs could also depend on other reasons; these include, but are not limited to, the emergence of inhibitor treatment-resistant mTOR mutations [159], intratumor signaling network heterogeneity [80,160] due to the uneven clonal evolution of cancer [137,161] or an acidic tumor microenvironment [162].

Preclinical data strongly indicate that identifying combinations, either with targeted agents or with chemotherapy, might be the key to unleashing the full potential of mTOR inhibitors in T-ALL patients, as we have highlighted in this review. Early clinical data support this claim in other cancer types [163–165], although it will have to be conclusively documented that better responses are not accompanied by unacceptable toxicities [166]. Allosteric mTOR inhibitors have been tested in a limited number of clinical trials for treating relapsed/refractory ALL patients in combination with polychemotherapy. These trials have revealed that this class of drugs was also quite well tolerated in childhood patients in general, except for one study. Nevertheless, well-known adverse effects of everolimus and temsirolimus include hyperglycemia, dyslipidemia, mouth ulceration, stomatitis, increased susceptibility to infections, interstitial pneumonitis, vomiting, and diarrhea [97,167–169].

The depth and duration of target inhibition as well as the safety profiles of these inhibitors might be improved through the use of intermittent dosing schedules, which could lead to a better drug exposure with more effective target inhibition and fewer adverse effects, as seen in other cancer types [170–172].

A key issue in the field of targeted therapy is the identification of biomarkers that could predict accurately inhibitor efficacy. Regarding the field of mTOR inhibitors, our knowledge is virtually non-existent, as potential biomarkers that were identified in preclinical studies unfortunately have not been subsequently validated in clinical trials [173]. Techniques such as kinase activity profiling [174,175], computational analysis [176], and next-generation sequencing [177] should provide a deeper insight into active signal transduction networks and point out critical signaling hubs, new potential druggable targets, as well as drug-sensitive and drug-resistant T-ALL patients. However, it is likely that an integrated approach comprising drug sensitivity, proteomic, phosphoproteomic, and genotypic analyses of primary leukemic cells could be the key for identifying the determinants of sensitivity to targeted compounds [178].

A better understanding of the effects of targeted inhibitors on the immunosuppressive leukemic microenvironment could improve therapeutic approaches [179]. Indeed, recent evidence pointed out that B-ALL cells induced the inhibition of Akt/mTORC1 signaling and glucose metabolism that drove T-cell functional impairment, while an enforced Akt/mTORC1 signaling rescued T-cell metabolism and partially improved anti-leukemia immunity [180]. Therefore, the use of mTOR inhibitors could further blunt immunological responses against leukemic cells. However, another recent report demonstrated that an Akt inhibitor counteracted Th17 cell-induced resistance to daunorubicin in a preclinical model of B-ALL [181].

Targeted therapy is one of the mainstays of personalized cancer medicine, which also includes companion diagnostic [182–184]. However, the implementation of targeted agents in T-ALL therapy remains a difficult challenge due to a wide variety of disease-specific and patient-specific factors, such as the co-existence of multiple driver mutations, interconnected signal transduction pathways, age, comorbidities, psychosocial health, and socio-economic status [182]. For example, aberrant NOTCH1 signaling is considered a very promising target for the innovative treatment of T-ALL patients [185]. However, there is a paucity of published studies regarding the clinical use of NOTCH1 inhibitors in T-ALL [186,187], and the same holds true for mTOR inhibitors.

Nevertheless, the field of anti-tumor mTORC1/mTORC2-targeted therapies has progressed rapidly over the past 10 years. We are confident that, as our knowledge of mTOR biology continuously evolves, so too will our capacity to refine these novel treatments for ameliorating T-ALL patient outcomes.

Author Contributions: All of the authors contributed to writing of the article.

Funding: J.A.M. was partially funded by East Carolina University Grants numbers 111104 and 111110-668715-0000.

Conflicts of Interest: The authors declare no conflict of interest. The founding sponsors had no role in the design of the study; in the collection, analyses, or interpretation of data; in the writing of the manuscript, and in the decision to publish the results.

Abbreviations

4E-BP1	Eukaryotic translation initiation factor 4E-binding protein 1
Bcl-2	B-cell lymphoma-2
BIM	Bcl-2-like protein 11
CCR	C-C chemokine receptor
CDK	Cyclin dependent kinase
CK2	Casein kinase 2
c-Myc	c-Myelocytomatosis oncogene protein
Cn	Calcineurin
CVAD	Cyclophosphamide, vincristine, adriamycin, dexamethasone
CXCR	C-X-C chemokine receptor
DCs	Dendritic cells
DEP	Dishevelled, Egl-10 and Pleckstrin
Deptor	DEP domain-containing mTOR-interacting protein
DNMT	DNA methyltransferase
EGR1	Early Growth Response 1
eIF4E	Eukaryotic translation initiation factor 4E
ERK	Extracellular signal-regulated kinase
ETP	Early T-cell-progenitor
EZH2	Enhancer of Zeste 2
FAT	FRAP, ATM, TRRAP
FoxO1/3a	Forkhead box O1/3a
GAP	GTP-ase activing protein
GCs	Glucocorticoids
GSI	γ-secretase inhibitor
Grb2	Growth factor receptor-bound protein 2
GSK3β	Glycogen synthase kinase 3β
H-RAS	Harvey-RAS
HER2	human epidermal growth factor receptor 2
HES1	Hairy and enhancer of split-1
HSP90	Heat shock protein 90
JAK3	Janus kinase 3
ICN1	Intracellular polypeptide of NOTCH1
IGF-1	Insulin-like growth factor-1
IGF1R	Insulin-like growth factor-1 receptor
IL	Interleukin
IL7R	Interleukin 7 receptor
IRS1/2	Insulin receptor substrate 1/2
K-RAS	Kirsten-RAS
MAML1	Mastermind like transcriptional coactivator 1
MCL-1	Myeloid leukemia cell differentiation
MEK	Mitogen-activated protein kinase kinase
mLST8	Mammalian lethal with SEC13 protein 8
MNKs	Mitogen-activated protein kinase interacting kinases
mSin1	Mammalian Stress-activated protein kinase interacting protein 1
mTOR	Mechanistic target of rapamycin
mTORC1	mTOR complex 1

N-RAS	Neuroblastoma-RAS
NF-κb	Nuclear factor κ-light-chain-enhancer of activated B cells
NOTCH1	Neurogenic locus notch homolog protein 1
NSG	NOD-SCID IL2Rγ^{null}
NTRK2	Neurotrophic tyrosine receptor kinase
p70S6K1	p70 Ribosomal protein S6 kinase 1
p90RSK1	p90 ribosomal S6 kinase 1
PDK1	Phosphoinositide-dependent kinase 1
PH	Pleckstrin homology
PI3K	Phosphatidylinositol 3-kinase
PIKK	PI3K-related kinase
PIP2	Phosphatidylinositol 4,5 bisphosphate
PIP3	Phosphatidylinositol 3,4,5 trisphosphate
PKC	Protein kinase C
Pol	RNA polymerase
PP2A	Protein phosphatase 2A
PPP	Prednisone poor responders
PRAS40	Proline-rich Akt substrate 1 40
Protor	Protein observed with Rictor
PTEN	Phosphatase and tensin deleted on chromosome 10
PUMA	p53 upregulated modulator of apoptosis
Raf	Rapidly accelerated fibrosarcoma
Raptor	Regulatory associated protein of mTOR
RAS	Rat sarcoma
RAS-GAP	RAS GTPase activating protein
RASGRP1	RAS guanine nucleotide-releasing protein 1
Rb	Retinoblastoma protein
Rheb	RAS homolog enriched in brain
Rictor	Rapamycin independent companion of tor
RTK	Receptor tyrosine kinase
S6RP	S6 ribosomal protein
SGK1	Serum and glucocorticoid-activated kinase 1
SOS	Son of sevenless homolog
T-ALL	T-cell acute lymphoblastic leukemia
TORKIs	ATP-competitive mTOR kinase inhibitors
TSC1	Tuberous scelerosis complex 1
TSC2	Tuberous sclerosis complex 2
Tti1	Tel2-interacting protein 1

References

1. Paul, S.; Kantarjian, H.; Jabbour, E.J. Adult acute lymphoblastic leukemia. *Mayo Clin. Proc.* **2016**, *91*, 1645–1666. [CrossRef] [PubMed]
2. Vadillo, E.; Dorantes-Acosta, E.; Pelayo, R.; Schnoor, M. T cell acute lymphoblastic leukemia (T-ALL): New insights into the cellular origins and infiltration mechanisms common and unique among hematologic malignancies. *Blood Rev.* **2018**, *32*, 36–51. [CrossRef] [PubMed]
3. Belver, L.; Ferrando, A. The genetics and mechanisms of T cell acute lymphoblastic leukaemia. *Nat. Rev. Cancer* **2016**, *16*, 494–507. [CrossRef] [PubMed]
4. Raetz, E.A.; Teachey, D.T. T-cell acute lymphoblastic leukemia. *Hematol. Am. Soc. Hematol. Educ. Program* **2016**, *2016*, 580–588. [CrossRef] [PubMed]
5. Gianfelici, V.; Chiaretti, S.; Demeyer, S.; Di Giacomo, F.; Messina, M.; La Starza, R.; Peragine, N.; Paoloni, F.; Geerdens, E.; Pierini, V.; et al. RNA sequencing unravels the genetics of refractory/relapsed T-cell acute lymphoblastic leukemia. Prognostic and therapeutic implications. *Haematologica* **2016**, *101*, 941–950. [CrossRef] [PubMed]

6. Richter-Pechanska, P.; Kunz, J.B.; Hof, J.; Zimmermann, M.; Rausch, T.; Bandapalli, O.R.; Orlova, E.; Scapinello, G.; Sagi, J.C.; Stanulla, M.; et al. Identification of a genetically defined ultra-high-risk group in relapsed pediatric T-lymphoblastic leukemia. *Blood Cancer J.* **2017**, *7*, e523. [CrossRef] [PubMed]

7. Teepen, J.C.; van Leeuwen, F.E.; Tissing, W.J.; van Dulmen-den Broeder, E.; van den Heuvel-Eibrink, M.M.; van der Pal, H.J.; Loonen, J.J.; Bresters, D.; Versluys, B.; Neggers, S.; et al. Long-term risk of subsequent malignant neoplasms after treatment of childhood cancer in the DCOG LATER study cohort: Role of chemotherapy. *J. Clin. Oncol.* **2017**, *35*, 2288–2298. [CrossRef] [PubMed]

8. Oliveira, M.L.; Akkapeddi, P.; Alcobia, I.; Almeida, A.R.; Cardoso, B.A.; Fragoso, R.; Serafim, T.L.; Barata, J.T. From the outside, from within: Biological and therapeutic relevance of signal transduction in T-cell acute lymphoblastic leukemia. *Cell. Signal.* **2017**, *38*, 10–25. [CrossRef] [PubMed]

9. Evangelisti, C.; Evangelisti, C.; Chiarini, F.; Lonetti, A.; Buontempo, F.; Bressanin, D.; Cappellini, A.; Orsini, E.; McCubrey, J.A.; Martelli, A.M. Therapeutic potential of targeting mTOR in T-cell acute lymphoblastic leukemia. *Int. J. Oncol.* **2014**, *45*, 909–918. [CrossRef] [PubMed]

10. Khanna, A.; Bhushan, B.; Chauhan, P.S.; Saxena, S.; Gupta, D.K.; Siraj, F. High mTOR expression independently prognosticates poor clinical outcome to induction chemotherapy in acute lymphoblastic leukemia. *Clin. Exp. Med.* **2018**, *18*, 221–227. [CrossRef] [PubMed]

11. Lench, N.J.; Macadam, R.; Markham, A.F. The human gene encoding FKBP-rapamycin associated protein (FRAP) maps to chromosomal band 1p36.2. *Hum. Genet.* **1997**, *99*, 547–549. [CrossRef] [PubMed]

12. Lempiainen, H.; Halazonetis, T.D. Emerging common themes in regulation of PIKKs and PI3Ks. *EMBO J.* **2009**, *28*, 3067–3073. [CrossRef] [PubMed]

13. Saxton, R.A.; Sabatini, D.M. mTOR signaling in growth, metabolism, and disease. *Cell* **2017**, *169*, 361–371. [CrossRef] [PubMed]

14. Hara, K.; Maruki, Y.; Long, X.; Yoshino, K.; Oshiro, N.; Hidayat, S.; Tokunaga, C.; Avruch, J.; Yonezawa, K. Raptor, a binding partner of target of rapamycin (TOR), mediates TOR action. *Cell* **2002**, *110*, 177–189. [CrossRef]

15. Wang, L.; Harris, T.E.; Lawrence, J.C., Jr. Regulation of proline-rich Akt substrate of 40 kDa (PRAS40) function by mammalian target of rapamycin complex 1 (mTORC1)-mediated phosphorylation. *J. Biol. Chem.* **2008**, *283*, 15619–15627. [CrossRef] [PubMed]

16. Dibble, C.C.; Cantley, L.C. Regulation of mTORC1 by PI3K signaling. *Trends Cell Biol.* **2015**, *25*, 545–555. [CrossRef] [PubMed]

17. Potter, C.J.; Pedraza, L.G.; Xu, T. Akt regulates growth by directly phosphorylating Tsc2. *Nat. Cell Biol.* **2002**, *4*, 658–665. [CrossRef] [PubMed]

18. Yoshida, S.; Hong, S.; Suzuki, T.; Nada, S.; Mannan, A.M.; Wang, J.; Okada, M.; Guan, K.L.; Inoki, K. Redox regulates mammalian target of rapamycin complex 1 (mTORC1) activity by modulating the TSC1/TSC2-Rheb GTPase pathway. *J. Biol. Chem.* **2011**, *286*, 32651–32660. [CrossRef] [PubMed]

19. Yang, H.; Jiang, X.; Li, B.; Yang, H.J.; Miller, M.; Yang, A.; Dhar, A.; Pavletich, N.P. Mechanisms of mTORC1 activation by RHEB and inhibition by PRAS40. *Nature* **2017**, *552*, 368–373. [CrossRef] [PubMed]

20. Fonseca, B.D.; Alain, T.; Finestone, L.K.; Huang, B.P.; Rolfe, M.; Jiang, T.; Yao, Z.; Hernandez, G.; Bennett, C.F.; Proud, C.G. Pharmacological and genetic evaluation of proposed roles of mitogen-activated protein kinase/extracellular signal-regulated kinase kinase (MEK), extracellular signal-regulated kinase (ERK), and p90(RSK) in the control of mTORC1 protein signaling by phorbol esters. *J. Biol. Chem.* **2011**, *286*, 27111–27122. [CrossRef] [PubMed]

21. Carriere, A.; Cargnello, M.; Julien, L.A.; Gao, H.; Bonneil, E.; Thibault, P.; Roux, P.P. Oncogenic MAPK signaling stimulates mTORC1 activity by promoting RSK-mediated raptor phosphorylation. *Curr. Biol.* **2008**, *18*, 1269–1277. [CrossRef] [PubMed]

22. Rad, E.; Murray, J.T.; Tee, A.R. Oncogenic signalling through mechanistic target of rapamycin (mTOR): A driver of metabolic transformation and cancer progression. *Cancers* **2018**, *10*, 5. [CrossRef] [PubMed]

23. Ben-Sahra, I.; Manning, B.D. mTORC1 signaling and the metabolic control of cell growth. *Curr. Opin. Cell Biol.* **2017**, *45*, 72–82. [CrossRef] [PubMed]

24. Paquette, M.; El-Houjeiri, L.; Pause, A. mTOR pathways in cancer and autophagy. *Cancers* **2018**, *10*, 18. [CrossRef] [PubMed]

25. Sarbassov, D.D.; Ali, S.M.; Kim, D.H.; Guertin, D.A.; Latek, R.R.; Erdjument-Bromage, H.; Tempst, P.; Sabatini, D.M. Rictor, a novel binding partner of mTOR, defines a rapamycin-insensitive and

raptor-independent pathway that regulates the cytoskeleton. *Curr. Biol.* **2004**, *14*, 1296–1302. [CrossRef] [PubMed]

26. Jacinto, E.; Facchinetti, V.; Liu, D.; Soto, N.; Wei, S.; Jung, S.Y.; Huang, Q.; Qin, J.; Su, B. SIN1/MIP1 maintains rictor-mTOR complex integrity and regulates Akt phosphorylation and substrate specificity. *Cell* **2006**, *127*, 125–137. [CrossRef] [PubMed]

27. Liu, P.; Gan, W.; Chin, Y.R.; Ogura, K.; Guo, J.; Zhang, J.; Wang, B.; Blenis, J.; Cantley, L.C.; Toker, A.; et al. PtdIns(3,4,5)P3-dependent activation of the mTORC2 kinase complex. *Cancer Discov.* **2015**, *5*, 1194–1209. [CrossRef] [PubMed]

28. Pearce, L.R.; Sommer, E.M.; Sakamoto, K.; Wullschleger, S.; Alessi, D.R. Protor-1 is required for efficient mTORC2-mediated activation of SGK1 in the kidney. *Biochem. J.* **2011**, *436*, 169–179. [CrossRef] [PubMed]

29. Pearce, L.R.; Komander, D.; Alessi, D.R. The nuts and bolts of AGC protein kinases. *Nat. Rev. Mol. Cell Biol.* **2010**, *11*, 9–22. [CrossRef] [PubMed]

30. Sarbassov, D.D.; Guertin, D.A.; Ali, S.M.; Sabatini, D.M. Phosphorylation and regulation of Akt/PKB by the rictor-mTOR complex. *Science* **2005**, *307*, 1098–1101. [CrossRef] [PubMed]

31. Arias, E.; Koga, H.; Diaz, A.; Mocholi, E.; Patel, B.; Cuervo, A.M. Lysosomal mTORC2/PHLPP1/Akt regulate chaperone-mediated autophagy. *Mol. Cell* **2015**, *59*, 270–284. [CrossRef] [PubMed]

32. Guri, Y.; Colombi, M.; Dazert, E.; Hindupur, S.K.; Roszik, J.; Moes, S.; Jenoe, P.; Heim, M.H.; Riezman, I.; Riezman, H.; et al. mTORC2 promotes tumorigenesis via lipid synthesis. *Cancer Cell* **2017**, *32*, 807.e12–823.e12. [CrossRef] [PubMed]

33. McCubrey, J.A.; Steelman, L.S.; Chappell, W.H.; Abrams, S.L.; Franklin, R.A.; Montalto, G.; Cervello, M.; Libra, M.; Candido, S.; Malaponte, G.; et al. Ras/Raf/MEK/ERK and PI3K/PTEN/Akt/mTOR cascade inhibitors: How mutations can result in therapy resistance and how to overcome resistance. *Oncotarget* **2012**, *3*, 1068–1111. [CrossRef] [PubMed]

34. McCubrey, J.A.; Steelman, L.S.; Chappell, W.H.; Abrams, S.L.; Montalto, G.; Cervello, M.; Nicoletti, F.; Fagone, P.; Malaponte, G.; Mazzarino, M.C.; et al. Mutations and deregulation of Ras/Raf/MEK/ERK and PI3K/PTEN/Akt/mTOR cascades which alter therapy response. *Oncotarget* **2012**, *3*, 954–987. [CrossRef] [PubMed]

35. Haddadi, N.; Lin, Y.; Travis, G.; Simpson, A.M.; McGowan, E.M.; Nassif, N.T. PTEN/PTENP1: 'Regulating the regulator of RTK-dependent PI3K/Akt signalling', new targets for cancer therapy. *Mol. Cancer* **2018**, *17*, 37. [CrossRef] [PubMed]

36. Mendes, R.D.; Cante-Barrett, K.; Pieters, R.; Meijerink, J.P. The relevance of PTEN-AKT in relation to NOTCH1-directed treatment strategies in T-cell acute lymphoblastic leukemia. *Haematologica* **2016**, *101*, 1010–1017. [CrossRef] [PubMed]

37. Tesio, M.; Trinquand, A.; Macintyre, E.; Asnafi, V. Oncogenic PTEN functions and models in T-cell malignancies. *Oncogene* **2016**, *35*, 3887–3896. [CrossRef] [PubMed]

38. Petit, A.; Trinquand, A.; Chevret, S.; Ballerini, P.; Cayuela, J.M.; Grardel, N.; Touzart, A.; Brethon, B.; Lapillonne, H.; Schmitt, C.; et al. Oncogenetic mutations combined with MRD improve outcome prediction in pediatric T-cell acute lymphoblastic leukemia. *Blood* **2018**, *131*, 289–300. [CrossRef] [PubMed]

39. Silva, A.; Yunes, J.A.; Cardoso, B.A.; Martins, L.R.; Jotta, P.Y.; Abecasis, M.; Nowill, A.E.; Leslie, N.R.; Cardoso, A.A.; Barata, J.T. PTEN posttranslational inactivation and hyperactivation of the PI3K/Akt pathway sustain primary T cell leukemia viability. *J. Clin. Investig.* **2008**, *118*, 3762–3774. [CrossRef] [PubMed]

40. Buontempo, F.; McCubrey, J.A.; Orsini, E.; Ruzzene, M.; Cappellini, A.; Lonetti, A.; Evangelisti, C.; Chiarini, F.; Evangelisti, C.; Barata, J.T.; et al. Therapeutic targeting of CK2 in acute and chronic leukemias. *Leukemia* **2018**, *32*, 1–10. [CrossRef] [PubMed]

41. Buontempo, F.; Orsini, E.; Martins, L.R.; Antunes, I.; Lonetti, A.; Chiarini, F.; Tabellini, G.; Evangelisti, C.; Evangelisti, C.; Melchionda, F.; et al. Cytotoxic activity of the casein kinase 2 inhibitor CX-4945 against T-cell acute lymphoblastic leukemia: Targeting the unfolded protein response signaling. *Leukemia* **2014**, *28*, 543–553. [CrossRef] [PubMed]

42. Di Maira, G.; Brustolon, F.; Pinna, L.A.; Ruzzene, M. Dephosphorylation and inactivation of Akt/PKB is counteracted by protein kinase CK2 in HEK 293T cells. *Cell. Mol. Life Sci.* **2009**, *66*, 3363–3373. [CrossRef] [PubMed]

43. Yuan, T.; Yang, Y.; Chen, J.; Li, W.; Li, W.; Zhang, Q.; Mi, Y.; Goswami, R.S.; You, J.Q.; Lin, D.; et al. Regulation of PI3K signaling in T-cell acute lymphoblastic leukemia: A novel PTEN/Ikaros/miR-26b mechanism reveals a critical targetable role for PIK3CD. *Leukemia* **2017**, *31*, 2355–2364. [CrossRef] [PubMed]

44. Yuzugullu, H.; Von, T.; Thorpe, L.M.; Walker, S.R.; Roberts, T.M.; Frank, D.A.; Zhao, J.J. NTRK2 activation cooperates with PTEN deficiency in T-ALL through activation of both the PI3K-AKT and JAK-STAT3 pathways. *Cell Discov.* **2016**, *2*, 16030. [CrossRef] [PubMed]

45. Efimenko, E.; Dave, U.P.; Lebedeva, I.V.; Shen, Y.; Sanchez-Quintero, M.J.; Diolaiti, D.; Kung, A.; Lannutti, B.J.; Chen, J.; Realubit, R.; et al. PI3Kg/d and NOTCH1 cross-regulate pathways that define the T-cell acute lymphoblastic leukemia disease signature. *Mol. Cancer Ther.* **2017**, *16*, 2069–2082. [CrossRef] [PubMed]

46. Sanchez-Martin, M.; Ferrando, A. The NOTCH1-MYC highway toward T-cell acute lymphoblastic leukemia. *Blood* **2017**, *129*, 1124–1133. [CrossRef] [PubMed]

47. Palomero, T.; Sulis, M.L.; Cortina, M.; Real, P.J.; Barnes, K.; Ciofani, M.; Caparros, E.; Buteau, J.; Brown, K.; Perkins, S.L.; et al. Mutational loss of PTEN induces resistance to NOTCH1 inhibition in T-cell leukemia. *Nat. Med.* **2007**, *13*, 1203–1210. [CrossRef] [PubMed]

48. Hales, E.C.; Orr, S.M.; Larson Gedman, A.; Taub, J.W.; Matherly, L.H. Notch1 receptor regulates AKT protein activation loop (Thr308) dephosphorylation through modulation of the PP2A phosphatase in phosphatase and tensin homolog (PTEN)-null T-cell acute lymphoblastic leukemia cells. *J. Biol. Chem.* **2013**, *288*, 22836–22848. [CrossRef] [PubMed]

49. Mavrakis, K.J.; Wolfe, A.L.; Oricchio, E.; Palomero, T.; de Keersmaecker, K.; McJunkin, K.; Zuber, J.; James, T.; Khan, A.A.; Leslie, C.S.; et al. Genome-wide RNA-mediated interference screen identifies miR-19 targets in Notch-induced T-cell acute lymphoblastic leukaemia. *Nat. Cell Biol.* **2010**, *12*, 372–379. [CrossRef] [PubMed]

50. Gutierrez, A.; Grebliunaite, R.; Feng, H.; Kozakewich, E.; Zhu, S.; Guo, F.; Payne, E.; Mansour, M.; Dahlberg, S.E.; Neuberg, D.S.; et al. Pten mediates Myc oncogene dependence in a conditional zebrafish model of T cell acute lymphoblastic leukemia. *J. Exp. Med.* **2011**, *208*, 1595–1603. [CrossRef] [PubMed]

51. Chan, S.M.; Weng, A.P.; Tibshirani, R.; Aster, J.C.; Utz, P.J. Notch signals positively regulate activity of the mTOR pathway in T-cell acute lymphoblastic leukemia. *Blood* **2007**, *110*, 278–286. [CrossRef] [PubMed]

52. Ravitz, M.J.; Chen, L.; Lynch, M.; Schmidt, E.V. c-myc Repression of TSC2 contributes to control of translation initiation and Myc-induced transformation. *Cancer Res.* **2007**, *67*, 11209–11217. [CrossRef] [PubMed]

53. Lee, K.; Nam, K.T.; Cho, S.H.; Gudapati, P.; Hwang, Y.; Park, D.S.; Potter, R.; Chen, J.; Volanakis, E.; Boothby, M. Vital roles of mTOR complex 2 in Notch-driven thymocyte differentiation and leukemia. *J. Exp. Med.* **2012**, *209*, 713–728. [CrossRef] [PubMed]

54. Buonamici, S.; Trimarchi, T.; Ruocco, M.G.; Reavie, L.; Cathelin, S.; Mar, B.G.; Klinakis, A.; Lukyanov, Y.; Tseng, J.C.; Sen, F.; et al. CCR7 signalling as an essential regulator of CNS infiltration in T-cell leukaemia. *Nature* **2009**, *459*, 1000–1004. [CrossRef] [PubMed]

55. Lang, S.A.; Hackl, C.; Moser, C.; Fichtner-Feigl, S.; Koehl, G.E.; Schlitt, H.J.; Geissler, E.K.; Stoeltzing, O. Implication of RICTOR in the mTOR inhibitor-mediated induction of insulin-like growth factor-I receptor (IGF-IR) and human epidermal growth factor receptor-2 (Her2) expression in gastrointestinal cancer cells. *Biochim. Biophys. Acta* **2010**, *1803*, 435–442. [CrossRef] [PubMed]

56. Hua, C.; Guo, H.; Bu, J.; Zhou, M.; Cheng, H.; He, F.; Wang, J.; Wang, X.; Zhang, Y.; Wang, Q.; et al. Rictor/mammalian target of rapamycin 2 regulates the development of Notch1 induced murine T-cell acute lymphoblastic leukemia via forkhead box O3. *Exp. Hematol.* **2014**, *42*, 1031.e4–1040.e4. [CrossRef] [PubMed]

57. Hayashi, H.; Kume, T. Forkhead transcription factors regulate expression of the chemokine receptor CXCR4 in endothelial cells and CXCL12-induced cell migration. *Biochem. Biophys. Res. Commun.* **2008**, *367*, 584–589. [CrossRef] [PubMed]

58. Hu, Y.; Su, H.; Liu, C.; Wang, Z.; Huang, L.; Wang, Q.; Liu, S.; Chen, S.; Zhou, J.; Li, P.; et al. DEPTOR is a direct NOTCH1 target that promotes cell proliferation and survival in T-cell leukemia. *Oncogene* **2017**, *36*, 1038–1047. [CrossRef] [PubMed]

59. Varusai, T.M.; Nguyen, L.K. Dynamic modelling of the mTOR signalling network reveals complex emergent behaviours conferred by DEPTOR. *Sci. Rep.* **2018**, *8*, 643. [CrossRef] [PubMed]

60. Tamburini, J.; Chapuis, N.; Bardet, V.; Park, S.; Sujobert, P.; Willems, L.; Ifrah, N.; Dreyfus, F.; Mayeux, P.; Lacombe, C.; et al. Mammalian target of rapamycin (mTOR) inhibition activates phosphatidylinositol 3-kinase/Akt by up-regulating insulin-like growth factor-1 receptor signaling in acute myeloid leukemia: Rationale for therapeutic inhibition of both pathways. *Blood* **2008**, *111*, 379–382. [CrossRef] [PubMed]

61. Prior, I.A.; Lewis, P.D.; Mattos, C. A comprehensive survey of Ras mutations in cancer. *Cancer Res.* **2012**, *72*, 2457–2467. [CrossRef] [PubMed]

62. Cox, A.D.; Fesik, S.W.; Kimmelman, A.C.; Luo, J.; Der, C.J. Drugging the undruggable RAS: Mission possible? *Nat. Rev. Drug Discov.* **2014**, *13*, 828–851. [CrossRef] [PubMed]

63. Kano, Y.; Cook, J.D.; Lee, J.E.; Ohh, M. New structural and functional insight into the regulation of Ras. *Semin. Cell Dev. Biol.* **2016**, *58*, 70–78. [CrossRef] [PubMed]

64. Danis, E.; Yamauchi, T.; Echanique, K.; Zhang, X.; Haladyna, J.N.; Riedel, S.S.; Zhu, N.; Xie, H.; Orkin, S.H.; Armstrong, S.A.; et al. Ezh2 Controls an early hematopoietic program and growth and survival signaling in early T cell precursor acute lymphoblastic leukemia. *Cell Rep.* **2016**, *14*, 1953–1965. [CrossRef] [PubMed]

65. Kindler, T.; Cornejo, M.G.; Scholl, C.; Liu, J.; Leeman, D.S.; Haydu, J.E.; Frohling, S.; Lee, B.H.; Gilliland, D.G. K-RasG12D-induced T-cell lymphoblastic lymphoma/leukemias harbor Notch1 mutations and are sensitive to g-secretase inhibitors. *Blood* **2008**, *112*, 3373–3382. [CrossRef] [PubMed]

66. Kong, G.; Du, J.; Liu, Y.; Meline, B.; Chang, Y.I.; Ranheim, E.A.; Wang, J.; Zhang, J. Notch1 gene mutations target KRAS G12D-expressing CD8+ cells and contribute to their leukemogenic transformation. *J. Biol. Chem.* **2013**, *288*, 18219–18227. [CrossRef] [PubMed]

67. Cramer, S.D.; Hixon, J.A.; Andrews, C.; Porter, R.J.; Rodrigues, G.O.L.; Wu, X.; Back, T.; Czarra, K.; Michael, H.; Cam, M.; et al. Mutant IL-7Ra and mutant NRas are sufficient to induce murine T cell acute lymphoblastic leukemia. *Leukemia* **2018**. [CrossRef] [PubMed]

68. Von Lintig, F.C.; Huvar, I.; Law, P.; Diccianni, M.B.; Yu, A.L.; Boss, G.R. Ras activation in normal white blood cells and childhood acute lymphoblastic leukemia. *Clin. Cancer Res.* **2000**, *6*, 1804–1810. [PubMed]

69. Zhang, J.; Ding, L.; Holmfeldt, L.; Wu, G.; Heatley, S.L.; Payne-Turner, D.; Easton, J.; Chen, X.; Wang, J.; Rusch, M.; et al. The genetic basis of early T-cell precursor acute lymphoblastic leukaemia. *Nature* **2012**, *481*, 157–163. [CrossRef] [PubMed]

70. Yokota, S.; Nakao, M.; Horiike, S.; Seriu, T.; Iwai, T.; Kaneko, H.; Azuma, H.; Oka, T.; Takeda, T.; Watanabe, A.; et al. Mutational analysis of the N-ras gene in acute lymphoblastic leukemia: A study of 125 Japanese pediatric cases. *Int. J. Hematol.* **1998**, *67*, 379–387. [CrossRef]

71. Perentesis, J.P.; Bhatia, S.; Boyle, E.; Shao, Y.; Shu, X.O.; Steinbuch, M.; Sather, H.N.; Gaynon, P.; Kiffmeyer, W.; Envall-Fox, J.; et al. RAS oncogene mutations and outcome of therapy for childhood acute lymphoblastic leukemia. *Leukemia* **2004**, *18*, 685–692. [CrossRef] [PubMed]

72. Wiemels, J.L.; Zhang, Y.; Chang, J.; Zheng, S.; Metayer, C.; Zhang, L.; Smith, M.T.; Ma, X.; Selvin, S.; Buffler, P.A.; et al. RAS mutation is associated with hyperdiploidy and parental characteristics in pediatric acute lymphoblastic leukemia. *Leukemia* **2005**, *19*, 415–419. [CrossRef] [PubMed]

73. Jain, N.; Lamb, A.V.; O'Brien, S.; Ravandi, F.; Konopleva, M.; Jabbour, E.; Zuo, Z.; Jorgensen, J.; Lin, P.; Pierce, S.; et al. Early T-cell precursor acute lymphoblastic leukemia/lymphoma (ETP-ALL/LBL) in adolescents and adults: A high-risk subtype. *Blood* **2016**, *127*, 1863–1869. [CrossRef] [PubMed]

74. Hoshii, T.; Kasada, A.; Hatakeyama, T.; Ohtani, M.; Tadokoro, Y.; Naka, K.; Ikenoue, T.; Ikawa, T.; Kawamoto, H.; Fehling, H.J.; et al. Loss of mTOR complex 1 induces developmental blockage in early T-lymphopoiesis and eradicates T-cell acute lymphoblastic leukemia cells. *Proc. Natl. Acad. Sci. USA* **2014**, *111*, 3805–3810. [CrossRef] [PubMed]

75. Hartzell, C.; Ksionda, O.; Lemmens, E.; Coakley, K.; Yang, M.; Dail, M.; Harvey, R.C.; Govern, C.; Bakker, J.; Lenstra, T.L.; et al. Dysregulated RasGRP1 responds to cytokine receptor input in T cell leukemogenesis. *Sci. Signal.* **2013**, *6*, ra21. [CrossRef] [PubMed]

76. Ksionda, O.; Melton, A.A.; Bache, J.; Tenhagen, M.; Bakker, J.; Harvey, R.; Winter, S.S.; Rubio, I.; Roose, J.P. RasGRP1 overexpression in T-ALL increases basal nucleotide exchange on Ras rendering the Ras/PI3K/Akt pathway responsive to protumorigenic cytokines. *Oncogene* **2016**, *35*, 3658–3668. [CrossRef] [PubMed]

77. Biagi, C.; Astolfi, A.; Masetti, R.; Serravalle, S.; Franzoni, M.; Chiarini, F.; Melchionda, F.; Pession, A. Pediatric early T-cell precursor leukemia with NF1 deletion and high-sensitivity in vitro to tipifarnib. *Leukemia* **2010**, *24*, 1230–1233. [CrossRef] [PubMed]

78. Lubeck, B.A.; Lapinski, P.E.; Oliver, J.A.; Ksionda, O.; Parada, L.F.; Zhu, Y.; Maillard, I.; Chiang, M.; Roose, J.; King, P.D. Cutting Edge: Codeletion of the Ras GTPase-activating proteins (RasGAPs) neurofibromin 1 and p120 RasGAP in T cells results in the development of T cell acute lymphoblastic leukemia. *J. Immunol.* **2015**, *195*, 31–35. [CrossRef] [PubMed]

79. Mues, M.; Roose, J.P. Distinct oncogenic Ras signals characterized by profound differences in flux through the RasGDP/RasGTP cycle. *Small GTPases* **2017**, *8*, 20–25. [CrossRef] [PubMed]

80. Ksionda, O.; Mues, M.; Wandler, A.M.; Donker, L.; Tenhagen, M.; Jun, J.; Ducker, G.S.; Matlawska-Wasowska, K.; Shannon, K.; Shokat, K.M.; et al. Comprehensive analysis of T cell leukemia signals reveals heterogeneity in the PI3 kinase-Akt pathway and limitations of PI3 kinase inhibitors as monotherapy. *PLoS ONE* **2018**, *13*, e0193849. [CrossRef] [PubMed]

81. Gusscott, S.; Jenkins, C.E.; Lam, S.H.; Giambra, V.; Pollak, M.; Weng, A.P. IGF1R Derived PI3K/AKT signaling maintains growth in a subset of human T-cell acute lymphoblastic leukemias. *PLoS ONE* **2016**, *11*, e0161158. [CrossRef] [PubMed]

82. Medyouf, H.; Gusscott, S.; Wang, H.; Tseng, J.C.; Wai, C.; Nemirovsky, O.; Trumpp, A.; Pflumio, F.; Carboni, J.; Gottardis, M.; et al. High-level IGF1R expression is required for leukemia-initiating cell activity in T-ALL and is supported by Notch signaling. *J. Exp. Med.* **2011**, *208*, 1809–1822. [CrossRef] [PubMed]

83. Trimarchi, T.; Bilal, E.; Ntziachristos, P.; Fabbri, G.; Dalla-Favera, R.; Tsirigos, A.; Aifantis, I. Genome-wide mapping and characterization of Notch-regulated long noncoding RNAs in acute leukemia. *Cell* **2014**, *158*, 593–606. [CrossRef] [PubMed]

84. Gusscott, S.; Kuchenbauer, F.; Humphries, R.K.; Weng, A.P. Notch-mediated repression of miR-223 contributes to IGF1R regulation in T-ALL. *Leuk. Res.* **2012**, *36*, 905–911. [CrossRef] [PubMed]

85. Triplett, T.A.; Cardenas, K.T.; Lancaster, J.N.; Hu, Z.; Selden, H.J.; Jasso, G.J.; Balasubramanyam, S.; Chan, K.; Li, L.; Chen, X.; et al. Endogenous dendritic cells from the tumor microenvironment support T-ALL growth via IGF1R activation. *Proc. Natl. Acad. Sci. USA* **2016**, *113*, E1016–E1025. [CrossRef] [PubMed]

86. Li, Y.; Buijs-Gladdines, J.G.; Cante-Barrett, K.; Stubbs, A.P.; Vroegindeweij, E.M.; Smits, W.K.; van Marion, R.; Dinjens, W.N.; Horstmann, M.; Kuiper, R.P.; et al. IL-7 receptor mutations and steroid resistance in pediatric T cell acute lymphoblastic leukemia: A genome sequencing study. *PLoS Med.* **2016**, *13*, e1002200. [CrossRef] [PubMed]

87. Melao, A.; Spit, M.; Cardoso, B.A.; Barata, J.T. Optimal interleukin-7 receptor-mediated signaling, cell cycle progression and viability of T-cell acute lymphoblastic leukemia cells rely on casein kinase 2 activity. *Haematologica* **2016**, *101*, 1368–1379. [CrossRef] [PubMed]

88. Cante-Barrett, K.; Spijkers-Hagelstein, J.A.; Buijs-Gladdines, J.G.; Uitdehaag, J.C.; Smits, W.K.; van der Zwet, J.; Buijsman, R.C.; Zaman, G.J.; Pieters, R.; Meijerink, J.P. MEK and PI3K-AKT inhibitors synergistically block activated IL7 receptor signaling in T-cell acute lymphoblastic leukemia. *Leukemia* **2016**, *30*, 1832–1843. [CrossRef] [PubMed]

89. Gonzalez-Garcia, S.; Garcia-Peydro, M.; Alcain, J.; Toribio, M.L. Notch1 and IL-7 receptor signalling in early T-cell development and leukaemia. *Curr. Top. Microbiol. Immunol.* **2012**, *360*, 47–73. [CrossRef] [PubMed]

90. Keely, P.J. Mechanisms by which the extracellular matrix and integrin signaling act to regulate the switch between tumor suppression and tumor promotion. *J. Mammary Gland Biol. Neoplasia* **2011**, *16*, 205–219. [CrossRef] [PubMed]

91. Liao, Y.X.; Zhou, C.H.; Zeng, H.; Zuo, D.Q.; Wang, Z.Y.; Yin, F.; Hua, Y.Q.; Cai, Z.D. The role of the CXCL12-CXCR4/CXCR7 axis in the progression and metastasis of bone sarcomas. *Int. J. Mol. Med.* **2013**, *32*, 1239–1246. [CrossRef] [PubMed]

92. Naci, D.; Aoudjit, F. a2b1 integrin promotes T cell survival and migration through the concomitant activation of ERK/Mcl-1 and p38 MAPK pathways. *Cell. Signal.* **2014**, *26*, 2008–2015. [CrossRef] [PubMed]

93. Piovan, E.; Tosello, V.; Amadori, A.; Zanovello, P. Chemotactic Cues for NOTCH1-Dependent Leukemia. *Front. Immunol.* **2018**, *9*, 633. [CrossRef] [PubMed]

94. Karakas, B.; Bachman, K.E.; Park, B.H. Mutation of the PIK3CA oncogene in human cancers. *Br. J. Cancer* **2006**, *94*, 455–459. [CrossRef] [PubMed]

95. Forbes, S.A.; Beare, D.; Gunasekaran, P.; Leung, K.; Bindal, N.; Boutselakis, H.; Ding, M.; Bamford, S.; Cole, C.; Ward, S.; et al. COSMIC: Exploring the world's knowledge of somatic mutations in human cancer. *Nucleic Acids Res.* **2015**, *43*, D805–D811. [CrossRef] [PubMed]

96. Gutierrez, A.; Sanda, T.; Grebliunaite, R.; Carracedo, A.; Salmena, L.; Ahn, Y.; Dahlberg, S.; Neuberg, D.; Moreau, L.A.; Winter, S.S.; et al. High frequency of PTEN, PI3K, and AKT abnormalities in T-cell acute lymphoblastic leukemia. *Blood* **2009**, *114*, 647–650. [CrossRef] [PubMed]

97. Martelli, A.M.; Buontempo, F.; McCubrey, J.A. Drug discovery targeting the mTOR pathway. *Clin. Sci. (Lond.)* **2018**, *132*, 543–568. [CrossRef] [PubMed]

98. Grabiner, B.C.; Nardi, V.; Birsoy, K.; Possemato, R.; Shen, K.; Sinha, S.; Jordan, A.; Beck, A.H.; Sabatini, D.M. A diverse array of cancer-associated MTOR mutations are hyperactivating and can predict rapamycin sensitivity. *Cancer Discov.* **2014**, *4*, 554–563. [CrossRef] [PubMed]

99. Ghosh, A.P.; Marshall, C.B.; Coric, T.; Shim, E.H.; Kirkman, R.; Ballestas, M.E.; Ikura, M.; Bjornsti, M.A.; Sudarshan, S. Point mutations of the mTOR-RHEB pathway in renal cell carcinoma. *Oncotarget* **2015**, *6*, 17895–17910. [CrossRef] [PubMed]

100. Schubbert, S.; Cardenas, A.; Chen, H.; Garcia, C.; Guo, W.; Bradner, J.; Wu, H. Targeting the MYC and PI3K pathways eliminates leukemia-initiating cells in T-cell acute lymphoblastic leukemia. *Cancer Res.* **2014**, *74*, 7048–7059. [CrossRef] [PubMed]

101. Meyer, J.; Rhein, M.; Schiedlmeier, B.; Kustikova, O.; Rudolph, C.; Kamino, K.; Neumann, T.; Yang, M.; Wahlers, A.; Fehse, B.; et al. Remarkable leukemogenic potency and quality of a constitutively active neurotrophin receptor, DTrkA. *Leukemia* **2007**, *21*, 2171–2180. [CrossRef] [PubMed]

102. Schwarzer, A.; Holtmann, H.; Brugman, M.; Meyer, J.; Schauerte, C.; Zuber, J.; Steinemann, D.; Schlegelberger, B.; Li, Z.; Baum, C. Hyperactivation of mTORC1 and mTORC2 by multiple oncogenic events causes addiction to eIF4E-dependent mRNA translation in T-cell leukemia. *Oncogene* **2015**, *34*, 3593–3604. [CrossRef] [PubMed]

103. Siddiqui, N.; Sonenberg, N. Signalling to eIF4E in cancer. *Biochem. Soc. Trans.* **2015**, *43*, 763–772. [CrossRef] [PubMed]

104. Wang, W.; Li, J.; Wen, Q.; Luo, J.; Chu, S.; Chen, L.; Qing, Z.; Xie, G.; Xu, L.; Alnemah, M.M.; et al. 4EGI-1 induces apoptosis and enhances radiotherapy sensitivity in nasopharyngeal carcinoma cells via DR5 induction on 4E-BP1 dephosphorylation. *Oncotarget* **2016**, *7*, 21728–21741. [CrossRef] [PubMed]

105. Kosciuczuk, E.M.; Saleiro, D.; Platanias, L.C. Dual targeting of eIF4E by blocking MNK and mTOR pathways in leukemia. *Cytokine* **2017**, *89*, 116–121. [CrossRef] [PubMed]

106. Sabatini, D.M. Twenty-five years of mTOR: Uncovering the link from nutrients to growth. *Proc. Natl. Acad. Sci. USA* **2017**, *114*, 11818–11825. [CrossRef] [PubMed]

107. Steelman, L.S.; Martelli, A.M.; Cocco, L.; Libra, M.; Nicoletti, F.; Abrams, S.L.; McCubrey, J.A. The therapeutic potential of mTOR inhibitors in breast cancer. *Br. J. Clin. Pharmacol.* **2016**, *82*, 1189–1212. [CrossRef] [PubMed]

108. Martelli, A.M.; Chiarini, F.; Evangelisti, C.; Cappellini, A.; Buontempo, F.; Bressanin, D.; Fini, M.; McCubrey, J.A. Two hits are better than one: Targeting both phosphatidylinositol 3-kinase and mammalian target of rapamycin as a therapeutic strategy for acute leukemia treatment. *Oncotarget* **2012**, *3*, 371–394. [CrossRef] [PubMed]

109. Lee, J.S.; Vo, T.T.; Fruman, D.A. Targeting mTOR for the treatment of B cell malignancies. *Br. J. Clin. Pharmacol.* **2016**, *82*, 1213–1228. [CrossRef] [PubMed]

110. Barata, J.T.; Cardoso, A.A.; Nadler, L.M.; Boussiotis, V.A. Interleukin-7 promotes survival and cell cycle progression of T-cell acute lymphoblastic leukemia cells by down-regulating the cyclin-dependent kinase inhibitor p27(kip1). *Blood* **2001**, *98*, 1524–1531. [CrossRef] [PubMed]

111. Batista, A.; Barata, J.T.; Raderschall, E.; Sallan, S.E.; Carlesso, N.; Nadler, L.M.; Cardoso, A.A. Targeting of active mTOR inhibits primary leukemia T cells and synergizes with cytotoxic drugs and signaling inhibitors. *Exp. Hematol.* **2011**, *39*, 457.e3–472.e3. [CrossRef] [PubMed]

112. Oda, K.; Arakawa, H.; Tanaka, T.; Matsuda, K.; Tanikawa, C.; Mori, T.; Nishimori, H.; Tamai, K.; Tokino, T.; Nakamura, Y.; et al. p53AIP1, a potential mediator of p53-dependent apoptosis, and its regulation by Ser-46-phosphorylated p53. *Cell* **2000**, *102*, 849–862. [CrossRef]

113. Li, H.; Kong, X.; Cui, G.; Ren, C.; Fan, S.; Sun, L.; Zhang, Y.; Cao, R.; Li, Y.; Zhou, J. Rapamycin restores p14, p15 and p57 expression and inhibits the mTOR/p70S6K pathway in acute lymphoblastic leukemia cells. *Int. J. Hematol.* **2015**, *102*, 558–568. [CrossRef] [PubMed]

114. Zhang, Y.P.; Huang, Y.T.; Huang, T.S.; Pang, W.; Zhu, J.J.; Liu, Y.F.; Tang, R.Z.; Zhao, C.R.; Yao, W.J.; Li, Y.S.; et al. The mammalian target of rapamycin and DNA methyltransferase 1 axis mediates vascular endothelial dysfunction in response to disturbed flow. *Sci. Rep.* **2017**, *7*, 14996. [CrossRef] [PubMed]

115. Avellino, R.; Romano, S.; Parasole, R.; Bisogni, R.; Lamberti, A.; Poggi, V.; Venuta, S.; Romano, M.F. Rapamycin stimulates apoptosis of childhood acute lymphoblastic leukemia cells. *Blood* **2005**, *106*, 1400–1406. [CrossRef] [PubMed]

116. Wu, K.N.; Zhao, Y.M.; He, Y.; Wang, B.S.; Du, K.L.; Fu, S.; Hu, K.M.; Zhang, L.F.; Liu, L.Z.; Hu, Y.X.; et al. Rapamycin interacts synergistically with idarubicin to induce T-leukemia cell apoptosis in vitro and in a mesenchymal stem cell simulated drug-resistant microenvironment via Akt/mammalian target of rapamycin and extracellular signal-related kinase signaling pathways. *Leuk. Lymphoma* **2014**, *55*, 668–676. [CrossRef] [PubMed]

117. Zhang, Y.; Hua, C.; Cheng, H.; Wang, W.; Hao, S.; Xu, J.; Wang, X.; Gao, Y.; Zhu, X.; Cheng, T.; et al. Distinct sensitivity of CD8+ CD4− and CD8+ CD4+ leukemic cell subpopulations to cyclophosphamide and rapamycin in Notch1-induced T-ALL mouse model. *Leuk. Res.* **2013**, *37*, 1592–1601. [CrossRef] [PubMed]

118. Teachey, D.T.; Sheen, C.; Hall, J.; Ryan, T.; Brown, V.I.; Fish, J.; Reid, G.S.; Seif, A.E.; Norris, R.; Chang, Y.J.; et al. mTOR inhibitors are synergistic with methotrexate: An effective combination to treat acute lymphoblastic leukemia. *Blood* **2008**, *112*, 2020–2023. [CrossRef] [PubMed]

119. Gu, L.; Zhou, C.; Liu, H.; Gao, J.; Li, Q.; Mu, D.; Ma, Z. Rapamycin sensitizes T-ALL cells to dexamethasone-induced apoptosis. *J. Exp. Clin. Cancer Res.* **2010**, *29*, 150. [CrossRef] [PubMed]

120. Zhang, C.; Ryu, Y.K.; Chen, T.Z.; Hall, C.P.; Webster, D.R.; Kang, M.H. Synergistic activity of rapamycin and dexamethasone in vitro and in vivo in acute lymphoblastic leukemia via cell-cycle arrest and apoptosis. *Leuk. Res.* **2012**, *36*, 342–349. [CrossRef] [PubMed]

121. Serafin, V.; Capuzzo, G.; Milani, G.; Minuzzo, S.A.; Pinazza, M.; Bortolozzi, R.; Bresolin, S.; Porcu, E.; Frasson, C.; Indraccolo, S.; et al. Glucocorticoid resistance is reverted by LCK inhibition in pediatric T-cell acute lymphoblastic leukemia. *Blood* **2017**, *130*, 2750–2761. [CrossRef] [PubMed]

122. Schrappe, M.; Valsecchi, M.G.; Bartram, C.R.; Schrauder, A.; Panzer-Grumayer, R.; Moricke, A.; Parasole, R.; Zimmermann, M.; Dworzak, M.; Buldini, B.; et al. Late MRD response determines relapse risk overall and in subsets of childhood T-cell ALL: Results of the AIEOP-BFM-ALL 2000 study. *Blood* **2011**, *118*, 2077–2084. [CrossRef] [PubMed]

123. Wei, G.; Twomey, D.; Lamb, J.; Schlis, K.; Agarwal, J.; Stam, R.W.; Opferman, J.T.; Sallan, S.E.; den Boer, M.L.; Pieters, R.; et al. Gene expression-based chemical genomics identifies rapamycin as a modulator of MCL1 and glucocorticoid resistance. *Cancer Cell* **2006**, *10*, 331–342. [CrossRef] [PubMed]

124. Guo, X.; Zhou, C.Y.; Li, Q.; Gao, J.; Zhu, Y.P.; Gu, L.; Ma, Z.G. Rapamycin sensitizes glucocorticoid resistant acute lymphoblastic leukemia CEM-C1 cells to dexamethasone induced apoptosis through both mTOR suppression and up-regulation and activation of glucocorticoid receptor. *Biomed. Environ. Sci.* **2013**, *26*, 371–381. [CrossRef] [PubMed]

125. Cullion, K.; Draheim, K.M.; Hermance, N.; Tammam, J.; Sharma, V.M.; Ware, C.; Nikov, G.; Krishnamoorthy, V.; Majumder, P.K.; Kelliher, M.A. Targeting the Notch1 and mTOR pathways in a mouse T-ALL model. *Blood* **2009**, *113*, 6172–6181. [CrossRef] [PubMed]

126. Iacovelli, S.; Ricciardi, M.R.; Allegretti, M.; Mirabilii, S.; Licchetta, R.; Bergamo, P.; Rinaldo, C.; Zeuner, A.; Foa, R.; Milella, M.; et al. Co-targeting of Bcl-2 and mTOR pathway triggers synergistic apoptosis in BH3 mimetics resistant acute lymphoblastic leukemia. *Oncotarget* **2015**, *6*, 32089–32103. [CrossRef] [PubMed]

127. Akers, L.J.; Fang, W.; Levy, A.G.; Franklin, A.R.; Huang, P.; Zweidler-McKay, P.A. Targeting glycolysis in leukemia: A novel inhibitor 3-BrOP in combination with rapamycin. *Leuk. Res.* **2011**, *35*, 814–820. [CrossRef] [PubMed]

128. Pikman, Y.; Alexe, G.; Roti, G.; Conway, A.S.; Furman, A.; Lee, E.S.; Place, A.E.; Kim, S.; Saran, C.; Modiste, R.; et al. Synergistic drug combinations with a CDK4/6 inhibitor in T-cell acute lymphoblastic leukemia. *Clin. Cancer Res.* **2017**, *23*, 1012–1024. [CrossRef] [PubMed]

129. Chilosi, M.; Doglioni, C.; Yan, Z.; Lestani, M.; Menestrina, F.; Sorio, C.; Benedetti, A.; Vinante, F.; Pizzolo, G.; Inghirami, G. Differential expression of cyclin-dependent kinase 6 in cortical thymocytes and T-cell lymphoblastic lymphoma/leukemia. *Am. J. Pathol.* **1998**, *152*, 209–217. [PubMed]

130. Mulligan, C.G.; Phillips, L.A.; Su, X.; Ma, J.; Miller, C.B.; Shurtleff, S.A.; Downing, J.R. Genomic analysis of the clonal origins of relapsed acute lymphoblastic leukemia. *Science* **2008**, *322*, 1377–1380. [CrossRef] [PubMed]

131. Li, X.; Gounari, F.; Protopopov, A.; Khazaie, K.; von Boehmer, H. Oncogenesis of T-ALL and nonmalignant consequences of overexpressing intracellular NOTCH1. *J. Exp. Med.* **2008**, *205*, 2851–2861. [CrossRef] [PubMed]

132. Joshi, I.; Minter, L.M.; Telfer, J.; Demarest, R.M.; Capobianco, A.J.; Aster, J.C.; Sicinski, P.; Fauq, A.; Golde, T.E.; Osborne, B.A. Notch signaling mediates G1/S cell-cycle progression in T cells via cyclin D3 and its dependent kinases. *Blood* **2009**, *113*, 1689–1698. [CrossRef] [PubMed]

133. Sawai, C.M.; Freund, J.; Oh, P.; Ndiaye-Lobry, D.; Bretz, J.C.; Strikoudis, A.; Genesca, L.; Trimarchi, T.; Kelliher, M.A.; Clark, M.; et al. Therapeutic targeting of the cyclin D3:CDK4/6 complex in T cell leukemia. *Cancer Cell* **2012**, *22*, 452–465. [CrossRef] [PubMed]

134. Klein, M.E.; Kovatcheva, M.; Davis, L.E.; Tap, W.D.; Koff, A. CDK4/6 Inhibitors: The mechanism of action may not be as simple as once thought. *Cancer Cell* **2018**. [CrossRef] [PubMed]

135. Knudsen, E.S.; Witkiewicz, A.K. The strange case of CDK4/6 inhibitors: Mechanisms, resistance, and combination strategies. *Trends Cancer* **2017**, *3*, 39–55. [CrossRef] [PubMed]

136. Ku, B.M.; Yi, S.Y.; Koh, J.; Bae, Y.H.; Sun, J.M.; Lee, S.H.; Ahn, J.S.; Park, K.; Ahn, M.J. The CDK4/6 inhibitor LY2835219 has potent activity in combination with mTOR inhibitor in head and neck squamous cell carcinoma. *Oncotarget* **2016**, *7*, 14803–14813. [CrossRef] [PubMed]

137. Faes, S.; Demartines, N.; Dormond, O. Resistance to mTORC1 inhibitors in cancer therapy: From kinase mutations to intratumoral heterogeneity of kinase activity. *Oxid. Med. Cell. Longev.* **2017**, *2017*, 1726078. [CrossRef] [PubMed]

138. Chiarini, F.; Fala, F.; Tazzari, P.L.; Ricci, F.; Astolfi, A.; Pession, A.; Pagliaro, P.; McCubrey, J.A.; Martelli, A.M. Dual inhibition of class IA phosphatidylinositol 3-kinase and mammalian target of rapamycin as a new therapeutic option for T-cell acute lymphoblastic leukemia. *Cancer Res.* **2009**, *69*, 3520–3528. [CrossRef] [PubMed]

139. Chiarini, F.; Grimaldi, C.; Ricci, F.; Tazzari, P.L.; Evangelisti, C.; Ognibene, A.; Battistelli, M.; Falcieri, E.; Melchionda, F.; Pession, A.; et al. Activity of the novel dual phosphatidylinositol 3-kinase/mammalian target of rapamycin inhibitor NVP-BEZ235 against T-cell acute lymphoblastic leukemia. *Cancer Res.* **2010**, *70*, 8097–8107. [CrossRef] [PubMed]

140. Gazi, M.; Moharram, S.A.; Marhall, A.; Kazi, J.U. The dual specificity PI3K/mTOR inhibitor PKI-587 displays efficacy against T-cell acute lymphoblastic leukemia (T-ALL). *Cancer Lett.* **2017**, *392*, 9–16. [CrossRef] [PubMed]

141. Shepherd, C.; Banerjee, L.; Cheung, C.W.; Mansour, M.R.; Jenkinson, S.; Gale, R.E.; Khwaja, A. PI3K/mTOR inhibition upregulates NOTCH-MYC signalling leading to an impaired cytotoxic response. *Leukemia* **2013**, *27*, 650–660. [CrossRef] [PubMed]

142. Schult, C.; Dahlhaus, M.; Glass, A.; Fischer, K.; Lange, S.; Freund, M.; Junghanss, C. The dual kinase inhibitor NVP-BEZ235 in combination with cytotoxic drugs exerts anti-proliferative activity towards acute lymphoblastic leukemia cells. *Anticancer Res.* **2012**, *32*, 463–474. [PubMed]

143. Hall, C.P.; Reynolds, C.P.; Kang, M.H. Modulation of glucocorticoid resistance in pediatric T-cell acute lymphoblastic leukemia by increasing BIM expression with the PI3K/mTOR inhibitor BEZ235. *Clin. Cancer Res.* **2016**, *22*, 621–632. [CrossRef] [PubMed]

144. Tosello, V.; Saccomani, V.; Yu, J.; Bordin, F.; Amadori, A.; Piovan, E. Calcineurin complex isolated from T-cell acute lymphoblastic leukemia (T-ALL) cells identifies new signaling pathways including mTOR/AKT/S6K whose inhibition synergize with calcineurin inhibition to promote T-ALL cell death. *Oncotarget* **2016**, *7*, 45715–45729. [CrossRef] [PubMed]

145. Hogan, P.G. Calcium-NFAT transcriptional signalling in T cell activation and T cell exhaustion. *Cell Calcium* **2017**, *63*, 66–69. [CrossRef] [PubMed]

146. Passaro, D.; Irigoyen, M.; Catherinet, C.; Gachet, S.; Da Costa De Jesus, C.; Lasgi, C.; Tran Quang, C.; Ghysdael, J. CXCR4 is required for leukemia-initiating cell activity in T cell acute lymphoblastic leukemia. *Cancer Cell* **2015**, *27*, 769–779. [CrossRef] [PubMed]

147. Gachet, S.; Genesca, E.; Passaro, D.; Irigoyen, M.; Alcalde, H.; Clemenson, C.; Poglio, S.; Pflumio, F.; Janin, A.; Lasgi, C.; et al. Leukemia-initiating cell activity requires calcineurin in T-cell acute lymphoblastic leukemia. *Leukemia* **2013**, *27*, 2289–2300. [CrossRef] [PubMed]

148. Feldman, M.E.; Apsel, B.; Uotila, A.; Loewith, R.; Knight, Z.A.; Ruggero, D.; Shokat, K.M. Active-site inhibitors of mTOR target rapamycin-resistant outputs of mTORC1 and mTORC2. *PLoS Biol.* **2009**, *7*, e38. [CrossRef] [PubMed]

149. Willems, L.; Chapuis, N.; Puissant, A.; Maciel, T.T.; Green, A.S.; Jacque, N.; Vignon, C.; Park, S.; Guichard, S.; Herault, O.; et al. The dual mTORC1 and mTORC2 inhibitor AZD8055 has anti-tumor activity in acute myeloid leukemia. *Leukemia* **2012**, *26*, 1195–1202. [CrossRef] [PubMed]

150. Evangelisti, C.; Ricci, F.; Tazzari, P.; Tabellini, G.; Battistelli, M.; Falcieri, E.; Chiarini, F.; Bortul, R.; Melchionda, F.; Pagliaro, P.; et al. Targeted inhibition of mTORC1 and mTORC2 by active-site mTOR inhibitors has cytotoxic effects in T-cell acute lymphoblastic leukemia. *Leukemia* **2011**, *25*, 781–791. [CrossRef] [PubMed]

151. Park, S.; Sim, H.; Lee, K. Rapamycin-resistant and torin-sensitive mTOR signaling promotes the survival and proliferation of leukemic cells. *BMB Rep.* **2016**, *49*, 63–68. [CrossRef] [PubMed]

152. Zhang, L.N.; Li, J.Y.; Xu, W. A review of the role of Puma, Noxa and Bim in the tumorigenesis, therapy and drug resistance of chronic lymphocytic leukemia. *Cancer Gene Ther.* **2013**, *20*, 1–7. [CrossRef] [PubMed]

153. Roy, A.; Banerjee, S. p27 and leukemia: Cell cycle and beyond. *J. Cell. Physiol.* **2015**, *230*, 504–509. [CrossRef] [PubMed]

154. Yun, S.; Vincelette, N.D.; Knorr, K.L.; Almada, L.L.; Schneider, P.A.; Peterson, K.L.; Flatten, K.S.; Dai, H.; Pratz, K.W.; Hess, A.D.; et al. 4EBP1/c-MYC/PUMA and NF-κB/EGR1/BIM pathways underlie cytotoxicity of mTOR dual inhibitors in malignant lymphoid cells. *Blood* **2016**, *127*, 2711–2722. [CrossRef] [PubMed]

155. Kantarjian, H.M.; O'Brien, S.; Smith, T.L.; Cortes, J.; Giles, F.J.; Beran, M.; Pierce, S.; Huh, Y.; Andreeff, M.; Koller, C.; et al. Results of treatment with hyper-CVAD, a dose-intensive regimen, in adult acute lymphocytic leukemia. *J. Clin. Oncol.* **2000**, *18*, 547–561. [CrossRef] [PubMed]

156. Daver, N.; Boumber, Y.; Kantarjian, H.; Ravandi, F.; Cortes, J.; Rytting, M.E.; Kawedia, J.D.; Basnett, J.; Culotta, K.S.; Zeng, Z.; et al. A phase I/II study of the mTOR inhibitor everolimus in combination with HyperCVAD chemotherapy in patients with relapsed/refractory acute lymphoblastic leukemia. *Clin. Cancer Res.* **2015**, *21*, 2704–2714. [CrossRef] [PubMed]

157. Rheingold, S.R.; Tasian, S.K.; Whitlock, J.A.; Teachey, D.T.; Borowitz, M.J.; Liu, X.; Minard, C.G.; Fox, E.; Weigel, B.J.; Blaney, S.M. A phase 1 trial of temsirolimus and intensive re-induction chemotherapy for 2nd or greater relapse of acute lymphoblastic leukaemia: A Children's Oncology Group study (ADVL1114). *Br. J. Haematol.* **2017**, *177*, 467–474. [CrossRef] [PubMed]

158. Place, A.E.; Pikman, Y.; Stevenson, K.E.; Harris, M.H.; Pauly, M.; Sulis, M.L.; Hijiya, N.; Gore, L.; Cooper, T.M.; Loh, M.L.; et al. Phase I trial of the mTOR inhibitor everolimus in combination with multi-agent chemotherapy in relapsed childhood acute lymphoblastic leukemia. *Pediatr. Blood Cancer* **2018**, *65*, e27062. [CrossRef] [PubMed]

159. Rodrik-Outmezguine, V.S.; Okaniwa, M.; Yao, Z.; Novotny, C.J.; McWhirter, C.; Banaji, A.; Won, H.; Wong, W.; Berger, M.; de Stanchina, E.; et al. Overcoming mTOR resistance mutations with a new-generation mTOR inhibitor. *Nature* **2016**, *534*, 272–276. [CrossRef] [PubMed]

160. Gerlinger, M.; Rowan, A.J.; Horswell, S.; Math, M.; Larkin, J.; Endesfelder, D.; Gronroos, E.; Martinez, P.; Matthews, N.; Stewart, A.; et al. Intratumor heterogeneity and branched evolution revealed by multiregion sequencing. *N. Engl. J. Med.* **2012**, *366*, 883–892. [CrossRef] [PubMed]

161. Ferrando, A.A.; Lopez-Otin, C. Clonal evolution in leukemia. *Nat. Med.* **2017**, *23*, 1135–1145. [CrossRef] [PubMed]

162. Faes, S.; Duval, A.P.; Planche, A.; Uldry, E.; Santoro, T.; Pythoud, C.; Stehle, J.C.; Horlbeck, J.; Letovanec, I.; Riggi, N.; et al. Acidic tumor microenvironment abrogates the efficacy of mTORC1 inhibitors. *Mol. Cancer* **2016**, *15*, 78. [CrossRef] [PubMed]

163. Andre, F.; O'Regan, R.; Ozguroglu, M.; Toi, M.; Xu, B.; Jerusalem, G.; Masuda, N.; Wilks, S.; Arena, F.; Isaacs, C.; et al. Everolimus for women with trastuzumab-resistant, HER2-positive, advanced breast cancer (BOLERO-3): A randomised, double-blind, placebo-controlled phase 3 trial. *Lancet Oncol.* **2014**, *15*, 580–591. [CrossRef]

164. Moscetti, L.; Vici, P.; Gamucci, T.; Natoli, C.; Cortesi, E.; Marchetti, P.; Santini, D.; Giuliani, R.; Sperduti, I.; Mauri, M.; et al. Safety analysis, association with response and previous treatments of everolimus and exemestane in 181 metastatic breast cancer patients: A multicenter Italian experience. *Breast* **2016**, *29*, 96–101. [CrossRef] [PubMed]

165. Gatzka, M.V. Targeted tumor therapy remixed-an update on the use of small-molecule drugs in combination therapies. *Cancers* **2018**, *10*, 155. [CrossRef] [PubMed]

166. Baselga, J.; Im, S.A.; Iwata, H.; Cortes, J.; De Laurentiis, M.; Jiang, Z.; Arteaga, C.L.; Jonat, W.; Clemons, M.; Ito, Y.; et al. Buparlisib plus fulvestrant versus placebo plus fulvestrant in postmenopausal, hormone receptor-positive, HER2-negative, advanced breast cancer (BELLE-2): A randomised, double-blind, placebo-controlled, phase 3 trial. *Lancet Oncol.* **2017**, *18*, 904–916. [CrossRef]

167. Davies, M.; Saxena, A.; Kingswood, J.C. Management of everolimus-associated adverse events in patients with tuberous sclerosis complex: A practical guide. *Orphanet J. Rare Dis.* **2017**, *12*, 35. [CrossRef] [PubMed]

168. Morviducci, L.; Rota, F.; Rizza, L.; Di Giacinto, P.; Ramponi, S.; Nardone, M.R.; Tubili, C.; Lenzi, A.; Zuppi, P.; Baldelli, R. Everolimus is a new anti-cancer molecule: Metabolic side effects as lipid disorders and hyperglycemia. *Diabetes Res. Clin. Pract.* **2018**. [CrossRef] [PubMed]

169. Eiden, A.M.; Zhang, S.; Gary, J.M.; Simmons, J.K.; Mock, B.A. Molecular pathways: Increased susceptibility to infection is a complication of mTOR inhibitor use in cancer therapy. *Clin. Cancer Res.* **2016**, *22*, 277–283. [CrossRef] [PubMed]

170. Guichard, S.M.; Curwen, J.; Bihani, T.; D'Cruz, C.M.; Yates, J.W.; Grondine, M.; Howard, Z.; Davies, B.R.; Bigley, G.; Klinowska, T.; et al. AZD2014, an inhibitor of mTORC1 and mTORC2, is highly effective in ER⁺ breast cancer when administered using intermittent or continuous schedules. *Mol. Cancer Ther.* **2015**, *14*, 2508–2518. [CrossRef] [PubMed]

171. Tolcher, A.W.; LoRusso, P.; Arzt, J.; Busman, T.A.; Lian, G.; Rudersdorf, N.S.; Vanderwal, C.A.; Waring, J.F.; Yang, J.; Holen, K.D.; et al. Safety, efficacy, and pharmacokinetics of navitoclax (ABT-263) in combination with irinotecan: Results of an open-label, phase 1 study. *Cancer Chemother. Pharmacol.* **2015**, *76*, 1041–1049. [CrossRef] [PubMed]

172. Yates, J.W.; Dudley, P.; Cheng, J.; D'Cruz, C.; Davies, B.R. Validation of a predictive modeling approach to demonstrate the relative efficacy of three different schedules of the AKT inhibitor AZD5363. *Cancer Chemother. Pharmacol.* **2015**, *76*, 343–356. [CrossRef] [PubMed]

173. Yi, Z.; Ma, F. Biomarkers of everolimus sensitivity in hormone receptor-positive breast cancer. *J. Breast Cancer* **2017**, *20*, 321–326. [CrossRef]

174. Casado, P.; Rodriguez-Prados, J.C.; Cosulich, S.C.; Guichard, S.; Vanhaesebroeck, B.; Joel, S.; Cutillas, P.R. Kinase-substrate enrichment analysis provides insights into the heterogeneity of signaling pathway activation in leukemia cells. *Sci. Signal.* **2013**, *6*, rs6. [CrossRef] [PubMed]

175. Wu, X.; Xing, X.; Dowlut, D.; Zeng, Y.; Liu, J.; Liu, X. Integrating phosphoproteomics into kinase-targeted cancer therapies in precision medicine. *J. Proteom.* **2018**. [CrossRef] [PubMed]

176. Van der Sligte, N.E.; Scherpen, F.J.; Meeuwsen-de Boer, T.G.; Lourens, H.J.; Ter Elst, A.; Diks, S.H.; Guryev, V.; Peppelenbosch, M.P.; van Leeuwen, F.N.; de Bont, E.S. Kinase activity profiling reveals active signal transduction pathways in pediatric acute lymphoblastic leukemia: A new approach for target discovery. *Proteomics* **2015**, *15*, 1245–1254. [CrossRef] [PubMed]

177. Montano, A.; Forero-Castro, M.; Marchena-Mendoza, D.; Benito, R.; Hernandez-Rivas, J.M. New challenges in targeting signaling pathways in acute lymphoblastic leukemia by NGS approaches: An update. *Cancers* **2018**, *10*, 110. [CrossRef] [PubMed]

178. Casado, P.; Wilkes, E.H.; Miraki-Moud, F.; Hadi, M.M.; Rio-Machin, A.; Rajeeve, V.; Pike, R.; Iqbal, S.; Marfa, S.; Lea, N.; et al. Proteomic and genomic integration identifies kinase and differentiation determinants of kinase inhibitor sensitivity in leukemia cells. *Leukemia* **2018**. [CrossRef] [PubMed]

179. Binnewies, M.; Roberts, E.W.; Kersten, K.; Chan, V.; Fearon, D.F.; Merad, M.; Coussens, L.M.; Gabrilovich, D.I.; Ostrand-Rosenberg, S.; Hedrick, C.C.; et al. Understanding the tumor immune microenvironment (TIME) for effective therapy. *Nat. Med.* **2018**, *24*, 541–550. [CrossRef] [PubMed]

180. Siska, P.J.; van der Windt, G.J.; Kishton, R.J.; Cohen, S.; Eisner, W.; MacIver, N.J.; Kater, A.P.; Weinberg, J.B.; Rathmell, J.C. Suppression of Glut1 and glucose metabolism by decreased Akt/mTORC1 signaling drives T cell impairment in B cell leukemia. *J. Immunol.* **2016**, *197*, 2532–2540. [CrossRef] [PubMed]

181. Bi, L.; Wu, J.; Ye, A.; Wu, J.; Yu, K.; Zhang, S.; Han, Y. Increased Th17 cells and IL-17A exist in patients with B cell acute lymphoblastic leukemia and promote proliferation and resistance to daunorubicin through activation of Akt signaling. *J. Transl. Med.* **2016**, *14*, 132. [CrossRef] [PubMed]

182. Brinda, B.; Khan, I.; Parkin, B.; Konig, H. The rocky road to personalized medicine in acute myeloid leukaemia. *J. Cell. Mol. Med.* **2018**, *22*, 1411–1427. [CrossRef] [PubMed]

183. Harris, E.E.R. Precision medicine for breast cancer: The paths to truly individualized diagnosis and treatment. *Int. J. Breast Cancer* **2018**, *2018*, 4809183. [CrossRef] [PubMed]

184. Yang, W.; Freeman, M.R.; Kyprianou, N. Personalization of prostate cancer therapy through phosphoproteomics. *Nat. Rev. Urol.* **2018**. [CrossRef] [PubMed]

185. Gao, L.; Yuan, K.; Ding, W.; Lin, M. Notch signaling: A potential therapeutic target for hematologic malignancies. *Crit. Rev. Eukaryot. Gene Expr.* **2016**, *26*, 239–246. [CrossRef] [PubMed]

186. Knoechel, B.; Bhatt, A.; Pan, L.; Pedamallu, C.S.; Severson, E.; Gutierrez, A.; Dorfman, D.M.; Kuo, F.C.; Kluk, M.; Kung, A.L.; et al. Complete hematologic response of early T-cell progenitor acute lymphoblastic leukemia to the γ-secretase inhibitor BMS-906024: Genetic and epigenetic findings in an outlier case. *Cold Spring Harb. Mol. Case Stud.* **2015**, *1*, a000539. [CrossRef] [PubMed]

187. Papayannidis, C.; DeAngelo, D.J.; Stock, W.; Huang, B.; Shaik, M.N.; Cesari, R.; Zheng, X.; Reynolds, J.M.; English, P.A.; Ozeck, M.; et al. A Phase 1 study of the novel gamma-secretase inhibitor PF-03084014 in patients with T-cell acute lymphoblastic leukemia and T-cell lymphoblastic lymphoma. *Blood Cancer J.* **2015**, *5*, e350. [CrossRef] [PubMed]

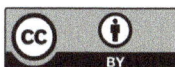

International Journal of
Molecular Sciences

MDPI

Article

mTOR Pathway in Papillary Thyroid Carcinoma: Different Contributions of mTORC1 and mTORC2 Complexes for Tumor Behavior and *SLC5A5* mRNA Expression

Catarina Tavares [1,2,3], Catarina Eloy [1,2,3], Miguel Melo [1,2,4,5], Adriana Gaspar da Rocha [1,2,6], Ana Pestana [1,2,3], Rui Batista [1,2,3], Luciana Bueno Ferreira [1,2,7], Elisabete Rios [1,2,3,8,9], Manuel Sobrinho Simões [1,2,3,8,9] and Paula Soares [1,2,3,8,*]

[1] Instituto de Investigação e Inovação em Saúde (i3S), Universidade do Porto, Porto 4099-002, Portugal; ctavares@ipatimup.pt (C.T.); celoy@ipatimup.pt (C.E.); jmiguelmelo@live.com.pt (M.M.); adrianar@ipatimup.pt (A.G.d.R.); apestana@ipatimup.pt (A.P.); rbatista@ipatimup.pt (R.B.); lferreira@ipatimup.pt (L.B.F.); erios@ipatimup.pt (E.R.); ssimoes@ipatimup.pt (M.S.S.)
[2] Institute of Molecular Pathology and Immunology of the University of Porto (IPATIMUP), Porto 4099-002, Portugal
[3] Faculty of Medicine, Porto University, Porto 4099-002, Portugal
[4] Department of Endocrinology, Diabetes and Metabolism, University and Hospital Center of Coimbra, 3000-075 Coimbra, Portugal
[5] Faculty of Medicine, University of Coimbra, Coimbra 3004-504, Portugal
[6] Public Health Unit, ACeS Baixo Mondego, Coimbra 3000-075, Portugal
[7] Programa de Oncobiologia Celular e Molecular, Instituto Nacional de Câncer, Rio de Janeiro 20230-130, Brasil
[8] Department of Pathology, Medical Faculty of the University of Porto, Porto 4099-002, Portugal
[9] Department of Pathology, Hospital de S. João, Porto 4200-319, Portugal
*   Correspondence: psoares@ipatimup.pt; Tel.: +351-22-040-8800

Received: 2 May 2018; Accepted: 7 May 2018; Published: 13 May 2018

Abstract: The mammalian target of rapamycin (mTOR) pathway is overactivated in thyroid cancer (TC). We previously demonstrated that phospho-mTOR expression is associated with tumor aggressiveness, therapy resistance, and lower mRNA expression of *SLC5A5* in papillary thyroid carcinoma (PTC), while phospho-S6 (mTORC1 effector) expression was associated with less aggressive clinicopathological features. The distinct behavior of the two markers led us to hypothesize that mTOR activation may be contributing to a preferential activation of the mTORC2 complex. To approach this question, we performed immunohistochemistry for phospho-AKT Ser473 (mTORC2 effector) in a series of 182 PTCs previously characterized for phospho-mTOR and phospho-S6 expression. We evaluated the impact of each mTOR complex on *SLC5A5* mRNA expression by treating cell lines with RAD001 (mTORC1 blocker) and Torin2 (mTORC1 and mTORC2 blocker). Phospho-AKT Ser473 expression was positively correlated with phospho-mTOR expression. Nuclear expression of phospho-AKT Ser473 was significantly associated with the presence of distant metastases. Treatment of cell lines with RAD001 did not increase *SLC5A5* mRNA levels, whereas Torin2 caused a ~6 fold increase in *SLC5A5* mRNA expression in the TPC1 cell line. In PTC, phospho-mTOR activation may lead to the activation of the mTORC2 complex. Its downstream effector, phospho-AKT Ser473, may be implicated in distant metastization, therapy resistance, and downregulation of *SLC5A5* mRNA expression.

Keywords: mTOR; thyroid cancer; sodium iodide symporter (NIS)/*SLC5A5*

Int. J. Mol. Sci. **2018**, *19*, 1448

1. Introduction

Thyroid cancer (TC) is the most common endocrine neoplasia. Differentiated thyroid carcinoma (DTC) arises from thyroid follicular cells and represents more than 90% of all cases of TC. DTC comprises papillary thyroid carcinoma (PTC) and follicular thyroid carcinoma (FTC), PTC being the most prevalent type [1,2]. PTC can be further subdivided into the so-called classic PTC (cPTC) and the follicular variant of PTC (fvPTC) [1].

PTC carries an overall good, or even very good, prognosis (overall survival rates of >95% at 25 years) [3] after being treated with surgery followed by radioactive iodine (RAI) therapy at adequate levels [4]. Due to poorly understood reasons, a subgroup of TC patients (10–15%) become resistant to RAI treatment [4], leading to recurrence and/or metastization and a significant reduction of 10-year survival rate [5,6]. The molecular mechanism behind this resistance relies, at least in part, on the loss of sodium iodide symporter (NIS) expression and/or function. NIS is codified by the *SLC5A5* (Solute Carrier Family 5 Member 5) gene, being normally expressed in the basolateral membrane of thyroid follicular cells. It is the gateway of iodine into the interior of the follicular cells as it becomes further incorporated in thyroid hormones. Usually, PTCs maintain NIS expression and function allowing the incorporation of ^{131}I causing tumor cell death, a very efficient targeted radiotherapy [7].

The mTOR pathway can be activated by diverse stimuli, such as growth factors, nutrients, energy, stress signals, and other essential signaling pathways, such as phosphoinositide 3-kinase (PI3K) and mitogen-activated protein kinase (MAPK) [8–10]. It is overactivated in a variety of human neoplasms [10], including TC [9,11,12]. mTOR can associate with distinct proteins and form two distinct complexes: mTORC1 and mTORC2. The complexes have different downstream effectors and physiological functions: mTORC1 effectors are S6K1 and 4EBP1, which participate in cellular growth, proliferation, and survival, whereas mTORC2 can phosphorylate protein kinase C-α (PKC-α) and AKT (Ser 473) and regulates the actin cytoskeleton and cell migration [8,10].

A recent study by our group demonstrated that phospho-mTOR is a marker of aggressiveness in PTC; its expression was associated with aggressive clinicopathological features, including distant metastases, resistance to ^{131}I therapy and, consequently, worse prognosis [13]. In the same study, we observed that phospho-S6 expression was associated with clinicopathological features of low aggressiveness and we did not find a significant correlation between phospho-mTOR and phospho-S6 expression in the tumors [13]. The absence of correlation between the two proteins and their divergent behavior led us to hypothesize that, in PTC, the activation of phospho-mTOR might be contributing preferentially to the activation of the mTORC2 complex, and consequently to AKT phosphorylation (phospho-AKT Ser473) [13], as it has been observed in other tumor models [14–17]. Phospho-AKT is upregulated in PTC [9,11,12,18], but its role in PTC clinical behavior and resistance to therapy needs to be further explored.

Previous studies showed that NIS expression increases when the mTOR pathway is inhibited [6], however, such studies only explored the role of mTORC1 complex [19,20]. As far as we are aware, the role of mTORC2 on *SLC5A5* mRNA expression has not been previously analyzed. So far, it is only known that dual inhibition of mTORC1 and mTORC2 complexes by Torin2 in TC models causes a decrease in cell growth [21,22] and inhibits metastization [22]. In this study, we intended to understand the relevance of mTORC2 complex activation in PTC, by exploring the role of phospho-AKT Ser473 in PTC clinical behavior and the response of TC derived cell lines to Torin2 dual inhibition of mTORC1 and mTORC2 complexes.

2. Results

2.1. Immunoexpression of Phospho-AKT Ser473 in PTC

The expression of phospho-AKT Ser473 was negative in 49.5% of cases. 50.5% of positive cases were distributed throughout the score values (Table 1). In the group of positive cases, immunostaining was detected only in the cytoplasm in 40/92 of cases, and concurrently in the cytoplasm and nucleus in 52/92 of cases.

Among the positive cases, phospho-AKT Ser473 was more intense and preferentially located at the invasive front in 44% of the tumors (Figure 1). Once in the tumor's periphery, phospho-AKT Ser473 was more frequently located in the nucleus (67.6% of the cases with phospho-AKT Ser473 in the invasive areas of the tumor displayed nuclear staining) (Figure 1).

Table 1. Distribution of phospho-AKT score throughout the series.

Phospho-AKT Score	Frequency	%
0	90	49.5
1	18	9.9
2	15	8.2
3	6	3.3
4	8	4.4
6	14	7.7
8	11	6.0
9	6	3.3
12	14	7.7
Total	182	100

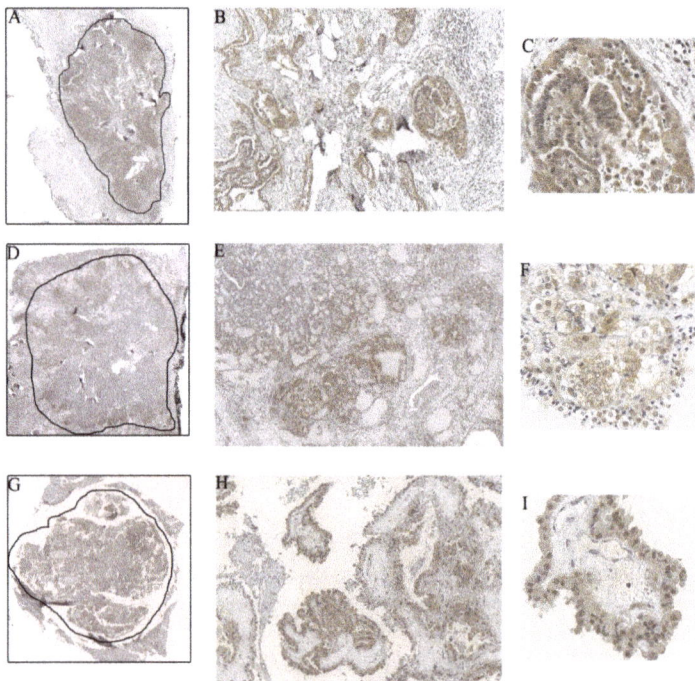

Figure 1. (**A–C**) Intensification of the immunostaining and phospho-AKT Ser473 nuclear expression in the invasive front of a classic papillary thyroid carcinoma (cPTC); (A) 0.44×, (B) 10×, and (C) 40× magnification; (**D–F**) Preferential phospho-AKT Ser473 expression in the tumor periphery, another example in a cPTC. Notice that, in this case, the nuclear translocation was not so intense compared to the previous one; (D) 0.44×, (E) 4×, and (F) 40× magnification; (**G–I**) Strong and disseminated phospho-AKT Ser473 nuclear expression in a hobnail variant of papillary thyroid carcinoma (PTC); (G) 0.44×, (H) 10×, and (I) 40× magnification. The drawn lines, at 0.44× magnification (Figure 1A,D,G), circumscribe the tumor.

2.2. Relationship between the Phospho-AKT Ser473 Expression and Clinicopathological and Molecular Features

Phospho-AKT Ser473 total expression (cytoplasm plus nuclear) was positively correlated with phospho-mTOR expression (r(168) = 0.2, p = 0.02) but not with phospho-S6 expression (r(139) = 0.02, p = 0.8).

Phospho-AKT Ser473 was significantly more expressed in PTCs harboring the *BRAF*V600E mutation than in *BRAF* wild type (WT) PTC (p = 0.04) (Table 2); when divided by histological variant this significant association was maintained in the cPTC group but was lost in the fvPTC group. There were no significant associations between phospho-AKT Ser473 total expression and the following features: age, tumor size, tumor capsule, multifocality, lymphocytic infiltrate, vascular invasion, lymph node metastases, tumor margins (well circumscribed vs. infiltrative), distant metastases, staging, *NRAS* and *TERT*p status, number of ^{131}I therapies or cumulative dose of radioactive iodine, additional treatments, disease-free status at one year, and disease-free status at the end of follow-up.

Table 2. Association between phospho-AKT score and *BRAF* status.

BRAF	Phospho-AKT Score	p Value
WT (n = 106)	2.2 ± 3.3	0.04
V600E (n = 74)	3.4 ± 4.4	

WT: wild type

The nuclear expression of phospho-AKT Ser473 was more often detected in cases with distant metastases compared with cases without distant metastases (p = 0.04) (Table 3). We did not find any significant association between phospho-AKT Ser473 nuclear expression and other clinicopathological or molecular features (all PTCs, and cPTC or fvPTC subgroups).

Table 3. Association between phospho-AKT nuclear expression and distant metastases.

Nuclear Expression	Distant Metastases		p Value
	Yes	No	
Yes	9 (81.82%)	19 (47.5%)	
No	2 (18.18%)	21 (52.5%)	0.04
Total	11	40	51

2.3. Contribution of mTORC1 and mTORC2 Complexes in the Regulation of SLC5A5 mRNA Expression

To study the role of both mTORC1 and mTORC2 complexes on *SLC5A5* mRNA expression, we performed treatments of the TPC1 and K1 cell lines with RAD001 (mTORC1 inhibitor) and Torin 2 (mTORC1 and mTORC2 dual inhibitor) for 60 and 72 h.

We confirmed the efficacy of the drugs in the activity of mTOR complexes through the evaluation of phospho-S6 Ser235/236 expression as a read-out of mTORC1 activity and phospho-AKT Ser473 as read-out of mTORC2 activity. After 72 h of treatment, RAD001 caused a significant downregulation of the mTORC1 complex and did not affect the activity of the mTORC2 complex (significant decrease of phospho-S6 expression and no differences in phospho-AKT Ser473 expression) (Figure 2A,B). Torin2 treatment led to a significant and concurrent downregulation of mTORC1 and mTORC2 complex activity (significant decrease of phospho-S6 and phospho-AKT Ser473 expression) (Figure 2A,B). These effects were also observed after 60 h of treatment in both cell lines.

At 72h, RAD001 treatment did not affect *SLC5A5* mRNA expression in the TPC1 cell line and caused a slight decrease in the K1 cell line. Torin2 treatment caused a significant increase in *SLC5A5* mRNA expression (~6 fold, p = 0.02) in the TPC-1 cell line but had no effect on the K1 cell line (Figure 3). *SLC5A5* mRNA expression was not altered in either cell line after 60 h of treatment with both drugs (except for a slight decrease of *SLC5A5* mRNA expression in the K1cell line after 60 h of treatment with RAD001).

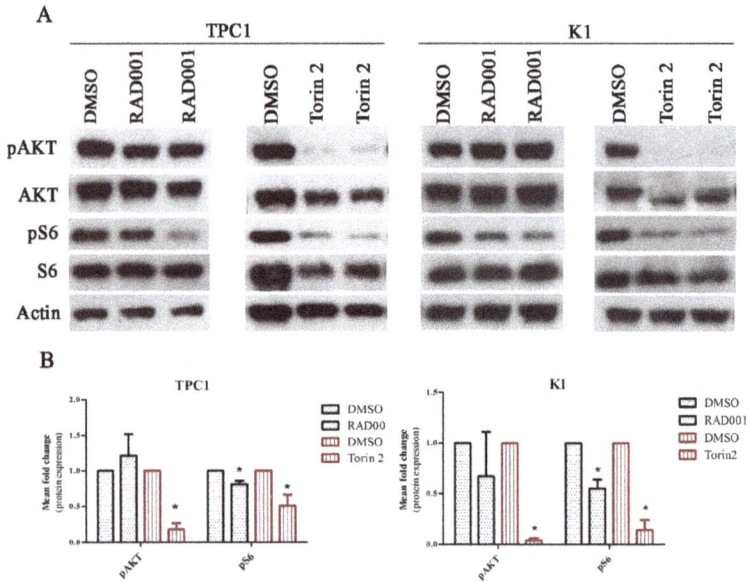

Figure 2. RAD001 and Torin2 effect on TPC1 and K1 cell lines. (**A**) Cells were treated with 20 nM of RAD001 and 450 nM of Torin2 for 72 h. Western blot analysis of RAD001 and Torin2 effect on the activation status of mTORC1 and mTORC2 complexes was evaluated by phospho-S6 Ser235/236 and phospho-AKT Ser473 expression, respectively. Representative actin expression is shown. Protein level in treated cells was evaluated in duplicate. (**B**) Mean fold change of protein expression observed in TPC1 cell line treated with 20 nM of RAD001 and 450 nM of Torin2 in comparison to cells treated with DMSO. Phosphorylated proteins were normalized by the levels of their correspondent total proteins. Results are shown as mean expression value of three independent experiments ±SEM. * $p < 0.05$ (unpaired Student's *t* test).

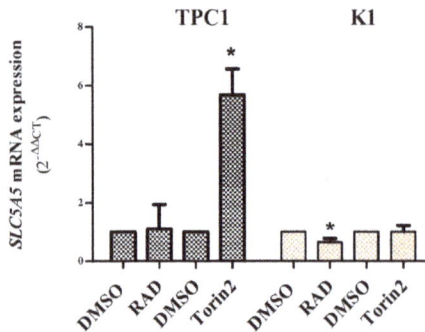

Figure 3. *SLC5A5* expression in TPC1 and K1 cell lines after treatment with RAD001 (20 nM) and Torin2 (450 nM) for 72 h. Mean fold change of *SLC5A5* mRNA expression observed in TPC1 and K1 cell lines after treatment in comparison to cells treated with DMSO. Treatment with RAD001 did not affect *SLC5A5* expression in the TPC1 cell line and caused a slight decrease in the K1 cell line. Treatment with Torin2 caused a significant increase (~6 fold) in *SLC5A5* expression in the TPC1 cell line but not in the K1 cell line. Bars represent mean expression ± SEM. * $p < 0.05$. Results are shown as mean expression values of three independent experiments.

2.4. BRAF Regulation of SLC5A5 mRNA Expression and of mTORC1 and mTORC2 Status in K1 Cell Line

Given the lack of effect of Torin2 to increase *SLC5A5* mRNA expression in the K1 cell line, we hypothesized that it may be related to the fact that the K1 cell line presents the *BRAF*V600E mutation (known to decrease *SLC5A5* mRNA expression [23]). In order explore this hypothesis we performed *BRAF* down-regulation by siRNA (24 h and 72 h). As observed in Figure 4, *BRAF*-C2 siRNA led to a significant downregulation of *BRAF* and pERKs, confirming the downregulation of the MAPK pathway. *BRAF* silencing in the K1 cell line caused a significant increase in *SLC5A5* mRNA expression (~3 fold increase) (Figure 5).

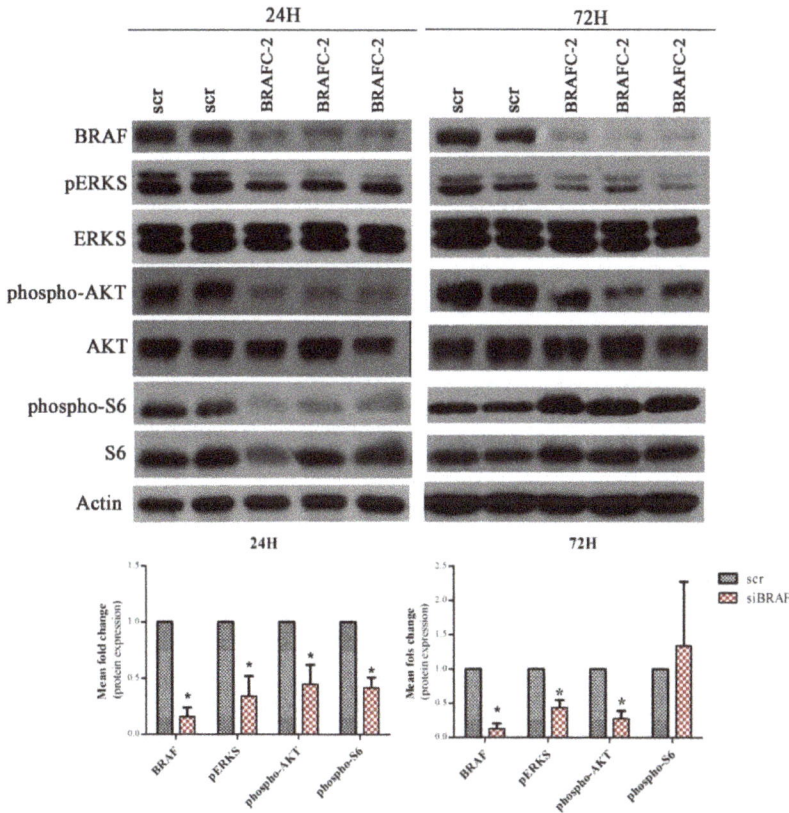

Figure 4. *BRAF*, pERKS, ERKS, phospho-AKT Ser473, AKT, phospho-S6 Ser235/236, and S6 expression in the K1 cell line after *BRAF* silencing. Western blot for *BRAF*, pERKS, ERKS, phospho-AKT Ser473, AKT, phospho-S6 Ser235/236, S6 expression and actin in K1 cell line treated with *BRAF*-C2 siRNA (50 nM) after 24 and 72 h. The levels of *BRAF* were analyzed for control of silencing efficiency and the levels of pERKS as a readout of MAPK pathway activity. Representative actin expression pattern is shown. Protein level, in scramble siRNA treated cells, was evaluated in duplicate (Scr), whereas in *BRAF* siRNA treated cells, it was analyzed in triplicate. The graphics depicts the mean fold change of protein expression observed in K1 cell line treated with *BRAF*-C2 siRNA in comparison to cells treated with scramble siRNA. Phosphorylated proteins were normalized by the levels of their correspondent total proteins, all others were normalized by the levels of control protein (actin). Results are shown as mean expression value of two independent experiments ±SEM. * $p < 0.05$ (unpaired Student's t test).

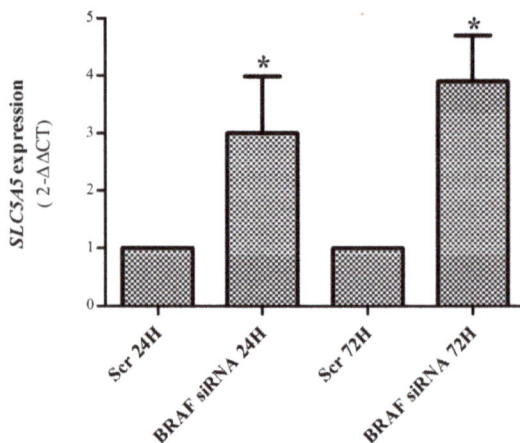

Figure 5. *SLC5A5* mRNA expression in K1 cell line after *BRAF* silencing (50 nM, 24 and 72 h). *BRAF* silencing caused a significant (~3 fold) increase in *SLC5A5* mRNA expression at both time points. Bars represent mean expression $\pm$ SEM. * $p < 0.05$. Results are shown as mean expression values of two independent experiments, each one with three replicates.

Since we observed, in our tumor samples, that PTCs harboring the *BRAF*V600E mutation presented higher levels of phospho-AKT Ser473, we were also interested in the effect of the *BRAF*V600E mutation in the activation status of each mTOR complex. To address this issue, we also evaluated phospho-AKT Ser473 and phospho-S6 expression (mTORC1 and mTORC2 readout, respectively) after *BRAF* silencing. After 24 h of *BRAF* silencing, both phospho-S6 Ser235/236 and phospho-AKT Ser473 expression were significantly decreased, however after 72 h of silencing, phospho-AKT Ser473 expression remained significantly lower while phospho-S6 Ser235/236 expression increased and became higher in silenced cells compared to scramble cells.

3. Discussion

In a recent study by our group we demonstrated that phospho-mTOR is a marker of aggressiveness in PTC, as its expression is associated with aggressive clinicopathological features, including distant metastases, resistance to ^{131}I therapy, and, consequently, worse prognosis [13]. Paradoxically, in the same study, we did not find a significant correlation between phospho-mTOR and phospho-S6 expression [13]. This led us to hypothesize that, in PTC, the activation of phospho-mTOR might be contributing preferentially to the activation of the mTORC2 complex, and consequently, to AKT phosphorylation (phospho-AKT Ser473) [13]. In the present study, we observed a positive and significant correlation between phospho-mTOR and phospho-AKT Ser473 expression, indicating that PTCs that expressed higher levels of phospho-mTOR also expressed higher levels of phospho-AKT Ser473. We also demonstrated that phospho-AKT Ser473 nuclear expression is associated with the presence of distant metastases. These results support our hypothesis that, in PTC, mTOR phosphorylation may lead to the preferential activation of the mTORC2 complex and its downstream effector phospho-AKT Ser473, which seems to play a role in distant metastization.

Preferential formation of the mTORC2 complex was previously observed in other human malignancies and is usually associated with increased cell motility [14–17]. In TC, both mTORC1 and mTORC2 complexes are overexpressed compared to normal tissues [9,21], but the contribution of each complex to tumor behavior and prognosis still needs further investigation. Previous studies showed that phospho-AKT Ser473 is overexpressed in TC [9,11,12,24], and its expression has been associated with metastization in animal models of TC [25,26]. Recently, a study by Matson et al. [18] demonstrated that the depletion of AKT1 expression in TC cell lines was able to decrease invasion.

Our results indicate that the activation of phospho-AKT Ser473 plays a role in TC distant metastization. We observed that phospho-AKT Ser473 expression was associated with distant metastasis only when nuclear expression was considered. It seems that phospho-AKT Ser473 nuclear translocation is of major importance to migration and distant metastization of TC. Vasko et al. [12] demonstrated that phospho-AKT Ser473 was expressed in the cytoplasm of PTC throughout the tumor, but the immunostaining was more intense and localized in the nucleus of cells located in the invasive regions. We also observed that when phospho-AKT Ser473 staining was more concentrated in the invasive front of the tumor, it was preferentially located in the nucleus. Moreover, in an animal model of TC, phospho-AKT Ser473 expression was localized primarily in the nucleus of cells from metastatic lesions, while in the respective primary tumors it was located in the cytoplasm and nucleus of cells. These results suggest that phospho-AKT Ser473 nuclear distribution may be relevant for promoting metastization [26].

As previously mentioned, these results contrast with the lack of correlation between phospho-mTOR and phospho-S6 expression, as well as the distinct behavior associated with the expression of each marker observed in our previous study [13]. One possible interpretation is the fact that phospho-S6 can be phosphorylated (at Ser235/236) in an mTORC1 independent manner. For instance, S6K1-/-/2-/- knock-out mice were found to display no phosphorylation of phospho-S6 Ser240/244 but present persistent phosphorylation at phospho-S6 Ser235/236, revealing the presence of another in vivo phospho-S6 kinase, p90 ribosomal S6 kinase (RSK) [27], which can phosphorylate S6 in response to the RAS/ERK pathway, serum, and growth factors independently of mTORC1 [28]. Furthermore, in some situations, the equal activation of both mTOR complexes may not coexist, since it has already been shown that mTORC1 inhibition can increase mTORC2 activation. Inhibition of mTOR/S6K1 can induce phospho-AKT S473 phosphorylation (by a negative feedback loop) through the activation of insulin receptor substrate-1 (IRS1) function, a mediator of the insulin receptor-dependent activation of PI3K [29].

We also found that phospho-AKT Ser473 expression (cytoplasmic and nuclear) was significantly higher in PTCs harboring the *BRAF*V600E mutation compared to *BRAF*WT PTCs (Table 2). In our previous study we observed that *BRAF*V600E mutated PTCs expressed similar high levels of phospho-mTOR but significantly lower levels of phospho-S6 compared to *BRAF*WT PTCs [13]. Altogether, the results of both studies suggest that PTCs harboring a *BRAF*V600E mutation display a preferential activation of the mTORC2 complex in comparison to mTORC1 (Figure 6). Our in vitro results reinforce this assumption: After 24 h of *BRAF* silencing we observed a significant decrease of phospho-S6 Ser235/236 and phospho-AKT Ser473 expression, nevertheless after 72 h, even though *BRAF* was still silenced and pERKS diminished, phospho-S6 Ser235/236 expression increased while phospho-AKT Ser 473 protein levels remained significantly decreased. These results suggest that *BRAF*V600E might have a long-lasting effect in the regulation of phospho-AKT Ser 473 expression (mTORC2) compared to phospho-S6 Ser235/236 expression (mTORC1).

Recent studies explored the role of the mTOR pathway in NIS expression/function in rat thyroid cells [19] and in human TC cell lines (8505C, TPC1, and BCPAP) [20], demonstrating that treatments with rapamycin, a mTORC1 inhibitor, were able to restore NIS expression and function in some cell lines, but not in TPC-1 [19,20]. Loss of NIS expression and function has been indicated as the molecular mechanism responsible for radioactive iodine therapy resistance and metastatic progression in TC [7]. Since our results indicated preferential mTORC2 activation in PTCs, we have also become interested in exploring the role of mTORC2 in the NIS protein and *SLC5A5* mRNA expression. We performed our study in TPC1 and K1 cell lines. RAD001 caused a decrease in phospho-S6 expression, but it did not alter phospho-AKT Ser473 nor *SLC5A5* expression in both cell lines (as it was already observed for the TPC1 cell line) [20]. On the other hand, Torin2 treatment caused a decrease of phospho-S6 and phospho-AKT Ser473 expression in both cell lines, and a significant increase in *SLC5A5* mRNA expression, but only in the TPC1 cell line (Figures 2 and 3). These results demonstrate that the inhibition of the mTORC2 complex may be of major importance in the restoration of *SLC5A5* mRNA expression, highlighting its role as a potential therapeutic target. To the best of our knowledge, the impact of Torin2 in *SLC5A5* mRNA expression or NIS protein function has not been previously addressed. Of note, patients with PTC that developed recurrences and/or distant metastases presented lower levels of *SLC5A5* mRNA expression compared to patients without tumor progression [30]. This information is in line with our present results indicating that mTORC2 (phospho-AKT Ser 473) can be implicated in distant metastization as well as in the regulation of *SLC5A5* mRNA expression.

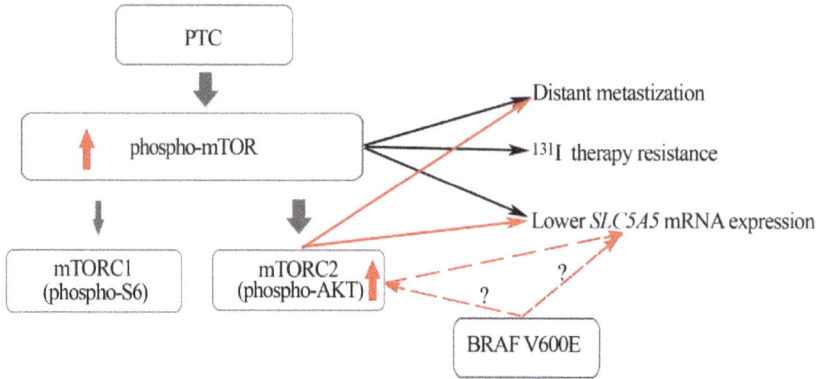

Figure 6. mTOR can be found in two distinct complexes: mTORC1 and mTORC2, each one with different downstream effectors, pS6 and pAKT, respectively. In PTCs, MTOR activation (high phosphor-mTOR expression) and the mTORC2 downstream effector (nuclear phospho-AKT Ser473) are associated with aggressive features (distant metastization). PTCs harboring *BRAFV600E* also present higher levels of pAKT. The impact of *BRAF* V600E on *SLC5A5* mRNA expression can be direct or mediated by activation of pAKT. The red dotted arrows refers to different possibilities.

The different responses to Torin2 treatment, in terms of *SLC5A5* mRNA expression, of the two cell lines, led us to focus on the differences between them. One major difference is the genetic background: the TPC1 cell line harbors rearranged during transfection proto-oncogene *RET/PTC1* rearrangement, while the K1 cell line harbors the *BRAFV600E* point mutation [31]. It is well established that, at variance to *RET/PTC* rearrangement, *BRAFV600E* mutation impairs *SLC5A5* mRNA expression, as well as NIS trafficking to the basolateral membrane in patients and cell lines [23,32]. The molecular mechanism behind this impairment is not fully understood yet, and even though the *BRAFV600E* mutation activates the MAPK pathway, its effect on NIS impairment does not seem to be mediated by the MAPK pathway [23]. Taking this information into consideration, we performed *BRAF* silencing in the K1 cell line to evaluate if *BRAF* was interfering with *SLC5A5* mRNA expression. In fact, after *BRAF* silencing, we observed a significant increase in *SLC5A5* mRNA expression, as well as a decrease in phosphor AKT Ser 473 expression. Gathering the literature [23,32] together with our present results, we hypothesize that in a *BRAFV600E* context, the concurrent mTORC1 and mTORC2 downregulation may not be sufficient to induce *SLC5A5* mRNA expression, thus explaining the absence of an increase in *SLC5A5* mRNA expression in the K1cell line after Torin2 treatment.

Summing up, we have demonstrated that the mTORC2 pathway is activated in PTC, especially in those PTC harboring the *BRAFV600E* mutation. We have also shown that in the mTORC2 downstream effector phospho-AKT Ser473, nuclear translocation may play a role in distant metastization, and, possibly, in *SLC5A5* mRNA downregulation. We propose that, in PTC, the mTORC2 complex may be preferentially activated (phospho-AKT473), and that this specific complex may be implicated in the distant metastization, decrease in *SLC5A5* mRNA expression, and therapy resistance.

4. Materials and Methods

4.1. Patient Tissue Samples

One hundred and eighty-two formalin-fixed, paraffin-embedded representative tissue samples of PTCs were collected from files of the Institute of Molecular Pathology and Immunology of the University of Porto (IPATIMUP, Porto, Portugal), corresponding to 182 patients followed in two university hospitals in Portugal. In 115 cases we had access to follow-up data. The histology of all tumors samples was revised (CE, ER, MSS) according to the World Health Organization criteria [33]. Epidemiological, clinical, and molecular data of the 182 cases are summarized in Table 4. This work was approved by the Ethic Committee for Health (CES) of the Hospital Center of São João (CHSJ)/Faculty of Medicine of the University of Porto (FMUP) (CES 137 284-13, 2014) and by the Ethics Committee of the Faculty of Medicine of the University of Coimbra (n °1309, 2010). All procedures described in this study were in accordance with National Ethical Standards (Law n° 12/2005) and the Helsinki Declaration.

Table 4. Epidemiologic, histologic, and clinical data of the patients.

Patients		Total and %		
		cPTC	fvPTC	Other PTC Variants
Gender	F n = 150	94 (82.5)	41 (87.2)	15 (71.4)
	M n = 32	20 (17.5)	6 (12.8)	6 (28.6)
Age	<45 years n = 94	62 (54.9)	21 (45.7)	11 (55.0)
	≥45 years n = 85	51 (45.1)	25 (54.3)	9 (45.0)
Tumor size	<2cm n = 64	39 (36.8)	17 (37.0)	8 (40.0)
	≥2cm n = 108	67 (63.2)	29 (63.0)	12 (60.0)
Tumor capsule	Present n = 83	42 (39.6)	32 (71.1)	9 (42.9)
	Absent n = 89	64 (60.4)	13 (28.9)	12 (57.1)
Tumor capsule Invasion	Yes n = 64	35 (89.7)	22 (68.8)	7 (100)
	No n = 14	4 (10.3)	10 (31.3)	0 (0)
Extra thyroid invasion	Yes n = 73	50 (48.1)	12 (27.3)	11 (55.0)
	No n = 95	54 (51.9)	32 (72.7)	9 (45.0)
Multifocality	Single n = 104	58 (54.7)	32 (68.1)	14 (70.0)
	Multiple n = 69	48 (45.3)	15 (31.9)	6 (30.0)
Lymphocytic infiltrate	Present n = 108	77 (70.6)	19 (41.3)	12 (60.0)
	Absent n = 67	32 (29.4)	27 (58.7)	8 (40.0)
Vascular invasion	Present n = 59	42 (40.4)	10 (22.2)	7 (35.0)
	Absent n = 110	62 (59.6)	35 (77.8)	13 (65.0)
Lymph node metastases	Present n = 57	40 (43.0)	12 (34.3)	5 (29.4)
	Absent n = 88	53 (57.0)	23 (65.7)	12 (70.6)
Tumor margins	Infiltrative n = 78	57 (79.2)	13 (46.4)	8 (72.7)
	Well defined n = 33	15 (20.8)	15 (53.6)	3 (27.3)
Distant metastases	Yes n = 17	9 (11.8)	5 (17.9)	3 (30.0)
	No n = 97	67 (88.2)	23 (82.1)	7 (70.0)
One year disease free survival	Yes n = 64	41 (56.2)	19 (67.9)	4 (40.0)
	No n = 47	32 (43.8)	9 (32.1)	6 (60.0)
Disease free (at the end of follow up)	Yes n = 70	44 (59.5)	19 (67.9)	7 (70.0)
	No n = 42	30 (40.5)	9 (32.1)	3 (30.0)
Deaths	Yes n = 5	2 (2.6)	2 (7.1)	1 (9.1)
	No n = 110	74 (97.4)	26 (92.9)	10 (90.9)
BRAF	WT n = 106	56 (49.1)	37 (82.2)	13 (61.9)
	V600E n = 74	58 (50.9)	8 (17.8)	8 (38.1)
NRAS	WT n = 162	108 (99.1)	38 (90.5)	16 (80.0)
	Mut n = 9	1 (0.9)	4 (9.5)	4 (20.0)
TERTp	WT n = 152	95 (96.0)	40 (95.2)	17 (100.0)
	Mut n = 6	4 (4.0)	2 (4.8)	0 (0.0)
RET/PTC	WT n = 56	29 (78.4)	18 (94.7)	9 (90.0)
	Rearrangment n = 10	8 (21.6)	1 (5.3)	1 (10.0)
Staging	I n = 64	45 (64.3)	15 (60.0)	4 (50.0)
	II n = 6	3 (4.3)	3 (12.0)	0 (0.0)
	III n = 24	19 (27.1)	3 (12.0)	2 (25.0)
	IV n = 9	3 (4.3)	4 (16.0)	2 (25.0)

4.2. Patient's Follow Up

Patients were treated and followed in accordance with the international protocols available at the time. Data regarding the number of radioiodine treatments and cumulative activity were retrieved from hospital records. Patients were considered as being disease free at the end of follow-up if they had undetectable stimulated thyroglobulin (in the absence of thyroglobulin antibodies) and no imagiological evidence of the disease. The mean time of follow up was 8.0 ± 6.8 years. The number of ^{131}I treatments varied between 1 and 5 (mean 1.8) and cumulative dose of RAI totalized values were between 30 and 1146 mCi (mean 245.2 mCi). For statistical analysis, we defined the category "additional treatments", in which we included other treatment modalities in addition to radioiodine, including extra surgery, external beam irradiation, and treatment with tyrosine kinase inhibitors.

4.3. Immunohistochemistry

Immunohistochemistry was performed as previously described [9]. Briefly, sections were subjected to heat-induced antigen retrieval in 10 mM sodium citrate buffer (pH 6.0). Endogenous peroxidase activity was blocked with 3% of H_2O_2 and nonspecific binding with Large Volume Ultra V Block reagent (Thermo Scientific/Lab Vision, Waltham, MA, USA). Sections were then incubated overnight at 4 °C with anti-phospho-AKT Ser473 antibody (clone 736E11) (Cell Signaling Technology, Danvers, MA, USA) (1:50). The detection was performed with a labeled streptavidin-biotin immunoperoxidase detection system (Thermo Scientific/Lab Vision, Waltham, MA, USA) followed by 3,3'-diaminobenzidine (Dako, Glostrup, Denmark) reaction and counterstained with hematoxylin.

The immunostaining evaluation was done according to our previous work [9]. Slides were evaluated by two independent observers and semiquantitatively scored in terms of percentage of tumor stained cells (0: <5%; 1: 5–25%; 2: 25–50%; 3: 50–75%; 4: >75%) and staining intensity (0—negative; 1—weak; 2—intermediate; 3—strong). An immunohistochemical score was calculated by multiplying the proportion of positive cells by the intensity of the staining, 12 being the maximum score. The distribution of cases within the scores is summarized in Table 4. The cellular localization was also evaluated as membrane and/or cytoplasmic and/or nuclear. To be considered positive for nuclear expression, tumors must display phospho-AKT Ser473 immunostaining in at least 5% of tumor cells. As a positive control, we used a breast carcinoma known to be positive for phospho-AKT Ser473, for a negative control, we used the same carcinoma and omitted the primary antibody (Figure S1). Slides were observed using a Axioskop 2 Zeiss microscope. Representative slides were scanned using a DSight Viewer (Menarini, Florence, Italy) and photographs were obtained through snapshots from DSight Viewer Software (Menarini). From the 182 cases characterized for phospho-AKT Ser473, 170 have been previously characterized for phospho-mTOR Ser2448 and 141 for phospho-S6 Ser235/236 [13].

4.4. DNA Extraction, PCR and Sanger Sequencing

The genetic characterization (PCR and sequencing) of the tumors regarding *BRAF*, *NRAS*, *RET/PTC*, and *TERT* promoter (*TERTp*) mutations were screened as previously described [34–38], and in part as had been previously reported [13].

4.5. Cell Lines, Treatments with RAD001 and Torin2 and Transfection Assays

The TPC1 cell line was kindly provided by Doctor Dumont JE and Doctor Marell M, and the K1 cell line was provided by Dr. Wynford-Thomas D [31]. Both cell lines were derived from papillary thyroid carcinoma. They have already been characterized at the molecular and genotypic level, TPC1 cell line harbors the *RET/PTC1* rearrangement and *TERT*p mutation (-124 G>A). The K1 cell line harbors the *BRAF*V600E and *PI3K*E542K mutations and also the *TERT*p mutation (-124 G>A) [31,38]. Cell lines were maintained in RPMI supplemented with antibiotics; 1% (*v*/*v*) Pen Strep and 0.5% fungizone (*v*/*v*) (Biowest, Nuaillé, France) and 10% (*v*/*v*) of fetal bovine serum (FBS) (GIBCO, Thermo Fisher Scientific Waltham, MA, USA). Cells were grown in a humidified incubator with 5% CO_2 at 37 °C.

For treatment purposes, cell were plated in six well plates, TPC1 (1×10^5 cells per well) and K1 (2×10^5 cells per well), 24 h later cells were treated with RAD001 (20 nM) or Torin2 (450 nM) (Selleckchem, Houston, TX, USA). Treatments lasted for 60 h and 72 h. Treatments were performed in triplicate, each experiment had two replicates of the treatment.

Small interfering RNAS (siRNA) assays were performed as previously reported [39], using 50 nM of oligo *BRAF* (BRAF-C2), cell lysates were obtained after 24 h and 72 h. Silencing was performed in duplicate (two independent experiments), each experiment had two replicates of the scramble and tree replicates of the silencing.

4.6. RNA Extraction, Reverse Transcription and Real Time PCR

Total RNA was extracted from TPC1 and K1 cell lines using a Trizol commercial kit (Thermo Scientific/GIBCO, Waltham, MA, USA) according to the manufacturer's protocol. RNA was quantified by spectrophotometry, and its quality was checked by analysis of 260/280 nm and 260/230 nm ratios. For cDNA preparation, 1 µg of total RNA was reverse transcribed using the RevertAid first strand cDNA synthesis kit (Thermo Scientific/Fermentas, Waltham, MA, USA).

Reverse transcription products were amplified for *SLC5A5* by qPCR (IDT:Integrated DNA Technologies, Leuven, Belgium; no. HS.PT.56a.40789288) using a TaqMan PCR Master Mix (Applied Biosystems, Foster City, CA, USA) with the TBP gene (TATA-binding protein) as an endogenous control (Applied Biosystems; no. 4326322E-0705006). The ABI PRISM 7500 Fast Sequence Detection System (Applied Biosystems, Foster City, CA, USA) was used and was programmed to an initial step of 20 s at 50 °C, 10 min at 95° C, followed by 40 cycles of 95 °C for 15 s and 60 °C for 1 min. For each sample, TBP and *SLC5A5* amplifications were done in triplicate using 1 µL of cDNA (~25 ng).

The relative quantification of target genes was determined using the $2^{-\Delta\Delta CT}$ method. Similar efficiencies of both assays were confirmed using Livak's Linear Regression Method [40] (slope −0.4).

4.7. Western Blot Analysis

Cells were lysed in RIPA buffer supplemented with phosphatase and protease inhibitors. Proteins were quantified using DC™ Protein Assay (Bio-RAD, CA, USA), then were resolved by SDS-PAGE and transferred onto nitrocellulose membranes (GE Healthcare, Little Chalfont, UK). The primary antibodies were: phospho-S6 Ser235/236, S6, phospho-AKTSer473, AKT, pERKS, ERKS (1:1000), and *BRAF* (1:500) (Santa Cruz Biotechnology, Santa Cruz, CA, USA), all antibodies were acquired from Cell Signaling Technology (Danvers, MA, USA).

Protein was detected using a horseradish peroxidase-conjugated antibody (Santa Cruz Biotechnology, Santa Cruz, CA, USA) and a luminescence system (Perkin-Elmer, Waltham, MA, USA). For the protein loading control, membranes were incubated with an antiactin Santa Cruz Biotechnology (Santa Cruz, CA, USA) antibody. Protein expression was quantified using the Bio-Rad Quantity One 1-D Analysis software (Bio-Rad Laboratories, Inc., Hercules, CA, USA). The levels of phosphorylated proteins: phospho-S6 Ser235/236, phospho-AKT Ser 473, and pERKS were normalized by the levels of their corresponding total protein (total, S6, and AKT), all others were normalized by loading control (actin). The levels of expression of phosphorylated proteins and their corresponding total protein were evaluated in the same gel, furthermore, the antibodies used for the total proteins recognize all forms of the phosphorylated proteins.

4.8. Statistical Analysis

Statistical analysis was conducted with SPSS version 21.00 (SPSS Inc). The expression of phospho-AKT Ser473 is expressed as mean ± standard deviation. An independent sample Student's t test was used to evaluate possible associations between phospho-AKT Ser 473 expression and clinicopathological and molecular features to compare protein expression (analyzed by western blot) between groups. A Pearson Correlation was used to evaluate the correlation between phospho-AKT Ser473, phospho-mTOR Ser2448, and phospho-S6 Ser235/236 expression. A Chi-square test was used to evaluate possible associations between phospho-AKT Ser 473 nuclear expression and clinicopathological and molecular features. Results were considered statistically significant at $p \leq 0.05$.

Supplementary Materials: Supplementary materials can be found at http://www.mdpi.com/1422-0067/19/5/1448/s1.

Author Contributions: C.T. and P.S. conceived and designed the experiments; C.T., A.P., R.B., A.G., and D.R. performed the experiments; C.T., P.S., M.M., C.E., and L.B.F. analyzed the data; M.S.S., C.E., and E.R. performed the histological revision of the cases; C.T. and P.S. wrote the paper; P.S. and M.S.S. revised the paper.

Acknowledgments: This study was supported by FCT ("Portuguese Foundation for Science and Technology") through PhD grants to Catarina Tavares (SFRH/BD/87887/2012), Ana Pestana (SFRH/BD/110617/2015), and Rui Batista (SFRH/BD/111321/2015) and by a CNPq PhD grant ("National Counsel of Technological and Scientific Development", Brazil), Science without Borders, Process n# 237322/2012-9 for Luciana Ferreira. Miguel Melo received a grant from Genzyme for the research project "Molecular biomarkers of prognosis and response to therapy in differentiated thyroid carcinomas". Further funding was obtained from FEDER—Fundo Europeu de Desenvolvimento Regional funds through the COMPETE 2020—Operational Program for Competitiveness and Internationalization (POCI), Portugal 2020, and by Portuguese funds through FCT—Fundação para a Ciência e a Tecnologia/Ministério da Ciência, Tecnologia e Inovação in the framework of the project "Institute for Research and Innovation in Health Sciences" (POCI-01-0145-FEDER-007274), and by the project "Advancing cancer research: from basic acknowledgement to application"; NORTE-01-0145-FEDER-000029; "Projetos Estruturados de I&D&I, funded by Norte 2020-Programa Operacional Regional do Norte. This work was also financed by Sociedade Portuguesa de Endocrinologia Diabetes e Metabolismo through a grant "Prof. E. Limbert Sociedade Portuguesa de Endocrinologia Diabetes e Metabolismo/Sanofi-Genzyme in thyroid pathology".

Conflicts of Interest: The authors declare no conflicts of interest.

Abbreviations

TC	thyroid cancer
PTC	papillary thyroid carcinoma
SLC5A5	Solute Carrier Family 5 Member 5
cPTC	classic PTC
fvPTC	follicular variant of PTC
NIS	sodium iodide symporter
RAI	radioactive iodine

References

1. Sipos, J.A.; Mazzaferri, E.L. Thyroid cancer epidemiology and prognostic variables. *Clin. Oncol.* **2010**, *22*, 395–404. [CrossRef] [PubMed]
2. Petrulea, M.S.; Plantinga, T.S.; Smit, J.W.; Georgescu, C.E.; Netea-Maier, R.T. PI3K/Akt/mTOR: A promising therapeutic target for non-medullary thyroid carcinoma. *Cancer Treat. Rev.* **2015**, *41*, 707–713. [CrossRef] [PubMed]
3. LiVolsi, V.A. Papillary thyroid carcinoma: An update. *Mod. Pathol.* **2011**, *24* (Suppl. 2), S1–S9. [CrossRef] [PubMed]
4. Soares, P.; Celestino, R.; Melo, M.; Fonseca, E.; Sobrinho-Simoes, M. Prognostic biomarkers in thyroid cancer. *Virchows Archiv Int. J. Pathol.* **2014**, *464*, 333–346. [CrossRef] [PubMed]
5. Durante, C.; Haddy, N.; Baudin, E.; Leboulleux, S.; Hartl, D.; Travagli, J.P.; Caillou, B.; Ricard, M.; Lumbroso, J.D.; De Vathaire, F.; et al. Long-term outcome of 444 patients with distant metastases from papillary and follicular thyroid carcinoma: Benefits and limits of radioiodine therapy. *J. Clin. Endocrinol. Metab.* **2006**, *91*, 2892–2899. [CrossRef] [PubMed]
6. Fallahi, P.; Mazzi, V.; Vita, R.; Ferrari, S.M.; Materazzi, G.; Galleri, D.; Benvenga, S.; Miccoli, P.; Antonelli, A. New therapies for dedifferentiated papillary thyroid cancer. *Int. J. Mol. Sci.* **2015**, *16*, 6153–6182. [CrossRef] [PubMed]
7. Vaisman, F.; Carvalho, D.P.; Vaisman, M. A new appraisal of iodine refractory thyroid cancer. *Endocr.-Relat. Cancer* **2015**, *22*, R301–R310. [CrossRef] [PubMed]
8. De Souza, E.C.L.; Freitas Ferreira, A.C.; de Carvalho, D.P. The mTOR protein as a target in thyroid cancer. *Expert Opin. Ther. Targets* **2011**, *15*, 1099–1112. [CrossRef] [PubMed]

9. Faustino, A.; Couto, J.P.; Populo, H.; Rocha, A.S.; Pardal, F.; Cameselle-Teijeiro, J.M.; Lopes, J.M.; Sobrinho-Simoes, M.; Soares, P. mTOR pathway overactivation in BRAF mutated papillary thyroid carcinoma. *J. Clin. Endocrinol. Metab.* **2012**, *97*, E1139–E1149. [CrossRef] [PubMed]

10. Populo, H.; Lopes, J.M.; Soares, P. The mTOR signalling pathway in human cancer. *Int. J. Mol. Sci.* **2012**, *13*, 1886–1918. [CrossRef] [PubMed]

11. Miyakawa, M.; Tsushimma, T.; Murakami, H.; Wakai, K.; Isozaki, O.; Takano, K. Increased expression of phosphorylated p70S6 kinase and Akt in papillary thyroid cancer tissues. *Endocr. J.* **2003**, *50*, 77–83. [CrossRef] [PubMed]

12. Vasko, V.; Saji, M.; Hardy, E.; Kruhlak, M.; Larin, A.; Savchenko, V.; Miyakawa, M.; Isozaki, O.; Murakami, H.; Tsushima, T.; et al. Akt activation and localisation correlate with tumour invasion and oncogene expression in thyroid cancer. *J. Med. Genet.* **2004**, *41*, 161–170. [CrossRef] [PubMed]

13. Tavares, C.; Coelho, M.J.; Melo, M.; da Rocha, A.G.; Pestana, A.; Batista, R.; Salgado, C.; Eloy, C.; Ferreira, L.; Rios, E.; et al. pmTOR is a marker of aggressiveness in papillary thyroid carcinomas. *Surgery* **2016**, *160*, 1582–1590. [CrossRef] [PubMed]

14. Gupta, S.; Hau, A.M.; Beach, J.R.; Harwalker, J.; Mantuano, E.; Gonias, S.L.; Egelhoff, T.T.; Hansel, D.E. Mammalian target of rapamycin complex 2 (mTORC2) is a critical determinant of bladder cancer invasion. *PLoS ONE* **2013**, *8*, e81081. [CrossRef] [PubMed]

15. Masri, J.; Bernath, A.; Martin, J.; Jo, O.D.; Vartanian, R.; Funk, A.; Gera, J. mTORC2 activity is elevated in gliomas and promotes growth and cell motility via overexpression of rictor. *Cancer Res.* **2007**, *67*, 11712–11720. [CrossRef] [PubMed]

16. Bian, Y.; Wang, Z.; Xu, J.; Zhao, W.; Cao, H.; Zhang, Z. Elevated Rictor expression is associated with tumor progression and poor prognosis in patients with gastric cancer. *Biochem. Biophys. Res. Commun.* **2015**, *21*, 534–540. [CrossRef] [PubMed]

17. Maru, S.; Ishigaki, Y.; Shinohara, N.; Takata, T.; Tomosugi, N.; Nonomura, K. Inhibition of mTORC2 but not mTORC1 up-regulates E-cadherin expression and inhibits cell motility by blocking HIF-2α expression in human renal cell carcinoma. *J. Urol.* **2013**, *189*, 1921–1929. [CrossRef] [PubMed]

18. Matson, D.R.; Hardin, H.; Buehler, D.; Lloyd, R.V. AKT activity is elevated in aggressive thyroid neoplasms where it promotes proliferation and invasion. *Exp. Mol. Pathol.* **2017**, *103*, 288–293. [CrossRef] [PubMed]

19. De Souza, E.C.; Padron, A.S.; Braga, W.M.; de Andrade, B.M.; Vaisman, M.; Nasciutti, L.E.; Ferreira, A.C.; de Carvalho, D.P. MTOR downregulates iodide uptake in thyrocytes. *J. Endocrinol.* **2010**, *206*, 113–120. [CrossRef] [PubMed]

20. Plantinga, T.S.; Heinhuis, B.; Gerrits, D.; Netea, M.G.; Joosten, L.A.; Hermus, A.R.; Oyen, W.J.; Schweppe, R.E.; Haugen, B.R.; Boerman, O.C.; et al. mTOR Inhibition promotes TTF1-dependent redifferentiation and restores iodine uptake in thyroid carcinoma cell lines. *J. Clin. Endocrinol. Metab.* **2014**, *99*, E1368–E1375. [CrossRef] [PubMed]

21. Ahmed, M.; Hussain, A.R.; Bavi, P.; Ahmed, S.O.; Al Sobhi, S.S.; Al-Dayel, F.; Uddin, S.; Al-Kuraya, K.S. High prevalence of mTOR complex activity can be targeted using Torin2 in papillary thyroid carcinoma. *Carcinogenesis* **2014**, *35*, 1564–1572. [CrossRef] [PubMed]

22. Sadowski, S.M.; Boufragech, M.; Zhang, L.; Mehta, A.; Kapur, P.; Zhang, Y.; Li, Z.; Shen, M.; Kebebew, E. Torin2 targets dysregulated pathways in anaplastic thyroid cancer and inhibits tumor growth and metastasis. *Oncotarget* **2015**, *6*, 18038–18049. [CrossRef] [PubMed]

23. Riesco-Eizaguirre, G.; Gutierrez-Martinez, P.; Garcia-Cabezas, M.A.; Nistal, M.; Santisteban, P. The oncogene BRAF V600E is associated with a high risk of recurrence and less differentiated papillary thyroid carcinoma due to the impairment of Na+/I− targeting to the membrane. *Endocr.-Relat. Cancer* **2006**, *13*, 257–269. [CrossRef] [PubMed]

24. Ringel, M.D.; Hayre, N.; Saito, J.; Saunier, B.; Schuppert, F.; Burch, H.; Bernet, V.; Burman, K.D.; Kohn, L.D.; Saji, M. Overexpression and overactivation of Akt in thyroid carcinoma. *Cancer Res.* **2001**, *61*, 6105–6111. [PubMed]

25. Saji, M.; Narahara, K.; McCarty, S.K.; Vasko, V.V.; la Perle, K.M.; Porter, K.; Jarjoura, D.; Cheng, S.-Y.; Lu, C.; Ringel, M.D. Akt deficiency delays tumor progression, vascular invasion, and distant metastases in a murine model of thyroid cancer. *Oncogene* **2011**, *30*, 4307–4315. [CrossRef] [PubMed]

26. Kim, C.S.; Vasko, V.V.; Kato, Y.; Kruhlak, M.; Saji, M.; Cheng, S.Y.; Ringel, M.D. AKT activation promotes metastasis in a mouse model of follicular thyroid carcinoma. *Endocrinology* **2005**, *146*, 4456–4463. [CrossRef] [PubMed]

27. Pende, M.; Um, S.H.; Mieulet, V.; Sticker, M.; Goss, V.L.; Mestan, J.; Mueller, M.; Fumagalli, S.; Kozma, S.C.; Thomas, G. S6K1−/−/S6K2−/− Mice Exhibit Perinatal Lethality and Rapamycin-Sensitive 5′-Terminal Oligopyrimidine mRNA Translation and Reveal a Mitogen-Activated Protein Kinase-Dependent S6 Kinase Pathway. *Mol. Cell Biol.* **2004**, *24*, 3112–3124. [CrossRef] [PubMed]

28. Roux, P.P.; Shahbazian, D.; Vu, H.; Holz, M.K.; Cohen, M.S.; Taunton, J.; Sonenberg, N.; Blenis, J. RAS/ERK signaling promotes site-specific ribosomal protein S6 phosphorylation via RSK and stimulates cap-dependent translation. *J. Biol. Chem.* **2007**, *282*, 14056–14064. [CrossRef] [PubMed]

29. Breuleux, M.; Klopfenstein, M.; Stephan, C.; Doughty, C.A.; Barys, L.; Maira, S.-M.; Kwiatkowski, D.; Lane, H.A. Increased AKT S473 phosphorylation after mTORC1 inhibition is rictor dependent and does not predict tumor cell response to PI3K/mTOR inhibition. *Mol. Cancer Ther.* **2009**, *8*, 742–753. [CrossRef] [PubMed]

30. Tavares, C.; Coelho, M.J.; Eloy, C.; Melo, M.; da Rocha, A.G.; Pestana, A.; Batista, R.; Ferreira, L.B.; Rios, E.; Selmi-Ruby, S.; et al. NIS expression in thyroid tumors, relation with prognosis clinicopathological and molecular features. *Endocr. Connect.* **2018**, *7*, 78–90. [CrossRef] [PubMed]

31. Meireles, A.M.; Preto, A.; Rocha, A.S.; Rebocho, A.P.; Maximo, V.; Pereira-Castro, I.; Moreira, S.; Feijao, T.; Botelho, T.; Marques, R.; et al. Molecular and genotypic characterization of human thyroid follicular cell carcinoma-derived cell lines. *Thyroid Off. J. Am. Thyroid Assoc.* **2007**, *17*, 707–715. [CrossRef] [PubMed]

32. Durante, C.; Puxeddu, E.; Ferretti, E.; Morisi, R.; Moretti, S.; Bruno, R.; Barbi, F.; Avenia, N.; Scipioni, A.; Verrienti, A.; et al. BRAF mutations in papillary thyroid carcinomas inhibit genes involved in iodine metabolism. *J. Clin. Endocrinol. Metab.* **2007**, *92*, 2840–2843. [CrossRef] [PubMed]

33. DeLellis, R.A.; Lloyd, R.V.; Heitz, P.U.; Eng, C.; WHO Classification of Tumours. *Pathology and Genetics of Tumours of Endocrine Organs*; IARC Press: Lyon, France, 2004.

34. Soares, P.; Trovisco, V.; Rocha, A.S.; Lima, J.; Castro, P.; Preto, A.; Maximo, V.; Botelho, T.; Seruca, R.; Sobrinho-Simoes, M. BRAF mutations and RET/PTC rearrangements are alternative events in the etiopathogenesis of PTC. *Oncogene* **2003**, *22*, 4578–4580. [CrossRef] [PubMed]

35. Trovisco, V.; Soares, P.; Preto, A.; de Castro, I.V.; Lima, J.; Castro, P.; Maximo, V.; Botelho, T.; Moreira, S.; Meireles, A.M.; et al. Type and prevalence of BRAF mutations are closely associated with papillary thyroid carcinoma histotype and patients' age but not with tumour aggressiveness. *Virchows Archiv Int. J. Pathol.* **2005**, *446*, 589–595. [CrossRef] [PubMed]

36. De Vries, M.M.; Celestino, R.; Castro, P.; Eloy, C.; Maximo, V.; van der Wal, J.E.; Plukker, J.T.; Links, T.P.; Hofstra, R.M.; Sobrinho-Simoes, M.; et al. RET/PTC rearrangement is prevalent in follicular Hurthle cell carcinomas. *Histopathology* **2012**, *61*, 833–843. [CrossRef] [PubMed]

37. Melo, M.; da Rocha, A.G.; Vinagre, J.; Batista, R.; Peixoto, J.; Tavares, C.; Celestino, R.; Almeida, A.; Salgado, C.; Eloy, C.; et al. TERT promoter mutations are a major indicator of poor outcome in differentiated thyroid carcinomas. *J. Clin. Endocrinol. Metab.* **2014**, *99*, E754–E765. [CrossRef] [PubMed]

38. Vinagre, J.; Almeida, A.; Populo, H.; Batista, R.; Lyra, J.; Pinto, V.; Coelho, R.; Celestino, R.; Prazeres, H.; Lima, L.; et al. Frequency of TERT promoter mutations in human cancers. *Nat. Commun.* **2013**, *4*, 2185. [CrossRef] [PubMed]

39. Preto, A.; Goncalves, J.; Rebocho, A.P.; Figueiredo, J.; Meireles, A.M.; Rocha, A.S.; Vasconcelos, H.M.; Seca, H.; Seruca, R.; Soares, P.; et al. Proliferation and survival molecules implicated in the inhibition of BRAF pathway in thyroid cancer cells harbouring different genetic mutations. *BMC Cancer* **2009**, *9*, 387. [CrossRef] [PubMed]

40. Livak, K.J.; Schmittgen, T.D. Analysis of relative gene expression data using real-time quantitative PCR and the 2(-Delta Delta C(T)) Method. *Methods* **2001**, *25*, 402–408. [CrossRef] [PubMed]

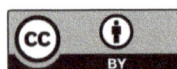

International Journal of
Molecular Sciences

MDPI

Article

NVP-BEZ235 Attenuated Cell Proliferation and Migration in the Squamous Cell Carcinoma of Oral Cavities and p70S6K Inhibition Mimics its Effect

Cheng-Ming Hsu [1,2], Pai-Mei Lin [3], Hsin-Ching Lin [4], Yao-Te Tsai [1], Ming-Shao Tsai [1], Shau-Hsuan Li [5], Ching-Yuan Wu [2,6], Yao-Hsu Yang [2,6], Sheng-Fung Lin [7,8,*] and Ming-Yu Yang [4,9,*]

[1] Department of Otolaryngology, Chiayi Chang Gung Memorial Hospital and Chang Gung University College of Medicine, Chiayi 61363, Taiwan; scm0031@adm.cgmh.org.tw (C.-M.H.); yaote1215@gmail.com (Y.-T.T.); b87401061@gmail.com (M.-S.T.)
[2] School of Traditional Chinese Medicine, College of Medicine, Chang Gung University, Taoyuan 33302, Taiwan; smbepigwu77@gmail.com (C.-Y.W.); r95841012@adm.cgmh.org.tw (Y.-H.Y.)
[3] Department of Nursing, I-Shou University, Kaohsiung 82445, Taiwan; paimei@isu.edu.tw
[4] Department of Otolaryngology, Kaohsiung Chang Gung Memorial Hospital and Chang Gung University College of Medicine, Kaohsiung 83301, Taiwan; hclin@cgmh.org.tw
[5] Division of Hematology-Oncology, Department of Internal Medicine, Kaohsiung Chang Gung Memorial Hospital and Chang Gung University College of Medicine, Kaohsiung 83301, Taiwan; lee0624@cgmh.org.tw
[6] Department of Chinese Medicine, Chiayi Chang Gung Memorial Hospital, Chiayi 61363, Taiwan
[7] Division of Hematology and Oncology, Department of Internal Medicine, E-Da Hospital, Kaohsiung 82445, Taiwan
[8] School of Medicine, I-Shou University, Kaohsiung 82445, Taiwan
[9] Graduate Institute of Clinical Medical Sciences, College of Medicine, Chang Gung University, Tao-Yuan 33302, Taiwan
* Correspondence: shlintw@yahoo.com.tw (S.-F.L.); yangmy@mail.cgu.edu.tw (M.-Y.Y.); Tel.: +886-7-7317125 (ext. 8865) (M.-Y.Y.); Fax: +886-7-7311696 (M.-Y.Y.)

Received: 9 October 2018; Accepted: 8 November 2018; Published: 10 November 2018

Abstract: NVP-BEZ235 or BEZ235 is a dual inhibitor of adenosine triphosphate (ATP)-competitive phosphoinositide 3-kinase (PI3K)/mammalian-target-of-rapamycin (mTOR) and is promising for cancer treatment. Because it targets more than one downstream effector, a dual approach is promising for cancer treatment. The aim of this study was to evaluate the efficacy of NVP-BEZ235 in treating oral cavity squamous cell carcinoma (OSCC). Two human OSCC cell lines, SCC-4 and SCC-25, were used in this study. PI3K-AKT signaling, proliferation, and cell migratory and invasion capabilities of OSCC cells were examined. In NVP-BEZ235-treated SCC-4 and SCC-25 cells, the phosphorylation of 70-kDa ribosomal S6 kinase (p70S6K), but not mTOR, decreased within 24 h. NVP-BEZ235 inhibited OSCC-cell proliferation, migration, and invasion possibly by directly deregulating the phosphorylation of p70S6K. The phospho-p70S6K inhibitor mimicked the effects of NVP-BEZ235 for preventing proliferation and weakening the migratory and invasion abilities of SCC-4 and SCC-25 cells. This study further confirmed the effect of NVP-BEZ235 on OSCC cells and provided a new strategy for controlling the proliferation, migration, and invasion of OSCC cells using the phopho-p70S6K inhibitor.

Keywords: oral cavity squamous cell carcinoma (OSCC); NVP-BEZ235; mTOR; p70S6K

1. Introduction

Squamous cell carcinoma of the head and neck (SCCHN) is the sixth most common malignancy worldwide. With a mortality rate of approximately 50%, it affects 600,000 new patients every year.

Oral cavity squamous cell carcinoma (OSCC) accounts for the vast majority of all SCCHN cases [1]. OSCC has the sixth highest cancer incidence in Taiwan and is the most common malignancy diagnosis for Taiwanese men aged 30 to 50 years [2,3]. Most treatment modalities are based on tumor (T) staging, and they include surgery and adjuvant therapy, such as chemotherapy and radiotherapy [4].

Even though progress has been made in cancer treatment, oral cancer has high rates of local recurrence, secondary primary malignancy, and morbidity [5]. Once patients with inoperable and recurrent OSCC, or distant metastasis, platinum-combination therapy is the standard first-line treatment [6,7]. However, if cis-diamminedichloridoplatinum (CDDP)-based chemotherapy fails and a patient's cancer is still inoperable, the therapeutic options are limited; moreover, most patients are only eligible to receive palliative radiation or supportive care [8–10].

With the advances of cancer research, target therapy has become the major trend for various malignant diseases as the first- or second-line treatment option, including OSCC [11]. Synergistic antitumor effects exerted by combination of targeted therapy with CDDP have been demonstrated in many preclinical studies [12,13]. The PI3K/AKT/mTOR intracellular signaling pathway plays a vital role in various physiological processes, such as cellular survival, migration, proliferation, and differentiation, as well as angiogenesis, protein synthesis, and glucose metabolism. Additionally, the PI3K/AKT/mTOR pathway is associated with various oncogenic processes, and is one of the signaling pathways most frequently dysregulated in cancer, including OSCC [14]. The PI3K/AKT/mTOR pathway and its downstream 70-kDa ribosomal S6 kinase (p70S6K) are constitutively activated in human tumor cells, providing unique opportunities for therapeutic intervention. Therefore, targeting PI3K/AKT/mTOR signaling could be a rational strategy for the treatment of OSCC, a disease—particularly when advanced—in which systemic therapy plays a crucial role. The ability of NVP-BEZ235 (dactolisib), a dual PI3K/mTOR inhibitor, to treat some cancer types is being evaluated in phase I/II clinical trials. NVP-BEZ235 is an imidazo [4] quinoline derivative. It binds to the ATP-binding cleft of enzymes and thus inhibits PI3K and mTOR kinase activity [5]. A dual approach that targets more than one downstream effector is promising because it may delay or even prevent therapy resistance [15]. NVP-BEZ235 has exhibited antitumor effects on lung cancer [16,17], human glioma cells [18,19], breast cancer [20,21], melanoma [22], pancreatic cancer [23,24], sarcoma [15,25], nasopharyngeal cancer [26,27], and hepatoma [28–30]. Additionally, NVP-BEZ235 demonstrated great promise for controlling solid tumors in a preclinical mouse model [15].

The p70S6K is a member of the protein kinase A, G, and C families (AGC) serine/threonine kinase family which contains more than 60 human proteins including Akt, protein kinase C, and 90-kDa ribosomal S6 kinase [31]. By increasing ribosomal production and mRNA translation, p70S6K can promote cell growth through global protein synthesis [31]. p70S6K is a downstream target of the mTOR signaling pathway, specifically mTOR complex 1 (mTORC1). p70S6K is also a downstream signal of mitogen activated protein kinase (MAPK)/extracellular-signal-regulated kinase (ERK) pathway. p70S6K involves in the cross-talk between mTOR and MAPK/ERK signaling pathways at various regulatory levels. Activation of p70S6K occurs via phosphorylation at serine-411 (Ser411), threonine-421 (Thr421), and Ser424 by endogenous mitogens such as epidermal growth factor, thrombin, and lysophosphatidic acid. The p70S6K pathway is also essential for signaling two filamentous actin (F-actin) microdomains in cells and regulating cell migration [32].

In the present study, we investigated the effect of NVP-BEZ235 on PI3K/AKT/mTOR signaling in OSCC cells in vitro. We first discovered that NVP-BEZ235 inhibited proliferation and attenuated cell migration in a subset of SCC-4 and SCC-25 cells and thus enhanced reduction of p70S6K expression. We also used a p70S6K inhibitor to investigate the possibility of substituting NVP-BEZ235, which has undesirable side effects.

2. Results

2.1. Analysis of mTOR Expression in OSCC Tissue Using Real-Time Quantitative Reverse Transcriptase—Polymerase Chain Reaction (qRT-PCR)

To clarify whether the expression levels of *mTOR* and *p70S6K* were different in cancerous tissue compared with noncancerous tissue, cancerous and noncancerous tissue samples taken from the 28 OSCC patients were examined using qRT-PCR to determine the expression of *mTOR* and *p70S6K*. Our data demonstrated that the expression levels of mTOR ($p < 0.05$) and p70S6K ($p < 0.01$) were significantly upregulated in OSCC (Figure 1A).

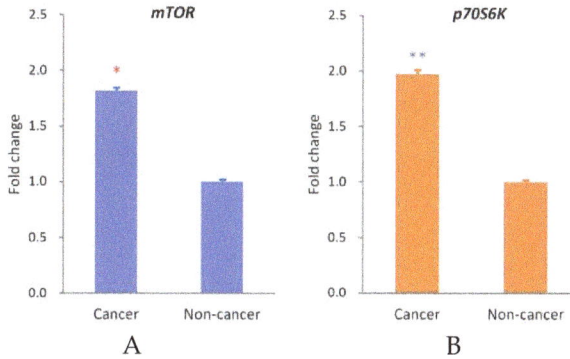

Figure 1. Expression *of mTOR* and *p70S6K* of squamous cell carcinoma (OSCC). Expression of *mTOR* (**A**) and *p70S6K* (**B**) was upregulated in the cancerous tissue of OSCC ($p < 0.05$ and 0.01, respectively). The y-axis represents the fold change in the *mTOR* or *p70S6K* expression level of cancerous relative to noncancerous tissues. The mean *mTOR* or *p70S6K* expression level in noncancerous tissues was assigned a value of 1 to obtain the fold change in expression in cancerous tissues. The mean ΔCt values for *mTOR* are 5.98 ± 0.26 (cancer parts) and 6.84 ± 0.22 (noncancer parts), and for *p70S6K* are 6.03 ± 0.31 (cancer parts) and 7.01 ± 0.19 (noncancer parts).The red * $p < 0.05$ and blue ** $p < 0.01$ indicate the statistical significance of differences between the cancer parts and noncancer parts.

2.2. NVP-BEZ235 Inhibited Cell Proliferation and Downregulated the PI3K/AKT/mTOR-Signaling Pathway of OSCC Cells, Resulting in the Suppression of Phospho-p70S6K

The antiproliferative potential of NVP-BEZ235 was assessed using 3-(4.5-dimethylthiazol-2-yl)-2,5-diphenyl-tetrazolium bromide (MTT) assay on SCC-4 and SCC-25 cells. After 72 h of treatment, NVP-BEZ235 had significantly inhibited the growth of SCC-4 (Figure 2A) and SCC-25 (Figure 2C) when it was used at concentrations of 7.5 nM and greater. The phosphorylation of p70S6K decreased within 24 h, and the phosphor-p70S6K was completely absent for at least 3 days when the 30 nM dose was administered (Figure 2B,D). However, the phosphorylation of mTOR did not reduce significantly up to 3 days.

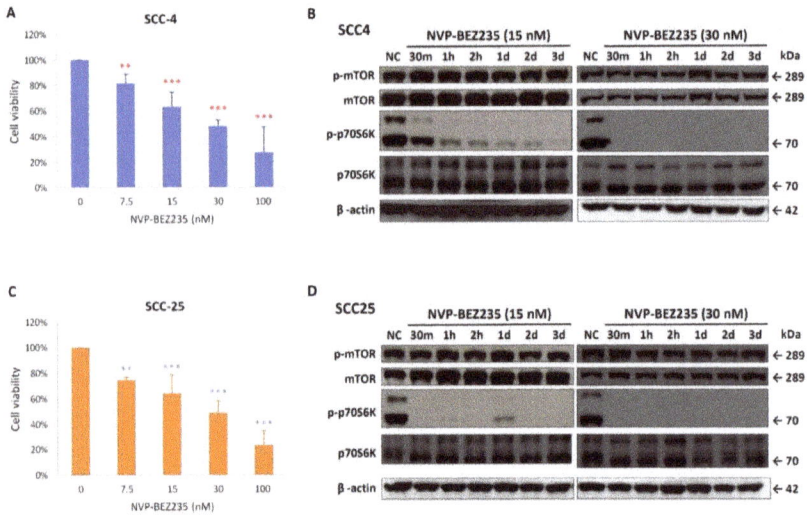

Figure 2. NVP-BEZ235 suppressed cell proliferation and reduced the expression of phospho-mTOR and phospho-p70S6K in SCC-4 and SCC-25 cells. The inhibitory effects of various doses (7.5, 15, 30, and 100 nM) of NVP-BEZ235 on SCC-4 (**A**) and SCC-25 (**C**) cells were assessed using MTT assay after 72 h of treatment. Data presented are the mean and standard error of the mean of three independent experiments. The ** $p < 0.01$ and *** $p < 0.001$ indicate the statistical significance of differences between the results for cells with and without treatment (red ** and *** for SCC-4 and blue ** and *** for SCC-25). As determined through Western blotting, NVP-BEZ235 reduced the expression of phospho-mTOR (p-mTOR) and phospho-p70S6K (p-p70S6K) in SCC-4 (**B**) and SCC-25 (**D**) cells. SCC-4 and SCC-25 cells were treated with 15 or 30 nM NVP-BEZ235 for 30 min (30 min), 1 h (1 h), 2 h (2 h), 1 day (1 d), 2 days (2 d), and 3 days (3 d) in six-well plates. Western blot analysis was performed to examine the expression levels of p-mTOR, mTOR, p-p70S6K, p70S6K, and β-actin.

2.3. NVP-BEZ235 Inhibited the Migratory and Invasion Abilities of SCC-4 and SCC-25 Cells

Weaker migratory ability was observed in SCC-4 and SCC-25 cells that had been treated with NVP-BEZ235 through the detection of the wound-healing assay (Figure 3A). In SCC-4 cells, migration was significantly slower in the cells that had been treated with NVP-BEZ235 for 4 to 24 h than in untreated cells. In SCC-25 cells, migration was significantly slower from 8 to 36 h after NVP-BEZ235 treatment. Weaker invasion ability was also observed in SCC-4 and SCC-25 cells that had been treated with NVP-BEZ235, as detected using the transwell cell migration assay (Figure 3B). After incubation for 24 h in transwell chambers, the number of cells that had migrated or invaded was markedly decreased in NVP-BEZ235-treated SCC-4 ($p < 0.01$) and SCC-25 ($p < 0.01$) cells.

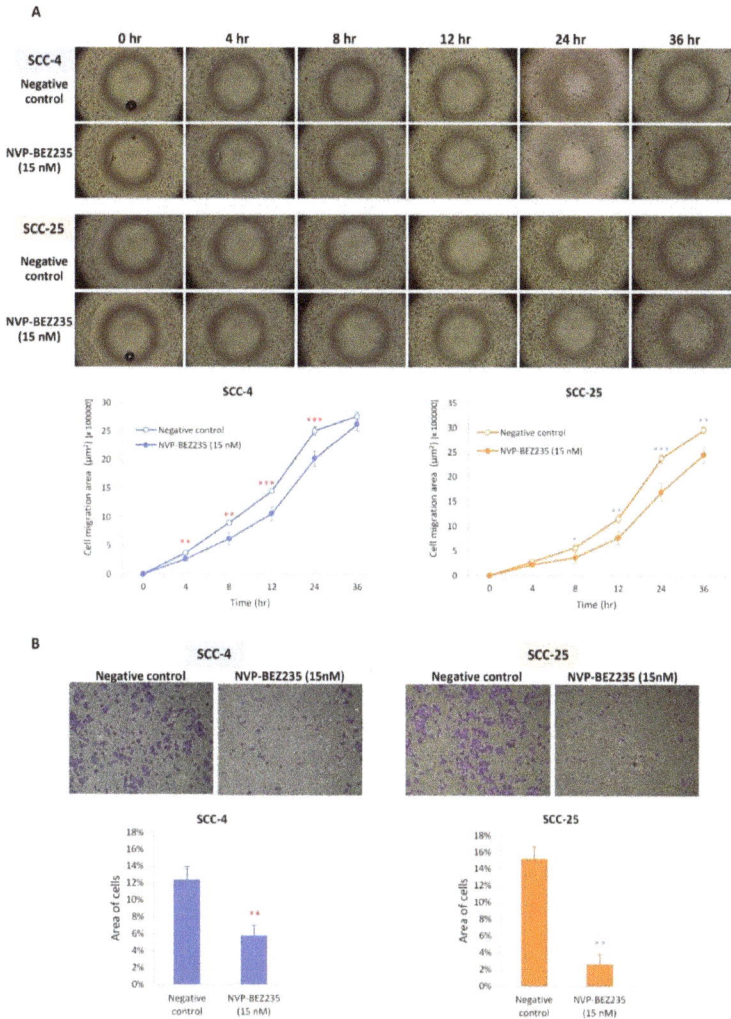

Figure 3. NVP-BEZ235 inhibited the migratory and invasion capabilities of SCC-4 and SCC-25 cells. (**A**) Wound-healing assay determined that SCC-4 and SCC-25 cells had shorter migration distances after NVP-BEZ235 treatment. * $p < 0.05$, ** $p < 0.01$, and *** $p < 0.001$ indicate the statistical significance of differences at one point in time between the results for cells with and without treatment. Hollow dots are for negative controls and solid dots are for NVP-BEZ235 treatments. (**B**) After incubating for 24 h (SCC-4) or 48 h (SCC-25) with transwell chambers, the area of migratory or invasive cells was markedly decreased in NVP-BEZ235-treated cells in comparison with cells without treatment. ** $p < 0.01$ indicates the statistical significance of the differences between cells with and without treatment (red ** for SCC-4 and blue ** for SCC-25).

2.4. Phospho-p70S6K Inhibitor 2-((4-(5-Ethylpyrimidin-4-yl)piperazin-1-yl)methyl)-5-(trifluoromethyl)-1H-benzo[d]imidazole (PF-4708671) Suppressed Proliferation and Inhibited the Expression of Phospho-mTOR and Phospho-p70S6K in SCC-4 and SCC-25 Cells

Because NVP-BEZ235 did not demonstrate proliferative abilities through phospho-p70S6K inhibition, we wondered if the direct suppression of phospho-p70S6K would achieve the same effect. PF-4708671, a phospho-p70S6K inhibitor, was used to evaluate its antiproliferative potential in SCC-4 and SCC-25 cells. As displayed in Figure 4A, the expression of phospho-p70S6K was completely abolished in SCC-4 (2 days) and SCC-25 (18 h) after PF-4708671 treatment. The expression of phosphor-mTOR was also downregulated by PF-4708671 treatment. MTT assays were also performed to determine the effects of PF-4708671 on cell growth. After 72 h of PF-4708671 treatment, the growth of SCC-4 and SCC-25 cells was significantly inhibited (Figure 4B). SCC-4 cells were more sensitive to PF-4708671 than SCC-25 cells were.

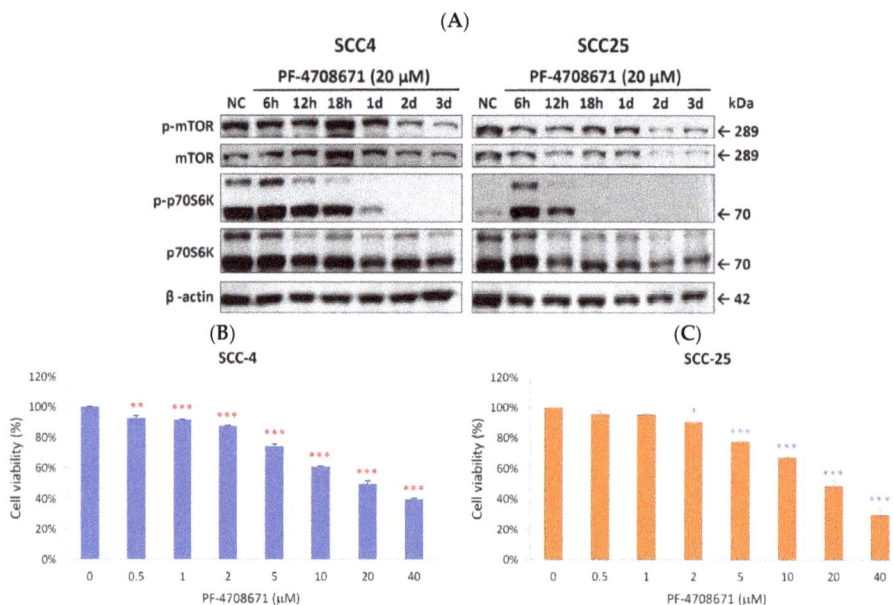

Figure 4. Phospho-p70S6K inhibitor (PF-4708671) suppressed phospho-p70S6K expression and cell proliferation in SCC-4 and SCC-25 cells. (**A**) As determined using Western blotting, the phospho-p70S6K (p-p70S6K) inhibitor (PF-4708671) reduced the expression of phospho-mTOR (p-mTOR) and p-p70S6K in SCC-4 and SCC-25 cells. SCC-4 and SCC-25 cells were not treated as negative control (NC) or treated with 20 μM PF-4708671 for 6 h (6 h), 12 h (12 h), 18 h (18 h), 1 day (1 d), 2 days (2 d), and 3 days (3 d). Western blot analysis was performed to examine the expression levels of p-mTOR, mTOR, p-p70S6K, p70S6K, and β-actin. (**B**) Inhibitory effects of various doses (0.5, 1, 2, 5, 10, 20, and 40 μM) of PF-4708671 on SCC-4 (**B**) and SCC-25 (**C**) cells were assessed using MTT assay after 72 h of treatment. Data presented are the mean and standard error of the mean of three independent experiments. * $p < 0.05$, ** $p < 0.01$, and *** $p < 0.001$ indicate the statistical significance of differences between cells with and without treatment. t (red ** and *** for SCC-4 and blue *, ** and *** for SCC-25).

2.5. Phospho-p70S6K Inhibitor (PF-4708671) also Suppressed Migration and Invasion as an NVP-BEZ235 in SCC-4 and SCC-25 Cells

The migratory and invasion abilities of SCC-4 and SCC-25 cells were also weakened by the phospho-p70S6K inhibitor (PF-4708671). In SCC-4 cells, migration was significantly slower in cells treated with PF-4708671 for 4 to 36 h than in untreated cells. In SCC-25 cells, migration was significantly slower at 24 and 36 h after PF-4708671 treatment (Figure 5A). After incubating for 24 h in transwell chambers, the number of migrated and invaded cells was markedly decreased in PF-4708671-treated SCC-4 ($p < 0.05$) and SCC-25 ($p < 0.05$) cells (Figure 5B).

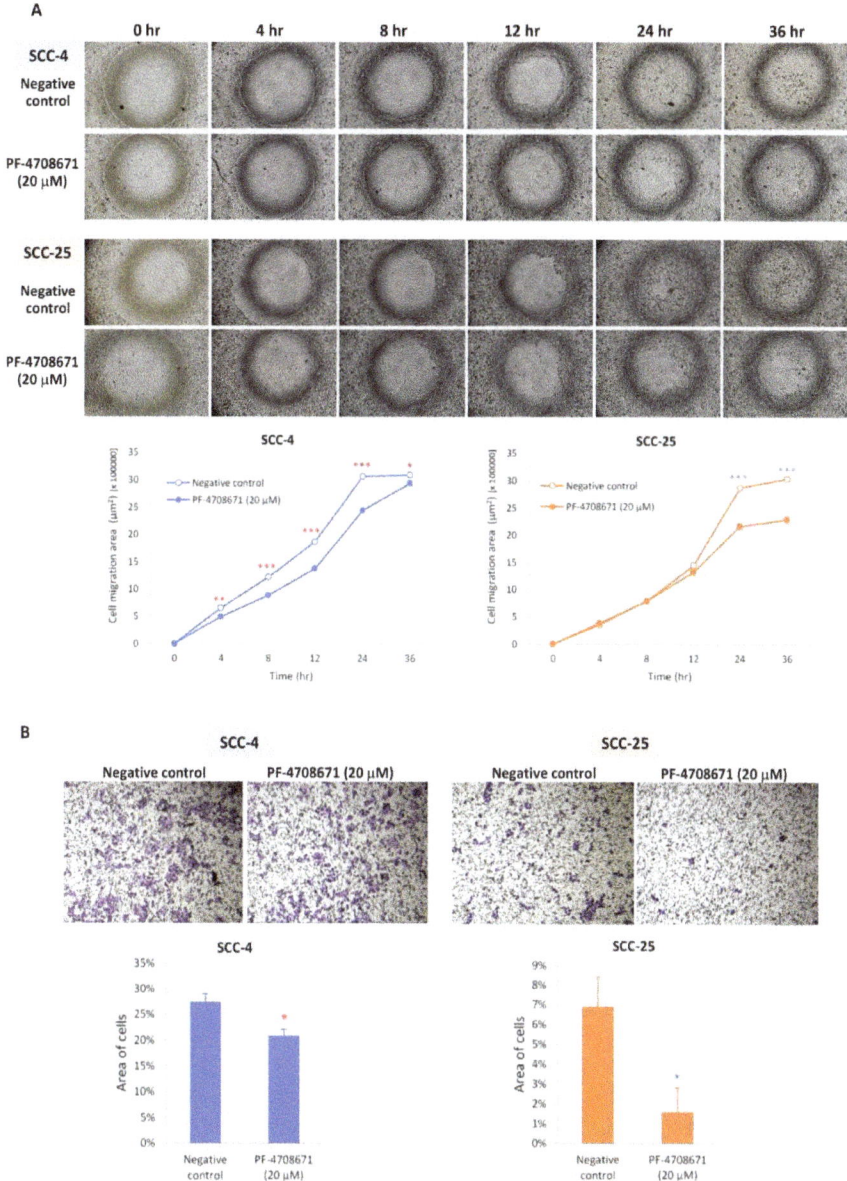

Figure 5. Phospho-p70S6K inhibitor (PF-4708671) inhibited the migratory and invasion activities of SCC-4 and SCC-25 cells. (**A**) Wound-healing assay revealed that SCC-4 and SCC-25 cells had shorter migration distances after PF-4708671 treatment. * $p < 0.05$, ** $p < 0.01$, and *** $p < 0.001$ indicate the statistical significance of the differences at one point in time between cells with and without treatment. (**B**) After incubating for 24 h (SCC-4) or 48 h (SCC-25) in transwell chambers, the area of migratory or invasive cells was markedly decreased in PF-4708671-treated cells compared with cells without treatment. * $p < 0.05$ indicates the statistical significance of differences between cells with and without treatment (red * for SCC-4 and blue * for SCC-25).

3. Discussion

This is the first study to investigate the effect of NVP-BEZ235 therapy in OSCC. NVP-BEZ235 is a novel, orally consumable dual PI3K/mTOR inhibitor that is currently being used in clinical trials [33]. The PI3K/AKT/mTOR signaling pathway and abnormal activation of this pathway reportedly play an essential role in the progression, metastasis, and chemoresistance of numerous tumor types [34]. Currently, NVP-BEZ235 is in phase I/II clinical trials and was demonstrated to control solid tumors in a preclinical mouse model [33].

In our patients with OSCC, the expression of *mTOR* and *p70S6K* was significantly upregulated (Figure 1). It has been reported that p70S6K plays an important role in metastasis within the mTOR signaling networks, including mTORC1 and mTORC2 [35]. Our in vitro results demonstrated that NVP-BEZ235 significantly reduced SCC-4 and SCC-25 proliferation. They also revealed that NVP-BEZ235 suppressed phospho-mTOR and phospho-p70S6K levels. S6 kinase proteins (S6K) has also been reported to influence apoptosis through different mechanisms [36,37]. In the PI3K/AKT/mTOR pathway, activation of mTOR results in the phosphorylation of numerous substrates, including the phosphorylation of S6K by mTORC1. The effect of NVP-BEZ235 on the apoptosis of OSCC cells may be associated with the phosphorylation of S6K. The antitumor effects of NVP-BEZ235 result not only from inhibiting the Akt survival pathway but also from promoting cell apoptosis. These effects raise the possibility that a combination treatment, once developed, would be a promising therapeutic strategy for enhancing the effects of chemotherapy and improving clinical outcomes for patients with OSCC. NVP-BEZ235 completely reduces phosphor-p70S6K activation and can inhibit phospho-mTOR activation. p70S6K has been reported to regulate cytoskeletal organization and cell motility induced by members of the Ras homologous (Rho) GTPase family, such as Ras homolog gene family, member A (Rho A), Ras-related C3 botulinum toxin substrate 1 (Rac1), and cell division control protein 42 homolog (cdc42) [38]. Therefore, NVP-BEZ235 affects not only cell proliferation but also cell migration (Figure 3). The rate of distant metastasis or regional lymph node metastasis of OSCC is possibly reduced by NVP-BEZ235.

The function of PI3K/Akt pathway is to promote cell survival and to inhibit apoptosis. When the intracellular signaling of PI3K/Akt pathway is altered, the cellular proliferation will be promoted and the upregulated glycolysis caused by the Warburg effect will be used to sustain the higher metabolic demand of transformed cells [39]. Carlo et al. reported grade 3–4 adverse effects of NVP-BEZ235 in 50% of patients (5 of 10) [40], without objective responses from subjects in the study group. The fatigue, diarrhea, nausea, and mucositis that has been reported with NVP-BEZ235 has limited the doses in which it is commonly prescribed, and it is unsurprising that combined PI3K and mTOR blockades resulted in frequent adverse effects [41]. Hence, caution is advised when taking NVP-BEZ235 orally.

According to our results, the p70S6K inhibitor could mimic the effects of NVP-BEZ235 and other mTOR inhibitors. The phospho-p70S6K inhibitor significantly inhibited the growth of SCC-4 and SCC-25 cells (Figure 4). Therefore, the phosphor-p70S6K inhibitor could weaken the Warburg effect and replace the mTOR inhibitor in the future. Indeed, the phospho-p70S6K inhibitor (PF-4708671) could suppress not only phospho-p70S6K but also phospho-mTOR, which is a result superior even to that obtained with NVP-BEZ235 (Figure 4).

In conclusion, proliferation and migration of OSCC cells could be effectively inhibited by NVP-BEZ235 through direct deregulation of phosphorylation of p70S6K. Even p70S6K is the downstream of PI3K/AKT/mTOR pathway, inhibition of phospho-p70S6K could still reduce the phosphorylation of mTOR. This study further confirmed the effect of NVP-BEZ235 on OSCC cells and provided a new strategy for controlling the migration and proliferation of OSCC cells by using the phopho-p70S6K inhibitor.

4. Materials and Methods

4.1. Patients and Samples

This study enrolled 28 patients (27 men and one female aged 31–75 years; mean ± standard deviation [SD]: 53.23 ± 10.98 years) diagnosed with OSCC who underwent surgery in the Department of Otolaryngology at Kaohsiung Chang Gung Memorial Hospital between 2009 and 2012. The clinical pathological characteristics—such as age; sex; tumor, neck lymph node, and metastasis staging; tumor size; and survival—of the patients are listed in Table 1. Tissues of tumor and adjacent nontumor parts were obtained from surgery and tissue samples were snap-frozen in liquid nitrogen immediately after resection. Prior to tissue acquisition, all the patients agreed and signed the informed consent. The Institutional Review Board of the Kaohsiung Chang Gung Memorial Hospital approved this study on August 01, 2012 (IRB No. 100-4455A3).

Table 1. Characteristics of patients with OSCC.

Characteristic	Number of Patients
Sex	
Male	27
Female	1
Median age year (range)	53.23 (31–75)
Staging [1]	
I	6
II	6
III	7
IV	9
Site	
Bucca	7
Gum	6
Palate	1
Tongue	12
Trigone	2
N stage [1]	
N0	20
N1	7
N2a	0
N2b	1
N2c	0
N3	0
Survival	
Expired	10 [2]
Survived	18

[1] The stage of OSCC is defined by the National Comprehensive Cancer Network (NCCN) clinical practice guideline 7th edition; [2] The patients died from disease after 5 years of follow-up.

4.2. Real-time Quantitative Reverse-transcriptase Polymerase Chain Reaction (qRT-PCR) Analysis

The total RNA of SCC-4 cells, SCC-25 cells, and cancerous and noncancerous tissues obtained from the patients with OSCC was extracted using a TRIzol reagent (Invitrogen; Life Technologies, Carlsbad, CA, USA), and the High-Capacity cDNA Reverse Transcription Kit (Applied Biosystems, Foster City, CA, USA) was used to synthesize complementary DNA (cDNA). The PCR reaction mixture contained 25 ng of cDNA; 0.5 µL of *mTOR* gene-expression assay (Hs00234508_m1, Applied Biosystems, Foster City, CA, USA) or β-actin (*ACTB*) gene-expression assay (Hs01060665_g1, Applied Biosystems, Foster City, CA, USA); and 5 µL of 2× TaqMan Universal PCR Master Mix (Applied Biosystems, Foster City, CA, USA). qPCR analysis was run in an ABI 7500 Fast Real-Time System (Applied

Biosystems, Foster City, CA, USA), and the thermal parameters were 1 cycle of 95 °C for 10 min and 40 cycles of 95 °C for 20 s and 60 °C for 1 min. The threshold cycle (Ct) of the *mTOR* gene or *p70S6K* gene was first normalized to the *ACTB* internal control to obtain the relative threshold cycle (ΔCt), and then the $2^{-\Delta\Delta Ct}$ method was used to calculate the relative expression of target gene.

4.3. Cell Culture

The two human SCCHN cell lines, SCC-4 and SCC-25, used in this study were purchased from the Food Industry Research and Development Institute in Taiwan. Both SCC-4 and SCC-25 cells are tongue squamous cell carcinoma. Cells were preserved and grown in a minimum essential medium (MEM)-F12 medium (Invitrogen, Life Technologies, Carlsbad, CA, USA) containing 0.4 µg/mL hydrocortisone (Sigma Aldrich, St. Louis, MO, USA) and 10% fetal bovine serum at 37 °C with 5% CO_2.

4.4. MTT Assay

The mitochondrial conversion of MTT to formazine was used to determine the percentage of metabolically active cells. Various concentrations of NVP-BEZ235 were used to treat SCC-4 and SCC-25 cells. Cells treated with phosphate-buffered saline (PBS) were used as negative control. The culture media were replaced with Dulbecco's Modified Eagle Medium/Nutrient Mixture F-12 (DMEM/F-12) (without phenol) containing 0.02% MTT (Sigma Aldrich, St. Louis, MO, USA) after different incubation times. After incubation for 4 h, the media containing MTT were then replaced with dimethyl sulfoxide (200 µL per well). The absorbance at a wavelength of 595 nm were measured using a DTX880 Multimode Detector (Beckman Coulter, Brea, CA, USA).

4.5. Western Blotting

Radioimmunoprecipitation assay buffer (20 mM Tris-HCl at pH 7.5, 150 mM NaCl, 1 mM Na2EDTA, 1 mM ethylene glycol tetraacetic acid (EGTA), 1% Nonidet P-40 (NP-40), 1% sodium deoxycholate, 2.5 mM sodium pyrophosphate, 1 mM β-glycerophosphate, 1 mM Na3VO4, and 1 µg/mL leupeptin) was added to samples for protein extraction. For Western blotting, 30 µg of the total lysates was separated using 6% to 15% sodium dodecyl sulfate–polyacrylamide gel electrophoresis and transferred to a polyvinylidene fluoride membrane (Millipore, Darmstadt, Germany). After blocking with dried nonfat milk for 1 h, the membrane was incubated overnight with primary antibodies at 1:3000 dilution. The primary antibodies and antibodies against phosphorylated epitopes used in this study were mTOR, phospho-mTOR (Ser2448), p70S6K, and phospho-p70S6K (all purchased from Cell Signaling Technologies, Danvers, MA, USA). β-actin (1:5000 dilution; Sigma Aldrich, St. Louis, MO, USA) was used as the internal control. Horseradish-peroxidase-conjugated goat anti-mouse IgG (Sigma Aldrich, St. Louis, MO, USA) and goat anti-rabbit Immunoglobulin G (IgG) (Sigma Aldrich, St. Louis, MO, USA) were used as secondary antibodies. Western Lightning® Plus-Enhanced Chemiluminescence (ECL) Substrates (PerkinElmer, Inc., Boston, MA, USA) were used to visualize the proteins.

4.6. Wound-Healing Assay

The migration activity of cells was analyzed using wound-healing assay. Cultures of SCC-4 and SCC-25 cells were optimized to ensure a homogeneous and viable cell monolayer prior to application of the wound-healing assay. One day before the assay, 2×10^5 cells were seeded in 6-well plates, and when cell confluence reached approximately 90%, a homogeneous wound was artificially created on the monolayer using a sterile, plastic, 200-µL-micropipette tip. After creating the wound, cells were washed with PBS to remove debris. Cells that had migrated into the wounded area were photographed using a Zeiss microscope (Zeiss, Gottingen, Germany) at 40× magnification, and the migration area was calculated using ImageJ free software, version 1.41o (NIH, Bethesda, MD, USA).

4.7. Transwell Assays

The migration ability of SCC-4 and SCC-25 cells was measured using a 24-pore transwell chamber (Corning Inc., Corning, NY, USA) with a polycarbonate membrane filter covered by a gelatin package. The bottom membranes (8-μm aperture) of the transwell chambers were coated with Matrigel (Sigma, St. Louis, MO, USA) for the determination of invasive ability. Cells (5×10^5 in 200 μL) were inoculated onto the upper chamber, and the lower chamber was filled with 600 μL of DMEM nutrient solution containing 10% fetal bovine serum (FBS). After a 24- to 48-h incubation at 37 °C with 5% CO_2, the wells were removed, fixed with methanol and glacial acetic acid (3:1), stained with 0.1% crystal violet, and finally mounted [33]. The areas of migratory or invasive cells were discerned by calculating five randomly selected fields of stained cells using ImageJ free software, version 1.41o (NIH, Bethesda, MD, USA) [42].

4.8. Statistical Analysis

The data sets for MTT assay, wound-healing assay, and transwell migration assay consisted of at least three biological replicates, and the data are expressed as a mean ± SD. For statistical analysis of the gene expression of qRT-PCR, ΔCt values were used. The statistical significance was determined using a two-sample *t*-test, and *p*-values < 0.05 mean if null hypotheses of no difference were rejected. All the statistical analyses in this study were performed using SPSS version 15.0 software (SPSS, Chicago, IL, USA).

Author Contributions: Conceptualization, C.-M.H., S.-F.L., and M.-Y.Y.; methodology, C.-M.H., P.-M.L., S.-F.L., and M.-Y.Y.; data acquisition, C.-M.H., H.-C.L., Y.-T.T., M.-S.T., S.-H.L., C.-Y.W., and Y.-H.Y.; statistical analysis, C.M.H., M.-S.T., and M.-Y.Y.; writing—original draft preparation, C.-M.H. and M.-Y.Y.; writing—review and editing, S.-F.L. and M.-Y.Y.; funding acquisition, C.-M.H. and M.-Y.Y.

Funding: Chang Gung Memorial Hospital, grant numbers CMRPG6G0521, CMRPG6G0341, CMRPG6H0411, CMRPG6F0511, CMRPD8F0761, and CMRPD8H0011.

Conflicts of Interest: The authors declare no conflicts of interest.

Abbreviations

CDDP	Cis-diamminedichloridoplatinum
cDNA	Complementary DNA
mTOR	Mammalian target of rapamycin
mTORC1	Mammalian target of rapamycin complex 1
MTT	3-(4,5-dimethylthiazol-2-yl)-2,5-diphenyl-tetrazolium bromide
OSCC	Oral cavity squamous cell carcinoma
p70S6K	70-kDa ribosomal S6 kinase
PBS	Phosphate-buffered saline
PI3K	Phosphoinositide 3-kinase
qRT-PCR	Real-time quantitative reverse transcriptase–polymerase chain reaction
S6K	S6 kinase proteins
SCCHN	Squamous cell carcinoma of the head and neck

References

1. Vigneswaran, N.; Williams, M.D. Epidemiologic trends in head and neck cancer and aids in diagnosis. *Oral Maxillofac. Surg. Clin. North Am.* **2014**, *26*, 123–141. [CrossRef] [PubMed]
2. Liao, C.T.; Chen, H.N.; Wen, Y.W.; Lee, S.R.; Ng, S.H.; Liu, T.W.; Tsai, S.T.; Tsai, M.H.; Lin, J.C.; Lou, P.J.; et al. Association between the diagnosis-to-treatment interval and overall survival in Taiwanese patients with oral cavity squamous cell carcinoma. *Eur. J. Cancer* **2017**, *72*, 226–234. [CrossRef] [PubMed]
3. Liao, C.T.; Lin, C.Y.; Fan, K.H.; Wang, H.M. The Optimal Treatment Modality for Taiwan Oral Cavity Cancer Patients-Experience of a Medical Center. *J. Cancer Res. Pract.* **2015**, *2*, 113–116.

4. Tangthongkum, M.; Kirtsreesakul, V.; Supanimitjaroenporn, P.; Leelasawatsuk, P. Treatment outcome of advance staged oral cavity cancer: Concurrent chemoradiotherapy compared with primary surgery. *Eur. Arch. Otorhinolaryngol.* **2017**, *274*, 2567–2572. [CrossRef] [PubMed]

5. Denaro, N.; Russi, E.G.; Adamo, V.; Merlano, M.C. State-of-the-art and emerging treatment options in the management of head and neck cancer: News from 2013. *Oncology* **2014**, *86*, 212–229. [CrossRef] [PubMed]

6. Vermorken, J.B.; Peyrade, F.; Krauss, J.; Mesía, R.; Remenar, E.; Gauler, T.C.; Keilholz, U.; Delord, J.P.; Schafhausen, P.; Erfán, J.; et al. Cisplatin, 5-fluorouracil, and cetuximab (PFE) with or without cilengitide in recurrent/metastatic squamous cell carcinoma of the head and neck: Results of the randomized phase I/II ADVANTAGE trial (phase II part). *Ann. Oncol.* **2014**, *25*, 682–688. [CrossRef] [PubMed]

7. Guo, Y.; Shi, M.; Yang, A.; Feng, J.; Zhu, X.; Choi, Y.J.; Hu, G.; Pan, J.; Hu, C.; Luo, R.; et al. Platinum-based chemotherapy plus cetuximab first-line for Asian patients with recurrent and/or metastatic squamous cell carcinoma of the head and neck: Results of an open-label, single-arm, multicenter trial. *Head Neck* **2015**, *37*, 1081–1087. [CrossRef] [PubMed]

8. Sosa, A.E.; Grau, J.J.; Feliz, L.; Pereira, V.; Alcaraz, D.; Muñoz-García, C.; Caballero, M. Outcome of patients treated with palliative weekly paclitaxel plus cetuximab in recurrent head and neck cancer after failure of platinum-based therapy. *Eur. Arch. Otorhinolaryngol.* **2014**, *271*, 373–378. [CrossRef] [PubMed]

9. Péron, J.; Ceruse, P.; Lavergne, E.; Buiret, G.; Pham, B.N.; Chabaud, S.; Favier, B.; Girodet, D.; Zrounba, P.; Ramade, A.; et al. Paclitaxel and cetuximab combination efficiency after the failure of a platinum-based chemotherapy in recurrent/metastatic head and neck squamous cell carcinoma. *Anticancer Drugs* **2012**, *23*, 996–1001. [CrossRef] [PubMed]

10. Chinn, S.B.; Darr, O.A.; Peters, R.D.; Prince, M.E. The role of head and neck squamous cell carcinoma cancer stem cells in tumorigenesis, metastasis, and treatment failure. *Front. Endocrinol. (Lausanne)* **2012**, *3*, 90. [CrossRef] [PubMed]

11. Moon, D.G.; Lee, S.E.; Oh, M.M.; Lee, S.C.; Jeong, S.J.; Hong, S.K.; Yoon, C.Y.; Byun, S.S.; Park, H.S.; Cheon, J. NVP-BEZ235, a dual PI3K/mTOR inhibitor synergistically potentiates the antitumor effects of cisplatin in bladder cancer cells. *Int. J. Oncol.* **2014**, *45*, 1027–1035. [CrossRef] [PubMed]

12. Sacchi, A.; Gasparri, A.; Gallo-Stampino, C.; Toma, S.; Curnis, F.; Corti, A. Synergistic antitumor activity of cisplatin, paclitaxel, and gemcitabine with tumor vasculature-targeted tumor necrosis factor-alpha. *Clin. Cancer Res.* **2006**, *12*, 175–182. [CrossRef] [PubMed]

13. Vassilopoulos, A.; Xiao, C.; Chisholm, C.; Chen, W.; Xu, X.; Lahusen, T.J.; Bewley, C.; Deng, C.X. Synergistic therapeutic effect of cisplatin and phosphatidylinositol 3-kinase (PI3K) inhibitors in cancer growth and metastasis of Brca1 mutant tumors. *J. Biol. Chem.* **2014**, *289*, 24202–24214. [CrossRef] [PubMed]

14. Simpson, D.R.; Mell, L.K.; Cohen, E.E. Targeting the PI3K/AKT/mTOR pathway in squamous cell carcinoma of the head and neck. *Oral Oncol.* **2015**, *51*, 291–298. [CrossRef] [PubMed]

15. Gobin, B.; Battaglia, S.; Lanel, R.; Chesneau, J.; Amiaud, J.; Rédini, F.; Ory, B.; Heymann, D. NVP-BEZ235, a dual PI3K/mTOR inhibitor, inhibits osteosarcoma cell proliferation and tumor development in vivo with an improved survival rate. *Cancer Lett.* **2014**, *344*, 291–298. [CrossRef] [PubMed]

16. Herrera, V.A.; Zeindl-Eberhart, E.; Jung, A.; Huber, R.M.; Bergner, A. The dual PI3K/mTOR inhibitor BEZ235 is effective in lung cancer cell lines. *Anticancer Res.* **2011**, *31*, 849–854. [PubMed]

17. Xu, C.X.; Li, Y.; Yue, P.; Owonikoko, T.K.; Ramalingam, S.S.; Khuri, F.R.; Sun, S.Y. The combination of RAD001 and NVP-BEZ235 exerts synergistic anticancer activity against non-small cell lung cancer in vitro and in vivo. *PLoS ONE* **2011**, *6*, e20899. [CrossRef] [PubMed]

18. Wang, W.J.; Long, L.M.; Yang, N.; Zhang, Q.Q.; Ji, W.J.; Zhao, J.H.; Qin, Z.H.; Wang, Z.; Chen, G.; Liang, Z.Q. NVP-BEZ235, a novel dual PI3K/mTOR inhibitor, enhances the radiosensitivity of human glioma stem cells in vitro. *Acta Pharmacol. Sin.* **2013**, *34*, 681–690. [CrossRef] [PubMed]

19. Gil del Alcazar, C.R.; Hardebeck, M.C.; Mukherjee, B.; Tomimatsu, N.; Gao, X.; Yan, J.; Xie, X.J.; Bachoo, R.; Li, L.; Habib, A.A.; et al. Inhibition of DNA double-strand break repair by the dual PI3K/mTOR inhibitor NVP-BEZ235 as a strategy for radiosensitization of glioblastoma. *Clin. Cancer Res.* **2014**, *20*, 1235–1248. [CrossRef] [PubMed]

20. Kuger, S.; Corek, E.; Polat, B.; Kammerer, U.; Flentje, M.; Djuzenova, C.S. Novel PI3K and mTOR Inhibitor NVP-BEZ235 Radiosensitizes Breast Cancer Cell Lines under Normoxic and Hypoxic Conditions. *Breast Cancer (Auckl)* **2014**, *8*, 39–49. [CrossRef] [PubMed]

21. Leung, E.; Kim, J.E.; Rewcastle, G.W.; Finlay, G.J.; Baguley, B.C. Comparison of the effects of the PI3K/mTOR inhibitors NVP-BEZ235 and GSK2126458 on tamoxifen-resistant breast cancer cells. *Cancer Biol. Ther.* **2011**, *11*, 938–946. [CrossRef] [PubMed]

22. Sznol, J.A.; Jilaveanu, L.B.; Kluger, H.M. Studies of NVP-BEZ235 in melanoma. *Curr. Cancer Drug Targets* **2013**, *13*, 165–174. [CrossRef] [PubMed]

23. Venkannagari, S.; Fiskus, W.; Peth, K.; Atadja, P.; Hidalgo, M.; Maitra, A.; Bhalla, K.N. Superior efficacy of co-treatment with dual PI3K/mTOR inhibitor NVP-BEZ235 and pan-histone deacetylase inhibitor against human pancreatic cancer. *Oncotarget* **2012**, *3*, 1416–1427. [CrossRef] [PubMed]

24. Awasthi, N.; Yen, P.L.; Schwarz, M.A.; Schwarz, R.E. The efficacy of a novel, dual PI3K/mTOR inhibitor NVP-BEZ235 to enhance chemotherapy and antiangiogenic response in pancreatic cancer. *J. Cell Biochem.* **2012**, *113*, 784–791. [CrossRef] [PubMed]

25. Manara, M.C.; Nicoletti, G.; Zambelli, D.; Ventura, S.; Guerzoni, C.; Landuzzi, L.; Lollini, P.L.; Maira, S.M.; García-Echeverría, C.; Mercuri, M.; et al. NVP-BEZ235 as a new therapeutic option for sarcomas. *Clin. Cancer Res.* **2010**, *16*, 530–540. [CrossRef] [PubMed]

26. Ma, B.B.; Lui, V.W.; Hui, C.W.; Lau, C.P.; Wong, C.H.; Hui, E.P.; Ng, M.H.; Cheng, S.H.; Tsao, S.W.; Tsang, C.M.; et al. Preclinical evaluation of the mTOR-PI3K inhibitor BEZ235 in nasopharyngeal cancer models. *Cancer Lett.* **2014**, *343*, 24–32. [CrossRef] [PubMed]

27. Yang, F.; Qian, X.J.; Qin, W.; Deng, R.; Wu, X.Q.; Qin, J.; Feng, G.K.; Zhu, X.F. Dual phosphoinositide 3-kinase/mammalian target of rapamycin inhibitor NVP-BEZ235 has a therapeutic potential and sensitizes cisplatin in nasopharyngeal carcinoma. *PLoS ONE* **2013**, *8*, e59879. [CrossRef] [PubMed]

28. Masuda, M.; Shimomura, M.; Kobayashi, K.; Kojima, S.; Nakatsura, T. Growth inhibition by NVP-BEZ235, a dual PI3K/mTOR inhibitor, in hepatocellular carcinoma cell lines. *Oncol. Rep.* **2011**, *26*, 1273–1279. [CrossRef] [PubMed]

29. Chang, Z.; Shi, G.; Jin, J.; Guo, H.; Guo, X.; Luo, F.; Song, Y.; Jia, X. Dual PI3K/mTOR inhibitor NVP-BEZ235-induced apoptosis of hepatocellular carcinoma cell lines is enhanced by inhibitors of autophagy. *Int. J. Mol. Med.* **2013**, *31*, 1449–1456. [CrossRef] [PubMed]

30. Kirstein, M.M.; Boukouris, A.E.; Pothiraju, D.; Buitrago-Molina, L.E.; Marhenke, S.; Schütt, J.; Orlik, J.; Kühnel, F.; Hegermann, J.; Manns, M.P.; et al. Activity of the mTOR inhibitor RAD001, the dual mTOR and PI3-kinase inhibitor BEZ235 and the PI3-kinase inhibitor BKM120 in hepatocellular carcinoma. *Liver Int.* **2013**, *33*, 780–793. [CrossRef] [PubMed]

31. Abe, Y.; Yoon, S.O.; Kubota, K.; Mendoza, M.C.; Gygi, S.P.; Blenis, J. p90 ribosomal S6 kinase and p70 ribosomal S6 kinase link phosphorylation of the eukaryotic chaperonin containing TCP-1 to growth factor, insulin, and nutrient signaling. *J. Biol. Chem.* **2009**, *284*, 14939–14948. [CrossRef] [PubMed]

32. Berven, L.A.; Willard, F.S.; Crouch, M.F. Role of the p70(S6K) pathway in regulating the actin cytoskeleton and cell migration. *Exp. Cell Res.* **2004**, *296*, 183–195. [CrossRef] [PubMed]

33. Wise-Draper, T.M.; Moorthy, G.; Salkeni, M.A.; Karim, N.A.; Thomas, H.E.; Mercer, C.A.; Beg, M.S.; O'Gara, S.; Olowokure, O.; Fathallah, H.; et al. A phase Ib study of the dual PI3K/mTOR inhibitor Dactolisib (BEZ235) combined with Everolimus in patients with advanced solid malignancies. *Target Oncol.* **2017**, *12*, 323–332. [CrossRef] [PubMed]

34. Broek, R.V.; Mohan, S.; Eytan, D.F.; Chen, Z.; Van Waes, C. The PI3K/Akt/mTOR axis in head and neck cancer: Functions, aberrations, cross-talk, and therapies. *Oral Dis.* **2015**, *21*, 815–825. [CrossRef] [PubMed]

35. Magnuson, B.; Ekim, B.; Fingar, D.C. Regulation and function of ribosomal protein S6 kinase (S6K) within mTOR signalling networks. *Biochem. J.* **2012**, *441*, 1–21. [CrossRef] [PubMed]

36. Miwa, S.; Sugimoto, N.; Yamamoto, N.; Shirai, T.; Nishida, H.; Hayashi, K.; Kimura, H.; Takeuchi, A.; Igarashi, K.; Yachie, A.; et al. Caffeine induces apoptosis of osteosarcoma cells by inhibiting AKT/mTOR/S6K, NF-κB and MAPK pathways. *Anticancer Res.* **2012**, *32*, 3643–3649. [PubMed]

37. Tomioka, H.; Mukohara, T.; Kataoka, Y.; Ekyalongo, R.C.; Funakoshi, Y.; Imai, Y.; Kiyota, N.; Fujiwara, Y.; Minami, H. Inhibition of the mTOR/S6K signal is necessary to enhance fluorouracil-induced apoptosis in gastric cancer cells with HER2 amplification. *Int. J. Oncol.* **2012**, *41*, 551–558. [CrossRef] [PubMed]

38. Aslan, J.E.; Tormoen, G.W.; Loren, C.P.; Pang, J.; McCarty, O.J. S6K1 and mTOR regulate Rac1-driven platelet activation and aggregation. *Blood.* **2011**, *118*, 3129–3136. [CrossRef] [PubMed]

39. Warburg, O. On the origin of cancer cells. *Science* **1956**, *123*, 309–314. [CrossRef] [PubMed]

40. Carlo, M.I.; Molina, A.M.; Lakhman, Y.; Patil, S.; Woo, K.; DeLuca, J.; Lee, C.H.; Hsieh, J.J.; Feldman, D.R.; Motzer, R.J.; et al. A phase Ib study of BEZ235, a dual inhibitor of phosphatidylinositol 3-kinase (PI3K) and mammalian target of rapamycin (mTOR), in patients with advanced renal cell carcinoma. *Oncologist* **2016**, *21*, 787–788. [CrossRef] [PubMed]
41. Pongas, G.; Fojo, T. BEZ235: When promising science meets clinical reality. *Oncologist* **2016**, *21*, 1033–1034. [CrossRef] [PubMed]
42. Marshall, J. Transwell(®) invasion assays. *Methods Mol. Biol.* **2011**, *769*, 97–110. [CrossRef] [PubMed]

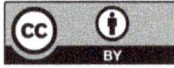

International Journal of
Molecular Sciences

MDPI

Review

mTOR Complexes as a Nutrient Sensor for Driving Cancer Progression

Mio Harachi [1], Kenta Masui [1,*], Yukinori Okamura [1], Ryota Tsukui [1], Paul S. Mischel [2] and Noriyuki Shibata [1]

[1] Department of Pathology, Division of Pathological Neuroscience, Tokyo Women's Medical University, Tokyo 162-8666, Japan; harachi.mio@twmu.ac.jp (M.H.); y.okamura.vtol.osprey@gmail.com (Y.O.); tsukuryo0525@gmail.com (R.T.); shibatan@twmu.ac.jp (N.S.)

[2] Ludwig Institute for Cancer Research, University of California San Diego, La Jolla, CA 92093, USA; pmischel@ucsd.edu

* Correspondence: masui-kn@twmu.ac.jp; Tel.: +81-3-3353-8111; Fax: +81-3-5269-7408

Received: 16 September 2018; Accepted: 14 October 2018; Published: 21 October 2018

Abstract: Recent advancement in the field of molecular cancer research has clearly revealed that abnormality of oncogenes or tumor suppressor genes causes tumor progression thorough the promotion of intracellular metabolism. Metabolic reprogramming is one of the strategies for cancer cells to ensure their survival by enabling cancer cells to obtain the macromolecular precursors and energy needed for the rapid growth. However, an orchestration of appropriate metabolic reactions for the cancer cell survival requires the precise mechanism to sense and harness the nutrient in the microenvironment. Mammalian/mechanistic target of rapamycin (mTOR) complexes are known downstream effectors of many cancer-causing mutations, which are thought to regulate cancer cell survival and growth. Recent studies demonstrate the intriguing role of mTOR to achieve the feat through metabolic reprogramming in cancer. Importantly, not only mTORC1, a well-known regulator of metabolism both in normal and cancer cell, but mTORC2, an essential partner of mTORC1 downstream of growth factor receptor signaling, controls cooperatively specific metabolism, which nominates them as an essential regulator of cancer metabolism as well as a promising candidate to garner and convey the nutrient information from the surrounding environment. In this article, we depict the recent findings on the role of mTOR complexes in cancer as a master regulator of cancer metabolism and a potential sensor of nutrients, especially focusing on glucose and amino acid sensing in cancer. Novel and detailed molecular mechanisms that amino acids activate mTOR complexes signaling have been identified. We would also like to mention the intricate crosstalk between glucose and amino acid metabolism that ensures the survival of cancer cells, but at the same time it could be exploitable for the novel intervention to target the metabolic vulnerabilities of cancer cells.

Keywords: mTOR complex; metabolic reprogramming; cancer; microenvironment; nutrient sensor

1. Introduction

Proliferating cells require not only adenosine triphosphate (ATP) as an essential energy source, but also intracellular building blocks including nucleotides, fatty acids, and proteins, and a reprogrammed metabolism could serve to support the synthesis of macromolecules [1,2]. The Warburg effect is a hallmark phenomenon of cancer metabolism and relies on aerobic glycolysis to generate the energy needed for an array of cellular processes in contrast to normal differentiated cells on mitochondrial oxidative phosphorylation [3,4]. In other words, cancer cells are heavily dependent and addicted to glucose metabolism for their survival. Amino acids are another major determinant to support cancer cell proliferation. For example, cancer cells take up glutamine to survive or proliferate by promoting the production of nucleotides, fatty acids, and proteins [5–7], an anaplerotic process that replenishes a metabolic cycle.

Cancer cells take up a large amount of amino acids and glucose from the extracellular environment as a carbon and nitrogen source for protein and nucleotide synthesis [1,8]. In the process of tumor initiation and progression, cancer cells are exposed to harsh conditions such as hypoxia or nutrient depletion in the tumor microenvironment. To survive in this severe environment, cancer cells must sense and respond to the status of nutrient availability in the extracellular environment to coordinately regulate the gene expression for sustaining the cell proliferation as well as everting the various stress that halts the cell proliferation and induce cell death [9–11]. Thus, unveiling the mechanisms how cancer cells gather the information on environmental nutrient and facilitate their survival would shed new light on the molecular pathogenesis of cancer progression, which could be harnessed to identify the unrecognized addiction and vulnerability.

Here, we focus on mammalian/mechanistic target of rapamycin (mTOR) complexes, essential regulator of cell proliferation and metabolism, as a potential key player to play a role in sensing nutrients to drive the intracellular tumor-promoting signaling cascade through metabolic reprogramming and epigenetic shift, and a key node which should be therapeutically targeted as a new mode of treatment to interfere with cancer cell metabolism.

2. Metabolic Reprogramming as an Essential Hallmark in Cancer

The hallmarks of cancer are composed of six biological capabilities, which are acquired during the multistep evolution of human neoplasms [12]. The complexities of neoplastic disease are well explained by fundamental principles of the cancer hallmarks. Metabolic reprogramming is an emerging core hallmark of cancer [12], and similar alterations are also observed in rapidly proliferating cells such as immune cells under patho-physiological conditions [13]. Various intrinsic and extrinsic molecular signaling shifts the intracellular metabolism to support the demands of rapidly proliferating cells, including ATP generation to maintain energy, biosynthesis of macromolecules, and maintenance of reduction-oxidation (redox) reaction. The central hallmark of this reprogramming lies in the phenomenon that cancer cells undergo glycolysis even in the presence of sufficient oxygen, termed "the Warburg effect," and there has been much interest in examining and comprehending the pathways that regulate the survival advantages conferred by this aerobic glycolysis [3]. Over the past decade, however, far more complex aspects of cancer metabolism have emerged, and the Warburg effect alone cannot well explain all the metabolic changes required for rapid cell growth, including aerobic glycolysis, glutaminolysis, altered lipid metabolism, de novo nucleic acid synthesis, and reactive oxygen species (ROS) management. For instance, as for ROS metabolism, nutrient deficiency, glucose deprivation and hypoxia induce ATP reduction and ROS overproduction, which could promote metabolic reprogramming in cancer cells [14]. Of interest, activated mTORC1 increased the level of ROS [15], suggesting that mTOR complex induces metabolic reprogramming via ROS production in response to unpreferable environments for cancer cells. On the contrary, mTORC1 regulates superoxide dismutase 1 (SOD1) activity through reversible phosphorylation in response to nutrients, which moderates ROS level and prevents oxidative DNA damage [16], and mTORC2 regulates the production of reduced form of nicotinamide adenine dinucleotide phosphate (NADPH) and glutathione (GSH), which could counteract the overproduction of ROS [17]. Further, epigenetic landscape including a shift in DNA and histone modifications are shaped and modulated by intermediary metabolites produced via metabolic reprogramming [13]. Therefore, the dynamic plasticity of metabolic reprogramming and epigenetic shift can converge to confer the survival advantage to cancer cells, but these alterations also render cancer cells vulnerable to interference with the metabolic and epigenetic network. Deciphering the molecular mechanism of the metabolic and epigenetic regulations in cancer could pave the way for therapeutic intervention, and the recent emerging evidences have revealed the essential regulatory role of mTOR complexes in metabolic reprogramming, the responsibility to microenvironments, and the subsequent epigenetic changes, which can result in cell survival in harsh metabolic conditions and provide therapeutic opportunities in cancer.

3. mTORC1 and mTORC2-Irreplaceable Partners in Cancer Metabolic Reprogramming

Genetic mutations to constitutively activate phosphoinositide 3-kinase (PI3K)-Akt-mTOR signaling are reported to reprogram cellular metabolism and tumorigenesis, including receptor tyrosine kinase (RTK) amplification and mutations, phosphatidylinositol 4,5-bisphosphate 3-kinase catalytic subunit alpha isoform (PIK3CA) mutation and phosphatase and tensin homolog deleted from chromosome 10 (PTEN) loss [18]. Among them, as a serine/threonine protein kinase essential for the cellular function, two distinct multi-protein complexes of mTOR associate the signaling from growth factor receptor with cell growth, proliferation, and survival. mTOR complex 1 (mTORC1), an established druggable target against cancer, phosphorylates and controls its substrates p70 ribosomal protein S6 kinase 1 (S6K1) and eukaryotic translation initiation factor 4E-binding protein 1 (4E-BP1) to promote protein translation as well as anabolic metabolism downstream of growth factor receptor-activated PI3K-Akt signaling [19,20]. The important role of mTOR complex 2 (mTORC2) has been gradually unraveled, especially in the field of metabolic homeostasis and cancer biology. mTORC2 has been considered to be responsive to growth factor signaling and the interaction of ribosome, and to function mainly through activating Akt by phosphorylating it on serine 473 (Ser473) [21,22]. It can also phosphorylate other AGC subfamily kinases including serum and glucocorticoid-inducible kinase 1 (SGK1) and protein kinase C (PKC). Recent studies demonstrated that mTORC2 regulates tumor progression, chemotherapy resistance, and genome DNA stability in cancer cells, playing an unrecognized, essential role in cancer biology [23,24]. Of note, these effects appear to be independent from canonical Akt-mediated signaling [25], indicating the importance of mTORC2 itself in cancer biology.

The structures of mTORC1 and mTORC2 are characterized by sharing some components: they share the catalytic mTOR subunit, as well as mammalian lethal with sec-13 (mLST8, also known as GβL) [26,27], the DEP domain containing mTOR-interacting protein (DEPTOR) [28], and the Tti1/Tel2 complex [29]. In contrast, regulatory-associated protein of mammalian target of rapamycin (raptor) [30,31] and proline-rich Akt substrate 40kDa (PRAS40) [32–35] are specific to mTORC1, while rapamycin-insensitive companion of mTOR (rictor) [26,36], mammalian stress-activated map kinase-interacting protein 1 (mSin1) [37,38], and protein observed with rictor 1 and 2 (protor1/2) [33, 39,40] are specific components of mTORC2.

Oncogenes and tumor suppressors are a key determinant in controlling cancer metabolism [41–43]. In various types of cancers, growth factor receptor signaling converges to an oncogenic transcription factor c-Myc, which promotes cell proliferation via metabolic reprogramming to connect nutrient uptake with intracellular biomass accumulation [44–46]. We recently identified that cancer cell metabolism was promoted through c-Myc which could be activated cooperatively by both mTORC1 and mTORC2 [47]. In glioblastoma (GBM, a malignant glial/astrocytic tumor) cells with activating epidermal growth factor receptor (EGFR) mutations, mTORC1 upregulates the heterogeneous nuclear ribonucleoprotein A1 (hnRNPA1) splicing factor, promoting the alternative splicing of Myc-associated factor X (Max) to generate Delta Max, thereby functionally augmenting Myc-dependent glycolytic metabolism and tumor cell proliferation [48]. mTORC2, on the other hand, increases the transcription of c-Myc through inhibitory phosphorylation of class IIa histone deacetylases (HDACs), resulting in inactivation of forkhead box O (FoxO) transcription factors through post-translational acetylation [47]. Therefore, growth factor receptor-PI3K signaling requires the synergistic action of mTORC1 and mTORC2 for c-Myc-dependent metabolic reprogramming by controlling both c-Myc transcription and its functional activity (Figure 1). Considering the essential and coupling roles of two mTOR complexes in reprogramming cancer cell metabolism, the next critical questions would be raised how mTOR complexes could sense the information on the source of metabolic reactions (i.e., nutrients) and subsequently respond to the microenvironmental condition to favor their survival.

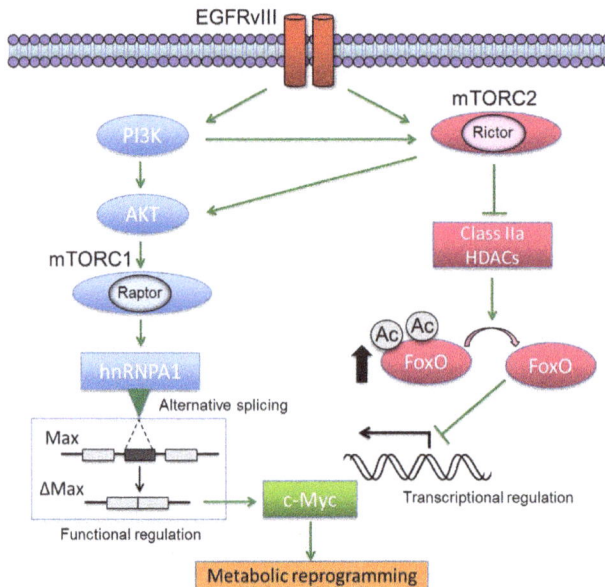

Figure 1. EGFRvIII controls c-Myc through two interlacing and synergistic mechanisms. EGFRvIII-mTORC1 signaling promotes glycolytic metabolism by activating hnRNPA1-dependent alternative splicing of a Myc-binding partner Delta Max, thereby functionally augmenting the oncogenic activity of c-Myc. Alternatively, EGFR-mTORC2 signaling controls c-Myc transcription, translation and protein level through FoxO acetylation, resulting in the enhancement of metabolic reprogramming. These findings point to the central role of c-Myc in regulating EGFRvIII-activated glycolytic metabolism. EGFRvIII: epidermal growth factor receptor variant III; PI3K: phosphoinositide 3-kinase; mTORC1/2: mammalian/mechanistic target of rapamycin complex 1/2; HDAC: histone deacetylase; hnRNPA1: heterogeneous nuclear ribonucleoprotein A1; Max: myc-associated factor X; FoxO: forkhead box O; Ac: acetyl-group.

4. mTORC1 as a Sensor of Amino Acids in Cancer Cells

mTORC1 is an evolutionarily conserved multi-protein complex that coordinates a network of signaling cascades and functions as a key mediator of protein translation, gene transcription, and autophagy [49–51]. mTORC1 is activated by growth factors such as insulin, and nutrients such as amino acids, which eventually promote cell growth and proliferation by regulating anabolic and catabolic processes and by driving cell cycle progression through phosphorylating its substrates [52,53]. However, when amino acid supplies become restricted, the activity of mTORC1 is significantly suppressed, and mammalian cells employ homeostatic mechanisms to rapidly inhibit processes such as protein synthesis, which demands high levels of amino acids. Additionally, mTORC1 supplies amino acid resource through releasing the suppression of autophagy under a starved state [54]. Of interest, the amino acid sensing mechanism that non-cancer cells use via mTORC1 could be exploited by cancer cells as described in the following sections, and the future endeavor should be directed to examine if there is actually a difference between cancer and non-cancer cells for amino acid sensing through mTORC1.

Leucine, one of the essential amino acids in human cells, mainly induces the recruitment of mTORC1 to the lysosomal membrane and its subsequent activation; that is, mTORC1 is activated in response to the level of leucine [55]. Leucine is also a signaling molecule that directly regulates animal physiology, including satiety [56], insulin secretion [57], and skeletal muscle anabolism [58,59]. Signal transduction through mTORC1, which is involved in cell growth through enhanced protein translation, is activated by extracellular leucine through Sestrin1/2, a GATOR2-interacting protein that inhibits mTORC1 signaling [55,60] (Figure 2). In addition to sensing leucine for its activation, CASTOR proteins were identified as a putative arginine sensor for the mTORC1 pathway, which is activated by extracellular arginine and interacts with GATOR2 and activate mTORC1 via promotion of the hetero-dimerization of GTP-RagA and GDP-RagC [61] (Figure 2).

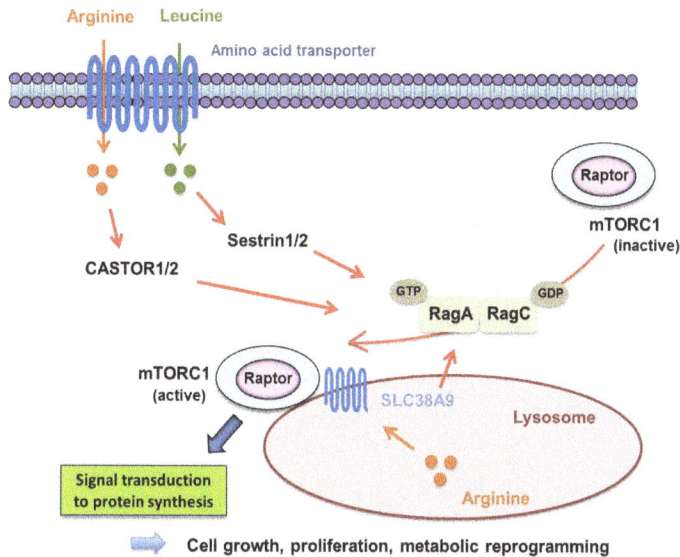

Figure 2. Mechanism of mTORC1 activation via Rag proteins by amino acids. mTORC1 is transferred to lysosome from cytosol by promoting heterodimerization of GTP-binding Rag proteins, which work as mediators of amino acid signaling to mTORC1. It is then activated by binding to GTP-bound Rheb on lysosome. Extracellular arginine and leucine activate RagA-RagC heterodimer, GTP-binding RagA, and GDP-binding RagC via amino acid transporter CASTOR1/2 and Sestrin1/2 to transfer mTORC1 to lysosome. Lysosomal arginine also activates Rag heterodimer via lysosomal amino acid transporter SLC38A9.

Recent studies also demonstrate the intriguing interaction of amino acid metabolism and mTORC1 signaling through the ubiquitin signaling systems, displaying that, in response to amino acids, the KLHL22 E3 ubiquitin ligase promotes K48-linked polyubiquitination, enabling mTORC1 signaling to promote tumorigenesis and aging [62]. Another interesting example is SAMTOR, which was reported to inhibit mTORC1 signaling by interacting with GATOR1, the GTPase activating protein (GAP) for RagA/B [63]. Notably, the methyl donor S-adenosylmethionine (SAM) disrupts the SAMTOR-GATOR1 complex, and methionine-induced activation of mTORC1 requires the SAM binding capacity of SAMTOR, indicating that mTORC1 is involved in methionine and one-carbon metabolism, which potentially control the epigenetic (methylation) shift in cancer. mTORC1 could thus respond to a range of amino acids and relevant metabolites, the mechanism of which could be involved in multiple human disease conditions including cancer. Importantly, the insufficiency for new protein synthesis is actively monitored by both prokaryotic and eukaryotic cells, and these amino acid sensing mechanisms described here might be an Achilles heel in cancer, which could be exploitable for the novel therapeutic strategies against cancer [64].

5. mTORC2 at the Intersection of Glucose and Amino Acid Metabolism

Cancer cells convert the majority of glucose into lactate even under ample oxygen (the Warburg effect), the products of which could be used as carbon-containing precursors for the macromolecule production by rapidly proliferating cells. This intriguing phenomenon necessitates the presence of "glucose sensor" in cancer cells to precisely catch the information on the glucose in the microenvironment for appropriately responding to the environment and ensuring their survival. In recent years, several fascinating reports have been published, referring to the relationship between mTORC2, metabolic reprogramming, and nutrient sensing in cancer cells. mTORC2 is activated on the high-glucose extracellular condition via acetylation of Rictor, the main component of mTORC2 in human GBM cells [65] (Figure 3). This is metabolically mediated by the increased production of acetyl-coenzyme A (acetyl-CoA), a well-known donor of the acetyl group to the protein [66]. The findings suggest the possibility that mTORC2 could work as a potential glucose sensor in cancer cells.

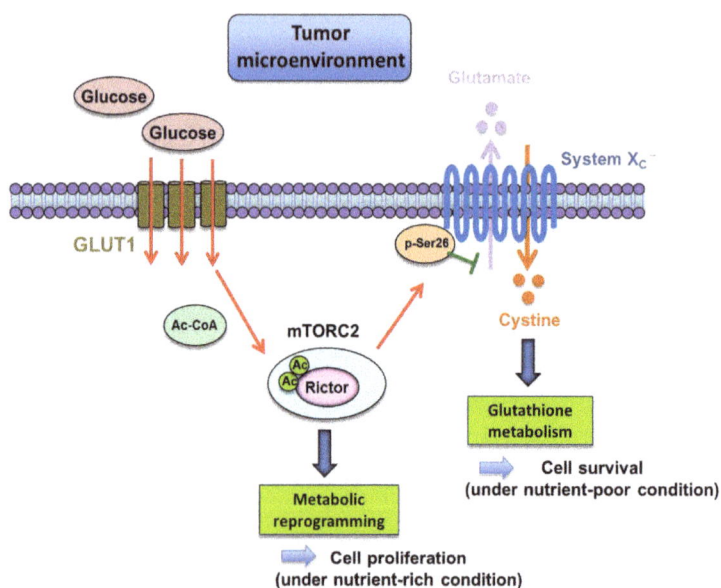

Figure 3. The function of mTORC2 as a sensor of glucose and amino acid. mTORC2 is activated by glucose through acetylation of Rictor, playing a role as a sensor of glucose. Phosphorylation of Ser26 of xCT by mTORC2 represses its function as glutamate-cystine anti-transporter. Under nutrient (glucose) poor conditions, lower mTORC2 signaling could tilt the balance from proliferation to survival by favoring glutamate efflux, cystine uptake, and glutathione synthesis to protect tumor cells from cellular stress.

Unlike mTORC1, which works as an amino acid sensor, the role of mTORC2 as a sensor of amino acid has yet to be clarified. However, using an unbiased proteomic screen, our recent work unraveled that mTORC2 could suppress the activity of the cystine-glutamate antiporter, system Xc transporter-related protein (xCT) via inhibitory phosphorylation of serine 26 of xCT's N terminus cytosolic domain [67] (Figure 3). These results identify an unanticipated mechanism regulating amino acid metabolism in cancer, indicating that genetic mutations and aberrant signal transduction in cancer cells could reprogram amino acid metabolism. Additionally, this novel system would implicate the new role of mTORC2 as a potential amino acid sensor. Glutamine uptake, promoted by aberrant growth factor receptor and c-Myc signaling, is important for tumor cell proliferation, since it is subsequently converted to glutamate essential for tricarboxylic acid (TCA) cycle anaplerosis to provide a carbon source for proliferating cancer cells [65,68]. Thus, when the levels of exogenous nutrient are sufficiently high to support cancer cell proliferation, it would be of disadvantage for cancer cells to secrete glutamate, which is necessary for their anaplerotic reactions. Recently identified mechanisms here enable glutamine-derived glutamate to be utilized primarily for tumor cell proliferation when nutrients are rich in the tumor microenvironment. On the other hand, it would be an advantage for cancer cells to increase xCT-dependent cystine uptake in exchange for glutamate efflux, enabling tumor cells to neutralize the cellular oxidative stresses by synthesizing glutathione from xCT-derived cysteine, when extracellular nutrients are lacking. Therefore, the mechanism on amino acid metabolism described here makes it possible for cancer cells to respond and adapt to a dynamic shift in nutrient levels in the tumor microenvironment.

An unexpected implication for cancer cell metabolism comes from these recent studies regarding the sensing mechanism of glucose and amino acid by mTORC2. Exogenous nutrients including glucose and acetate have been reported to activate mTORC2 to phosphorylate its downstream substrates as aforementioned [69], and this mTORC2-dependent glucose sensing mechanism would raise the possibility that, when extracellular nutrients become scarce, lower mTORC2 signaling could tilt the balance of tumor cell status from cell proliferation to cell survival, at least partly by preferring glutamate efflux, cystine uptake, and glutathione synthesis in order to protect tumor cells from the oxidative cellular stresses, the mechanism of which is based on the mTORC2-dependent regulation of xCT systems (Figure 3). The findings provide the challenging and promising ideas on the previously unrecognized interaction between glucose and amino acid metabolism through mTORC2 signaling, which enables cancer cells to promote their survival according to the level of nutrients in the microenvironment.

6. Epigenetic Modulation by mTOR-Dependent Metabolism in Cancer

Many enzymes that play important roles in epigenetic gene regulation utilize intermediary metabolites as co-substrates yielded by cellular metabolic reprogramming [70]. Indeed, epigenetic modifiers are sensitive to alterations in the levels of multiple intermediary metabolites, which can be regulated by PI3K/Akt/mTOR signaling.

Acetylation on the N-terminal lysine tail of histones leads to the neutralization of positively charged lysine with an open chromatin configuration facilitating transcription. On the other side of the coin, deacetylation of histones is associated with condensed chromatin and reduction of transcriptional activity. Acetyl-CoA is the substrate used to modify histone tails, and can be produced through a variety of metabolic pathways. Its primary generation sources are through the conversion of pyruvate from glycolysis and citrate from the TCA cycle. Intriguingly, some of the processes seem to be governed by the RTK/PI3K/Akt/mTOR pathway, thus possibly linking their metabolic processes to epigenetic status. Recent studies demonstrated that dynamic translocation of mitochondrial pyruvate dehydrogenase complex (PDC) to the nucleus provides a pathway for nuclear acetyl-CoA synthesis required for histone acetylation and epigenetic regulation [71]. Interestingly, the nuclear translocation of PDC seems to be facilitated by the stimulation of growth factor receptor signaling, and it may be mediated by mTOR pathway signaling. ATP citrate lyase (ACLY) is a key enzyme responsible for generating cytosolic acetyl-CoA and oxaloacetate. Akt enhances the phosphorylation and activation of ACLY, and ACLY inhibition results in tumor growth arrest [72]. ACLY is also regulated by growth factor stimulation, which is required for histone acetylation and gene expression [73]. Thus, recent discoveries that class IIa HDACs (HDAC4, 5, 7, and 9) are involved in glucogenic metabolic processes [74] and are regulated by mTORC2 [47] suggest that mTORC2 may affect histone acetylation directly or indirectly through the regulation of acetyl-CoA producing as well as histone modifying enzymes. Intracellular acetyl-CoA also derives from β-oxidation of fatty acids. Recent work has highlighted the importance of fatty acid catabolism in cellular energy homeostasis, and it may also affect the epigenetics through the production of acetyl-CoA. In cancer cells, a gene expressed only in the brain, carnitine palmitoyltransferase 1C, was reported to promote fatty acid oxidation and cell survival, and confer rapamycin resistance, indicating that this gene may act in parallel to mTOR-enhanced glycolysis [75].

In addition to histone acetylation, histone methylation is also important in defining the epigenetic state of chromatin as well as the methylation of DNA itself. A methyl-donor SAM derived from methionine is utilized by methyltransferases; thus, its metabolism can profoundly affect the DNA and histone methylation status. Methionine adenosyltransferase (MAT) is an essential enzyme responsible for SAM biosynthesis, and the function and subclass switch of MAT can be associated with PI3K/Akt signaling, affecting global DNA methylation and cell survival in cancer [76]. Recently, HDAC4 (class IIa HDAC) is reported to play a central role for histone methylation in response to cardiac load, revealing a new relationship between HDACs and histone methylation [77], so mTORC2 might be involved in the regulation of global histone methylation through the inhibition of class IIa HDACs [47].

Somatic mutation of the NADP(+)-dependent enzyme isocitrate dehydrogenase (IDH) is frequently found in cancer, and is shown to acquire a neomorphic enzymatic activity that converts α-ketoglutarate (α-KG) to 2-hydroxyglutarate (2-HG) [78]. Oncometabolite 2-HG was shown to affect the epigenetic status through the inhibition of α-KG-dependent dioxygenase/DNA demethylase (TET2) for DNA methylation and the Jumonji-domain-containing protein 2A (JMJD2A/KDM4A) for histone methylation, eventually contributing to the genome-wide methylator phenotype (CIMP: CpG island methylator phenotype). 2-HG also activates the EGLN1 prolyl hydroxylase and increases the degradation of HIF. The PI3K/Akt/mTOR pathway is relevant to HIF regulation [13], which might further connect metabolism to epigenetics through the control of epigenetic enzymes by HIF and counter-balance the IDH-mediated epigenetic changes. Intriguingly, recent reports demonstrated that DNA methylation landscape of cancer progression shows extensive heterogeneity in time and space [79,80], and further comprehension of these relationships will help our understanding of the mechanics of a variety of metabolic diseases including cancer.

7. Molecular Therapies Targeting mTOR-Dependent Signaling and Metabolism

Understanding the complex role of mTOR in regulating signal transduction is critical to developing more effective therapies to target metabolic reprogramming in cancer. Distinctly, rapamycin treatment (a macrolide antibiotic and immunosuppressive compound that inhibits mTORC1 signaling) leads to the release of Akt suppression (hence activation of mTORC2), due to the loss of negative feedback for attenuating PI3K signaling [81]. The PI3K pathway reactivation after rapamycin treatment indicates that dual PI3K/mTOR inhibitors function by preventing PI3K signaling reactivation and more effectively target mTORC2 (and mTORC1) signaling [82]. Our study further sheds light on the resistant mechanisms of GBM to targeted therapies, providing compelling rationale for the combined inhibition of PI3K/Akt and mTORC2 as a promising "combinatorial targeted therapy" for targeting cancer cell metabolism [83] (Figure 4). We recently demonstrated that EGFRvIII and loss of PTEN potently activate mTORC2, resulting in GBM cell growth and survival by activating NF-κB through SGK1. This study also identified a previously unsuspected role for mTORC2 in mediating chemotherapy resistance, and EGFRvIII-expressing GBMs are exquisitely resistant to cisplatin, temozolomide, and etoposide [24]. These results strongly suggest a critical role for drugs that target both mTORC1 and mTORC2, including in combination with chemotherapy.

mTOR also plays a critical role in integrating cellular metabolism with signal transduction. mTORC1 has emerged as a critical effector downstream of the tumor suppressor liver kinase B1 (LKB1). LKB1 is thought to suppress tumor formation by negatively regulating mTORC1 signaling through adenosine monophosphate (AMP)-activated protein kinase (AMPK). A study by our group demonstrated that the AMPK activator, 5-aminoimidazole-4-carboxamide-1-β-D-ribonucleoside (AICAR) effectively blocks the growth of EGFR-activated GBM primarily by inhibiting lipogenesis [84] (Figure 4). We also demonstrated that EGFR signaling promotes activation of the transcriptional regulator of fatty acid synthesis, sterol regulatory element-binding protein-1 (SREBP-1) [85]. Further investigation uncovered an EGFRvIII-activated, PI3K/SREBP-1-dependent tumor survival pathway through the low-density lipoprotein receptor (LDLR) [86]. Targeting LDLR with the liver X receptor (LXR) agonist caused an inducible degrader of LDLR (IDOL)-mediated LDLR degradation and increased expression of the ATP-binding cassette protein A1 (ABCA1) cholesterol efflux transporter, potently promoting tumor cell death in a GBM model (Figure 4). Further, GBM is remarkably dependent on cholesterol for survival, rendering these tumors sensitive to LXR agonist-dependent cell death, based on identifying and targeting tumor co-dependencies shaped both by aberrant EGFR-mTOR signaling and the brain's unique biochemical environment [87]. Recent reports also demonstrate a novel link between mTOR complexes and lipid metabolism. mTORC2 stimulated sphingolipid and glycerophospholipid synthesis, and inhibition of fatty acid or sphingolipid synthesis prevented tumor development, indicating a causal effect in tumorigenesis as well as a novel therapeutic opportunity [88]. Further, in addition to the role of mTOR a sensor of amino acids and glucose, a recent study reveals that mTOR also senses the presence of lipids through production of phosphatidic acid, expanding its role as a metabolic sensor in the cell [89]. Additionally, the combination of an xCT inhibitor erastin with Torin1 (mTOR kinase inhibitor, which blocks both mTORC1 and mTORC2 activity) resulted in significant GBM cell death, while cell survival was not affected by either drug alone, indicating that increased xCT activity has a major contribution to glutathione synthesis and GBM cell survival upon pharmacological mTOR kinase inhibition [67] (Figure 4). Thus, understanding the regulation of cellular metabolism with mTOR signaling may pave the way for the development of more effective treatment strategies.

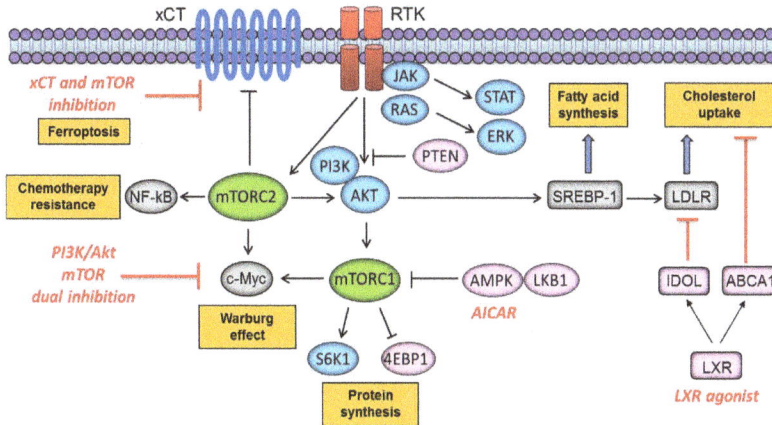

Figure 4. Potential molecular therapies targeting mTOR-dependent metabolic reprogramming in cancer cells. xCT: amino acid transport system Xc-; NF-κB: nuclear factor-kappa B; RTK: receptor tyrosine kinase; JAK: Janus kinase; STAT: signal transducers and activators of transcription; ERK: extracellular signal-regulated kinase; S6K1: ribosomal protein S6 kinase 1; 4EBP1: eukaryotic translation initiation factor 4E-binding protein 1; LKB1: liver kinase B1; AMPK: adenosine monophosphate-activated protein kinase; SREBP-1: sterol regulatory element-binding protein 1; LDLR: low density lipoprotein receptor; IDOL: inducible degrader of LDLR; ABCA1: ATP-binding cassette protein A1; LXR: liver X receptor.

8. Unanswered Questions on mTOR-Dependent Metabolism in Cancer

There have traditionally been plenty of the epidemiological studies endeavoring to reveal the statistic link between cancer incidence and metabolic factors including obesity, diabetes mellitus, and Western-type life style and diet. However, the relationship was not usually solid, partly because most of the studies did not touch on the tumor genotype. Future studies will be necessary to plan the mechanistic types of studies that will untangle the interaction between nutrients, metabolism, and cancer biology on a genetic and molecular basis, which will eventually reveal the impact of nutrient and metabolism on tumor pathogenesis, aggressiveness, and response/resistance to treatment. Thus, mTOR-dependent metabolism should be evaluated in the specific context of genotype-defined and nutrient/environment-restricted conditions.

We have proposed the questions on mTOR-dependent metabolism in cancer, which should be tackled in the future for achieving the goal of developing novel therapeutic and preventive strategies against cancer with facilitated metabolism. In order to determine whether accelerated cellular metabolism is not only a consequence reprogrammed by oncogenic signaling but also potentially affected by a specific tumor microenvironment, it will be necessary to regulate diet and nutrient levels in genotyped human and mouse tumor models to assess the impact of metabolism on signal activation, tumor progression, and response/resistance to treatment. The critical point here is to recognize that the status of specific nutrients in the tumor microenvironment are not merely a consequence of the diet but rather established by the intricate interaction between diet uptake, de novo/salvage synthesis, and cellular utilization [90]. Thus, directly measuring the levels of specific nutrient and tracing their uptake and utilization in tumor tissue in human and genetically engineered mouse models will be needed. Importantly, mTOR complexes are one of the critical hubs and nodes integrating nutrient status and altered growth factor receptor signaling, but understanding how they interact with other nutrient sensing pathways will also be important.

In addition, to test a hypothesis that mTOR complexes are a key node to integrate growth factor receptor signaling with nutrient availability, influencing tumor growth and response to treatment, it will be necessary to study the role of mTOR and its modulation by nutrients in various cancer types. Furthermore, to test the hypothesis that glucose or amino acid-derived intermediates including acetyl-CoA and SAM directly contribute to tumor growth and drug resistance, genetic studies will be needed particularly to confirm the hypothesized importance of histone acetylation, histone methylation, and DNA methylation and to determine if persistent mTOR signaling is sufficient to maintain tumor growth and cause drug resistance through metabolic reprogramming and subsequent epigenetic shifts, for example, by examining the impact of elevated acetyl-CoA and SAM levels on enhancer activation and transcriptional reprogramming.

9. Conclusions and Future Perspectives

The intricate orchestration of responses that enable cancer cells to meet their demands in a completely cell-autonomous fashion defines the specificity of metabolic reprogramming in cancer. A promising and less toxic therapeutic strategy for patients with cancer will be achieved by the development of inhibitors that target cancer-specific signal transduction and metabolism. However, that goal is unlikely to be achieved until the impact of cancer-causing driver mutations on metabolic reprogramming and epigenetic regulation are deeply comprehended, including the flexible ways in which tumor cells appropriately sense the nutrient status in microenvironment and adapt to changing conditions, so as to coordinately sustain the constitutive activation of downstream effectors necessary for tumor cell proliferation and survival. We have herein summarized the recent literature, clearly pointing out an unanticipated important role for both mTOR complexes in sensing essential nutrients including glucose and amino acids via cancer metabolic reprogramming, where they integrate aberrant signaling activities into biochemical reactions and potential transcriptional regulations that drive tumor progression. We have also highlighted an emerging role for mTORC2 in linking aerobic glycolytic metabolism with amino acid metabolism, which could potentially be a key mechanism to exquisitely tilt the balance between dichotomic cellular events essential for tumor cell survival including cell proliferation and cell protection from oxidative stress. Future endeavors should be directed to understand how driver mutations in cancer rewire intracellular signaling cascades to translate biochemical metabolic reactions into global epigenetic ensembles [17]. Cooperative, multidisciplinary, and translational approaches would be necessary to yield critical insights into the etiology and pathogenesis of cancer, shed new light on how tumor cells resist molecularly targeted therapies, and possibly pave the way for the development of more effective signaling-dependent metabolism-targeted treatments against cancer to achieve the goal of "precision medicine."

Funding: This research was funded by JSPS KAKENHI Grant Number 17K15672 and Grant-in-Aid from Takeda Science Foundation.

Acknowledgments: We thank Noriko Sakayori and Mizuho Karita (Department of pathology, Division of Pathological Neuroscience, Tokyo Women's Medical University) for their helpful assistance.

Conflicts of Interest: P.S.M. is a scientific co-founder and consultant for Pretzel Therapeutics, Inc.

References

1. DeBerardinis, R.J.; Lum, J.J.; Hatzivassiliou, G.; Thompson, C.B. The biology of cancer: Metabolic reprogramming fuels cell growth and proliferation. *Cell Metab.* **2008**, *7*, 11–20. [CrossRef] [PubMed]
2. Soga, T. Cancer metabolism: Key players in metabolic reprogramming. *Cancer Sci.* **2013**, *104*, 275–281. [CrossRef] [PubMed]
3. Vander Heiden, M.G.; Cantley, L.C.; Thompson, C.B. Understanding the warburg effect: The metabolic requirements of cell proliferation. *Science* **2009**, *324*, 1029–1033. [CrossRef] [PubMed]
4. Garber, K. Energy boost: The warburg effect returns in a new theory of cancer. *J. Natl. Cancer Inst. USA* **2004**, *96*, 1805–1806. [CrossRef] [PubMed]
5. Miyo, M.; Konno, M.; Nishida, N.; Sueda, T.; Noguchi, K.; Matsui, H.; Colvin, H.; Kawamoto, K.; Koseki, J.; Haraguchi, N.; et al. Metabolic adaptation to nutritional stress in human colorectal cancer. *Sci. Rep.* **2016**, *6*, 38415. [CrossRef] [PubMed]
6. Wise, D.R.; Thompson, C.B. Glutamine addiction: A new therapeutic target in cancer. *Trends Biochem. Sci.* **2010**, *35*, 427–433. [CrossRef] [PubMed]
7. Csibi, A.; Lee, G.; Yoon, S.O.; Tong, H.; Ilter, D.; Elia, I.; Fendt, S.M.; Roberts, T.M.; Blenis, J. The mTORC1/S6K1 pathway regulates glutamine metabolism through the eIF4B-dependent control of c-Myc translation. *Curr. Biol.* **2014**, *24*, 2274–2280. [CrossRef] [PubMed]
8. Yamamoto, N.; Ueda-Wakagi, M.; Sato, T.; Kawasaki, K.; Sawada, K.; Kawabata, K.; Akagawa, M.; Ashida, H. Measurement of glucose uptake in cultured cells. *Curr. Protoc. Pharmacol.* **2015**, *71*, 12.14.1–12.14.26. [PubMed]
9. Rock, C.L.; Doyle, C.; Demark-Wahnefried, W.; Meyerhardt, J.; Courneya, K.S.; Schwartz, A.L.; Bandera, E.V.; Hamilton, K.K.; Grant, B.; McCullough, M.; et al. Nutrition and physical activity guidelines for cancer survivors. *CA Cancer J. Clin.* **2012**, *62*, 243–274. [CrossRef] [PubMed]
10. Izuishi, K.; Kato, K.; Ogura, T.; Kinoshita, T.; Esumi, H. Remarkable tolerance of tumor cells to nutrient deprivation: Possible new biochemical target for cancer therapy. *Cancer Res.* **2000**, *60*, 6201–6207. [PubMed]
11. Davis, C.D. Nutritional interactions: Credentialing of molecular targets for cancer prevention. *Exp. Biol. Med. (Maywood)* **2007**, *232*, 176–183. [PubMed]
12. Hanahan, D.; Weinberg, R.A. Hallmarks of cancer: The next generation. *Cell* **2011**, *144*, 646–674. [CrossRef] [PubMed]
13. Pavlova, N.N.; Thompson, C.B. The emerging hallmarks of cancer metabolism. *Cell Metab.* **2016**, *23*, 27–47. [CrossRef] [PubMed]
14. Panieri, E.; Santoro, M.M. Ros homeostasis and metabolism: A dangerous liason in cancer cells. *Cell Death Dis.* **2016**, *7*, e2253. [CrossRef] [PubMed]
15. Chen, C.; Liu, Y.; Liu, R.; Ikenoue, T.; Guan, K.L.; Liu, Y.; Zheng, P. TSC-mTOR maintains quiescence and function of hematopoietic stem cells by repressing mitochondrial biogenesis and reactive oxygen species. *J. Exp. Med.* **2008**, *205*, 2397–2408. [CrossRef] [PubMed]
16. Tsang, C.K.; Chen, M.; Cheng, X.; Qi, Y.; Chen, Y.; Das, I.; Li, X.; Vallat, B.; Fu, L.W.; Qian, C.N.; et al. SOD1 phosphorylation by mTOR1 couples nutrient sensing and redox Regulation. *Mol. Cell* **2018**, *70*, 502–515. [CrossRef] [PubMed]
17. Masui, K.; Cavenee, W.K.; Mischel, P.S. mTORC2 in the center of cancer metabolic reprogramming. *Trends Endocrinol. Metab.* **2014**, *25*, 364–373. [CrossRef] [PubMed]
18. Lien, E.C.; Lyssiotis, C.A.; Cantley, L.C. Metabolic reprogramming by the PI3K-AKT-mTOR pathway in cancer. *Recent Results Cancer Res.* **2016**, *207*, 39–72. [PubMed]
19. Rabanal-Ruiz, Y.; Korolchuk, V.I. mTORC1 and nutrient homeostasis: The central role of the lysosome. *Int. J. Mol. Sci.* **2018**, *19*, 818. [CrossRef] [PubMed]
20. Fingar, D.C.; Richardson, C.J.; Tee, A.R.; Cheatham, L.; Tsou, C.; Blenis, J. mTOR controls cell cycle progression through its cell growth effectors S6K1 and 4E-BP1/eukaryotic translation initiation factor 4E. *Mol. Cell. Biol.* **2004**, *24*, 200–216. [CrossRef] [PubMed]

21. Lee, S.L.; Chou, C.C.; Chuang, H.C.; Hsu, E.C.; Chiu, P.C.; Kulp, S.K.; Byrd, J.C.; Chen, C.S. Functional role of mTORC2 versus integrin-linked kinase in mediating ser473-akt phosphorylation in pten-negative prostate and breast cancer cell lines. *PLoS ONE* **2013**, *8*, e67149. [CrossRef] [PubMed]

22. Lin, A.; Piao, H.L.; Zhuang, L.; Sarbassov dos, D.; Ma, L.; Gan, B. FoxO transcription factors promote AKT Ser473 phosphorylation and renal tumor growth in response to pharmacologic inhibition of the PI3K-AKT pathway. *Cancer Res.* **2014**, *74*, 1682–1693. [CrossRef] [PubMed]

23. Im-aram, A.; Farrand, L.; Bae, S.M.; Song, G.; Song, Y.S.; Han, J.Y.; Tsang, B.K. The mTORC2 component rictor contributes to cisplatin resistance in human ovarian cancer cells. *PLoS ONE* **2013**, *8*, e75455. [CrossRef] [PubMed]

24. Tanaka, K.; Babic, I.; Nathanson, D.; Akhavan, D.; Guo, D.; Gini, B.; Dang, J.; Zhu, S.; Yang, H.; De Jesus, J.; et al. Oncogenic EGFR signaling activates an mTORC2-NF-kappaB pathway that promotes chemotherapy resistance. *Cancer Discov.* **2011**, *1*, 524–538. [CrossRef] [PubMed]

25. Wick, W.; Blaes, J.; Weiler, M. mTORC 2:1 for chemotherapy sensitization in glioblastoma. *Cancer Discov.* **2011**, *1*, 475–476. [CrossRef] [PubMed]

26. Jacinto, E.; Loewith, R.; Schmidt, A.; Lin, S.; Ruegg, M.A.; Hall, A.; Hall, M.N. Mammalian tor complex 2 controls the actin cytoskeleton and is rapamycin insensitive. *Nat. Cell Biol.* **2004**, *6*, 1122–1128. [CrossRef] [PubMed]

27. Kim, S.G.; Buel, G.R.; Blenis, J. Nutrient regulation of the mTOR complex 1 signaling pathway. *Mol. Cells* **2013**, *35*, 463–473. [CrossRef] [PubMed]

28. Peterson, T.R.; Laplante, M.; Thoreen, C.C.; Sancak, Y.; Kang, S.A.; Kuehl, W.M.; Gray, N.S.; Sabatini, D.M. Deptor is an mTOR inhibitor frequently overexpressed in multiple myeloma cells and required for their survival. *Cell* **2009**, *137*, 873–886. [CrossRef] [PubMed]

29. Kaizuka, T.; Hara, T.; Oshiro, N.; Kikkawa, U.; Yonezawa, K.; Takehana, K.; Iemura, S.; Natsume, T.; Mizushima, N. Tti1 and Tel2 are critical factors in mammalian target of rapamycin complex assembly. *J. Biol. Chem.* **2010**, *285*, 20109–20116. [CrossRef] [PubMed]

30. Hara, K.; Maruki, Y.; Long, X.; Yoshino, K.; Oshiro, N.; Hidayat, S.; Tokunaga, C.; Avruch, J.; Yonezawa, K. Raptor, a binding partner of target of rapamycin (TOR), mediates tor action. *Cell* **2002**, *110*, 177–189. [CrossRef]

31. Kim, D.H.; Sarbassov, D.D.; Ali, S.M.; King, J.E.; Latek, R.R.; Erdjument-Bromage, H.; Tempst, P.; Sabatini, D.M. mTOR interacts with raptor to form a nutrient-sensitive complex that signals to the cell growth machinery. *Cell* **2002**, *110*, 163–175. [CrossRef]

32. Sancak, Y.; Thoreen, C.C.; Peterson, T.R.; Lindquist, R.A.; Kang, S.A.; Spooner, E.; Carr, S.A.; Sabatini, D.M. PRAS40 is an insulin-regulated inhibitor of the mTORC1 protein kinase. *Mol. Cell* **2007**, *25*, 903–915. [CrossRef] [PubMed]

33. Thedieck, K.; Polak, P.; Kim, M.L.; Molle, K.D.; Cohen, A.; Jeno, P.; Arrieumerlou, C.; Hall, M.N. PRAS40 and PRR5-like protein are new mTOR interactors that regulate apoptosis. *PLoS ONE* **2007**, *2*, e1217. [CrossRef] [PubMed]

34. Vander Haar, E.; Lee, S.I.; Bandhakavi, S.; Griffin, T.J.; Kim, D.H. Insulin signalling to mTOR mediated by the AKT/PKB substrate PRAS40. *Nat. Cell Biol.* **2007**, *9*, 316–323. [CrossRef] [PubMed]

35. Wang, L.; Harris, T.E.; Roth, R.A.; Lawrence, J.C., Jr. PRAS40 regulates mTORC1 kinase activity by functioning as a direct inhibitor of substrate binding. *J. Biol. Chem.* **2007**, *282*, 20036–20044. [CrossRef] [PubMed]

36. Sarbassov, D.D.; Ali, S.M.; Kim, D.H.; Guertin, D.A.; Latek, R.R.; Erdjument-Bromage, H.; Tempst, P.; Sabatini, D.M. Rictor, a novel binding partner of mTOR, defines a rapamycin-insensitive and raptor-independent pathway that regulates the cytoskeleton. *Curr. Biol.* **2004**, *14*, 1296–1302. [CrossRef] [PubMed]

37. Frias, M.A.; Thoreen, C.C.; Jaffe, J.D.; Schroder, W.; Sculley, T.; Carr, S.A.; Sabatini, D.M. Msin1 is necessary for AKT/PKB phosphorylation, and its isoforms define three distinct mTORC2s. *Curr. Biol.* **2006**, *16*, 1865–1870. [CrossRef] [PubMed]

38. Jacinto, E.; Facchinetti, V.; Liu, D.; Soto, N.; Wei, S.; Jung, S.Y.; Huang, Q.; Qin, J.; Su, B. SIN1/MIP1 maintains rictor-mTOR complex integrity and regulates AKT phosphorylation and substrate specificity. *Cell* **2006**, *127*, 125–137. [CrossRef] [PubMed]

39. Pearce, L.R.; Huang, X.; Boudeau, J.; Pawlowski, R.; Wullschleger, S.; Deak, M.; Ibrahim, A.F.; Gourlay, R.; Magnuson, M.A.; Alessi, D.R. Identification of protor as a novel rictor-binding component of mTOR complex-2. *Biochem. J.* **2007**, *405*, 513–522. [CrossRef] [PubMed]

40. Pearce, L.R.; Sommer, E.M.; Sakamoto, K.; Wullschleger, S.; Alessi, D.R. Protor-1 is required for efficient mTORC2-mediated activation of sgk1 in the kidney. *Biochem. J.* **2011**, *436*, 169–179. [CrossRef] [PubMed]

41. Iurlaro, R.; Leon-Annicchiarico, C.L.; Munoz-Pinedo, C. Regulation of cancer metabolism by oncogenes and tumor suppressors. *Methods Enzymol.* **2014**, *542*, 59–80. [PubMed]

42. Nagarajan, A.; Malvi, P.; Wajapeyee, N. Oncogene-directed alterations in cancer cell metabolism. *Trends Cancer* **2016**, *2*, 365–377. [CrossRef] [PubMed]

43. Kim, E.S.; Samanta, A.; Cheng, H.S.; Ding, Z.; Han, W.; Toschi, L.; Chang, Y.T. Effect of oncogene activating mutations and kinase inhibitors on amino acid metabolism of human isogenic breast cancer cells. *Mol. Biosyst.* **2015**, *11*, 3378–3386. [CrossRef] [PubMed]

44. Stine, Z.E.; Walton, Z.E.; Altman, B.J.; Hsieh, A.L.; Dang, C.V. MYC, metabolism, and cancer. *Cancer Discov.* **2015**, *5*, 1024–1039. [CrossRef] [PubMed]

45. Dang, C.V.; Le, A.; Gao, P. MYC-induced cancer cell energy metabolism and therapeutic opportunities. *Clin. Cancer Res.* **2009**, *15*, 6479–6483. [CrossRef] [PubMed]

46. Ischenko, I.; Zhi, J.; Moll, U.M.; Nemajerova, A.; Petrenko, O. Direct reprogramming by oncogenic ras and myc. *Proc. Natl. Acad. Sci. USA* **2013**, *110*, 3937–3942. [CrossRef] [PubMed]

47. Masui, K.; Tanaka, K.; Akhavan, D.; Babic, I.; Gini, B.; Matsutani, T.; Iwanami, A.; Liu, F.; Villa, G.R.; Gu, Y.; et al. mTOR complex 2 controls glycolytic metabolism in glioblastoma through foxo acetylation and upregulation of c-myc. *Cell Metab.* **2013**, *18*, 726–739. [CrossRef] [PubMed]

48. Babic, I.; Anderson, E.S.; Tanaka, K.; Guo, D.; Masui, K.; Li, B.; Zhu, S.; Gu, Y.; Villa, G.R.; Akhavan, D.; et al. EGFR mutation-induced alternative splicing of max contributes to growth of glycolytic tumors in brain cancer. *Cell Metab.* **2013**, *17*, 1000–1008. [CrossRef] [PubMed]

49. Zhang, Y.; Nicholatos, J.; Dreier, J.R.; Ricoult, S.J.; Widenmaier, S.B.; Hotamisligil, G.S.; Kwiatkowski, D.J.; Manning, B.D. Coordinated regulation of protein synthesis and degradation by mTORC1. *Nature* **2014**, *513*, 440–443. [CrossRef] [PubMed]

50. Goodman, C.A. The role of mTORC1 in regulating protein synthesis and skeletal muscle mass in response to various mechanical stimuli. *Rev. Physiol. Biochem. Pharmacol.* **2014**, *166*, 43–95. [PubMed]

51. Martina, J.A.; Chen, Y.; Gucek, M.; Puertollano, R. mTORC1 functions as a transcriptional regulator of autophagy by preventing nuclear transport of TFEB. *Autophagy* **2012**, *8*, 903–914. [CrossRef] [PubMed]

52. Dibble, C.C.; Manning, B.D. Signal integration by mTORC1 coordinates nutrient input with biosynthetic output. *Nat. Cell Biol.* **2013**, *15*, 555–564. [CrossRef] [PubMed]

53. Shimobayashi, M.; Hall, M.N. Making new contacts: The mTOR network in metabolism and signalling crosstalk. *Nat. Rev. Mol. Cell Biol.* **2014**, *15*, 155–162. [CrossRef] [PubMed]

54. Blommaart, E.F.; Luiken, J.J.; Blommaart, P.J.; van Woerkom, G.M.; Meijer, A.J. Phosphorylation of ribosomal protein s6 is inhibitory for autophagy in isolated rat hepatocytes. *J. Biol. Chem.* **1995**, *270*, 2320–2326. [CrossRef] [PubMed]

55. Wolfson, R.L.; Chantranupong, L.; Saxton, R.A.; Shen, K.; Scaria, S.M.; Cantor, J.R.; Sabatini, D.M. Sestrin2 is a leucine sensor for the mTORC1 pathway. *Science* **2016**, *351*, 43–48. [CrossRef] [PubMed]

56. Potier, M.; Darcel, N.; Tome, D. Protein, amino acids and the control of food intake. *Curr. Opin. Clin. Nutr. Metab. Care* **2009**, *12*, 54–58. [CrossRef] [PubMed]

57. Panten, U.; Christians, J.; von Kriegstein, E.; Poser, W.; Hasselblatt, A. Studies on the mechanism of l-leucine-and alpha-ketoisocaproic acid-induced insulin release from perifused isolated pancreatic islets. *Diabetologia* **1974**, *10*, 149–154. [CrossRef] [PubMed]

58. Greiwe, J.S.; Kwon, G.; McDaniel, M.L.; Semenkovich, C.F. Leucine and insulin activate p70 s6 kinase through different pathways in human skeletal muscle. *Am. J. Physiol. Endocrinol. Metab.* **2001**, *281*, E466–E471. [CrossRef] [PubMed]

59. Nair, K.S.; Schwartz, R.G.; Welle, S. Leucine as a regulator of whole body and skeletal muscle protein metabolism in humans. *Am. J. Physiol.* **1992**, *263*, E928–E934. [CrossRef] [PubMed]

60. Lee, M.; Kim, J.H.; Yoon, I.; Lee, C.; Fallahi Sichani, M.; Kang, J.S.; Kang, J.; Guo, M.; Lee, K.Y.; Han, G.; et al. Coordination of the leucine-sensing Rag GTPase cycle by leucyl-tRNA synthetase in the mTORC1 signaling pathway. *Proc. Natl. Acad. Sci. USA* **2018**, *115*, E5279–E5288. [CrossRef] [PubMed]

61. Chantranupong, L.; Scaria, S.M.; Saxton, R.A.; Gygi, M.P.; Shen, K.; Wyant, G.A.; Wang, T.; Harper, J.W.; Gygi, S.P.; Sabatini, D.M. The castor proteins are arginine sensors for the mTORC1 pathway. *Cell* **2016**, *165*, 153–164. [CrossRef] [PubMed]

62. Chen, J.; Ou, Y.; Yang, Y.; Li, W.; Xu, Y.; Xie, Y.; Liu, Y. Klhl22 activates amino-acid-dependent mTORC1 signalling to promote tumorigenesis and ageing. *Nature* **2018**, *557*, 585–589. [CrossRef] [PubMed]

63. Gu, X.; Orozco, J.M.; Saxton, R.A.; Condon, K.J.; Liu, G.Y.; Krawczyk, P.A.; Scaria, S.M.; Harper, J.W.; Gygi, S.P.; Sabatini, D.M. SAMTOR is an S-adenosylmethionine sensor for the mTORc1 pathway. *Science* **2017**, *358*, 813–818. [CrossRef] [PubMed]

64. Lamb, R.F. Amino acid sensing mechanisms: An achilles heel in cancer? *FEBS J.* **2012**, *279*, 2624–2631. [CrossRef] [PubMed]

65. Masui, K.; Tanaka, K.; Ikegami, S.; Villa, G.R.; Yang, H.; Yong, W.H.; Cloughesy, T.F.; Yamagata, K.; Arai, N.; Cavenee, W.K.; et al. Glucose-dependent acetylation of rictor promotes targeted cancer therapy resistance. *Proc. Natl. Acad. Sci. USA* **2015**, *112*, 9406–9411. [CrossRef] [PubMed]

66. Korkes, S.; Del Campillo, A.; Ochoa, S. Pyruvate oxidation system of heart muscle. *J. Biol. Chem.* **1952**, *195*, 541–547. [PubMed]

67. Gu, Y.; Albuquerque, C.P.; Braas, D.; Zhang, W.; Villa, G.R.; Bi, J.; Ikegami, S.; Masui, K.; Gini, B.; Yang, H.; et al. mTORC2 regulates amino acid metabolism in cancer by phosphorylation of the cystine-glutamate antiporter XCT. *Mol. Cell* **2017**, *67*, 128–138.e7. [CrossRef] [PubMed]

68. Altman, B.J.; Stine, Z.E.; Dang, C.V. From Krebs to clinic: Glutamine metabolism to cancer therapy. *Nat. Rev. Cancer* **2016**, *16*, 619–634. [CrossRef] [PubMed]

69. Masui, K.; Cavenee, W.K.; Mischel, P.S. mTORC2 and metabolic reprogramming in gbm: At the interface of genetics and environment. *Brain Pathol.* **2015**, *25*, 755–759. [CrossRef] [PubMed]

70. Kaelin, W.G., Jr.; McKnight, S.L. Influence of metabolism on epigenetics and disease. *Cell* **2013**, *153*, 56–69. [CrossRef] [PubMed]

71. Sutendra, G.; Kinnaird, A.; Dromparis, P.; Paulin, R.; Stenson, T.H.; Haromy, A.; Hashimoto, K.; Zhang, N.; Flaim, E.; Michelakis, E.D. A nuclear pyruvate dehydrogenase complex is important for the generation of acetyl-CoA and histone acetylation. *Cell* **2014**, *158*, 84–97. [CrossRef] [PubMed]

72. Migita, T.; Narita, T.; Nomura, K.; Miyagi, E.; Inazuka, F.; Matsuura, M.; Ushijima, M.; Mashima, T.; Seimiya, H.; Satoh, Y.; et al. Atp citrate lyase: Activation and therapeutic implications in non-small cell lung cancer. *Cancer Res.* **2008**, *68*, 8547–8554. [CrossRef] [PubMed]

73. Wellen, K.E.; Hatzivassiliou, G.; Sachdeva, U.M.; Bui, T.V.; Cross, J.R.; Thompson, C.B. Atp-citrate lyase links cellular metabolism to histone acetylation. *Science* **2009**, *324*, 1076–1080. [CrossRef] [PubMed]

74. Mihaylova, M.M.; Vasquez, D.S.; Ravnskjaer, K.; Denechaud, P.D.; Yu, R.T.; Alvarez, J.G.; Downes, M.; Evans, R.M.; Montminy, M.; Shaw, R.J. Class iia histone deacetylases are hormone-activated regulators of foxo and mammalian glucose homeostasis. *Cell* **2011**, *145*, 607–621. [CrossRef] [PubMed]

75. Zaugg, K.; Yao, Y.; Reilly, P.T.; Kannan, K.; Kiarash, R.; Mason, J.; Huang, P.; Sawyer, S.K.; Fuerth, B.; Faubert, B.; et al. Carnitine palmitoyltransferase 1c promotes cell survival and tumor growth under conditions of metabolic stress. *Genes Dev.* **2011**, *25*, 1041–1051. [CrossRef] [PubMed]

76. Frau, M.; Feo, F.; Pascale, R.M. Pleiotropic effects of methionine adenosyltransferases deregulation as determinants of liver cancer progression and prognosis. *J. Hepatol.* **2013**, *59*, 830–841. [CrossRef] [PubMed]

77. Hohl, M.; Wagner, M.; Reil, J.C.; Müller, S.A.; Tauchnitz, M.; Zimmer, A.M.; Lehmann, L.H.; Thiel, G.; Böhm, M.; Backs, J.; et al. Hdac4 controls histone methylation in response to elevated cardiac load. *J. Clin. Investig.* **2013**, *123*, 1359–1370. [CrossRef] [PubMed]

78. Masui, K.; Cavenee, W.K.; Mischel, P.S. Cancer metabolism as a central driving force of glioma pathogenesis. *Brain Tumor Pathol.* **2016**, *33*, 161–168. [CrossRef] [PubMed]

79. Klughammer, J.; Kiesel, B.; Roetzer, T.; Fortelny, N.; Nemc, A.; Nenning, K.H.; Furtner, J.; Sheffield, N.C.; Datlinger, P.; Peter, N.; et al. The DNA methylation landscape of glioblastoma disease progression shows extensive heterogeneity in time and space. *Nat. Med.* **2018**. [CrossRef] [PubMed]

80. Ceccarelli, M.; Barthel, F.P.; Malta, T.M.; Sabedot, T.S.; Salama, S.R.; Murray, B.A.; Morozova, O.; Newton, Y.; Radenbaugh, A.; Pagnotta, S.M.; et al. Molecular profiling reveals biologically discrete subsets and pathways of progression in diffuse glioma. *Cell* **2016**, *164*, 550–563. [CrossRef] [PubMed]

81. Cloughesy, T.F.; Yoshimoto, K.; Nghiemphu, P.; Brown, K.; Dang, J.; Zhu, S.; Hsueh, T.; Chen, Y.; Wang, W.; Youngkin, D.; et al. Antitumor activity of rapamycin in a phase I trial for patients with recurrent PTEN-deficient glioblastoma. *PLoS Med.* **2008**, *5*, e8. [CrossRef] [PubMed]

82. Fan, Q.W.; Knight, Z.A.; Goldenberg, D.D.; Yu, W.; Mostov, K.E.; Stokoe, D.; Shokat, K.M.; Weiss, W.A. A dual pi3 Kinase/mTOR inhibitor reveals emergent efficacy in glioma. *Cancer Cell* **2006**, *9*, 341–349. [CrossRef] [PubMed]

83. Masui, K.; Cavenee, W.K.; Mischel, P.S. mTORC2 dictates warburg effect and drug resistance. *Cell Cycle* **2014**, *13*, 1053–1054. [CrossRef] [PubMed]

84. Guo, D.; Hildebrandt, I.J.; Prins, R.M.; Soto, H.; Mazzotta, M.M.; Dang, J.; Czernin, J.; Shyy, J.Y.; Watson, A.D.; Phelps, M.; et al. The ampk agonist aicar inhibits the growth of egfrviii-expressing glioblastomas by inhibiting lipogenesis. *Proc. Natl. Acad. Sci. USA* **2009**, *106*, 12932–12937. [CrossRef] [PubMed]

85. Guo, D.; Prins, R.M.; Dang, J.; Kuga, D.; Iwanami, A.; Soto, H.; Lin, K.Y.; Huang, T.T.; Akhavan, D.; Hock, M.B.; et al. EGFR signaling through an AKT-SREBP-1-dependent, rapamycin-resistant pathway sensitizes glioblastomas to antilipogenic therapy. *Sci. Signal.* **2009**, *2*, ra82. [CrossRef] [PubMed]

86. Guo, D.; Reinitz, F.; Youssef, M.; Hong, C.; Nathanson, D.; Akhavan, D.; Kuga, D.; Amzajerdi, A.N.; Soto, H.; Zhu, S.; et al. An LXR agonist promotes glioblastoma cell death through inhibition of an EGFR/AKT/SREBP-1/LDLR-dependent pathway. *Cancer Discov.* **2011**, *1*, 442–456. [CrossRef] [PubMed]

87. Villa, G.R.; Hulce, J.J.; Zanca, C.; Bi, J.; Ikegami, S.; Cahill, G.L.; Gu, Y.; Lum, K.M.; Masui, K.; Yang, H.; et al. An lxr-cholesterol axis creates a metabolic co-dependency for brain cancers. *Cancer Cell* **2016**, *30*, 683–693. [CrossRef] [PubMed]

88. Guri, Y.; Colombi, M.; Dazert, E.; Hindupur, S.K.; Roszik, J.; Moes, S.; Jenoe, P.; Heim, M.H.; Riezman, I.; Riezman, H.; et al. mTORC2 promotes tumorigenesis via lipid synthesis. *Cancer Cell* **2017**, *32*, 807–823. [CrossRef] [PubMed]

89. Menon, D.; Salloum, D.; Bernfeld, E.; Gorodetsky, E.; Akselrod, A.; Frias, M.A.; Sudderth, J.; Chen, P.H.; DeBerardinis, R.; Foster, D.A. Lipid sensing by mTOR complexes via de novo synthesis of phosphatidic acid. *J. Biol. Chem.* **2017**, *292*, 6303–6311. [CrossRef] [PubMed]

90. Masui, K.; Shibata, N.; Cavenee, W.K.; Mischel, P.S. mTORC2 activity in brain cancer: Extracellular nutrients are required to maintain oncogenic signaling. *Bioessays* **2016**, *38*, 839–844. [CrossRef] [PubMed]

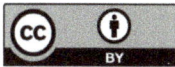

International Journal of
Molecular Sciences

MDPI

Article

Resistance to the Antiproliferative In Vitro Effect of PI3K-Akt-mTOR Inhibition in Primary Human Acute Myeloid Leukemia Cells Is Associated with Altered Cell Metabolism

Ina Nepstad [1], Håkon Reikvam [2], Annette K. Brenner [1,2], Øystein Bruserud [1,2] and Kimberley J. Hatfield [1,3,*]

[1]   Department of Clinical Science, University of Bergen, 5021 Bergen, Norway; ina.nepstad@uib.no (I.N.); annette.brenner@uib.no (A.K.B.); Oystein.Bruserud@uib.no (Ø.B.)
[2]   Department of Medicine, Haukeland University Hospital, 5021 Bergen, Norway; Hakon.Reikvam@uib.no
[3]   Department of Immunology and Transfusion Medicine, Haukeland University Hospital, 5021 Bergen, Norway
*   Correspondence: Kimberley.Hatfield@uib.no; Tel.: +47-55-973037

Received: 6 December 2017; Accepted: 23 January 2018; Published: 27 January 2018

Abstract: Constitutive signaling through the phosphatidylinositol-3-kinase-Akt-mechanistic target of rapamycin (PI3K-Akt-mTOR) pathway is present in acute myeloid leukemia (AML) cells. However, AML is a heterogeneous disease, and we therefore investigated possible associations between cellular metabolism and sensitivity to PI3K-Akt-mTOR pathway inhibitors. We performed non-targeted metabolite profiling to compare the metabolome differences of primary human AML cells derived from patients susceptible or resistant to the in vitro antiproliferative effects of mTOR and PI3K inhibitors. In addition, the phosphorylation status of 18 proteins involved in PI3K-Akt-mTOR signaling and the effect of the cyclooxygenase inhibitor indomethacin on their phosphorylation status was investigated by flow cytometry. Strong antiproliferative effects by inhibitors were observed only for a subset of patients. We compared the metabolite profiles for responders and non-responders towards PI3K-mTOR inhibitors, and 627 metabolites could be detected. Of these metabolites, 128 were annotated and 15 of the annotated metabolites differed significantly between responders and non-responders, including metabolites involved in energy, amino acid, and lipid metabolism. To conclude, leukemia cells that are susceptible or resistant to PI3K-Akt-mTOR inhibitors differ in energy, amino acid, and arachidonic acid metabolism, and modulation of arachidonic acid metabolism alters the activation of mTOR and its downstream mediators.

Keywords: acute myeloid leukemia; metabolism; mTOR; PI3K; phosphorylation

---

1. Introduction

Acute myeloid leukemia (AML) is a heterogeneous malignancy characterized by proliferating myeloblasts in the bone marrow [1,2]. Abnormal constitutive signaling through intracellular pathways is often observed in AML, including the phosphatidylinositol-3-kinase-Akt-mechanistic/mammalian target of rapamycin (PI3K-Akt-mTOR) pathway that seems to be important both in normal and leukemic hematopoiesis [3–5]. This pathway is important for regulation of proliferation, apoptosis, differentiation, and metabolism [6,7].

Constitutive signaling through the PI3K-Akt-mTOR pathway is found in 50–80% of AML patients and correlates with poor prognosis [4,8]. This abnormal signaling may be initiated by various mechanisms, e.g., oncogenes or mutated receptor tyrosine kinases, cell adhesion molecules, G-protein-coupled receptors, or other cytokine or hormonal receptors.

When signaling is initiated in response to extracellular stimuli, scaffolding proteins are recruited and bind to the regulatory subunit of PI3K. Sequentially, PI3K phosphorylates phosphatidylinositol (4,5)-bisphosphate (PIP2) to generate phosphatidylinositol (3,4,5)-trisphosphate (PIP3), which facilitates recruitment and binding of proteins containing pleckstrin–homology domains, including Akt and its upstream activator 3'phosphoinositide-dependent kinase 1 (PDK1) [9]. PDK1 phosphorylates Akt at T308, leading to its partial activation. However, a subsequent phosphorylation at S473 is required for full enzymatic activation of Akt [9,10], and this can be achieved by mTOR complex 2 (mTORC2) or DNA-dependent protein kinase (DNA-PK) [10,11]. The mTOR kinase is part of two complexes, mTORC1 and mTORC2 with different biochemical structures and substrate specificity. The interactions between Akt and mTORC1/2 are complex. Akt phosphorylates the inhibitor of mTORC1 and proline-rich Akt-substrate-40 (PRAS40), preventing the suppression of mTORC1 signaling. Additionally, an Akt-driven inactivation of tuberous sclerosis complex (TSC) 1/2, leads to activation of mTORC1 through Ras homolog enriched in brain (RHEB). mTORC1 is an important regulator of cellular metabolism and protein synthesis through phosphorylation and activation of both the S6 ribosomal protein kinase (S6PK) and the repressor of messenger RNA (mRNA) translation initiation factor 4E-binding protein 1 (4EBP1) [6].

The PI3K-Akt-mTOR signaling pathway is one of the most frequently dysregulated pathways in human malignancies, including AML [12,13]. Though PI3K-Akt-mTOR is rarely mutated in AML, these patients harbor several mutations that may activate the pathway [12,14] and, hence, contribute to chemoresistance [4,15]. Based on extensive experimental studies, this pathway has been regarded as a possible therapeutic target in human AML [3,16]. However, despite this evidence, the initial clinical studies suggest that the tested mTOR inhibitors have only a modest antileukemic effect [16]. However, it should be emphasized that previous experimental studies also suggest that therapeutic targeting of the PI3K-Akt-mTOR pathway will be effective only for a subset of patients [17], and pathway inhibition may be more effective when using combined treatment strategies [18].

As discussed in a recent review, previous studies of resistance towards PI3K-Akt-mTOR inhibitors have focused on the possible hyperactivation of upstream mediators through feedback loops (e.g., PI3K and Akt) and compensatory activation of other pathways [16]. However, this cannot be the only explanation because chemoresistance is also seen for inhibitors upstream to Akt [17]. Our present study is to the best of our knowledge the first to suggest that metabolic alterations are a part of the therapy-resistant AML cell phenotype, and the metabolic differences seem to involve pathways that are involved in cellular energy and amino acid metabolism.

2. Results

2.1. Selection of Patients for the Metabolomics Comparison of Primary Human Acute Myeloid Leukemia (AML) Cells

We investigated the antiproliferative effect of four PI3K-Akt-mTOR inhibitors on primary human AML cell proliferation in the presence of exogenous cytokines [17]. The antiproliferative effects of the inhibitors differed considerably between the 56 patient cell samples studied, and for a subset of patients, even increased proliferation was seen in the presence of pathway inhibitors. In contrast, these previous studies showed that pathway inhibitors had only minor effects on the spontaneous stress-induced in vitro apoptosis that occurs during culture of primary human AML cells [19], and only minor differences could then be detected between different patients [17]. Patient subsets could thus be identified based solely on differences in our proliferation assay, i.e., these cells survived for 6 days in the presence of the pathway inhibitors and could still proliferate and incorporate ^{3}H-thymidine during the period from day 6 to day 7 of the in vitro culture. This means that our subclassification was based on the pharmacological effects on a cell subset within the hierarchically organized AML cell population that were able to both survive and still be able to proliferate.

We also investigated the effects of pathway inhibitors on the in vitro proliferation of primary human AML cells for a second and larger cohort including 76 additional consecutive patients; in these experiments, we only examined the effects of rapamycin and GDC-0941. The overall results are presented in Figure 1. The studies of this second cohort confirmed that the antiproliferative effects of PI3K-Akt-mTOR pathway inhibition varied among individual patients, and a variation of the effect between the two drugs was observed. We also investigated the susceptibility to stress-induced or spontaneous in vitro apoptosis for these 76 patients, but we could not observe any correlation between this susceptibility to apoptosis and the antiproliferative effects of the two pathway inhibitors. Taken together, our results from the two patient cohorts showed that neither the general regulation of apoptosis, as reflected in the degree of spontaneous in vitro apoptosis, nor the viability of the AML cell population after in vitro exposure to pathway inhibitors showed any significant association with the variation in antiproliferative effects of pathway inhibitors that was detected in our proliferation assay.

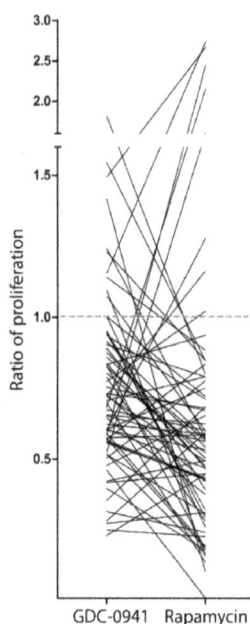

Figure 1. The effect of phosphatidylinositol-3-kinase-mechanistic target of rapamycin (PI3K-mTOR) inhibitors on cytokine-dependent in vitro acute myeloid leukemia (AML) cell proliferation. Leukemic cell proliferation was assayed as ^{3}H-thymidine incorporation after six days of culture. We compared the proliferation of primary human AML cells cultured in the presence of the PI3K-inhibitor GDC-0941 and the mTOR-inhibitor rapamycin. The results are presented as the ratio of proliferation, i.e., nuclear incorporation of ^{3}H-thymidine in drug-exposed cells relative to the incorporation in corresponding drug-free control cultures. The patient cohort included 76 patients, but detectable proliferation was only seen for the 68 AML patients whose results are presented in the figure. Each line represents the results for one patient. The dashed line indicates a ratio of 1.0, i.e., no change in proliferation.

The data presented in Figure 1 clearly illustrate that pathway inhibitors can increase AML cell proliferation for a subset of patients, whereas for other patients, a strong inhibition corresponding to more than 50% inhibition could be detected for different mediators. For further analysis of the possible association between metabolic characteristics and the antiproliferative effects of pathway inhibitors on primary human AML cells, we compared two contrasting groups of selected patients based on the studies of the two patient cohorts. We then selected 15 patient samples with significantly decreased proliferation after inhibition with both rapamycin and GDC-0941; these samples are referred to as responders to the treatment. The other group included 15 patient samples showing no significant alteration of proliferation (corresponding to <10% inhibition) or even growth enhancement in the presence of pathway inhibitors. These are referred to as non-responders to treatment.

2.2. Patient Samples with Different Drug Sensitivity towards PI3K-mTOR Inhibitors Also Differ in Energy, Amino Acid and Arachidonic Acid Metabolism

Previous studies suggest that metabolic regulation of chronic myeloid leukemia cells is important for their susceptibility towards targeted therapy with kinase inhibitors [20]. We compared the metabolic profiles of the two contrasting patient groups that were sensitive and insensitive to PI3K-Akt-mTOR inhibition in vitro. As described above, these groups were selected based on their susceptibility to the antiproliferative effect of PI3K and mTOR inhibitors [17]. The metabolic analysis of the AML cells detected a total of 627 metabolites, and 128 of these metabolites were annotated. A principal component analysis was performed to illustrate the variance between the different sample groups. The responders and non-responders showed a great overlap in the plot, though four of the non-responders clustered separately from the rest (Figure 2). Thus, responders and non-responders could not be separated by an analysis of the overall metabolic profile, and non-responder patients seem to be heterogeneous with regard to their global metabolite profiles even though they show a similar resistance to PI3K-Akt-mTOR pathway inhibition.

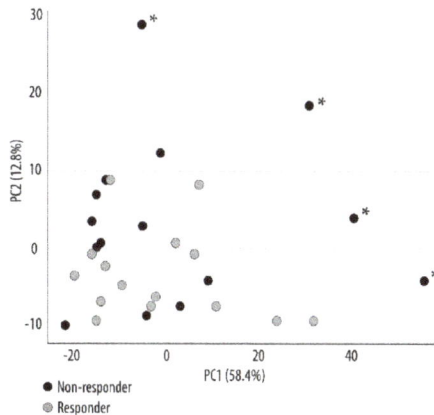

Figure 2. Principal component analysis (PCA) comparing the metabolic profiles of responders and non-responders to PI3K-mTOR inhibitors. The analysis was performed to generate an overview of the metabolic variance among the entire set of samples. Prior to this analysis, primary AML cells from 30 patients were separated into two contrasting groups based on their susceptibility to the in vitro antiproliferative effect of pathway inhibitors. The metabolic profiles for the primary AML cells derived from patients being susceptible (15 responders; grey circle) or resistant (15 non-responders; black circle) to PI3K-mTOR inhibitors were compared. The PCA depicts 71.2% (58.4 + 12.8% as indicated at the *X* and *Y* axis) of all variances in the data set. A separation of four non-responders (indicated by the asterisks *) from the rest of the sample was seen. Each circle represents the results for one patient.

Of the 627 detected metabolites, 23 metabolites differed significantly between the two contrasting groups of responders and non-responders, and among these, 15 were annotated (Table 1). These significantly altered metabolites are involved in energy (citric acid, isocitric acid, glutamine), amino acid (proline, glutamine, taurine), and lipid metabolism (two phosphatidylinositols (PI), the arachidonic acid metabolites 4,7,10,13-eicosatetraenoic acid, and 4,7,10,13,16-docosapentaenoic acid).

We did a metabolic pathway mapping based on the identified metabolites for further characterization of differences between responders and non-responders based on the 80 top-ranked metabolites. Purine metabolism (including the annotated metabolites glutamine, glutamic acid, glycine, and hypoxanthine) and Warburg effect (i.e., energy metabolism; including the annotated metabolites NAD, glutamic acid, glutamine citric acid, and isocitric acid) were then the two highest-ranked terms. This metabolic pathway mapping analysis further supports our conclusion that responders and non-responders to PI3K-mTOR inhibitors show metabolic differences.

2.3. Responders and Non-Responders to PI3K-Akt-mTOR Inhibition Could Be Identified Based on Metabolic Differences

No single metabolite could be used to identify responders and non-responders. However, a decision tree analysis was performed showing that samples can be differentiated based on the levels of cysteinyl-cysteine and threonic acid (Table 1). The patient subset sensitive to PI3K/mTOR inhibitors in vitro was then characterized by low levels of both these metabolites (Figure 3). Cysteinyl-cysteine is a dipeptide composed of two cysteine residues and an incomplete breakdown product of protein catabolism, whereas threonic acid is probably derived from glycated proteins or degradation of ascorbic acid (Human Metabolome Database). This additional and alternative analysis of our metabolomic data further illustrates that our contrasting groups of responder and non-responder AML cells show metabolic differences.

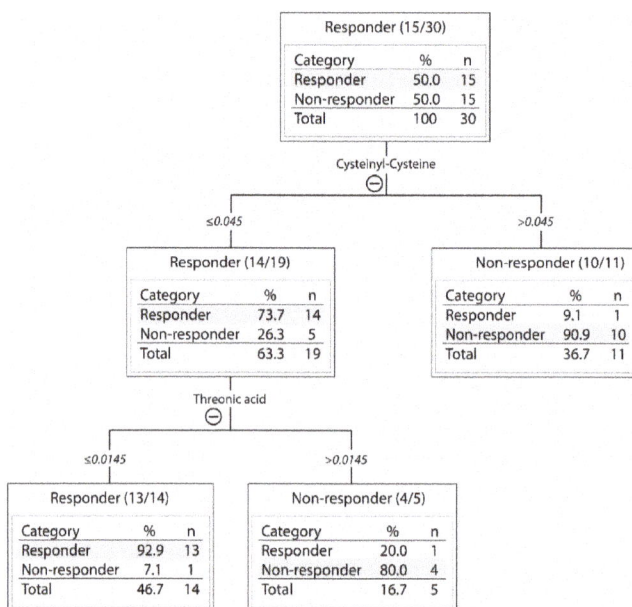

Figure 3. A decision tree analysis of the metabolic differences between 15 responders and 15 non-responders to PI3K-Akt-mTOR inhibition. The levels of two metabolites, cysteinyl-cysteine and threonic acid, allowed for discrimination between responders and non-responders. The 30 patients (see the upper box) were first classified into two subsets based on their cysteinyl-cysteine levels ($\leq$ or >0.045). In the box with high cysteinyl-cysteine (>0.045; right box), there were 10 non-responders and 1 responder. The 19 patients (14 responders and 5 non-responders) with low levels of cysteinyl-cysteine ($\leq$0.045; left box) were further subclassified into two subsets based on the level of threonic acid ($\leq$ or >0.0145). Thirteen of the 14 responders with low levels of cysteinyl-cysteine also showed low levels of threonic acid ($\leq$0.0145; left box). Whereas four of five non-responders among the 19 patients with low levels of cysteinyl-cysteine showed high levels of threonic acid (>0.0145; right box). Approximately ninety percent of patients were then correctly classified as responders or non-responders.

Table 1. A description of annotated metabolites that differed significantly between the two patient groups and were sensitive (responders) or insensitive (non-responders) to the *in vitro* antiproliferative effect of phosphatidylinositol-3-kinase-Akt-mechanistic/mammalian target of rapamycin (PI3K-Akt-mTOR) inhibition.

Metabolite	p-Value	Ratio * Responder versus Non-Responder	Short Description
↓Allose	0.037	−0.875	Sugar metabolism. Possibly involved in cell cycle regulation.
↓Citric acid	0.005	−1.262	Energy metabolism, citric acid cycle.
↓Cysteinyl-cysteine	0.006	−1.471	Dipeptide
↓Glutamine	0.029	−0.737	Non-essential amino acid, important for nucleic acid synthesis. Energy metabolism, conditionally essential during catabolic states.
↓Indoleacrylic acid	0.047	−0.426	Involved in tryptophan metabolism.
↓Isocitric acid	0.029	−0.698	Substrate of the citric acid cycle.
↑Phosphatidyl inositol (18:0/0:0)	0.040	0.765	Lipid metabolism, cell membrane constituents.
↑Phosphatidyl inositol (15:1(9Z)/22:6(4Z,7Z,10Z,13Z16Z19Z))	0.025	0.809	Lipid metabolism, cell membrane constituents.
↓Phosphonic acid (8:0/8:0)	0.009	−1.660	Lipid metabolism
↓Proline	0.046	−0.611	Non-essential amino acid, synthesized from glutamic acid and also other amino acids, energy metabolism.
↓Taurine	0.035	−1.0524	Sulfur amino acid not incorporated into protein; adults can synthesize taurine from cysteine. Stabilizes cell membranes, regulates ion transport.
↓2-amino-4-hydroxy-propiophenone	0.021	−0.744	Lipid metabolism
↓4-phenyl-1,2,3-thiadiazole	0.041	−1.024	Inhibitor of cytochrome P450 enzymes that regulate arachidonic acid metabolism.
↓4,7,10,13-eicosatetraenoic acid	0.021	−0.983	Arachidonic acid metabolite, possibly influencing the leukotriene B4 (LTB4) pathway; expression of the LTB4 receptor (BLT1) may be altered in myeloid leukemia cells.
↓4,7,10,13,16-docosapentaenoic acid	0.042	−0.766	Fatty acid and arachidonic acid metabolism, an intermediate between eicosapentaenoic acid and docosahexaenoic acid, precursor of prostanoids that are only formed from docosapentaenoic acid.

* Responders versus non-responders were compared as the $\log_2$-ratio. The arrows to the left in the table indicate whether the mean metabolite levels were decreased (↓) or increased (↑) in responder cells relative to the non-responder cells. The information in this table is based on PubChem and Human Metabolome databases.

2.4. Modulation of Arachidonic Acid Metabolism Alters PI3K-Akt-mTOR Signaling

In a previous study, we used Western blot to analyze phosphorylation mediators downstream of mTOR in a small group of patients treated with PI3K-mTOR inhibitors [17]. Even though these results have to be interpreted with great care as few patients were studied, the observations suggested that (i) patients differed considerably with respect to the degree of constitutive signaling through the PI3K-Akt-mTOR pathway; and (ii) the heterogeneous antiproliferative effects of PI3K-mTOR inhibitors seen among patients could not be explained by differences in constitutive pathway activation.

Arachidonic acid metabolism seems to be important for survival and proliferation of various cells, including myeloid cells [21,22]. Arachidonic acid can be metabolized by cyclooxygenase, lipoxygenase, or the cytochrome P450 pathways into a number of metabolites, referred to as eicosanoids. These arachidonic acid derived eicosanoids belong to a complex family of lipid signaling mediators that control many important cellular processes, including cell proliferation, apoptosis, and cell metabolism [21,23]. Therefore, we wanted to investigate whether modulation of the balance between the various pathways of arachidonic acid metabolism would influence PI3K-Akt-mTOR signaling in primary human AML cells.

In these experiments, we modulated the balance of arachidonic acid metabolism by incubating the cells with indomethacin (a nonselective cyclooxygenase 1/2 inhibitor), and we investigated the effects of this inhibitor on PI3K-Akt-mTOR signaling in primary AML cells derived from five patients showing constitutive signaling throughout this pathway. These five patients showed a wide variation in constitutive pathway activation; this activation was also observed in previous Western blot analyses of the downstream mTOR mediators P70SK6 and p4E-BP1 (see above) [17]. Thus, a variation in the degree of constitutive pathway activation can be detected by both Western blot and phospho-flow, and, therefore, we selected five patient samples with a constitutive, though wide variation of signaling. The variation between these five patients was, in addition, reproduced/documented in independent analysis of cells derived from separate freezing ampullas.

Using a flow cytometry technique, we explored the effects of indomethacin of the PI3K-Akt-mTOR pathway (10 μg/mL, 15-min incubation) for cells incubated in medium alone (i.e., constitutive signaling) and medium supplemented with insulin 10 μg/mL (Figures 4 and 5). Insulin was studied because PI3K-Akt-mTOR is an important pathway downstream of the insulin receptor [24,25], and in vitro studies have shown that insulin is an important growth factor for primary AML cells for a major subset of patients [26]. When performing an unsupervised hierarchical clustering of the overall results, we observed that the four combinations tested (medium alone ± indomethacin, insulin ± indomethacin) for each individual patient sample generally clustered together; showing that differences in pathway signaling between patients were maintained even in the presence of cyclooxygenase inhibition. An indomethacin-induced decrease of mTOR pS2448, S6 pS235 pS236, and S6 pS244 was seen for all patients in insulin-free and/or insulin-supplemented cultures, and for four of the five patients a decrease was seen for Akt pS473 and S6 pS240 (Figure 4).

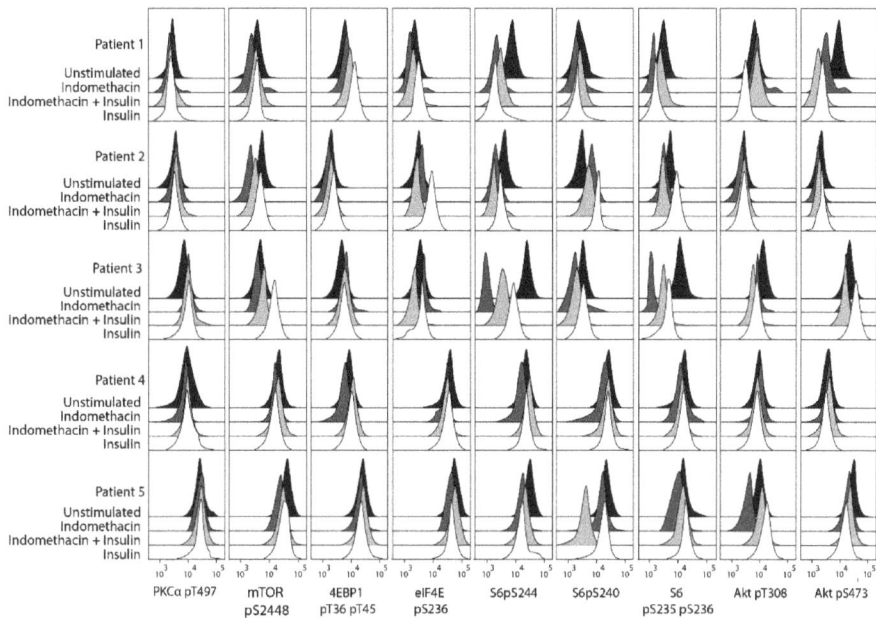

Figure 4. In vitro phospho-signaling analysis of primary AML cells derived from five patients to explore the effects of indomethacin on the PI3K-Akt-mTOR pathway. AML cells were incubated in medium alone, in medium supplemented with 10 μg/mL of either indomethacin or insulin, and in medium supplemented with the combination of insulin and indomethacin. Phosphorylation status of nine mediators were examined. An indomethacin-induced decrease of mTOR pS2448, S6 pS235 pS236, and S6 pS244 was seen for all patients in insulin-free and/or insulin-supplemented cultures, and a decrease of S6 pS240 and Akt pS473 was seen for four of the five patients. The *X*-axis is a log-scale for fluorescence intensity; the *Y*-axis indicates the number of cells.

Based on our current observations, we conclude that modulation of arachidonic acid metabolism by exposure to indomethacin has only minor effects on the phosphorylation of certain mediators in the PI3K-Akt-mTOR pathway; a similar conclusion can be made also for insulin. Only minor effects were observed on the overall pathway activation profile compared with the observed wide variation in constitutive pathway activation between different patients. Accordingly, our results in Figure 5 illustrate that the wide variation between patients in constitutive pathway activation seems to be maintained also after exposure of the leukemic cells to insulin, as well as after drug-induced modulation of arachidonic acid metabolism, i.e., samples from an individual patient cluster together whereas samples from insulin/indomethacin exposed cells do not cluster together.

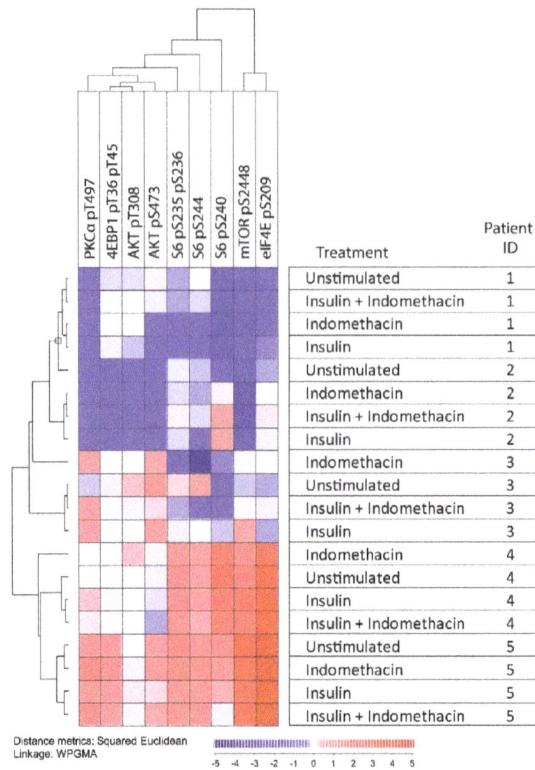

Figure 5. The effect of indomethacin on the activation of PI3K-Akt-mTOR signaling. We investigated the effects of indomethacin on PI3K-Akt-mTOR signaling in primary AML cells derived from five patients. For each sample, we tested AML cells incubated in medium alone, with only indomethacin 10 μg/mL, in medium supplemented with 10 μg/mL insulin, and with the combination of insulin and indomethacin. Phosphorylation status of nine mediators were examined. Red indicates high and blue indicates low phosphorylation/expression of the mediators. All combinations tested for each patient sample also clustered together in the same subclusters for all patients. All values from the flow cytometric analyses were calculated using fold change on the Inverse hyperbolic sine (Arcsinh) scale.

3. Discussion

The PI3K-Akt-mTOR signaling network shows constitutive activation in human AML [12]. However, previous experimental studies [17] suggest that the antileukemic effects of pathway inhibitors differ between patients, and the aim of the present study was to further characterize this patient heterogeneity with regard to constitutive PI3K-Akt-mTOR activation/signaling, pathway inhibition, and metabolic regulation.

For younger patients receiving the most intensive chemotherapy, the overall long-term AML-free survival is only 40–50%. However, the large group of patients above 70–75 years of age are not able to receive this intensive therapy, and are therefore, treated with AML-stabilizing treatment [27]. Many of these elderly patients, as well as younger unfit patients, have an expected survival of only 1–3 months. Thus, new therapeutic strategies are needed both for younger as well as for elderly and unfit patients who can only receive AML-stabilizing treatment; combination therapy including PI3K-Akt-mTOR inhibitors may then be an alternative therapeutic strategy [3,16,18]. However, due to the short survival of many elderly and unfit patients [28,29], they may get only one chance of antileukemic therapy because of the rapid disease progression if this first treatment fails. For this reason, pretreatment identification of patients with high risk of resistant disease will be important. Our present study suggests that metabolic characterization should be further explored as a possible strategy to identify patients with a high risk of resistance to PI3K-Akt-mTOR inhibition, and such patients should then try an alternative strategy as their initial treatment.

In vitro cultured hierarchically organized AML cell populations show spontaneous apoptosis during the first 4–5 days of culture; for most patients, this is an extensive process [19]. Our previous study showed that PI3K-mTOR inhibitors only have weak influence on this spontaneous or stress-induced in vitro apoptosis, and the variation between patients is limited so that it cannot be used for subset classification [17]. However, a wide variation between patients can be detected when using our ^{3}H-thymidine incorporation assay after six days of in vitro culture, i.e., an analysis of the AML cell minority that has been able to survive the initial six days of in vitro culture and still are able to proliferate. Inhibitors of the PI3K-Akt-mTOR pathway were added at the start of the cultures. Our patient classification reflects a combined effect of pathway inhibitors on both survival and proliferation, i.e., the presence of the drug during the initial six days characterized by spontaneous in vitro apoptosis and the ability of the remaining viable cells to still show cytokine-dependent proliferation in the presence of the pathway inhibitors when ^{3}H-thymidine incorporation is assayed from day six to seven of in vitro culture.

We investigated the effect of insulin on phosphorylation of the PI3K-Akt-mTOR-pathway as this pathway is important for insulin signaling [24,25], and insulin is also an important growth factor for in vitro cultured primary human AML cells for a large subset of patients [26]. Our present studies showed that insulin altered the activation/phosphorylation of several mediators; however, the effects were minor and differed between patients. Also, the wide variation in PI3K-Akt-mTOR pathway activation between patients was maintained in the presence of insulin (i.e., the samples exposed to insulin did not cluster together with each other but rather together with the corresponding insulin-free control (Figures 4 and 5)).

Even though constitutive activation of PI3K-Akt-mTOR signaling in the enriched leukemic cells is seen for most AML patients, resistance to the antiproliferative effect of pathway inhibitors is relatively common. In our present study, we show that resistant patient-derived leukemia cells differ with regard to their metabolomic profile, including the metabolites involved in amino acid and arachidonic acid metabolism. Similar abnormalities are also associated with chemoresistance in other myeloid malignancies [30].

Arachidonic acid metabolism is important for survival and proliferation of hematopoietic cells [21,23,31–33] and several of its metabolites can influence activation/signaling through the PI3K-Akt-mTOR pathway, e.g., pathway-activating prostaglandins and eicosatetraenoic acid derivatives [31–35]. Our comparison of the metabolite profiles of cell samples representing either responders or non-responders to PI3K-Akt-mTOR inhibition supports the hypothesis that arachidonic acid metabolism is important with regard to susceptibility to these inhibitors. This hypothesis was also supported by our observed effects of modulated arachidonic acid metabolism by indomethacin on mediator phosphorylation, and previous studies in both human chronic myeloid leukemia and in animal models of leukemic stem cells indicating that arachidonic acid metabolism is important for both leukemogenesis and chemosensitivity [20,36].

For other cell types, there are functional links between redox balance, purine metabolism, NADH, proline, and glutamine metabolism, and the citric acid cycle [37–41]. Even though few studies of myeloid cells are available, observations in other cell types suggest links between such metabolic steps and PI3K-Akt-mTOR signaling. Firstly, arachidonic acid metabolites can function as regulators of the PI3K-Akt-mTOR pathway [21,23,42,43], and our present results suggest that this may also be true in human AML. Secondly, there are links between PI3K-Akt-mTOR signaling via free oxygen radicals/redox homeostasis to the NAD/NADH/proline/glutamine/glutamate system [44,45]. Thirdly, proline and glutamine are interconvertible, and glutamine is an important substrate for the energy metabolism in many malignant cells; a link between arachidonic acid and energy metabolism/the citric acid cycle is therefore possible [37,39]. Finally, both arachidonic acid metabolism and PI3K-Akt-mTOR signaling are important for regulation of the peroxisome proliferator activated receptors, a group of transcription factors [21,40]. However, additional studies are needed to clarify the possible contributions of these various steps in human AML.

Previous experimental studies suggest that altered proline metabolism can be important for the development of cancer chemoresistance, and proline oxidase has been suggested as a possible target in cancer treatment [37,39,41,46]. Our present study suggests that proline/glutamine metabolism may also contribute to resistance of PI3K-mTOR inhibitors in human AML. Our observation of increased levels of eicosatetraenoic acid and docosapentaenoic acid indicates that arachidonic acid may be one of these interacting factors. However, an alternative explanation could be that effects on proline/glutamine only reflect differences in energy metabolisms, and differences in arachidonic acid metabolites may reflect the altered energy/lipid metabolism. This is further supported by previous studies showing that arachidonic acid metabolism is important in murine leukemogenesis and for chemoresistance in human chronic myeloid leukemia [20,36]. The PI3K-Akt-mTOR pathway may represent a link between these two systems through the effect of arachidonic acid metabolites on this pathway and the regulatory effect of mTOR on proline oxidase.

The role of arachidonic acid and its metabolites in normal and malignant hematopoiesis has been reviewed previously [21]. Increased expression of lipoxygenase enzymes has been detected in malignant myeloid cells, and products from this pathway of arachidonic acid metabolism often seem to mediate growth-enhancing and antiapoptotic effects. Our present observations of increased levels of eicosanoids in cells that are resistant to PI3K-Akt-mTOR inhibitors suggest that these metabolites may have such a role in human AML. Furthermore, the effect of arachidonic acid itself seems to differ between cell lines, but proapoptotic effects have been described. Finally, a previous study of primary human AML cells showed that even low levels of indomethacin could reduce the AML cell levels of prostaglandin E_2, and in their model PGE_2, could enhance both the spontaneous proliferation as well as Toll like receptor mediated growth enhancement of primary human AML cells [47].

4. Materials and Methods

4.1. AML Patients

The study was approved by the Regional Ethics Committee (REK) (REK III 060.02, 10 June 2002; REK Vest 215.03, 12 March 04; REK III 231.06, 15 March 2007; REK Vest 2013/634, 19 March 2013; REK Vest 2015/1410, 19 June 2015), The Norwegian Data Protection Authority 02/1118-5, 22 October 2002, and The Norwegian Ministry of Health 03/05340 HRA/ASD, 16 February 2004. All AML cell samples were collected after written informed consent.

The clinical and biological characteristics of those 30 patients included in the metabolic studies are summarized in Table 2. All patients had a high number and/or percentage of peripheral blood blasts; leukemic peripheral blood mononuclear cells could, therefore, be isolated by density gradient separation alone (Lymphoprep, Axis-Shield, Oslo, Norway) and generally contained at least 95% leukemic blasts. The contaminating cells were small lymphocytes. These enriched AML cells were stored in liquid nitrogen until used in the experiments [48]. All the 15 responder patients selected for metabolic profiling had a strong inhibition (i.e. >50% inhibition) of cytokine-dependent AML cell proliferation by both PI3K and mTOR inhibitors, whereas PI3K and mTOR inhibition either increased the proliferation or had a weak antiproliferative effect corresponding to <10% inhibition for the 15 non-responders.

Table 2. Important clinical and biological characteristics of responders and non-responders to phosphatidylinositol-3-kinase- mechanistic/mammalian target of rapamycin (PI3K-mTOR) inhibitors.

ID	Gender	Age	Previous Hematological Malignancy or Chemotherapy	FAB	CD34	Karyotype Abnormality	Karyotype Classification	Flt3 Mutation	NPM-1 Mutation
					Responders				
1	F	45	Chemotherapy	M4	Negative	Normal	Normal	wt	ins
2	F	63		M4	Positive	Normal	Normal	ITD	wt
3	M	72		M5	Negative	Normal	Normal	wt	ins
4	M	29	Relapse	M4	Positive	Normal	Normal	ITD	ins
5	F	80		M2	Positive	Complex	Adverse	wt	wt
6	F	36		M4	Positive	Normal	Normal	wt	nt
7	F	75		M1	Positive	nt		ITD	wt
8	M	71	Relapse	M2	Negative	Normal	Normal	G835	
9	M	35		M2	Positive	Normal	Normal	wt	wt
10	M	72	Myelodysplastic syndrome	M1	Positive	Complex	Adverse	wt	
11	F	64	Chemotherapy	M2	Negative	Normal	Normal	ITD	ins
12	F	59	Chemotherapy	M5	Negative	Normal	Normal	ITD	ins
13	M	58		M5	Positive	Normal	Normal	wt	wt
14	F	59	Chemotherapy	M4	Negative	Normal	Normal	ITD	ins
15	F	75		M4	Positive	Normal	Normal	ITD	wt
					Non-responders				
16	F	29	Chemotherapy	M5	Positive	Normal	Normal	ITD+Asp835	wt
17	M	24		M2	Positive	Multiple	Adverse	nt	wt
18	F	82		M4	Positive	Normal	Normal	ITD	wt
19	F	77		M1	Negative	nt		nt	ins
20	M	84		M1	Positive	Multiple	Adverse	wt	wt
21	M	53		M0	Positive	13	Intermediate	wt	wt
22	M	65		M5	Negative	Normal	Normal	ITD	ins
23	F	46		M1	Positive	inv(16)	Favorable	wt	wt
24	F	70		M4	Negative	nt		wt	ins
25	M	33	Chemotherapy	M1	Positive	Normal	Normal	wt	wt
26	F	77		M1	Positive	nt		nt	wt
27	M	76		M0	Positive	Normal	Normal	wt	wt
28	M	60		M4	Positive	Normal	Normal	ITD	wt
29	M	36		M5	Positive	+8, +22, inv(16)	Favorable	ITD	wt
30	F	67		M5	Negative	t(9,11), +19	Intermediate	wt	wt

The table shows the gender (M, male; F, female) and age (years) of the individual patients at diagnosis. The FAB classification was used to classify morphological and/or histochemical signs of differentiation. Cytogenetic abnormalities were classified according to the medical research council (MRC) criteria. The detection of Fms like tyrosine kinase 3 (Flt3) (ITD, internal tandem duplications) or nucleophosmin (NPM)-1 insertions (ins) is also indicated in the table. Complex karyotype means at least three abnormalities [1]. FAB: The French-American-British (FAB) classification system; nt: not tested; wt: wild type.

4.2. Drugs

Drugs used in this study included the mTOR inhibitor rapamycin (LC Laboratories, Woburn, MA, USA), the PI3K class I specific inhibitor GDC-0941 (Axon Medchem BV, Groningen, The Netherlands), human insulin (Sigma-Aldrich, St. Louis, MO, USA), and the nonselective cyclooxygenase 1/2 inhibitor indomethacin (Sigma-Aldrich; dissolved in dimethyl sulfoxide (DMSO)). Stock solutions were sterile filtered and stored at −20 °C until used in experiments, thawed only once, and diluted with their respective solvents to obtain the desired final concentrations.

Indomethacin (Sigma-Aldrich) was tested at a final concentration of 10 µg/mL (corresponding to 28 µM). Previous studies in human as well as murine AML cells often used indomethacin concentrations in the range of 10–50 µM (3.6–18 µg/mL) [49–51], and the conventional cyclooxygenase-blocking concentration of indomethacin is considered to be 10–20 µM (for original reference see [50]). However, even indomethacin concentrations as low as 1 µM (0.4 µg/mL) will decrease the in vitro prostaglandin production by primary human acute leukemia cells [47]. Our use of indomethacin 10 µg/mL was based on these previous studies. Finally, in pilot experiments we investigated pharmacological effects after incubation for 7, 10, 15, 30, and 45 min before analyzing the PI3K-Akt-mTOR pathway activation. We decided to incubate cells with the drugs for 15 min because additional effects could not be detected when using longer incubations.

4.3. Analysis of PI3K-Akt-mTOR Activation

Flow cytometry was used to examine the basal expression of 18 mediators in the PI3K-Akt-mTOR pathway/network in the AML cells. Cryopreserved and thawed primary leukemic cells were incubated for 20 min in RPMI-1640 (Sigma-Aldrich) before being directly fixed in 1.5% paraformaldehyde (PFA) and permeabilized with 100% methanol. The cells were subsequently rehydrated by adding 2 mL phosphate-buffered saline (PBS), gently re-suspended, and then centrifuged. The cell pellet was washed twice with 2 mL PBS and resuspended in 150 µL PBS supplemented with 0.1% bovine serum albumin (BSA) (Sigma-Aldrich). Washed cells were blocked with immunoglobulin (Octagam; Octapharma, Jessheim, Norway) and 1% BSA, and then split evenly into nineteen new tubes (1 × 10^5 cells per sample) before staining. All staining panels included the same live/dead discriminator, either FITC or Alexa Fluor® 647 Mouse anti-Cleaved PARP (Asp214); an unstained sample was also included. Three directly conjugated dyes were used: (i) Alexa Fluor® 647 was used for PTEN, PDPK1 pS241, PKCα, PKCα pT497, Akt pS473, 4EBP1 pT36 pT45, eIF4E pS209, S6 pS244, and mTOR; (ii) phycoerythrin (PE) for Akt total, Akt pT308, mTOR pS2448, and S6 pS240; and (iii) V450 for S6 pS235 pS236. Antibodies were purchased from BD Pharmingen (Franklin Lakes, NJ, USA), except for anti-mTOR that was purchased from Cell Signal Technology (Danvers, MA, USA). Four of the antibodies were unconjugated (anti Raptor, Tuberin, FKBP38, and RHEB; all from Abcam; Cambridge, UK) and required secondary antibody-conjugated Alexa Fluor® 647 (BD Pharmingen). Together these mediators represent the main steps in the PI3K-Akt-mTOR pathway and they were selected to provide an extended phosphorylation profile of this pathway. Finally, in our pharmacological studies, AML cells were incubated with human insulin 10 µg/mL (Sigma-Aldrich) and/or indomethacin 10 µg/mL (Sigma-Aldrich; dissolved in DMSO); final concentration in the medium 0.5%) or a DMSO control solution for 15 min before flow cytometric analysis as described above. Flow cytometry analysis was acquired on a BD FACS Verse 8-color flow cytometer (BD Biosciences, San Jose, CA, USA) and data analysis performed using FlowJo 10.0.7 software (Tree Star, Inc., Ashland, OR, USA).

4.4. Analysis of Cytokine-Dependent Proliferation in Presence of PI3K-mTOR Inhibitors

As described in detail previously [52,53]; AML cells (5 × 10^4 cells/well) were cultured in flat-bottomed microtiter plates (150 µL/well) in Stem Span SFEM™ serum-free medium (Stem Cell Technologies; Vancouver, BC, Canada) alone or in medium supplemented with granulocyte-macrophage colony-stimulation factor (GM-CSF), stem cell factor (SCF) and Fms like tyrosine kinase 3 ligand

Int. J. Mol. Sci. **2018**, *19*, 382

(Flt3L) [54]. All cytokines were purchased from Peprotech (Rocky Hill, NJ, USA) and used at 20 ng/mL. All drugs were added on the first day of culture, whereas 37 kBq/well of ^{3}H-thymidine (Perkin Elmer; Waltham, MA, USA) was added after 6 days, and nuclear incorporation was assayed after seven days of culture. The mTOR inhibitor rapamycin and the PI3K inhibitor GDC-0941 were added at a final concentration of 100 nM on the first day of culture [55].

4.5. Metabolomic Analysis

The metabolomic analyses and sample preparations were performed by Metabolomic Discoveries GmbH (Potsdam, Germany) [56]. Briefly, non-targeted metabolite profiling of cells included analyses by gas chromatography/mass spectrometry (GC-MS) and Liquid Chromatography Quadrupole-Time of Flight (LC-QTOF)/MS; metabolites could then be analyzed in the range of 50–1700 Da with an accuracy up to 1–2 ppm and a resolution of mass/Δmass = 40,000. Metabolites measured in the LC were annotated according to their accurate mass and subsequent sum formula prediction. Metabolite profiles were explored by the platforms of Metabolomic Discoveries and Small Molecule Pathway Database (BioVariance, Munich, Germany). The lists of the 627 detected and the 128 annotated metabolites are presented in the Supplementary Materials presenting the identity/accurate mass@retention time, the *p*-value, and responder/non-responder ratio.

4.6. Bioinformatical and Statistical Analyses

Bioinformatic analyses were performed using the J-Express 2012 software (MolMine AS, Bergen, Norway). For hierarchical clustering analysis, all values from cytometric analyses were calculated using fold change on the Inverse hyperbolic sine (Arcsinh) scale. The median signal for each phospho-protein was used as reference value for the calculation of basal phosphorylation. Complete linkage and Squared Euclidean correlation were used as linkage method and distance measurement, respectively. Statistical analyses were performed using the IBM Statistical Package for the Social Sciences (SPSS) version 23 (Chicago, IL, USA), and *p*-values < 0.05 were regarded as statistically significant.

5. Conclusions

Despite the metabolic heterogeneity of the non-responders to PI3K-Akt-mTOR inhibitors, there are distinct metabolic differences between responders and non-responders. Our present results are consistent with the hypothesis that differences in arachidonic acid metabolism together with differences in proline and/or energy metabolism are associated with differences in susceptibility to pathway inhibitors. The possible importance of such differences should be considered when planning or analyzing future clinical studies with PI3K-Akt-mTOR inhibitors and when designing combination therapy for various AML patient subsets [57].

Supplementary Materials: Supplementary materials can be found at http://www.mdpi.com/1422-0067/19/2/382/s1.

Acknowledgments: The technical assistance of Marie Hagen and Kristin Paulsen Rye is gratefully acknowledged.

Author Contributions: Øystein Bruserud is responsible for the AML biobanks. Ina Nepstad established the flow-cytometric methodology. All flow-cytometric analyses of PI3K-Akt-mTOR activation in primary human AML cells were performed by Ina Nepstad. Annette K. Brenner did the proliferation studies presented in Figure 1. Håkon Reikvam and Annette K. Brenner performed statistical analyses regarding AML cell proliferation. Kimberley J. Hatfield contributed to preparing samples for metabolic studies. Bioinformatic and statistical analyses were performed by Ina Nepstad, Håkon Reikvam, and Øystein Bruserud. Ina Nepstad, Øystein Bruserud, and Kimberley J. Hatfield contributed to writing the manuscript. All authors read and approved the final manuscript.

Conflicts of Interest: The authors declare no conflict of interest.

Abbreviations

4EBP1	Translation initiation factor 4E-binding protein 1
AML	Acute myeloid leukemia
DMSO	Dimethyl sulfoxide
DNA-PK	DNA-dependent protein kinase
FAB	The French-American-British () classification system
Flt3	Fms like tyrosine kinase 3
Flt3L	Flt3 ligand
GC-MS	Gas chromatography-mass spectrometry
GM-CSF	Granulocyte-macrophage colony-stimulation factor
ins	Insertions
ITD	Internal tandem duplications
LC-QTOF/MS	Liquid Chromatography Quadrupole-Time of Flight MS
mRNA	Messenger RNA
mTOR	Mechanistic/mammalian target of rapamycin
mTORC	mTOR complex
NPM	Nucleophosmin
PBS	Phosphate-buffered saline
PCA	Principal component analysis
PDK1	3′phosphoinositide-dependent kinase 1
PFA	Paraformaldehyde
PI3K	Phosphatidylinositol-3-kinase
PIP2	Phosphatidylinositol (4,5)-bisphosphate
PIP3	Phosphatidylinositol (3,4,5)-trisphosphate
PRAS40	Proline-rich Akt-substrate-40
RHEB	Ras homolog enriched in brain
S6PK	S6 ribosomal protein kinase
SCF	Stem cell factor
SPSS	Statistical Package for the Social Sciences
TSC	Tuberous sclerosis complex
elF4E pS209	eukaryotic translation Initiation Factor 4E
PKCα	Protein kinase C α
PTEN	Phosphatase and tensin homolog

References

1. Döhner, H.; Weisdorf, D.J.; Bloomfield, C.D. Acute myeloid leukemia. *N. Engl. J. Med.* **2015**, *373*, 1136–1152. [CrossRef] [PubMed]
2. Papaemmanuil, E.; Gerstung, M.; Bullinger, L.; Gaidzik, V.I.; Paschka, P.; Roberts, N.D.; Potter, N.E.; Heuser, M.; Thol, F.; Bolli, N.; et al. Genomic classification and prognosis in acute myeloid leukemia. *N. Engl. J. Med.* **2016**, *374*, 2209–2221. [CrossRef] [PubMed]
3. Brenner, A.K.; Andersson Tvedt, T.H.; Bruserud, O. The complexity of targeting PI3K-Akt-mTOR signalling in human acute myeloid leukaemia: The importance of leukemic cell heterogeneity, neighbouring mesenchymal stem cells and immunocompetent cells. *Molecules* **2016**, *21*, 1512. [CrossRef] [PubMed]
4. Martelli, A.M.; Evangelisti, C.; Chiarini, F.; McCubrey, J.A. The phosphatidylinositol 3-kinase/Akt/mTOR signaling network as a therapeutic target in acute myelogenous leukemia patients. *Oncotarget* **2010**, *1*, 89–103. [PubMed]
5. Polak, R.; Buitenhuis, M. The PI3K/PKB signaling module as key regulator of hematopoiesis: Implications for therapeutic strategies in leukemia. *Blood* **2012**, *119*, 911–923. [CrossRef] [PubMed]
6. Guertin, D.A.; Sabatini, D.M. Defining the role of mTOR in cancer. *Cancer Cell* **2007**, *12*, 9–22. [CrossRef] [PubMed]
7. Vivanco, I.; Sawyers, C.L. The phosphatidylinositol 3-Kinase AKT pathway in human cancer. *Nat. Rev. Cancer* **2002**, *2*, 489–501. [CrossRef] [PubMed]

8. Kornblau, S.M.; Tibes, R.; Qiu, Y.H.; Chen, W.; Kantarjian, H.M.; Andreeff, M.; Coombes, K.R.; Mills, G.B. Functional proteomic profiling of AML predicts response and survival. *Blood* **2009**, *113*, 154–164. [CrossRef] [PubMed]

9. Bellacosa, A.; Testa, J.R.; Moore, R.; Larue, L. A portrait of AKT kinases: Human cancer and animal models depict a family with strong individualities. *Cancer Biol. Ther.* **2004**, *3*, 268–275. [CrossRef] [PubMed]

10. Sarbassov, D.D.; Guertin, D.A.; Ali, S.M.; Sabatini, D.M. Phosphorylation and regulation of Akt/PKB by the rictor-mTOR complex. *Science* **2005**, *307*, 1098–1101. [CrossRef] [PubMed]

11. Feng, J.H.; Park, J.; Cron, P.; Hess, D.; Hemmings, B.A. Identification of a PKB/Akt hydrophobic motif Ser-473 kinase as DNA-dependent protein kinase. *J. Biol. Chem.* **2004**, *279*, 41189–41196. [CrossRef] [PubMed]

12. Engelman, J.A.; Luo, J.; Cantley, L.C. The evolution of phosphatidylinositol 3-kinases as regulators of growth and metabolism. *Nat. Rev. Genet.* **2006**, *7*, 606–619. [CrossRef] [PubMed]

13. Fransecky, L.; Mochmann, L.H.; Baldus, C.D. Outlook on PI3K/Akt/mTOR inhibition in acute leukemia. *Mol. Cell. Ther.* **2015**, *3*. [CrossRef] [PubMed]

14. Samuels, Y.; Ericson, K. Oncogenic PI3K and its role in cancer. *Curr. Opin. Oncol.* **2006**, *18*, 77–82. [CrossRef] [PubMed]

15. Wee, S.; Jagani, Z.; Xiang, K.X.Q.; Loo, A.; Dorsch, M.; Yao, Y.M.; Sellers, W.R.; Lengauer, C.; Stegmeier, F. PI3K pathway activation mediates resistance to MEK inhibitors in KRAS mutant cancers. *Cancer Res.* **2009**, *69*, 4286–4293. [CrossRef] [PubMed]

16. Herschbein, L.; Liesveld, J.L. Dueling for dual inhibition: Means to enhance effectiveness of PI3K/Akt/mTOR inhibitors in AML. *Blood Rev.* **2017**. [CrossRef] [PubMed]

17. Reikvam, H.; Tamburini, J.; Skrede, S.; Holdhus, R.; Poulain, L.; Ersvaer, E.; Hatfield, K.J.; Bruserud, O. Antileukaemic effect of PI3K-mTOR inhibitors in acute myeloid leukaemia-gene expression profiles reveal CDC25B expression as determinate of pharmacological effect. *Br. J. Haematol.* **2014**, *164*, 200–211. [CrossRef] [PubMed]

18. Su, Y.; Li, X.; Ma, J.; Zhao, J.; Liu, S.; Wang, G.; Edwards, H.; Taub, J.W.; Lin, H.; Ge, Y. Targeting PI3K, mTOR, ERK, and BCL-2 signaling network shows superior antileukemic activity against AML ex vivo. *Biochem. Pharmacol.* **2018**, *148*, 13–26. [CrossRef] [PubMed]

19. Ryningen, A.; Ersvaer, E.; Oyan, A.M.; Kalland, K.H.; Vintermyr, O.K.; Gjertsen, B.T.; Bruserud, Ø. Stress-induced in vitro apoptosis of native human acute myelogenous leukemia (AML) cells shows a wide variation between patients and is associated with low BCL-2:Bax ratio and low levels of heat shock protein 70 and 90. *Leuk. Res.* **2006**, *30*, 1531–1540. [CrossRef] [PubMed]

20. Lucas, C.M.; Harris, R.J.; Giannoudis, A.; McDonald, E.; Clark, R.E. Low leukotriene B4 receptor 1 leads to ALOX5 downregulation at diagnosis of chronic myeloid leukemia. *Haematologica* **2014**, *99*, 1710–1715. [CrossRef] [PubMed]

21. Rizzo, M.T. The role of arachidonic acid in normal and malignant hematopoiesis. *Prostaglandins Leukot. Essent. Fat. Acids* **2002**, *66*, 57–69. [CrossRef] [PubMed]

22. Sinclair, H.M. Essential fatty acids in perspective. *Hum. Nutr. Clin. Nutr.* **1984**, *38*, 245–260. [PubMed]

23. Hoggatt, J.; Pelus, L.M. Eicosanoid regulation of hematopoiesis and hematopoietic stem and progenitor trafficking. *Leukemia* **2010**, *24*, 1993–2002. [CrossRef] [PubMed]

24. Yoon, M.S. The role of mammalian target of rapamycin (mTOR) in insulin signaling. *Nutrients* **2017**, *9*, 1176. [CrossRef] [PubMed]

25. Haeusler, R.A.; McGraw, T.E.; Accili, D. Biochemical and cellular properties of insulin receptor signalling. *Nat. Rev. Mol. Cell Biol.* **2018**, *19*, 31–44. [CrossRef] [PubMed]

26. Salem, M.; Delwel, R.; Touw, I.; Mahmoud, L.; Lowenberg, B. Human AML colony growth in serum-free culture. *Leuk. Res.* **1988**, *12*, 157–165. [CrossRef]

27. Döhner, H.; Estey, E.; Grimwade, D.; Amadori, S.; Appelbaum, F.R.; Buchner, T.; Dombret, H.; Ebert, B.L.; Fenaux, P.; Larson, R.A.; et al. Diagnosis and management of AML in adults: 2017 ELN recommendations from an international expert panel. *Blood* **2017**, *129*, 424–447. [CrossRef] [PubMed]

28. Fredly, H.; Ersvaer, E.; Kittang, A.O.; Tsykunova, G.; Gjertsen, B.T.; Bruserud, O. The combination of valproic acid, all-trans retinoic acid and low-dose cytarabine as disease-stabilizing treatment in acute myeloid leukemia. *Clin. Epigenet.* **2013**, *5*. [CrossRef] [PubMed]

29. Fredly, H.; Gjertsen, B.T.; Bruserud, O. Histone deacetylase inhibition in the treatment of acute myeloid leukemia: The effects of valproic acid on leukemic cells, and the clinical and experimental evidence for combining valproic acid with other antileukemic agents. *Clin. Epigenet.* **2013**, *5*. [CrossRef] [PubMed]

30. Jiye, A.; Qian, S.; Wang, G.; Yan, B.; Zhang, S.; Huang, Q.; Ni, L.; Zha, W.; Liu, L.; Cao, B.; et al. Chronic myeloid leukemia patients sensitive and resistant to imatinib treatment show different metabolic responses. *PLoS ONE* **2010**, *5*, e13186.

31. Zhang, B.; Cao, H.; Rao, G.N. 15(*S*)-hydroxyeicosatetraenoic acid induces angiogenesis via activation of PI3K-Akt-mTOR-S6K1 signaling. *Cancer Res.* **2005**, *65*, 7283–7291. [CrossRef] [PubMed]

32. Durand, E.M.; Zon, L.I. Newly emerging roles for prostaglandin E2 regulation of hematopoiesis and hematopoietic stem cell engraftment. *Curr. Opin. Hematol.* **2010**, *17*, 308–312. [CrossRef] [PubMed]

33. Harris, R.E.; Beebe-Donk, J.; Doss, H.; Burr Doss, D. Aspirin, ibuprofen, and other non-steroidal anti-inflammatory drugs in cancer prevention: A critical review of non-selective COX-2 blockade. *Oncol. Rep.* **2005**, *13*, 559–583. [CrossRef] [PubMed]

34. Bertrand, J.; Liagre, B.; Ghezali, L.; Beneytout, J.L.; Leger, D.Y. Cyclooxygenase-2 positively regulates Akt signalling and enhances survival of erythroleukemia cells exposed to anticancer agents. *Apoptosis* **2013**, *18*, 836–850. [CrossRef] [PubMed]

35. Soumya, S.J.; Binu, S.; Helen, A.; Reddanna, P.; Sudhakaran, P.R. 15(*S*)-hete-induced angiogenesis in adipose tissue is mediated through activation of PI3K/Akt/mTOR signaling pathway. *Biochem. Cell Biol.* **2013**, *91*, 498–505. [CrossRef] [PubMed]

36. Chen, Y.; Hu, Y.; Zhang, H.; Peng, C.; Li, S. Loss of the *Alox5* gene impairs leukemia stem cells and prevents chronic myeloid leukemia. *Nat. Genet.* **2009**, *41*, 783–792. [CrossRef] [PubMed]

37. Phang, J.M.; Liu, W.; Hancock, C.N.; Fischer, J.W. Proline metabolism and cancer: Emerging links to glutamine and collagen. *Curr. Opin. Clin. Nutr. Metab. Care* **2015**, *18*, 71–77. [CrossRef] [PubMed]

38. Liu, W.; Phang, J.M. Proline dehydrogenase (oxidase) in cancer. *Biofactors* **2012**, *38*, 398–406. [CrossRef] [PubMed]

39. Phang, J.M.; Liu, W. Proline metabolism and cancer. *Front. Biosci.* **2012**, *17*, 1835–1845. [CrossRef]

40. Phang, J.M.; Liu, W.; Zabirnyk, O. Proline metabolism and microenvironmental stress. *Annu. Rev. Nutr.* **2010**, *30*, 441–463. [CrossRef] [PubMed]

41. Phang, J.M.; Donald, S.P.; Pandhare, J.; Liu, Y. The metabolism of proline, a stress substrate, modulates carcinogenic pathways. *Amino Acids* **2008**, *35*, 681–690. [CrossRef] [PubMed]

42. Markworth, J.F.; Cameron-Smith, D. Prostaglandin F2α stimulates PI3K/ERK/mTOR signaling and skeletal myotube hypertrophy. *Am. J. Physiol. Cell Physiol.* **2011**, *300*, C671–C682. [CrossRef] [PubMed]

43. Arvisais, E.W.; Romanelli, A.; Hou, X.; Davis, J.S. AKT-independent phosphorylation of TSC2 and activation of mTOR and ribosomal protein S6 kinase signaling by prostaglandin F2α. *J. Biol. Chem.* **2006**, *281*, 26904–26913. [CrossRef] [PubMed]

44. Wang, J.; Yang, X.; Zhang, J. Bridges between mitochondrial oxidative stress, ER stress and mTOR signaling in pancreatic β cells. *Cell Signal* **2016**, *28*, 1099–1104. [CrossRef] [PubMed]

45. Testa, U.; Labbaye, C.; Castelli, G.; Pelosi, E. Oxidative stress and hypoxia in normal and leukemic stem cells. *Exp. Hematol.* **2016**, *44*, 540–560. [CrossRef] [PubMed]

46. Kononczuk, J.C.U.; Moczydlowska, J.; Surażyński, A.; Palka, J.; Miltyk, W. Proline oxidase (POX) as a target for cancer therapy. *Curr. Drug Targets* **2015**, *16*, 1464–1469. [CrossRef] [PubMed]

47. Truffinet, V.; Donnard, M.; Vincent, C.; Faucher, J.L.; Bordessoule, D.; Turlure, P.; Trimoreau, F.; Denizot, Y. Cyclooxygenase-1, but not -2, in blast cells of patients with acute leukemia. *Int. J. Cancer* **2007**, *121*, 924–927. [CrossRef] [PubMed]

48. Bruserud, O.; Gjertsen, B.T.; Von Volkman, H.L. In vitro culture of human acute myelogenous leukemia (AML) cells in serum-free media: Studies of native AML blasts and AML cell lines. *J. Hematother. Stem Cell* **2000**, *9*, 923–932. [CrossRef] [PubMed]

49. Song, J.H.; Kim, S.H.; Kim, H.J.; Hwang, S.Y.; Kim, T.S. Alleviation of the drug-resistant phenotype in idarubicin and cytosine arabinoside double-resistant acute myeloid leukemia cells by indomethacin. *Int. J. Oncol.* **2008**, *32*, 931–936. [CrossRef] [PubMed]

50. Condino-Neto, A.; Whitney, C.; Newburger, P.E. Dexamethasone but not indomethacin inhibits human phagocyte nicotinamide adenine dinucleotide phosphate oxidase activity by down-regulating expression of genes encoding oxidase components. *J. Immunol.* **1998**, *161*, 4960–4967. [PubMed]

51. Draper, M.P.; Martell, R.L.; Levy, S.B. Indomethacin-mediated reversal of multidrug resistance and drug efflux in human and murine cell lines overexpressing MRP, but not P-glycoprotein. *Br. J. Cancer* **1997**, *75*, 810–815. [CrossRef] [PubMed]

52. Brenner, A.K.; Reikvam, H.; Bruserud, O. A subset of patients with acute myeloid leukemia has leukemia cells characterized by chemokine responsiveness and altered expression of transcriptional as well as angiogenic regulators. *Front. Immunol.* **2016**, *7*. [CrossRef] [PubMed]

53. Reikvam, H.; Oyan, A.M.; Kalland, K.H.; Hovland, R.; Hatfield, K.J.; Bruserud, O. Differences in proliferative capacity of primary human acute myelogenous leukaemia cells are associated with altered gene expression profiles and can be used for subclassification of patients. *Cell Prolif.* **2013**, *46*, 554–562. [CrossRef] [PubMed]

54. Brenner, A.K.; Reikvam, H.; Rye, K.P.; Hagen, K.M.; Lavecchia, A.; Bruserud, O. CDC25 inhibition in acute myeloid leukemia-a study of patient heterogeneity and the effects of different inhibitors. *Molecules* **2017**, *22*, 446. [CrossRef] [PubMed]

55. Reikvam, H.; Nepstad, I.; Bruserud, Ø.; Hatfield, K.J. Pharmacological targeting of the PI3K/mTOR pathway alters the release of angioregulatory mediators both from primary human acute myeloid leukemia cells and their neighboring stromal cells. *Oncotarget* **2013**, *4*, 830–843. [CrossRef] [PubMed]

56. Evans, A.M.; Bridgewater, B.R.; Liu, Q.; Mitchell, M.W.; Robinson, R.J.; Dai, H.; Stewart, S.J.; DeHaven, C.D.; Miller, L.A.D. High resolution mass spectrometry improves data quantity and quality as compared to unit mass resolution mass spectrometry in high-throughput profiling metabolomics. *Metabolomics* **2014**, *4*. [CrossRef]

57. Chen, W.L.; Wang, J.H.; Zhao, A.H.; Xu, X.; Wang, Y.H.; Chen, T.L.; Li, J.M.; Mi, J.Q.; Zhu, Y.M.; Liu, Y.F.; et al. A distinct glucose metabolism signature of acute myeloid leukemia with prognostic value. *Blood* **2014**, *124*, 1645–1654. [CrossRef] [PubMed]

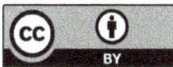

International Journal of
Molecular Sciences

MDPI

Review

Current Coverage of the mTOR Pathway by Next-Generation Sequencing Oncology Panels

Rita Seeboeck [1,2,†], Victoria Sarne [2,†] and Johannes Haybaeck [3,4,5,6,*]

1   Clinical Institute of Pathology, University Hospital St. Poelten, Karl Landsteiner University of Health Sciences, 3100 St. Pölten, Austria; rita.seeboeck@stpoelten.lknoe.at
2   Department Life Sciences, IMC University of Applied Sciences Krems, 3500 Krems, Austria; victoria.sarne@fh-krems.ac.at
3   Department of Pathology, Medical Faculty, Otto-von-Guericke University Magdeburg, 39106 Magdeburg, Germany
4   Department of Pathology, Neuropathology, and Molecular Pathology, Medical University of Innsbruck, 6020 Innsbruck, Austria
5   Department of Neuropathology, Diagnostic & Research Center for Molecular BioMedicine, Institute of Pathology, Medical University of Graz, 8036 Graz, Austria
6   German Center for Neurodegenerative Diseases (DZNE), 39120 Magdeburg, Germany
*   Correspondence: johannes.haybaeck@med.ovgu.de; Tel.: +49-391-67-15817
†   These authors contributed equally to this work.

Received: 16 January 2019; Accepted: 29 January 2019; Published: 5 February 2019

Abstract: The mTOR pathway is in the process of establishing itself as a key access-point of novel oncological drugs and targeted therapies. This is also reflected by the growing number of mTOR pathway genes included in commercially available next-generation sequencing (NGS) oncology panels. This review summarizes the portfolio of medium sized diagnostic, as well as research destined NGS panels and their coverage of the mTOR pathway, including 16 DNA-based panels and the current gene list of Foundation One as a major reference entity. In addition, we give an overview of interesting, mTOR-associated somatic mutations that are not yet incorporated. Especially eukaryotic translation initiation factors (eIFs), a group of mTOR downstream proteins, are on the rise as far as diagnostics and drug targeting in precision medicine are concerned. This review aims to raise awareness for the true coverage of NGS panels, which should be valuable in selecting the ideal platform for diagnostics and research.

Keywords: mTOR; NGS; illumina; IonTorrent; eIFs

1. Introduction

1.1. mTOR Pathway

The mTOR protein, a serine-threonine kinase of the phosphoinositide 3-kinase (PI3K)-related family, is part of two distinct complexes, mTORC1 and mTORC2. It regulates the cells in all catabolic and anabolic processes dependent on nutrients. Major components of the signaling network are summarized in Table 1 and introduced in the following chapters. Being an anchor point of cell growth, mTOR signaling is a critical target of genetic variation in cancer, and when affected it is frequently associated with carcinogenesis and tumor progression. As its term "mechanistic target of rapamycin" implies, mTOR is the target of the rapamycin-FKB12 complex [1]. mTOR is the catalytic subunit of two protein complexes, known as mTORC1 and mTORC2, acquiring different substrate specificities [2]. mTORC1 consists of a total of five components, apart from mTOR, regulatory-associated protein of mTOR (Raptor), mammalian lethal with Sec13 protein eight (mLST8, also referred to as GβL), proline-rich AKT substrate 40 kDa (PRAS40) and DEP-domain-containing mTOR-interacting protein (Deptor) [2].

Raptor is required for the correct subcellular localization of mTOR and facilitates substrate recruitment to mTOR by binding to the TOR signaling (TOS) motif on mTORC1 substrates [1–3]. mLST8 has been proposed to associate with the catalytic domain of the complex and to stabilize the kinase loop [4]. Despite these findings, it was also reported that mLST8 is not essential for mTORC1 signaling [5].

The remaining two subunits, PRAS40 and Deptor, have been characterized as negative regulators [6,7]. In this manner, when mTORC1 activity is reduced, the two subunits are recruited to the complex and promote the inhibition of mTORC1. Furthermore, it has been proposed that PRAS40 functions as a regulator of mTORC1 kinase activity by direct inhibition of substrate binding [8]. When mTORC1 is activated, it phosphorylates PRAS40 and Deptor, thereby reducing the physical interaction with mTORC1 and further activating the complex [7,8].

The second complex, mTORC2, shares some of the same subunits: mTOR, mLST8, and Deptor. Additionally, it consists of the rapamycin-insensitive companion of mTOR (Rictor), mammalian stress-activated protein kinase interacting protein (mSIN1), and protein observed with Rictor-1 (Protor-1). Deptor, again, has been shown to negatively regulate the activity of the complex [7]. In contrast, mLST8 seems to play a crucial role in maintaining mTORC2 function [5]. Rictor and mSIN1 have been reported to stabilize each other, thereby providing the structural foundation of mTORC2 [9,10]. mSIN1 additionally contains a phosphoinositide-binding PH domain that is critical for the insulin-dependent regulation of mTORC2 activity [1]. Rictor has also been shown to interact with Protor-1, but the physiological function of this interaction is not yet clear [11,12].

When considering the upstream signaling of these two complexes, it is important to mention, even though not relevant in physiological conditions, that mTORC1 is considered to be rapamycin-sensitive, whereas TOCR2 is not [13]. When rapamycin enters the cell, it binds to FK506-binding protein 12 kDa (FKBP12) and interacts with the FKBP12 binding domain (FBD) of mTOR. This interaction inhibits the function of mTORC1. On the contrary, rapamycin-FKBP12 cannot acutely inhibit mTORC2 [13]. However, it has been shown that, in some cases, chronic rapamycin treatment can inhibit mTORC2 activity after all [14]. Furthermore, it has been reported that rapamycin does not inhibit all functions of mTORC1 [15].

mTORC1 can be regulated by a variety of signals, such as growth factors (GFs), energy status, oxygen, DNA damage, and amino acids [16]. Multiple different GF pathways converge on one of the most important factors regulating mTORC1, the tuberous sclerosis complex (TSC). TSC is a heterotrimer that consists of TSC1, TSC2, and TBC1D7 [17]. This complex functions as a GTPase activation protein (GAP) for the Ras homolog enriched in brain (Rheb), converting it to its inactive, GDP-bound state. Active, GTP-bound Rheb directly interacts with mTORC1 and stimulates its activity. Hence, TSC1/2 negatively regulates mTORC1 [6,16,18]. GF pathways regulating mTORC1 include the insulin/insulin-like growth factor-1 (IGF-1) pathway, receptor-tyrosine kinase-dependent Ras signaling pathway, as well as Wnt and TNFα signaling. IGF-1 causes AKT-dependent phosphorylation of TSC2 [1,19]. Ras signaling also activates mTORC1 via TSC2 phosphorylation, which is achieved through the MAP kinase ERK and its effector p90RSK [1,16,20]. Additionally, AKT activation can activate mTORC1 in a TSC1/2-independent manner, by the promotion of the dissociation of PRAS40 from mTORC1 [6,8,21]. Wnt and TNFα, on the other hand, exert their influence on mTORC1 via the inhibition of TSC1 [22,23].

Intracellular and extracellular stress signals can also regulate mTORC1. In this manner, a reduction in cellular energy activates AMPK, which inhibits mTORC1 through the phosphorylation of Raptor and the activation of TSC2 [1,22]. Hypoxia also activates AMPK, but affects mTORC1 additionally through the induction of REDD1, which activates TSC [24]. DNA damage inhibits the mTORC1 complex via the induction of p53 target genes which, in turn, increase TSC activity [25]. Amino acid sensing by mTORC1 is mediated by Rags, which are heterodimers consisting of RagA or RagB with

RagC or RagD [26]. These dimers are tethered to the lysosomal membrane [27,28]. Upon amino acid stimulation, Rags are activated and bind Raptor, leading to the recruitment of mTORC1 to the lysosomal membrane where Rheb is located as well [28]. mTORC1 signaling only takes place when both Rheb and Rags are activated [1].

Compared to the mTORC1 upstream network, mTORC2 seems to be less complex. The complex primarily functions as an effector of insulin/PI3K signaling [1]. The PH domain of mSIN1 inhibits the catalytic function of mTORC2 in the absence of insulin. Upon binding to PI3K-generated PIP3, this inhibition is relieved [29]. Furthermore, AKT can phosphorylate mSIN1, suggesting the presence of a positive feedback loop in which partial AKT activation promotes mTORC2 activation, which then fully activates AKT [30]. Another regulator of mTORC2 is mTORC1, mediated by a negative feedback loop between mTORC1 and insulin/PI3K signaling [1,31]. The upstream network, as described here, is illustrated in Figure 1A.

The downstream signaling of mTORC1 is as diverse as its upstream paths. It plays a crucial role in the balance between anabolism and catabolism by promoting lipid, protein, and nucleotide production while simultaneously suppressing autophagy [1].

Lipid synthesis is promoted by mTORC1 through the sterol responsive element binding protein (SREBP) transcription factors. These control the expression of metabolic genes [1,32]. Usually SREPB is activated due to low sterol levels. However, mTORC1 can activate SREPB independent of sterol levels in a p70S6 Kinase 1 (S6K1)-dependent manner or via the phosphorylation of another substrate, Lipin1. In the absence of mTORC1, Lipin1 inhibits SERBP [33,34].

mTORC1 mostly promotes protein synthesis via S6K1 phosphorylation and eukaryotic initiation factor 4E (eIF4E) Binding Protein-1 (4EBP-1). By phosphorylating S6K1, mTORC1 enables its subsequent activation by PDK1. The active S6K1 then activates factors in favor of mRNA translation initiation, including eIF4B, which is a positive regulator of the 5' cap binding eIF4F complex [35]. S6K1 is known to phosphorylate, thereby promoting the degradation of PDCD4, an inhibitor of eIF4B [36]. 4EBP inhibits translation by binding eIF4E, which prevents the assembly of the eIF4F complex. However, mTORC1 phosphorylates 4EBP and thereby causes its dissociation from eIF4E. This allows eIF4E to promote cap-dependent translation [37–39]. This tremendous regulatory power of translation initiation links these two molecular processes and requires a consideration of further eIF subunits, when looking at the overall impact of mTOR signaling. Taking all subunits into consideration, this protein family comprises more than 30 members [40].

The synthesis of nucleotides is also promoted by mTORC1 signaling. Thus, mTORC1 induces purine synthesis through the increased expression of MTHFD2, which controls the mitochondrial tetrahydrofolate cycle [41]. In a similar vein, S6K1 phosphorylates carbamoyl-phosphate synthetase (CAD), which catalyzes the initial steps of de-novo pyrimidine synthesis [42]. mTORC1 has also been shown to increase the translation of HIF1α, which leads to the expression of glycolytic enzymes such as PFK [33]. The activation of SREBP by mTORC1 additionally leads to an increase in the pentose phosphate pathway (PPP). These mechanisms lead to a shift in glucose metabolism towards glycolysis, which facilitates growth [1]. All these anabolic processes support cell growth, however, mTORC1 also supports growth by the suppression of catabolic processes, the most notable process being autophagy [1]. An important transcription factor that drives the expression of genes for autophagy and lysosomal biogenesis is the transcription factor EB (TFEB). This transcription factor can be phosphorylated by mTORC1, which subsequently inhibits its nuclear translocation [43]. Furthermore, another important step in autophagy can be inhibited by mTORC1, which is the autophagosome formation. ULK1, a kinase that normally forms a complex with a number of other components, drives the autophagosome formation. However, under nutrient-rich conditions, mTORC1 phosphorylates ULK1 and thereby disrupts the interaction between ULK1 and AMPK, which is an activator of autophagy [44].

Similar to the upstream processes, the downstream processes of mTORC2 are considered to be less complex. Most probably, mTORC2 plays a key role in the phosphorylation of AKT [1]. AKT is a key effector protein of the insulin/PI3K signaling pathway and can be activated by mTORC2 [45]. When active, AKT promotes cell proliferation, survival and growth through the inhibition of various substrates, including but not limited to the FoxO1/3a TFs; GSK3ß, a metabolic regulator; and TSC2 [45]. Nevertheless, studies have shown that mTORC2 is not crucial to the phosphorylation of all substrates of Akt, for example, TSC can be phosphorylated by Akt without mTORC2 [5]. However, it has been reported to be essential for the phosphorylation of other substrates, such as FoxO1/3a [10]. mTORC2 phosphorylates several members of the AGC (PKA/PKG/PKC) family and thereby controls proliferation and survival [46,47]. One major cellular process influenced by mTORC2 is the actin cytoskeleton. Several PKC family members have been reported to be phosphorylated by mTORC2, all of which are involved in the regulation of cytoskeletal remodeling and cell migration [46–49]. Furthermore, mTORC2 can also activate SGK1, which is an AGC-kinase that regulates ion transport and cell survival [50].

The downstream processes of mTOR signaling are shown in Figure 1B. All proteins involved in mTOR signaling are summarized in Table 1.

Table 1. mTOR pathway-associated proteins, divided into mTOR complex components and upstream/downstream modules. Where applicable, protein activity is denoted as anabolic or catabolic.

Abbreviation	Full Name	Function	↑↓
	mTORC 1	Stimulating/Inhibiting Signal	
mTOR	mechanistic target of rapamycin	Serine-threonine kinase	-
Raptor	regulatory-associated protein of mTOR	Localization of mTOR, substrate recruitment to mTOR [1,3,4]	↑
mLST8	mammalian lethal with Sec13 protein 8	Stabilizing kinase loop [5]; not essential to TORC1 function [6]	-
PRAS40	proline rich AKT substrate 40 kDa	Inhibitory [7]; inhibits substrate binding, phosphorylated by active mTORC1 [9]	↓
Deptor	DEP-domain-containing mTOR-interacting protein	Inhibitory [8], phosphorylated by active mTORC1	↓
	mTORC 2	Stimulating/Inhibiting Signal	
mTOR	mechanistic target of rapamycin	serine-threonine kinase of the phosphoinositide 3-kinase (PI3K)-related family	
mLST8	mammalian lethal with Sec13 protein 8	Essential for stability and function of mTORC2 [6]	↑
Deptor	DEP-domain-containing mTOR-interacting protein	Inhibitory [8]	↓
Rictor	rapamycin-insensitive companion of mTOR	Stabilization [10,11]; shown to interact with Protor-1 [12,13]	↑
mSIN1	mammalian stress-activated protein kinase interacting protein	Stabilization [10,11], phosphoinositide-binding PH domain: critical for insulin dependent mTORC2 function, inhibits mTORC2 function in absence of insulin [1]	↑/↓
Protor-1	protein observed with Rictor-1	shown to interact with Rictor [12,13]	
	mTORC 1 Upstream	Stimulating/Inhibiting Signal	
-	rapamycin	Enters cell and binds FKBP12 [2]; when bound inhibits mTORC 1, but not all functions [15]	↓
FKBP12	FK506-binding protein 12 kDa	Is bound by rapamycin, interacts with FBD on mTOR [2]; when bound inhibits mTORC 1, but not all functions [15]; cannot acutely inhibit mTORC2 [2]	-
TSC	tuberous sclerosis complex	Consists of TC1, TC2, TBC1D7, negatively regulates mTORC1 via inactivation of Rheb [17], phosphorylated by AKT (mTORC2 independent) [6]	↓
Rheb	Ras homolog enriched in brain	Stimulates mTOCR1 activity when active [7,16,18]	↑
IGF-1 pathway	insulin/insulin like growth factor 1 pathway	Causes AKT dependent phosphorylation of TSC2 [1,19]	↑
Ras pathway	Rat Sarcoma Pathway	Causes TSC2 phosphorylation via ERK and p90rsk [1,16,20]	↑
AKT	AKT serine/threonine kinase	Phosphorylates TSC2 [1,19]; key effector protein of the insulin/PI3K signaling pathway, and can be activated by mTORC2 [45]; promotes dissociation of PRAS40 from mTORC1. [7,9,21]	↑
-	Wnt	Inhibits TSC1 [22]	↑
TNFα	tumor necrosis factor α	Inhibits TSC1 [23]	↑
AMPK	5'-AMP-activated protein kinase	Inhibits mTORC1 (in response to reduced cellular energy or hypoxia) by phosphorylating Raptor and activation of TSC2 [1,22,24]; activator of autophagy, activates ULK1 [44]	↓
REDD1	regulated in development and DNA damage responses 1	Activates TSC in response to hypoxia [24]	↓
-	p53 target genes	Increase TSC activity upon DNA damage [25]	↓

Table 1. *Cont.*

Abbreviation	Full Name	Function	↑↓
	mTORC 2 Upstream	Stimulating/Inhibiting Signal	
	Rapamycin	Enters cell and binds FKBP12 [2];	↓
FKBP12	FKBP prolyl isomerase	Is bound by rapamycin, interacts with FBD on mTOR cannot acutely inhibit mTORC2 [2]; chronic treatment can inhibit mTORC2 [14]	-
PIP3	Phosphatidylinositol (3,4,5)-trisphosphate	PI3K generated PIP3 binds to PH domain o mSIN1 and relieves inhibition of mTORC2 [29]	↑
AKT	AKT serine/threonine kinase	Phosphorylates mSIN1, positive feedback loop [30]	↑
mTORC1	mammalian target of rapamycin complex 1	Negative feedback loop between mTORC1 and insulin/PI3K signaling [1,31]	↓
	mTORC1 downstream	Stimulating/Inhibiting Signal	
SREBP	sterol responsive element binding protein	Activated by low sterol levels, in control of expression of metabolic genes, can be activated by mTORC1 independently via S6K1 or Lipin1 [1,32]; expression by mTORC1 increases PPP [1]	↑
S6K1	p70S6 Kinase 1	Can activate SREBP [33,34], when phosphorylated by mTORC1 can be activated by PDK1, promotes mRNA translation intitation [35]; promotes degradation of PDCD4 [36]; phosphorylates CAD (catalyzes first steps in de-novo pyrimidine synthesis) [42]	↑
-	Lipin1	Inhibits SREBP in absence of mTORC1, activates when mTORC1 is present [33,34]	↑
4EBP	eukaryotic initiation factor 4E binding protein	Inhibits translation by binding eIF4E → prevents assembly of eIF4F complex; when phosphorylated by mTORC1 → dissociates from eIF4e → allows assembly [37–39]	↑
eIF4B	eukaryotic translation initiation factor 4B	Positive regulator of the 5'-cap binding eIF4F complex, activated by S6K1 [35], inhibitor: PDCD4 [36]	↑
eIF4F complex	eukaryotic translation initiation factor 4F	Positively regulated by eIF4B, 5'-cap binding complex,	↑
MTHFD2	methylenetetrahydrofolate dehydrogenase	Controls the mitochondrial tetrahydrofolate cycle, expression increased bymTORC1 induction of purine synthesis [41]	↑
HIF1α	hypoxia inducible factor 1	Translation increased by mTORC1 → expression of glycolytic enzymes [33]	↑
TFEB	Transcription factor EB	expression of genes for autophagy and lysosomal biogenesis, when phosphorylated by mTORC1 →cannot translocate to nucleus [43]	↓
ULK1	unc-51 like autophagy activating kinase 1	Drives autophagosome formation, when phosphorylated by mTORC1 → no interaction with AMPK → no activation [44]	↓
AMPK	AMP-activated protein kinase	Inhibits mTORC1 (in response to reduced cellular energy or hypoxia) by phosphorylating Raptor and activation of TSC2 [1,22]; activator of autophagy, activates ULK1 [44]	↓
	mTORC2 downstream	Stimulating/Inhibiting Signal	
AKT	AKT serine/threonine kinase	Phosphorylated by mTORC2 [1]; phosphorylates TSC2; key effector protein of the insulin/PI3K signaling pathway [45]; activation by mTORC2 not crucial for the phosphorylation of all, but some of its substrates [6,11]	-
FoxO1/3a	Forkhead box protein O1	TFs, phosphorylated by AKT (mTORC2 dependent) [11]	-
GSK3ß	Glycogen synthase kinase 3β	Metabolic regulator, phosphorylated by AKT [6]	-
-	AGC (PKA/PKB/PKC) Family	Several members phosphorylated by mTORC2 for regulation of proliferation, survival and cytoskeleton [1,46–49]	-

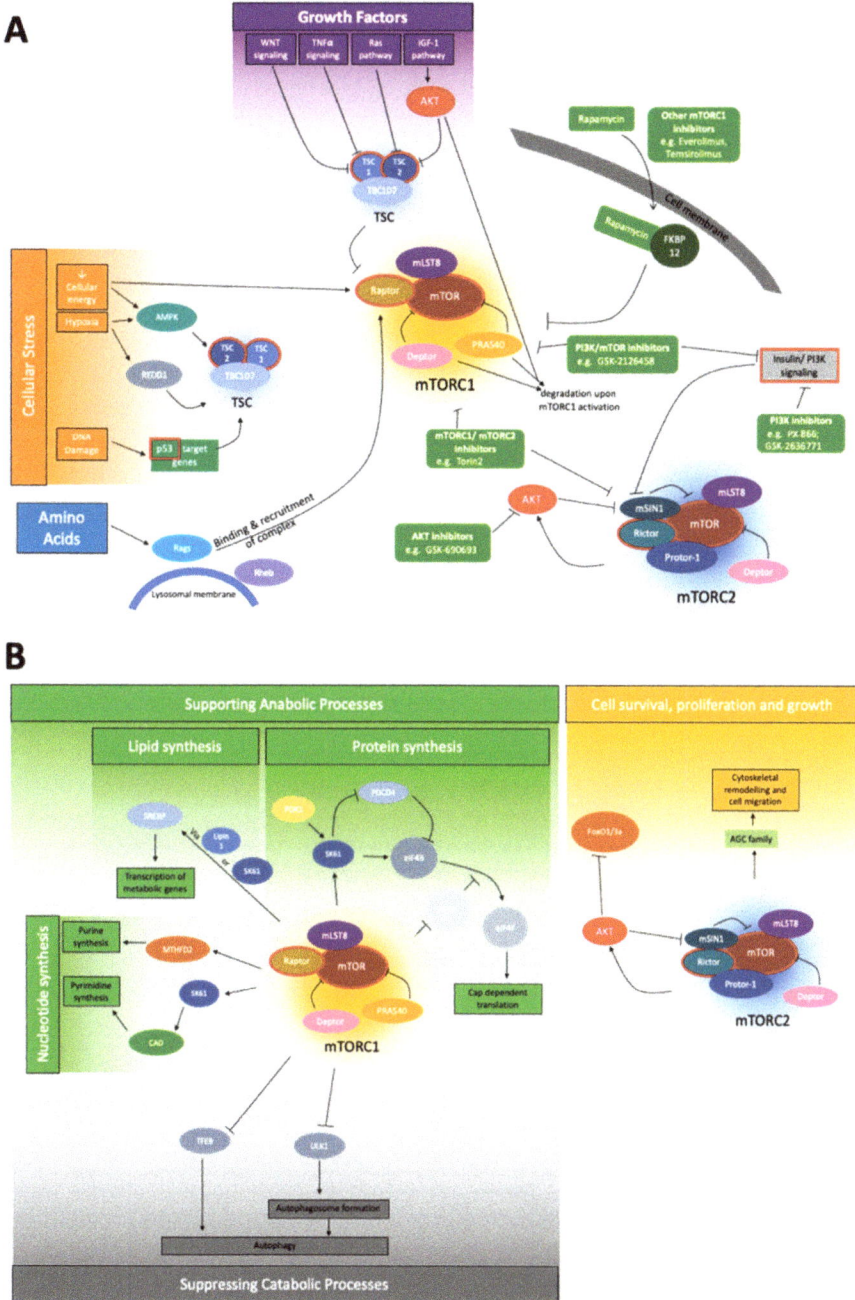

Figure 1. Schematic depiction of the mTOR signaling network. (**A**) The most important upstream signals of mTOR signaling are cellular stress, growth factors, and amino acids for the mTORC1 complex, and the insulin/PI3K pathway for mTORC2. Genes of special interest for NGS, due to their mutation frequency, are shown with a red border. No prominent pattern of a section specifically affected by these

mutations is obvious. To the best of our best knowledge, no companion diagnostic between a specific mutation and treatment is currently applicable. However, a variety of inhibitors (green) affecting the network at different points are known: Inhibitors affecting AKT, mTORC1/mTORC2, PI3K, PI3K/mTOR, and mTORC1 inhibitors like rapamycin and rapalogs [51,52]; and (**B**) the widespread downstream network of mTORC1 and mTORC2 is shown. mTORC1 is involved both in supporting anabolic processes via influencing nucleotide, lipid and protein synthesis, as well as suppressing catabolic processes, mainly autophagy. mTORC2, under the coregulation of AKT, is known to mainly affect cell survival, proliferation and growth, and the specifically the regulation of the cytoskeleton.

1.2. mTOR Signaling in Cancer

Considering how involved the mTOR signaling pathway is, it comes as no surprise that it also plays a crucial role in human disease, particularly cancer. The complex most commonly associated with cell proliferation and cancer progression when deregulated is the mTORC1 complex [53,54]. A number of signaling components both upstream and downstream of mTOR are frequently deregulated or altered in human cancer [53]. Through alterations in one or multiple of these elements, mTOR signaling is activated in many cancer types, suggesting mTOR as a potent target for cancer therapy. Due to this fact, mTOR pathway inhibitors have been of prime interest in recent years. These inhibitors include rapamycin and its analogs (rapalogs) and, more recently, mTOR kinase domain inhibitors [55]. Despite showing promise, rapalog monotherapy has been proven mostly insufficient in causing tumor regression, with notable exceptions of tumors showing mutations in mTOR itself, LOF mutations in TSC1 or TSC2 [55–59]. Broadrange reports correlating mTOR pathway mutations to drug response are yet missing, but there are studies towards that aim that are very promising. Specifically, a study identified 33 *MTOR* mutations that lead to pathway hyperactivity in cancer [58]. A heightened rapamycin sensitivity in cells harboring these hyperactivating mTOR mutations suggests that they convey mTOR pathway dependency. These results are supported by the report of an extraordinary responder with two activating mTOR mutations in urothelial carcinoma and an exceptional response to rapalog treatment in combination with a TKI [58,59].

Furthermore, patients with the genetic disorder tuberous sclerosis complex (TSC) (mutations in the *TSC1* or *TSC2* gene), commonly develop tumors like astrocytomas or angiomyolipomas as well as the related lung disorder Lymphangioleiomyomatosis (LAM). Treatment with rapalogs has been shown to improve clinical outcomes and cause tumor regression in TSC patients with astrocytomas or sporadic LAM, again suggesting a dependence on mTOR signaling for tumor growth [60–62]. A phase II clinical trial found a 50% response rate in TSC patients with angiomyolipomas or sporadic LAM [63]. Furthermore, heightened treatment sensitivity was associated with TSC1 or TSC2 LOF mutations, as reported in bladder and thyroid cancer [56,57]. Other responders have been reported in one pancreatic cancer with loss of suppression of mTOR signaling and three patients with perivascular epithelioid cell tumors with the loss of TSC2 [64,65]. However, in the thyroid cancer extraordinary responder case study, the tumor gained resistance to rapalog treatment as it acquired a mutation in mTOR, which prevented the binding of the rapalog, as well as a nonsense mutation in TSC2 [57]. Further literature regarding rapamycin and rapalogs as monotherapy includes References [66] and [67]. These specific cases show the importance of rapamycin and rapalogs, as well as the development of reliable biomarkers, for precision medicine. Apart from these cases, it has been shown that, while not very potent on its own, mTORC1 inhibition might be necessary to achieve a proper response to drugs that target the primary oncogenic pathway in the given cancer. On top of that, sustained mTORC1 activation is proposed to be a major mechanism of resistance to targeted therapies [55–59,68].

Furthermore, mTORC1 is, as mentioned above, not only involved in stimulating growth but also in regulating autophagy. Autophagy has been described as double-edged sword in the modulation of cancer, since both inhibition and induction of autophagy have been shown to be both pro and anti-tumorigenic [54–59,68,69]. Even though a better understanding of the individual factors contributing to the effect autophagy has on cancer is needed, mTORC1 and its associated regulators of autophagy, ULK1 and AMPK, represent attractive targets for cancer therapy [54].

1.3. Next-Generation-Sequencing

DNA sequence analysis has come a long way since the establishment of the Sanger chain termination method in 1977 [70]. From then on, scientists have developed reliable and reproducible ways of DNA sequencing, steadily decreasing the costs and increasing output. Output, which was formerly one read of one gene at a time, is now more adequately given in gigabases per run, reflecting the parallel analysis of multiple genes with read depths (i.e., the number of reads covering a genetic locus) of 20 up to 1000 or more, depending on the application [71]. Next Generation Sequencing (NGS) is the most common name of the second-generation, deep-sequencing techniques. All platforms are following a three-step procedure: (1) Library-preparation, (2) Cluster/Bridge Amplification, and (3) sequencing, i.e., strands of fragmented DNA are amplified and immobilized on a surface or bead, then nucleotide bases are added sequentially using DNA polymerase; excess reagent is washed out to enable correct imaging according to the base incorporated; this process repeats for each base. The actual sequence analysis is for, e.g., Illumina based on fluorescent signaling, while Ion Torrent technology relies on pH changes detected by semiconductors [72–74].

2. Summary and Comparison of Oncological NGS Panels and Their Coverage of the mTOR Pathway

In the following, we summarize commercially available NGS gene panels that cover a number of genes reasonable for research and clinical applications, i.e., covering a medium number of gene loci, excluding large scale screening panels. We included the gold standard genetic analysis panel Foundation One as a reference. In a next step, we look at the coverage of the mTOR pathway by the various panels. Therefore, we submerged a 78-item list of mTOR signaling-relevant genes. This list is based on the publicly available "mTOR Pathway—Gene List", generated with the help of David Sabatini, a leading expert in the field [75]. We extended the list by a number of genes, among them the complete eIF3 and eIF4 protein families, representing a more general field of mTOR impact (Supplementary Table S1).

Oncological NGS Gene Panels

The growing capacity of NGS devices, with an increasing number of genes and read depth has initiated a trend towards whole exome and whole genome sequencing. These techniques will be state of the art in the near future. Today, bioinformatic and data storage issues also limit the application of global analyses and make panels comprising 10–150 genes to the standards in the field. Most of these panels run on Illumina MiniSeq, MiSeq, and iSeq devices or on the Ion Torrent S5 Series devices by Applied Biosystems [76]. Supplementary Table S1 shows a collection of 16 different gene panels for oncological application and the full gene lists together with the gene list of Foundation One. The gene panels and number of genes are summarized in Table 2. As already mentioned, we consider only ready-made gene panles with a low-medium number of genes analyzed. All these panels are based on DNA only, as DNA material is sufficient to detect genetic mutations. RNA sequencing would add a surplus on information on e.g. gene fusions or gene expression, but RNA is more difficult to isolate from especially FFPE tissue in an adequate quality [77] and besides that hardly any gene panels covering RNA targets are available to date. One of the available gene panels with DNA and RNA pools is the Ion AmpliSeq/AmpliSeq for Illumina Focus Panel, which is also considered in this review. This Focus Panel targets 40 DNA sites and additional 23 RNA sites, among the latter is also the mTOR-relevant AKT3 [78].

Table 2. Oncologically relevant, predesigned NGS gene panels, with number of genes covered and the names of covered genes relevant to mTOR signaling.

Panel Name	Number of Genes Covered	mTOR Relevant Genes Covered
Foundation One	305	AKT1/2/3; CCND1; GSK3B; MDM2; MTOR; NF1; PDK1; PIK3C2; PIK3CA/B; PIK3R1; PTEN; RICTOR, RPTOR; SGK1; TNFAIP3; TP53; TSC1/2; VHL
Agilent ClearSeq Comprehensive Cancer Panel	150	AKT1/2/3; NF1; MTOR; PIK3R1; PIK3CA; PTEN; TP53; VHL
Qiagen Human Cancer Predisposition GeneRead DNAseq Targeted Panel V2	143	AKT1; NF1; PIK3CA; PTEN; TP53; TSC1/2; VHL
Integrated DNA Technologies (IDT) xGen Pan-Cancer Panel	127	AKT1; CCND1; EIF4A2; MTOR; NF1; PIK3CA; PIK3CG; PIK3R1; PTEN; TP53; VHL
Archer VariantPlex Solid Tumor	67	AKT1; CCND1; MDM2; PIK3CA; PIK3R1; PTEN; TP53; VHL
Swift Biosciences Accel-Amplicon 56G Oncology Panel v2	56	AKT1; PIK3CA; PTEN; TP53; TSC1; VHL
NEBNExt Direct Cancer HotSpot Panel	50	AKT1; PIK3CA; PTEN; TP53; VHL
AmpliSeq Cancer Hotspot Panel v2	49	AKT1; PIK3CA; PTEN; TP53; VHL
TruSeq Amplicon Cancer Panel	48	AKT1; PIK3CA; PTEN; TP53; VHL
AmpliSeq for Illumina Focus Panel	40	AKT1; CCND1; MTOR; PIK3CA
Archer VariantPlex Comprehensive Thyroid and Lung Kit	31	AKT1; CCND1; MDM2; PIK3CA; PTEN; TP53
TruSight Tumor 26	26	AKT1; PIK3CA; PTEN; TP53
Agilent SureMASTR Tumor Hotspot	25	AKT; PIK3CA; PTEN
Qiagen Human Clinically Relevant Tumor GeneRead DNAseq Targeted Panel V2	24	AKT1; PIK3CA; PTEN; TP53
Asuragen QuantideX NGS DNA Hotspot 21 Kit	21	AKT1/2; PIK3CA
TruSight Tumor 15	15	AKT1; PIK3CA; TP53
Qiagen Human Tumor Actionable Mutations GeneRead DNAseq Targeted Panel v2	8	-

The mTOR-relevant genes covered by the oncological NGS panels primarily consist of mTOR upstream AKT and PIK3CA. To elucidate the relevance for the signaling pathway, we collected data from the catalog of somatic mutations in cancer (COSMIC; cancer.sanger.ac.uk/cosmic) on mutational frequency and associated drug sensitivity/resistances (Table 3).

Table 3. COSMIC data for mTOR pathway-associated genes. The mutational frequencies are highlighted in grey, if >1%. If a gene mutation alters the sensitivity to drug treatment, the gene name is written in bold letters.

Gene	Frequency of Mutation in Cancer
4E-BP	<0.1%
AKT1	1.1%
AKT2	0.4%
AKT3	0.5%
CCND1	0.3%
Deptor	0.3%
eIF3a	0.8%
eIF3b	0.4%
eIF3c	<0.1%
eIF3d	0.3%
eIF3e	0.3%
eIF3f	0.2%
eIF3g	0.2%
eIF3h	0.2%
eIF3i	0.2%
eIF3j	0.1%
eIF3k	0.1%

Table 3. *Cont.*

Gene	Frequency of Mutation in Cancer
eIF3l	0.3%
eIF3m	0.2%
eIF4a	0.3%
eIF4b	0.3%
eIF4E	0.2%
eIF4g	1.0%
eIF4h	0.2%
FOXO	0.4%
GBL/mLST8	0.2%
GSK3A	0.2%
GSK3B	0.4%
HIF1α	0.5%
LKB1	0.5%
MDM2	0.4%
mSin1 = MAPKAP1	0.2%
MTHFD2	0.1%
mTOR	2.1%
NF1	**3.8%**
PDK1	0.2%
PIK3CA	**9.7%**
PIK3CB	0.7%
PIK3CD	0.7%
PIK3CG	1.6%
PIK3R1	**1.4%**
PIK3R2	0.5%
PIK3R3	0.3%
PIK3R4	0.7%
PIK3R5	0.7%
PIK3R6	0.6%
PIP3	0.4%
PKC alpha	0.4%
PKC beta	1.0%
PKC delta	0.4%
PKC epsilon	0.5%
PKC eta	0.5%
PKC gamma	0.7%
PKC iota	0.4%
PKC theta	0.7%
PKC zeta	0.4%
PRAS40 = AKT1S1	0.2%
Protor = PRR5	0.3%
PTEN	**5.0%**
Raptor	1.0%
REDD1 = DDIT4	0.1%
Rheb	0.1%
Rictor	1.0%
RRAGA	0.1%
RRAGB	0.2%
RRAGC	0.2%
RRAGD	0.2%
S6K	0.2%
SGK	0.4%
SREBP	0.5%
TFEB	0.3%
TNFα	0.3%
TP53	**25.2%**
TSC1	1.2%
TSC2	1.7%
ULK1	0.7%
VHL	4.5%
Wnt	0.3%

Of the genes analyzed here, TP53 was identified by this catalog as the by far most commonly mutated gene in cancer (25.2%), followed by PIK3CA (9.7%) and PTEN (5%). According to the catalog, none of the genes harbor drug-associated resistance mutations, but indeed, mutations were associated with altered sensitivity. In this manner, mutations of NF1 alter the sensitivity to the drug Nutlin-3a, which is targeting MDM2. Mutations in PIK3CA are associated with altered sensitivity to Pictilisib and GSK690693, targeting PI3K and AKT1/2/3, respectively. Mutations in PIK3R1 are associated with altered sensitivity to Dacinostat, targeting HDAC1. Mutations in PTEN are associated with altered sensitivity to GSK690693. Mutations in TP53 are associated with altered sensitivity to the following seven drugs: 5-Fluorouracil (5-FU, antimetabolite), Rucaparib (targeting PARP1/2), CX-5461 (acts on RNA polymerase 1), (5Z)-7-Oxozeaenol (targeting TAK1), Bleomycin (acts by induction of dsDNA breaks and DNA damage repair), Dabrafenib (targeting BRAF), and Nutlin-3a [79].

The most frequently mutated genes, together with affected tissues and actual occurring mutations, are listed in Table 4.

Table 4. Summary of most frequently mutated mTOR related genes and affected tissues. The mutational frequencies are highlighted in grey, if >1%.

Gene	Frequency of Mutation in Cancer	Most Common Genetic Mutations	Tissue	Reference
AKT1	1.1%	E17K, Q79K, L52R	breast, skin, urinary tract	[80,81]
eIF4g	1.0%	T436fs * 86; K643R	colon, lung (overexpression w/o genetic mutation)	[80,82,83]
mTOR	2.1%	S2215Y, S2215F, E1799K, T1977K, L1460P	colon, endometrium, skin, kidney	[80,84]
NF1	3.8%	R2450 *, R440 *, R1534 *	skin, soft tissue, urinary tract, lung, colon	[80,85,86]
PIK3CA	9.7%	H1047R, E545K, E542K, H1047L, Q546K, R88Q, N345K, C420L	breast, endometrium, urinary tract, colon	[80,87–89]
PIK3CG	1.6%	V759I, V165I, R472C, E267K, A84V	skin, colon, lung	[80,90,91]
PIK3R1	1.4%	N564D, R348 *, K567E, G376R	breast, endometrium, prostate, leukemia	[80,92]
PKC beta	1.0%	D427N, D630N, E533K	lung, skin, colon	[80,93]
PTEN	5.0%	R130G, R130Q, R233 *, R130 *	breast, endometrium, prostate, leukemia	[80,94,95]
Raptor	1.0%	R718C, R139H, Q1264fs * 4, T1121M	various	[80]
Rictor	1.0%	S1101L, R401C	lung, breast	[80,96]
TP53	25.2%	R175H, R248Q, R273H, R282W, R213 *, G245S, R249S, Y220C, R196 *, R342 *	solid cancer, leukemia, lymphoma, melanoma	[80,97,98]
TSC1	1.2%	M322T, P1143L	skin, urinary tract, liver	[80,99–101]
TSC2	1.7%	F690fs * 8, R1417fs * 59, S1364fs * 50, K1638 *	liver, breast	[80,101]
VHL	4.5%	kidney, neuroendocrine tumors	R161 *, L89H, S65 *	[80,102,103]

3. Discussion and Conclusions

We have shown that mTOR-associated genes generally show low mutational frequencies in cancer. Only TP53, with 25.2% is a frequent target of mutations, and is known to interact with numerous signaling cascades besides the mTOR pathway. PIK3CA with 9.7% and PTEN with 5% mutational frequency are especially interesting, as they are also associated with drug sensitivities. In fact, a ranking of genes according to their associated drug sensitivity also shows a better representation of the mTOR pathway than with actual number of mutated samples. When looking at all described genes, it becomes evident that very little awareness is drawn to mTOR downstream, e.g., eIFs, with low mutational frequencies throughout and no reported drug sensitivity alterations. This results in a ambivalent situation; on the one hand the high importance of mTOR pathway and translational control for carcinogenesis and growth control of tumor cells, is emphasized by a growing number of research as well as clinical reports, on the other hand, NGS and following the information of tumor mutational burden, generated by NGS analyses show only limited applicability in terms of mTOR pathway associated readouts. For the here featured pathway, it will be critical to employ RNA-sequencing and nanopore sequencing techniques, which will allow for an evaluation of gene expression next to mutational status, thereby multiplying the information on mTOR signaling in cancer. By those means well described predictive as well as prognostic tumor markers can be evaluated by their expression levels. This is changing the view on our gene panel, which holds numerous marker genes that are known to have great impact on disease progression and prognosis, even though they are poorly covered by NGS and are rarely mutated. Important examples of these markers are the eIF subunits [104–106].

Supplementary Materials: Supplementary materials can be found at http://www.mdpi.com/1422-0067/20/3/690/s1.

Conflicts of Interest: The authors declare no conflict of interest.

References

1. Saxton, R.A.; Sabatini, D.M. mTOR Signaling in Growth, Metabolism, and Disease. *Cell* **2017**, *168*, 960–976. [CrossRef] [PubMed]
2. Guertin, D.A.; Sabatini, D.M. Defining the role of mTOR in cancer. *Cancer Cell* **2007**, *12*, 9–22. [CrossRef] [PubMed]
3. Schalm, S.S.; Fingar, D.C.; Sabatini, D.M.; Blenis, J. TOS motif-mediated raptor binding regulates 4E-BP1 multisite phosphorylation and function. *Curr. Biol.* **2003**, *13*, 797–806. [CrossRef]
4. Nojima, H.; Tokunaga, C.; Eguchi, S.; Oshiro, N.; Hidayat, S.; Yoshino, K.; Hara, K.; Tanaka, N.; Avruch, J.; Yonezawa, K. The mammalian target of rapamycin (mTOR) partner, raptor, binds the mTOR substrates p70 S6 kinase and 4E-BP1 through their TOR signaling (TOS) motif. *J. Biol. Chem.* **2003**, *278*, 15461–15464. [CrossRef] [PubMed]
5. Yang, H.; Rudge, D.G.; Koos, J.D.; Vaidialingam, B.; Yang, H.J.; Pavletich, N.P. mTOR kinase structure, mechanism and regulation. *Nature* **2013**, *497*, 217–223. [CrossRef] [PubMed]
6. Guertin, D.A.; Stevens, D.M.; Thoreen, C.C.; Burds, A.A.; Kalaany, N.Y.; Moffat, J.; Brown, M.; Fitzgerald, K.J.; Sabatini, D.M. Ablation in mice of the mTORC components raptor, rictor, or mLST8 reveals that mTORC2 is required for signaling to Akt-FOXO and PKCalpha, but not S6K1. *Dev. Cell* **2006**, *11*, 859–871. [CrossRef] [PubMed]
7. Sancak, Y.; Thoreen, C.C.; Peterson, T.R.; Lindquist, R.A.; Kang, S.A.; Spooner, E.; Carr, S.A.; Sabatini, D.M. PRAS40 is an insulin-regulated inhibitor of the mTORC1 protein kinase. *Mol. Cell* **2007**, *25*, 903–915. [CrossRef] [PubMed]
8. Peterson, T.R.; Laplante, M.; Thoreen, C.C.; Sancak, Y.; Kang, S.A.; Kuehl, W.M.; Gray, N.S.; Sabatini, D.M. DEPTOR is an mTOR inhibitor frequently overexpressed in multiple myeloma cells and required for their survival. *Cell* **2009**, *137*, 873–886. [CrossRef] [PubMed]
9. Wang, L.; Harris, T.E.; Roth, R.A.; Lawrence, J.C., Jr. PRAS40 regulates mTORC1 kinase activity by functioning as a direct inhibitor of substrate binding. *J. Biol. Chem.* **2007**, *282*, 20036–20044. [CrossRef]
10. Frias, M.A.; Thoreen, C.C.; Jaffe, J.D.; Schroder, W.; Sculley, T.; Carr, S.A.; Sabatini, D.M. mSin1 is necessary for Akt/PKB phosphorylation, and its isoforms define three distinct mTORC2s. *Curr. Biol.* **2006**, *16*, 1865–1870. [CrossRef] [PubMed]
11. Jacinto, E.; Facchinetti, V.; Liu, D.; Soto, N.; Wei, S.; Jung, S.Y.; Huang, Q.; Qin, J.; Su, B. SIN1/MIP1 maintains rictor-mTOR complex integrity and regulates Akt phosphorylation and substrate specificity. *Cell* **2006**, *127*, 125–137. [CrossRef] [PubMed]
12. Woo, S.Y.; Kim, D.H.; Jun, C.B.; Kim, Y.M.; Haar, E.V.; Lee, S.I.; Hegg, J.W.; Bandhakavi, S.; Griffin, T.J. PRR5, a novel component of mTOR complex 2, regulates platelet-derived growth factor receptor beta expression and signaling. *J. Biol. Chem.* **2007**, *282*, 25604–25612. [CrossRef] [PubMed]

13. Thedieck, K.; Polak, P.; Kim, M.L.; Molle, K.D.; Cohen, A.; Jeno, P.; Arrieumerlou, C.; Hall, M.N. PRAS40 and PRR5-like protein are new mTOR interactors that regulate apoptosis. *PLoS ONE* **2007**, *2*, e1217. [CrossRef] [PubMed]

14. Sarbassov, D.D.; Ali, S.M.; Sengupta, S.; Sheen, J.H.; Hsu, P.P.; Bagley, A.F.; Markhard, A.L.; Sabatini, D.M. Prolonged rapamycin treatment inhibits mTORC2 assembly and Akt/PKB. *Mol. Cell* **2006**, *22*, 159–168. [CrossRef] [PubMed]

15. Thoreen, C.C.; Kang, S.A.; Chang, J.W.; Liu, Q.; Zhang, J.; Gao, Y.; Reichling, L.J.; Sim, T.; Sabatini, D.M.; Gray, N.S. An ATP-competitive mammalian target of rapamycin inhibitor reveals rapamycin-resistant functions of mTORC1. *J. Biol. Chem.* **2009**, *284*, 8023–8032. [CrossRef] [PubMed]

16. Laplante, M.; Sabatini, D.M. mTOR signaling at a glance. *J. Cell Sci.* **2009**, *122*, 3589–3594. [CrossRef] [PubMed]

17. Dibble, C.C.; Elis, W.; Menon, S.; Qin, W.; Klekota, J.; Asara, J.M.; Finan, P.M.; Kwiatkowski, D.J.; Murphy, L.O.; Manning, B.D. TBC1D7 is a third subunit of the TSC1-TSC2 complex upstream of mTORC1. *Mol. Cell* **2012**, *47*, 535–546. [CrossRef]

18. Long, X.; Lin, Y.; Ortiz-Vega, S.; Yonezawa, K.; Avruch, J. Rheb binds and regulates the mTOR kinase. *Curr. Biol.* **2005**, *15*, 702–713. [CrossRef]

19. Inoki, K.; Li, Y.; Zhu, T.; Wu, J.; Guan, K.L. TSC2 is phosphorylated and inhibited by Akt and suppresses mTOR signalling. *Nat. Cell Biol.* **2002**, *4*, 648–657. [CrossRef]

20. Ma, L.; Chen, Z.; Erdjument-Bromage, H.; Tempst, P.; Pandolfi, P.P. Phosphorylation and functional inactivation of TSC2 by Erk implications for tuberous sclerosis and cancer pathogenesis. *Cell* **2005**, *121*, 179–193. [CrossRef]

21. Vander Haar, E.; Lee, S.I.; Bandhakavi, S.; Griffin, T.J.; Kim, D.H. Insulin signalling to mTOR mediated by the Akt/PKB substrate PRAS40. *Nat. Cell Biol.* **2007**, *9*, 316–323. [CrossRef] [PubMed]

22. Inoki, K.; Ouyang, H.; Zhu, T.; Lindvall, C.; Wang, Y.; Zhang, X.; Yang, Q.; Bennett, C.; Harada, Y.; Stankunas, K.; et al. TSC2 integrates Wnt and energy signals via a coordinated phosphorylation by AMPK and GSK3 to regulate cell growth. *Cell* **2006**, *126*, 955–968. [CrossRef] [PubMed]

23. Lee, D.F.; Kuo, H.P.; Chen, C.T.; Hsu, J.M.; Chou, C.K.; Wei, Y.; Sun, H.L.; Li, L.Y.; Ping, B.; Huang, W.C.; et al. IKK beta suppression of TSC1 links inflammation and tumor angiogenesis via the mTOR pathway. *Cell* **2007**, *130*, 440–455. [CrossRef] [PubMed]

24. Brugarolas, J.; Lei, K.; Hurley, R.L.; Manning, B.D.; Reiling, J.H.; Hafen, E.; Witters, L.A.; Ellisen, L.W.; Kaelin, W.G., Jr. Regulation of mTOR function in response to hypoxia by REDD1 and the TSC1/TSC2 tumor suppressor complex. *Genes Dev.* **2004**, *18*, 2893–2904. [CrossRef] [PubMed]

25. Feng, Z.; Hu, W.; de Stanchina, E.; Teresky, A.K.; Jin, S.; Lowe, S.; Levine, A.J. The regulation of AMPK beta1, TSC2, and PTEN expression by p53: Stress, cell and tissue specificity, and the role of these gene products in modulating the IGF-1-AKT-mTOR pathways. *Cancer Res.* **2007**, *67*, 3043–3053. [CrossRef] [PubMed]

26. Kim, E.; Goraksha-Hicks, P.; Li, L.; Neufeld, T.P.; Guan, K.L. Regulation of TORC1 by Rag GTPases in nutrient response. *Nat. Cell Biol.* **2008**, *10*, 935–945. [CrossRef]

27. Sancak, Y.; Bar–Peled, L.; Zoncu, R.; Markhard, A.L.; Nada, S.; Sabatini, D.M. Ragulator-Rag complex targets mTORC1 to the lysosomal surface and is necessary for its activation by amino acids. *Cell* **2010**, *141*, 290–303. [CrossRef]

28. Bar-Peled, L.; Schweitzer, L.D.; Zoncu, R.; Sabatini, D.M. Ragulator is a GEF for the rag GTPases that signal amino acid levels to mTORC1. *Cell* **2012**, *150*, 1196–1208. [CrossRef]

29. Liu, P.; Gan, W.; Chin, Y.R.; Ogura, K.; Guo, J.; Zhang, J.; Wang, B.; Blenis, J.; Cantley, L.C.; Toker, A.; et al. PtdIns(3,4,5)P3-Dependent Activation of the mTORC2 Kinase Complex. *Cancer Discov.* **2015**, *5*, 1194–1209. [CrossRef]

30. Yang, G.; Murashige, D.S.; Humphrey, S.J.; James, D.E. A Positive Feedback Loop between Akt and mTORC2 via SIN1 Phosphorylation. *Cell Rep.* **2015**, *12*, 937–943. [CrossRef]

31. Hsu, P.P.; Kang, S.A.; Rameseder, J.; Zhang, Y.; Ottina, K.A.; Lim, D.; Peterson, T.R.; Choi, Y.; Gray, N.S.; Yaffe, M.B.; et al. The mTOR-regulated phosphoproteome reveals a mechanism of mTORC1-mediated inhibition of growth factor signaling. *Science* **2011**, *332*, 1317–1322. [CrossRef] [PubMed]

32. Porstmann, T.; Santos, C.R.; Griffiths, B.; Cully, M.; Wu, M.; Leevers, S.; Griffiths, J.R.; Chung, Y.L.; Schulze, A. SREBP activity is regulated by mTORC1 and contributes to Akt-dependent cell growth. *Cell Metab.* **2008**, *8*, 224–236. [CrossRef]

33. Duvel, K.; Yecies, J.L.; Menon, S.; Raman, P.; Lipovsky, A.I.; Souza, A.L.; Triantafellow, E.; Ma, Q.; Gorski, R.; Cleaver, S.; et al. Activation of a metabolic gene regulatory network downstream of mTOR complex 1. *Mol. Cell* **2010**, *39*, 171–183. [CrossRef] [PubMed]

34. Peterson, T.R.; Sengupta, S.S.; Harris, T.E.; Carmack, A.E.; Kang, S.A.; Balderas, E.; Guertin, D.A.; Madden, K.L.; Carpenter, A.E.; Finck, B.N.; et al. mTOR complex 1 regulates lipin 1 localization to control the SREBP pathway. *Cell* **2011**, *146*, 408–420. [CrossRef]

35. Holz, M.K.; Ballif, B.A.; Gygi, S.P.; Blenis, J. mTOR and S6K1 mediate assembly of the translation preinitiation complex through dynamic protein interchange and ordered phosphorylation events. *Cell* **2005**, *123*, 569–580. [CrossRef] [PubMed]

36. Dorrello, N.V.; Peschiaroli, A.; Guardavaccaro, D.; Colburn, N.H.; Sherman, N.E.; Pagano, M. S6K1- and betaTRCP-mediated degradation of PDCD4 promotes protein translation and cell growth. *Science* **2006**, *314*, 467–471. [CrossRef] [PubMed]

37. Brunn, G.J.; Hudson, C.C.; Sekulic, A.; Williams, J.M.; Hosoi, H.; Houghton, P.J.; Lawrence, J.C., Jr.; Abraham, R.T. Phosphorylation of the translational repressor PHAS-I by the mammalian target of rapamycin. *Science* **1997**, *277*, 99–101. [CrossRef]

38. Gingras, A.C.; Gygi, S.P.; Raught, B.; Polakiewicz, R.D.; Abraham, R.T.; Hoekstra, M.F.; Aebersold, R.; Sonenberg, N. Regulation of 4E-BP1 phosphorylation: A novel two-step mechanism. *Genes Dev.* **1999**, *13*, 1422–1437. [CrossRef]

39. Richter, J.D.; Sonenberg, N. Regulation of cap-dependent translation by eIF4E inhibitory proteins. *Nature* **2005**, *433*, 477–480. [CrossRef]

40. Spilka, R.; Ernst, C.; Mehta, A.K.; Haybaeck, J. Eukaryotic translation initiation factors in cancer development and progression. *Cancer Lett.* **2013**, *340*, 9–21. [CrossRef]

41. Ben-Sahra, I.; Hoxhaj, G.; Ricoult, S.J.H.; Asara, J.M.; Manning, B.D. mTORC1 induces purine synthesis through control of the mitochondrial tetrahydrofolate cycle. *Science* **2016**, *351*, 728–733. [CrossRef] [PubMed]

42. Ben-Sahra, I.; Howell, J.J.; Asara, J.M.; Manning, B.D. Stimulation of de novo pyrimidine synthesis by growth signaling through mTOR and S6K1. *Science* **2013**, *339*, 1323–1328. [CrossRef] [PubMed]

43. Roczniak-Ferguson, A.; Petit, C.S.; Froehlich, F.; Qian, S.; Ky, J.; Angarola, B.; Walther, T.C.; Ferguson, S.M. The transcription factor TFEB links mTORC1 signaling to transcriptional control of lysosome homeostasis. *Sci. Signal.* **2012**, *5*, ra42. [CrossRef] [PubMed]

44. Kim, J.; Kundu, M.; Viollet, B.; Guan, K.L. AMPK and mTOR regulate autophagy through direct phosphorylation of Ulk1. *Nat. Cell Biol.* **2011**, *13*, 132–141. [CrossRef] [PubMed]

45. Sarbassov, D.D.; Guertin, D.A.; Ali, S.M.; Sabatini, D.M. Phosphorylation and regulation of Akt/PKB by the rictor-mTOR complex. *Science* **2005**, *307*, 1098–1101. [CrossRef] [PubMed]

46. Sarbassov, D.D.; Ali, S.M.; Kim, D.H.; Guertin, D.A.; Latek, R.R.; Erdjument-Bromage, H.; Tempst, P.; Sabatini, D.M. Rictor, a novel binding partner of mTOR, defines a rapamycin-insensitive and raptor-independent pathway that regulates the cytoskeleton. *Curr. Biol.* **2004**, *14*, 1296–1302. [CrossRef] [PubMed]

47. Gan, X.; Wang, J.; Wang, C.; Sommer, E.; Kozasa, T.; Srinivasula, S.; Alessi, D.; Offermanns, S.; Simon, M.I.; Wu, D. PRR5L degradation promotes mTORC2-mediated PKC-delta phosphorylation and cell migration downstream of Galpha12. *Nat. Cell Biol.* **2012**, *14*, 686–696. [CrossRef]

48. Li, X.; Gao, T. mTORC2 phosphorylates protein kinase Czeta to regulate its stability and activity. *EMBO Rep.* **2014**, *15*, 191–198.

49. Thomanetz, V.; Angliker, N.; Cloetta, D.; Lustenberger, R.M.; Schweighauser, M.; Oliveri, F.; Suzuki, N.; Ruegg, M.A. Ablation of the mTORC2 component rictor in brain or Purkinje cells affects size and neuron morphology. *J. Cell Biol.* **2013**, *201*, 293–308. [CrossRef]

50. Garcia-Martinez, J.M.; Alessi, D.R. mTOR complex 2 (mTORC2) controls hydrophobic motif phosphorylation and activation of serum- and glucocorticoid-induced protein kinase 1 (SGK1). *Biochem. J.* **2008**, *416*, 375–385. [CrossRef]

51. Fumarola, C.; Bonelli, M.A.; Petronini, P.G.; Alfieri, R.R. Targeting PI3K/AKT/mTOR pathway in non small cell lung cancer. *Biochem. Pharmacol.* **2014**, *90*, 197–207. [CrossRef] [PubMed]

52. Knight, S.D.; Adams, N.D.; Burgess, J.L.; Chaudhari, A.M.; Darcy, M.G.; Donatelli, C.A.; Luengo, J.I.; Newlander, K.A.; Parrish, C.A.; Ridgers, L.H.; et al. Discovery of GSK2126458, a Highly Potent Inhibitor of PI3K and the Mammalian Target of Rapamycin. *ACS Med. Chem. Lett.* **2010**, *1*, 39–43. [CrossRef] [PubMed]

53. Populo, H.; Lopes, J.M.; Soares, P. The mTOR signalling pathway in human cancer. *Int. J. Mol. Sci.* **2012**, *13*, 1886–1918. [CrossRef] [PubMed]

54. Paquette, M.; El-Houjeiri, L.; Pause, A. mTOR Pathways in Cancer and Autophagy. *Cancers* **2018**, *10*, 18. [CrossRef]

55. Ilagan, E.; Manning, B.D. Emerging role of mTOR in the response to cancer therapeutics. *Trends Cancer* **2016**, *2*, 241–251. [CrossRef] [PubMed]

56. Iyer, G.; Hanrahan, A.J.; Milowsky, M.I.; Al-Ahmadie, H.; Scott, S.N.; Janakiraman, M.; Pirun, M.; Sander, C.; Socci, N.D.; Ostrovnaya, I.; et al. Genome sequencing identifies a basis for everolimus sensitivity. *Science* **2012**, *338*, 221. [CrossRef] [PubMed]

57. Wagle, N.; Grabiner, B.C.; Van Allen, E.M.; Amin-Mansour, A.; Taylor-Weiner, A.; Rosenberg, M.; Gray, N.; Barletta, J.A.; Guo, Y.; Swanson, S.J.; et al. Response and acquired resistance to everolimus in anaplastic thyroid cancer. *N. Engl. J. Med.* **2014**, *371*, 1426–1433. [CrossRef]

58. Grabiner, B.C.; Nardi, V.; Birsoy, K.; Possemato, R.; Shen, K.; Sinha, S.; Jordan, A.; Beck, A.H.; Sabatini, D.M. A diverse array of cancer-associated MTOR mutations are hyperactivating and can predict rapamycin sensitivity. *Cancer Discov.* **2014**, *4*, 554–563. [CrossRef]

59. Wagle, N.; Grabiner, B.C.; Van Allen, E.M.; Hodis, E.; Jacobus, S.; Supko, J.G.; Stewart, M.; Choueiri, T.K.; Gandhi, L.; Cleary, J.M.; et al. Activating mTOR mutations in a patient with an extraordinary response on a phase I trial of everolimus and pazopanib. *Cancer Discov.* **2014**, *4*, 546–553. [CrossRef]

60. Bissler, J.J.; McCormack, F.X.; Young, L.R.; Elwing, J.M.; Chuck, G.; Leonard, J.M.; Schmithorst, V.J.; Laor, T.; Brody, A.S.; Bean, J.; et al. Sirolimus for Angiomyolipoma in Tuberous Sclerosis Complex or Lymphangioleiomyomatosis. *N. Engl. J. Med.* **2008**, *358*, 140–151. [CrossRef]

61. Krueger, D.A.; Care, M.M.; Holland, K.; Agricola, K.; Tudor, C.; Mangeshkar, P.; Wilson, K.A.; Byars, A.; Sahmoud, T.; Franz, D.N. Everolimus for subependymal giant-cell astrocytomas in tuberous sclerosis. *N. Engl. J. Med.* **2010**, *363*, 1801–1811. [CrossRef] [PubMed]

62. Franz, D.N.; Leonard, J.; Tudor, C.; Chuck, G.; Care, M.; Sethuraman, G.; Dinopoulos, A.; Thomas, G.; Crone, K.R. Rapamycin causes regression of astrocytomas in tuberous sclerosis complex. *Ann. Neurol.* **2006**, *59*, 490–498. [CrossRef]

63. Davies, D.M.; de Vries, P.J.; Johnson, S.R.; McCartney, D.L.; Cox, J.A.; Serra, A.L.; Watson, P.C.; Howe, C.J.; Doyle, T.; Pointon, K.; et al. Sirolimus therapy for angiomyolipoma in tuberous sclerosis and sporadic lymphangioleiomyomatosis: A phase 2 trial. *Clin. Cancer Res.* **2011**, *17*, 4071–4081. [CrossRef] [PubMed]

64. Klümpen, H.J.; Queiroz, K.C.; Spek, C.A.; van Noesel, C.J.; Brink, H.C.; de Leng, W.W.; de Wilde, R.F.; Mathus-Vliegen, E.M.; Offerhaus, G.J.A.; Alleman, M.A.; et al. mTOR Inhibitor Treatment of Pancreatic Cancer in a Patient With Peutz-Jeghers Syndrome. *J. Clin. Oncol.* **2011**, *29*, e150–e153. [CrossRef] [PubMed]

65. Wagner, A.J.; Malinowska-Kolodziej, I.; Morgan, J.A.; Qin, W.; Fletcher, C.D.; Vena, N.; Ligon, A.H.; Antonescu, C.R.; Ramaiya, N.H.; Demetri, G.D.; et al. Clinical Activity of mTOR Inhibition With Sirolimus in Malignant Perivascular Epithelioid Cell Tumors: Targeting the Pathogenic Activation of mTORC1 in Tumors. *J. Clin. Oncol.* **2010**, *28*, 835–840. [CrossRef] [PubMed]

66. Meng, L.; Zheng, X.S. Toward rapamycin analog (rapalog)-based precision cancer therapy. *Acta Pharmacol. Sin.* **2015**, *36*, 1163–1169. [CrossRef] [PubMed]

67. Li, J.; Kim, S.G.; Blenis, J. Rapamycin: One Drug, Many Effects. *Cell Metab.* **2014**, *19*, 373–379. [CrossRef]

68. Kelsey, I.; Manning, B.D. mTORC1 status dictates tumor response to targeted therapeutics. *Sci. Signal.* **2013**, *6*, pe31. [CrossRef]

69. White, E.; DiPaola, R.S. The double–edged sword of autophagy modulation in cancer. *Clin. Cancer Res.* **2009**, *15*, 5308–5316. [CrossRef]

70. Sanger, F.; Nicklen, S.; Coulson, A.R. DNA sequencing with chain–terminating inhibitors. *Proc. Natl. Acad. Sci. USA* **1977**, *74*, 5463–5467. [CrossRef]

71. Muzzey, D.; Evans, E.A.; Lieber, C. Understanding the Basics of NGS: From Mechanism to Variant Calling. *Curr. Genet. Med. Rep.* **2015**, *3*, 158–165. [CrossRef]

72. Ku, C.S.; Roukos, D.H. From next–generation sequencing to nanopore sequencing technology: paving the way to personalized genomic medicine. *Exp. Rev. Med. Devices* **2013**, *10*, 1–6. [CrossRef] [PubMed]

73. Lahens, N.F.; Ricciotti, E.; Smirnova, O.; Toorens, E.; Kim, E.J.; Baruzzo, G.; Hayer, K.E.; Ganguly, T.; Schug, J.; Grant, G.R. A comparison of Illumina and Ion Torrent sequencing platforms in the context of differential gene expression. *BMC Genom.* **2017**, *18*, 602. [CrossRef]

74. Kamps, R.; Brandao, R.D.; Bosch, B.J.; Paulussen, A.D.; Xanthoulea, S.; Blok, M.J.; Romano, A. Next–Generation Sequencing in Oncology: Genetic Diagnosis, Risk Prediction and Cancer Classification. *Int. J. Mol. Sci.* **2017**, *18*. [CrossRef] [PubMed]

75. mTOR Pathway. Available online: http://www.addgene.org/cancer/mtor--pathway/#gene--list (accessed on 20 December 2018).

76. Del Vecchio, F.; Mastroiaco, V.; Di Marco, A.; Compagnoni, C.; Capece, D.; Zazzeroni, F.; Capalbo, C.; Alesse, E.; Tessitore, A. Next–generation sequencing: Recent applications to the analysis of colorectal cancer. *J. Transl. Med.* **2017**, *15*, 246. [CrossRef] [PubMed]

77. Landolt, L.; Marti, H.P.; Beisland, C.; Flatberg, A.; Eikrem, O.S. RNA extraction for RNA sequencing of archival renal tissues. *Scand. J. Clin. Lab. Investig.* **2016**, *76*, 426–434. [CrossRef] [PubMed]

78. AmpliSeq for Illumina Focus Panel Data Sheet. Available online: https://science--docs.illumina.com/documents/LibraryPrep/ampliseq--focus--panel--data--sheet--770--2017--027/Content/Source/Library--Prep/AmpliSeq/focus--panel/ampliseq--focus--panel--data--sheet.htm (accessed on 20 December 2018).

79. Forbes, S.A.; Beare, D.; Boutselakis, H.; Bamford, S.; Bindal, N.; Tate, J.; Cole, C.G.; Ward, S.; Dawson, E.; Ponting, L.; et al. COSMIC: somatic cancer genetics at high–resolution. *Nucleic Acids Res* **2017**, *45*, D777–D783. [CrossRef]

80. COSMIC—Catalogue of Somatic Mutations in Cancer. Available online: https://cancer.sanger.ac.uk/cosmic (accessed on 24 January 2019).

81. Hyman, D.M.; Smyth, L.M.; Donoghue, M.T.A.; Westin, S.N.; Bedard, P.L.; Dean, E.J.; Bando, H.; El–Khoueiry, A.B.; Perez–Fidalgo, J.A.; Mita, A.; et al. AKT Inhibition in Solid Tumors with AKT1 Mutations. *J. Clin. Oncol.* **2017**, *35*, 2251–2259. [CrossRef]

82. Comtesse, N.; Keller, A.; Diesinger, I.; Bauer, C.; Kayser, K.; Huwer, H.; Lenhof, H.P.; Meese, E. Frequent overexpression of the genes FXR1, CLAPM1 and EFI4G located on amplicon 3q26-27 in squamous cell carcinoma of the lung. *Int. J. Cancer* **2007**, *120*, 2538–2544. [CrossRef]

83. Cheng, F.; Zhao, J.; Hanker, A.B.; Brewer, M.R.; Arteaga, C.L.; Zhao, Z. Transcriptome- and proteome-oriented identification of dysregulated eIF4G, STAT3 and Hippo pathways altered by PIK3CA H1047R in HER2/ER-positive breast cancer. *Breast Cancer Res. Treat.* **2016**, *160*, 457–474. [CrossRef]

84. Sato, T.; Nakashima, A.; Guo, L.; Coffman, K.; Tamanoi, F. Single amino-acid changes that confer constitutive activation of mTOR are discovered in human cancer. *Oncogene* **2010**, *29*, 2746–2752. [CrossRef] [PubMed]

85. Philpott, C.; Tovell, H.; Frayling, I.M.; Cooper, D.N.; Upadhyaya, M. The NF1 somatic mutational landscape in sporadic human cancers. *Hum. Genom.* **2017**, *11*, 13. [CrossRef] [PubMed]

86. Kiuru, M.; Busam, K.J. The NF1 gene in tumor syndromes and melanoma. *Lab. Investig.* **2017**, *97*, 146–157. [CrossRef] [PubMed]

87. Sawa, K.; Koh, Y.; Kawaguchi, T.; Kambayashi, S.; Asai, K.; Mitsuoka, S.; Kimura, T.; Yoshimura, N.; Yoshimoto, N.; Kubo, A.; et al. PIK3CA mutation as a distinctive genetic feature of non-small cell lung cancer with chronic obstructive pulmonary disease: A comprehensive mutational analysis from a multi-institutional cohort. *Lung Cancer* **2017**, *112*, 96–101. [CrossRef]

88. Mei, Z.B.; Duan, C.Y.; Li, C.B.; Cui, L.; Ogino, S. Prognostic role of tumor PIK3CA mutation in colorectal cancer: A systematic review and meta-analysis. *Ann. Oncol.* **2016**, *27*, 1836–1848. [CrossRef]

89. Dirican, E.; Akkiprik, M.; Ozer, A. Mutation distribution and clinical correlations of PIK3CA gene mutations in breast cancer. *Tumour Biol.* **2016**, *37*, 7033–7045. [CrossRef]

90. Lim, S.M.; Park, H.S.; Kim, S.; Ali, S.M.; Greenbowe, J.R.; Yang, I.S.; Kwon, N.J.; Lee, J.L.; Ryu, M.H.; Ahn, J.H.; et al. Next-generation sequencing reveals somatic mutations that conver exceptional response to everolimus. *Oncotarget* **2016**, *7*, 10547–10556. [CrossRef] [PubMed]

91. Liu, P.; Morrison, C.; Wang, L.; Xiong, D.; Vedell, P.; Cui, P.; Hua, X.; Ding, F.; Lu, Y.; James, M.; et al. Identification of somatic mutations in non-small cell lung carcinomas using whole-exome sequencing. *Carcinogenesis* **2012**, *33*, 1270–1276. [CrossRef]

92. Cheung, L.W.; Mills, G.B. Targeting therapeutic liabilities engendered by PIK3R1 mutations for cancer treatment. *Pharmacogenomics* **2016**, *17*, 297–307. [PubMed]

93. Isakov, N. Protein Kinase C (PKC) isoforms in cancer, tumor promotion and tumor suppression. *Semin. Cancer Biol.* **2018**, *48*, 36–52. [CrossRef] [PubMed]

94. Smith, I.N.; Briggs, J.M. Structural mutation analysis of PTEN and its genotype-phenotype correlations in endometriosis and cancer. *Proteins* **2016**, *84*, 1625–1643. [PubMed]

95. Malaney, P.; Uversky, V.N.; Dave, V. PTEN proteoforms in biology and disease. *Cell. Mol. Life Sci.* **2017**, *74*, 2783–2794. [CrossRef] [PubMed]

96. Javle, M.; Rashid, A.; Churi, C.; Kar, S.; Zuo, M.; Eterovic, A.K.; Nogueras–Gonzalez, G.M.; Janku, F.; Shroff, R.T.; Aloia, T.A.; et al. Molecular characterization of gallbladder cancer using somatic mutation profiling. *Hum. Pathol.* **2014**, *45*, 701–708. [CrossRef] [PubMed]

97. Kamp, W.M.; Wang, P.Y.; Hwang, P.M. TP53 mutation, mitochondria and cancer. *Curr. Opin. Genet. Dev.* **2016**, *38*, 16–22. [CrossRef] [PubMed]

98. Te Raa, G.D.; Kater, A.P. TP53 dysfunction in CLL: Implications for prognosis and treatment. *Best Pract. Res. Clin. Haematol.* **2016**, *29*, 90–99. [CrossRef] [PubMed]

99. Ho, D.W.H.; Chan, L.K.; Chiu, Y.T.; Xu, I.M.J.; Poon, R.T.P.; Cheung, T.T.; Tang, C.N.; Tang, V.W.L.; Lo, I.L.O.; Lam, P.W.Y.; et al. TSC1/2 mutations define a molecular subset of HCC with aggressive behaviour and treatment implication. *Gut* **2017**, *66*, 1496–1506. [CrossRef] [PubMed]

100. Ma, M.; Dai, J.; Xu, T.; Yu, S.; Yu, H.; Tang, H.; Yan, J.; Wu, X.; Yu, J.; Chi, Z.; et al. Analysis of TSC1 mutation spectrum in mucosal melanoma. *J. Cancer Res. Clin. Oncol.* **2018**, *144*, 257–267. [CrossRef]

101. Martin, K.R.; Zhou, W.; Bowman, M.J.; Shih, J.; Au, K.S.; Dittenhafer-Reed, K.E.; Sisson, K.A.; Koeman, J.; Weisenberger, D.J.; Cottingham, S.L.; et al. The genomic landscape of tuberous sclerosis complex. *Nat. Commun.* **2017**, *8*, 15816. [CrossRef]

102. Kim, W.Y.; Kaelin, W.G. Role of VHL gene mutation in human cancer. *J. Clin. Oncol.* **2004**, *22*, 4991–5004. [CrossRef]

103. Xu, J.; Pham, C.G.; Albanese, S.K.; Dong, Y.; Oyama, T.; Lee, C.H.; Rodrik–Outmezguine, V.; Yao, Z.; Han, S.; Chen, D.; et al. Mechanistically distinct cancer-associated mTOR activation clusters predict sensitivity to rapamycin. *J. Clin. Investig.* **2016**, *126*, 3526–3540. [CrossRef]

104. Golob–Schwarzl, N.; Schweiger, C.; Koller, C.; Krassnig, S.; Gogg–Kamerer, M.; Gantenbein, N.; Toeglhofer, A.M.; Wodlej, C.; Bergler, H.; Pertschy, B.; et al. Separation of low and high grade colon and rectum carcinoma by eukaryotic translation initiation factors 1, 5 and 6. *Oncotarget* **2017**, *8*, 101224–101243. [CrossRef] [PubMed]

105. Spilka, R.; Laimer, K.; Bachmann, F.; Spizzo, G.; Vogetseder, A.; Wieser, M.; Muller, H.; Haybaeck, J.; Obrist, P. Overexpression of eIF3a in Squamous Cell Carcinoma of the Oral Cavity and Its Putative Relation to Chemotherapy Response. *J. Oncol.* **2012**, *2012*, 901956. [CrossRef] [PubMed]

106. Spilka, R.; Ernst, C.; Bergler, H.; Rainer, J.; Flechsig, S.; Vogetseder, A.; Lederer, E.; Benesch, M.; Brunner, A.; Geley, S.; et al. eIF3a is over–expressed in urinary bladder cancer and influences its phenotype independent of translation initiation. *Cell. Oncol. (Dordrecht)* **2014**, *37*, 253–267. [CrossRef] [PubMed]

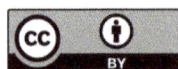

International Journal of
Molecular Sciences

MDPI

Review

Role of mTOR Signaling in Tumor Microenvironment: An Overview

Fabiana Conciatori [1], **Chiara Bazzichetto** [1,2], **Italia Falcone** [1], **Sara Pilotto** [3], **Emilio Bria** [4], **Francesco Cognetti** [1], **Michele Milella** [1] and **Ludovica Ciuffreda** [1,*]

1   Medical Oncology 1, IRCCS Regina Elena National Cancer Institute, Rome 00144, Italy; fabiana.conciatori@ifo.gov.it (F.C.); chiara.bazzichetto@ifo.gov.it (C.B.); italia.falcone@ifo.gov.it (I.F.); francesco.cognetti@ifo.gov.it (F.C.); michele.milella@ifo.gov.it (M.M.)
2   Department of Molecular Medicine, University of Rome, La Sapienza, Rome 00185, Italy
3   Department Medical Oncology Unit, Azienda Ospedaliera Universitaria Integrata, University of Verona, Verona 37100, Italy; sara.pilotto.85@gmail.com
4   Medical Oncology, Fondazione Policlinico Universitario "A. Gemelli" IRCCS Università Cattolica del Sacro Cuore, Rome 00168, Italy; emilio.bria@unicat.it
*   Correspondence: ludovica.ciuffreda@ifo.gov.it; Tel.: +39-06-5266-5185

Received: 11 July 2018; Accepted: 15 August 2018; Published: 19 August 2018

Abstract: The mammalian target of rapamycin (mTOR) pathway regulates major processes by integrating a variety of exogenous cues, including diverse environmental inputs in the tumor microenvironment (TME). In recent years, it has been well recognized that cancer cells co-exist and co-evolve with their TME, which is often involved in drug resistance. The mTOR pathway modulates the interactions between the stroma and the tumor, thereby affecting both the tumor immunity and angiogenesis. The activation of mTOR signaling is associated with these pro-oncogenic cellular processes, making mTOR a promising target for new combination therapies. This review highlights the role of mTOR signaling in the characterization and the activity of the TME's elements and their implications in cancer immunotherapy.

Keywords: mTOR; tumor microenvironment; angiogenesis; immunotherapy

1. Introduction

The mammalian target of rapamycin (mTOR) forms two functionally and structurally distinct multi-component complexes, named mTOR complex 1 (mTORC1) and mTOR complex 2 (mTORC2). These two complexes regulate several physiological processes, such as protein synthesis, biosynthesis of macromolecules, cytoskeleton remodeling, angiogenesis, homeostasis, survival, metabolism, autophagy, and response to stress [1]. Because of its key role in cell growth and differentiation, its deregulation is implicated in pathological conditions including neoplastic transformation and progression, such as in breast, gastrointestinal, liver, and prostate cancers [2].

Moreover, the mTOR pathway is involved in the differentiation, function, and metabolic regulation of adaptive/innate immune cells, as demonstrated by the use of rapamycin in clinical practice as an immune suppressant in organ transplant patients. Indeed, mTOR may regulate the activity of immune cells, such as macrophages and T cells, by regulating the expression of the inflammatory factors, such as cytokines/chemokines (i.e., interleukin (IL)-10, transforming growth factor (TGF)-β) and/or membrane receptors (i.e., Cytotoxic T-Lymphocyte protein 4 (CTLA-4) and Programmed Death 1 (PD-1)) [3]. The immune cells, recruited in the tumor microenvironment (TME) by the cytokines/chemokines-cytokines/chemokines receptor interactions, could exert the anti-tumor functions or promote cancer cells' growth. Thus, inflammation plays a central role in the tumor dynamic and represents one of the hallmarks of cancer [4].

Along with the immune system, tumor vasculature is a key component of TME and can influence the tumor behavior and drug treatment; mTOR is involved in the regulation of tumor-related vascular formation, through the promotion of angiogenesis [5]. One of the most prominent effects of mTOR under a hypoxic condition is the translation of hypoxia-inducible factor (HIF) 1-2. The HIF transcription factors lead to the expression of the hypoxic stress response genes, including angiogenic growth factors such as vascular endothelial growth factor (VEGF), TGF-α, and platelet-derived growth factor β (PDGF-β) [6].

The mTOR-mediated cellular metabolism is implicated in the cancer cells'–TME interactions during the tumor progression and drug resistance, suggesting that phosphoinositide 3-kinase (PI3K)-/protein kinase B (AKT)-/mTOR-blockade may have the dual benefit of reducing the cells' proliferation, migration, and survival, and enhancing the tumor immunosurveillance through both the downregulation of the immunosuppressive pathways and the activation of anti-tumor immune activities.

In this review, we describe the role of mTOR in tumor and non-tumor cells in order to better analyze the mechanisms of cancer progression and metastasis as well as drug resistance development.

2. mTOR Signaling

mTOR is an evolutionarily conserved serine/threonine kinase belonging to the PI3K-related kinase family, which integrates a variety of exogenous cues to coordinate several cellular processes, including cell growth and metabolism (Figure 1) [2,7,8].

mTOR forms two functional multiprotein complexes, mTORC1 and mTORC2, which are characterized by the different binding partners that confer distinguishing functions upon them. mTORC1 includes mTOR, raptor, proline-rich AKT substrate 40 (PRAS40), DEP domain-containing mTOR interacting protein (DEPTOR), mammalian lethal with sec13 protein 8 (mLST8), Rac1, GRp58, Tel2-interacting protein 1 (Tti1) and Telomere maintenance 2 (Tel2), while mTORC2 includes rictor, mammalian stress-activated protein kinase interacting protein 1 (mSIN1), protein observed with rictor (Protor) 1/2, proline-rich protein 5 (PRR5), and heat shock protein 70 (Hsp70), in addition to mTOR, DEPTOR, mLST8, Rac1, GRp58, and Tti1 and Tel2 [1]. In both complexes, the mTOR kinase acts as the central catalytic component, whereas the scaffolding protein mLST8, the regulatory subunit DEPTOR, and Tti1/Tel2 act as important regulators of assembly and stability. Furthermore, each complex is composed of specific components that contribute to complex regulation, substrate specificity, and subcellular localization [1].

mTORC1 is rapamycin-sensitive and its main targets are the proteins involved in mRNA translation, including the p70^{S6K1} and 4EBP-1. Conversely, mTORC2 is insensitive to rapamycin and the promotes phosphorylation of the hydrophobic motif of protein kinase B (AKT), serum and glucocorticoid kinase (SGK), and protein kinase C (PKC) [9]. The mTORC1 activity depends on diverse positive signals, such as energy levels, oxygen, amino acids, or growth factors, and regulates several processes required for cell growth and metabolism, including ribosomal biogenesis, protein translation, and autophagy. mTORC2 has been characterized as a downstream effector of the insulin/insulin growth factor (IGF)-1 signaling pathway and it is involved in the regulation of proliferation, survival, cytoskeletal remodeling, and cell migration [9–11]. In response to the insulin or growth factors, mTORC1 is mainly activated by PI3K/AKT signaling [12]; similarly, PI3K is also a key modulator of mTORC2, by promoting the binding of mTORC2 to ribosome [13]. PI3K is activated by receptor tyrosine kinases, G protein-coupled receptors, and RAS, and it acts as a kinase on the lipid second messenger phosphatidylinositol 4,5-bisphosphate (PIP2) to produce phosphatidylinositol 3,4,5-trisphosphate (PIP3), which recruits the phosphoinositide-dependent kinase-1 (PDK1) and AKT to the plasma membrane and thus activating the mTOR signaling [14]. Phosphatase and tensin homolog on chromosome 10 (PTEN) is a classical tumor suppressor and it acts as a phosphatase, by dephosphorylating PIP3 to PIP2 and thus reversing the action of PI3K and its downstream functions [15,16].

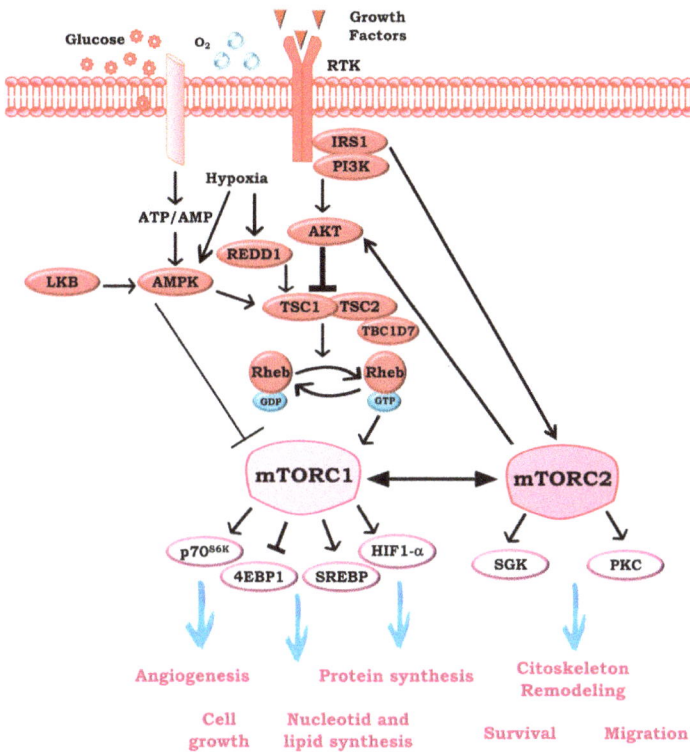

Figure 1. The mammalian target of rapamycin (mTOR) pathway. mTOR signaling is activated by extracellular signals like growth factors, nutrient, and oxygen levels via the phosphoinositide 3-kinase (PI3K)/protein kinase B (AKT) pathways. Extracellular signals may both inhibit the tuberous sclerosis complexes 1–2 (TSC1–2) to promote the accumulation of RAS homolog enriched in brain (Rheb)-GTP and the subsequent activation of mTOR complex 1 (mTORC1), and activate TSC1–2 complex to block mTORC1 by Rheb. Activation of 5′-AMP activated protein kinase β (AMPK-β) by low levels of energy results in direct phosphorylation and activation of the TSC1–2 complex. mTOR complex 1 (mTORC1) activation leads to the phosphorylation and activation of mTORC1 effector proteins ribosomal protein S6 kinase (p70^{S6K1}) and 4E-Binding Protein 1 (4EBP-1), thus resulting in initiation of specific cap-dependent translation events. Then, mTORC1 regulates cell growth and protein translation through p70^{S6K1} and 4EBP-1, as well as lipid synthesis through SREBP1, while angiogenesis through hypoxia-inducible factor (HIF)-1. The function and activation of mTORC2 is less well understood. It is thought to be activated by growth factors through the PI3K pathway and mTORC1. mTORC2 influences the cytoskeletal organization survival and migration.

Because of the key role of mTOR signaling in regulating these fundamental biological processes, the deregulation of the PI3K-AKT-mTOR pathway is tightly connected to cancer initiation and progression, and several biological investigations have focused on targeting this pathway in cancer cells, also within therapeutic combinations [1]. Interestingly, recent evidence shows that treatment with PI3K-AKT-mTOR signaling inhibitors not only affects the tumor progression, but also tumor immunosurveillance within the TME [17].

3. Tumor Microenvironment

TME is composed of the stroma and its components, different cells types, and paracrine factors (Figure 2) [18]. Mounting evidence suggests the involvement of TME in cancer progression and drug resistance; indeed, in physiological conditions, the stroma acts as a physical barrier, whereas, during carcinogenesis, the presence of tumor cells induce changes that convert the adjacent TME into a pathological entity [18,19].

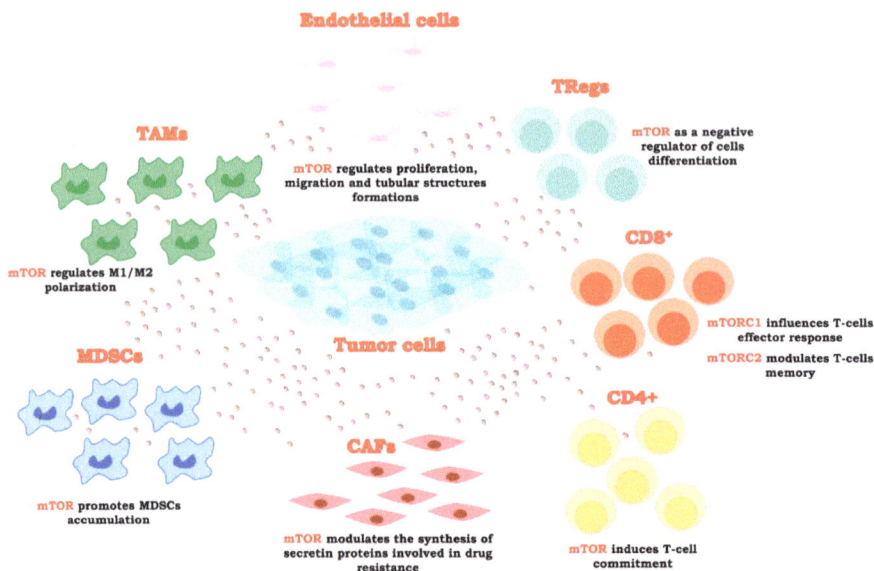

Figure 2. mTOR in characterization and the activity of the tumor microenvironment (TME) elements. mTOR signaling is involved in the modulation of several environmental inputs in TME, mainly composed by regulatory T cells (Treg), CD8+ and CD4+ lymphocytes, myeloid-derived suppressor cells (MDSCs), tumor-associated macrophages (TAMs), endothelial cells, and fibroblasts.

Several cell types contribute to the characterization of TME, including cancer and non-cancer cells [20]. Non-malignant components consist of cancer-associated fibroblasts (CAF), myeloid-derived suppressor cells (MDSCs), tumor-associated macrophages (TAM), and regulatory T cells (Treg); they all have a dynamic and tumor-promoting function during the carcinogenesis process [21,22]. CAFs are the major components of cancer stroma and promote tumorigenesis by both remodeling the extracellular matrix (ECM) and secreting cytokines [20]. The MDSCs are myeloid cells, involved in the inhibition of immune cells by releasing IL-10 and in the polarization of TAM towards a tumor-promoting phenotype [20]. Indeed, the TAMs usually display pro-tumorigenic properties and they are the major contributor to tumor angiogenesis [23]. The TAMs represent the prominent leukocytic infiltrate component in cancers and can comprise up to 50% of the cell tumor mass [24]. The cytokines in the TME directly regulate the phenotype switching of macrophages into M1 and M2 polarization, thus leading to the acquisition of distinct functional features; the M1 macrophages predominantly secrete pro-inflammatory mediators, whereas the M2 secrete the anti-inflammatory ones [25]. Numerous evidence suggest that infiltrating the macrophages switches their phenotype from the anti-tumoral M1 to pro-tumoral M2 during cancer progression, even if the TAMs are the unique polarized macrophages that express both M1 and M2 marker genes [25]. Tregs exert their suppressive activity via cell-to-cell contact (i.e., PD-1 and CTLA-4) or via the expression of soluble factors, such as TGF-β and IL-10 [26].

The ECM consists not only of a physical scaffold for TAM cells (fibrous and matricellular proteins and glycosaminoglycans), but also of the growth factors, cytokines, and hormones secreted by the stromal and tumor cells. ECM is characterized by biochemical properties specific for each tissue, and may be involved in overcoming the host's immune surveillance [18,27–29].

In TME, the complex and dynamic network of cytokines, chemokines, and growth factors drive the inter- and intra-cellular communication that may modulate tumor/stroma interaction, including immune responses; indeed, the chemokines–chemokine receptors interactions recruit different immune cells into the TME and they regulate the tumor immune responses in a spatiotemporal regulated manner [30].

The cytokines are low-molecular-weight proteins, released by cancer, immune cells, and stromal cells, such as fibroblasts and endothelial cells, in order to regulate the cell proliferation, survival, migration, and death [31]. The chemokines are a type of cytokine with chemo-attractant properties and are divided in four subfamilies (C, CC, CXC, and CX3C), based on their primary structure and function; all have the main cysteine residues in their N-terminal regions [32]. The data obtained in our laboratories have suggested that the hyperactivation of the PI3K-AKT-mTOR pathway is involved in the up-regulation of specific cyto- and chemo-kines expression (i.e., IL-8 and VEGF), thus directly affecting the TME components [33,34]. De la Iglesia, et al. demonstrated that in PTEN-loss glioblastoma, the unphosphorylated signal transducer and activator of Signal transducer and activator of transcription 3 (STAT3), which transcriptionally represses IL-8, does not bind the IL-8 promoter, thus leading to an increased transcription and expression of IL-8 gene; in this way, IL-8 promotes the glioblastoma cell proliferation and invasiveness only in a genetic PTEN-loss context [35]. This relationship between PTEN-loss and a selective upregulation of IL-8 signaling has also been demonstrated in prostate carcinoma [36].

4. Immunoregulatory Functions of mTOR

Recent studies have established an important role for mTOR in the modulation of both innate and adaptive immunity, integrating different environmental inputs within the TME. Indeed, mTOR is involved in the regulation of many immune cellular functions promoting differentiation, activation of T cells, TAMs, and antigen-presenting cells (Figure 2) [37,38]. The effects of the mTOR complexes' activation in the TME elements are summarized in Table 1.

Table 1. Role of mammalian target of rapamycin (mTOR) complexes in tumor microenvironment (TME) elements. TAM—tumor-associated macrophages (TAM); MDSC—myeloid-derived suppressor cells; CAF—cancer-associated fibroblasts; IL—interleukin; mTORC1—mTOR complex 1; ↓ indicates a decrease of activity; ↑ indicates an increase of activity.

Element of TME.	mTORC1/2 Modulation	Effects of Modulation	References
CD8+	↓ mTORC1	↓ Effector ↑ Memory	[39,40]
	↓ mTORC2	↓ Memory	[39]
CD4+	↑ mTORC1/2	↑ Th1, 2, 17 differentiation	[41–43]
Treg	↑ mTORC1	↑ Differentiation in effector-like T cells	[44]
	↑ mTORC2	↓ Differentiation	[45,46]
TAM	↑ mTORC1/2	↑ M2 polarization	[47,48]
MDSC	↓↑ mTORC1	Variable effects	[49–51]
Endothelial cells	↑ mTORC1	↑ Proliferation	[52,53]
CAF	↓ mTORC1	↓ IL-6 secretion	[54]

It is actually known that the PI3K/mTOR inhibitors have an important immunomodulatory impact on the tumor microenvironment and angiogenesis. The modulation in the number and/or function of the specific TME cells involved in tumor progression is often associated with a better outcome in cancer therapy, and for this reason, the selective inhibition of the PI3K/mTOR axis correlates not only with the efficacy in leukemias, but also improves the immunotherapy in different solid cancer [27,55]. Recent studies showed that the inhibition of different hub of PI3K/mTOR pathways impacts the different TME components (Table 2).

Table 2. mTOR-axis inhibitors and potential therapeutic benefit. PI3K—phosphoinositide 3-kinase; Treg—regulatory T cells.

Drug(s)	Target Cell Population	Functional Implication	Potential Therapeutic Benefit	References
mTOR/p110β/pan-PI3K inhibitors	CD8+	↑ CD8+ infiltration in tumor	↑ Significant survival benefit	[39,56,57]
mTORC1 inhibitor	CD4+	↓ number of CD4+	↑ Significant survival benefit	[58]
mTOR/pan-AKT inhibitors	Treg	↓ Tregs selectively	↑ Significant survival benefit	[58,59]
PI3K inhibitors	TAM	↓ TAM recruitment	Variable effects	[60]
mTOR inhibitors	MDSC	Variable effects	Variable effects	[49,51]
mTOR inhibitors	Endothelial cells	↓ proliferation, migration and tubular structures formation ↑ apoptosis	↓Angiogenesis	[33,61–63]
mTORC1 inhibitor	CAF	↓ CAF-secreted cytokines	↓ Of cell migration, invasion, and metastasis	[64]

4.1. T Lymphocytes

Emerging evidence highlights a central role for mTOR in bridging the immune signals and metabolic cues to direct lymphocyte proliferation, differentiation, and survival [65].

The lymphocyte activation increases protein, nucleotide, and lipid biosynthesis and utilizes aerobic glycolysis to generate ATP during the rapid proliferation [40,66]. The metabolic programs regulated by mTORC1 make it an important link between metabolism and immune function [40,49].

4.1.1. CD8+

CD8+ cytotoxic T cells, derived from naïve CD8+ T cells, are the major antitumor mechanism of the immune system because of their ability to target and kill cancer cells and maintain a memory response. Recently, mTOR has been identified as a regulator of memory CD8+ T cells differentiation [67]. It has been demonstrated that rapamycin modulates the CD8+ T cells induced by viral infection, showing that mTOR regulates the memory CD8+ T cells differentiation [68]. Indeed, it has been reported that mTORC1 negatively modulates the memory T cells formation [40].

Moreover, Pollizzi et al. [39] have demonstrated that mTORC1 and mTORC2 may play a different role in the regulation of CD8+ cells; mTORC1 positively influences the CD8+ T cells effector responses and glycolytic phenotype, while the mTORC2 activity is involved in the CD8+ T cells memory up-regulation. Moreover, the direct modulation of the mTOR-mediated lipid metabolism by the inactivation of the sterol regulatory element binding proteins (SREBP) pathway inhibits CD8+ T-cell proliferation in vitro [69].

4.1.2. CD4+

The activation of naïve T cells can result in the simultaneous expression of the tumor specific antigens, Th (T helper) 1, 17, and 2, and it is now clear that mTORC1 and mTORC2 promote T cells commitment [42]. Indeed, Delgoffe and collaborators demonstrated that the mTOR-deficient CD4+ T cells failed to differentiate into Th1, Th17, or Th2 effector cells in vitro or in vivo; the loss of Rheb, an upstream activator of mTORC1, inhibits the differentiation of both the Th1 and Th17 cells, whereas the Th2 cells differentiation requires mTORC1 activation but not Rheb [41,42]. The loss of Raptor induces Th17 cells differentiation [70]. According to the key role of mTOR in Th differentiation, Templeton and collaborators have demonstrated that treatment with everolimus induces a statistically significant reduction in the numbers of CD4+ and an increase in the Treg population, in a dose dependent manner in metastatic prostate cancer patients, with an increase in progression free survival [58].

Recent studies have shown that antigen stimulation causes T cells to transit from catabolism to anabolism, and mTOR regulates this process by enhancing the T cells metabolic activity [71]. In antigen-stimulated T cells, the mTOR activates the glycolytic program inducing the expression of MYC and HIF-1α, which in turn mediates the expression of glycolytic enzymes and transporters [72,73].

4.1.3. Treg

The forkhead box 3+ (FOXO3+) Tregs suppress inflammation and have an important role in tumor immunity through their role as a suppressor of the effector T cells. High numbers of Treg and a reduction of the CD8+ numbers in the tumor infiltrate are associated with a poor prognosis [40]. The reduction of mTOR signaling induces Treg expansion through the FOXO3 expression; in fact, as opposed to the CD4+ T cells, the mTOR axis regulates the lineage commitment between effector and regulatory T cells through the STAT transcription factor activation [41,74]. Despite the well-known role of the PI3K-AKTpathway in T-cell proliferation, the AKT and PI3K blockade selectively inhibits the Tregs' proliferation with minimal effect on the other T cells' population (CD4+ and CD8+). Indeed, the in vitro and in vivo studies display that the Tregs have an increased dependence on the PI3K-AKT signaling pathway, as compared to the other T cells [59].

Interestingly, mTOR may mediate different Treg functions, as demonstrated by the pharmacological and genetic modulation of the mTOR network. Indeed, the reduction of mTORC1 activity, by the deletion of Raptor, reduces the Treg function, and conversely, the over-activation of mTORC1 reduces the FOXO3 expression and converts Treg into effettor-like T cells, in TSC1-deficient models [44]. Moreover, the activation of mTORC2 in the PTEN-loss Tregs induces a reduction in their stability and their ability to differentiate [45,46]. It has been also demonstrated that the programming of the Treg suppressive functions is dependent on mTORC1; indeed, Zeng et al. have demonstrated that mTORC1 acts as a link between the immunological signals via the T cell receptor (TCR) and IL-2 to lipogenic pathways [75].

Recently, it has been reported that mTOR also modulates the role of PD-L1 as a regulator of the development, maintenance, and function of the induced regulatory T cells [76]. PD-1 is highly expressed on Treg cells and PD-L1 is widely expressed in several stroma non-hematopoietic cells and in various tumors; Lastwika and collaborators have shown that the activation of the mTOR pathway regulates the PD-L1 expression in vitro and in vivo in lung carcinoma [77,78].

4.2. TAMs

TAMs are a class of immune cells that are present in high numbers in the TME and are recruited by soluble factors (cytokines and/or chemokines) or derived from tissue-resident macrophages. TAMs are generally classified into M1 and M2, depending on their polarization; M1 TAMs are involved in phagocyte-dependent inflammation and in antitumor response, whereas M2 TAMs inhibit the phagocytic function thereby being more tolerant towards tumor growth. However, it has been demonstrated that this is a simplification of the TAM's classification; Qian et al. showed that TAMs can share both M1 and M2 phenotype and functions, thus resulting in a difficult interpretation of their role in TME [40,79,80].

Early evidence highlights the role of mTOR signaling in macrophage activation and differentiation. Indeed, Byles et al. showed that the loss of TSC1 activity in the macrophage leads to constitutive mTORC1 activation, and the consequent decrease in IL-4 production induces M2 polarization [47]. Consistent with these results, different studies demonstrated that the mTORC1 downregulation by different pharmacological and genetic approaches results in both decreased proinflammatory cytokine production by macrophages, with a consequent reduction of inflammation, and unbalances in macrophages M1 polarization [48,81]. Moreover, the role of the mTOR pathway in macrophage activity is involved not only in M1/M2 polarization, but also in processes, such as autophagy, which could indirectly influence the outcome of tumor progression. Indeed, Shan and collaborators demonstrated that rapamycin both reduces the M2 macrophage polarization by down-regulating pSTAT3 on the Tyr705 expression, and increases the autophagy [82].

Polarized macrophages also differ in terms of the cyto-/chemo-kines production, and M2 macrophages also exert their pro-tumoral activities by releasing specific cyto-/chemo-kines, which are involved in the key mechanisms in the tumor progression, such as angiogenesis [80]. Indeed, the M2 macrophages release IL-10, which in turn promotes VEGF production, and it has been demonstrated that rapamycin reduces angiogenesis by down-regulating the IL-10 and VEGF secretion [83].

mTORC2 also plays a critical role in M2 macrophages polarization; indeed, the inhibition of mTORC2 signaling in macrophages, by the deletion of rictor, reduces the differentiations of the M2 macrophages [84]. More recently, Shrivastava and colleagues demonstrated that mTORC2 up-regulates the M2 surface markers, CD206 and CD163, through the AKT axis, thus leading to an increase of the invasion and metastasis in mammary tumor models, both in in vitro and in mice [85].

4.3. MDSCs

MDSCs are a heterogeneous group of immature myeloid cells at various stages of differentiation, including precursors of macrophages, granulocytes, and dendritic cells (DC). Even if understanding the phenotypic and functional characteristics of the MDSCs is controversial, MDSCs can be classified in granulocyte or monocyte, based on the expression of Ly6C and Ly6G molecules, and play critical roles in primary and metastatic cancer progression. mTOR signaling is involved in the modulation of the MDSCs recruitment in TME, both in cancer cells and MDSCs; indeed, in cancer cells, the mTOR axis regulates the release of the soluble factors involved in the MDSCs recruitment, whereas in MDSCs, mTOR signaling affects the expression of specific antigen on their surface.

Welte et al. demonstrated that mTOR signaling promotes MDSCs accumulation by up-regulating granulocyte colony-stimulating factor (G-CSF) in breast cancer cells. Indeed, both the rapamycin treatment and the deletion of Raptor reduce the G-CSF levels [86]. Another soluble factor involved in the recruitment of MDSCs in TME is TGF-β, a cytokine that directly promotes the expression of CD39$^+$/CD73$^+$ on the surface of myeloid cells, thereby exerting tumor-promoting roles [87]. Several studies in mouse models have demonstrated that the expression of these two ectonucleotidases leads to tumor cells' evasion from cytotoxic T cells responses, and that mTOR plays a critical role in the regulation of the CD39/CD73 expression. Indeed, it has been reported that rapamycin abrogates the TGF-β-mediated induction of CD39/CD73 expression, by HIF-1α [50].

Despite the role of mTOR, described above, in enhancing pro-tumoral MDSCs accumulation, other groups demonstrate an opposite aspect of the MDSCs recruitment mTOR-mediated, highlighting the controversial function of the MDSCs in TME. Indeed, it has been demonstrated that the rapamycin treatment upregulates the recruitment and the induction of MDSCs' immunosuppressive ability, by enhancing the production of IL-1 and IL-2, and by upregulating the expression of their effectors, arginase-1 and inducible nitric oxide synthase, which prevents T-cell proliferation [51].

Moreover, MDSCs can also affect tumor progression by modulating the commitment of the TME' components. Indeed, preliminary in vitro studies indicate a potential role of MDSCs in mTOR-mediated CD8[+] T cells differentiation into effector populations [88].

5. mTOR and Angiogenesis

TME is composed not only of the cells of the immune system, but also of tumor vasculature, and angiogenesis has long been recognized as a hallmark of cancer [89]. Angiogenesis represents the mechanism by which new blood vessels develop, and it is a dynamic and tightly regulated process, mainly induced by hypoxia [27]. During the tumor progression, pathological angiogenesis is driven by the presence of pro-angiogenic factors in TME, such as VEGF-A and IL-8. Several cells, including tumor and tumor-associated stromal cells (such as endothelial cell and macrophages), are involved in this process, in part, by secreting growth factors and cytokines [27].

The VEGF/VEGF receptor (VEGFR) axis is one of the key regulators of angiogenesis, as demonstrated by the use of anti-VEGF/VEGFR drugs, to inhibit angiogenesis in cancer therapy, and it is regulated, among others, by the PI3K-AKT-mTOR signaling pathway [33,90]. Indeed, mTORC1 regulates the HIF-1/HIF-2, which are the transcription factors for the hypoxic stress response genes, including VEGF and TGF-α [6,91]. HIF-1, the predominant form, is a heterodimer consisting of HIF-1α and HIF-1β subunits; although HIF-1β is constitutively expressed, the stability of HIF-1α is dependent on oxygen levels [92]. In the presence of O_2, the ubiquitination of HIF-1α induces its degradation by the 26S proteasome, whereas under hypoxic conditions, the accumulation of the HIF-1α subunit is because of a decrease in the rate of proteolytic degradation [92].

In addition to the HIF protein stability regulation, other mechanisms of the HIF-1α expression have been proposed at different levels, such as mRNA transcription and translation [93]. Recently, Dodd and colleagues demonstrated that mTORC1 enhances the transcription of HIF-1α mRNA, by directly phosphorylating STAT3 at Ser727 [94]. The same group also showed that mTORC1 regulates the HIF-1α translation, through the activity of both p70^{S6K1} and elongation initiation factor (EIF)-4E binding protein 1 (4E-BP1) [94]. Conversely, several studies reported that long-lasting hypoxic conditions downregulate mTORC1 activity, by activating the negative mTORC1 regulators tuberous sclerosis complex TSC1–2 or 5′-AMP activated protein Kinase β (AMPK-β), which in turn phosphorylates Raptor on Ser722/792 [95,96].

This tight connection between the mTOR pathway and angiogenesis regulation is also maintained in endothelial cells, as demonstrated by the effects of the mTOR inhibitors. Indeed, several groups showed that rapamycin displays anti-angiogenic properties in terms of a reduction of the proliferation, migration, tubular structures formation and an increase of apoptosis [61–63]. Our previous data also demonstrated that the mTOR inhibitor temsirolimus inhibits serum- and/or VEGF-driven endothelial cell proliferation and vessel formation in vitro and in vivo [33]. Specific knock-down experiments of mTORC1/2 interactors in endothelial cells confirmed the role of mTOR in angiogenesis; indeed, knocking-down TSC1, a negative regulator of mTORC1, increases the proliferation of endothelial cells, whereas the deletion of rictor, a positive regulator of mTORC1, reduces cell proliferation [52,53].

As reviewed by De Palma and others, hematopoietic-derived tumor-infiltrating cells also regulate angiogenesis, by releasing growth factors and inflammatory cytokines in the TME [27]. Among them, TAMs play a critical role in tumor angiogenesis, because they exert a dual role, in both the inhibition and activation of angiogenesis [97]. Interestingly, even in TAMs, the mTOR activity displays a key role in promoting angiogenesis and polarization into the M1 phenotype [81]. Moreover, macrophages secrete pro-angiogenic factors such as VEGF-A, IL-1β, IL-8, and metalloproteases (MMP) 2 and 9, which are released also by other tumor infiltrating cells, such as neutrophils, eosinophils, natural killers, and CAFs [27]. O_2 deprivation in specific tumor areas is a critical cue for the accumulation of TAMs, which are recruited by a hypoxia-induced chemoattractant gradient, such as VEGF, and endothelins [24].

Even if mTOR is a key regulator of HIF-1, the activation of other signaling pathways, which converge on the targets shared with the PI3K network, can also promote tumor angiogenesis. For example, the epidermal growth factor receptor (EGFR) activation increases the transcription of VEGF via the PI3K pathway, but not dependently on HIF-1, in glioblastoma cells; moreover, the EGFR amplification has an additive effect with a PTEN loss of function in increasing the VEGF levels, by enhancing the VEGF promoter activity [98,99]. Zundel and colleagues have demonstrated that in glioblastoma cell lines, a loss of PTEN results in HIF-1 stabilization which in turn causes the up-regulation of VEGF expression [100]. The loss of PTEN is a common mechanism of PI3K activation in several cancers, and its association with higher levels of secreted VEGF was observed also in other cancer cell lines with a different histological origin, such as pancreatic and prostate cancer cells, suggesting that PTEN plays a critical role in angiogenesis and tumorigenesis [101,102].

6. mTOR in CAFs Regulation

CAFs are cellular components of the stroma derived from the activated quiescent fibroblasts surrounding cancer cells, that directly promote tumor initiation, progression and metastasis by secreting growth factors, cytokines, and a large number of metabolites [103–105]. Moreover, the CAFs regulate normal epithelial differentiation and homeostasis, and cancer progression, particularly in stroma-rich tumors, like pancreatic cancers [106]. Indeed, in pancreatic ductal adenocarcinoma (PDAC), the stroma forms more than 80% of the tumor mass, and the CAFs express α-SMA (alpha-smooth muscle actin) and are also called activated pancreatic stellate cells [106]. Several studies demonstrated that CAFs display pro-tumorigenic properties by promoting invasion and metastasis in a non-vascular manner [107,108].

Similarly, recent evidence has showed that pancreatic CAFs may be involved in resistance to anticancer drugs [109,110]. Indeed, Duluc et al. demonstrated that, in pancreatic CAFs, the PI3K/mTOR pathway is activated by the autocrine secretion of PDGF and Janus kinase (JAK)2-dependent cytokines [54]. The CAFs also express the sst1 somatostatin receptor, whose activation inhibits the mTOR/4E-BP1 pathway, which in turn modulates the synthesis of the secreted proteins involved in the resistance to cancer drug therapies, including IL-6 and STAT3, and could be a possible upstream regulator of the IL-6 expression. These results suggest that counteracting the mTOR/IL-6 driven resistance might increase the effectiveness of the anticancer therapy [54,111]. Moreover, the specific inhibition of mTORC1 can also reverse the CAF-induced resistance through JAK/STAT3-, ERK- and AKT-signaling. Everolimus treatment, indeed, induces a significant reduction of the secretion of cytokines, such as IL-8, IL-13, and MCP-1, which are involved in the promotion of tumor cells' proliferation and migration [64].

Wang et al. demonstrated that CAFs promoted irradiated cancer cell recovery through the increase of autophagy, thus causing a tumor relapse after radiation therapy. Indeed, they ensured that CAFs, through the production of IGF1/2, IL-12, and β-hydroxybutyrate, were capable of inducing autophagy in cancer cells post-radiation, thus increasing the level of reactive oxygen species (ROS), which in turn enhances protein phosphatase 2 (PP2)A activity, blocks mTORC1 activation, and induces autophagy in cancer cells [112].

7. Implications in Cancer Immunotherapy

In addition to the central role of the PI3K/AKT/mTOR signaling network dysregulation in cancer cells, recent evidence highlights that targeting this pathway can also impact on the host immunity [17]. In the past years, the host's immune system has become a target for the development of new therapeutic strategies, such as immunomodulatory drugs or monoclonal antibodies, and cancer immunotherapy has achieved remarkable clinical efficacy in the treatment of many cancer patients, by promoting the antitumor activity of the immune system [4]. More specifically, two immune checkpoints have achieved the most attention so far, as follows: the cell surface protein PD-1 is expressed by activated T cells and the binding with its two ligands, PD-L1 and PD-L2, attenuates the activity of the T cells and the effector responses; CTLA-4 is a negative regulator of T cells, by competing with the co-stimulatory molecule CD28 for the binding to the ligands CD80 and CD86 [113]. The recruitment of regulatory immune cells can also mediate immune suppression; indeed, the modulation of T cell-mediated antitumor responses represents another therapeutic strategy [114]. Although blocking these checkpoints and the T cell-mediated immunotherapy exhibit clinical success, the majority of patients still fail to respond to immunotherapy, thus understanding the molecular mechanisms of resistance remains crucial to select a specific subset of patients and improve the overall survival [115].

As highlighted above, mTOR plays a central role in coordinating the environmental stimuli and cell metabolic responses, also because of its function in immune cell homeostasis and activation, and thus represents a potential target for cancer immunotherapy [116]. The first evidence of the tight connection between mTOR and immune regulatory targets was demonstrated by the immunosuppressive properties of the mTOR inhibitor rapamycin, because of its ability to block T cells proliferation [117]. In the last years, PD-L1 regulation has become the focus of many studies and several groups demonstrated that the PI3K/AKT/mTOR pathway regulates PD-L1 in different tumors, such as in non-small cell lung cancer [78]. As PI3K activation may occur via the loss of PTEN, it has been further reported that the loss of this tumor suppressor may induce the overexpression of PD-L1 and immunoresistance in several tumors of different histological origin (i.e., glioma, leiomyosarcoma, colorectal, breast cancer, and PDAC [118–122]. Mittendorf and her group also demonstrated that treatments with either the AKT inhibitor, MK-2206, or the mTOR inhibitor, rapamycin, significantly decreases the PD-L1 mRNA transcripts in the PTEN-mutant triple-negative breast cancer cell lines [121]. More recently, it has been also demonstrated that a loss of the PTEN expression correlates with a decrease of CD8$^+$ T cells' infiltration in melanoma and poor outcomes to immunotherapies, regardless of BRAF and NRAS status [56]. As opposed to PTEN, mTORC1 displays a controversial role in CD8$^+$ T cells; indeed, the mTORC1 activity is required for their effector functions, and the inhibiting mTORC1 activity displays paradoxical immune stimulating effects by promoting memory CD8$^+$ generation in a dose- and duration-dependent manner, as well [40].

CD8$^+$ T cells are not the only regulators of the adaptive immune response involved in cancer immunotherapy; the dysregulation of CD4$^+$ Treg cells are also involved in several pathological immune diseases and drug resistance. The mTOR and dual PI3K/mTOR inhibitors have been shown to induce Tregs' expansion and their immunosuppressive activity, thus correlating with a poor prognosis in cancer patients [123]. Encouragingly, Huijts and her group showed that the PI3K inhibition alone allows for the expansion of Tregs, but without affecting their overall suppressive activity [124].

In addition to the upregulation of Treg into tumor tissues, mTOR signaling stimulates also the infiltration of MDSCs, thus allowing for it to combine immunotherapy with PI3K-AKT-mTOR pathway inhibitors. The activation of toll-like receptors (TLR) on DCs leads to their maturation, and the TLR signaling activates PI3K; this evidence highlights the synergistic effects of the combined PI3K inhibitors with TLR agonists in mouse models [125].

8. Conclusions

The PI3K/AKT/mTOR network plays a significant role in the regulation of several processes in tumor initiation and progression, by controlling the protein synthesis, proliferation, growth, and survival in cancer cells on the one hand, and by affecting the characterization and the activity of the TME's elements on the other hand. The involvement of TME in cancer progression and drug resistance is well recognized, thus leading to a necessity to better investigate the molecular mechanisms of tumor-stroma interactions (TSI). Thus, targeting the molecular mediators of TSIs, such the elements of the mTOR network, may provide an excellent strategy for therapeutic opportunities.

Funding: This research was funded by the Italian Association for Cancer Research (AIRC) (Michele Milella, IG18622; Emilio Bria IG20583), the Fondazione Cariverona (Emilio Bria and Sara Pilotto, 2015.0872), and the International Association for the Study of Lung Cancer (IASLC, Emilio Bria and Sara Pilotto).

Int. J. Mol. Sci. **2018**, *19*, 2453

Acknowledgments: Chiara Bazzichetto is a PhD student at the Doctoral School in Immunological, Hematological, and Rheumatologic Sciences.

Conflicts of Interest: The authors declare no conflict of interest.

Abbreviations

AMPK-β	$5'$-AMP activated protein kinase β
CAF	cancer-associated fibroblasts
CTLA-4	cytotoxic t-lymphocyte protein 4
DC	dendridic cell
DEPTOR	DEP domain-containing mTOR interacting protein
ECM	extracellular matrix
EGFR	epidermal growth factor receptor
FOXO	forkhead box
G-CSF	granulocyte colony-stimulating factor
HIF	hypoxia-inducible factor
Hsp70	heat shock protein 70
IGF	insulin growth factor
IL	interleukin
JAK	Janus kinase
MDSC	myeloid-derived suppressor cells
mLST8	mammalian lethal with sec13 protein 8
MMP	metalloproteases
mSIN1	mammalian stress-activated protein kinase interacting protein 1
mTOR	mammalian target of rapamycin
mTORC	mTOR complex
PD-1	programmed death 1
PDAC	pancreatic ductal adenocarcinoma
PDGF	plated-derived growth factor
PDK1	phosphoinositide-dependent kinase-1
PIP2	phosphatidylinositol 4,5-bisphosphate
PIP3	phosphatidylinositol 3,4,5-trisphosphate
PI3K	phosphoinositide 3-kinase
PKC	protein kinase C
PP2	protein phosphatase 2
PRAS40	proline-rich AKT substrate 40
PRR	proline-rich protein
Protor	protein observed with rictor
PTEN	phosphatase and tensin homolog on chromosome 10
$p70^{S6K1}$	p70 ribosomal protein S6 kinase 1
ROS	reactive oxygen species
SGK	serum and glucocorticoid kinase
SREBP	sterol regulatory element binding proteins
STAT	signal transducer and activator of transcription
TAM	tumor-associated macrophages
TCR	T cell receptor
Tel2	telomere maintenance 2
TGF	trasforming growth factor
Th	T helper
TLR	tool-like receptor
TME	tumor microenvironment
Treg	regulatory T cells
TSC	tuberous sclerosis complexes
TSI	tumor-stroma interactions

Tti1   tel2-interacting protein 1
VEGF   vascular endothelial growth factor
VEGFR   VEGF receptor
4EBP-1   4E binding protein-1

References

1. Conciatori, F.; Ciuffreda, L.; Bazzichetto, C.; Falcone, I.; Pilotto, S.; Bria, E.; Cognetti, F.; Milella, M. mTOR Cross-Talk in Cancer and Potential for Combination Therapy. *Cancers (Basel)* **2018**, *10*, 23. [CrossRef] [PubMed]

2. Saxton, R.A.; Sabatini, D.M. mTOR Signaling in Growth, Metabolism, and Disease. *Cell* **2017**, *169*, 361–371. [CrossRef] [PubMed]

3. Kim, L.C.; Cook, R.S.; Chen, J. mTORC1 and mTORC2 in cancer and the tumor microenvironment. *Oncogene* **2017**, *36*, 2191–2201. [CrossRef] [PubMed]

4. Schaaf, M.B.; Garg, A.D.; Agostinis, P. Defining the role of the tumor vasculature in antitumor immunity and immunotherapy. *Cell Death Dis.* **2018**, *9*, 115. [CrossRef] [PubMed]

5. Karar, J.; Maity, A. PI3K/AKT/mTOR Pathway in Angiogenesis. *Front. Mol. Neurosci.* **2011**, *4*, 51. [CrossRef] [PubMed]

6. Laughner, E.; Taghavi, P.; Chiles, K.; Mahon, P.C.; Semenza, G.L. HER2 (neu) signaling increases the rate of hypoxia-inducible factor 1alpha (HIF-1alpha) synthesis: Novel mechanism for HIF-1-mediated vascular endothelial growth factor expression. *Mol. Cell Biol.* **2001**, *21*, 3995–4004. [CrossRef] [PubMed]

7. Brown, E.J.; Albers, M.W.; Shin, T.B.; Ichikawa, K.; Keith, C.T.; Lane, W.S.; Schreiber, S.L. A mammalian protein targeted by G1-arresting rapamycin-receptor complex. *Nature* **1994**, *369*, 756–758. [CrossRef] [PubMed]

8. Chiu, M.I.; Katz, H.; Berlin, V. RAPT1, a mammalian homolog of yeast Tor, interacts with the FKBP12/rapamycin complex. *Proc. Natl. Acad. Sci. USA* **1994**, *91*, 12574–12578. [CrossRef] [PubMed]

9. Jacinto, E.; Loewith, R.; Schmidt, A.; Lin, S.; Ruegg, M.A.; Hall, A.; Hall, M.N. Mammalian TOR complex 2 controls the actin cytoskeleton and is rapamycin insensitive. *Nat. Cell Biol.* **2004**, *6*, 1122–1128. [CrossRef] [PubMed]

10. Sarbassov, D.D.; Ali, S.M.; Kim, D.H.; Guertin, D.A.; Latek, R.R.; Erdjument-Bromage, H.; Tempst, P.; Sabatini, D.M. Rictor, a novel binding partner of mTOR, defines a rapamycin-insensitive and raptor-independent pathway that regulates the cytoskeleton. *Curr. Biol.* **2004**, *14*, 1296–1302. [CrossRef] [PubMed]

11. Thomanetz, V.; Angliker, N.; Cloetta, D.; Lustenberger, R.M.; Schweighauser, M.; Oliveri, F.; Suzuki, N.; Ruegg, M.A. Ablation of the mTORC2 component rictor in brain or Purkinje cells affects size and neuron morphology. *J. Cell Biol.* **2013**, *201*, 293–308. [CrossRef] [PubMed]

12. Zhang, H.; Bajraszewski, N.; Wu, E.; Wang, H.; Moseman, A.P.; Dabora, S.L.; Griffin, J.D.; Kwiatkowski, D.J. PDGFRs are critical for PI3K/Akt activation and negatively regulated by mTOR. *J. Clin. Investig.* **2007**, *117*, 730–738. [CrossRef] [PubMed]

13. Willems, L.; Tamburini, J.; Chapuis, N.; Lacombe, C.; Mayeux, P.; Bouscary, D. PI3K and mTOR signaling pathways in cancer: New data on targeted therapies. *Curr. Oncol. Rep.* **2012**, *14*, 129–138. [CrossRef] [PubMed]

14. Sarbassov, D.D.; Guertin, D.A.; Ali, S.M.; Sabatini, D.M. Phosphorylation and regulation of Akt/PKB by the rictor-mTOR complex. *Science* **2005**, *307*, 1098–1101. [CrossRef] [PubMed]

15. Milella, M.; Falcone, I.; Conciatori, F.; Cesta Incani, U.; Del Curatolo, A.; Inzerilli, N.; Nuzzo, C.M.; Vaccaro, V.; Vari, S.; Cognetti, F.; et al. PTEN: Multiple Functions in Human Malignant Tumors. *Front. Oncol.* **2015**, *5*, 24. [CrossRef] [PubMed]

16. Ciuffreda, L.; McCubrey, J.A.; Milella, M. Signaling intermediates (PI3K/PTEN/AKT/mTOR and RAF/MEK/ERK pathways) as therapeutic targets for anti-cancer and anti-angiogenesis treatments. *Curr. Signal. Transd. Ther.* **2009**, *4*, 130–143. [CrossRef]

17. Xue, G.; Zippelius, A.; Wicki, A.; Mandala, M.; Tang, F.; Massi, D.; Hemmings, B.A. Integrated Akt/PKB signaling in immunomodulation and its potential role in cancer immunotherapy. *J. Natl. Cancer Inst.* **2015**, *107*, 7. [CrossRef] [PubMed]

18. Wang, M.; Zhao, J.; Zhang, L.; Wei, F.; Lian, Y.; Wu, Y.; Gong, Z.; Zhang, S.; Zhou, J.; Cao, K.; et al. Role of tumor microenvironment in tumorigenesis. *J. Cancer* **2017**, *8*, 761–773. [CrossRef] [PubMed]

19. Kenny, P.A.; Lee, G.Y.; Bissell, M.J. Targeting the tumor microenvironment. *Front. Biosci.* **2007**, *12*, 3468–3474. [CrossRef] [PubMed]

20. Balkwill, F.R.; Capasso, M.; Hagemann, T. The tumor microenvironment at a glance. *J. Cell Sci.* **2012**, *125*, 5591–5596. [CrossRef] [PubMed]

21. Hanahan, D.; Coussens, L.M. Accessories to the crime: Functions of cells recruited to the tumor microenvironment. *Cancer Cell* **2012**, *21*, 309–322. [CrossRef] [PubMed]

22. Chen, F.; Zhuang, X.; Lin, L.; Yu, P.; Wang, Y.; Shi, Y.; Hu, G.; Sun, Y. New horizons in tumor microenvironment biology: Challenges and opportunities. *BMC Med.* **2015**, *13*, 45. [CrossRef] [PubMed]

23. Zumsteg, A.; Christofori, G. Corrupt policemen: Inflammatory cells promote tumor angiogenesis. *Curr. Opin. Oncol.* **2009**, *21*, 60–70. [CrossRef] [PubMed]

24. Murdoch, C.; Giannoudis, A.; Lewis, C.E. Mechanisms regulating the recruitment of macrophages into hypoxic areas of tumors and other ischemic tissues. *Blood* **2004**, *104*, 2224–2234. [CrossRef] [PubMed]

25. Lawrence, T.; Natoli, G. Transcriptional regulation of macrophage polarization: Enabling diversity with identity. *Nat. Rev. Immunol.* **2011**, *11*, 750–761. [CrossRef] [PubMed]

26. Chaudhary, B.; Elkord, E. Regulatory T Cells in the Tumor Microenvironment and Cancer Progression: Role and Therapeutic Targeting. *Vaccines (Basel)* **2016**, *4*, 28. [CrossRef] [PubMed]

27. De Palma, M.; Biziato, D.; Petrova, T.V. Microenvironmental regulation of tumour angiogenesis. *Nat. Rev. Cancer* **2017**, *17*, 457–474. [CrossRef] [PubMed]

28. Gattazzo, F.; Urciuolo, A.; Bonaldo, P. Extracellular matrix: A dynamic microenvironment for stem cell niche. *Biochim. Biophys. Acta* **2014**, *1840*, 2506–2519. [CrossRef] [PubMed]

29. Popovic, Z.V.; Sandhoff, R.; Sijmonsma, T.P.; Kaden, S.; Jennemann, R.; Kiss, E.; Tone, E.; Autschbach, F.; Platt, N.; Malle, E.; et al. Sulfated glycosphingolipid as mediator of phagocytosis: SM4s enhances apoptotic cell clearance and modulates macrophage activity. *J. Immunol.* **2007**, *179*, 6770–6782. [CrossRef] [PubMed]

30. Nagarsheth, N.; Wicha, M.S.; Zou, W. Chemokines in the cancer microenvironment and their relevance in cancer immunotherapy. *Nat. Rev. Immunol.* **2017**, *17*, 559–572. [CrossRef] [PubMed]

31. Landskron, G.; De la Fuente, M.; Thuwajit, P.; Thuwajit, C.; Hermoso, M.A. Chronic inflammation and cytokines in the tumor microenvironment. *J. Immunol. Res.* **2014**, *2014*, 149185. [CrossRef] [PubMed]

32. Zlotnik, A.; Yoshie, O. Chemokines: A new classification system and their role in immunity. *Immunity* **2000**, *12*, 121–127. [CrossRef]

33. Del Bufalo, D.; Ciuffreda, L.; Trisciuoglio, D.; Desideri, M.; Cognetti, F.; Zupi, G.; Milella, M. Antiangiogenic potential of the Mammalian target of rapamycin inhibitor temsirolimus. *Cancer Res.* **2006**, *66*, 5549–5554. [CrossRef] [PubMed]

34. Milella, M.; Falcone, I.; Conciatori, F.; Matteoni, S.; Sacconi, A.; De Luca, T.; Bazzichetto, C.; Corbo, V.; Simbolo, M.; Sperduti, I.; et al. PTEN status is a crucial determinant of the functional outcome of combined MEK and mTOR inhibition in cancer. *Sci. Rep.* **2017**, *7*, 43013. [CrossRef] [PubMed]

35. De la Iglesia, N.; Konopka, G.; Lim, K.L.; Nutt, C.L.; Bromberg, J.F.; Frank, D.A.; Mischel, P.S.; Louis, D.N.; Bonni, A. Deregulation of a STAT3-interleukin 8 signaling pathway promotes human glioblastoma cell proliferation and invasiveness. *J. Neurosci.* **2008**, *28*, 5870–5878. [CrossRef] [PubMed]

36. Maxwell, P.J.; Coulter, J.; Walker, S.M.; McKechnie, M.; Neisen, J.; McCabe, N.; Kennedy, R.D.; Salto-Tellez, M.; Albanese, C.; Waugh, D.J. Potentiation of inflammatory CXCL8 signalling sustains cell survival in PTEN-deficient prostate carcinoma. *Eur. Urol.* **2013**, *64*, 177–188. [CrossRef] [PubMed]

37. Weichhart, T.; Hengstschlager, M.; Linke, M. Regulation of innate immune cell function by mTOR. *Nat. Rev. Immunol.* **2015**, *15*, 599–614. [CrossRef] [PubMed]

38. Thomson, A.W.; Turnquist, H.R.; Raimondi, G. Immunoregulatory functions of mTOR inhibition. *Nat. Rev. Immunol.* **2009**, *9*, 324–337. [CrossRef] [PubMed]

39. Pollizzi, K.N.; Patel, C.H.; Sun, I.H.; Oh, M.H.; Waickman, A.T.; Wen, J.; Delgoffe, G.M.; Powell, J.D. mTORC1 and mTORC2 selectively regulate CD8(+) T cell differentiation. *J. Clin. Investig.* **2015**, *125*, 2090–2108. [CrossRef] [PubMed]

40. Zeng, H. mTOR signaling in immune cells and its implications for cancer immunotherapy. *Cancer Lett.* **2017**, *408*, 182–189. [CrossRef] [PubMed]

41. Delgoffe, G.M.; Kole, T.P.; Zheng, Y.; Zarek, P.E.; Matthews, K.L.; Xiao, B.; Worley, P.F.; Kozma, S.C.; Powell, J.D. The mTOR kinase differentially regulates effector and regulatory T cell lineage commitment. *Immunity* **2009**, *30*, 832–844. [CrossRef] [PubMed]

42. Delgoffe, G.M.; Pollizzi, K.N.; Waickman, A.T.; Heikamp, E.; Meyers, D.J.; Horton, M.R.; Xiao, B.; Worley, P.F.; Powell, J.D. The kinase mTOR regulates the differentiation of helper T cells through the selective activation of signaling by mTORC1 and mTORC2. *Nat. Immunol.* **2011**, *12*, 295–303. [CrossRef] [PubMed]

43. Lee, K.; Gudapati, P.; Dragovic, S.; Spencer, C.; Joyce, S.; Killeen, N.; Magnuson, M.A.; Boothby, M. Mammalian target of rapamycin protein complex 2 regulates differentiation of Th1 and Th2 cell subsets via distinct signaling pathways. *Immunity* **2010**, *32*, 743–753. [CrossRef] [PubMed]

44. Park, Y.; Jin, H.S.; Lopez, J.; Elly, C.; Kim, G.; Murai, M.; Kronenberg, M.; Liu, Y.C. TSC1 regulates the balance between effector and regulatory T cells. *J. Clin. Investig.* **2013**, *123*, 5165–5178. [CrossRef] [PubMed]

45. Huynh, A.; DuPage, M.; Priyadharshini, B.; Sage, P.T.; Quiros, J.; Borges, C.M.; Townamchai, N.; Gerriets, V.A.; Rathmell, J.C.; Sharpe, A.H.; et al. Control of PI(3) kinase in Treg cells maintains homeostasis and lineage stability. *Nat. Immunol.* **2015**, *16*, 188–196. [CrossRef] [PubMed]

46. Shrestha, S.; Yang, K.; Guy, C.; Vogel, P.; Neale, G.; Chi, H. Treg cells require the phosphatase PTEN to restrain TH1 and TFH cell responses. *Nat. Immunol.* **2015**, *16*, 178–187. [CrossRef] [PubMed]

47. Byles, V.; Covarrubias, A.J.; Ben-Sahra, I.; Lamming, D.W.; Sabatini, D.M.; Manning, B.D.; Horng, T. The TSC-mTOR pathway regulates macrophage polarization. *Nat. Commun.* **2013**, *4*, 2834. [CrossRef] [PubMed]

48. Jiang, H.; Westerterp, M.; Wang, C.; Zhu, Y.; Ai, D. Macrophage mTORC1 disruption reduces inflammation and insulin resistance in obese mice. *Diabetologia* **2014**, *57*, 2393–2404. [CrossRef] [PubMed]

49. Guri, Y.; Nordmann, T.M.; Roszik, J. mTOR at the Transmitting and Receiving Ends in Tumor Immunity. *Front. Immunol.* **2018**, *9*, 578. [CrossRef] [PubMed]

50. Li, J.; Wang, L.; Chen, X.; Li, L.; Li, Y.; Ping, Y.; Huang, L.; Yue, D.; Zhang, Z.; Wang, F.; et al. CD39/CD73 upregulation on myeloid-derived suppressor cells via TGF-beta-mTOR-HIF-1 signaling in patients with non-small cell lung cancer. *Oncoimmunology* **2017**, *6*, e1320011. [CrossRef] [PubMed]

51. Zhang, C.; Wang, S.; Li, J.; Zhang, W.; Zheng, L.; Yang, C.; Zhu, T.; Rong, R. The mTOR signal regulates myeloid-derived suppressor cells differentiation and immunosuppressive function in acute kidney injury. *Cell Death Dis.* **2017**, *8*, e2695. [CrossRef] [PubMed]

52. Sun, S.; Chen, S.; Liu, F.; Wu, H.; McHugh, J.; Bergin, I.L.; Gupta, A.; Adams, D.; Guan, J.L. Constitutive Activation of mTORC1 in Endothelial Cells Leads to the Development and Progression of Lymphangiosarcoma through VEGF Autocrine Signaling. *Cancer Cell* **2015**, *28*, 758–772. [CrossRef] [PubMed]

53. Wang, S.; Amato, K.R.; Song, W.; Youngblood, V.; Lee, K.; Boothby, M.; Brantley-Sieders, D.M.; Chen, J. Regulation of endothelial cell proliferation and vascular assembly through distinct mTORC2 signaling pathways. *Mol. Cell. Biol.* **2015**, *35*, 1299–1313. [CrossRef] [PubMed]

54. Duluc, C.; Moatassim-Billah, S.; Chalabi-Dchar, M.; Perraud, A.; Samain, R.; Breibach, F.; Gayral, M.; Cordelier, P.; Delisle, M.B.; Bousquet-Dubouch, M.P.; et al. Pharmacological targeting of the protein synthesis mTOR/4E-BP1 pathway in cancer-associated fibroblasts abrogates pancreatic tumour chemoresistance. *EMBO Mol. Med.* **2015**, *7*, 735–753. [CrossRef] [PubMed]

55. Ahmad, S.; Abu-Eid, R.; Shrimali, R.; Webb, M.; Verma, V.; Doroodchi, A.; Berrong, Z.; Samara, R.; Rodriguez, P.C.; Mkrtichyan, M.; et al. Differential PI3Kdelta Signaling in CD4(+) T-cell Subsets Enables Selective Targeting of T Regulatory Cells to Enhance Cancer Immunotherapy. *Cancer Res.* **2017**, *77*, 1892–1904. [CrossRef] [PubMed]

56. Peng, W.; Chen, J.Q.; Liu, C.; Malu, S.; Creasy, C.; Tetzlaff, M.T.; Xu, C.; McKenzie, J.A.; Zhang, C.; Liang, X.; et al. Loss of PTEN Promotes Resistance to T Cell-Mediated Immunotherapy. *Cancer Discov.* **2016**, *6*, 202–216. [CrossRef] [PubMed]

57. Dong, Y.; Richards, J.A.; Gupta, R.; Aung, P.P.; Emley, A.; Kluger, Y.; Dogra, S.K.; Mahalingam, M.; Wajapeyee, N. PTEN functions as a melanoma tumor suppressor by promoting host immune response. *Oncogene* **2014**, *33*, 4632–4642. [CrossRef] [PubMed]

58. Templeton, A.J.; Dutoit, V.; Cathomas, R.; Rothermundt, C.; Bartschi, D.; Droge, C.; Gautschi, O.; Borner, M.; Fechter, E.; Stenner, F.; et al. Swiss Group for Clinical Cancer, R., Phase 2 trial of single-agent everolimus in chemotherapy-naive patients with castration-resistant prostate cancer (SAKK 08/08). *Eur. Urol.* **2013**, *64*, 150–158. [CrossRef] [PubMed]

59. Abu-Eid, R.; Samara, R.N.; Ozbun, L.; Abdalla, M.Y.; Berzofsky, J.A.; Friedman, K.M.; Mkrtichyan, M.; Khleif, S.N. Selective inhibition of regulatory T cells by targeting the PI3K-Akt pathway. *Cancer Immunol. Res.* **2014**, *2*, 1080–1089. [CrossRef] [PubMed]

60. Schmid, M.C.; Avraamides, C.J.; Dippold, H.C.; Franco, I.; Foubert, P.; Ellies, L.G.; Acevedo, L.M.; Manglicmot, J.R.; Song, X.; Wrasidlo, W.; et al. Receptor tyrosine kinases and TLR/IL1Rs unexpectedly activate myeloid cell PI3kgamma, a single convergent point promoting tumor inflammation and progression. *Cancer Cell* **2011**, *19*, 715–727. [CrossRef] [PubMed]

61. Vinals, F.; Chambard, J.C.; Pouyssegur, J. p70 S6 kinase-mediated protein synthesis is a critical step for vascular endothelial cell proliferation. *J. Biol. Chem.* **1999**, *274*, 26776–26782. [CrossRef] [PubMed]

62. Dormond, O.; Madsen, J.C.; Briscoe, D.M. The effects of mTOR-Akt interactions on anti-apoptotic signaling in vascular endothelial cells. *J. Biol. Chem.* **2007**, *282*, 23679–23686. [CrossRef] [PubMed]

63. Shinohara, E.T.; Cao, C.; Niermann, K.; Mu, Y.; Zeng, F.; Hallahan, D.E.; Lu, B. Enhanced radiation damage of tumor vasculature by mTOR inhibitors. *Oncogene* **2005**, *24*, 5414–5422. [CrossRef] [PubMed]

64. Heits, N.; Heinze, T.; Bernsmeier, A.; Kerber, J.; Hauser, C.; Becker, T.; Kalthoff, H.; Egberts, J.H.; Braun, F. Influence of mTOR-inhibitors and mycophenolic acid on human cholangiocellular carcinoma and cancer associated fibroblasts. *BMC Cancer* **2016**, *16*, 322. [CrossRef] [PubMed]

65. Zeng, H.; Chi, H. mTOR and lymphocyte metabolism. *Curr. Opin. Immunol.* **2013**, *25*, 347–355. [CrossRef] [PubMed]

66. Deberardinis, R.J.; Sayed, N.; Ditsworth, D.; Thompson, C.B. Brick by brick: Metabolism and tumor cell growth. *Curr. Opin. Genet. Dev.* **2008**, *18*, 54–61. [CrossRef] [PubMed]

67. Araki, K.; Ahmed, R. AMPK: A metabolic switch for CD8+ T-cell memory. *Eur. J. Immunol.* **2013**, *43*, 878–881. [CrossRef] [PubMed]

68. Araki, K.; Turner, A.P.; Shaffer, V.O.; Gangappa, S.; Keller, S.A.; Bachmann, M.F.; Larsen, C.P.; Ahmed, R. mTOR regulates memory CD8 T-cell differentiation. *Nature* **2009**, *460*, 108–112. [CrossRef] [PubMed]

69. Kidani, Y.; Elsaesser, H.; Hock, M.B.; Vergnes, L.; Williams, K.J.; Argus, J.P.; Marbois, B.N.; Komisopoulou, E.; Wilson, E.B.; Osborne, T.F.; et al. Sterol regulatory element-binding proteins are essential for the metabolic programming of effector T cells and adaptive immunity. *Nat. Immunol.* **2013**, *14*, 489–499. [CrossRef] [PubMed]

70. Kurebayashi, Y.; Nagai, S.; Ikejiri, A.; Ohtani, M.; Ichiyama, K.; Baba, Y.; Yamada, T.; Egami, S.; Hoshii, T.; Hirao, A.; et al. PI3K-Akt-mTORC1-S6K1/2 axis controls Th17 differentiation by regulating Gfi1 expression and nuclear translocation of RORgamma. *Cell Rep.* **2012**, *1*, 360–373. [CrossRef] [PubMed]

71. Yang, K.; Chi, H. mTOR and metabolic pathways in T cell quiescence and functional activation. *Semin. Immunol.* **2012**, *24*, 421–428. [CrossRef] [PubMed]

72. Wang, R.; Dillon, C.P.; Shi, L.Z.; Milasta, S.; Carter, R.; Finkelstein, D.; McCormick, L.L.; Fitzgerald, P.; Chi, H.; Munger, J.; et al. The transcription factor Myc controls metabolic reprogramming upon T lymphocyte activation. *Immunity* **2011**, *35*, 871–882. [CrossRef] [PubMed]

73. Shi, L.Z.; Wang, R.; Huang, G.; Vogel, P.; Neale, G.; Green, D.R.; Chi, H. HIF1alpha-dependent glycolytic pathway orchestrates a metabolic checkpoint for the differentiation of TH17 and Treg cells. *J. Exp. Med.* **2011**, *208*, 1367–1376. [CrossRef] [PubMed]

74. Battaglia, M.; Stabilini, A.; Migliavacca, B.; Horejs-Hoeck, J.; Kaupper, T.; Roncarolo, M.G. Rapamycin promotes expansion of functional CD4+CD25+FOXP3+ regulatory T cells of both healthy subjects and type 1 diabetic patients. *J. Immunol.* **2006**, *177*, 8338–8347. [CrossRef] [PubMed]

75. Zeng, H.; Yang, K.; Cloer, C.; Neale, G.; Vogel, P.; Chi, H. mTORC1 couples immune signals and metabolic programming to establish T(reg)-cell function. *Nature* **2013**, *499*, 485–490. [CrossRef] [PubMed]

76. Francisco, L.M.; Salinas, V.H.; Brown, K.E.; Vanguri, V.K.; Freeman, G.J.; Kuchroo, V.K.; Sharpe, A.H. PD-L1 regulates the development, maintenance, and function of induced regulatory T cells. *J. Exp. Med.* **2009**, *206*, 3015–3029. [CrossRef] [PubMed]

77. Keir, M.E.; Butte, M.J.; Freeman, G.J.; Sharpe, A.H. PD-1 and its ligands in tolerance and immunity. *Annu. Rev. Immunol.* **2008**, *26*, 677–704. [CrossRef] [PubMed]

78. Lastwika, K.J.; Wilson, W.; Li, Q.K.; Norris, J.; Xu, H.; Ghazarian, S.R.; Kitagawa, H.; Kawabata, S.; Taube, J.M.; Yao, S.; et al. Control of PD-L1 Expression by Oncogenic Activation of the AKT-mTOR Pathway in Non-Small Cell Lung Cancer. *Cancer Res.* **2016**, *76*, 227–238. [CrossRef] [PubMed]

79. Qian, B.Z.; Pollard, J.W. Macrophage diversity enhances tumor progression and metastasis. *Cell* **2010**, *141*, 39–51. [CrossRef] [PubMed]

80. Mantovani, A.; Sozzani, S.; Locati, M.; Allavena, P.; Sica, A. Macrophage polarization: Tumor-associated macrophages as a paradigm for polarized M2 mononuclear phagocytes. *Trends Immunol.* **2002**, *23*, 549–555. [CrossRef]

81. Mercalli, A.; Calavita, I.; Dugnani, E.; Citro, A.; Cantarelli, E.; Nano, R.; Melzi, R.; Maffi, P.; Secchi, A.; Sordi, V.; et al. Rapamycin unbalances the polarization of human macrophages to M1. *Immunology* **2013**, *140*, 179–190. [CrossRef] [PubMed]

82. Shan, M.; Qin, J.; Jin, F.; Han, X.; Guan, H.; Li, X.; Zhang, J.; Zhang, H.; Wang, Y. Autophagy suppresses isoprenaline-induced M2 macrophage polarization via the ROS/ERK and mTOR signaling pathway. *Free Radic. Biol. Med.* **2017**, *110*, 432–443. [CrossRef] [PubMed]

83. Chen, W.; Ma, T.; Shen, X.N.; Xia, X.F.; Xu, G.D.; Bai, X.L.; Liang, T.B. Macrophage-induced tumor angiogenesis is regulated by the TSC2-mTOR pathway. *Cancer Res.* **2012**, *72*, 1363–1372. [CrossRef] [PubMed]

84. Hallowell, R.W.; Collins, S.L.; Craig, J.M.; Zhang, Y.; Oh, M.; Illei, P.B.; Chan-Li, Y.; Vigeland, C.L.; Mitzner, W.; Scott, A.L.; et al. mTORC2 signalling regulates M2 macrophage differentiation in response to helminth infection and adaptive thermogenesis. *Nat. Commun.* **2017**, *8*, 14208. [CrossRef] [PubMed]

85. Shrivastava, R.; Asif, M.; Singh, V.; Dubey, P.; Ahmad Malik, S.; Lone, M.U.; Tewari, B.N.; Baghel, K.S.; Pal, S.; Nagar, G.K.; et al. M2 polarization of macrophages by Oncostatin M in hypoxic tumor microenvironment is mediated by mTORC2 and promotes tumor growth and metastasis. *Cytokine* **2018**. [CrossRef] [PubMed]

86. Welte, T.; Kim, I.S.; Tian, L.; Gao, X.; Wang, H.; Li, J.; Holdman, X.B.; Herschkowitz, J.I.; Pond, A.; Xie, G.; et al. Oncogenic mTOR signalling recruits myeloid-derived suppressor cells to promote tumour initiation. *Nat. Cell Biol.* **2016**, *18*, 632–644. [CrossRef] [PubMed]

87. Ryzhov, S.V.; Pickup, M.W.; Chytil, A.; Gorska, A.E.; Zhang, Q.; Owens, P.; Feoktistov, I.; Moses, H.L.; Novitskiy, S.V. Role of TGF-beta signaling in generation of CD39+CD73+ myeloid cells in tumors. *J. Immunol.* **2014**, *193*, 3155–3164. [CrossRef] [PubMed]

88. Raber, P.L.; Sierra, R.A.; Thevenot, P.T.; Shuzhong, Z.; Wyczechowska, D.D.; Kumai, T.; Celis, E.; Rodriguez, P.C. T cells conditioned with MDSC show an increased anti-tumor activity after adoptive T cell based immunotherapy. *Oncotarget* **2016**, *7*, 17565–17578. [CrossRef] [PubMed]

89. Hanahan, D.; Weinberg, R.A. Hallmarks of cancer: The next generation. *Cell* **2011**, *144*, 646–674. [CrossRef] [PubMed]

90. Hicklin, D.J.; Ellis, L.M. Role of the vascular endothelial growth factor pathway in tumor growth and angiogenesis. *J. Clin. Oncol.* **2005**, *23*, 1011–1027. [CrossRef] [PubMed]

91. Advani, S.H. Targeting mTOR pathway: A new concept in cancer therapy. *Indian J. Med. Paediatr. Oncol.* **2010**, *31*, 132–136. [CrossRef] [PubMed]

92. Semenza, G.L. Hydroxylation of HIF-1: Oxygen sensing at the molecular level. *Physiology (Bethesda)* **2004**, *19*, 176–182. [CrossRef] [PubMed]

93. Faes, S.; Santoro, T.; Demartines, N.; Dormond, O. Evolving Significance and Future Relevance of Anti-Angiogenic Activity of mTOR Inhibitors in Cancer Therapy. *Cancers (Basel)* **2017**, *9*, 152. [CrossRef] [PubMed]

94. Dodd, K.M.; Tee, A.R. STAT3 and mTOR: Co-operating to drive HIF and angiogenesis. *Oncoscience* **2015**, *2*, 913–914. [PubMed]

95. DeYoung, M.P.; Horak, P.; Sofer, A.; Sgroi, D.; Ellisen, L.W. Hypoxia regulates TSC1/2-mTOR signaling and tumor suppression through REDD1-mediated 14-3-3 shuttling. *Genes Dev.* **2008**, *22*, 239–251. [CrossRef] [PubMed]

96. Gwinn, D.M.; Shackelford, D.B.; Egan, D.F.; Mihaylova, M.M.; Mery, A.; Vasquez, D.S.; Turk, B.E.; Shaw, R.J. AMPK phosphorylation of raptor mediates a metabolic checkpoint. *Mol. Cell* **2008**, *30*, 214–226. [CrossRef] [PubMed]

97. Squadrito, M.L.; De Palma, M. Macrophage regulation of tumor angiogenesis: Implications for cancer therapy. *Mol. Aspects Med.* **2011**, *32*, 123–145. [CrossRef] [PubMed]

98. Maity, A.; Pore, N.; Lee, J.; Solomon, D.; O'Rourke, D.M. Epidermal growth factor receptor transcriptionally up-regulates vascular endothelial growth factor expression in human glioblastoma cells via a pathway involving phosphatidylinositol 3'-kinase and distinct from that induced by hypoxia. *Cancer Res.* **2000**, *60*, 5879–5886. [PubMed]

99. Pore, N.; Liu, S.; Haas-Kogan, D.A.; O'Rourke, D.M.; Maity, A. PTEN mutation and epidermal growth factor receptor activation regulate vascular endothelial growth factor (VEGF) mRNA expression in human glioblastoma cells by transactivating the proximal VEGF promoter. *Cancer Res.* **2003**, *63*, 236–241. [PubMed]

100. Zundel, W.; Schindler, C.; Haas-Kogan, D.; Koong, A.; Kaper, F.; Chen, E.; Gottschalk, A.R.; Ryan, H.E.; Johnson, R.S.; Jefferson, A.B.; et al. Loss of PTEN facilitates HIF-1-mediated gene expression. *Genes Dev.* **2000**, *14*, 391–396. [PubMed]

101. Fang, J.; Ding, M.; Yang, L.; Liu, L.Z.; Jiang, B.H. PI3K/PTEN/AKT signaling regulates prostate tumor angiogenesis. *Cell Signal.* **2007**, *19*, 2487–2497. [CrossRef] [PubMed]

102. Ma, X.M.; Blenis, J. Molecular mechanisms of mTOR-mediated translational control. *Nat. Rev. Mol. Cell Biol.* **2009**, *10*, 307–318. [CrossRef] [PubMed]

103. Orimo, A.; Gupta, P.B.; Sgroi, D.C.; Arenzana-Seisdedos, F.; Delaunay, T.; Naeem, R.; Carey, V.J.; Richardson, A.L.; Weinberg, R.A. Stromal fibroblasts present in invasive human breast carcinomas promote tumor growth and angiogenesis through elevated SDF-1/CXCL12 secretion. *Cell* **2005**, *121*, 335–348. [CrossRef] [PubMed]

104. Bhowmick, N.A.; Neilson, E.G.; Moses, H.L. Stromal fibroblasts in cancer initiation and progression. *Nature* **2004**, *432*, 332–337. [CrossRef] [PubMed]

105. Grum-Schwensen, B.; Klingelhofer, J.; Berg, C.H.; El-Naaman, C.; Grigorian, M.; Lukanidin, E.; Ambartsumian, N. Suppression of tumor development and metastasis formation in mice lacking the S100A4(mts1) gene. *Cancer Res.* **2005**, *65*, 3772–3780. [CrossRef] [PubMed]

106. Apte, M.V.; Pirola, R.C.; Wilson, J.S. Pancreatic stellate cells: A starring role in normal and diseased pancreas. *Front. Physiol.* **2012**, *3*, 344. [CrossRef] [PubMed]

107. Kumar, V.; Donthireddy, L.; Marvel, D.; Condamine, T.; Wang, F.; Lavilla-Alonso, S.; Hashimoto, A.; Vonteddu, P.; Behera, R.; Goins, M.A.; et al. Cancer-Associated Fibroblasts Neutralize the Anti-tumor Effect of CSF1 Receptor Blockade by Inducing PMN-MDSC Infiltration of Tumors. *Cancer Cell* **2017**, *32*, 654–668. [CrossRef] [PubMed]

108. Shan, T.; Chen, S.; Chen, X.; Lin, W.R.; Li, W.; Ma, J.; Wu, T.; Cui, X.; Ji, H.; Li, Y.; et al. Cancer-associated fibroblasts enhance pancreatic cancer cell invasion by remodeling the metabolic conversion mechanism. *Oncol. Rep.* **2017**, *37*, 1971–1979. [CrossRef] [PubMed]

109. Erkan, M. Understanding the stroma of pancreatic cancer: Co-evolution of the microenvironment with epithelial carcinogenesis. *J. Pathol.* **2013**, *231*, 4–7. [CrossRef] [PubMed]

110. Von Ahrens, D.; Bhagat, T.D.; Nagrath, D.; Maitra, A.; Verma, A. The role of stromal cancer-associated fibroblasts in pancreatic cancer. *J. Hematol. Oncol.* **2017**, *10*, 76. [CrossRef] [PubMed]

111. Kumari, N.; Dwarakanath, B.S.; Das, A.; Bhatt, A.N. Role of interleukin-6 in cancer progression and therapeutic resistance. *Tumour Biol.* **2016**, *37*, 11553–11572. [CrossRef] [PubMed]

112. Wang, Y.; Gan, G.; Wang, B.; Wu, J.; Cao, Y.; Zhu, D.; Xu, Y.; Wang, X.; Han, H.; Li, X.; et al. Cancer-associated Fibroblasts Promote Irradiated Cancer Cell Recovery Through Autophagy. *EBioMedicine* **2017**, *17*, 45–56. [CrossRef] [PubMed]

113. Chen, D.S.; Mellman, I. Elements of cancer immunity and the cancer-immune set point. *Nature* **2017**, *541*, 321–330. [CrossRef] [PubMed]

114. Bethune, M.T.; Joglekar, A.V. Personalized T cell-mediated cancer immunotherapy: Progress and challenges. *Curr. Opin. Biotechnol.* **2017**, *48*, 142–152. [CrossRef] [PubMed]

115. Pancione, M.; Giordano, G.; Parcesepe, P.; Cerulo, L.; Coppola, L.; Curatolo, A.D.; Conciatori, F.; Milella, M.; Porras, A. Emerging Insight into MAPK Inhibitors and Immunotherapy in Colorectal Cancer. *Curr. Med. Chem.* **2017**, *24*, 1383–1402. [CrossRef] [PubMed]

116. O'Donnell, J.S.; Massi, D.; Teng, M.W.L.; Mandala, M. PI3K-AKT-mTOR inhibition in cancer immunotherapy, redux. *Semin. Cancer Biol.* **2018**, *48*, 91–103. [CrossRef] [PubMed]

117. Saunders, R.N.; Metcalfe, M.S.; Nicholson, M.L. Rapamycin in transplantation: A review of the evidence. *Kidney Int.* **2001**, *59*, 3–16. [CrossRef] [PubMed]

118. Parsa, A.T.; Waldron, J.S.; Panner, A.; Crane, C.A.; Parney, I.F.; Barry, J.J.; Cachola, K.E.; Murray, J.C.; Tihan, T.; Jensen, M.C.; et al. Loss of tumor suppressor PTEN function increases B7-H1 expression and immunoresistance in glioma. *Nat. Med.* **2007**, *13*, 84–88. [CrossRef] [PubMed]

119. George, S.; Miao, D.; Demetri, G.D.; Adeegbe, D.; Rodig, S.J.; Shukla, S.; Lipschitz, M.; Amin-Mansour, A.; Raut, C.P.; Carter, S.L.; et al. Loss of PTEN Is Associated with Resistance to Anti-PD-1 Checkpoint Blockade Therapy in Metastatic Uterine Leiomyosarcoma. *Immunity* **2017**, *46*, 197–204. [CrossRef] [PubMed]

120. Song, M.; Chen, D.; Lu, B.; Wang, C.; Zhang, J.; Huang, L.; Wang, X.; Timmons, C.L.; Hu, J.; Liu, B.; et al. PTEN loss increases PD-L1 protein expression and affects the correlation between PD-L1 expression and clinical parameters in colorectal cancer. *PLoS ONE* **2013**, *8*, e65821. [CrossRef] [PubMed]

121. Mittendorf, E.A.; Philips, A.V.; Meric-Bernstam, F.; Qiao, N.; Wu, Y.; Harrington, S.; Su, X.; Wang, Y.; Gonzalez-Angulo, A.M.; Akcakanat, A.; et al. PD-L1 expression in triple-negative breast cancer. *Cancer Immunol. Res.* **2014**, *2*, 361–370. [CrossRef] [PubMed]

122. Zhao, L.; Li, C.; Liu, F.; Zhao, Y.; Liu, J.; Hua, Y.; Liu, J.; Huang, J.; Ge, C. A blockade of PD-L1 produced antitumor and antimetastatic effects in an orthotopic mouse pancreatic cancer model via the PI3K/Akt/mTOR signaling pathway. *Onco Targets Ther.* **2017**, *10*, 2115–2126. [CrossRef] [PubMed]

123. Chapman, N.M.; Chi, H. mTOR signaling, Tregs and immune modulation. *Immunotherapy* **2014**, *6*, 1295–1311. [CrossRef] [PubMed]

124. Huijts, C.M.; Santegoets, S.J.; Quiles Del Rey, M.; de Haas, R.R.; Verheul, H.M.; de Gruijl, T.D.; van der Vliet, H.J. Differential effects of inhibitors of the PI3K/mTOR pathway on the expansion and functionality of regulatory T cells. *Clin. Immunol.* **2016**, *168*, 47–54. [CrossRef] [PubMed]

125. Marshall, N.A.; Galvin, K.C.; Corcoran, A.M.; Boon, L.; Higgs, R.; Mills, K.H. Immunotherapy with PI3K inhibitor and Toll-like receptor agonist induces IFN-gamma+IL-17+ polyfunctional T cells that mediate rejection of murine tumors. *Cancer Res.* **2012**, *72*, 581–591. [CrossRef] [PubMed]

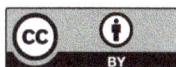

International Journal of
Molecular Sciences

MDPI

Review
mTOR and Tumor Cachexia

Adrian P. Duval, Cheryl Jeanneret, Tania Santoro and Olivier Dormond *

Department of Visceral Surgery, Lausanne University Hospital, 1011 Lausanne, Switzerland;
adrian.duval@chuv.ch (A.P.D.); cheryl.jeanneret@unil.ch (C.J.); tania.santoro@chuv.ch (T.S.)
* Correspondence: olivier.dormond@chuv.ch; Tel.: +41-79-556-0340

Received: 3 July 2018; Accepted: 25 July 2018; Published: 30 July 2018

Abstract: Cancer cachexia affects most patients with advanced forms of cancers. It is mainly characterized by weight loss, due to muscle and adipose mass depletion. As cachexia is associated with increased morbidity and mortality in cancer patients, identifying the underlying mechanisms leading to cachexia is essential in order to design novel therapeutic strategies. The mechanistic target of rapamycin (mTOR) is a major intracellular signalling intermediary that participates in cell growth by upregulating anabolic processes such as protein and lipid synthesis. Accordingly, emerging evidence suggests that mTOR and mTOR inhibitors influence cancer cachexia. Here, we review the role of mTOR in cellular processes involved in cancer cachexia and highlight the studies supporting the contribution of mTOR in cancer cachexia.

Keywords: tumour cachexia; mTOR; signalling; metabolism; proteolysis; lipolysis

1. Introduction

Cancer is a leading cause of death worldwide with nearly 600,000 cancer related deaths projected to occur in 2018 in the United States [1]. Most cancer related deaths are observed in patients with metastasized tumours. Indeed, at least two factors contribute to lethality from metastasis. Firstly, tumour-secreted factors profoundly modify cancer patients' homeostasis, increasing their susceptibility to infections and thrombo-embolic events, with major morbid and mortal consequences [2,3]. Secondly, organ invasion by neoplastic cells can lead to organ failure.

Tumour secreted factors promote tumour cachexia, a multifactorial condition characterized by decreased body weight due to losses of skeletal muscle and adipose tissue mass [4]. Nearly 80% of all cancer patients are affected by tumour cachexia, which significantly contributes to cancer-related morbidity and mortality. In particular, cachexia is associated with poor performance status, reduced tolerance to therapies and a high mortality rate [5,6]. The incidence of cachexia varies according to tumour type and is highly associated with cancers of the oesophagus, stomach, liver and lung. Cachexia may precede clinical diagnosis of cancer and may be present with small primary tumours. Since treatment options against tumour cachexia are so far very limited, a greater understanding of the underlying mechanisms is necessary.

The mechanistic target of rapamycin (mTOR) is an ubiquitously expressed serine-threonine kinase that is part of two different protein complexes named mTORC1 and mTORC2 [7]. Both complexes participate in cell proliferation and survival and, accordingly, represent a target in cancer therapy. Indeed, drugs which inhibit mTOR, named rapalogs, have proven clinical benefits in cancer patients and were approved for the treatment of different advanced neoplasias. Of note, mTORC1 is a major signalling intermediary, which stimulates anabolic processes, including protein, lipid and nucleotide synthesis and represses catabolic pathways such as autophagy. Emerging evidence demonstrated the importance of mTORC1 in stimulating skeletal muscle growth and in facilitating adipogenesis and lipogenesis [8]. This suggests that mTOR might be involved in tumour-related cachexia and, conversely, that mTOR inhibitors during cancer treatments might contribute to tumour cachexia.

Here, we review the putative roles played by mTOR in cellular processes relevant to tumour cachexia and highlight the experimental evidence of mTOR signalling importance in these processes. We further speculate on the consequences of mTOR inhibition in the development of cancer cachexia.

2. Cancer Cachexia

Patients with advanced forms of cancer are frequently affected by a multifactorial syndrome named cachexia. It results from a negative balance of energy caused by reduced caloric intake and altered metabolism including inflammation, elevated catabolism and excess energy expenditure [9,10]. Consequently, patients affected by cachexia present body weight loss, with predominant decrease of skeletal muscle and adipose tissue mass, eliciting reduced response to treatment, reduced quality of life and decreased survival. Altered energy balance is a major feature of tumour cachexia with reduced energy intake and increased resting energy expenditure [11]. Whereas the central nervous system is mainly responsible for reduced caloric intake, the increased energy expenditure relies on different causes, including tumour metabolism, inflammation and metabolic cycling [9].

Cachexia is driven by multiple mediators produced by cancer cells and cells within the tumour microenvironment [12]. Among these mediators are pro-inflammatory cytokines such as prostaglandin E_2, IL-6, TNF, IFNγ, TRAF6, IL-1α, IL-1β and other tumour-derived catabolic factors such as activin and myostatin [12]. These molecules directly promote catabolism in target tissues including skeletal and cardiac muscles as well as adipose tissue (Figure 1). In addition, they produce central nervous system alterations leading to reduced caloric intake and increased catabolic neural outputs [9].

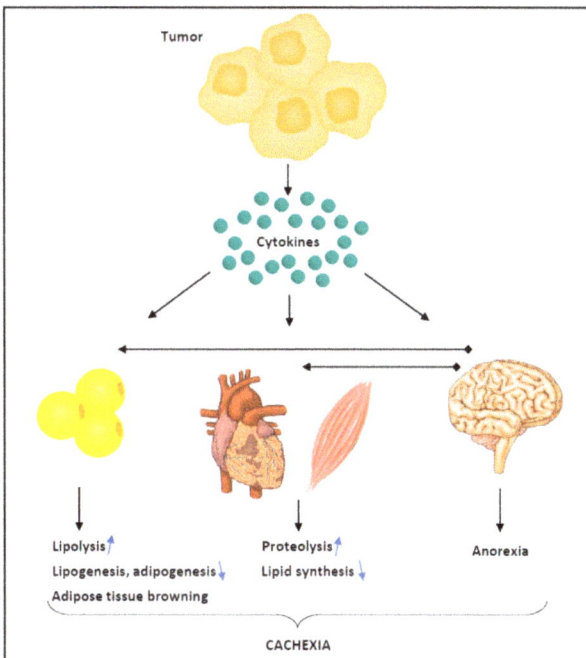

Figure 1. Mechanisms involved in cancer cachexia. Tumour-derived catabolic factors such as pro-inflammatory cytokines act on target tissues to elicit excess catabolism. Alteration of the central nervous system results in reduced food intake and increased catabolic neural outputs. Proteolysis is induced in skeletal and cardiac muscles through up-regulation of the ubiquitin-proteasome system and autophagy. Reduced protein synthesis has also been reported. Loss of adipose tissue results from increased lipolysis, decreased lipogenesis and adipogenesis and white adipose tissue browning.

In skeletal muscle, the majority of these factors activate intracellular signals that lead to transcription of genes encoding components of the autophagy and ubiquitin-proteasome systems (UPS) [13]. Once activated, these systems selectively destroy myofibrillar proteins resulting in muscle atrophy [9]. Several studies highlighted the importance of UPS in degradation of muscular proteins [14–17]. Furthermore, more recent studies demonstrated increased proteasome activity in numerous murine models of cancer cachexia and showed that proteasome inhibitors improve cachexia in tumour bearing mice [18]. In contrast to pre-clinical studies, the role of UPS during loss of skeletal muscle in cancer patients is not clear. Whereas some studies showed increased expression of UPS components [19–21], others failed to detect any changes [22,23]. Besides UPS, autophagic processes contribute to protein degradation in tumour cachexia [24]. In C26 tumour bearing mice, autophagy is induced in muscular cells at initial and advanced stages of cachexia. Similar observations were made in mice transplanted with Lewis lung carcinoma and in rats bearing hepatomas [24], showing that this phenomenon was not specific of C26 tumours.

In addition to catabolic processes, reduced protein synthesis also participates in muscle atrophy in cancer cachexia [25–27]. Under physiological conditions, insulin-like growth factor 1 (IGF1)/PI3K/AKT/mTOR signalling pathway embodies the main anabolic pathway [28]. In the context of tumour cachexia however, contrasting results were reported as both increased and decreased AKT activity was observed in different models [29–31]. Hence, additional studies are needed to assess the role of reduced protein synthesis in cancer cachexia.

Besides loss of skeletal muscle, cardiac muscle atrophy is also associated with cancer cachexia [32]. The pathogenesis of cardiac atrophy remains poorly explored but seems to share similar mechanisms with skeletal muscle atrophy. Indeed, reduced protein synthesis and increased protein degradation in hearts of cachectic rodents were detected [33,34]. In addition, cardiomyocytes apoptosis was also observed in AH-130 tumour-bearing rats and C26 tumour bearing mice cachectic models [35,36].

Finally, as mentioned previously, tumour cachexia is also characterized by loss of adipose tissue [37]. In contrast to skeletal muscle loss, little is known about the role of fat shrinkage in cancer. Nevertheless, an association between fat loss and poor outcomes was identified in advanced cancer patients [38,39]. Several mechanisms are responsible for the loss of adipose tissue including reduced food intake, increased lipolysis, decreased lipogenesis, impaired adipogenesis and decreased lipid deposition [37,40]. In particular, lipolysis represents a major cause of adipose tissue loss in cancer, as cachectic cancer patients present increased expression of hormone sensitive lipases compared to weight stable cancer patients [41,42]. In addition, cachectic patients exhibit increased expression of receptors of lipolytic hormones on adipocytes [42]. Furthermore, besides hormone-sensitive lipases, adipose triglyceride lipase (ATGL) contributes to lipolysis in cancer patients, as ATGL-deficient tumour bearing mice did not show increased lipolysis [43].

Enhanced lipolysis generates excess fatty acids that are subsequently oxidized by mitochondria. Accordingly, up-regulation of genes regulating mitochondrial lipid oxidation was observed in animal models and in patients with cachexia [40,44]. Additionally, recent studies also found that white adipose tissue browning contributes to fatty acid catabolism [45,46]. This process uncouples mitochondrial respiration toward thermogenesis instead of ATP synthesis, resulting in increased lipid mobilization and energy expenditure [47].

Finally, in addition to augmented lipolysis and fat oxidation, loss of fat mass in cancer patients relies on reduced lipid deposition and lipogenesis. Decreased activity of fatty acid synthase and lipoprotein lipase was shown in adipose tissue of cancer patients [48] and adipogenesis, a process essential to form mature adipocytes, is impaired in experimental models of cancer cachexia with reduced expression of adipogenic transcription factors [44,49,50].

3. mTOR Signalling Pathway

The mechanistic target of rapamycin (mTOR) is an ubiquitously expressed and well conserved serine/threonine kinase belonging to the PI3K-related kinases family [7]. mTOR is one of the main component of two protein complexes named mTOR complex 1 and mTOR complex 2 (respectively mTORC1 and mTORC2), which are involved in cell growth regulation (Figure 2) [7].

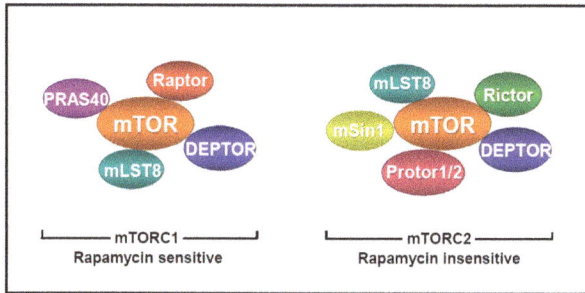

Figure 2. Components of mTORC1 and mTORC2. Specific components of mTORC1 are Raptor and PRAS40 and specific components of mTORC2 are Rictor, mSin1 and Protor1/2.

mTORC1 is composed of mTOR, raptor (Regulatory-associated protein of mTOR) [51], mLST8 (mammalian lethal with Sec13 protein 8) [52] and two inhibitory proteins PRAS40 (proline-rich AKT substrate 40 kDa) [53] and Deptor (Dishevelled, Egl-10 and Pleckstrin domain-containing mTOR-interacting protein) [54]. In presence of favourable extracellular conditions, mTORC1 coordinates cell growth by stimulating protein, lipid and nucleotide synthesis and repressing autophagy [7]. Several factors regulate mTORC1 activity including growth factors, hormones, amino acids, energy level, oxygen and stress. The intracellular signalling pathways leading to mTORC1 activation by growth factors and hormones were identified and can be summarized as follows (Figure 3). Ensuing binding and activation of their specific receptors, two major signalling pathways are stimulated; the Ras/Raf/Mek/Erk as well as the PI3K/AKT signalling pathways. In turn, activated AKT or Erk and its downstream effector p90^{RSK} phosphorylate tuberous sclerosis complex 2 (TSC2) resulting in its dissociation from TSC1 and TBC1D7. This results in the inactivation of the TSC complex by dissociation from the lysosomal membrane where it exerts its inhibition on the GTPase Rheb [55–59]. Since the TSC complex converts the GTPase Rheb to its inactive form, TSC complex inhibition elicits Rheb activation, which strongly enhances mTORC1 activity. In addition to its effect on TSC2, AKT enhances mTORC1 activity by phosphorylating and inactivating PRAS40 [53]. Besides growth factors, energetic modulations also regulate mTORC1 activity via the TSC axis [60]. Indeed, reduced levels of ATP following energy deprivation lead to the activation of the AMP-activated protein kinase (AMPK), which in turn activates TSC2 by phosphorylation, resulting in enhanced inhibition of Rheb and consequently of mTORC1. Moreover, AMPK reduces mTORC1 activity by phosphorylating raptor [61]. Hypoxia also downregulates mTORC1 activity either by activating AMPK or by inducing the expression of REDD1 which inactivates mTORC1 by activating the TSC complex [62]. Finally, mTORC1 activity is regulated by amino acid levels. In this context, amino acids signalling to mTORC1 involve recruitment of mTORC1 at the surface of the lysosomes. In turn, mTORC1 associates with Rag GTPases which promote its interaction with the lysosomal pool of Rheb [63,64].

Once activated mTORC1 regulates diverse cellular functions needed for cell growth and proliferation. In particular, mTORC1 promotes protein synthesis directly by phosphorylating S6K1 and 4EBP. S6K1 phosphorylates several substrates to promote mRNA translation initiation [65]. Phosphorylation of 4EBP by mTORC1 leads to its dissociation from eIF4E and results in 5′ cap-dependent mRNA translation [66]. Besides protein, mTORC1 also promotes nucleotide synthesis required for DNA replication and up-regulates glycolysis, leading to newly generated biomass [67–69]. Finally, and as discussed in more detail later, mTORC1 stimulates lipid synthesis [70].

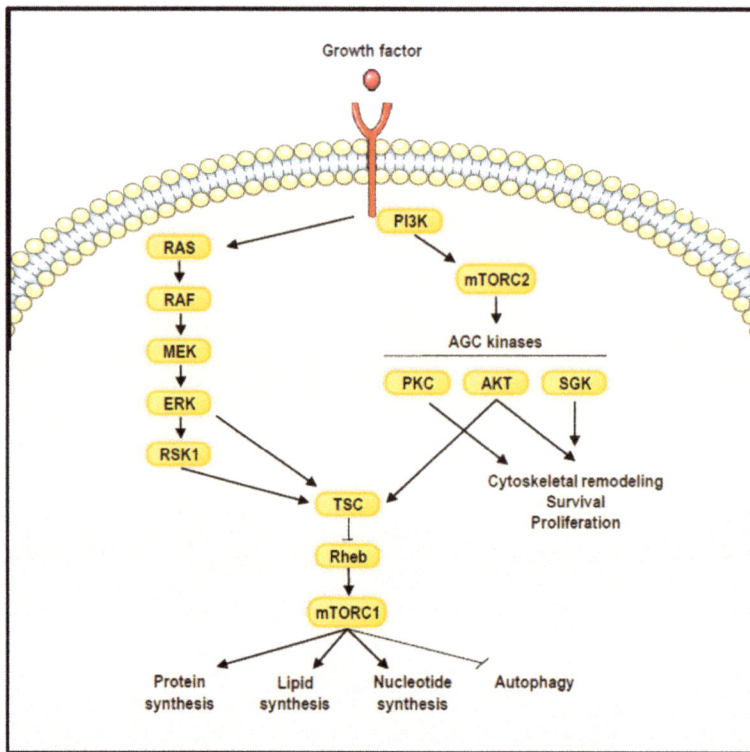

Figure 3. Activation of mTOR signalling pathway by growth factors. Upon stimulation of growth factor receptors, mTORC1 is activated via the PI3K/AKT and Ras/Raf/Mek/Erk signalling pathways and stimulates anabolic processes and represses autophagy. mTORC2 activation requires PI3K. Once activated mTORC2 regulates cytoskeletal organization, cell proliferation and survival by phosphorylating members of the AGC kinases family.

Interestingly, activated mTORC1 is able to signal back to the plasma membrane to inhibit growth factor signalling, protecting from pathway over activation [71]. Two different mechanisms were identified in this process. Firstly, mTORC1 and S6K1 promote insulin receptor substrate-1 degradation [72]. Secondly, mTORC1 stabilizes Grb10, which acts as an endogenous inhibitor of receptor tyrosine kinases [73,74].

mTORC2 comprises mTOR, Rictor (rapamycin insensitive companion of mTOR) [75], mLST8, DEPTOR, mSin1 (mammalian stress-activated protein kinase-interacting protein) [76,77] and Protor1/2 (protein observed with rictor 1 and 2) (Figure 2) [78]. Upstream regulators of mTORC2 are mainly growth factors and PI3K [79]. Upon binding of the PH domain of mSin1 to phosphoinositides generated by PI3K, the inhibitory effect of mSin1 PH domain on mTORC2 is relieved, leading to mTORC2 activation [80]. Additionally, PI3K stimulates mTORC2 activity by inducing its association to ribosomes, which probably represent another cellular pool of mTORC2 [81]. Following activation, mTORC2 functions as a kinase of several members of the AGC family of protein kinases, including PKC, AKT and SGK1 [79]. By activating members of the PKC family including PKCα, PKCδ, PKCγ and PKCζ, mTORC2 regulates cytoskeletal remodelling and cell migration [75,82–84]. More importantly, mTORC2 also phosphorylates AKT, which regulates cell proliferation and survival and appears to provide substrate specificity to AKT [85].

Several genetic mutations have been reported that lead to PI3K/AKT/mTOR pathway activation in cancer. Activating mutations of PI3K, AKT, mTOR as well as inactivating mutations of TSC1, TSC2 or PTEN are commonly observed in several types of cancers [86,87]. More recently, an extensive study of more than 11,000 human cancers confirmed the high prevalence of genetic mutations of components of mTOR signalling pathway [87]. In addition, activation of the pathway without genetic mutations was also found suggesting alternate mechanisms for pathway activation [87].

Since mTOR signalling controls both cell growth and proliferation and since activating mutations of components of this pathway are frequently found in cancer, many studies addressed the effects of mTOR inhibitors in cancer therapy [88–90]. Initially, mTOR inhibition was achieved with rapamycin or its derivatives named rapalogs. Rapamycin associates to FKBP12, which bind together to the FRB domain of mTOR, partially occluding the access of substrates to its kinase domain [91]. Inhibition of mTORC1 by rapalogs is however incomplete as some protein residues phosphorylated by mTORC1 are rapamycin resistant [92]. Furthermore, rapalogs do not provide an immediate inhibition of mTORC2. Indeed, mTORC2 is classically rapalog-insensitive in most cancer cell types [93]. Only a limited number of cell types with prolonged exposure to rapalogs show mTORC2 inhibition, presumably from the inability to generate novel mTORC2 complexes from rapalog-bound mTOR [94]. To overcome these limitations, a second generation of mTOR inhibitors was developed to directly target the kinase domain of mTOR. Accordingly, compared to rapalogs, kinase inhibitors of mTOR inhibit mTORC2 and provide a complete inhibition of mTORC1 [95].

To date only rapalogs are approved for the treatment of various advanced cancers including renal cell carcinoma [96,97], advanced pancreatic neuroendocrine tumours [98], postmenopausal hormone receptor-positive advanced breast cancer in combination with exemestane [99], advanced non-functional neuroendocrine tumours of the lung or gastrointestinal tract [100] and refractory mantle cell lymphoma [101]. The anti-cancer efficacy of rapalogs is however limited failing to provide long lasting benefits.

4. mTOR in Muscle and Lipid Metabolism

mTOR signalling is an important anabolic pathway in skeletal muscle growth [102]. Indeed, genetic and pharmacologic experiments support a major role of mTOR in this process. Muscle-specific deletion of mTOR causes weight loss with a strong decrease of fast-twitch glycolytic muscles leading to premature death [103]. mTOR deficient muscles further display metabolic alterations including decreased oxidative capacity, altered mitochondrial regulation and glycogen accumulation. A similar phenotype is observed in raptor but not in rictor deficient muscles, indicating that mTORC1 disruption likely accounts for these changes [104]. Consistent with these findings, muscle depletion of S6K1, a direct downstream target of mTORC1, causes muscle atrophy [105]. Interestingly, chronic activation of mTORC1 also results in muscle atrophy and low body mass [106]. In this case, loss of muscle mass is primarily due to inhibition of autophagy by mTORC1 activity. Besides genetic gain and loss of function experiments, the role of mTOR signalling in skeletal muscle was demonstrated with chemical inhibition of mTOR. For instance, skeletal muscle hypertrophy induced by muscle overload was inhibited by rapamycin [107]. Of note, rapamycin does not induce muscle atrophy in control muscles. Rapamycin also inhibits muscle growth induced by the expression of a constitutive active mutant of AKT [108]. Early studies identified IGF-I and leucine as a major stimulator of mTORC1 in skeletal muscle [28,109]. In addition, mechanical stimulus promotes mTORC1 activity in part independently of IGF-I [110,111]. In particular, mechanical stimulation induced multisite phosphorylation of raptor resulting in up-regulated mTORC1 activity, promoting the lysosomal association of mTOR and abolishing the lysosomal association of TSC2 [112].

mTOR also influences various aspects of lipid metabolism including lipogenesis, adipogenesis, lipolysis and lipid oxidation [70]. mTORC1 is a particularly important mediator of lipid biogenesis by controlling the expression of many lipogenic genes. Sterol regulatory element-binding proteins (SREBPs) are components of a family of transcription factors that induce lipid synthesis and that are positively regulated by mTORC1 [113,114]. Several studies demonstrated that rapamycin decreases the expression of lipogenic genes by affecting SREBPs processing and activation [115–117]. Depletion of raptor but not rictor downregulates the expression of lipogenic genes confirming that mTORC1 and not mTORC2 is mainly involved in this process [116]. In contrast to these observations, recent studies highlighted the critical role of mTORC2 in lipid synthesis. Liver depletion of rictor results in reduced SREBP activity and expression of lipogenic genes [118,119]. On top of lipogenesis, mTOR is also involved in adipogenesis regulation. Indeed, rapamycin inhibits adipocyte differentiation in vitro [120,121] and adipogenesis was also abrogated in 3T3-L1 preadipocytes following raptor deletion [122]. Likewise, the potential of raptor null mouse embryonic fibroblasts to differentiate into adipocytes is impaired [122]. The role of mTORC1 in adipogenesis was also addressed in vivo; specific knock-down of raptor in adipocytes limits lipid accumulation in adipocytes and protects mice from obesity induced by diet [122]. Similarly, rapamycin treated mice accumulate less adipose tissue [123,124]. However, although AKT plays an important role in adipogenesis, deletion of rictor in adipose tissue does not affect adipose tissue accumulation [125–128]. Hence, mTORC2-mediated AKT phosphorylation on Ser473 is not necessary for AKT to transmit pro-adipogenic signals. Nevertheless, deletion of rictor in white adipocyte progenitors is associated with less adipose tissue suggesting that mTORC2 is required for early adipogenesis [129].

mTOR further participates in adipose mass accumulation by inhibiting catabolic processes such as lipolysis. Indeed, circulating free fatty acids are elevated in humans treated with rapamycin [130] and higher lipolysis intensity was recorded in isolated adipocytes treated with rapamycin [131,132]. Finally, increasing mTORC1 activation via overexpression of Rheb inhibits lipolysis in 3T3-L1 adipocytes [131]. Regarding mTORC2, its activity also affects lipolysis, but contrasting results were found regarding the role of rictor in this process [127,128].

5. mTOR and Tumour Cachexia

mTORC1 involvement in tumour cachexia was evidenced in $Apc^{Min/+}$ mice, a model of colorectal cancer that develops cachexia that is dependent on interleukin-6 [133]. Analysis of the gastrocnemius muscle of $Apc^{Min/+}$ mice revealed a progressive decrease of mTORC1 activity from the initiation of cachexia to extreme body weight loss [134]. mTORC1 inhibition was mediated via the activation of AMPK by IL-6, which was further confirmed in C2C12 myoblasts [135]. This study suggests that reduction of anabolic mTORC1 signalling in skeletal muscle contributes to loss of muscle mass during cachexia. Accordingly, treadmill exercise restoring mTORC1 activity in skeletal muscle prevents cachexia in $Apc^{Min/+}$ mice [136]. The anti-cachectic role of mTORC1 was further substantiated in mice bearing Lewis cell carcinoma. In this model, cachexia was also associated with reduced mTORC1 signalling in the gastrocnemius muscle [137]. Furthermore, in vitro in C2C12 myoblasts, studies showed that stretch-induced mTORC1 activation was inhibited by media containing cachectic factors derived from Lewis cell carcinoma [138]. Finally, salidroside, a major phenylpropanoid glycosides found in *Rhodiola rosea* L., prevented tumour cachexia in CT-26 colon cancer and Lewis lung carcinoma and restored levels of muscle phospho-mTOR, used as a read-out of mTORC1 activity [139]. Hence, in these models, prevention of tumour cachexia is associated with restored mTORC1 activity. Finally, as mentioned earlier, activation of UPS is a major process that leads to skeletal muscle loss in cancer cachexia [10]. Recently, two studies demonstrated that mTOR inhibition leads to proteolysis via the UPS, suggesting that mTOR prevents protein loss by repressing anabolic processes [140,141]. Nevertheless, additional studies are needed to investigate it in the context of tumour cachexia.

In contrast to these results, mTORC1 inhibition was also reported to prevent loss of muscle mass in tumour cachexia [142]. In fact, colon cancer tumour-bearing mice and tumour patients display altered autophagic markers, suggesting that autophagy flux proceed at a slower rate. Pharmaceutical intervention with rapamycin in these mice restored autophagy in skeletal muscles and prevented tumour cachexia [142]. Similarly, treatment with an AMPK activator or aerobic exercise counteracted tumour cachexia-induced weight loss which was associated with increased autophagy. In addition, rapamycin prevented C2C12 myoblasts atrophy induced by colon carcinoma preconditioned media. This effect was abrogated following inhibition of autophagy, further suggesting that rapamycin-induced autophagy prevents loss of muscle during tumour cachexia [142]. Consistent with these observations, it was demonstrated that muscle-specific deletion of a crucial autophagy gene, Atg7, resulted in profound muscle atrophy and exacerbated muscle loss during denervation and fasting [143]. Taken together, these results suggest that autophagy can prevent muscle loss during tumour cachexia and that targeting mTORC1 to induce autophagy represent a treatment strategy to prevent cachexia.

Besides inducing autophagy, another mechanism was proposed to explain the anti-cachectic properties of mTOR inhibitors. In a transgenic murine lymphoma model, mice developed a cachectic syndrome characterized by reduced appetite, severe body weight loss, complete depletion of adipose tissue mass and significant loss of muscle mass [144]. This phenotype was associated with increased levels of cachexia mediators in particular interleukin-10. Administration of rapamycin in these mice prevented the development of cachexia and decreased IL-10 levels, suggesting that the production of pro-cachectic factors are regulated by mTOR. In particular, rapamycin improved appetite and reduced the severity of fat loss. Similarly, everolimus, a specific mTOR inhibitor, reduced IL-6 levels and alleviated the cachectic phenotype of CT-26 colon cancer bearing mice in which IL-6 is the main cachectic driver [144,145]. CT-26 tumours induced a significant decrease in the weight of tibialis anterior, gastrocnemius-soleus-plantaris complex and quadriceps muscles, which was prevented by everolimus treatment. Of note, everoliums did not induce muscle loss in non-tumour bearing control mice [145]. Therefore, suppression of cytokine production by targeting mTOR represents a treatment strategy to ameliorate tumour cachexia.

The effect of mTOR inhibition on tumour cachexia in cancer patients remains poorly investigated. Nevertheless, a retrospective study analysed the consequences of long-term treatment with rapalogs on cancer patients' muscle mass. Twenty patients, treated with rapalogs as monotherapy for at least 6 months, were investigated by CT-scan [146]. A significant decrease of skeletal muscle area without affecting body weight nor adipose tissue was observed in these patients. However, as this study did not involve an untreated control group of patients, the presence of other regulating factors cannot be excluded. This study suggests at least that cancer patients treated with mTOR inhibitors do not experience adipose tissue loss.

Pivotal phase III studies that tested rapalogs in cancer patients did not address specifically cancer cachexia. Nevertheless, parameters that are associated with cancer cachexia were reported. In a multicentre double-blind study patients with advanced pancreatic neuroendocrine tumours were randomly assigned to the rapalog everolimus, 10 mg daily, or placebo. Two hundred and four patients received everolimus versus 203 placebos. Sixteen percent of patients receiving everolimus experienced weight loss compared to 4% in the placebo group [98]. Decreased appetite was also more frequently reported in the everolimus group (20% vs. 7%). Similar findings were found in a phase III randomized trial comparing everolimus with exemestane to placebo with exemestane in patients with hormone receptor positive advanced breast cancer [99]. Of the 485 patients in the everolimus group, 19% had decreased weight versus 5% in the placebo group. In addition, 29% displayed decreased appetite under everolimus treatment compared to 10% of patients receiving placebo. Reduced appetite in patients treated with rapalog was observed in three additional phase III studies [100,101,147]. Taken together, these results show that patients treated with mTOR inhibitors present more frequently signs and symptoms that are either part of tumour cachexia or specific to mTOR inhibitors and in this case, that may worsen cachexia. In addition, they further show that some patients are more sensitive to the side effects generated by mTOR inhibitors. Hence, in the context of cachexia, it will be important to be able to detect these patients early in the course of treatment.

6. Conclusions

Tumour cachexia, characterized by weight loss due to decreased skeletal muscle and lipid mass, is a severe condition in cancer patients with limited therapeutic options. Initial studies demonstrate the complex and contrasting role played by mTOR in this process. On one hand, mTORC1 activity is significantly reduced in skeletal muscles and lipid tissue of cachectic mice suggesting that loss of mTORC1 activity results in reduced protein and lipid synthesis. On the other hand, inhibition of mTORC1 protects from tumour cachexia by up-regulating autophagy and by inhibiting production of pro-cachectic factors. Hence mTORC1 plays a dual role in tumour cachexia that needs to be fully characterized. In addition, clinical trials that specifically address the effects of mTOR inhibitors on tumour cachexia are needed.

Author Contributions: Conceptualization, O.D. and A.P.D.; Writing—Original Draft Preparation, A.P.D., C.J., T.S., O.D.

Funding: This work was supported by research grants of the Swiss National Science Foundation (310030_160125).

Conflicts of Interest: The authors declare no conflict of interest.

Abbreviations

4EBP	Eukaryotic translation initiation factor 4E-binding protein
AMPK	AMP activated protein kinase
Erk	Extracellular signal-regulated kinase
Grb10	Growth factor receptor-bound protein 10
IL	Interleukin
IGF-1	Insulin-like growth factor-1
mTOR	Mechanistic target of rapamycin
PI3K	Phosphatidylinositol 3-kinase
Raptor	Regulatory associated protein of mTOR
Rheb	RAS homolog enriched in brain
Rictor	Rapamycin insensitive companion of mTOR
TSC	Tuberous sclerosis complex
UPS	Ubiquitin proteasome system

References

1. Siegel, R.L.; Miller, K.D.; Jemal, A. Cancer statistics, 2018. *CA Cancer J. Clin.* **2018**, *68*, 7–30. [CrossRef] [PubMed]
2. Ambrus, J.L.; Ambrus, C.M.; Mink, I.B.; Pickren, J.W. Causes of death in cancer patients. *J. Med.* **1975**, *6*, 61–64. [PubMed]
3. Inagaki, J.; Rodriguez, V.; Bodey, G.P. Proceedings: Causes of death in cancer patients. *Cancer* **1974**, *33*, 568–573. [CrossRef]
4. Fearon, K.; Arends, J.; Baracos, V. Understanding the mechanisms and treatment options in cancer cachexia. *Nat. Rev. Clin. Oncol.* **2013**, *10*, 90–99. [CrossRef] [PubMed]
5. Dewys, W.D.; Begg, C.; Lavin, P.T.; Band, P.R.; Bennett, J.M.; Bertino, J.R.; Cohen, M.H.; Douglass, H.O., Jr.; Engstrom, P.F.; Ezdinli, E.Z.; et al. Prognostic effect of weight loss prior to chemotherapy in cancer patients. Eastern cooperative oncology group. *Am. J. Med.* **1980**, *69*, 491–497. [CrossRef]
6. Bachmann, J.; Heiligensetzer, M.; Krakowski-Roosen, H.; Buchler, M.W.; Friess, H.; Martignoni, M.E. Cachexia worsens prognosis in patients with resectable pancreatic cancer. *J. Gastrointest. Surg.* **2008**, *12*, 1193–1201. [CrossRef] [PubMed]
7. Saxton, R.A.; Sabatini, D.M. Mtor signalling in growth, metabolism and disease. *Cell* **2017**, *168*, 960–976. [CrossRef] [PubMed]
8. Yoon, M.S. Mtor as a key regulator in maintaining skeletal muscle mass. *Front. Physiol.* **2017**, *8*, 788. [CrossRef] [PubMed]

9. Baracos, V.E.; Martin, L.; Korc, M.; Guttridge, D.C.; Fearon, K.C.H. Cancer-associated cachexia. *Nat. Rev. Dis. Prim.* **2018**, *4*, 17105. [CrossRef] [PubMed]

10. Petruzzelli, M.; Wagner, E.F. Mechanisms of metabolic dysfunction in cancer-associated cachexia. *Genes Dev.* **2016**, *30*, 489–501. [CrossRef] [PubMed]

11. Hall, K.D.; Baracos, V.E. Computational modeling of cancer cachexia. *Curr. Opin. Clin. Nutr. Metab. Care* **2008**, *11*, 214–221. [CrossRef] [PubMed]

12. Fearon, K.C.; Glass, D.J.; Guttridge, D.C. Cancer cachexia: Mediators, signalling and metabolic pathways. *Cell Metab.* **2012**, *16*, 153–166. [CrossRef] [PubMed]

13. Mueller, T.C.; Bachmann, J.; Prokopchuk, O.; Friess, H.; Martignoni, M.E. Molecular pathways leading to loss of skeletal muscle mass in cancer cachexia—Can findings from animal models be translated to humans? *BMC Cancer* **2016**, *16*, 75. [CrossRef] [PubMed]

14. Attaix, D.; Combaret, L.; Tilignac, T.; Taillandier, D. Adaptation of the ubiquitin-proteasome proteolytic pathway in cancer cachexia. *Mol. Biol. Rep.* **1999**, *26*, 77–82. [CrossRef] [PubMed]

15. Lazarus, D.D.; Destree, A.T.; Mazzola, L.M.; McCormack, T.A.; Dick, L.R.; Xu, B.; Huang, J.Q.; Pierce, J.W.; Read, M.A.; Coggins, M.B.; et al. A new model of cancer cachexia: Contribution of the ubiquitin-proteasome pathway. *Am. J. Physiol.* **1999**, *277*, E332–E341. [CrossRef] [PubMed]

16. Khal, J.; Wyke, S.M.; Russell, S.T.; Hine, A.V.; Tisdale, M.J. Expression of the ubiquitin-proteasome pathway and muscle loss in experimental cancer cachexia. *Br. J. Cancer* **2005**, *93*, 774–780. [CrossRef] [PubMed]

17. Combaret, L.; Ralliere, C.; Taillandier, D.; Tanaka, K.; Attaix, D. Manipulation of the ubiquitin-proteasome pathway in cachexia: Pentoxifylline suppresses the activation of 20s and 26s proteasomes in muscles from tumour-bearing rats. *Mol. Biol. Rep.* **1999**, *26*, 95–101. [CrossRef] [PubMed]

18. Zhang, L.; Tang, H.; Kou, Y.; Li, R.; Zheng, Y.; Wang, Q.; Zhou, X.; Jin, L. Mg132-mediated inhibition of the ubiquitin-proteasome pathway ameliorates cancer cachexia. *J. Cancer Res. Clin. Oncol.* **2013**, *139*, 1105–1115. [CrossRef] [PubMed]

19. Williams, A.; Sun, X.; Fischer, J.E.; Hasselgren, P.O. The expression of genes in the ubiquitin-proteasome proteolytic pathway is increased in skeletal muscle from patients with cancer. *Surgery* **1999**, *126*, 744–749, discussion 749–750. [CrossRef]

20. Bossola, M.; Muscaritoli, M.; Costelli, P.; Bellantone, R.; Pacelli, F.; Busquets, S.; Argiles, J.; Lopez-Soriano, F.J.; Civello, I.M.; Baccino, F.M.; et al. Increased muscle ubiquitin mrna levels in gastric cancer patients. *Am. J. Physiol. Regul. Integr. Comp. Physiol.* **2001**, *280*, R1518–R1523. [CrossRef] [PubMed]

21. DeJong, C.H.; Busquets, S.; Moses, A.G.; Schrauwen, P.; Ross, J.A.; Argiles, J.M.; Fearon, K.C. Systemic inflammation correlates with increased expression of skeletal muscle ubiquitin but not uncoupling proteins in cancer cachexia. *Oncol. Rep.* **2005**, *14*, 257–263. [PubMed]

22. Jagoe, R.T.; Redfern, C.P.; Roberts, R.G.; Gibson, G.J.; Goodship, T.H. Skeletal muscle mrna levels for cathepsin b, but not components of the ubiquitin-proteasome pathway, are increased in patients with lung cancer referred for thoracotomy. *Clin. Sci. (Lond.)* **2002**, *102*, 353–361. [PubMed]

23. Op den Kamp, C.M.; Langen, R.C.; Minnaard, R.; Kelders, M.C.; Snepvangers, F.J.; Hesselink, M.K.; Dingemans, A.C.; Schols, A.M. Pre-cachexia in patients with stages i–iii non-small cell lung cancer: Systemic inflammation and functional impairment without activation of skeletal muscle ubiquitin proteasome system. *Lung Cancer* **2012**, *76*, 112–117. [CrossRef] [PubMed]

24. Penna, F.; Costamagna, D.; Pin, F.; Camperi, A.; Fanzani, A.; Chiarpotto, E.M.; Cavallini, G.; Bonelli, G.; Baccino, F.M.; Costelli, P. Autophagic degradation contributes to muscle wasting in cancer cachexia. *Am. J. Pathol.* **2013**, *182*, 1367–1378. [CrossRef] [PubMed]

25. Eley, H.L.; Tisdale, M.J. Skeletal muscle atrophy, a link between depression of protein synthesis and increase in degradation. *J. Biol. Chem.* **2007**, *282*, 7087–7097. [CrossRef] [PubMed]

26. Emery, P.W.; Lovell, L.; Rennie, M.J. Protein synthesis measured in vivo in muscle and liver of cachectic tumour-bearing mice. *Cancer Res.* **1984**, *44*, 2779–2784. [PubMed]

27. Emery, P.W.; Edwards, R.H.; Rennie, M.J.; Souhami, R.L.; Halliday, D. Protein synthesis in muscle measured in vivo in cachectic patients with cancer. *Br. Med. J. (Clin. Res. Ed.)* **1984**, *289*, 584–586. [CrossRef]

28. Rommel, C.; Bodine, S.C.; Clarke, B.A.; Rossman, R.; Nunez, L.; Stitt, T.N.; Yancopoulos, G.D.; Glass, D.J. Mediation of igf-1-induced skeletal myotube hypertrophy by pi(3)k/akt/mtor and pi(3)k/akt/gsk3 pathways. *Nat. Cell Biol.* **2001**, *3*, 1009–1013. [CrossRef] [PubMed]

29. Schmitt, T.L.; Martignoni, M.E.; Bachmann, J.; Fechtner, K.; Friess, H.; Kinscherf, R.; Hildebrandt, W. Activity of the akt-dependent anabolic and catabolic pathways in muscle and liver samples in cancer-related cachexia. *J. Mol. Med.* **2007**, *85*, 647–654. [CrossRef] [PubMed]

30. Stephens, N.A.; Skipworth, R.J.; Gallagher, I.J.; Greig, C.A.; Guttridge, D.C.; Ross, J.A.; Fearon, K.C. Evaluating potential biomarkers of cachexia and survival in skeletal muscle of upper gastrointestinal cancer patients. *J. Cachexia Sarcopenia Muscle* **2015**, *6*, 53–61. [CrossRef] [PubMed]

31. Penna, F.; Bonetto, A.; Muscaritoli, M.; Costamagna, D.; Minero, V.G.; Bonelli, G.; Rossi Fanelli, F.; Baccino, F.M.; Costelli, P. Muscle atrophy in experimental cancer cachexia: Is the igf-1 signalling pathway involved? *Int. J. Cancer* **2010**, *127*, 1706–1717. [CrossRef] [PubMed]

32. Murphy, K.T. The pathogenesis and treatment of cardiac atrophy in cancer cachexia. *Am. J. Physiol. Heart Circ. Physiol.* **2016**, *310*, H466–H477. [CrossRef] [PubMed]

33. Manne, N.D.; Lima, M.; Enos, R.T.; Wehner, P.; Carson, J.A.; Blough, E. Altered cardiac muscle mtor regulation during the progression of cancer cachexia in the apcmin/+ mouse. *Int. J. Oncol.* **2013**, *42*, 2134–2140. [CrossRef] [PubMed]

34. Tian, M.; Asp, M.L.; Nishijima, Y.; Belury, M.A. Evidence for cardiac atrophic remodeling in cancer-induced cachexia in mice. *Int. J. Oncol.* **2011**, *39*, 1321–1326. [PubMed]

35. Cosper, P.F.; Leinwand, L.A. Cancer causes cardiac atrophy and autophagy in a sexually dimorphic manner. *Cancer Res.* **2011**, *71*, 1710–1720. [CrossRef] [PubMed]

36. Springer, J.; Tschirner, A.; Haghikia, A.; von Haehling, S.; Lal, H.; Grzesiak, A.; Kaschina, E.; Palus, S.; Potsch, M.; von Websky, K.; et al. Prevention of liver cancer cachexia-induced cardiac wasting and heart failure. *Eur. Heart J.* **2014**, *35*, 932–941. [CrossRef] [PubMed]

37. Ebadi, M.; Mazurak, V.C. Evidence and mechanisms of fat depletion in cancer. *Nutrients* **2014**, *6*, 5280–5297. [CrossRef] [PubMed]

38. Murphy, R.A.; Wilke, M.S.; Perrine, M.; Pawlowicz, M.; Mourtzakis, M.; Lieffers, J.R.; Maneshgar, M.; Bruera, E.; Clandinin, M.T.; Baracos, V.E.; et al. Loss of adipose tissue and plasma phospholipids: Relationship to survival in advanced cancer patients. *Clin. Nutr.* **2010**, *29*, 482–487. [CrossRef] [PubMed]

39. Fouladiun, M.; Korner, U.; Bosaeus, I.; Daneryd, P.; Hyltander, A.; Lundholm, K.G. Body composition and time course changes in regional distribution of fat and lean tissue in unselected cancer patients on palliative care—Correlations with food intake, metabolism, exercise capacity and hormones. *Cancer* **2005**, *103*, 2189–2198. [CrossRef] [PubMed]

40. Dahlman, I.; Mejhert, N.; Linder, K.; Agustsson, T.; Mutch, D.M.; Kulyte, A.; Isaksson, B.; Permert, J.; Petrovic, N.; Nedergaard, J.; et al. Adipose tissue pathways involved in weight loss of cancer cachexia. *Br. J. Cancer* **2010**, *102*, 1541–1548. [CrossRef] [PubMed]

41. Agustsson, T.; Ryden, M.; Hoffstedt, J.; van Harmelen, V.; Dicker, A.; Laurencikiene, J.; Isaksson, B.; Permert, J.; Arner, P. Mechanism of increased lipolysis in cancer cachexia. *Cancer Res.* **2007**, *67*, 5531–5537. [CrossRef] [PubMed]

42. Cao, D.X.; Wu, G.H.; Yang, Z.A.; Zhang, B.; Jiang, Y.; Han, Y.S.; He, G.D.; Zhuang, Q.L.; Wang, Y.F.; Huang, Z.L.; et al. Role of beta1-adrenoceptor in increased lipolysis in cancer cachexia. *Cancer Sci.* **2010**, *101*, 1639–1645. [CrossRef] [PubMed]

43. Das, S.K.; Eder, S.; Schauer, S.; Diwoky, C.; Temmel, H.; Guertl, B.; Gorkiewicz, G.; Tamilarasan, K.P.; Kumari, P.; Trauner, M.; et al. Adipose triglyceride lipase contributes to cancer-associated cachexia. *Science* **2011**, *333*, 233–238. [CrossRef] [PubMed]

44. Bing, C.; Russell, S.; Becket, E.; Pope, M.; Tisdale, M.J.; Trayhurn, P.; Jenkins, J.R. Adipose atrophy in cancer cachexia: Morphologic and molecular analysis of adipose tissue in tumour-bearing mice. *Br. J. Cancer* **2006**, *95*, 1028–1037. [CrossRef] [PubMed]

45. Petruzzelli, M.; Schweiger, M.; Schreiber, R.; Campos-Olivas, R.; Tsoli, M.; Allen, J.; Swarbrick, M.; Rose-John, S.; Rincon, M.; Robertson, G.; et al. A switch from white to brown fat increases energy expenditure in cancer-associated cachexia. *Cell Metab.* **2014**, *20*, 433–447. [CrossRef] [PubMed]

46. Kir, S.; White, J.P.; Kleiner, S.; Kazak, L.; Cohen, P.; Baracos, V.E.; Spiegelman, B.M. Tumour-derived pth-related protein triggers adipose tissue browning and cancer cachexia. *Nature* **2014**, *513*, 100–104. [CrossRef] [PubMed]

47. Abdullahi, A.; Jeschke, M.G. White adipose tissue browning: A double-edged sword. *Trends Endocrinol. Metab.* **2016**, *27*, 542–552. [CrossRef] [PubMed]

48. Notarnicola, M.; Miccolis, A.; Tutino, V.; Lorusso, D.; Caruso, M.G. Low levels of lipogenic enzymes in peritumoral adipose tissue of colorectal cancer patients. *Lipids* **2012**, *47*, 59–63. [CrossRef] [PubMed]

49. Batista, M.L., Jr.; Neves, R.X.; Peres, S.B.; Yamashita, A.S.; Shida, C.S.; Farmer, S.R.; Seelaender, M. Heterogeneous time-dependent response of adipose tissue during the development of cancer cachexia. *J. Endocrinol.* **2012**, *215*, 363–373. [CrossRef] [PubMed]

50. Tsoli, M.; Schweiger, M.; Vanniasinghe, A.S.; Painter, A.; Zechner, R.; Clarke, S.; Robertson, G. Depletion of white adipose tissue in cancer cachexia syndrome is associated with inflammatory signaling and disrupted circadian regulation. *PLoS ONE* **2014**, *9*, e92966. [CrossRef] [PubMed]

51. Hara, K.; Maruki, Y.; Long, X.; Yoshino, K.; Oshiro, N.; Hidayat, S.; Tokunaga, C.; Avruch, J.; Yonezawa, K. Raptor, a binding partner of target of rapamycin (tor), mediates tor action. *Cell* **2002**, *110*, 177–189. [CrossRef]

52. Kim, D.H.; Sarbassov, D.D.; Ali, S.M.; Latek, R.R.; Guntur, K.V.; Erdjument-Bromage, H.; Tempst, P.; Sabatini, D.M. Gbetal, a positive regulator of the rapamycin-sensitive pathway required for the nutrient-sensitive interaction between raptor and mtor. *Mol. Cell* **2003**, *11*, 895–904. [CrossRef]

53. Sancak, Y.; Thoreen, C.C.; Peterson, T.R.; Lindquist, R.A.; Kang, S.A.; Spooner, E.; Carr, S.A.; Sabatini, D.M. Pras40 is an insulin-regulated inhibitor of the mtorc1 protein kinase. *Mol. Cell* **2007**, *25*, 903–915. [CrossRef] [PubMed]

54. Peterson, T.R.; Laplante, M.; Thoreen, C.C.; Sancak, Y.; Kang, S.A.; Kuehl, W.M.; Gray, N.S.; Sabatini, D.M. Deptor is an mtor inhibitor frequently overexpressed in multiple myeloma cells and required for their survival. *Cell* **2009**, *137*, 873–886. [CrossRef] [PubMed]

55. Dibble, C.C.; Elis, W.; Menon, S.; Qin, W.; Klekota, J.; Asara, J.M.; Finan, P.M.; Kwiatkowski, D.J.; Murphy, L.O.; Manning, B.D. Tbc1d7 is a third subunit of the tsc1-tsc2 complex upstream of mtorc1. *Mol. Cell* **2012**, *47*, 535–546. [CrossRef] [PubMed]

56. Manning, B.D.; Tee, A.R.; Logsdon, M.N.; Blenis, J.; Cantley, L.C. Identification of the tuberous sclerosis complex-2 tumor suppressor gene product tuberin as a target of the phosphoinositide 3-kinase/akt pathway. *Mol. Cell* **2002**, *10*, 151–162. [CrossRef]

57. Long, X.; Lin, Y.; Ortiz-Vega, S.; Yonezawa, K.; Avruch, J. Rheb binds and regulates the mtor kinase. *Curr. Biol.* **2005**, *15*, 702–713. [CrossRef] [PubMed]

58. Inoki, K.; Li, Y.; Zhu, T.; Wu, J.; Guan, K.L. Tsc2 is phosphorylated and inhibited by akt and suppresses mtor signalling. *Nat. Cell Biol.* **2002**, *4*, 648–657. [CrossRef] [PubMed]

59. Roux, P.P.; Ballif, B.A.; Anjum, R.; Gygi, S.P.; Blenis, J. Tumor-promoting phorbol esters and activated ras inactivate the tuberous sclerosis tumor suppressor complex via p90 ribosomal s6 kinase. *Proc. Natl. Acad. Sci. USA* **2004**, *101*, 13489–13494. [CrossRef] [PubMed]

60. Inoki, K.; Zhu, T.; Guan, K.L. Tsc2 mediates cellular energy response to control cell growth and survival. *Cell* **2003**, *115*, 577–590. [CrossRef]

61. Gwinn, D.M.; Shackelford, D.B.; Egan, D.F.; Mihaylova, M.M.; Mery, A.; Vasquez, D.S.; Turk, B.E.; Shaw, R.J. Ampk phosphorylation of raptor mediates a metabolic checkpoint. *Mol. Cell* **2008**, *30*, 214–226. [CrossRef] [PubMed]

62. Brugarolas, J.; Lei, K.; Hurley, R.L.; Manning, B.D.; Reiling, J.H.; Hafen, E.; Witters, L.A.; Ellisen, L.W.; Kaelin, W.G., Jr. Regulation of mtor function in response to hypoxia by redd1 and the tsc1/tsc2 tumor suppressor complex. *Genes Dev.* **2004**, *18*, 2893–2904. [CrossRef] [PubMed]

63. Sancak, Y.; Bar-Peled, L.; Zoncu, R.; Markhard, A.L.; Nada, S.; Sabatini, D.M. Ragulator-rag complex targets mtorc1 to the lysosomal surface and is necessary for its activation by amino acids. *Cell* **2010**, *141*, 290–303. [CrossRef] [PubMed]

64. Sancak, Y.; Peterson, T.R.; Shaul, Y.D.; Lindquist, R.A.; Thoreen, C.C.; Bar-Peled, L.; Sabatini, D.M. The rag gtpases bind raptor and mediate amino acid signaling to mtorc1. *Science* **2008**, *320*, 1496–1501. [CrossRef] [PubMed]

65. Holz, M.K.; Ballif, B.A.; Gygi, S.P.; Blenis, J. Mtor and s6k1 mediate assembly of the translation preinitiation complex through dynamic protein interchange and ordered phosphorylation events. *Cell* **2005**, *123*, 569–580. [CrossRef] [PubMed]

66. Brunn, G.J.; Hudson, C.C.; Sekulic, A.; Williams, J.M.; Hosoi, H.; Houghton, P.J.; Lawrence, J.C., Jr.; Abraham, R.T. Phosphorylation of the translational repressor phas-i by the mammalian target of rapamycin. *Science* **1997**, *277*, 99–101. [CrossRef] [PubMed]

67. Ben-Sahra, I.; Howell, J.J.; Asara, J.M.; Manning, B.D. Stimulation of de novo pyrimidine synthesis by growth signaling through mtor and s6k1. *Science* **2013**, *339*, 1323–1328. [CrossRef] [PubMed]

68. Robitaille, A.M.; Christen, S.; Shimobayashi, M.; Cornu, M.; Fava, L.L.; Moes, S.; Prescianotto-Baschong, C.; Sauer, U.; Jenoe, P.; Hall, M.N. Quantitative phosphoproteomics reveal mtorc1 activates de novo pyrimidine synthesis. *Science* **2013**, *339*, 1320–1323. [CrossRef] [PubMed]

69. Duvel, K.; Yecies, J.L.; Menon, S.; Raman, P.; Lipovsky, A.I.; Souza, A.L.; Triantafellow, E.; Ma, Q.; Gorski, R.; Cleaver, S.; et al. Activation of a metabolic gene regulatory network downstream of mtor complex 1. *Mol. Cell* **2010**, *39*, 171–183. [CrossRef] [PubMed]

70. Caron, A.; Richard, D.; Laplante, M. The roles of mtor complexes in lipid metabolism. *Annu. Rev. Nutr.* **2015**, *35*, 321–348. [CrossRef] [PubMed]

71. Efeyan, A.; Sabatini, D.M. Mtor and cancer: Many loops in one pathway. *Curr. Opin. Cell Biol.* **2010**, *22*, 169–176. [CrossRef] [PubMed]

72. Harrington, L.S.; Findlay, G.M.; Gray, A.; Tolkacheva, T.; Wigfield, S.; Rebholz, H.; Barnett, J.; Leslie, N.R.; Cheng, S.; Shepherd, P.R.; et al. The tsc1-2 tumor suppressor controls insulin-pi3k signaling via regulation of irs proteins. *J. Cell Biol.* **2004**, *166*, 213–223. [CrossRef] [PubMed]

73. Hsu, P.P.; Kang, S.A.; Rameseder, J.; Zhang, Y.; Ottina, K.A.; Lim, D.; Peterson, T.R.; Choi, Y.; Gray, N.S.; Yaffe, M.B.; et al. The mtor-regulated phosphoproteome reveals a mechanism of mtorc1-mediated inhibition of growth factor signaling. *Science* **2011**, *332*, 1317–1322. [CrossRef] [PubMed]

74. Yu, Y.; Yoon, S.O.; Poulogiannis, G.; Yang, Q.; Ma, X.M.; Villen, J.; Kubica, N.; Hoffman, G.R.; Cantley, L.C.; Gygi, S.P.; et al. Phosphoproteomic analysis identifies grb10 as an mtorc1 substrate that negatively regulates insulin signaling. *Science* **2011**, *332*, 1322–1326. [CrossRef] [PubMed]

75. Sarbassov, D.D.; Ali, S.M.; Kim, D.H.; Guertin, D.A.; Latek, R.R.; Erdjument-Bromage, H.; Tempst, P.; Sabatini, D.M. Rictor, a novel binding partner of mtor, defines a rapamycin-insensitive and raptor-independent pathway that regulates the cytoskeleton. *Curr. Biol.* **2004**, *14*, 1296–1302. [CrossRef] [PubMed]

76. Frias, M.A.; Thoreen, C.C.; Jaffe, J.D.; Schroder, W.; Sculley, T.; Carr, S.A.; Sabatini, D.M. Msin1 is necessary for akt/pkb phosphorylation and its isoforms define three distinct mtorc2s. *Curr. Biol.* **2006**, *16*, 1865–1870. [CrossRef] [PubMed]

77. Jacinto, E.; Facchinetti, V.; Liu, D.; Soto, N.; Wei, S.; Jung, S.Y.; Huang, Q.; Qin, J.; Su, B. Sin1/mip1 maintains rictor-mtor complex integrity and regulates akt phosphorylation and substrate specificity. *Cell* **2006**, *127*, 125–137. [CrossRef] [PubMed]

78. Pearce, L.R.; Huang, X.; Boudeau, J.; Pawlowski, R.; Wullschleger, S.; Deak, M.; Ibrahim, A.F.; Gourlay, R.; Magnuson, M.A.; Alessi, D.R. Identification of protor as a novel rictor-binding component of mtor complex-2. *Biochem. J.* **2007**, *405*, 513–522. [CrossRef] [PubMed]

79. Gaubitz, C.; Prouteau, M.; Kusmider, B.; Loewith, R. Torc2 structure and function. *Trends Biochem. Sci.* **2016**, *41*, 532–545. [CrossRef] [PubMed]

80. Liu, P.; Gan, W.; Chin, Y.R.; Ogura, K.; Guo, J.; Zhang, J.; Wang, B.; Blenis, J.; Cantley, L.C.; Toker, A.; et al. Ptdins(3,4,5)p3-dependent activation of the mtorc2 kinase complex. *Cancer Discov.* **2015**, *5*, 1194–1209. [CrossRef] [PubMed]

81. Zinzalla, V.; Stracka, D.; Oppliger, W.; Hall, M.N. Activation of mtorc2 by association with the ribosome. *Cell* **2011**, *144*, 757–768. [CrossRef] [PubMed]

82. Jacinto, E.; Loewith, R.; Schmidt, A.; Lin, S.; Ruegg, M.A.; Hall, A.; Hall, M.N. Mammalian tor complex 2 controls the actin cytoskeleton and is rapamycin insensitive. *Nat. Cell Biol.* **2004**, *6*, 1122–1128. [CrossRef] [PubMed]

83. Gan, X.; Wang, J.; Wang, C.; Sommer, E.; Kozasa, T.; Srinivasula, S.; Alessi, D.; Offermanns, S.; Simon, M.I.; Wu, D. Prr5l degradation promotes mtorc2-mediated pkc-delta phosphorylation and cell migration downstream of galpha12. *Nat. Cell Biol.* **2012**, *14*, 686–696. [CrossRef] [PubMed]

84. Thomanetz, V.; Angliker, N.; Cloetta, D.; Lustenberger, R.M.; Schweighauser, M.; Oliveri, F.; Suzuki, N.; Ruegg, M.A. Ablation of the mtorc2 component rictor in brain or purkinje cells affects size and neuron morphology. *J. Cell Biol.* **2013**, *201*, 293–308. [CrossRef] [PubMed]

85. Guertin, D.A.; Stevens, D.M.; Thoreen, C.C.; Burds, A.A.; Kalaany, N.Y.; Moffat, J.; Brown, M.; Fitzgerald, K.J.; Sabatini, D.M. Ablation in mice of the mtorc components raptor, rictor, or mlst8 reveals that mtorc2 is required for signaling to akt-foxo and pkcalpha, but not s6k1. *Dev. Cell* **2006**, *11*, 859–871. [CrossRef] [PubMed]

86. Faes, S.; Dormond, O. Pi3k and akt: Unfaithful partners in cancer. *Int. J. Mol. Sci.* **2015**, *16*, 21138–21152. [CrossRef] [PubMed]

87. Zhang, Y.; Kwok-Shing Ng, P.; Kucherlapati, M.; Chen, F.; Liu, Y.; Tsang, Y.H.; de Velasco, G.; Jeong, K.J.; Akbani, R.; Hadjipanayis, A.; et al. A pan-cancer proteogenomic atlas of pi3k/akt/mtor pathway alterations. *Cancer Cell* **2017**, *31*, 820.e3–832.e3. [CrossRef] [PubMed]

88. Guertin, D.A.; Sabatini, D.M. Defining the role of mtor in cancer. *Cancer Cell* **2007**, *12*, 9–22. [CrossRef] [PubMed]

89. Xie, J.; Wang, X.; Proud, C.G. Mtor inhibitors in cancer therapy. *F1000Research* **2016**, *5*. [CrossRef] [PubMed]

90. Faes, S.; Demartines, N.; Dormond, O. Resistance to mtorc1 inhibitors in cancer therapy: From kinase mutations to intratumoral heterogeneity of kinase activity. *Oxid. Med. Cell. Longev.* **2017**, *2017*, 1726078. [CrossRef] [PubMed]

91. Yang, H.; Rudge, D.G.; Koos, J.D.; Vaidialingam, B.; Yang, H.J.; Pavletich, N.P. Mtor kinase structure, mechanism and regulation. *Nature* **2013**, *497*, 217–223. [CrossRef] [PubMed]

92. Thoreen, C.C.; Kang, S.A.; Chang, J.W.; Liu, Q.; Zhang, J.; Gao, Y.; Reichling, L.J.; Sim, T.; Sabatini, D.M.; Gray, N.S. An atp-competitive mammalian target of rapamycin inhibitor reveals rapamycin-resistant functions of mtorc1. *J. Biol. Chem.* **2009**, *284*, 8023–8032. [CrossRef] [PubMed]

93. Sarbassov, D.D.; Ali, S.M.; Sengupta, S.; Sheen, J.H.; Hsu, P.P.; Bagley, A.F.; Markhard, A.L.; Sabatini, D.M. Prolonged rapamycin treatment inhibits mtorc2 assembly and akt/pkb. *Mol. Cell* **2006**, *22*, 159–168. [CrossRef] [PubMed]

94. Lamming, D.W.; Ye, L.; Katajisto, P.; Goncalves, M.D.; Saitoh, M.; Stevens, D.M.; Davis, J.G.; Salmon, A.B.; Richardson, A.; Ahima, R.S.; et al. Rapamycin-induced insulin resistance is mediated by mtorc2 loss and uncoupled from longevity. *Science* **2012**, *335*, 1638–1643. [CrossRef] [PubMed]

95. Benjamin, D.; Colombi, M.; Moroni, C.; Hall, M.N. Rapamycin passes the torch: A new generation of mtor inhibitors. *Nat. Rev. Drug Discov.* **2011**, *10*, 868–880. [CrossRef] [PubMed]

96. Hudes, G.; Carducci, M.; Tomczak, P.; Dutcher, J.; Figlin, R.; Kapoor, A.; Staroslawska, E.; Sosman, J.; McDermott, D.; Bodrogi, I.; et al. Temsirolimus, interferon alfa, or both for advanced renal-cell carcinoma. *N. Engl. J. Med.* **2007**, *356*, 2271–2281. [CrossRef] [PubMed]

97. Motzer, R.J.; Escudier, B.; Oudard, S.; Hutson, T.E.; Porta, C.; Bracarda, S.; Grunwald, V.; Thompson, J.A.; Figlin, R.A.; Hollaender, N.; et al. Efficacy of everolimus in advanced renal cell carcinoma: A double-blind, randomised, placebo-controlled phase iii trial. *Lancet* **2008**, *372*, 449–456. [CrossRef]

98. Yao, J.C.; Shah, M.H.; Ito, T.; Bohas, C.L.; Wolin, E.M.; Van Cutsem, E.; Hobday, T.J.; Okusaka, T.; Capdevila, J.; de Vries, E.G.; et al. Everolimus for advanced pancreatic neuroendocrine tumors. *N. Engl. J. Med.* **2011**, *364*, 514–523. [CrossRef] [PubMed]

99. Baselga, J.; Campone, M.; Piccart, M.; Burris, H.A., 3rd; Rugo, H.S.; Sahmoud, T.; Noguchi, S.; Gnant, M.; Pritchard, K.I.; Lebrun, F.; et al. Everolimus in postmenopausal hormone-receptor-positive advanced breast cancer. *N. Engl. J. Med.* **2012**, *366*, 520–529. [CrossRef] [PubMed]

100. Yao, J.C.; Fazio, N.; Singh, S.; Buzzoni, R.; Carnaghi, C.; Wolin, E.; Tomasek, J.; Raderer, M.; Lahner, H.; Voi, M.; et al. Everolimus for the treatment of advanced, non-functional neuroendocrine tumours of the lung or gastrointestinal tract (radiant-4): A randomised, placebo-controlled, phase 3 study. *Lancet* **2016**, *387*, 968–977. [CrossRef]

101. Hess, G.; Herbrecht, R.; Romaguera, J.; Verhoef, G.; Crump, M.; Gisselbrecht, C.; Laurell, A.; Offner, F.; Strahs, A.; Berkenblit, A.; et al. Phase iii study to evaluate temsirolimus compared with investigator's choice therapy for the treatment of relapsed or refractory mantle cell lymphoma. *J. Clin. Oncol.* **2009**, *27*, 3822–3829. [CrossRef] [PubMed]

102. Schiaffino, S.; Dyar, K.A.; Ciciliot, S.; Blaauw, B.; Sandri, M. Mechanisms regulating skeletal muscle growth and atrophy. *FEBS J.* **2013**, *280*, 4294–4314. [CrossRef] [PubMed]

103. Risson, V.; Mazelin, L.; Roceri, M.; Sanchez, H.; Moncollin, V.; Corneloup, C.; Richard-Bulteau, H.; Vignaud, A.; Baas, D.; Defour, A.; et al. Muscle inactivation of mtor causes metabolic and dystrophin defects leading to severe myopathy. *J. Cell Biol.* **2009**, *187*, 859–874. [CrossRef] [PubMed]

104. Bentzinger, C.F.; Romanino, K.; Cloetta, D.; Lin, S.; Mascarenhas, J.B.; Oliveri, F.; Xia, J.; Casanova, E.; Costa, C.F.; Brink, M.; et al. Skeletal muscle-specific ablation of raptor, but not of rictor, causes metabolic changes and results in muscle dystrophy. *Cell Metab.* **2008**, *8*, 411–424. [CrossRef] [PubMed]

105. Ohanna, M.; Sobering, A.K.; Lapointe, T.; Lorenzo, L.; Praud, C.; Petroulakis, E.; Sonenberg, N.; Kelly, P.A.; Sotiropoulos, A.; Pende, M. Atrophy of s6k1(-/-) skeletal muscle cells reveals distinct mtor effectors for cell cycle and size control. *Nat. Cell Biol.* **2005**, *7*, 286–294. [CrossRef] [PubMed]

106. Castets, P.; Lin, S.; Rion, N.; Di Fulvio, S.; Romanino, K.; Guridi, M.; Frank, S.; Tintignac, L.A.; Sinnreich, M.; Ruegg, M.A. Sustained activation of mtorc1 in skeletal muscle inhibits constitutive and starvation-induced autophagy and causes a severe, late-onset myopathy. *Cell Metab.* **2013**, *17*, 731–744. [CrossRef] [PubMed]

107. Bodine, S.C.; Stitt, T.N.; Gonzalez, M.; Kline, W.O.; Stover, G.L.; Bauerlein, R.; Zlotchenko, E.; Scrimgeour, A.; Lawrence, J.C.; Glass, D.J.; et al. Akt/mtor pathway is a crucial regulator of skeletal muscle hypertrophy and can prevent muscle atrophy in vivo. *Nat. Cell Biol.* **2001**, *3*, 1014–1019. [CrossRef] [PubMed]

108. Pallafacchina, G.; Calabria, E.; Serrano, A.L.; Kalhovde, J.M.; Schiaffino, S. A protein kinase b-dependent and rapamycin-sensitive pathway controls skeletal muscle growth but not fiber type specification. *Proc. Natl. Acad. Sci. USA* **2002**, *99*, 9213–9218. [CrossRef] [PubMed]

109. Anthony, J.C.; Yoshizawa, F.; Anthony, T.G.; Vary, T.C.; Jefferson, L.S.; Kimball, S.R. Leucine stimulates translation initiation in skeletal muscle of postabsorptive rats via a rapamycin-sensitive pathway. *J. Nutr.* **2000**, *130*, 2413–2419. [CrossRef] [PubMed]

110. Baar, K.; Esser, K. Phosphorylation of p70(s6k) correlates with increased skeletal muscle mass following resistance exercise. *Am. J. Physiol.* **1999**, *276*, C120–C127. [CrossRef] [PubMed]

111. Spangenburg, E.E.; Le Roith, D.; Ward, C.W.; Bodine, S.C. A functional insulin-like growth factor receptor is not necessary for load-induced skeletal muscle hypertrophy. *J. Physiol.* **2008**, *586*, 283–291. [CrossRef] [PubMed]

112. Jacobs, B.L.; You, J.S.; Frey, J.W.; Goodman, C.A.; Gundermann, D.M.; Hornberger, T.A. Eccentric contractions increase the phosphorylation of tuberous sclerosis complex-2 (tsc2) and alter the targeting of tsc2 and the mechanistic target of rapamycin to the lysosome. *J. Physiol.* **2013**, *591*, 4611–4620. [CrossRef] [PubMed]

113. Bakan, I.; Laplante, M. Connecting mtorc1 signaling to srebp-1 activation. *Curr. Opin. Lipidol.* **2012**, *23*, 226–234. [CrossRef] [PubMed]

114. Horton, J.D.; Goldstein, J.L.; Brown, M.S. Srebps: Activators of the complete program of cholesterol and fatty acid synthesis in the liver. *J. Clin. Investig.* **2002**, *109*, 1125–1131. [CrossRef] [PubMed]

115. Mauvoisin, D.; Rocque, G.; Arfa, O.; Radenne, A.; Boissier, P.; Mounier, C. Role of the pi3-kinase/mtor pathway in the regulation of the stearoyl coa desaturase (scd1) gene expression by insulin in liver. *J. Cell Commun. Signal.* **2007**, *1*, 113–125. [CrossRef] [PubMed]

116. Porstmann, T.; Santos, C.R.; Griffiths, B.; Cully, M.; Wu, M.; Leevers, S.; Griffiths, J.R.; Chung, Y.L.; Schulze, A. Srebp activity is regulated by mtorc1 and contributes to akt-dependent cell growth. *Cell Metab.* **2008**, *8*, 224–236. [CrossRef] [PubMed]

117. Yecies, J.L.; Zhang, H.H.; Menon, S.; Liu, S.; Yecies, D.; Lipovsky, A.I.; Gorgun, C.; Kwiatkowski, D.J.; Hotamisligil, G.S.; Lee, C.H.; et al. Akt stimulates hepatic srebp1c and lipogenesis through parallel mtorc1-dependent and independent pathways. *Cell Metab.* **2011**, *14*, 21–32. [CrossRef] [PubMed]

118. Hagiwara, A.; Cornu, M.; Cybulski, N.; Polak, P.; Betz, C.; Trapani, F.; Terracciano, L.; Heim, M.H.; Ruegg, M.A.; Hall, M.N. Hepatic mtorc2 activates glycolysis and lipogenesis through akt, glucokinase and srebp1c. *Cell Metab.* **2012**, *15*, 725–738. [CrossRef] [PubMed]

119. Yuan, M.; Pino, E.; Wu, L.; Kacergis, M.; Soukas, A.A. Identification of akt-independent regulation of hepatic lipogenesis by mammalian target of rapamycin (mtor) complex 2. *J. Biol. Chem.* **2012**, *287*, 29579–29588. [CrossRef] [PubMed]

120. Yeh, W.C.; Bierer, B.E.; McKnight, S.L. Rapamycin inhibits clonal expansion and adipogenic differentiation of 3t3-l1 cells. *Proc. Natl. Acad. Sci. USA* **1995**, *92*, 11086–11090. [CrossRef] [PubMed]

121. Zhang, H.H.; Huang, J.; Duvel, K.; Boback, B.; Wu, S.; Squillace, R.M.; Wu, C.L.; Manning, B.D. Insulin stimulates adipogenesis through the akt-tsc2-mtorc1 pathway. *PLoS ONE* **2009**, *4*, e6189. [CrossRef] [PubMed]

122. Polak, P.; Cybulski, N.; Feige, J.N.; Auwerx, J.; Ruegg, M.A.; Hall, M.N. Adipose-specific knockout of raptor results in lean mice with enhanced mitochondrial respiration. *Cell Metab.* **2008**, *8*, 399–410. [CrossRef] [PubMed]

123. Chang, G.R.; Chiu, Y.S.; Wu, Y.Y.; Chen, W.Y.; Liao, J.W.; Chao, T.H.; Mao, F.C. Rapamycin protects against high fat diet-induced obesity in c57bl/6j mice. *J. Pharmacol. Sci.* **2009**, *109*, 496–503. [CrossRef] [PubMed]

124. Houde, V.P.; Brule, S.; Festuccia, W.T.; Blanchard, P.G.; Bellmann, K.; Deshaies, Y.; Marette, A. Chronic rapamycin treatment causes glucose intolerance and hyperlipidemia by upregulating hepatic gluconeogenesis and impairing lipid deposition in adipose tissue. *Diabetes* **2010**, *59*, 1338–1348. [CrossRef] [PubMed]

125. Magun, R.; Burgering, B.M.; Coffer, P.J.; Pardasani, D.; Lin, Y.; Chabot, J.; Sorisky, A. Expression of a constitutively activated form of protein kinase b (c-akt) in 3t3-l1 preadipose cells causes spontaneous differentiation. *Endocrinology* **1996**, *137*, 3590–3593. [CrossRef] [PubMed]

126. Nakae, J.; Kitamura, T.; Kitamura, Y.; Biggs, W.H., 3rd; Arden, K.C.; Accili, D. The forkhead transcription factor foxo1 regulates adipocyte differentiation. *Dev. Cell* **2003**, *4*, 119–129. [CrossRef]

127. Cybulski, N.; Polak, P.; Auwerx, J.; Ruegg, M.A.; Hall, M.N. Mtor complex 2 in adipose tissue negatively controls whole-body growth. *Proc. Natl. Acad. Sci. USA* **2009**, *106*, 9902–9907. [CrossRef] [PubMed]

128. Kumar, A.; Lawrence, J.C., Jr.; Jung, D.Y.; Ko, H.J.; Keller, S.R.; Kim, J.K.; Magnuson, M.A.; Harris, T.E. Fat cell-specific ablation of rictor in mice impairs insulin-regulated fat cell and whole-body glucose and lipid metabolism. *Diabetes* **2010**, *59*, 1397–1406. [CrossRef] [PubMed]

129. Yao, Y.; Suraokar, M.; Darnay, B.G.; Hollier, B.G.; Shaiken, T.E.; Asano, T.; Chen, C.H.; Chang, B.H.; Lu, Y.; Mills, G.B.; et al. Bsta promotes mtorc2-mediated phosphorylation of akt1 to suppress expression of foxc2 and stimulate adipocyte differentiation. *Sci. Signal.* **2013**, *6*, ra2. [CrossRef] [PubMed]

130. Morrisett, J.D.; Abdel-Fattah, G.; Kahan, B.D. Sirolimus changes lipid concentrations and lipoprotein metabolism in kidney transplant recipients. *Transpl. Proc.* **2003**, *35*, 143S–150S. [CrossRef]

131. Chakrabarti, P.; English, T.; Shi, J.; Smas, C.M.; Kandror, K.V. Mammalian target of rapamycin complex 1 suppresses lipolysis, stimulates lipogenesis and promotes fat storage. *Diabetes* **2010**, *59*, 775–781. [CrossRef] [PubMed]

132. Pereira, M.J.; Palming, J.; Rizell, M.; Aureliano, M.; Carvalho, E.; Svensson, M.K.; Eriksson, J.W. The immunosuppressive agents rapamycin, cyclosporin a and tacrolimus increase lipolysis, inhibit lipid storage and alter expression of genes involved in lipid metabolism in human adipose tissue. *Mol. Cell. Endocrinol.* **2013**, *365*, 260–269. [CrossRef] [PubMed]

133. Baltgalvis, K.A.; Berger, F.G.; Pena, M.M.; Davis, J.M.; Muga, S.J.; Carson, J.A. Interleukin-6 and cachexia in apcmin/+ mice. *Am. J. Physiol. Regul. Integr. Comp. Physiol.* **2008**, *294*, R393–R401. [CrossRef] [PubMed]

134. White, J.P.; Baynes, J.W.; Welle, S.L.; Kostek, M.C.; Matesic, L.E.; Sato, S.; Carson, J.A. The regulation of skeletal muscle protein turnover during the progression of cancer cachexia in the apc(min/+) mouse. *PLoS ONE* **2011**, *6*, e24650. [CrossRef] [PubMed]

135. White, J.P.; Puppa, M.J.; Gao, S.; Sato, S.; Welle, S.L.; Carson, J.A. Muscle mtorc1 suppression by il-6 during cancer cachexia: A role for ampk. *Am. J. Physiol. Endocrinol. Metab.* **2013**, *304*, E1042–E1052. [CrossRef] [PubMed]

136. Puppa, M.J.; White, J.P.; Velazquez, K.T.; Baltgalvis, K.A.; Sato, S.; Baynes, J.W.; Carson, J.A. The effect of exercise on il-6-induced cachexia in the apc (min/+) mouse. *J. Cachexia Sarcopenia Muscle* **2012**, *3*, 117–137. [CrossRef] [PubMed]

137. Puppa, M.J.; Gao, S.; Narsale, A.A.; Carson, J.A. Skeletal muscle glycoprotein 130's role in lewis lung carcinoma-induced cachexia. *FASEB J.* **2014**, *28*, 998–1009. [CrossRef] [PubMed]

138. Gao, S.; Carson, J.A. Lewis lung carcinoma regulation of mechanical stretch-induced protein synthesis in cultured myotubes. *Am. J. Physiol. Cell Physiol.* **2016**, *310*, C66–C79. [CrossRef] [PubMed]

139. Chen, X.; Wu, Y.; Yang, T.; Wei, M.; Wang, Y.; Deng, X.; Shen, C.; Li, W.; Zhang, H.; Xu, W.; et al. Salidroside alleviates cachexia symptoms in mouse models of cancer cachexia via activating mtor signalling. *J. Cachexia Sarcopenia Muscle* **2016**, *7*, 225–232. [CrossRef] [PubMed]

140. Zhao, J.; Zhai, B.; Gygi, S.P.; Goldberg, A.L. Mtor inhibition activates overall protein degradation by the ubiquitin proteasome system as well as by autophagy. *Proc. Natl. Acad. Sci. USA* **2015**, *112*, 15790–15797. [CrossRef] [PubMed]

141. Rousseau, A.; Bertolotti, A. An evolutionarily conserved pathway controls proteasome homeostasis. *Nature* **2016**, *536*, 184–189. [CrossRef] [PubMed]

142. Pigna, E.; Berardi, E.; Aulino, P.; Rizzuto, E.; Zampieri, S.; Carraro, U.; Kern, H.; Merigliano, S.; Gruppo, M.; Mericskay, M.; et al. Aerobic exercise and pharmacological treatments counteract cachexia by modulating autophagy in colon cancer. *Sci. Rep.* **2016**, *6*, 26991. [CrossRef] [PubMed]

143. Masiero, E.; Agatea, L.; Mammucari, C.; Blaauw, B.; Loro, E.; Komatsu, M.; Metzger, D.; Reggiani, C.; Schiaffino, S.; Sandri, M. Autophagy is required to maintain muscle mass. *Cell Metab.* **2009**, *10*, 507–515. [CrossRef] [PubMed]

144. Robert, F.; Mills, J.R.; Agenor, A.; Wang, D.; DiMarco, S.; Cencic, R.; Tremblay, M.L.; Gallouzi, I.E.; Hekimi, S.; Wing, S.S.; et al. Targeting protein synthesis in a myc/mtor-driven model of anorexia-cachexia syndrome delays its onset and prolongs survival. *Cancer Res.* **2012**, *72*, 747–756. [CrossRef] [PubMed]

145. Hatakeyama, S.; Summermatter, S.; Jourdain, M.; Melly, S.; Minetti, G.C.; Lach-Trifilieff, E. Actrii blockade protects mice from cancer cachexia and prolongs survival in the presence of anti-cancer treatments. *Skelet. Muscle* **2016**, *6*, 26. [CrossRef] [PubMed]

146. Gyawali, B.; Shimokata, T.; Honda, K.; Kondoh, C.; Hayashi, N.; Yoshino, Y.; Sassa, N.; Nakano, Y.; Gotoh, M.; Ando, Y. Muscle wasting associated with the long-term use of mtor inhibitors. *Mol. Clin. Oncol.* **2016**, *5*, 641–646. [CrossRef] [PubMed]

147. Motzer, R.J.; Escudier, B.; McDermott, D.F.; George, S.; Hammers, H.J.; Srinivas, S.; Tykodi, S.S.; Sosman, J.A.; Procopio, G.; Plimack, E.R.; et al. Nivolumab versus everolimus in advanced renal-cell carcinoma. *N. Engl. J. Med.* **2015**, *373*, 1803–1813. [CrossRef] [PubMed]

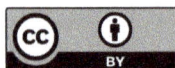

International Journal of
Molecular Sciences

MDPI

Review

mTOR-Related Brain Dysfunctions in Neuropsychiatric Disorders

Larisa Ryskalin [1], Fiona Limanaqi [1], Alessandro Frati [2], Carla L. Busceti [2] and Francesco Fornai [1,2,]

[1] Human Anatomy, Department of Translational Research and New Technologies in Medicine and Surgery, University of Pisa, Via Roma 55, 56126 Pisa, Italy; larisa.ryskalin@unipi.it (L.R.); f.limanaqi@studenti.unipi.it (F.L.)

[2] I.R.C.C.S. Neuromed, Via Atinense 18, 86077 Isernia, Italy; alessandro.frati@uniroma1.it (A.F.); clbusceti@libero.it (C.L.B.)

* Correspondence: francesco.fornai@med.unipi.it; Tel.: +39-050-221-8611

Received: 4 July 2018; Accepted: 27 July 2018; Published: 30 July 2018

Abstract: The mammalian target of rapamycin (mTOR) is an ubiquitously expressed serine-threonine kinase, which senses and integrates several intracellular and environmental cues to orchestrate major processes such as cell growth and metabolism. Altered mTOR signalling is associated with brain malformation and neurological disorders. Emerging evidence indicates that even subtle defects in the mTOR pathway may produce severe effects, which are evident as neurological and psychiatric disorders. On the other hand, administration of mTOR inhibitors may be beneficial for a variety of neuropsychiatric alterations encompassing neurodegeneration, brain tumors, brain ischemia, epilepsy, autism, mood disorders, drugs of abuse, and schizophrenia. mTOR has been widely implicated in synaptic plasticity and autophagy activation. This review addresses the role of mTOR-dependent autophagy dysfunction in a variety of neuropsychiatric disorders, to focus mainly on psychiatric syndromes including schizophrenia and drug addiction. For instance, amphetamines-induced addiction fairly overlaps with some neuropsychiatric disorders including neurodegeneration and schizophrenia. For this reason, in the present review, a special emphasis is placed on the role of mTOR on methamphetamine-induced brain alterations.

Keywords: mTOR; rapamycin; autophagy; protein aggregation; methamphetamine; schizophrenia

1. Introduction

The discovery of the mammalian target of rapamycin (mTOR) dates back to early 1970s with the collection of a soil sample of Easter Island (Rapa Nui) and the serendipitous identification of a lipophilic macrolide produced by the soil bacterium *Streptomyces hygroscopicus* [1]. This natural compound called rapamycin was initially developed as an antifungal drug, but it soon raised considerable interest because of its unexpected and, at that time, undesired immunosuppressive side effects. The discovery of rapamycin-mediated anti-proliferative effects on immune cells was a milestone in organ transplantation [2–6]. However, the finding of anti-proliferative activities, way beyond the immunosuppressive properties, disclosed novel potential therapeutic uses that fueled research on its mechanisms of action [7–10]. Nowadays, it is well established that rapamycin exerts its effects by forming a complex with FK506-binding protein 12 (FKBP12), which in turn inhibits the target of rapamycin (TOR). TOR is a large (289 kDa), evolutionarily highly conserved, serine/threonine kinase, which represents the catalytic domain of a multiprotein complex named TORC (target of rapamycin complex) [5,11–13]. The need of FKBP-12 to mediate the effects of rapamycin on TORC is demonstrated by a lack of effects induced by rapamycin when the binding between FKBP12 and rapamycin is occluded by a missense point mutations within the

FRB domain of TOR [14,15]. In mammals, TOR kinase, also known as mTOR (i.e., mammalian TOR), is ubiquitously expressed in all cell types and it assembles with several scaffolds and regulatory subunits to form two distinct multiprotein complexes, hereinafter referred as mTOR complex 1 (mTORC1) and mTOR complex 2 (mTORC2) [16–19]. These mTOR complexes share four components that are identical; they possess (i) a catalytic subunit, along with (ii) a small protein known as mLSt8, which represent the core of both complexes. These in turn are composed of two more components, namely (iii) the Tti1/Tel2 associated regulatory proteins, which create a scaffold for recruitment of substrates; and (iv) the negative regulator Deptor, which inhibits the substrate binding [20–22]. In addition, there are specific subunits depending on which mTOR complex is considered. In detail, mTORC1 contains the scaffold protein Raptor and the inhibitory subunit PRAS40 as key components, while mTORC2 specifically associates with the regulatory subunit Protor 1/2 and scaffold proteins Rictor and mSIN1, which help the complex assembly [20,23–28]. The mTOR complex represents a downstream substrate of the PI3K/PTEN/Akt pathway, which controls cell growth, proliferation, metabolism, and motility in response to bioenergetics and nutritional requests [29,30]. Extracellular and environmental stimuli are conveyed through mTOR via the PI3K/PTEN/Akt pathway. The binding of insulin and growth factors to tyrosine kinase receptors (RTKs) activates the lipid kinase PI3K, which phosphorylates phosphatidylinositol-4,5-phosphate (PIP2) to generate phosphatidylinositol-3,4,5-phosphate (PIP3). This second messenger recruits Akt, which promotes mTOR activity. This occurs via the phosphorylation of the tuberous sclerosis complex (TSC), which impairs its inhibitory activity on mTOR. TSC is a heterodimer that is composed of hamartin (TSC1) and tuberin (TSC2). In this way, the activation of PI3K/Akt signaling leads to the activation of mTOR through TSC inhibition. Once activated, mTOR promotes various activities including protein synthesis, ribosome, and lipid biogenesis [21,31] (Figure 1). Among these activities, mTOR inhibits autophagy [32]. In mammalian cells, three main autophagy pathways are described, all providing the lysosomal degradation of intracellular components: (i) micro-autophagy; (ii) macro-autophagy; and (iii) chaperone-mediated autophagy (CMA). In detail, micro-autophagy enwraps small portions of cytosol and proteins into lysosomes [33], while macro-autophagy sequesters "in bulk" cytosolic cargoes, including organelles, within autophagosomes to merge with lysosomes [34]. Finally, CMA is a rather selective process where proteins are bound to cytosolic chaperones (e.g., LAMP-2) to be recognized and translocated across the lysosomal membrane for degradation [35]. In the present review, we focus on macro-autophagy (hereinafter referred to as autophagy), which is mostly related to mTOR activity. In detail, mTOR inhibits autophagy by suppressing the ULK1 complex, which consists of several autophagy-related proteins (ULK1, Atg13, FIP200). In fact, by phosphorylating the ULK1 complex, mTOR inhibits early steps in the biogenesis of autophagosomes [36–39] (Figure 1). Conversely, rapamycin-induced mTOR inhibition strongly activates autophagy. In eukaryotic cells, autophagy represents the main cell clearing system. The autophagy pathway is initiated through a nascent double-layered membrane vacuole, which, at early stages, is not yet complete and is named phagophore. The maturation of the phagophore leads to seal the vacuole, which is then named autophagosome. At this stage, the vacuole stains for beclin-1 (the ortholog of yeast Atg6) and LC3 (Atg8), which are thus considered gold standard autophagy markers [40]. The autophagosome carries a variety of substrates to the lysosomal compartment, which possesses a rich enzymatic activity. In detail, when the autophagosome merges with the lysosome, the catalytic organelle autophagolysosome is generated, where degradation and recycling of sequestered cytosolic cargoes occurs. Autophagy can be tuned very finely to obtain either slight or robust effects based upon specific cell needs. For instance, autophagy is strongly induced by nutrient depletion, which occurs during cell starvation. In these conditions, enhanced protein degradation within lysosomes results in the generation of single amino acids. This is the prototype for extreme cell conditions when cell survival is jeopardized; however, a slight autophagy activation is needed in baseline conditions to keep steady the level of misfolded proteins that naturally occur within a living cell. An appropriate tuning of autophagy avoids the burden of aged structures within the cell. Along with degrading misfolded proteins, autophagy degrades altered subcellular organelles (mitochondria, endoplasmic reticulum, ribosomes, and even synaptic vesicles). Thus, when a mild failure in the autophagy pathway occurs, the cell still survives, though such a decreased protein turnover during prolonged time intervals is detrimental. In fact, this may alter a variety of cell activities and may even produce toxicity. This is why it takes time to appreciate the effects of a slight relenting of protein and organelle turnover due to a mild autophagy deficiency. In fact, in these conditions, the cell may easily cope with moderate energy demands. In contrast, when the production of altered structures exceeds a reduced autophagy activity, these accumulate and become visible over the years through intracellular deposits that contain altered protein aggregates. This is probably why an autophagy defect eventually leads to slowly developing neuronal inclusions. This is facilitated by the inner nature of specific proteins such as alpha synuclein, which is prone to aggregate because 30% of its native form undergoes spontaneous oligomerization independently of the metabolic conditions [41]. Thus, autophagy defects are expected to generate protein aggregates, which in turn promote toxicity and cell death [42]. This is kind of an oversimplification, but it helps to schematize the concept of autophagy as a cell clearing system beyond its powerful energetic effects. Unlike most cell types, neurons are extremely vulnerable to autophagy impairment. This is not surprising when considering that adult neuronal cells are post-mitotic. Therefore, neurons cannot profit from mitosis to dilute potential toxic waste within daughter cells. In fact, mice deficient for autophagy-related proteins, such as Atg5 or Atg7, show inclusion bodies and marked neuronal loss [43,44]. In line with this, mTOR-dependent impairment of autophagy is implicated in various neuropsychiatric disorders such as dementia, movement disorders, motor neuron disease, seizures, brain ischemia, autism, affective disorders, addiction, and schizophrenia [45–57]. While the involvement of autophagy in neurological disorders is intensely investigated, the evidence about an involvement of autophagy in psychiatric disorders is less clear. Therefore, the aim of the present manuscript is to mention the role of mTOR-dependent autophagy in neurodegeneration while emphasizing its role in methamphetamine (METH) addiction and psychiatric disorders, namely schizophrenia. Remarkably, a growing evidence shows that mTOR dysfunction may underlie a variety of psychiatric syndromes, including mood disorders, drug addiction, and schizophrenia. In fact, many psychotropic drugs including mood stabilizers and neuroleptics are powerful autophagy inducers [58–67]. In such an attempt, we hint to the role of mTOR-dependent autophagy as a hub in etiologically distinct brain disorders from neurodegeneration to METH abuse and schizophrenia.

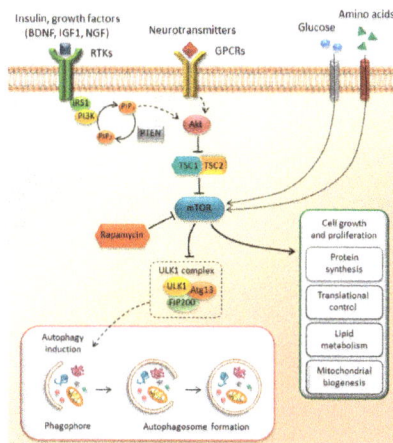

Figure 1. The mammalian target of rapamycin (mTOR) pathway. The cartoon summarizes the main up- and down-stream components of the mTOR pathway. Growth factors, glucose, and amino acids

activate mTOR, which in turn promotes protein synthesis, lipid metabolism, and mitochondrial biogenesis, while autophagy is under the negative control mTOR. GPCRs—G-protein coupled receptors. TSC—tuberous sclerosis complex; TSC1—hamartin; TSC2—tuberin; RTKs—receptor tyrosine kinase receptors; Akt—protein kinase B; PTEN—Phosphatase and Tensin Homolog; BDNF—Brain-derived neurotrophic factor; IGF—insulin-like growth factor; NGF—nerve growth factor.

2. A Short Overview on Autophagy Impairment in Neurodegenerative Disorders

Dysfunctional autophagy appears as a recurring feature in neurodegenerative disorders (NDDs), such as Parkinson's disease (PD) and Alzheimer's disease (AD), where a defect along the autophagy pathway occurs at different stages [68–76]. The accumulation of aggregate-prone proteins triggers the formation of cytoplasmic and/or extracellular neuronal inclusions within specific brain areas. This occurs in PD, where aggregate-prone alpha synuclein accumulates in the so-called Lewy bodies, which are mostly found within spared dopaminergic (DA) neurons of the substantia nigra pars compacta (SNpc) [77,78], as well as within extra-nigral neuronal populations [79]. Remarkably, genetic ablation of Atg7 specifically within dopamine (DA) neurons fully reproduces PD pathology, including the formation of Lewy bodies, which stain for alpha synuclein, pointing at a key role for autophagy in DA-related disorders [80]. Likewise, AD cortical pathology features abnormal intracellular hyperphosporylated tau protein, which forms fibrils known as neurofibrillary tangles (NFT) along with extracellular amyloid-β (Aβ) plaques [81]. Pathological TAR DNA-binding protein 43 (TDP-43) is a major component of inclusions that are found in most cases of amyotrophic lateral sclerosis (ALS) and in frontotemporal lobar degeneration (FTLD) [82,83]. Remarkably, further investigation on the autophagy pathway revealed that all these misfolded proteins are autophagy substrates depending on mTOR activity [84–88]. In an attempt to attribute a specific protein accumulation to the onset of a specific disorder within the aim of describing a sort of "precision medicine", investigators faced the hurdle that these protein aggregates may indeed be shared by different disorders and different proteins may aggregate in the same disease. In fact, TDP-43 positive inclusions are found within the very same neurons containing tau-positive NFTs and alpha synuclein-positive Lewy bodies of post-mortem brains from patients with AD and dementia with Lewy bodies (DLB), respectively [89]. In addition, most DLB patients show most features of AD (i.e., hyperphosphorylated tau deposits and Aβ) to various extents [90]. Moreover, alpha synuclein immunoreactivity often co-localizes within huntingtin polyglutamine-positive aggregates in brain sections from patients with late-stage Huntington's disease (HD) patients [91], or even within SOD1-positive inclusions, as revealed by immunohistochemical analysis performed in post-mortem brain and spinal cord from cases of familial ALS [92]. All this evidence challenges the concept of a protein-specific vulnerability to characterize each disease leading to clinically distinct neurological phenotypes. Such a contamination even overcomes the clear cut between neurodegenerative disorders and acute cerebral ischemia/chronic hypoperfusion [93]. A failure in autophagy-dependent handling of misfolded proteins impedes the clearance of these substrates that are likely to accumulate within the cell. Therefore, a common pathogenesis underlying all these NDDs disorders has been linked to autophagy inhibition due to mTOR hyperactivation [52,54,94–97]. For instance, an increased mTOR activity correlates with accumulation of Aβ and hyperphosphorylated tau in AD brains [98,99]. On the other hand, some evidence indicates that suppressing mTOR activity ameliorates AD cognitive defects by decreasing Aβ and tau pathology [100]. Again, rapamycin and rapalogs protect against toxicity produced by a number of misfolded proteins encompassing alpha synuclein, TDP43, and hyperphosphorylated tau [101–104]. Therefore, mTOR inhibitors, as such autophagy inducers, may be useful to boost relented cell clearing mechanisms by decreasing abnormal aggregate-prone proteins, which is supposed to ameliorate neurodegeneration.

3. Beyond Classic Neurodegeneration

The beneficial effects of mTOR inhibitors have been demonstrated in patients affected by neurodevelopmental disorders [105–108]. In fact, compounds belonging to the macrolides family, such as rapamycin and rapalogs, and ameliorate cognitive, affective, and overall psychiatric symptoms, which is in line with an Akt–mTOR-dependent antidepressant and mood stabilizing effect [105,109,110]. This is further supported by mounting evidence obtained in rodent models, which demonstrate that rapamycin normalizes impaired social interactions and reverses behavioral defects [61,109,111–114]. This appears indeed as a continuum rather than a concomitance of different effects, as patients affected by neurodegenerative disorders frequently develop psychiatric symptoms like mood alterations, depression, and schizophrenia, which may appear early during disease development and then may persist throughout the disease course [115–120]. As briefly reported, despite a high number of studies correlating mTOR and autophagy with neurological disorders [45–57], only a few studies addressed such an issue in psychiatric disorders such as schizophrenia [121,122]. This is likely to depend on the lower amount of biological and pathological investigations that are carried out in these patients and the scarce knowledge about the molecular neurobiology of disease-concerning psychiatric disorders. In schizophrenia, a progressive synaptic disorder is likely to promote neurodegeneration [123]. In support of this view, autoptic studies on schizophrenic brains have revealed the presence of neuronal inclusions (see Section 5), which may depend on dysfunctional mTOR-related cell clearing systems. Similarly, neuronal inclusions occur in METH abusers [124], confirming what was previously demonstrated in animal models [125,126]. As detailed in the following paragraph, METH exerts disruptive effects on DA neurotransmission, which translate into abnormal stimulation of post-synaptic DA receptors, mainly D1-type DA receptors (D1R), thus leading to non-canonical signaling cascades sustaining behavioral alterations that overlap with schizophrenia-like symptoms (i.e., visual and auditory hallucinations and delusions) [127–130]. Increased activity of D1R is considered as a major determinant of neuropsychiatric alterations occurring in both METH models/abusers and in schizophrenia [130–132]. This is key, because abnormal stimulation of D1R and subsequent signaling cascades were recently shown to produce an over-activation of mTOR and inhibition of the autophagy machinery [133]. In addition, several susceptibility genes for schizophrenia (e.g., *DISC1*, *NRG1/ErbB4*, and *CRMP2*), which are involved in either pre-synaptic DA release or post-synaptic D1R-related cascades, are similarly dysregulated by METH. Interestingly, they all converge on mTOR signaling (see Section 6, Table 1). In fact, mTOR-induced autophagy inhibition exacerbates the ultrastructural effects of METH [126,134–136], while rapamycin administration reverts both behavioral and morphological alterations induced by METH [137]. Such an issue will be further dealt with in the next paragraph. Here, we wish to point out that the detrimental effects of METH on both DA neurotransmission and mTOR-dependent cell clearing systems produce behavioral alterations that are reminiscent of schizophrenia. Thus, METH addicted brains may represent a bridge that connects neurodegenerative and psychiatric disorders. Understanding the molecular and cellular mechanisms that operate during METH toxicity is expected to increase our insight into the neurobiology of schizophrenia. Thus, in the next paragraph we discuss evidence on how altered mTOR and an impaired autophagy pathway may indeed represent a common hub between drug addiction and schizophrenia.

4. Bridging Neurodegeneration and Psychiatric Disorders: The Paradigm of Methamphetamine-Addicted Brains

METH is a widely abused drug that rapidly enters and persists within the central nervous system (CNS), thereby exerting powerful addictive effects [138–140]. In humans, the sensitizing effects of prolonged chronic METH intake are considered a major determinant to the occurrence and relapse of psychoses, which mirror those occurring in schizophrenic patients. In fact, METH-addicted patients commonly develop psychoses with positive symptoms similar to those of schizophrenia, which led to the use of METH as an experimental model of schizophrenia (Figure 2). In fact, psychotic patients are oversensitive to amphetamines [141,142]. Accordingly, clinical evidence points towards an elevation of pre-synaptic DA synthesis and release as a key event for schizophrenia [141,143,144]. Likewise, the psychostimulant effects experienced by METH-addicted patients rely on increased DA synthesis and massive DA release from nerve terminals within limbic areas as occurring in the schizophrenic brain [145–149]. Such an abnormal DA release produces peaks of extracellular DA, which cannot be taken up within nerve terminals, because METH inhibits and reverts the direction of the dopamine transporter (DAT). In line with this, recent studies suggest that DAT expression is significantly reduced in the midbrain of postmortem schizophrenic samples [150], which is reminiscent of the METH-addicted brain [151,152]. Upon METH administration, the massive amount of extracellular DA is followed by DA depletion, which translates into a pulsatile stimulation of post-synaptic DA receptors. This triggers non-canonical transduction pathways driving phenotypic changes at the level of post-synaptic neurons. The abnormal activity of DA receptors is an additional commonality between METH and schizophrenia, which is likely to represent the molecular mechanism underlying behavioral alterations [130–132]. Remarkably, mTOR over-activation was recently linked to METH-induced behavioral sensitization, while rapamycin prevents such an effect [137]. Likewise, rapamycin was found to be beneficial for ameliorating psychotic symptoms [109,112,114,153,154]. The relevance of autophagy for sustaining these mTOR-induced effects is confirmed by drugs inducing autophagy independently of mTOR activation. In fact, lithium is able to delay METH-induced sensitization, while being a powerful treatment in schizophrenia [155]. Behavioral alterations driven by abnormal DA receptor activity are widely dependent on the amount of DA released from pre-synaptic terminals. Noteworthy, genetic ablation of autophagy was shown to produce an extremely powerful DA release upon electrical stimuli, suggesting that autophagy is key to restrain DA release both upon basal neural activity and mostly after rapamycin-induced autophagy [156]. These findings strongly suggest that an autophagy dysfunction acts both at pre- and post-synaptic level to alter DA neurotransmission during both METH administration and schizophrenia (Figure 2). This confirms our previous studies showing that both genetic and pharmacological autophagy inhibition worsen the effects of METH administration [126]. Given the paucity of studies showing such a role in schizophrenia, dissecting the molecular mechanisms underlying autophagy dysfunction in METH may provide insights in the pathophysiology of schizophrenia. In line with this, METH produces ultrastructural alterations reflecting dysfunctional autophagy flux, which are DA-dependent. In fact, METH produces a massive increase of endogenous intra-cytosolic DA levels by inhibiting and reverting the direction of the vesicular monoamine transporter type 2 (VMAT-2), thus disrupting the physiological storage of DA. A reduction in VMAT-2 gene expression and protein levels in DA neurons occurs in both METH models and schizophrenic patients, marking quite impressively the overlap between these disorders [150,157,158]. It is worth mentioning that freely diffusible intra-cytosolic DA can readily undergo auto-oxidation and produce a cascade of oxidative-related damage, which is bound to the neurotoxic effects of high doses of METH [125,159–161]. In fact, DA auto-oxidation generates several toxic and highly reactive species such as DA-quinones, hydrogen peroxide, and superoxide radicals. Beyond METH, redox-related changes that result from an imbalance between reactive oxygen species (ROS) production and ROS clearance are implicated in schizophrenia [122]. As a result of an altered intracellular redox environment, proteins lose their native conformational fold and assume an aberrant, misfolded conformation with an abnormal tendency to aggregate into larger, often insoluble, inclusions [148,159,162]. This excessive amount of aggregate-prone proteins within DA axon terminals leads to an autophagy engulfment, which fuels a vicious cycle of oxidative stress, protein misfolding, and aggregation [125,126,148,162] (Figure 2). In fact, when administered both in vitro and in vivo, METH generates multi-lamellar whorls corresponding to stagnant autophagy vacuoles, which further develop into eosinophilic cytoplasmic inclusions within both nigral DA neurons and striatal cells [125,162,163]. These inclusions are reminiscent of PD-like Lewy bodies because they stain for typical PD markers such alpha synuclein [125,126,162,164,165]. The occurrence of analogous nigral inclusions was confirmed in human chronic METH abusers [124]. In addition, the occurrence of alpha synuclein gene (*SNCA*) polymorphisms is associated with human METH psychosis [166]. This is in line with genetic studies associating psychotic symptoms with *SNCA* multiplications [167]. As both DA neurotransmission and handling of misfolded proteins are directly bound to autophagy, it is likely that autophagy alterations represent a causative mechanism underling ongoing synaptic pathology, which could predispose to neurodegeneration. In the light of these findings, in the next paragraph, we provide evidence that ultrastructural changes related to autophagy alterations occur in schizophrenia as well.

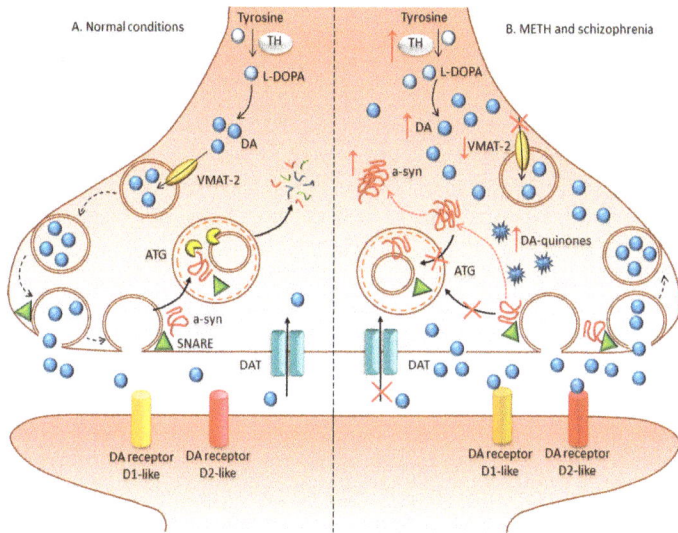

Figure 2. Overlap of dopamine-dependent molecular mechanisms underlying methamphetamine (METH) and schizophrenia. In normal conditions (**A**), the amount of intra-cytosolic dopamine is determined by the rate limiting enzyme tyrosine hydroxylase (TH), which converts tyrosine into L-dihydroxyphenylalanine (L-DOPA) and eventually dopamine (DA). DA is selectively taken-up into synaptic vesicles by the vesicular monoamine transporter type-2 (VMAT-2), which is key to surveil the physiological storage of vesicular DA. DA-containing synaptic vesicles are coated with soluble NSF (N-ethylmaleimide-sensitive factor) attachment protein receptor (SNARE) proteins co-chaperoned by alpha-synuclein, which mediate docking, priming, and release of DA-synaptic vesicles via exocytosis. Once exocytosis has occurred, synaptic vesicles and their associated proteins are endocytosed and sorted for autophagy (ATG) degradation. In this way, ATG monitors the amount of releasable DA synaptic vesicles, thus playing a key role in restraining DA release and in the turnover of synaptic proteins. In the synaptic cleft, the dopamine transporter (DAT) is key to take-up extracellular DA in order to guarantee a physiological stimulation of post-synaptic DA receptors. On the other hand, METH addicted and schizophrenic brains (**B**) feature alterations of DA metabolism and handling, which consist of the following: (i) increased levels of TH, which produces high levels of intra-cytosolic DA; (ii) a decrease in VMAT-2, which leads to a loss of DA vesicular storage and increases the amount freely diffusible intra-cytosolic DA; (iii) free cytosolic DA is highly prone to auto-oxidation into reactive DA-quinones, which produce structural modifications of presynaptic proteins such as alpha synuclein; (iv) a rapid and massive release of DA occurs via either exocytosis or efflux from the axoplasm; (v) extracellular DA rapidly accumulates as DAT is inhibited or downregulated, thus leading to abnormal stimulation of post-synaptic DA receptors, mainly D1-like receptors; (vi) dysfunctions in the ATG machinery, which cannot restrain DA release, are likely to play a key role in such a mechanism. In addition, impaired ATG cannot handle the oxidatively modified alpha-synuclein, thus leading to a progressive accumulation of alpha-synuclein aggregates fueling synaptic pathology.

5. Cytoskeletal Abnormalities and Neuronal Inclusions in Schizophrenia

Neuropathological evidence showing cytoarchitectural abnormalities and neuronal inclusions in schizophrenic patients date back to the late 1990s from post-mortem studies. In detail, ultrastructural alterations encompassing reduction and swelling of DA terminals, mitochondrial alterations, and multi-lamellar structures were reported within DA terminals of the SNpc [168]. Interestingly, these ultrastructural abnormalities are highly reminiscent of those induced by METH. In addition, cytoskeletal derangement appears as a prominent feature of the ultrastructural pathology of schizophrenia [169]. Cytoskeleton organization and dynamics depend on the fine control of microtubule assembly, which relies on the interaction of microtubules with a specific class of proteins known as microtubule-associated protein (MAP). These proteins represent a sort of cytoskeletal regulatory elements that bind microtubules to ensure their stability and integrity. Among various identified MAPs, microtubule-associated protein 2 (MAP2), which belongs to the MAP2/Tau family, is enriched in the brain and especially in dendrites, where it contributes to microtubule stabilization and overall dendritic architecture. Alterations in MAP2 immunoreactivity within the subiculum, entorhinal cortex, hippocampus, and prefrontal cortex have been suggested as the primary array of cytoskeletal abnormalities, which in turn result in impaired neurotransmission observed in schizophrenia [170–173]. Notably, a marked reduction in MAP2 immunoreactivity, along with a decrease in dendritic arbor, is reported in the primary auditory cortex (BA41) of schizophrenic subjects compared with healthy controls [174]. These structural abnormalities observed in the post-mortem auditory cortex of schizophrenic individuals may underlie altered auditory information processing, which in turn may manifest as auditory hallucinations. Moreover, pathological deposition of hyperphosphorylated MAP-tau (MAPT), which is the hallmark of several neurodegenerative disorders such as AD and frontotemporal dementia (FTD), has been described in elderly subjects with schizophrenia [175–177]. However, this issue is still under debate, because some autopsy studies do not report any significant difference in the prevalence of AD pathology between elderly schizophrenic patients and age-matched healthy controls [178–181]. Momeni and colleagues (2010) recently reported two relatives with an early age at onset (27 and 29 years) of schizophrenic symptoms showing a marked neuronal tau deposition, as confirmed at pathological examination [182]. Remarkably, this familial behavioral variant of frontotemporal lobar degeneration (FTLD) was associated with a novel exon 12 mutation in the conserved microtubule binding region of microtubule-associated protein tau (*MAPT*) gene, thus suggesting that disturbances in proteins involved in regulation of microtubule stability and overall cytoskeletal dynamics may accelerate tau deposition, leading to early disease onset. Notably, post-mortem analysis performed in the prefrontal cortex of schizophrenic patients revealed oligodendrocyte ultrastructural abnormalities [183]. Similarly, cytoskeletal derangements within nigro-striatal DA neurons and axons were recently evidenced in another cohort of schizophrenic brains [184]. Remarkably, a very recent neuropathological examination provided evidence for TDP-43-positive cytosolic inclusions and dystrophic neurites in the brain of a patient diagnosed with FTLD presenting brief psychotic episodes and catatonia, which is a syndrome related to schizophrenia [120]. Preliminary in vitro studies demonstrated that two proteins, namely DISC1 and dysbindin-1, which are encoded by two susceptibility genes for schizophrenia, can form insoluble protein aggregates that are reminiscent of those occurring in neurodegenerative disorders [185–188]. Intriguingly, the interactome analysis of both DISC1, dysbindin-1, and CRMP2, which is another susceptibility gene for schizophrenia, revealed common protein interactions with microtubules, actin cytoskeleton, and proteins involved in intracellular transport [189,190]. In particular, CRMP2 is a cytosolic protein enriched in the CNS, which has been implicated in microtubule stabilization, and thus in the regulation of cytoskeletal dynamics and vesicle trafficking. Remarkably, multiple proteomic studies of postmortem brains show altered CRMP2 protein levels in schizophrenic patients compared with healthy subjects [191–194]. These findings suggest that all these schizophrenia risk genes may encompass cytoskeletal stability and organization. It is worth mentioning that the reciprocal modulation between cytoskeleton dynamics and autophagy is emerging as a crucial point for neuronal homeostasis. Inhibition of the physiological microtubule transport is known to associate with an impaired shuttling of protein aggregates towards autophagy vacuoles, as well as impaired intracellular vesicle trafficking. Such an effect contributes to dysfunction in both the autophagy and secretory pathway leading to altered transmission of axonal information to and from the somato-dendritic domain [195]. The biological implication behind an impairment of microtubule dynamics is confirmed in post-mortem schizophrenic brain samples, as well as in mouse models of schizophrenia, where mTOR-dependent autophagy dysfunction is accompanied by an altered gene expression and protein levels of the microtubule-associated protein 6 (MAP6) [196,197]. These findings suggest that a close interplay between cytoskeletal dynamics and mTOR signaling is key in early axonal transport defects and altered synaptic transmission, a common pathological hallmark in schizophrenia [144,198–201].

6. mTOR Modulation of Dopamine Transmission in Methamphetamine and Schizophrenia

Despite some epidemiological evidence concerning risk factors for schizophrenia, which represents a chronic debilitating condition, the identification of the molecular mechanisms underlying its pathogenesis is still challenging. Interestingly, as has emerged from review of the literature published in the last few years, a novel scenario begins to delineate in which a dysfunctional mTOR pathway may be a key mechanism in the chain of events for the development of schizophrenia (Figure 3). In line with this, a number of genetic studies linked mTOR-related genetic alterations to schizophrenia. This is the case of the disrupted in schizophrenia 1 (*DISC1*) gene, a schizophrenia-related gene, originally discovered in a large Scottish family with a high incidence of psychiatric symptoms [202]. This gene encodes for the DISC1 ubiquitous protein, which is implicated in neurogenesis, neuronal migration, axon/dendrite, and synapse formation [203–206]. Remarkably, DISC1 plays a key role in DA neurotransmission [207]. In line with this, experimental models of DISC1 deficiency treated with METH show a significant potentiation of DA release, along with increased expression of D1R in the ventral striatum when compared with controls [208]. Mutations of DISC1 in the striatum associate with increased METH-induced behavioral sensitization suggesting that DISC1 represents a hub underlying alterations in those DA-dependent molecular mechanisms that modulate reward and sensitization in both drug abuse and mental disorders [209]. In addition, these findings strongly suggest that DISC1 alterations may increase the risk of schizophrenia by dysregulating DA release. In support of this view, DISC1 alterations are associated with pathological stress and converge in producing early alterations in DA neurotransmission during adolescence. This is a critical life-time for the development of schizophrenia [210,211]. Noteworthy, both DISC1 deficiency and over-stimulated D1Rs up-regulate the Akt–mTOR pathway [133,153,212], which highlights the impressive overlap between pathways that modulate DA neurotransmission and cell clearing systems. In particular, DISC1 acts by blocking KIAA1212, an Akt-binding partner, which directly interacts with Akt and strengthens the activation of this kinase, which represents a major mediator of the mTOR pathway. Therefore, the binding between DISC1 and KIAA1212 prevents KIAA1212-dependent Akt activation (Figure 3). This decreases Akt activity, which in turn dampens mTOR signaling [212]. Therefore, disruption of DISC1 activity, due to genetic rearrangements (i.e., balanced (1;11) (q42;q14) chromosomal translocation) or missense mutations, produces schizophrenic-like behavior, which is bound to enhanced Akt activity, over-activation of mTOR signaling, and depressed autophagy [213–215]. Likewise, administration of either D1R agonists or METH enhances Akt activity and over-activates mTOR signaling [133,137,216]. Remarkably, inhibition of mTOR with rapamycin reverses the effects occurring in both DISC1-shRNA and METH-treated mice, while ameliorating behavioral alterations [137,153,212]. Again, an impaired Akt signaling, achieved by neuronal deletion of rictor, a key regulatory subunit of mTORC2, contributes to schizophrenia-like phenotypes in rictor-null (KO) mice [217]. Dysregulation in Akt signaling and altered Akt protein levels were found in the frontal cortex and hippocampus of post-mortem brain samples from individuals affected by schizophrenia [218]. Since the first report by Emamian et al. (2004) [218], numerous subsequent studies further confirmed the genetic association of *AKT1* gene variants with schizophrenia, supporting the key role of impaired Akt–mTOR signaling in the pathogenesis of this psychiatric disorder [219–224]. In line with this, increased *AKT1* gene expression, due to increased hypomethylation of *AKT1* gene promoter, was detected in human METH abusers [225].

Furthermore, genetic linkage and association studies led to the identification of two additional susceptibility factors related to schizophrenia, such as neuregulin-1 (*NRG1*) and its receptor *ErbB4* [226,227]. NRG1 is a family of trophic factors that is synthesized as trans-membrane proteins displaying an extracellular epidermal growth factor (EGF)-like domain that is essential for ErbB4 receptor binding. Upon proteolytic processing, the soluble N-terminal moieties that contain the EGF-like domain is released and it acts by stimulating the ErbB4 receptor. Alterations in the NRG1/ErbB4 signaling are reported in schizophrenic brains [228]. In particular, NRG1, which is mostly involved in regulating neurodevelopment and neurotransmission, acts by binding ErbB4, a type I transmembrane receptor tyrosine kinase belonging to the family of ErbB proteins, which contain a binding site for PI3K kinase, an AKT upstream effector, in the C-terminal cytoplasmic tail (CYT) [229]. The binding between ErbB4 and PI3K activates this latter kinase, which in turn can phosphorylate and activate its downstream target Akt. Thus, changes in NRG1/ErbB4 signaling leads to a cascade of events that culminate in a dysregulation of the Akt–mTOR pathway (Figure 3). Moreover, it has been demonstrated that NRG1 also regulates DISC1 expression [230], thus further worsening the aberrancy of the Akt–mTOR pathway and the pathogenesis of schizophrenia and related behaviors. Noteworthy, NRG1/ErbB4 signaling plays a key role in DA-related behaviors by increasing DA release within the hippocampus, striatum, and prefrontal cortex [231]. In mice harboring mutated ErbB4, D1R's levels and binding activity are significantly increased [232], suggesting that ErbB4 may be another putative protein linking increased DA activity to increased mTOR activity and depressed autophagy.

Another identified susceptibility gene for schizophrenia is the dihydropyrimidinase-like 2 (*DPYSL2*) gene. This gene is located on chromosome 8p21 and it encodes the cytosolic microtubule-associated protein CRMP2 (collapsin response mediator protein-2), which is highly expressed in the CNS and plays a role in axonal growth [233]. Several *DPYSL2* single-nucleotide polymorphisms (SNPs) have been associated with the development to schizophrenia [234,235]. Although in mammals there are three DPYSL2 transcripts (i.e., DPYSL2A, DPYSL2B, and DPYSL2C), which differ in their first exon sequence, most of the studies have focused on the DPYSL2B transcript, also known as "short" transcript [236]. Multiple functional sequence variants were identified both in and around *DPYSL2B*, including three single-nucleotide polymorphisms (SNPs) in the proximal promoter and two SNPs in intron 1, which were significantly associated with schizophrenia [236]. In vitro functional luciferase assays in both neuronal (mouse primary cortical neurons) and non-neuronal (HEK293) cell types demonstrated that in the presence of increasing concentrations of rapamycin, a polymorphic di-nucleotide repeat (DNR) in the 5′-UTR of the *DPYSL2B* gene dose-dependently decreases allele expression at translation level, suggesting a functional link between this schizophrenia high-risk allele (13 DNRs) and mTOR signaling [236]. The relationship between the *DPYSL2* gene and susceptibility to schizophrenia was recently confirmed in vivo in rats exposed to prenatal stress (PNS), which indeed is frequently reported as an environmental risk factor for developing schizophrenia in adults [237]. Remarkably, immunohistochemical and Western blot analyses performed in the prefrontal cortex and hippocampus revealed a decreased DPYSL2 expression in the PNS group compared with non-stressed control offspring [238]. CRMP2 protein levels are significantly altered by METH administration [239]. In turn, CRMP2-KO mice show altered levels of proteins and genes involved in GABA-, glutamate-, and neurotrophin-signaling pathways, which are related to both schizophrenia and METH-induced sensitization [240]. Once again, such an overlap between altered molecular mechanisms occurring in both schizophrenia and METH may be key to decipher those early events linking CRMP2 and DA activity. In line with this, the dendritic spine-regulating activity of CRMP2 is under the control of the cyclin-dependent kinase 5 (CDK5) [241]. CDK5 is a key second messenger participating in METH-induced behavioral sensitization [130,242,243]. Both administration of amphetamines and stimulation of D1R induce a significant increase of *CDK5* gene expression and protein levels, which, at molecular level, associates with increased dendritic spine density and hyper-phosphorylation of the cytoskeletal tau protein [244–246]. In detail, the activation of CDK5 by D1R occurs via proteolysis of p35, the binding partner of CDK5. Remarkably, the marked reduction of p35 levels in schizophrenic brains, which mirrors enhanced CDK5 activity [247], suggests a role for CDK5-CRMP2-dependent alterations of cytoskeleton architecture and psychiatric behavior.

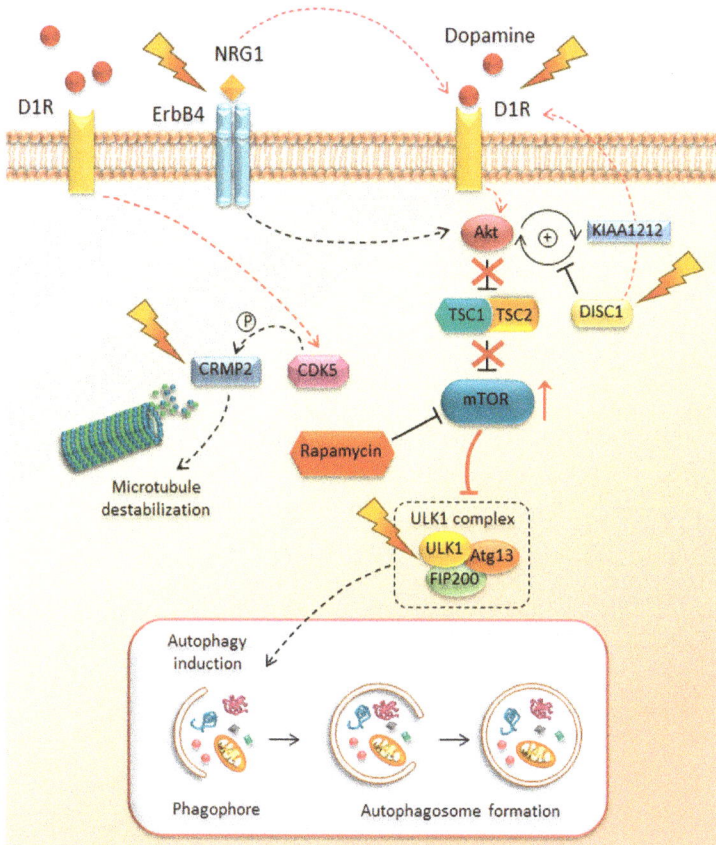

Figure 3. The Akt/mTOR pathway in schizophrenia. The cartoon summarizes key proteins involved in schizophrenia (lightning bolts), which converge on the overactivation of the Akt/mTOR pathway. These include disrupted in schizophrenia 1 (DISC1), neuregulin-1 (NRG1)/avian erythroblastosis oncogene B4-like protein (ErbB4), and collapsin response mediator protein 2 (CRMP2), as well as dopamine D1 receptors (D1R), which in turn are modulated by DISC1 and NRG1/ErbB4.

Table 1. Altered proteins converging on the mammalian target of rapamycin (mTOR) pathway during schizophrenia and methamphetamine addiction. DISC1—disrupted in schizophrenia 1; Akt—protein kinase B; NGR1—neuregulin-1; ErbB4—avian erythroblastosis oncogene B4-like protein; CRMP2—collapsin response mediator protein 2; CDK5—cyclin-dependent kinase 5.

Protein	Schizophrenia	Methamphetamine
DISC1	[153,212–215]	[208,209]
Akt	[218–224]	[225]
NRG1/ErbB4	[228,230,232]	[231]
CRMP2	[236,238]	[239,240]
CDK5/p35	[247]	[130,242,243]

7. A Step Forward about a Role of Autophagy in the Pathophysiology of Schizophrenia

While recent advances in molecular psychiatry have identified several mTOR-related schizophrenia risk genes, the role of autophagy in schizophrenia has been recently investigated. Remarkably, the identification of rare genetic variants of *ULK1* in a cohort of schizophrenic patients by means of exome sequence analysis strengthens the idea of a key role of both disrupted mTOR signaling and autophagy in the pathophysiology and susceptibility to schizophrenia [248] (Figure 3). The first evidence of a dysregulation of autophagy in schizophrenia was provided in 2011 by the Horesh group, who performed gene expression profile analysis in different brain areas of post-mortem schizophrenic patients compared with healthy controls, with no evidence of concomitant dementia [249]. The study revealed profound differences between the two groups, especially when looking at Broadman area 22 (BA 22), which is associated with positive symptoms, mainly auditory-verbal hallucinations or "hearing voices" [250,251]. In particular, at BA 22, the vast majority of abnormally expressed genes referred to key autophagy genes (i.e., *BECN1*, *ULK2*, *ATG3*), which were significantly down-regulated compared with controls [249]. A few months later, another transcriptomic study reported a BA 22-specific down-regulation in several autophagy-related genes, thus strengthening the link between impaired autophagy and schizophrenia positive symptoms [252]. Furthermore, the transcriptional analysis performed on the very same post-mortem samples demonstrated no substantial changes in the mRNA levels of the above-mentioned autophagy-related genes within the anterior prefrontal cortex (BA 10), which is mainly involved in schizophrenic negative symptoms and cognitive dysfunction, thus reinforcing the involvement of an impaired autophagy in mediating positive symptoms. Later on, further analysis reported a disruption of the autophagy pathway also in the hippocampus of post-mortem schizophrenic patients [197]. In detail, the analysis of mRNA expression of a key protein for autophagy initiation, namely beclin1, revealed a significant region-specific reduction in hippocampal samples from 12 schizophrenic patients compared with 12 age-matched healthy controls. The deficiency in hippocampal beclin1 transcript levels matches those observed in haploinsufficient mice for the activity-dependent neuroprotective protein (ADNP) (ADNP$^{+/-}$ mice), a transgenic model of schizophrenia [197]. ADNP is an essential protein for brain development and it has been shown to physically interact with a key protein in autophagosome biogenesis and maturation, namely LC3 [253]. Remarkably, a co-immunoprecipitation assay performed in a hippocampal protein fraction from ADNP$^{+/-}$ mice showed a dramatic reduction in the ADNP–LC3 protein interaction, which correlates with decreased ADNP expression [197]. A reduction of ADNP and its homologous protein, ADNP2, is observed in schizophrenic patients [254], and it is recapitulated in Map6-deficient (Map6$^{+/-}$) mice, another transgenic model of schizophrenia [196]. Immuno-histochemical analysis showed a three-fold decrease in the number of beclin1-positive cells in Map6$^{+/-}$ mice. These results were confirmed at transcriptional level by demonstrating a reduced expression of BECN1 mRNA. On the other hand, chronic treatment with an eight-amino-acid peptide snippet from ADNP (NAP), also known as davunetide, restored both Beclin1 and ADNP mRNA levels along with ADNP-LC3 interaction, thus providing neuroprotection while ameliorating schizophrenic-like behavioral and cognitive deficits in Map6$^{+/-}$ mice [196]. A recent phase II, multicenter, double-blind, randomized clinical trial has shown an improvement in cognitive performance of schizophrenic patients treated with NAP (AL-108; 5 and 30 mg/day, intranasally) versus placebo-treated patients [255]. These pieces of evidence corroborate findings showing that several autophagy inducers, such as lithium, rapamycin, and Food and Drug Administration (FDA) approved antipsychotic drugs are effective to treat psychosis including schizophrenia [59–62,109,256–260]. Notably, high-throughput image-based screens performed by Zhang et al. (2007) [60] on a human glioblastoma H4 cell line expressing human LC3 coupled with green fluorescent protein (GFP) led us to disclose that three typical antipsychotic drugs (fluspirilene, trifluoperazine, and pimozide) are effective autophagy inducers. In particular, pimozide provides an mTOR-independent autophagy induction, because it directly activates AMPK1, which in turn promotes autophagy through the phosphorylation of ULK1 [260]. In contrast, chlorpromazine, which is a typical antipsychotic agent, induces autophagy by inhibiting the Akt/mTOR pathway [59]. Recently, in vitro studies on the effects of second-generation, atypical antipsychotics demonstrated that sertindole and clozapine are potent autophagy inducers in both neuronal and non-neuronal cell lines [257,261]. Similar to pimozide, clozapine activates the autophagy process via the AMPK–ULK1–Beclin1 pathway, as evidenced by increased levels of autophagy markers (i.e., LC3-II and Atg5–Atg12 conjugate); increased phosphorylation of AMPK and its downstream substrates, namely ULK1 and beclin1; and an increased number of autophagosomes in the frontal cortex in clozapine-treated rats [259]. Most reports evidenced autophagy induction by neuroleptics indirectly, only by measuring the degradation of autophagy-dependent substrates. For instance, the increase in autophagy flux induced by pimozide occurs along with a depression of phosphorylated tau in a transgenic mouse model of AD [260]. Again, the effects of two typical antipsychotics, trifluoperazine and haloperidol, on autophagy have been demonstrated indirectly [262,263]. For instance, haloperidol occludes huntingtin aggregation [262]. Chronic clozapine treatment (20 mg/kg/day) reduces Aβ deposition [264]. Although typical and atypical antipsychotics may alleviate diseases featuring aberrant protein misfolding and accumulation, in vivo systematic investigations regarding the efficacy and the molecular mechanisms of these drugs on autophagy have been questioned [265]. This issue is biased by the routine intake of neuroleptics by most schizophrenic patients for long time intervals, sometimes lasting decades.

8. Conclusions and Future Perspectives

The exponential development in the past few years of genome-wide linkage studies and high-throughput genotyping technologies has led to the identification of many other susceptibility genes for schizophrenia, and this list is expected to grow further. However, the molecular mechanisms underlying schizophrenia are far from being deciphered. Up-to-date neuropathological studies performed on post-mortem schizophrenic brains appear to be scattered and they have not yielded to the identification of a distinct neuropathological hallmark. This is due to the limited sample availability and confounding interpretation of pathological data when comparing antipsychotic-treated and non-treated patients. This contrasts with classic neurodegenerative disorders where the accumulation of misfolded or aggregated proteins within neurons may imply a dysregulation of autophagy. Again, most experimental models available so far fail at large to reproduce most features of schizophrenia. Thus, methamphetamine remains an appropriate model compared with genetic manipulation to decipher the molecular progression underlying the pathophysiology of schizophrenia. In fact, METH bridges autophagy alterations with altered DA transmission and degeneration that is reminiscent of schizophrenia.

The present manuscript reviewed genetic and biochemical evidence that suggests that autophagy impairment may be involved in early DA neurotransmission, leading to synaptic dysfunction, which underlies some psychiatric disorders. An ongoing and persistent autophagy dysfunction that occludes handling of misfolded proteins while fueling synaptic alterations predisposes to the onset of degeneration. This scenario, depicting schizophrenia as an autophagy-dependent progressive synaptic pathology, may be a ground for planning the use of mTOR inhibitors and autophagy inducers as early treatment intervention.

Funding: This research was funded by MINISTERO DELLA SALUTE (RICERCA CORRENTE 2018).

Conflicts of Interest: The authors declare no conflict of interest.

Abbreviations

AD	Alzheimer's disease
ADNP	activity-dependent neuroprotective protein
Akt	protein kinase B
ALS	Amyotrophic lateral sclerosis
Aβ	amyloid-β
BA 22	Broadman area 22
BA41	Broadman area 41
CDK5	cyclin-dependent kinase 5
CMA	chaperone-mediated autophagy
CNS	central nervous system
CRMP2	collapsin response mediator protein 2
D1R	dopamine receptor type 1
DA	dopamine/dopaminergic
DAT	dopamine transporter
DISC1	disrupted in schizophrenia 1
DLB	Dementia with Lewy bodies
DNR	di-nucleotide repeat
DPYSL2	dihydropyrimidinase-like 2
ErbB4	avian erythroblastosis oncogene B4-like protein
FRKBP12	FK506-binding protein 12
FTD	Frontotemporal dementia
FTLD	Frontotemporal lobar degeneration
GFP	green fluorescent protein
GPCRs	G-protein coupled receptors
HD	Huntington's disease
MAP	microtubule-associated protein
MAPT	microtubule-associated protein tau
METH	methamphetamine
mTOR	mammalian Target Of Rapamycin
mTORC1	mammalian Target Of Rapamycin complex 1
mTORC2	mammalian Target Of Rapamycin complex 2
NDDs	neurodegenerative disorders
NFT	neurofibrillary tangles
NRG1	neuregulin-1
PD	Parkinson's disease
PI3k	phosphatidylinositol-3-Kinase
PIP2	phosphatidylinositol-4,5-phosphate
PIP3	phosphatidylinositol-3,4,5-phosphate
PNS	prenatal stress
ROS	reactive oxygen species
RTKs	receptor tyrosine kinase receptors
SNARE	Soluble NSF (N-ethylmaleimide-sensitive factor) attachment protein receptor
SNCA	alpha synuclein gene
SNpc	substantia nigra pars compacta
SNPs	single-nucleotide polymorphisms

SOD1	superoxide dismutase 1
TDP-43	TAR DNA-binding protein 43
TEM	transmission electron microscopy
TORC	target of rapamycin complex
TSC	tuberous sclerosis complex
TSC1	hamartin
TSC2	tuberin
VMAT-2	vesicular monoamine transporter type 2

References

1. Vezina, C.; Kudelski, A.; Sehgal, S.N. Rapamycin (AY-22,989), a new antifungal antibiotic. I. Taxonomy of the producing streptomycete and isolation of the active principle. *J. Antibiot.* **1975**, *28*, 721–726. [CrossRef] [PubMed]
2. Calne, R.Y.; Collier, D.S.; Lim, S.; Pollard, S.G.; Samaan, A.; White, D.J.; Thiru, S. Rapamycin for immunosuppression in organ allografting. *Lancet* **1989**, *2*, 227. [CrossRef]
3. Starzl, T.E.; Schreiber, S.L.; Albers, M.W.; Porter, K.A.; Foglieni, C.S.; Francavilla, A. Hepatotrophic properties in dogs of human FKBP, the binding protein for FK506 and rapamycin. *Transplantation* **1991**, *52*, 751–753. [PubMed]
4. Watson, C.J.; Friend, P.J.; Jamieson, N.V.; Frick, T.W.; Alexander, G.; Gimson, A.E.; Calne, R. Sirolimus: A potent new immunosuppressant for liver transplantation. *Transplantation* **1999**, *67*, 505–509. [CrossRef] [PubMed]
5. Loewith, R.; Jacinto, E.; Wullschleger, S.; Lorberg, A.; Crespo, J.L.; Bonenfant, D.; Oppliger, W.; Jenoe, P.; Hall, M.N. Two TOR complexes, only one of which is rapamycin sensitive, have distinct roles in cell growth control. *Mol. Cell* **2002**, *10*, 457–468. [CrossRef]
6. Sehgal, S.N. Sirolimus: Its discovery, biological properties, and mechanism of action. *Transplant. Proc.* **2003**, *35*, 7S–14S. [CrossRef]
7. Heitman, J.; Movva, N.R.; Hall, M.N. Targets for cell cycle arrest by the immunosuppressant rapamycin in yeast. *Science* **1991**, *253*, 905–909. [CrossRef] [PubMed]
8. Zhang, H.; Stallock, J.P.; Ng, J.C.; Reinhard, C.; Neufeld, T.P. Regulation of cellular growth by the Drosophila target of rapamycin dTOR. *Genes Dev.* **2000**, *14*, 2712–2724. [CrossRef] [PubMed]
9. Garber, K. Rapamycin's resurrection: A new way to target the cancer cell cycle. *J. Natl. Cancer Inst.* **2001**, *93*, 1517–1519. [CrossRef] [PubMed]
10. Hay, N.; Sonenberg, N. Upstream and downstream of mTOR. *Genes Dev.* **2004**, *18*, 1926–1945. [CrossRef] [PubMed]
11. Fingar, D.C.; Blenis, J. Target of rapamycin (TOR): An integrator of nutrient and growth factor signals and coordinator of cell growth and cell cycle progression. *Oncogene* **2004**, *23*, 3151–3171. [CrossRef] [PubMed]
12. Soulard, A.; Cohen, A.; Hall, M.N. TOR signaling in invertebrates. *Curr. Opin. Cell Biol.* **2009**, *21*, 825–836. [CrossRef] [PubMed]
13. Katz, L.A. Origin and diversification of eukaryotes. *Annu. Rev. Microbiol.* **2012**, *66*, 411–427. [CrossRef] [PubMed]
14. Koltin, Y.; Faucette, L.; Bergsma, D.J.; Levy, M.A.; Cafferkey, R.; Koser, P.L.; Johnson, R.K.; Livi, G.P. Rapamycin sensitivity in *Saccharomyces cerevisiae* is mediated by a peptidyl-prolyl cis-trans isomerase related to human FK506-binding protein. *Mol. Cell. Biol.* **1991**, *11*, 1718–1723. [CrossRef] [PubMed]
15. Lorenz, M.C.; Heitman, J. TOR mutations confer rapamycin resistance by preventing interaction with FKBP12-rapamycin. *J. Biol. Chem.* **1995**, *270*, 27531–27537. [CrossRef] [PubMed]
16. Guertin, D.A.; Sabatini, D.M. An expanding role for mTOR in cancer. *Trends Mol. Med.* **2005**, *11*, 353–361. [CrossRef] [PubMed]
17. Sarbassov, D.D.; Ali, S.M.; Sabatini, D.M. Growing roles for the mTOR pathway. *Curr. Opin. Cell Biol.* **2005**, *17*, 596–603. [CrossRef] [PubMed]
18. Wullschleger, S.; Loewith, R.; Hall, M.N. TOR signaling in growth and metabolism. *Cell* **2006**, *124*, 471–484. [CrossRef] [PubMed]

19. Laplante, M.; Sabatini, D.M. MTOR signaling in growth control and disease. *Cell* **2012**, *149*, 274–293. [CrossRef] [PubMed]

20. Guertin, D.A.; Stevens, D.M.; Thoreen, C.C.; Burds, A.A.; Kalaany, N.Y.; Moffat, J.; Brown, M.; Fitzgerald, K.J.; Sabatini, D.M. Ablation in mice of the mTORC components raptor, rictor, or mLST8 reveals that mTORC2 is required for signaling to Akt-FOXO and PKCalpha, but not S6K1. *Dev. Cell* **2006**, *11*, 859–871. [CrossRef] [PubMed]

21. Laplante, M.; Sabatini, D.M. mTOR signaling at a glance. *J. Cell Sci.* **2009**, *122*, 3589–3594. [CrossRef] [PubMed]

22. Peterson, T.R.; Laplante, M.; Thoreen, C.C. DEPTOR is an mTOR inhibitor frequently overexpressed in multiple myeloma cells and required for their survival. *Cell* **2009**, *137*, 873–886. [CrossRef] [PubMed]

23. Sarbassov, D.D.; Ali, S.M.; Kim, D.H.; Guertin, D.A.; Latek, R.R.; Erdjument-Bromage, H.; Tempst, P.; Sabatini, D.M. Rictor, a novel binding partner of mTOR, defines a rapamycin-insensitive and raptor-independent pathway that regulates the cytoskeleton. *Curr. Biol.* **2004**, *14*, 1296–1302. [CrossRef] [PubMed]

24. Frias, M.A.; Thoreen, C.C.; Jaffe, J.D.; Schroder, W.; Sculley, T.; Carr, S.A.; Sabatini, D.M. mSin1 is necessary for Akt/PKB phosphorylation, and its isoforms define three distinct mTORC2s. *Curr. Biol.* **2006**, *16*, 1865–1870. [CrossRef] [PubMed]

25. Pearce, L.R.; Huang, X.; Boudeau, J.; Pawłowski, R.; Wullschleger, S.; Deak, M.; Ibrahim, A.F.M.; Gourlay, R.; Magnuson, M.A.; Alessi, D.R. Identification of protor as a novel Rictor-binding component ofmTOR complex-2. *Biochem. J.* **2007**, *405*, 513–522. [CrossRef] [PubMed]

26. Sancak, Y.; Thoreen, C.C.; Peterson, T.R.; Lindquist, R.A.; Kang, S.A.; Spooner, E.; Carr, S.A.; Sabatini, D.M. PRAS40 is an insulin-regulated inhibitor of the mTORC1 protein kinase. *Mol. Cell* **2007**, *25*, 903–915. [CrossRef] [PubMed]

27. Wang, L.; Harris, T.E.; Roth, R.A.; Lawrence, J.C., Jr. PRAS40 regulates mTORC1 kinase activity by functioning as a direct inhibitor of substrate binding. *J. Biol. Chem.* **2007**, *282*, 20036–20044. [CrossRef] [PubMed]

28. Kaizuka, T.; Hara, T.; Oshiro, N.; Kikkawa, U.; Yonezawa, K.; Takehana, K.; Iemura, S.; Natsume, T.; Mizushima, N. Tti1 and Tel2 are critical factors in mammalian target of rapamycin complex assembly. *J. Biol. Chem.* **2010**, *285*, 20109–20116. [CrossRef] [PubMed]

29. Zoncu, R.; Efeyan, A.; Sabatini, D.M. mTOR: From growth signal integration to cancer, diabetes and ageing. *Nat. Rev. Mol. Cell Biol.* **2011**, *12*, 21–35. [CrossRef] [PubMed]

30. Haissaguerre, M.; Saucisse, N.; Cota, D. Influence of mTOR in energy and metabolic homeostasis. *Mol. Cell. Endocrinol.* **2014**, *397*, 67–77. [CrossRef] [PubMed]

31. Ma, X.M.; Blenis, J. Molecular mechanisms of mTOR-mediated translational control. *Nat. Rev. Mol. Cell Biol.* **2009**, *10*, 307–318. [CrossRef] [PubMed]

32. Meijer, A.J.; Codogno, P. Signalling and autophagy regulation in health, aging and disease. *Mol. Asp. Med.* **2006**, *27*, 411–425. [CrossRef] [PubMed]

33. Ahlberg, J.; Marzella, L.; Glaumann, H. Uptake and degradation of proteins by isolated rat liver lysosomes. Suggestion of a microautophagic pathway of proteolysis. *Lab. Investig.* **1982**, *47*, 523–532. [PubMed]

34. Klionsky, D.J.; Emr, S.D. Autophagy as a regulated pathway of cellular degradation. *Science* **2000**, *290*, 1717–1721. [CrossRef] [PubMed]

35. Dice, J.F. Chaperone-mediated autophagy. *Autophagy* **2007**, *3*, 295–299. [CrossRef] [PubMed]

36. Hara, T.; Takamura, A.; Kishi, C.; Iemura, S.; Natsume, T.; Guan, J.L.; Mizushima, N. FIP200, a ULK-interacting protein, is required for autophagosome formation in mammalian cells. *J. Cell Biol.* **2008**, *181*, 497–510. [CrossRef] [PubMed]

37. Ganley, I.G.; Lam du, H.; Wang, J.; Ding, X.; Chen, S.; Jiang, X. ULK1.ATG13.FIP200 complex mediates mTOR signaling and is essential for autophagy. *J. Biol. Chem.* **2009**, *284*, 12297–12305. [CrossRef] [PubMed]

38. Hosokawa, N.; Hara, T.; Kaizuka, T.; Kishi, C.; Takamura, A.; Miura, Y.; Iemura, S.; Natsume, T.; Takehana, K.; Yamada, N.; et al. Nutrient-dependent mTORC1 association with the ULK1–Atg13–FIP200 complex required for autophagy. *Mol. Biol. Cell* **2009**, *20*, 1981–1991. [CrossRef] [PubMed]

39. Jung, C.H.; Jun, C.B.; Ro, S.H.; Kim, Y.M.; Otto, N.M.; Cao, J.; Kundu, M.; Kim, D.H. ULK–Atg13–FIP200 complexes mediate mTOR signaling to the autophagy machinery. *Mol. Biol. Cell* **2009**, *20*, 1992–2003. [CrossRef] [PubMed]

40. Bernard, A.; Klionsky, D.J. Defining the membrane precursor supporting the nucleation of the phagophore. *Autophagy* **2014**, *10*, 1–2. [CrossRef] [PubMed]

41. Burré, J.; Vivona, S.; Diao, J.; Sharma, M.; Brunger, A.T.; Südhof, T.C. Properties of native brain α-synuclein. *Nature* **2013**, *498*, E4–E6; discussion E6–E7. [CrossRef] [PubMed]

42. Nixon, R.A. The role of autophagy in neurodegenerative disease. *Nat. Med.* **2013**, *19*, 983–997. [CrossRef] [PubMed]

43. Hara, T.; Nakamura, K.; Matsui, M.; Yamamoto, A.; Nakahara, Y.; Suzuki-Migishima, R.; Yokoyama, M.; Mishima, K.; Saito, I.; Okano, H.; et al. Suppression of basal autophagy in neural cells causes neurodegenerative disease in mice. *Nature* **2006**, *441*, 885–889. [CrossRef] [PubMed]

44. Komatsu, M.; Waguri, S.; Chiba, T.; Murata, S.; Iwata, J.; Tanida, I.; Ueno, T.; Koike, M.; Uchiyama, Y.; Kominami, E.; et al. Loss of autophagy in the central nervous system causes neurodegeneration in mice. *Nature* **2006**, *441*, 880–884. [CrossRef] [PubMed]

45. Mariño, G.; López-Otín, C. Autophagy: Molecular mechanisms, physiological functions and relevance in human pathology. *Cell. Mol. Life Sci.* **2004**, *61*, 1439–1454. [CrossRef] [PubMed]

46. Fornai, F.; Longone, P.; Ferrucci, M.; Lenzi, P.; Isidoro, C.; Ruggieri, S.; Paparelli, A. Autophagy and amyotrophic lateral sclerosis: The multiple roles of lithium. *Autophagy* **2008**, *4*, 527–530. [CrossRef] [PubMed]

47. Fornai, F.; Longone, P.; Cafaro, L.; Kastsiuchenka, O.; Ferrucci, M.; Manca, M.L.; Lazzeri, G.; Spalloni, A.; Bellio, N.; Lenzi, P.; et al. Lithium delays progression of amyotrophic lateral sclerosis. *Proc. Natl. Acad. Sci. USA* **2008**, *105*, 2052–2057. [CrossRef] [PubMed]

48. Carloni, S.; Buonocore, G.; Balduini, W. Protective role of autophagy in neonatal hypoxia-ischemia induced brain injury. *Neurobiol. Dis.* **2008**, *32*, 329–339. [CrossRef] [PubMed]

49. Akhavan, D.; Cloughesy, T.F.; Mischel, P.S. mTOR signaling in glioblastoma: Lessons learned from bench to bedside. *Neuro Oncol.* **2010**, *12*, 882–889. [CrossRef] [PubMed]

50. Fan, Q.W.; Weiss, W.A. Inhibition of PI3K-Akt-mTOR signaling in glioblastoma by mTORC1/2 inhibitors. *Methods Mol. Biol.* **2012**, *821*, 349–359. [PubMed]

51. Arcella, A.; Biagioni, F.; Antonietta Oliva, M.; Bucci, D.; Frati, A.; Esposito, V.; Cantore, G.; Giangaspero, F.; Fornai, F. Rapamycin inhibits the growth of glioblastoma. *Brain Res.* **2013**, *1495*, 37–51. [CrossRef] [PubMed]

52. Heras-Sandoval, D.; Pérez-Rojas, J.M.; Hernández-Damián, J.; Pedraza-Chaverri, J. The role of PI3K/AKT/mTOR pathway in the modulation of autophagy and the clearance of protein aggregates in neurodegeneration. *Cell. Signal.* **2014**, *26*, 2694–2701. [CrossRef] [PubMed]

53. Giorgi, F.S.; Biagioni, F.; Lenzi, P.; Frati, A.; Fornai, F. The role of autophagy in epileptogenesis and in epilepsy-induced neuronal alterations. *J. Neural Transm.* **2015**, *122*, 849–862. [CrossRef] [PubMed]

54. Tramutola, A.; Triplett, J.C.; Di Domenico, F.; Niedowicz, D.M.; Murphy, M.P.; Coccia, R.; Perluigi, M.; Butterfield, D.A. Alteration of mTOR signaling occurs early in the progression of Alzheimer disease (AD): Analysis of brain from subjects with pre-clinical AD, amnestic mild cognitive impairment and late-stage AD. *J. Neurochem.* **2015**, *133*, 739–749. [CrossRef] [PubMed]

55. Ferrucci, M.; Biagioni, F.; Lenzi, P.; Gambardella, S.; Ferese, R.; Calierno, M.T.; Falleni, A.; Grimaldi, A.; Frati, A.; Esposito, V.; et al. Rapamycin promotes differentiation increasing βIII-tubulin, NeuN, and NeuroD while suppressing nestin expression in glioblastoma cells. *Oncotarget* **2017**, *8*, 29574–29599. [CrossRef] [PubMed]

56. Ryskalin, L.; Lazzeri, G.; Flaibani, M.; Biagioni, F.; Gambardella, S.; Frati, A.; Fornai, F. mTOR-Dependent Cell Proliferation in the Brain. *Biomed. Res. Int.* **2017**, *2017*, 7082696. [CrossRef] [PubMed]

57. Ryskalin, L.; Limanaqi, F.; Biagioni, F.; Frati, A.; Esposito, V.; Calierno, M.T.; Lenzi, P.; Fornai, F. The emerging role of m-TOR up-regulation in brain Astrocytoma. *Histol. Histopathol.* **2017**, *32*, 413–431. [PubMed]

58. Williams, R.S.; Cheng, L.; Mudge, A.W.; Harwood, A.J. A common mechanism of action for three mood-stabilizing drugs. *Nature* **2002**, *417*, 292–295. [CrossRef] [PubMed]

59. Sarkar, S.; Floto, R.A.; Berger, Z.; Imarisio, S.; Cordenier, A.; Pasco, M.; Cook, L.J.; Rubinsztein, D.C. Lithium induces autophagy by inhibiting inositol monophosphatase. *J. Cell Biol.* **2005**, *170*, 1101–1111. [CrossRef] [PubMed]

60. Zhang, L.; Yu, J.; Pan, H.; Hu, P.; Hao, Y.; Cai, W.; Zhu, H.; Yu, A.D.; Xie, X.; Ma, D.; et al. Small molecule regulators of autophagy identified by an image-based high-throughput screen. *Proc. Natl. Acad. Sci. USA* **2007**, *104*, 19023–19028. [CrossRef] [PubMed]

61. Kara, N.Z.; Toker, L.; Agam, G.; Anderson, G.W.; Belmaker, R.H.; Einat, H. Trehalose induced antidepressant-like effects and autophagy enhancement in mice. *Psychopharmacology* **2013**, *229*, 367–375. [CrossRef] [PubMed]

62. Shin, S.Y.; Lee, K.S.; Choi, Y.K.; Lim, H.J.; Lee, H.G.; Lim, Y.; Lee, Y.H. The antipsychotic agent chlorpromazine induces autophagic cell death by inhibiting the Akt/mTOR pathway in human U-87MG glioma cells. *Carcinogenesis* **2013**, *34*, 2080–2089. [CrossRef] [PubMed]

63. Vucicevic, L.; Misirkic-Marjanovic, M.; Paunovic, V.; Kravic-Stevovic, T.; Martinovic, T.; Ciric, D.; Maric, N.; Petricevic, S.; Harhaji-Trajkovic, L.; Bumbasirevic, V.; et al. Autophagy inhibition uncovers the neurotoxic action of the antipsychotic drug olanzapine. *Autophagy* **2014**, *10*, 2362–2378. [CrossRef] [PubMed]

64. Li, Y.; McGreal, S.; Zhao, J.; Huang, R.; Zhou, Y.; Zhong, H.; Xia, M.; Ding, W.X. A cell-based quantitative high-throughput image screening identified novel autophagy modulators. *Pharmacol. Res.* **2016**, *110*, 35–49. [CrossRef] [PubMed]

65. Gould, T.D.; O'Donnell, K.C.; Dow, E.R.; Du, J.; Chen, G.; Manji, H.K. Involvement of AMPA receptors in the antidepressant-like effects of lithium in the mouse tail suspension test and forced swim test. *Neuropharmacology* **2008**, *54*, 577–587. [CrossRef] [PubMed]

66. Einat, H.; Yuan, P.; Szabo, S.T.; Dogra, S.; Manji, H.K. Protein kinase C inhibition by tamoxifen antagonizes manic-like behavior in rats: Implications for the development of novel therapeutics for bipolar disorder. *Neuropsychobiology* **2007**, *55*, 123–131. [CrossRef] [PubMed]

67. Zarate, C.A., Jr.; Singh, J.B.; Carlson, P.J.; Quiroz, J.; Jolkovsky, L.; Luckenbaugh, D.A.; Manji, H.K. Efficacy of a protein kinase C inhibitor (tamoxifen) in the treatment of acute mania: A pilot study. *Bipolar Disord.* **2007**, *9*, 561–570. [CrossRef] [PubMed]

68. Anglade, P.; Vyas, S.; Javoy-Agid, F.; Herrero, M.T.; Michel, P.P.; Marquez, J.; Mouatt-Prigent, A.; Ruberg, M.; Hirsch, E.C.; Agid, Y. Apoptosis and autophagy in nigral neurons of patients with Parkinson's disease. *Histol. Histopathol.* **1997**, *12*, 25–31. [PubMed]

69. Nixon, R.A.; Wegiel, J.; Kumar, A.; Yu, W.H.; Peterhoff, C.; Cataldo, A.; Cuervo, A.M. Extensive involvement of autophagy in Alzheimer disease: An immuno-electron microscopy study. *J. Neuropathol. Exp. Neurol.* **2005**, *64*, 113–122. [CrossRef] [PubMed]

70. Rudnicki, D.D.; Pletnikova, O.; Vonsattel, J.P.; Ross, C.A.; Margolis, R.L. A comparison of huntington disease and huntington disease-like 2 neuropathology. *J. Neuropathol. Exp. Neurol.* **2008**, *67*, 366–374. [CrossRef] [PubMed]

71. Madeo, F.; Eisenberg, T.; Kroemer, G. Autophagy for the avoidance of neurodegeneration. *Genes Dev.* **2009**, *23*, 2253–2259. [CrossRef] [PubMed]

72. Pasquali, L.; Longone, P.; Isidoro, C.; Ruggieri, S.; Paparelli, A.; Fornai, F. Autophagy, lithium, and amyotrophic lateral sclerosis. *Muscle Nerve* **2009**, *40*, 173–194. [CrossRef] [PubMed]

73. Pasquali, L.; Ruggieri, S.; Murri, L.; Paparelli, A.; Fornai, F. Does autophagy worsen or improve the survival of dopaminergic neurons? *Parkinsonism Relat. Disord.* **2009**, *15*, S24–S27. [CrossRef]

74. Ferrucci, M.; Fulceri, F.; Toti, L.; Soldani, P.; Siciliano, G.; Paparelli, A.; Fornai, F. Protein clearing pathways in ALS. *Arch. Ital. Biol.* **2011**, *149*, 121–149. [PubMed]

75. Sasaki, S. Autophagy in spinal cord motor neurons in sporadic amyotrophic lateral sclerosis. *J. Neuropathol. Exp. Neurol.* **2011**, *70*, 349–359. [CrossRef] [PubMed]

76. Natale, G.; Lenzi, P.; Lazzeri, G.; Falleni, A.; Biagioni, F.; Ryskalin, L.; Fornai, F. Compartment-dependent mitochondrial alterations in experimental ALS, the effects of mitophagy and mitochondriogenesis. *Front. Cell. Neurosci.* **2015**, *9*, 434. [CrossRef] [PubMed]

77. Spillantini, M.G.; Schmidt, M.L.; Lee, V.M.; Trojanowski, J.Q.; Jakes, R.; Goedert, M. α-synuclein in Lewy bodies. *Nature* **1997**, *388*, 839–840. [CrossRef] [PubMed]

78. Shults, C.W. Lewy bodies. *Proc. Natl. Acad. Sci. USA* **2006**, *103*, 1661–1668. [CrossRef] [PubMed]

79. Roberts, R.F.; Wade-Martins, R.; Alegre-Abarrategui, J. Direct visualization of alpha-synuclein oligomers reveals previously undetected pathology in Parkinson's disease brain. *Brain* **2015**, *138*, 1642–1657. [CrossRef] [PubMed]

80. Sato, S.; Hattori, N. Dopaminergic Neuron-Specific Autophagy-Deficient Mice. *Methods Mol. Biol.* **2018**. [CrossRef]

81. Hyman, B.T.; Phelps, C.H.; Beach, T.G.; Bigio, E.H.; Cairns, N.J.; Carrillo, M.C.; Dickson, D.W.; Duyckaerts, C.; Frosch, M.P.; Masliah, E.; et al. National institute on aging-Alzheimer's association guidelines for the neuropathologic assessment of Alzheimer's disease. *Alzheimers Dement.* **2012**, *8*, 1–13. [CrossRef] [PubMed]

82. Neumann, M.; Sampathu, D.M.; Kwong, L.K.; Truax, A.C.; Micsenyi, M.C.; Chou, T.T.; Bruce, J.; Schuck, T.; Grossman, M.; Clark, C.M.; et al. Ubiquitinated TDP-43 in frontotemporal lobar degeneration and amyotrophic lateral sclerosis. *Science* **2006**, *314*, 130–133. [CrossRef] [PubMed]

83. Grossman, M.; Wood, E.M.; Moore, P.; Neumann, M.; Kwong, L.; Forman, M.S.; Clark, C.M.; McCluskey, L.F.; Miller, B.L.; Lee, V.M.; et al. TDP-43 pathologic lesions and clinical phenotype in frontotemporal lobar degeneration with ubiquitin-positive inclusions. *Arch. Neurol.* **2007**, *64*, 1449–1454. [CrossRef] [PubMed]

84. Ravikumar, B.; Vacher, C.; Berger, Z.; Davies, J.E.; Luo, S.; Oroz, L.G.; Scaravilli, F.; Easton, D.F.; Duden, R.; O'Kane, C.J.; et al. Inhibition of mTOR induces autophagy and reduces toxicity of polyglutamine expansions in fly and mouse models of Huntington disease. *Nat. Genet.* **2004**, *36*, 585–595. [CrossRef] [PubMed]

85. Berger, Z.; Ravikumar, B.; Menzies, F.M.; Oroz, L.G.; Underwood, B.R.; Pangalos, M.N.; Schmitt, I.; Wullner, U.; Evert, B.O.; O'Kane, C.J.; et al. Rapamycin alleviates toxicity of different aggregate-prone proteins. *Hum. Mol. Genet.* **2006**, *15*, 433–442. [CrossRef] [PubMed]

86. Spencer, B.; Potkar, R.; Trejo, M.; Rockenstein, E.; Patrick, C.; Gindi, R.; Adame, A.; Wyss-Coray, T.; Masliah, E. Beclin 1 gene transfer activates autophagy and ameliorates the neurodegenerative pathology in alpha-synuclein models of Parkinson's and Lewy body diseases. *J. Neurosci.* **2009**, *29*, 13578–13588. [CrossRef] [PubMed]

87. Tian, Y.; Chang, J.C.; Fan, E.Y.; Flajolet, M.; Greengard, P. Adaptor complex AP2/PICALM, through interaction with LC3, targets Alzheimer's APP-CTF for terminal degradation via autophagy. *Proc. Natl. Acad. Sci. USA* **2013**, *110*, 17071–17076. [CrossRef] [PubMed]

88. Jo, C.; Gundemir, S.; Pritchard, S.; Jin, Y.N.; Rahman, I.; Johnson, G.V. Nrf2 reduces levels of phosphorylated tau protein by inducing autophagy adaptor protein NDP52. *Nat. Commun.* **2014**, *5*, 3496. [CrossRef] [PubMed]

89. Higashi, S.; Iseki, E.; Yamamoto, R.; Minegishi, M.; Hino, H.; Fujisawa, K.; Togo, T.; Katsuse, O.; Uchikado, H.; Furukawa, Y.; et al. Concurrence of TDP-43, tau and alpha-synuclein pathology in brains of Alzheimer's disease and dementia with Lewy bodies. *Brain Res.* **2007**, *1184*, 284–294. [CrossRef] [PubMed]

90. Colom-Cadena, M.; Gelpi, E.; Charif, S.; Belbin, O.; Blesa, R.; Martí, M.J.; Clarimón, J.; Lleó, A. Confluence of α-synuclein, tau, and β-amyloid pathologies in dementia with Lewy bodies. *J. Neuropathol. Exp. Neurol.* **2013**, *72*, 1203–1212. [CrossRef] [PubMed]

91. Charles, V.; Mezey, E.; Reddy, P.H.; Dehejia, A.; Young, T.A.; Polymeropoulos, M.H.; Brownstein, M.J.; Tagle, D.A. α-synuclein immunoreactivity of huntingtin polyglutamine aggregates in striatum and cortex of Huntington's disease patients and transgenic mouse models. *Neurosci. Lett.* **2000**, *289*, 29–32. [CrossRef]

92. Takei, Y.; Oguchi, K.; Koshihara, H.; Hineno, A.; Nakamura, A.; Ohara, S. α-Synuclein coaggregation in familial amyotrophic lateral sclerosis with SOD1 gene mutation. *Hum. Pathol.* **2013**, *44*, 1171–1176. [CrossRef] [PubMed]

93. Zhao, Y.; Gong, C.X. From chronic cerebral hypoperfusion to Alzheimer-like brain pathology and neurodegeneration. *Cell. Mol. Neurobiol.* **2015**, *35*, 101–110. [CrossRef] [PubMed]

94. Spilman, P.; Podlutskaya, N.; Hart, M.J.; Debnath, J.; Gorostiza, O.; Bredesen, D.; Richardson, A.; Strong, R.; Galvan, V. Inhibition of mTOR by rapamycin abolishes cognitive deficits and reduces amyloid-beta levels in a mouse model of Alzheimer's disease. *PLoS ONE* **2010**, *5*, e9979. [CrossRef] [PubMed]

95. Bové, J.; Martínez-Vicente, M.; Vila, M. Fighting neurodegeneration with rapamycin: Mechanistic insights. *Nat. Rev. Neurosci.* **2011**, *12*, 437–452. [CrossRef] [PubMed]

96. Roscic, A.; Baldo, B.; Crochemore, C.; Marcellin, D.; Paganetti, P. Induction of autophagy with catalytic mTOR inhibitors reduces huntingtin aggregates in a neuronal cell model. *J. Neurochem.* **2011**, *119*, 398–407. [CrossRef] [PubMed]

97. Pryor, W.M.; Biagioli, M.; Shahani, N.; Swarnkar, S.; Huang, W.C.; Page, D.T.; MacDonald, M.E.; Subramaniam, S. Huntingtin promotes mTORC1 signaling in the pathogenesis of Huntington's disease. *Sci. Signal.* **2014**, *7*, ra103. [CrossRef] [PubMed]

98. An, W.L.; Cowburn, R.F.; Li, L.; Braak, H.; Alafuzoff, I.; Iqbal, K.; Iqbal, I.G.; Winblad, B.; Pei, J.J. Up-regulation of phosphorylated/activated p70 S6 kinase and its relationship to neurofibrillary pathology in Alzheimer's disease. *Am. J. Pathol.* **2003**, *163*, 591–607. [CrossRef]

99. Li, X.; Alafuzoff, I.; Soininen, H.; Winblad, B.; Pei, J.J. Levels of mTOR and its downstream targets 4E-BP1, eEF2, and eEF2 kinase in relationships with tau in Alzheimer's disease brain. *FEBS J.* **2005**, *272*, 4211–4220. [CrossRef] [PubMed]

100. Caccamo, A.; Maldonado, M.A.; Majumder, S.; Medina, D.X.; Holbein, W.; Magri, A.; Oddo, S. Naturally secreted amyloid-β increases mammalian target of rapamycin (mTOR) activity via a PRAS40-mediated mechanism. *J. Biol. Chem.* **2011**, *286*, 8924–8932. [CrossRef] [PubMed]

101. Ozcelik, S.; Fraser, G.; Castets, P.; Schaeffer, V.; Skachokova, Z.; Breu, K.; Clavaguera, F.; Sinnreich, M.; Kappos, L.; Goedert, M.; et al. Rapamycin attenuates the progression of tau pathology in P301S tau transgenic mice. *PLoS ONE* **2013**, *8*, e62459. [CrossRef] [PubMed]

102. Barmada, S.J.; Serio, A.; Arjun, A.; Bilican, B.; Daub, A.; Ando, D.M.; Tsvetkov, A.; Pleiss, M.; Li, X.; Peisach, D.; et al. Autophagy induction enhances TDP43 turnover and survival in neuronal ALS models. *Nat. Chem. Biol.* **2014**, *10*, 677–685. [CrossRef] [PubMed]

103. Jiang, T.; Yu, J.T.; Zhu, X.C.; Tan, M.S.; Wang, H.F.; Cao, L.; Zhang, Q.Q.; Shi, J.Q.; Gao, L.; Qin, H.; et al. Temsirolimus promotes autophagic clearance of amyloid-β and provides protective effects in cellular and animal models of Alzheimer's disease. *Pharmacol. Res.* **2014**, *81*, 54–63. [CrossRef] [PubMed]

104. Frederick, C.; Ando, K.; Leroy, K.; Heraud, C.; Suain, V.; Buee, L.; Brion, J.P. Rapamycin ester analog CCI-779/Temsirolimus alleviates tau pathology and improves motor deficit in mutant tau transgenic mice. *J. Alzheimers Dis.* **2015**, *44*, 1145–1156. [CrossRef] [PubMed]

105. Lang, U.E.; Heger, J.; Willbring, M.; Domula, M.; Matschke, K.; Tugtekin, S.M. Immunosuppression using the mammalian target of rapamycin (mTOR) inhibitor everolimus: Pilot study shows significant cognitive and affective improvement. *Transplant. Proc.* **2009**, *41*, 4285–4288. [CrossRef] [PubMed]

106. Ehninger, D.; Silva, A.J. Rapamycin for treating Tuberous sclerosis and Autism spectrum disorders. *Trends Mol. Med.* **2011**, *17*, 78–87. [CrossRef] [PubMed]

107. Hwang, S.K.; Lee, J.H.; Yang, J.E.; Lim, C.S.; Lee, J.A.; Lee, Y.S.; Lee, K.; Kaang, B.K. Everolimus improves neuropsychiatric symptoms in a patient with tuberous sclerosis carrying a novel TSC2 mutation. *Mol. Brain* **2016**, *9*, 56. [CrossRef] [PubMed]

108. Kilincaslan, A.; Kok, B.E.; Tekturk, P.; Yalcinkaya, C.; Ozkara, C.; Yapici, Z. Beneficial Effects of Everolimus on Autism and Attention-Deficit/Hyperactivity Disorder Symptoms in a Group of Patients with Tuberous Sclerosis Complex. *J. Child Adolesc. Psychopharmacol.* **2017**, *27*, 383–388. [CrossRef] [PubMed]

109. Cleary, C.; Linde, J.A.; Hiscock, K.M.; Hadas, I.; Belmaker, R.H.; Agam, G.; Flaisher-Grinberg, S.; Einat, H. Antidepressive-like effects of rapamycin in animal models: Implications for mTOR inhibition as a new target for treatment of affective disorders. *Brain Res. Bull.* **2008**, *76*, 469–473. [CrossRef] [PubMed]

110. Bou Khalil, R. Is there any place for macrolides in mood disorders? *Med. Hypotheses* **2012**, *78*, 86–87. [CrossRef] [PubMed]

111. Ehninger, D.; Han, S.; Shilyansky, C.; Zhou, Y.; Li, W.; Kwiatkowski, D.J.; Ramesh, V.; Silva, A.J. Reversal of learning deficits in a Tsc2$^{+/-}$ mouse model of tuberous sclerosis. *Nat. Med.* **2008**, *14*, 843–848. [CrossRef] [PubMed]

112. Sato, A.; Kasai, S.; Kobayashi, T.; Takamatsu, Y.; Hino, O.; Ikeda, K.; Mizuguchi, M. Rapamycin reverses impaired social interaction in mouse models of tuberous sclerosis complex. *Nat. Commun.* **2012**, *3*, 1292. [CrossRef] [PubMed]

113. Tang, G.; Gudsnuk, K.; Kuo, S.H.; Cotrina, M.L.; Rosoklija, G.; Sosunov, A.; Sonders, M.S.; Kanter, E.; Castagna, C.; Yamamoto, A.; et al. Loss of mTOR-dependent macroautophagy causes autistic-like synaptic pruning deficits. *Neuron* **2014**, *83*, 1131–1143. [CrossRef] [PubMed]

114. Kara, N.Z.; Flaisher-Grinberg, S.; Anderson, G.W.; Agam, G.; Einat, H. Mood-stabilizing effects of rapamycin and its analog temsirolimus: Relevance to autophagy. *Behav. Pharmacol.* **2018**, *29*, 379–384. [CrossRef] [PubMed]

115. Chaudhuri, K.R.; Healy, D.G.; Schapira, A.H.; National Institute for Clinical Excellence. Non-motor symptoms of Parkinson's disease: Diagnosis and management. *Lancet Neurol.* **2006**, *5*, 235–245. [CrossRef]

116. Velakoulis, D.; Walterfang, M.; Mocellin, R.; Pantelis, C.; McLean, C. Frontotemporal dementia presenting as schizophrenia-like psychosis in young people: Clinicopathological series and review of cases. *Br. J. Psychiatry* **2009**, *194*, 298–305. [CrossRef] [PubMed]

117. Lyketsos, C.G.; Carrillo, M.C.; Ryan, J.M.; Khachaturian, A.S.; Trzepacz, P.; Amatniek, J.; Cedarbaum, J.; Brashear, R.; Miller, D.S. Neuropsychiatric symptoms in Alzheimer's disease. *Alzheimers Dement.* **2011**, *7*, 532–539. [CrossRef] [PubMed]

118. Fornai, F.; Frati, A.; Gesi, M.; Fulceri, F.; Paparelli, S.; Falleni, A.; Ruggieri, S. Neurobiology and neuroanatomy of psychiatric symptoms in parkinsonism. *Arch. Ital. Biol.* **2013**, *151*, 179–191. [PubMed]

119. Aarsland, D.; Kramberger, M.G. Neuropsychiatric Symptoms in Parkinson's Disease. *J. Parkinsons Dis.* **2015**, *5*, 659–667. [CrossRef] [PubMed]

120. Watanabe, R.; Kawakami, I.; Onaya, M.; Higashi, S.; Arai, N.; Akiyama, H.; Hasegawa, M.; Arai, T. Frontotemporal dementia with trans-activation response DNA-binding protein 43 presenting with catatonic syndrome. *Neuropathology* **2018**, *38*, 281–287. [CrossRef] [PubMed]

121. Gururajan, A.; van den Buuse, M. Is the mTOR-signalling cascade disrupted in Schizophrenia? *J. Neurochem.* **2014**, *129*, 377–387. [CrossRef] [PubMed]

122. Maas, D.A.; Vallès, A.; Martens, G.J.M. Oxidative stress, prefrontal cortex hypomyelination and cognitive symptoms in schizophrenia. *Transl. Psychiatry* **2017**, *7*, 1–10. [CrossRef] [PubMed]

123. Khan, B.K.; Woolley, J.D.; Chao, S.; See, T.; Karydas, A.M.; Miller, B.L.; Rankin, K.P. Schizophrenia or neurodegenerative disease prodrome? Outcome of a first psychotic episode in a 35-year-old woman. *Psychosomatics* **2012**, *53*, 280–284. [CrossRef] [PubMed]

124. Quan, L.; Ishikawa, T.; Michiue, T.; Li, D.R.; Zhao, D.; Oritani, S.; Zhu, B.L.; Maeda, H. Ubiquitin-immunoreactive structures in the midbrain of methamphetamine abusers. *Leg. Med.* **2005**, *3*, 144–150. [CrossRef] [PubMed]

125. Fornai, F.; Lenzi, P.; Gesi, M.; Soldani, P.; Ferrucci, M.; Lazzeri, G.; Capobianco, L.; Battaglia, G.; De Blasi, A.; Nicoletti, F.; et al. Methamphetamine produces neuronal inclusions in the nigrostriatal system and in PC12 cells. *J. Neurochem.* **2004**, *88*, 114–123. [CrossRef] [PubMed]

126. Castino, R.; Lazzeri, G.; Lenzi, P.; Bellio, N.; Follo, C.; Ferrucci, M.; Fornai, F.; Isisoro, C. Suppression of autophagy precipitates neuronal cell death following low doses of methamphetamine. *J. Neurochem.* **2008**, *106*, 1426–1439. [CrossRef] [PubMed]

127. Yui, K.; Ikemoto, S.; Goto, K.; Nishijima, K.; Yoshino, T.; Ishiguro, T. Spontaneous recurrence of methamphetamine-induced paranoid-hallucinatory states in female subjects: Susceptibility to psychotic states and implications for relapse of schizophrenia. *Pharmacopsychiatry* **2002**, *35*, 62–71. [CrossRef] [PubMed]

128. Fasihpour, B.; Molavi, S.; Shariat, S.V. Clinical features of inpatients with methamphetamine induced psychosis. *J. Ment. Health* **2013**, *22*, 341–349. [CrossRef] [PubMed]

129. McKetin, R. Methamphetamine psychosis: Insights from the past. *Addiction* **2018**, *113*, 1522–1527. [CrossRef] [PubMed]

130. Limanaqi, F.; Gambardella, S.; Biagioni, F.; Busceti, C.; Fornai, F. Epigenetic effects induced by methamphetamine and methamphetamine-dependent oxidative stress. *Oxid. Med. Cell. Longev.* **2018**, *2018*, 4982453. [CrossRef]

131. Abi-Dargham, A.; Moore, H. Prefrontal DA transmission at D1 receptors and the pathology of schizophrenia. *Neuroscientist* **2003**, *9*, 404–416. [CrossRef] [PubMed]

132. Perreault, M.L.; Hasbi, A.; Alijaniaram, M.; Fan, T.; Varghese, G.; Fletcher, P.J.; Seeman, P.; O'Dowd, B.F.; George, S.R. The dopamine D1-D2 receptor heteromer localizes in dynorphin/enkephalin neurons: Increased high affinity state following amphetamine and in schizophrenia. *J. Biol. Chem.* **2010**, *285*, 36625–36634. [CrossRef] [PubMed]

133. Wang, D.; Ji, X.; Liu, J.; Li, Z.; Zhang, X. Dopamine Receptor Subtypes Differentially Regulate Autophagy. *Int. J. Mol. Sci.* **2018**, *19*, 1540. [CrossRef] [PubMed]

134. Pasquali, L.; Lazzeri, G.; Isidoro, C.; Ruggieri, S.; Paparelli, A.; Fornai, F. Role of autophagy during methamphetamine neurotoxicity. *Ann. N. Y. Acad. Sci.* **2008**, *1139*, 191–196. [CrossRef] [PubMed]

135. Lin, M.; Chandramani-Shivalingappa, P.; Jin, H.; Ghosh, A.; Anantharam, V.; Ali, S.; Kanthasamy, A.G.; Kanthasamy, A. Methamphetamine-induced neurotoxicity linked to ubiquitin-proteasome system dysfunction and autophagy-related changes that can be modulated by protein kinase C delta in dopaminergic neuronal cells. *Neuroscience* **2012**, *210*, 308–332. [CrossRef] [PubMed]

136. Aki, T.; Funakoshi, T.; Unuma, K.; Uemura, K. Impairment of autophagy: From hereditary disorder to drug intoxication. *Toxicology* **2013**, *311*, 205–215. [CrossRef] [PubMed]

137. Huang, S.H.; Wu, W.R.; Lee, L.M.; Huang, P.R.; Chen, J.C. mTOR signaling in the nucleus accumbens mediates behavioral sensitization to methamphetamine. *Prog. Neuropsychopharmacol. Biol. Psychiatry* **2018**, *86*, 331–339. [CrossRef] [PubMed]

138. Meredith, C.W.; Jaffe, C.; Ang-Lee, K.; Saxon, A.J. Implications of chronic methamphetamine use: A literature review. *Harv. Rev. Psychiatry* **2005**, *13*, 141–154. [CrossRef] [PubMed]

139. Homer, B.D.; Solomon, T.M.; Moeller, R.W.; Mascia, A.; DeRaleau, L.; Halkitis, P.N. Methamphetamine abuse and impairment of social functioning: A review of the underlying neurophysiological causes and behavioral implications. *Psychol. Bull.* **2008**, *134*, 301–310. [CrossRef] [PubMed]

140. Volkow, N.D.; Fowler, J.S.; Wang, G.J.; Shumay, E.; Telang, F.; Thanos, P.K.; Alexoff, D. Distribution and Pharmacokinetics of Methamphetamine in the Human Body: Clinical Implications. *PLoS ONE* **2010**, *5*, e15269. [CrossRef] [PubMed]

141. Laruelle, M.; Abi-Dargham, A.; Gil, R.; Kegeles, L.; Innis, R. Increased dopamine transmission in schizophrenia: Relationship to illness phases. *Biol. Psychiatry* **1999**, *46*, 56–72. [CrossRef]

142. Weidenauer, A.; Bauer, M.; Sauerzopf, U.; Bartova, L.; Praschak-Rieder, N.; Sitte, H.H.; Kasper, S.; Willeit, M. Making Sense of: Sensitization in Schizophrenia. *Int. J. Neuropsychopharmacol.* **2016**, *20*, 1–10. [CrossRef] [PubMed]

143. Dean, B. Neurochemistry of schizophrenia: The contribution of neuroimaging postmortem pathology and neurochemistry in schizophrenia. *Curr. Top. Med. Chem.* **2012**, *12*, 2375–2392. [CrossRef] [PubMed]

144. Howes, O.D.; Kambeitz, J.; Kim, E.; Stahl, D.; Slifstein, M.; Abi-Dargham, A.; Kapur, S. The nature of dopamine dysfunction in schizophrenia and what this means for treatment. *Arch. Gen. Psychiatry* **2012**, *69*, 776–786. [CrossRef] [PubMed]

145. Abekawa, T.; Ohmori, T.; Koyama, T. Effects of repeated administration of a high dose of methamphetamine on dopamine and glutamate release in rat striatum and nucleus accumbens. *Brain Res.* **1994**, *643*, 276–281. [CrossRef]

146. Stephans, S.E.; Yamamoto, B.Y. Effect of repeated methamphetamine administrations on dopamine and glutamate efflux in rat prefrontal cortex. *Brain Res.* **1995**, *700*, 99–106. [CrossRef]

147. Nishijima, K.; Kashiwa, A.; Hashimoto, A.; Iwama, H.; Umino, A.; Nishikawa, T. Differential effects of phencyclidine and methamphetamine on dopamine metabolism in rat frontal cortex and striatum as revealed by in vivo dialysis. *Synapse* **1996**, *22*, 304–312. [CrossRef]

148. Larsen, K.E.; Fon, E.A.; Hastings, T.G.; Edwards, R.H.; Sulzer, D. Methamphetamine-induced degeneration of dopaminergic neurons involves autophagy and upregulation of dopamine synthesis. *J. Neurosci.* **2002**, *22*, 8951–8960. [CrossRef] [PubMed]

149. Uehara, T.; Sumiyoshi, T.; Itoh, H.; Kurachi, M. Inhibition of dopamine synthesis with alpha-methyl-p-tyrosine abolishes the enhancement of methamphetamine-induced extracellular dopamine levels in the amygdala of rats with excitotoxic lesions of the entorhinal cortex. *Neurosci. Lett.* **2004**, *356*, 21–24. [CrossRef] [PubMed]

150. Purves-Tyson, T.D.; Owens, S.J.; Rothmond, D.A.; Halliday, G.M.; Double, K.L.; Stevens, J.; McCrossin, T.; Shannon Weickert, C. Putative presynaptic dopamine dysregulation in schizophrenia is supported by molecular evidence from post-mortem human midbrain. *Transl. Psychiatry* **2017**, *7*, e1003. [CrossRef] [PubMed]

151. Volkow, N.D.; Chang, L.; Wang, G.J.; Fowler, J.S.; Leonido-Yee, M.; Franceschi, D.; Sedler, M.J.; Gatley, S.J.; Hitzemann, R.; Ding, Y.S.; et al. Association of dopamine transporter reduction with psychomotor impairment in methamphetamine abusers. *Am. J. Psychiatry* **2001**, *158*, 377–382. [CrossRef] [PubMed]

152. German, C.L.; Hanson, G.R.; Fleckenstein, A.E. Amphetamine and methamphetamine reduce striatal dopamine transporter function without concurrent dopamine transporter relocalization. *J. Neurochem.* **2012**, *123*, 288–297. [CrossRef] [PubMed]

153. Zhou, M.; Li, W.; Huang, S.; Song, J.; Kim, J.Y.; Tian, X.; Kang, E.; Sano, Y.; Liu, C.; Balaji, J.; et al. mTOR Inhibition ameliorates cognitive and affective deficits caused by Disc1 knockdown in adult-born dentate granule neurons. *Neuron* **2013**, *77*, 647–654. [CrossRef] [PubMed]

154. Wesseling, H.; Elgersma, Y.; Bahn, S. A brain proteomic investigation of rapamycin effects in the $Tsc1^{+/-}$ mouse model. *Mol. Autism* **2017**, *8*, 41. [CrossRef] [PubMed]

155. Beaulieu, J.M.; Sotnikova, T.D.; Yao, W.D.; Kockeritz, L.; Woodgett, J.R.; Gainetdinov, R.R.; Caron, M.G. Lithium antagonizes dopamine-dependent behaviors mediated by an AKT/glycogen synthase kinase 3 signaling cascade. *Proc. Natl. Acad. Sci. USA* **2004**, *101*, 5099–5104. [CrossRef] [PubMed]

156. Hernandez, D.; Torres, C.A.; Setlik, W.; Cebrián, C.; Mosharov, E.V.; Tang, G.; Cheng, H.C.; Kholodilov, N.; Yarygina, O.; Burke, R.E.; et al. Regulation of presynaptic neurotransmission by macroautophagy. *Neuron* **2012**, *74*, 277–284. [CrossRef] [PubMed]

157. Hogan, K.A.; Staal, R.G.; Sonsalla, P.K. Analysis of VMAT2 binding after methamphetamine or MPTP treatment: Disparity between homogenates and vesicle preparations. *J. Neurochem.* **2000**, *74*, 2217–2220. [CrossRef] [PubMed]

158. Guillot, T.S.; Shepherd, K.R.; Richardson, J.R.; Wang, M.Z.; Li, Y.; Emson, P.C.; Miller, G.W. Reduced vesicular storage of dopamine exacerbates methamphetamine-induced neurodegeneration and astrogliosis. *J. Neurochem.* **2008**, *106*, 2205–2217. [CrossRef] [PubMed]

159. Cubells, J.F.; Rayport, S.; Rajendran, G.; Sulzer, D. Methamphetamine neurotoxicity involves vacuolation of endocytic organelles and dopamine-dependent intracellular oxidative stress. *J. Neurosci.* **1994**, *14*, 2260–2271. [CrossRef] [PubMed]

160. Fornai, F.; Chen, K.; Giorgi, F.S.; Gesi, M.; Alessandri, M.G.; Shih, J.C. Striatal dopamine metabolism in monoamine oxidase B-deficient mice: A brain dialysis study. *J. Neurochem.* **1999**, *73*, 2434–2440. [CrossRef] [PubMed]

161. Gesi, M.; Santinami, A.; Ruffoli, R.; Conti, G.; Fornai, F. Novel aspects of dopamine oxidative metabolism (confounding outcomes take place of certainties). *Pharmacol. Toxicol.* **2001**, *89*, 217–224. [CrossRef] [PubMed]

162. Lazzeri, G.; Lenzi, P.; Busceti, C.L.; Ferrucci, M.; Falleni, A.; Bruno, V.; Paparelli, A.; Fornai, F. Mechanisms involved in the formation of dopamine-induced intracellular bodies within striatal neurons. *J. Neurochem.* **2007**, *101*, 1414–1427. [CrossRef] [PubMed]

163. Fornai, F.; Lenzi, P.; Frenzilli, G.; Gesi, M.; Ferrucci, M.; Lazzeri, G.; Biagioni, F.; Nigro, M.; Falleni, A.; Giusiani, M.; et al. DNA damage and ubiquitinated neuronal inclusions in the substantia nigra and striatum of mice following MDMA (ecstasy). *Psychopharmacology* **2004**, *173*, 353–363. [CrossRef] [PubMed]

164. Butler, B.; Gamble-George, J.; Prins, P.; North, A.; Clarke, J.T.; Khoshbouei, H. Chronic Methamphetamine Increases Alpha-Synuclein Protein Levels in the Striatum and Hippocampus but not in the Cortex of Juvenile Mice. *J. Addict. Prev.* **2014**, *2*, 6. [PubMed]

165. Ferrucci, M.; Ryskalin, L.; Biagioni, F.; Gambardella, S.; Busceti, C.L.; Falleni, A.; Lazzeri, G.; Fornai, F. Methamphetamine increases Prion Protein and induces dopamine-dependent expression of protease resistant PrPsc. *Arch. Ital. Biol.* **2017**, *155*, 81–97. [PubMed]

166. Kobayashi, H.; Ide, S.; Hasegawa, J.; Ujike, H.; Sekine, Y.; Ozaki, N.; Inada, T.; Harano, M.; Komiyama, T.; Yamada, M.; et al. Study of association between α-synuclein gene polymorphism and methamphetamine psychosis/dependence. *Ann. N. Y. Acad. Sci.* **2004**, *1025*, 325–334. [CrossRef] [PubMed]

167. Fuchs, J.; Nilsson, C.; Kachergus, J.; Munz, M.; Larsson, E.M.; Schüle, B.; Langston, J.W.; Middleton, F.A.; Ross, O.A.; Hulihan, M.; et al. Phenotypic variation in a large Swedish pedigree due to SNCA duplication and triplication. *Neurology* **2007**, *68*, 916–922. [CrossRef] [PubMed]

168. Kolomeets, N.S.; Uranova, N.A. Synaptic contacts in schizophrenia: Study with immunocytochemical identification of dopaminergic neurons. *Zhurnal Nevrol. Psikhiatrii Imeni S. S. Korsakova* **1997**, *97*, 39–43. [CrossRef]

169. Uranova, N.A.; Levité, O.I. Ultrastructure of the substantia nigra in schizophrenia. *Zhurnal Nevrol. Psikhiatrii Imeni S. S. Korsakova* **1987**, *87*, 1017–1024.

170. Arnold, S.E.; Lee, V.M.; Gur, R.E.; Trojanowski, J.Q. Abnormal expression of two microtubule-associated proteins (MAP2 and MAP5) in specific subfields of the hippocampal formation in schizophrenia. *Proc. Natl. Acad. Sci. USA* **1991**, *88*, 10850–10854. [CrossRef] [PubMed]

171. Cotter, D.; Kerwin, R.; Doshi, B.; Martin, C.S.; Everall, I.P. Alterations in hippocampal non-phosphorylated MAP2 protein expression in schizophrenia. *Brain Res.* **1997**, *765*, 238–246. [CrossRef]

172. Rosoklija, G.; Keilp, J.G.; Toomayan, G.; Mancevski, B.; Haroutunian, V.; Liu, D.; Malespina, D.; Hays, A.P.; Sadiq, S.; Latov, N.; et al. Altered subicular MAP2 immunoreactivity in schizophrenia. *Prilozi* **2005**, *26*, 13–34. [PubMed]

173. Somenarain, L.; Jones, L.B. A comparative study of MAP2 immunostaining in areas 9 and 17 in schizophrenia and Huntington chorea. *J. Psychiatr. Res.* **2010**, *44*, 694–699. [CrossRef] [PubMed]

174. Shelton, M.A.; Newman, J.T.; Gu, H.; Sampson, A.R.; Fish, K.N.; MacDonald, M.L.; Moyer, C.E.; DiBitetto, J.V.; Dorph-Petersen, K.A.; Penzes, P.; et al. Loss of Microtubule-Associated Protein 2 Immunoreactivity Linked to Dendritic Spine Loss in Schizophrenia. *Biol. Psychiatry* **2015**, *78*, 374–385. [CrossRef] [PubMed]

175. Soustek, Z. Ultrastructure of cortical synapses in the brain of schizophrenics. *Zentralbl. Allg. Pathol.* **1989**, *135*, 25–32. [PubMed]

176. Prohovnik, I.; Dwork, A.J.; Kaufman, M.A.; Willson, N. Alzheimer-type neuropathology in elderly schizophrenia patients. *Schizophr. Bull.* **1993**, *19*, 805–816. [CrossRef] [PubMed]

177. Wisniewski, H.M.; Constantinidis, J.; Wegiel, J.; Bobinski, M.; Tarnawski, M. Neurofibrillary pathology in brains of elderly schizophrenics treated with neuroleptics. *Alzheimer Dis. Assoc. Disord.* **1994**, *8*, 211–227. [CrossRef] [PubMed]

178. Arnold, S.E.; Trojanowski, J.Q.; Gur, R.E.; Blackwell, P.; Han, L.Y.; Choi, C. Absence of neurodegeneration and neural injury in the cerebral cortex in a sample of elderly patients with schizophrenia. *Arch. Gen. Psychiatry* **1998**, *55*, 225–232. [CrossRef] [PubMed]

179. Purohit, D.P.; Perl, D.P.; Haroutunian, V.; Powchik, P.; Davidson, M.; Davis, K.L. Alzheimer disease and related neurodegenerative diseases in elderly patients with schizophrenia: A postmortem neuropathologic study of 100 cases. *Arch. Gen. Psychiatry* **1998**, *55*, 205–211. [CrossRef] [PubMed]

180. Falke, E.; Han, L.Y.; Arnold, S.E. Absence of neurodegeneration in the thalamus and caudate of elderly patients with schizophrenia. *Psychiatry Res.* **2000**, *93*, 103–110. [CrossRef]

181. Bozikas, V.P.; Kövari, E.; Bouras, C.; Karavatos, A. Neurofibrillary tangles in elderly patients with late onset schizophrenia. *Neurosci. Lett.* **2002**, *324*, 109–112. [CrossRef]

182. Momeni, P.; Wickremaratchi, M.M.; Bell, J.; Arnold, R.; Beer, R.; Hardy, J.; Revesz, T.; Neal, J.W.; Morris, H.R. Familial early onset frontotemporal dementia caused by a novel S356T MAPT mutation, initially diagnosed as schizophrenia. *Clin. Neurol. Neurosurg.* **2010**, *112*, 917–920. [CrossRef] [PubMed]

183. Uranova, N.A.; Vikhreva, O.V.; Rachmanova, V.I.; Orlovskaya, D.D. Ultrastructural alterations of myelinated fibers and oligodendrocytes in the prefrontal cortex in schizophrenia: A postmortem morphometric study. *Schizophr. Res. Treat.* **2011**, *2011*, 325789. [CrossRef] [PubMed]

184. Walker, C.K.; Roche, J.K.; Sinha, V.; Roberts, R.C. Substantia nigra ultrastructural pathology in schizophrenia. *Schizophr. Res.* **2017**. [CrossRef] [PubMed]

185. Leliveld, S.R.; Bader, V.; Hendriks, P.; Prikulis, I.; Sajnani, G.; Requena, J.R.; Korth, C. Insolubility of disrupted-in-schizophrenia 1 disrupts oligomer-dependent interactions with nuclear distribution element 1 and is associated with sporadic mental disease. *J. Neurosci.* **2008**, *28*, 3839–3845. [CrossRef] [PubMed]

186. Ottis, P.; Bader, V.; Trossbach, S.V.; Kretzschmar, H.; Michel, M.; Leliveld, S.R.; Korth, C. Convergence of two independent mental disease genes on the protein level: Recruitment of dysbindin to cell-invasive disrupted-in-schizophrenia 1 aggresomes. *Biol. Psychiatry* **2011**, *70*, 604–610. [CrossRef] [PubMed]

187. Atkin, T.; Kittler, J. DISC1 and the aggresome: A disruption to cellular function? *Autophagy* **2012**, *8*, 851–852. [CrossRef] [PubMed]

188. Xu, Y.; Sun, Y.; Ye, H.; Zhu, L.; Liu, J.; Wu, X.; Wang, L.; He, T.; Shen, Y.; Wu, J.Y.; et al. Increased dysbindin-1B isoform expression in schizophrenia and its propensity in aggresome formation. *Cell Discov.* **2015**, *1*, 15032. [CrossRef] [PubMed]

189. Camargo, L.M.; Collura, V.; Rain, J.C.; Mizuguchi, K.; Hermjakob, H.; Kerrien, S.; Bonnert, T.P.; Whiting, P.J.; Brandon, N.J. Disrupted in Schizophrenia 1 Interactome: Evidence for the close connectivity of risk genes and a potential synaptic basis for schizophrenia. *Mol. Psychiatry* **2007**, *12*, 74–86. [CrossRef] [PubMed]

190. Martins-de-Souza, D.; Cassoli, J.S.; Nascimento, J.M.; Hensley, K.; Guest, P.C.; Pinzon-Velasco, A.M.; Turck, C.W. The protein interactome of collapsin response mediator protein-2 (CRMP2/DPYSL2) reveals novel partner proteins in brain tissue. *Proteom. Clin. Appl.* **2015**, *9*, 817–831. [CrossRef] [PubMed]

191. Edgar, P.F.; Douglas, J.E.; Cooper, G.J.; Dean, B.; Kydd, R.; Faull, R.L. Comparative proteome analysis of the hippocampus implicates chromosome 6q in schizophrenia. *Mol. Psychiatry* **2000**, *5*, 85–90. [CrossRef] [PubMed]

192. Johnston-Wilson, N.L.; Sims, C.D.; Hofmann, J.P.; Anderson, L.; Shore, A.D.; Torrey, E.F.; Yolken, R.H. Disease-specific alterations in frontal cortex brain proteins in schizophrenia, bipolar disorder, and major depressive disorder. The Stanley Neuropathology Consortium. *Mol. Psychiatry* **2000**, *5*, 142–149. [CrossRef] [PubMed]

193. Beasley, C.L.; Pennington, K.; Behan, A.; Wait, R.; Dunn, M.J.; Cotter, D. Proteomic analysis of the anterior cingulate cortex in the major psychiatric disorders: Evidence for disease-associated changes. *Proteomics* **2006**, *6*, 3414–3425. [CrossRef] [PubMed]

194. Martins-de-Souza, D.; Gattaz, W.F.; Schmitt, A.; Maccarrone, G.; Hunyadi-Gulyás, E.; Eberlin, M.N.; Souza, G.H.; Marangoni, S.; Novello, J.C.; Turck, C.W.; et al. Proteomic analysis of dorsolateral prefrontal cortex indicates the involvement of cytoskeleton, oligodendrocyte, energy metabolism and new potential markers in schizophrenia. *J. Psychiatr. Res.* **2009**, *43*, 978–986. [CrossRef] [PubMed]

195. Vijayan, V.; Verstreken, P. Autophagy in the presynaptic compartment in health and disease. *J. Cell Biol.* **2017**, *216*, 1895–1906. [CrossRef] [PubMed]

196. Merenlender-Wagner, A.; Shemer, Z.; Touloumi, O.; Lagoudaki, R.; Giladi, E.; Andrieux, A.; Grigoriadis, N.C.; Gozes, I. New horizons in schizophrenia treatment: Autophagy protection is coupled with behavioral improvements in a mouse model of schizophrenia. *Autophagy* **2014**, *10*, 2324–2332. [CrossRef] [PubMed]

197. Merenlender-Wagner, A.; Malishkevich, A.; Shemer, Z.; Udawela, M.; Gibbons, A.; Scarr, E.; Dean, B.; Levine, J.; Agam, G.; Gozes, I. Autophagy has a key role in the pathophysiology of schizophrenia. *Mol. Psychiatry* **2015**, *20*, 126–132. [CrossRef] [PubMed]

198. Morfini, G.A.; Burns, M.; Binder, L.I.; Kanaan, N.M.; LaPointe, N.; Bosco, D.A.; Brown, R.H., Jr.; Brown, H.; Tiwari, A.; Hayward, L.; et al. Axonal transport defects in neurodegenerative diseases. *J. Neurosci.* **2009**, *29*, 12776–12786. [CrossRef] [PubMed]

199. Daoust, A.; Bohic, S.; Saoudi, Y.; Debacker, C.; Gory-Fauré, S.; Andrieux, A.; Barbier, E.L.; Deloulme, J.C. Neuronal transport defects of the MAP6 KO mouse—A model of schizophrenia- and alleviation by Epothilone D treatment, as observed using MEMRI. *Neuroimage* **2014**, *96*, 133–142. [CrossRef] [PubMed]

200. Calabrese, F.; Riva, M.A.; Molteni, R. Synaptic alterations associated with depression and schizophrenia: Potential as a therapeutic target. *Expert Opin. Ther. Targets* **2016**, *20*, 1195–1207. [CrossRef] [PubMed]

201. Bridi, J.C.; Hirth, F. Mechanisms of α-Synuclein Induced Synaptopathy in Parkinson's Disease. *Front. Neurosci.* **2018**, *12*, 80. [CrossRef] [PubMed]

202. St Clair, D.; Blackwood, D.; Muir, W.; Carothers, A.; Walker, M.; Spowart, G.; Gosden, C.; Evans, H.J. Association within a family of a balanced autosomal translocation with major mental illness. *Lancet* **1990**, *336*, 13–16. [CrossRef]

203. Schurov, I.L.; Handford, E.J.; Brandon, N.J.; Whiting, B.J. Expression of disrupted in schizophrenia 1 (DISC1) protein in the adult and developing mouse brain indicates its role in neurodevelopment. *Mol. Psychiatry* **2004**, *9*, 1100–1110. [CrossRef] [PubMed]

204. Brandon, N.J.; Sawa, A. Linking neurodevelopmental and synaptic theories of mental illness through DISC1. *Nat. Rev. Neurosci.* **2011**, *12*, 707–722. [CrossRef] [PubMed]

205. Hikida, T.; Gamo, N.J.; Sawa, A. DISC1 as a therapeutic target for mental illnesses. *Expert Opin. Ther. Targets* **2012**, *16*, 1151–1160. [CrossRef] [PubMed]

206. Lipska, B.K.; Mitkus, S.N.; Mathew, S.V.; Fatula, R.; Hyde, T.M.; Weinberger, D.R.; Kleinman, J.E. Functional genomics in postmortem human brain: Abnormalities in a DISC1 molecular pathway in schizophrenia. *Dialogues Clin. Neurosci.* **2006**, *8*, 353–357. [PubMed]

207. Dahoun, T.; Trossbach, S.V.; Brandon, N.J.; Korth, C.; Howes, O.D. The impact of Disrupted-in-Schizophrenia 1 (DISC1) on the dopaminergic system: A systematic review. *Transl. Psychiatry* **2017**, *7*, e1015. [CrossRef] [PubMed]

208. Nakai, T.; Nagai, T.; Wang, R.; Yamada, S.; Kuroda, K.; Kaibuchi, K.; Yamada, K. Alterations of GABAergic and dopaminergic systems in mutant mice with disruption of exons 2 and 3 of the Disc1 gene. *Neurochem. Int.* **2014**, *74*, 74–83. [CrossRef] [PubMed]

209. Pogorelov, V.M.; Nomura, J.; Kim, J.; Kannan, G.; Ayhan, Y.; Yang, C.; Taniguchi, Y.; Abazyan, B.; Valentine, H.; Krasnova, I.N.; et al. Mutant DISC1 affects methamphetamine-induced sensitization and conditioned place preference: A comorbidity model. *Neuropharmacology* **2012**, *62*, 1242–1251. [CrossRef] [PubMed]

210. Niwa, M.; Lee, R.S.; Tanaka, T.; Okada, K.; Kano, S.; Sawa, A. A critical period of vulnerability to adolescent stress: Epigenetic mediators in mesocortical dopaminergic neurons. *Hum. Mol. Genet.* **2016**, *25*, 1370–1381. [CrossRef] [PubMed]

211. Owen, M.J.; Sawa, A.; Mortensen, P.B. Schizophrenia. *Lancet* **2016**, *388*, 86–97. [CrossRef]

212. Kim, J.Y.; Duan, X.; Liu, C.Y.; Jang, M.H.; Guo, J.U.; Pow-anpongkul, N.; Kang, E.; Song, H.; Ming, G.L. DISC1 regulates new neuron development in the adult brain via modulation of AKT-mTOR signaling through KIAA1212. *Neuron* **2009**, *63*, 761–773. [CrossRef] [PubMed]

213. Blackwood, D.H.; Fordyce, A.; Walker, M.T.; St Clair, D.M.; Porteous, D.J.; Muir, W.J. Schizophrenia and affective disorders—Cosegregation with a translocation at chromosome 1q42 that directly disrupts brain-expressed genes: Clinical and P300 findings in a family. *Am. J. Hum. Genet.* **2001**, *69*, 428–433. [CrossRef] [PubMed]

214. Clapcote, S.J.; Lipina, T.V.; Millar, J.K.; Mackie, S.; Christie, S.; Ogawa, F.; Lerch, J.P.; Trimble, K.; Uchiyama, M.; Sakuraba, Y.; et al. Behavioral phenotypes of Disc1 missense mutations in mice. *Neuron* **2007**, *54*, 387–402. [CrossRef] [PubMed]

215. Chubb, J.E.; Bradshaw, N.J.; Soares, D.C.; Porteous, D.J.; Millar, J.K. The DISC locus in psychiatric illness. *Mol. Psychiatry* **2008**, *13*, 36–64. [CrossRef] [PubMed]

216. Gangarossa, G.; Ceolin, L.; Paucard, A.; Lerner-Natoli, M.; Perroy, J.; Fagni, L.; Valjent, E. Repeated stimulation of dopamine D1-like receptor and hyperactivation of mTOR signaling lead to generalized seizures, altered dentate gyrus plasticity, and memory deficits. *Hippocampus* **2014**, *24*, 1466–1481. [CrossRef] [PubMed]

217. Siuta, M.A.; Robertson, S.D.; Kocalis, H.; Saunders, C.; Gresch, P.J.; Khatri, V.; Shiota, C.; Kennedy, J.P.; Lindsley, C.W.; Daws, L.C.; et al. Dysregulation of the norepinephrine transporter sustains cortical hypodopaminergia and schizophrenia-like behaviors in neuronal rictor null mice. *PLoS Biol.* **2010**, *8*, e1000393. [CrossRef] [PubMed]

218. Emamian, E.S.; Hall, D.; Birnbaum, M.J.; Karayiorgou, M.; Gogos, J.A. Convergent evidence for impaired AKT1-GSK3β signaling in schizophrenia. *Nat. Genet.* **2004**, *36*, 131–137. [CrossRef] [PubMed]

219. Ikeda, M.; Iwata, N.; Suzuki, T.; Kitajima, T.; Yamanouchi, Y.; Kinoshita, Y.; Inada, T.; Ozaki, N. Association of AKT1 with schizophrenia confirmed in a Japanese population. *Biol. Psychiatry* **2004**, *56*, 698–700. [CrossRef] [PubMed]

220. Schwab, S.G.; Hoefgen, B.; Hanses, C.; Hassenbach, M.B.; Albus, M.; Lerer, B.; Trixler, M.; Maier, W.; Wildenauer, D.B. Further evidence for association of variants in the AKT1 gene with schizophrenia in a sample of European sib-pair families. *Biol. Psychiatry* **2005**, *58*, 446–450. [CrossRef] [PubMed]

221. Bajestan, S.N.; Sabouri, A.H.; Nakamura, M.; Takashima, H.; Keikhaee, M.R.; Behdani, F.; Fayyazi, M.R.; Sargolzaee, M.R.; Bajestan, M.N.; Sabouri, Z.; et al. Association of AKT1 haplotype with the risk of schizophrenia in Iranian population. *Am. J. Med. Genet. B Neuropsychiatr. Genet.* **2006**, *141*, 383–386. [CrossRef] [PubMed]

222. Xu, M.Q.; Xing, Q.H.; Zheng, Y.L.; Li, S.; Gao, J.J.; He, G.; Guo, T.W.; Feng, G.Y.; Xu, F.; He, L. Association of AKT1 gene polymorphisms with risk of schizophrenia and with response to antipsychotics in the Chinese population. *J. Clin. Psychiatry* **2007**, *68*, 1358–1367. [CrossRef] [PubMed]

223. Thiselton, D.L.; Vladimirov, V.I.; Kuo, P.H.; McClay, J.; Wormley, B.; Fanous, A.; O'Neill, F.A.; Walsh, D.; Van den Oord, E.J.; Kendler, K.S.; et al. AKT1 is associated with schizophrenia across multiple symptom dimensions in the Irish study of high density schizophrenia families. *Biol. Psychiatry* **2008**, *63*, 449–457. [CrossRef] [PubMed]

224. Karege, F.; Méary, A.; Perroud, N.; Jamain, S.; Leboyer, M.; Ballmann, E.; Fernandez, R.; Malafosse, A.; Schürhoff, F. Genetic overlap between schizophrenia and bipolar disorder: A study with AKT1 gene variants and clinical phenotypes. *Schizophr. Res.* **2012**, *135*, 8–14. [CrossRef] [PubMed]

225. Nohesara, S.; Ghadirivasfi, M.; Barati, M.; Ghasemzadeh, M.R.; Narimani, S.; Mousavi-Behbahani, Z.; Joghataei, M.; Soleimani, M.; Taban, M.; Mehrabi, S.; et al. Methamphetamine-induced psychosis is associated with DNA hypomethylation and increased expression of AKT1 and key dopaminergic genes. *Am. J. Med. Genet. B Neuropsychiatr. Genet.* **2016**, *171*, 1180–1189. [CrossRef] [PubMed]

226. Petryshen, T.L.; Middleton, F.A.; Kirby, A.; Aldinger, K.A.; Purcell, S.; Tahl, A.R.; Morley, C.P.; McGann, L.; Gentile, K.L.; Rockwell, G.N.; et al. Support for involvement of neuregulin 1 in schizophrenia pathophysiology. *Mol. Psychiatry* **2005**, *10*, 366–374. [CrossRef] [PubMed]

227. Law, A.J.; Kleinman, J.E.; Weinberger, D.R.; Weickert, C.S. Disease-associated intronic variants in the ErbB4 gene are related to altered ErbB4 splice-variant expression in the brain in schizophrenia. *Hum. Mol. Genet.* **2007**, *16*, 129–141. [CrossRef] [PubMed]

228. Hahn, C.G.; Wang, H.Y.; Cho, D.S.; Talbot, K.; Gur, R.E.; Berrettini, W.H.; Bakshi, K.; Kamins, J.; Borgmann-Winter, K.E.; Siegel, S.J.; et al. Altered neuregulin 1-erbB4 signaling contributes to NMDA receptor hypofunction in schizophrenia. *Nat. Med.* **2006**, *12*, 824–828. [CrossRef] [PubMed]

229. Mei, L.; Xiong, W.C. Neuregulin 1 in neural development, synaptic plasticity and schizophrenia. *Nat. Rev.* **2008**, *9*, 437–452. [CrossRef] [PubMed]

230. Seshadri, S.; Kamiya, A.; Yokota, Y.; Prikulis, I.; Kano, S.; Hayashi-Takagi, A.; Stanco, A.; Eom, T.Y.; Rao, S.; Ishizuka, K.; et al. Disrupted-in-Schizophrenia-1 expression is regulated by beta-site amyloid precursor protein cleaving enzyme-1-neuregulin cascade. *Proc. Natl. Acad. Sci. USA* **2010**, *107*, 5622–5627. [CrossRef] [PubMed]

231. Skirzewski, M.; Karavanova, I.; Shamir, A.; Erben, L.; Garcia-Olivares, J.; Shin, J.H.; Vullhorst, D.; Alvarez, V.A.; Amara, S.G.; Buonanno, A. ErbB4 Signaling in Dopaminergic Axonal Projections Increases Extracellular Dopamine Levels and Regulates Spatial/Working Memory Behaviors. *Mol. Psychiatry* **2017**. [CrossRef] [PubMed]

232. Roy, K.; Murtie, J.C.; El-Khodor, B.F.; Edgar, N.; Sardi, S.P.; Hooks, B.M.; Benoit-Marand, M.; Chen, C.; Moore, H.; O'Donnell, P.; et al. Loss of erbB signaling in oligodendrocytes alters myelin and dopaminergic function, a potential mechanism for neuropsychiatric disorders. *Proc. Natl. Acad. Sci. USA* **2007**, *104*, 8131–8136. [CrossRef] [PubMed]

233. Zhao, X.; Tang, R.; Xiao, Z.; Shi, Y.; Feng, G.; Gu, N.; Shi, J.; Xing, Y.; Yan, L.; Sang, H.; et al. An investigation of the dihydropyrimidinase-like 2 (DPYSL2) gene in schizophrenia: Genetic association study and expression analysis. *Int. J. Neuropsychopharmacol.* **2006**, *9*, 705–712. [CrossRef] [PubMed]

234. Nakata, K.; Ujike, H.; Sakai, A.; Takaki, M.; Imamura, T.; Tanaka, Y.; Kuroda, S. The human dihydropyrimidinase-related protein 2 gene on chromosome 8p21 is associated with paranoid-type schizophrenia. *Biol. Psychiatry* **2003**, *53*, 571–576. [CrossRef]

235. Fallin, M.D.; Lasseter, V.K.; Liu, Y.; Avramopoulos, D.; McGrath, J.; Wolyniec, P.S.; Nestadt, G.; Liang, K.Y.; Chen, P.L.; Valle, D.; et al. Linkage and association on 8p21.2-p21.1 in schizophrenia. *Am. J. Med. Genet. B Neuropsychiatr. Genet.* **2011**, *156*, 188–197. [CrossRef] [PubMed]

236. Liu, Y.; Pham, X.; Zhang, L.; Chen, P.L.; Burzynski, G.; McGaughey, D.M.; He, S.; McGrath, J.A.; Wolyniec, P.; Fallin, M.D.; et al. Functional variants in DPYSL2 sequence increase risk of schizophrenia and suggest a link to mTOR signaling. *G3* **2014**, *5*, 61–72. [CrossRef] [PubMed]

237. Lim, C.; Chong, S.A.; Keefe, R. Psychosocial factors in the neurobiology of schizophrenia: A selective review. *Ann. Acad. Med. Singap.* **2009**, *38*, 402–406. [PubMed]

238. Lee, H.; Joo, J.; Nah, S.S.; Kim, J.W.; Kim, H.K.; Kwon, J.T.; Lee, H.Y.; Kim, Y.O.; Kim, H.J. Changes in Dpysl2 expression are associated with prenatally stressed rat offspring and susceptibility to schizophrenia in humans. *Int. J. Mol. Med.* **2015**, *35*, 1574–1586. [CrossRef] [PubMed]

239. Kobeissy, F.H.; Warren, M.W.; Ottens, A.K.; Sadasivan, S.; Zhang, Z.; Gold, M.S.; Wang, K.K. Psychoproteomic analysis of rat cortex following acute methamphetamine exposure. *J. Proteome Res.* **2008**, *7*, 1971–1983. [CrossRef] [PubMed]

240. Nakamura, H.; Yamashita, N.; Kimura, A.; Kimura, Y.; Hirano, H.; Makihara, H.; Kawamoto, Y.; Jitsuki-Takahashi, A.; Yonezaki, K.; Takase, K.; et al. Comprehensive behavioral study and proteomic analyses of CRMP2-deficient mice. *Genes Cells* **2016**, *21*, 1059–1079. [CrossRef] [PubMed]

241. Jin, X.; Sasamoto, K.; Nagai, J.; Yamazaki, Y.; Saito, K.; Goshima, Y.; Inoue, T.; Ohshima, T. Phosphorylation of CRMP2 by Cdk5 Regulates Dendritic Spine Development of Cortical Neuron in the Mouse Hippocampus. *Neural Plast.* **2016**, *2016*, 6790743. [CrossRef] [PubMed]

242. Benavides, D.R.; Bibb, J.A. Role of Cdk5 in drug abuse and plasticity. *Ann. N. Y. Acad. Sci.* **2004**, *1025*, 335–344. [CrossRef] [PubMed]

243. Mlewski, E.C.; Arias, C.; Paglini, G. Association between the expression of amphetamine-induced behavioral sensitization and Cdk5/p35 activity in dorsal striatum. *Behav. Neurosci.* **2016**, *130*, 114–122. [CrossRef] [PubMed]

244. Lebel, M.; Patenaude, C.; Allyson, J.; Massicotte, G.; Cyr, M. Dopamine D1 receptor activation induces tau phosphorylation via Cdk5 and GSK3 signaling pathways. *Neuropharmacology* **2009**, *57*, 392–402. [CrossRef] [PubMed]

245. Cantrup, R.; Sathanantham, K.; Rushlow, W.J.; Rajakumar, N. Chronic hyperdopaminergic activity of schizophrenia is associated with increased ΔFosB levels and cdk-5 signaling in the nucleus accumbens. *Neuroscience* **2012**, *222*, 124–135. [CrossRef] [PubMed]
246. Ferreras, S.; Fernández, G.; Danelon, V.; Pisano, M.V.; Masseroni, L.; Chapleau, C.A.; Krapacher, F.A.; Mlewski, E.C.; Mascó, D.H.; Arias, C.; et al. Cdk5 Is Essential for Amphetamine to Increase Dendritic Spine Density in Hippocampal Pyramidal Neurons. *Front. Cell. Neurosci.* **2017**, *11*, 372. [CrossRef] [PubMed]
247. Engmann, O.; Hortobágyi, T.; Pidsley, R.; Troakes, C.; Bernstein, H.G.; Kreutz, M.R.; Mill, J.; Nikolic, M.; Giese, K.P. Schizophrenia is associated with dysregulation of a Cdk5 activator that regulates synaptic protein expression and cognition. *Brain* **2011**, *134*, 2408–2421. [CrossRef] [PubMed]
248. Al Eissa, M.M.; Fiorentino, A.; Sharp, S.I.; O'Brien, N.L.; Wolfe, K.; Giaroli, G.; Curtis, D.; Bass, N.J.; McQuillin, A. Exome sequence analysis and follow up genotyping implicates rare ULK1 variants to be involved in susceptibility to schizophrenia. *Ann. Hum. Genet.* **2018**, *82*, 88–92. [CrossRef] [PubMed]
249. Horesh, Y.; Katsel, P.; Haroutunian, V.; Domany, E. Gene expression signature is shared by patients with Alzheimer's disease and schizophrenia at the superior temporal gyrus. *Eur. J. Neurol.* **2011**, *18*, 410–424. [CrossRef] [PubMed]
250. Woodruff, P.W.; Wright, I.C.; Bullmore, E.T.; Brammer, M.; Howard, R.J.; Williams, S.C.; Shapleske, J.; Rossell, S.; David, A.S.; McGuire, P.K.; et al. Auditory hallucinations and the temporal cortical response to speech in schizophrenia: A functional magnetic resonance imaging study. *Am. J. Psychiatry* **1997**, *154*, 1676–1682. [CrossRef] [PubMed]
251. Allen, P.; Larøi, F.; McGuire, P.K.; Aleman, A. The hallucinating brain: A review of structural and functional neuroimaging studies of hallucinations. *Neurosci. Biobehav. Rev.* **2008**, *32*, 175–191. [CrossRef] [PubMed]
252. Barnes, M.R.; Huxley-Jones, J.; Maycox, P.R.; Lennon, M.; Thornber, A.; Kelly, F.; Bates, S.; Taylor, A.; Reid, J.; Jones, N.; et al. Transcription and pathway analysis of the superior temporal cortex and anterior prefrontal cortex in schizophrenia. *J. Neurosci. Res.* **2011**, *89*, 1218–1227. [CrossRef] [PubMed]
253. Vinayagam, A.; Stelzl, U.; Foulle, R.; Plassmann, S.; Zenkner, M.; Timm, J.; Assmus, H.E.; Andrade-Navarro, M.A.; Wanker, E.E. A directed protein interaction network for investigating intracellular signal transduction. *Sci. Signal.* **2011**, *4*, rs8. [CrossRef] [PubMed]
254. Dresner, E.; Agam, G.; Gozes, I. Activity-dependent neuroprotective protein (ADNP) expression level is correlated with the expression of the sister protein ADNP2: Deregulation in schizophrenia. *Eur. Neuropsychopharmacol.* **2011**, *21*, 355–361. [CrossRef] [PubMed]
255. Javitt, D.C.; Buchanan, R.W.; Keefe, R.S.; Kern, R.; McMahon, R.P.; Green, M.F.; Lieberman, J.; Goff, D.C.; Csernansky, J.G.; McEvoy, J.P.; et al. Effect of the neuroprotective peptide davunetide (AL-108) on cognition and functional capacity in schizophrenia. *Schizophr. Res.* **2012**, *136*, 25–31. [CrossRef] [PubMed]
256. Sarkar, S.; Krishna, G.; Imarisio, S.; Saili, S.; O'Kane, C.J.; Rubinsztein, D.C. A rational mechanism for combination treatment of Huntington's disease using lithium and rapamycin. *Hum. Mol. Genet.* **2008**, *17*, 170–178. [CrossRef] [PubMed]
257. Yin, Y.C.; Lin, C.C.; Chen, T.T.; Chen, J.Y.; Tsai, H.J.; Wang, C.Y.; Chen, S.Y. Clozapine induces autophagic cell death in non-small cell lung cancer cells. *Cell. Physiol. Biochem.* **2015**, *35*, 945–956. [CrossRef] [PubMed]
258. Sade, Y.; Toker, L.; Kara, N.Z.; Einat, H.; Rapoport, S.; Moechars, D.; Berry, G.T.; Bersudsky, Y.; Agam, G. IP3 accumulation and/or inositol depletion: Two downstream lithium's effects that may mediate its behavioral and cellular changes. *Transl. Psychiatry* **2016**, *6*, e968. [CrossRef] [PubMed]
259. Kim, S.H.; Park, S.; Yu, H.S.; Ko, K.H.; Park, H.G.; Kim, Y.S. The antipsychotic agent clozapine induces autophagy via the AMPK-ULK1-Beclin1 signaling pathway in the rat frontal cortex. *Prog. Neuropsychopharmacol. Biol. Psychiatry* **2018**, *81*, 96–104. [CrossRef] [PubMed]
260. Kim, Y.D.; Jeong, E.I.; Nah, J.; Yoo, S.M.; Lee, W.J.; Kim, Y.; Moon, S.; Hong, S.H.; Jung, Y.K. Pimozide reduces toxic forms of tau in TauC3 mice via 5' adenosine monophosphate-activated protein kinase-mediated autophagy. *J. Neurochem.* **2017**, *142*, 734–746. [CrossRef] [PubMed]
261. Shin, J.H.; Park, S.J.; Kim, E.S.; Jo, Y.K.; Hong, J.; Cho, D.H. Sertindole, a potent antagonist at dopamine D$_2$ receptors, induces autophagy by increasing reactive oxygen species in SH-SY5Y neuroblastoma cells. *Biol. Pharm. Bull.* **2012**, *35*, 1069–1075. [CrossRef] [PubMed]
262. Charvin, D.; Roze, E.; Perrin, V.; Deyts, C.; Betuing, S.; Pagès, C.; Régulier, E.; Luthi-Carter, R.; Brouillet, E.; Déglon, N.; et al. Haloperidol protects striatal neurons from dysfunction induced by mutated huntingtin in vivo. *Neurobiol. Dis.* **2008**, *29*, 22–29. [CrossRef] [PubMed]

263. Höllerhage, M.; Goebel, J.N.; de Andrade, A.; Hildebrandt, T.; Dolga, A.; Culmsee, C.; Oertel, W.H.; Hengerer, B.; Höglinger, G.U. Trifluoperazine rescues human dopaminergic cells from wild-type α-synuclein-induced toxicity. *Neurobiol. Aging* **2014**, *35*, 1700–1711. [CrossRef] [PubMed]

264. Choi, Y.; Jeong, H.J.; Liu, Q.F.; Oh, S.T.; Koo, B.S.; Kim, Y.; Chung, I.W.; Kim, Y.S.; Jeon, S. Clozapine Improves Memory Impairment and Reduces Aβ Level in the Tg-APPswe/PS1dE9 Mouse Model of Alzheimer's Disease. *Mol. Neurobiol.* **2017**, *54*, 450–460. [CrossRef] [PubMed]

265. Park, J.; Chung, S.; An, H.; Kim, J.; Seo, J.; Kim, D.H.; Yoon, S.Y. Haloperidol and clozapine block formation of autophagolysosomes in rat primary neurons. *Neuroscience* **2012**, *209*, 64–73. [CrossRef] [PubMed]

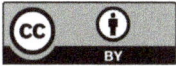

International Journal of
Molecular Sciences

MDPI

Review

Balancing mTOR Signaling and Autophagy in the Treatment of Parkinson's Disease

Zhou Zhu [1], Chuanbin Yang [1], Ashok Iyaswamy [1], Senthilkumar Krishnamoorthi [1], Sravan Gopalkrishnashetty Sreenivasmurthy [1], Jia Liu [1], Ziying Wang [1], Benjamin Chun-Kit Tong [1], Juxian Song [2], Jiahong Lu [3], King-Ho Cheung [1] and Min Li [1,*]

[1] Mr. and Mrs. Ko Chi Ming Centre for Parkinson's Disease Research, School of Chinese Medicine, Hong Kong Baptist University, Hong Kong SAR 999077, China; zzhou1022@gmail.com (Z.Z.); nkyangchb@gmail.com (C.Y.); ashokenviro@gmail.com (A.I.); senthilnslab@gmail.com (S.K.); sravans@gmail.com (S.G.S.); liujiatheone@hotmail.com (J.L.); wangziying.12@163.com (Z.W.); benjamintck@gmail.com (B.C.-K.T.); kingho@hkbu.edu.hk (K.-H.C.)
[2] Medical College of Acupuncture-Moxibustion and Rehabilitation, Guangzhou University of Chinese Medicine, Guangzhou 510006, China; juxian.song@gmail.com
[3] State Key Laboratory of Quality Research in Chinese Medicine, Institute of Chinese Medical Sciences, University of Macau, Taipa, Macau SAR 999078, China; jiahonglu@um.edu.mo
* Correspondence: limin@hkbu.edu.hk; Tel: +852-3411-2919

Received: 15 January 2019; Accepted: 1 February 2019; Published: 8 February 2019

Abstract: The mammalian target of rapamycin (mTOR) signaling pathway plays a critical role in regulating cell growth, proliferation, and life span. mTOR signaling is a central regulator of autophagy by modulating multiple aspects of the autophagy process, such as initiation, process, and termination through controlling the activity of the unc51-like kinase 1 (ULK1) complex and vacuolar protein sorting 34 (VPS34) complex, and the intracellular distribution of TFEB/TFE3 and proto-lysosome tubule reformation. Parkinson's disease (PD) is a serious, common neurodegenerative disease characterized by dopaminergic neuron loss in the substantia nigra pars compacta (SNpc) and the accumulation of Lewy bodies. An increasing amount of evidence indicates that mTOR and autophagy are critical for the pathogenesis of PD. In this review, we will summarize recent advances regarding the roles of mTOR and autophagy in PD pathogenesis and treatment. Further characterizing the dysregulation of mTOR pathway and the clinical translation of mTOR modulators in PD may offer exciting new avenues for future drug development.

Keywords: mTOR; autophagy; Parkinson's disease

---

1. Introduction of mTOR

The target of rapamycin (TOR) was first identified as a target protein of rapamycin, encoded by TOR1 and TOR2 alleles, through screening of rapamycin-resistant mutant yeast [1]. This study showed rapamycin could form a complex with FK506-binding protein (FKBP), leading to cell cycle arrest in the G1 phase, which is mediated by TOR1 and TOR2 [1]. Subsequent studies of mammalian cells found homologous proteins, termed mammalian targets of rapamycin (mTOR), which shared more than 40% consistency in amino acid sequence with yeast TOR1 and TOR2 [2]. In addition, the function of mTOR was also related to the rapamycin-FKBP12 induced cell cycle arrest [2,3].

mTOR, which is also termed as FKBP12-rapamycin complex-associated protein (FRAP), is a conserved serine/threonine protein kinase, and mTOR belongs to the phosphoinositide-3-kinase (PI3K)-related kinase family of protein kinases [4]. mTOR constitutes the catalytic component of two distinct multiprotein complexes: mTOR complex 1 (mTORC1) and mTOR complex 2 (mTORC2) (Figure 1) [5].

mTORC1 contains mTOR, mammalian lethal with SEC13 protein 8 (mLST8), DEP (DVL, Egl-10, pleckstrin)-domain containing mTOR-interacting protein (DEPTOR), proline-rich Akt substrate of 40 kD (PRAS40), and regulatory associated protein of mammalian target of rapamycin (Raptor) (Figure 1) [6–10]. In this complex, mTOR-combined DEPTOR and PRAS40 can negatively regulate mTORC1 activity [6,10]. mTORC1 plays a key role in regulating cell growth, cell size, and proliferation [8,11,12]. mTORC1 is a core component in a series of signaling networks. Additionally, it senses different stimuli such as insulin level, energy level, and amino acid level, and is involved in protein synthesis, lipid metabolism, glycolytic metabolism, and autophagy [13,14].

mTORC2 consists of mTOR, mLST8, DEPTOR, rapamycin-insensitive companion of mTOR (Rictor), mammalian stress-activated map kinase-interacting protein 1 (mSIN1), and protein observed with Rictor (Protor) (Figure 1) [6,15–19]. mTORC2 also regulates many cellular processes, such as cell growth, proliferation, metabolism, and cell motility via the AGC kinase family member Akt, serum/glucocorticoid regulated kinase (SGK), protein kinase C (PKC), and filamin A [20–23]. The well-known substrate of mTORC2 is Akt. Akt can be fully activated when it is phosphorylated by 3-phosphoinositide dependent protein kinase-1 (PDK1) at Thr308 site, and subsequently phosphorylated by mTORC2 at Ser473 site [24,25]. Actually, Yang et al. found that mSIN1, a component of mTORC2, mediates a positive feedback loop between mTORC2 and Akt [26]. The phosphorylation of mSIN1 at Thr86 site, which is induced by phospho-Akt, enhances mTORC2 activity in response to growth factors [26,27].

The PI3K/Akt/mTOR signaling pathway has been extensively studied because it plays a crucial role in controlling cell growth, in maintaining cell viability, and in determining a cell's life span [28,29]. Insulin receptor substrate (IRS) activates phosphatidylinositol 3-kinase (PI3K) upon presence of growth factors, recruiting PIP2 to the plasma membrane, and enhancing transformation of PIP2 to PIP3. PIP3 promotes the phosphorylation of Akt on the Thr308 and Ser473 sites by PDK1 and mTORC2, respectively. Once being fully activated, Akt phosphorylates and inhibits tuberous sclerosis complex (TSC), which is the negative regulator of Ras homolog enriched in brain (Rheb) and finally leads to the activation of mTORC1 [30]. There are two well-established downstream effectors being phosphorylated by mTORC1, p70 ribosomal S6 kinase (P70S6K) and eukaryotic initiation factor 4E (eIF4E) binding protein 1 (4EBP1); both of them are main regulators of cap-dependent protein synthesis [31,32].

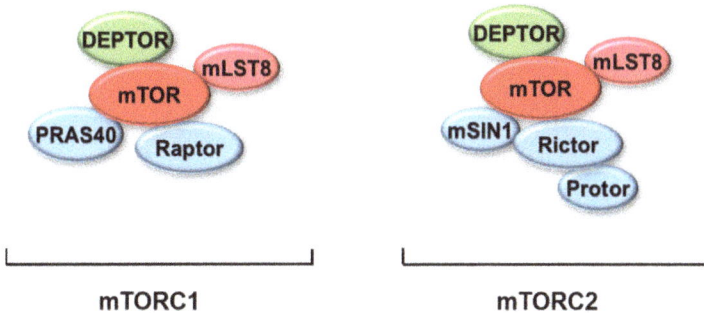

Figure 1. Protein components of mTORC1 and mTORC2. Both mTORC1 and mTORC2 include the same macromolecules such as mTOR, mLST8, and DEPTOR. Apart from these components, mTORC1 also contains PRAS40 and Raptor. Correspondingly, mTORC2 contains mSIN1, Rictor, and Protor. Abbreviation: mTORC1, mTOR complex 1; mTORC2, mTOR complex 2; mTOR, Mammalian targets of rapamycin; mLST8, Mammalian lethal with sec-13 protein 8; DEPTOR, DEP-domain containing mTOR-interacting protein; PRAS40, Proline-rich Akt substrate of 40 kDa; Raptor, Regulatory associated protein of mammalian target of rapamycin; mSIN1, Mammalian stress-activated map kinase-interacting protein 1, Rictor, Rapamycin-insensitive companion of mTOR; Protor, Protein observed with Rictor.

2. Role of mTOR in Autophagy

Autophagy is an evolutionarily conserved turnover process that exerts great importance on the clearance of long-lived proteins, aggregated protein, or dysfunctional organelles, and provides energy and macromolecular precursors in return [33]. Autophagy has been widely divided into three sorts: macro-autophagy, micro-autophagy, and chaperone-mediated autophagy [34,35]. The term "autophagy" in this review refers to macro-autophagy. The process of autophagy includes initiation, nucleation, elongation, and formation of a double-membrane autophagosome, followed by the fusion of the autophagosome with a lysosome to form autolysosomes to degrade and recycle autophagosome-sequestered substrates [33]. It has been reported that mTOR plays a complex role in the induction, process, and termination of autophagy. Here, we will briefly summarize several key mTOR-related pathways that regulate autophagy activity.

2.1. mTOR/AMPK/ULK1 Signaling

Unc51-like kinase 1 (ULK1) interacts with ATG13, ATG101 and focal adhesion kinase family interacting protein of 200 kD (FIP200), making up ULK1 complex (Figure 2) [36–38]. This complex is a critical initiator of autophagy, and its activity is mainly regulated by being phosphorylated at different sites by the combination of mTORC1 and AMP-activated protein kinase (AMPK) [39,40]. Normally, mTORC1 phosphorylates ULK1 on the P757 site and disrupts the interaction of AMPK and ULK1, inhibiting the initiation of autophagy [39]. Upon nutrient deprivation or other cellular stresses, ULK1 is released from mTORC1, which has been inhibited, and is activated through being phosphorylated by AMPK at multiple sites [39]. This phosphorylation by AMPK has been shown to induce autophagy in most cases [39,41]. ATG13, one component of ULK1 complex, also can be phosphorylated by activated mTOR, leading to the decreased activity of ULK1 complex and autophagy inhibition [42]. Thus, inhibition of mTORC1 induces ULK1 complex-mediated autophagy, which can be suppressed by inhibition or deficiency of ULK1 [43].

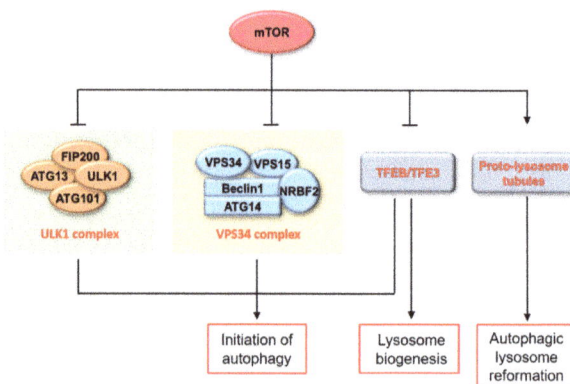

Figure 2. Role of mTOR in autophagy. mTOR plays a crucial role in the regulation of autophagy flux, including the formation of phagophore and autophagosome, the degradation of autolysosomes, and the reformation of autophagic lysosomes.

2.2. mTOR/VPS34-ATG14 Complex Signaling

Vacuolar protein sorting 34 (VPS34), also known as PIK3C3, is the catalytic subunit of type III PI3K. VPS34 plays an important role in endosome trafficking and pre-autophagosome formation with the function of converting phosphatidylinositol (PI) to phosphatidylinositol 3-phosphate (PI3P) [44]. VPS34, VPS15, and beclin 1 constitute core subunits of two VPS34 complexes, complex I and complex II, with ATG14 and UVRAG separately [38]. Among them, Atg14-containing VPS34 complex is involved in autophagy induction, facilitating the formation of isolation membrane on the endoplasmic reticulum (ER) membrane (Figure 2) [45–47]. Although it has been reported that VPS34 activates P70S6K phosphorylation in mammalian cells in the presence of nutrients, it remains unclear whether VPS34 influences mTOR activation directly [48,49]. Meanwhile, it has been reported that mTORC1 inhibits the activity of the VPS34 complex by directly phosphorylating ATG14 on a series of sites [50]. Mutation of these sites, which is resistant to inhibition by mTOR, could enhance autophagy flux [50]. In recent years, nuclear receptor binding factor 2 (NRBF2) has been reported to act as the fifth subunit of the Atg14-containing VPS34 complex [51]. NRBF2 is indispensable for the integrity of this complex [51–54] and has been implicated in neurodegenerative diseases such as Alzheimer's disease [55]. In addition, NRBF2 can be phosphorylated by mTORC1 at S113 and S120 and its dephosphorylated form enhances VPS34 complex assembly and activity, promoting autophagy flux [52].

2.3. mTOR/TFEB/TFE3

Both TFEB and TFE3 are members of the MiT-TFE family, belonging to helix-loop-helix leucine-zipper transcription factors [56,57]. TFEB is a master regulator of genes related to lysosomal biogenesis and autophagy, and recently TFE3 has also been found to regulate the transcription of genes that largely overlap with the ones regulated by TFEB [57,58]. The common mechanism underlying shuttling of transcription factors between nucleus and cytoplasm mainly depends on whether transcription factors are phosphorylated or not [57,58]. When nutrients are present, TFEB and TFE3 are recruited to the membranes of lysosomes and undergo mTOR-dependent phosphorylation, at S211 of TFEB and S321 of TFE3, creating a binding site for the chaperone 14-3-3 and thus sequestrating them in the cytosol [59]. Upon nutrient deprivation, together with mTOR inactivation, dephosphorylated TFEB and TFE3 translocate to the nucleus and induce lysosomal biogenesis and autophagy [59]. Additionally, TFEB nuclear export is induced by hierarchical phosphorylation of Ser142 and Ser138 by activated mTOR [60]. Thus, mTOR plays a critical role in both autophagic and lysosomal biogenesis through regulating TFEB and TFE3 nuclear-cytoplasmic shuttling.

2.4. mTOR in Autophagic Lysosome Reformation (ALR)

At the termination of autophagy, lysosomes are recycled from autolysosomes through a process termed ALR, which includes proto-lysosome tubules generation, elongation, and scission [61]. This process exerts great importance throughout autophagy. Inhibition of ALR increases cells' sensitivity to starvation and, over the long term, leads to death. [62]. During short-term food deprivation, mTOR is inhibited; while during long-term starvation, it is reactivated. This reactivation is essential for proto-lyosome tubule reformation [63]. What is more, mTOR is also initially inactivated and then reactivated in H_2O_2-induced autophagy, mediating the process ALR to regenerate functional lysosomes [64]. It has been found that mTOR inhibits VPS34 complex activity through phosphorylating UVRAG on Ser550 and Ser571 sites. It thereby reduces PI3P production, resulting in an increase in number and length of proto-lysosome tubules, due to impairment of tubule scission, and indicating the indispensable function of mTOR in the scission of proto-lysosome tubules [62].

3. Role of mTOR in Parkinson's Disease

Parkinson's disease (PD) is one of the most common neurodegenerative diseases in the world, characterized mainly by dopaminergic neuron loss in the substantia nigra pars compacta (SNpc) and the accumulation of α-synuclein-containing inclusions, named Lewy bodies. Genetic mutations are the leading cause of the disease, but it can also be caused by aging or dopaminergic neuron-specific toxins, such as 6-hydroxydopamine (6-OHDA), 1-methyl-4-phenyl-1,2,3,6 tetrahydropyridine (MPTP), and rotenone [65]. Among these toxins, MPTP has been widely used for developing the PD animal model [66]. Actually, MPTP itself is nontoxic and can penetrate the blood–brain barrier. While in the brain, it can be oxidized to MPP+, which is toxic to dopaminergic neurons [67]. Thus, MPTP is usually used for animal models of PD, and MPP$^+$ is used for cell models of PD. As mTOR signaling is a central hub of signaling networks in cells, it has been widely explored and has been found to have a complex relationship with PD. Both activation and inactivation of mTOR signaling are involved in the different stages of PD.

α-synuclein accumulation is a hallmark of PD, which has been implicated in the pathogenesis of sporadic and familial PD [68,69]. mTOR protein expression levels were increased in the temporal cortex of patients displaying α-synuclein accumulation [70]. Additionally, upon overexpression of α-synuclein, it can inhibit autophagy possibly through inducing mTOR activity and mimic the symptoms of PD [71]. Conversely, rapamycin, an inhibitor of mTOR, can restore the increased mTOR activity caused by α-synuclein overexpression [71]. What is more, A53T α-synuclein, a common mutation of α-synuclein in PD, upregulates mTOR/P70S6K signaling and impairs autophagy, contributing to the aggregation of toxic A53T α-synuclein [72]. On the other hand, depletion of mTOR results in the induction of autophagy, leading to clearance of A53T α-synuclein [72]. These findings indicate that mTOR activities are increased in PD and α-synuclein accumulation may contribute to this process.

RTP801/REDD1 is a stress-related protein, whose expression is markedly elevated in neurons of the SNpc in PD patients compared to control patients [73]. RTP801 interacts with TSC2, inhibiting activation of mTOR and thus leading to neuron cell death; this process may account for the neuron loss in the SNpc of PD patients [74,75]. An increase in RTP801 expression is also observed in cellular models of PD (6-OHDA, MPP$^+$ or rotenone) and in animal models of PD. In both cases, the increased RTP801 expression is accompanied by decreased mTOR activity [73].

It is well known that mTOR signaling is of great importance in cell proliferation and survival. The phosphorylation of Akt, the upstream kinase of mTOR, is decreased in the MPP$^+$-induced cellular model of PD, attenuating the activation of mTOR [76]. In addition, AMPK is a negative regulator of mTOR, which is activated in different cellular models of PD [77]. Thus, in PD models induced by toxins, both increased Akt and AMPK could negatively regulate the activity of mTOR, leading to the impairment of downstream 4EBP1 and P70S6K-related protein synthesis. This protein synthesis is essential for cell long-term survival. Furthermore, neuronal cell death induced by PD toxins can be partially restored via overexpression of functional mTOR [77].

4. Potential PD Treatment by Targeting mTOR

Since an increase in toxic protein aggregation and a loss of dopaminergic neurons are the symptoms of PD, symptomatic treatment and prevention of neuron death are the primary strategies in the therapy to manage features and progress of PD.

4.1. Treatment of PD by Combining L-DOPA with mTOR Inhibitors

The dopamine precursor drug, L-DOPA has been clinically used for the initial treatment of PD for more than 50 years [78]. L-DOPA compensates for reduced dopamine levels caused by the loss of dopaminergic neurons. However, with long-term L-DOPA treatment, most patients start to experience motor response fluctuations or dyskinesia [79,80]. By using a genetic association approach, Martin-Flores et al. have detected genetic variability in the mTOR pathway and found it involved in the development of L-DOPA-induced dyskinesia [81]. Persistent activation of mTOR signaling in the striatum has been found in L-DOPA-induced dyskinesia [82]. L-DOPA induces increased dopamine D1 receptor-mediated phosphorylation of mTOR downstream substrates, P70S6K and 4EBP1, indicating enhanced activity of mTOR signaling in medium spiny neurons; this increased mTOR signaling activity correlates positively with L-DOPA-induced dyskinesia [82]. Thus, inhibition of mTOR activity may function in the reduction of dyskinesia caused by L-DOPA. mTOR inhibitor rapamycin has been used on animal model of PD in combination with L-DOPA when it successfully prevents increased activity of mTOR and reduces dyskinesia produced by L-DOPA [82]. Similarly, depletion of Ras homolog enriched in striatum (Rhes) also reduces mTOR signaling and diminishes L-DOPA-induced dyskinesia [83]. Rhes is a highly enriched striatal-specific protein, which binds to and activates mTOR in the striatum [83]. Thus, reducing or depleting Rhes is another way to limit the activation of mTOR

Int. J. Mol. Sci. **2019**, *20*, 728

in the development of L-DOPA-induced dyskinesia. Taken together, as shown in Figure 3, inhibition of mTOR signaling, through pharmacological blockade of mTOR or reduction of Rhes, provides a beneficial effect on the L-DOPA therapy of PD [84].

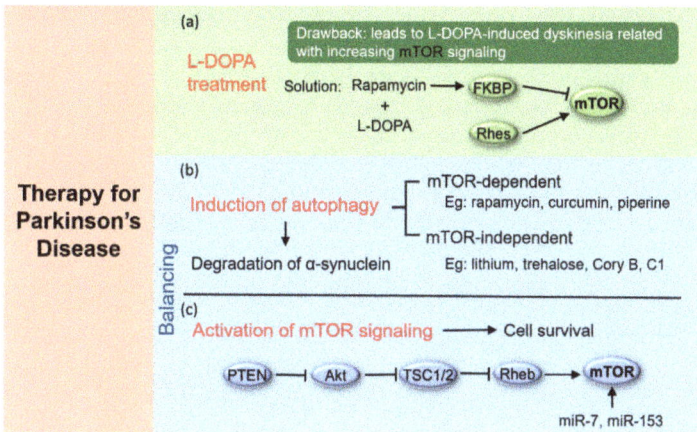

Figure 3. Potential for using mTOR in PD treatment. (**a**) Inhibition of mTOR signaling, through pharmacological blockade of mTOR or reduction of Rhes, provides a better stage for the L-DOPA therapy of PD. (**b**) The induction of autophagy by either mTOR-dependent or -independent pathway, enhances the degradation of toxic α-synuclein to alleviate the symptoms of PD. (**c**) Activation of Akt or Rheb, specific ablation of PTEN or overexpression of miR-7 and miR-153 could increase mTOR signaling to prevent neuron cell death. Furthermore, a balance between activation of mTOR signaling and enhancement of autophagy needs to be accurately managed in the treatment of PD. Abbreviations: PD, Parkinson's disease; Rhes, Ras homolog enriched in striatum; Rheb, Ras homolog enriched in brain; miR, MicroRNA.

4.2. Induction of Autophagy

Autophagy dysfunction has been reported to be associated with the pathogenesis of many neurodegenerative diseases including PD [85]. Genetic studies have identified mutations in genes which encode for components of the autophagy–lysosome pathway, including α-synuclein, leucine-rich repeat kinase 2 (LRRK2), glucosidase beta acid 1 (GBA1), scavenger receptor class B member 2 (SCARB2), Parkin, PTEN-induced putative kinase (PINK1), DJ-1, Fbxo7, and vacuolar protein sorting 35 (VPS35), and these mutations are associated with increasing risks for developing PD [86–88]. Pathological studies have observed decreased expression of autophagy–lysosome pathway-related proteins levels and lysosomal enzyme activity in PD patients [87]. For instance, lysosome depletion was indicated by decreased levels of LAMP1 in the SNpc of PD patients. Meanwhile, negative regulation of lysosomal enzymes, like GCase, have been demonstrated in different brain regions and cerebrospinal fluid of PD patients [89]. Importantly, TFEB expression in the nuclear compartment of dopaminergic neurons was significantly decreased in the postmortem SNpc of PD patients compared to controls, indicating that the subcellular localization of TFEB was changed [90]. Moreover, TFEB co-localized with Lewy bodies in the same region [90]. Given the fact that autophagy impairment is implicated in the pathogenesis of PD, autophagy is a key to the degradation of α-synuclein. It is proposed that autophagy-enhancing strategies have great potential as disease-modifying therapies for PD [91]. Indeed, genetic manipulations (such as TFEB or Beclin 1 overexpression) could enhance autophagy, thereby protecting nigral neurons from α-synuclein toxicity in PD animal models [90]. Similarly, rapamycin has been well studied for the treatment of PD in animal models; it has been found to enhance autophagy flux and degrade neurotoxic proteins partially by inhibiting mTOR, thereby boosting lysosome biogenesis and autophagosome formation [92]. In addition to enhancing degradation of aggregate-prone proteins in PD models with activated autophagy, rapamycin blocks the translation of RTP801 by selectively inhibiting actions of mTOR, restoring the mTORC2-dependent phosphorylation of Akt, and maintaining cellular metabolism [93,94]. By inhibiting RTP801 activity and stimulating autophagy, rapamycin exerts neuroprotective influence on animal models of PD induced by 6-OHDA and MPTP [93,94]. In addition, several small molecules have been reported to induce mTOR-dependent autophagy and enhance the degradation of A53T α-synuclein in neuron cells; the latter is toxic and known to accelerate the development of PD symptoms [72]. For example, curcumin, culinary spice, plays a neuroprotective role in an A53T α-synuclein cell model of PD by enhancing autophagic degradation of A53T α-synuclein via inhibiting mTOR/P70S6K signaling [72]. Piperine, an alkaloid that gives black pepper its pungency, inhibits mTOR via activation of PP2A and then induces autophagy, thereby rescuing neurons (whether in cell culture or in mice) from rotenone neurotoxicity [95].

However, mTOR-dependent autophagy enhancers may compromise cell growth because mTOR signaling is such a significant signaling hub, modulating both cell proliferation and survival. Moreover, mTOR is essential for cellular functions including synaptic plasticity, memory formation and retention [96,97]. Thus, in order to avoid the negative effects of mTOR inactivation, small molecules that enhance the activity of autophagy independent of mTOR inhibition may be advantageous for PD treatment. In vitro studies, including our studies, have demonstrated that several compounds, such as lithium [98], trehalose [99], Corynoxine B [100], and a synthesized curcumin derivative termed C1 [101], can activate autophagy independent of mTOR, still leading to enhanced degradation of α-synuclein associated with PD. It has been reported that autophagy can be boosted by lowering intracellular inositol 1,4,5-trisphosphate (IP3) level independent of mTOR signaling [98]. Sarkar et al. have found that lithium induces autophagy through inhibiting activity of inositol monophosphatase (IMPase), which is essential in the regulation of intracellular free inositol and IP3 levels [98]. This induction of autophagy by lithium contributes to the clearance of mutant α-synuclein in stable inducible PC12 cells via decreasing IP3 levels, but rapamycin does not affect IP3 levels. They also reported that induction of autophagy by combination of mTOR-dependent and -independent pathways has an additive effect on the clearance of mutant α-synuclein in PC12 cells by using both rapamycin and lithium [98,102]. Overall, induction of autophagy in a mTOR-dependent or -independent manner may serve as a promising therapeutic target to degrade α-synuclein in PD treatment.

4.3. Activation of mTOR Signaling

The hallmark of PD is the loss of dopaminergic neurons in the SNpc, accompanied by decreased levels of dopamine, making it important to prevent dopaminergic neuron death [103]. Since mTOR signaling is a key regulator of protein synthesis, cell proliferation and survival, and mTOR inhibition leads to progressive neuron degeneration and a PD-like phenotype, it is necessary to retain the activity of mTOR signaling for its protective role in neurons [104]. Activation of mTOR requires a GTP-charged form of Rheb [105]. And TSC1/2 is an upstream negative regulator of mTOR, which has GTPase-activating protein (GAP) activity for Rheb [106,107]. TSC1/2 is a downstream target negatively regulated by Akt-mediated phosphorylation [30,108]. The connection between these proteins establishes a wide stage for stimulation of mTOR signaling. For example, viral vector transduction of dopaminergic neurons with Akt or Rheb activates mTOR signaling and restores the neurons' ability to regenerate axons; this regenerative ability has valuable implications for the treatment of PD [109]. Moreover, the specific ablation of PTEN, an upstream negative regulator of Akt, contributes to activation of mTOR signaling and is neuroprotective in mouse models of PD [104].

MicroRNAs (miRs) are a class of small RNA molecules that play an essential role in the post-transcriptional regulation of gene expression via translational repression and mRNA degradation [110,111]. Recent studies have found that two miRs, miR-7, and miR-153, mainly expressed in neurons, negatively regulate α-synuclein expression [112]. In primary cortical neurons, overexpression of miR-7 and miR-153 promotes the mTOR/p70S6K signaling cascade and attenuates MPP$^+$-induced neurotoxicity, although the underlying mechanism remains elusive [113]. Thus, overexpression of miRs by viral transduction, thereby inhibiting neuron cell death, may provide another potential approach in the therapy of PD patients. Taken together, activation of mTOR to restore neuronal survival may serve as a promising therapeutic strategy for PD treatment.

5. Conclusions

mTOR plays an important role in regulating neuronal functions and autophagy. Given the importance of mTOR, targeting mTOR is a potentially effective therapeutic target for PD (Figure 3). In terms of therapy of PD, it is crucial to accelerate the clearance of aggregated toxic proteins in neurons. Autophagy is a key pathway for promoting degradation of α-synuclein; thus, enhancing autophagy flux seems to be an effective way for PD treatment. As the central role of mTOR in autophagy regulation, mTOR-dependent autophagy enhancers hold great promise for PD treatment. As such, on the one hand, inhibiting mTOR signaling appears to be a viable treatment strategy. On the other hand, maintaining a certain level of mTOR activity is necessary because mTOR signaling is essential for cellular survival and growth. Importantly, mTOR regulates multiple essential cellular functions including synaptic plasticity, memory formation, and retention in neuronal cells [96,97]. Too much or too little mTOR activity could be fatal to neurons. A balance between activation of mTOR signaling and enhancement of autophagy needs to be accurately managed, which may offer exciting new avenues for the development of therapeutic strategies for PD. Though targeting of the mTOR pathway has shown neuroprotective actions in a variety of in vivo and in vitro PD models, the therapeutic potential of mTOR inhibitors (such as to enhance autophagy by inhibiting mTOR) may be limited because mTOR regulates multiple cellular functions. Additionally, mTOR inhibitors, such as rapamycin, may have some side effects in clinical trials [114,115]. For example, rapamycin has been applied in treating patients with lymphangioleiomyomatosis, leading to some rapamycin levels-associated side effects, like apthous ulcers, nausea, and diarrhea [114]. Thus, the dosage of mTOR inhibitors in clinical trials should be continuously modified during the treatment period [114]. Although several fundamental questions need to be further addressed before these novel mTOR-targeting reagents could be applied in clinical trials, the research field of mTOR is developing quickly and clinically relevant updates on mTOR modulators may arise soon.

Author Contributions: Conceptualization, Z.Z., C.Y. and M.L.; Funding acquisition, C.Y. and M.L.; Investigation, Z.Z., C.Y., A.I., S.K., S.G.S., J.L., Z.W., J.S. and J.L.; Project administration, C.Y. and M.L.; Supervision, M.L.; Visualization, Z.Z., C.Y., A.I., S.K. and S.G.S.; Writing-original draft, Z.Z. and C.Y.; writing-review and editing, Z.Z., C.Y.,B.C.-K.T., K.-H.C. and M.L.

Funding: This study was supported by the National Natural Science Foundation of China (81703487 and 81773926), the Hong Kong General Research Fund (RGC/GRF/12100618, RGC/GRF/12101417), the Hong Kong Health and Medical Research Fund (HMRF/15163481, HMRF14150811) and the research fund from the Hong Kong Baptist University (HKBU/RC-IRCs/17-18/03, HKBU/RC-IRMS/15-16/04, FRGI/17-18/041, FRGII/17-18/021).

Conflicts of Interest: The authors declare no conflicts of interest.

Abbreviations

ALR	Autophagic lysosome reformation
AMPK	AMP-activated protein kinase
CLEAR	Coordinated lysosomal expression and regulation
DEPTOR	DEP-domain containing mTOR-interacting protein
ER	Endoplasmic reticulum
FIP200	Focal adhesion kinase family interacting protein of 200 kD
FKBP	FK506-binding protein
FRAP	FKBP12-rapamycin complex-associated protein
GAP	GTPase-activating protein
GBA1	Glucosidase beta acid 1

IMPase	Inositol monophosphatase
IP3	Inositol 1,4,5-trisphosphate
IRS	Insulin receptor substrate
LRRK2	Leucine-rich repeat kinase 2
miR	MicroRNA
mLST8	Mammalian lethal with sec-13 protein 8
MPTP	1-methyl-4-phenyl-1,2,3,6 tetrahydropyridine
mSIN1	Mammalian stress-activated map kinase-interacting protein 1
mTOR	Mammalian targets of rapamycin
mTORC1	mTOR complex 1
mTORC2	mTOR complex 2
NRBF2	Nuclear receptor binding factor 2
PD	Parkinson's disease
PDK1	3-Phosphoinositide dependent protein kinase-1
PI	Phosphatidylinositol
PINK1	PTEN-induced putative kinase 1
PI3K	Phosphatidylinositol 3-kinase
PI3P	Phosphatidylinositol 3-phosphate
PKC	Protein kinase C
PRAS40	Proline-rich Akt substrate of 40 kDa
Protor	Protein observed with Rictor
P70S6K	P70 ribosomal S6 kinase
Raptor	Regulatory associated protein of mammalian target of rapamycin
Rheb	Ras homolog enriched in brain
Rhes	Ras homolog enriched in striatum
Rictor	Rapamycin-insensitive companion of mTOR
SCARB2	Scavenger receptor class B member 2
SGK	Serum/glucocorticoid regulated kinase
SNpc	Substantia nigra pars compacta
TOR	Target of rapamycin
TSC	Tuberous sclerosis complex
ULK1	Unc51-like kinase 1
VPS34	Vacuolar protein sorting 34
VPS35	Vacuolar protein sorting 35
4EBP1	Eukaryotic initiation factor 4E (eIF4E) binding protein 1
6-OHDA	6-hydroxydopamine

References

1. Heitman, J.; Movva, N.R.; Hall, M.N. Targets for cell cycle arrest by the immunosuppressant rapamycin in yeast. *Science* **1991**, *253*, 905–909. [CrossRef] [PubMed]
2. Sabers, C.J.; Martin, M.M.; Brunn, G.J.; Williams, J.M.; Dumont, F.J.; Wiederrecht, G.; Abraham, R.T. Isolation of a protein target of the FKBP12-rapamycin complex in mammalian cells. *J. Biol. Chem.* **1995**, *270*, 815–822. [CrossRef] [PubMed]
3. Lorenz, M.C.; Heitman, J. TOR mutations confer rapamycin resistance by preventing interaction with FKBP12-rapamycin. *J. Biol. Chem.* **1995**, *270*, 27531–27537. [CrossRef] [PubMed]
4. Wullschleger, S.; Loewith, R.; Hall, M.N. TOR signaling in growth and metabolism. *Cell* **2006**, *124*, 471–484. [CrossRef]
5. Zheng, X.F.; Florentino, D.; Chen, J.; Crabtree, G.R.; Schreiber, S.L. TOR kinase domains are required for two distinct functions, only one of which is inhibited by rapamycin. *Cell* **1995**, *82*, 121–130. [CrossRef]
6. Peterson, T.R.; Laplante, M.; Thoreen, C.C.; Sancak, Y.; Kang, S.A.; Kuehl, W.M.; Gray, N.S.; Sabatini, D.M. DEPTOR is an mTOR inhibitor frequently overexpressed in multiple myeloma cells and required for their survival. *Cell* **2009**, *137*, 873–886. [CrossRef] [PubMed]

7. Hara, K.; Maruki, Y.; Long, X.; Yoshino, K.; Oshiro, N.; Hidayat, S.; Tokunaga, C.; Avruch, J.; Yonezawa, K. Raptor, a binding partner of target of rapamycin (TOR), mediates TOR action. *Cell* **2002**, *110*, 177–189. [CrossRef]

8. Kim, D.H.; Sarbassov, D.D.; Ali, S.M.; King, J.E.; Latek, R.R.; Erdjument-Bromage, H.; Tempst, P.; Sabatini, D.M. mTOR interacts with raptor to form a nutrient-sensitive complex that signals to the cell growth machinery. *Cell* **2002**, *110*, 163–175. [CrossRef]

9. Kim, D.H.; Sarbassov, D.D.; Ali, S.M.; Latek, R.R.; Guntur, K.V.; Erdjument-Bromage, H.; Tempst, P.; Sabatini, D.M. GbetaL, a positive regulator of the rapamycin-sensitive pathway required for the nutrient-sensitive interaction between raptor and mTOR. *Mol. Cell* **2003**, *11*, 895–904. [CrossRef]

10. Sancak, Y.; Thoreen, C.C.; Peterson, T.R.; Lindquist, R.A.; Kang, S.A.; Spooner, E.; Carr, S.A.; Sabatini, D.M. PRAS40 is an insulin-regulated inhibitor of the mTORC1 protein kinase. *Mol. Cell* **2007**, *25*, 903–915. [CrossRef]

11. Di Malta, C.; Siciliano, D.; Calcagni, A.; Monfregola, J.; Punzi, S.; Pastore, N.; Eastes, A.N.; Davis, O.; De Cegli, R.; Zampelli, A.; et al. Transcriptional activation of RagD GTPase controls mTORC1 and promotes cancer growth. *Science* **2017**, *356*, 1188–1192. [CrossRef] [PubMed]

12. Beirowski, B.; Wong, K.M.; Babetto, E.; Milbrandt, J. mTORC1 promotes proliferation of immature Schwann cells and myelin growth of differentiated Schwann cells. *Proc. Natl. Acad. Sci. USA* **2017**, *114*, e4261–e4270. [CrossRef] [PubMed]

13. Chiarini, F.; Evangelisti, C.; McCubrey, J.A.; Martelli, A.M. Current treatment strategies for inhibiting mTOR in cancer. *Trends Pharmacol. Sci.* **2015**, *36*, 124–135. [CrossRef]

14. Caron, A.; Richard, D.; Laplante, M. The Roles of mTOR Complexes in Lipid Metabolism. *Annu. Rev. Nutr.* **2015**, *35*, 321–348. [CrossRef] [PubMed]

15. Wang, B.; Jie, Z.; Joo, D.; Ordureau, A.; Liu, P.; Gan, W.; Guo, J.; Zhang, J.; North, B.J.; Dai, X.; et al. TRAF2 and OTUD7B govern a ubiquitin-dependent switch that regulates mTORC2 signalling. *Nature* **2017**, *545*, 365–369. [CrossRef] [PubMed]

16. Sarbassov, D.D.; Ali, S.M.; Kim, D.H.; Guertin, D.A.; Latek, R.R.; Erdjument-Bromage, H.; Tempst, P.; Sabatini, D.M. Rictor, a novel binding partner of mTOR, defines a rapamycin-insensitive and raptor-independent pathway that regulates the cytoskeleton. *Curr. Biol.* **2004**, *14*, 1296–1302. [CrossRef] [PubMed]

17. Frias, M.A.; Thoreen, C.C.; Jaffe, J.D.; Schroder, W.; Sculley, T.; Carr, S.A.; Sabatini, D.M. mSin1 is necessary for Akt/PKB phosphorylation, and its isoforms define three distinct mTORC2s. *Curr. Biol.* **2006**, *16*, 1865–1870. [CrossRef]

18. Jacinto, E.; Loewith, R.; Schmidt, A.; Lin, S.; Ruegg, M.A.; Hall, A.; Hall, M.N. Mammalian TOR complex 2 controls the actin cytoskeleton and is rapamycin insensitive. *Nat. Cell Biol.* **2004**, *6*, 1122–1128. [CrossRef]

19. Pearce, L.R.; Huang, X.; Boudeau, J.; Pawlowski, R.; Wullschleger, S.; Deak, M.; Ibrahim, A.F.; Gourlay, R.; Magnuson, M.A.; Alessi, D.R. Identification of Protor as a novel Rictor-binding component of mTOR complex-2. *Biochem. J.* **2007**, *405*, 513–522. [CrossRef]

20. Mizunuma, M.; Neumann-Haefelin, E.; Moroz, N.; Li, Y.J.; Blackwell, T.K. mTORC2-SGK-1 acts in two environmentally responsive pathways with opposing effects on longevity. *Aging Cell* **2014**, *13*, 869–878. [CrossRef]

21. Chantaravisoot, N.; Wongkongkathep, P.; Loo, J.A.; Mischel, P.S.; Tamanoi, F. Significance of filamin A in mTORC2 function in glioblastoma. *Mol. Cancer* **2015**, *14*, 127. [CrossRef]

22. Chen, B.W.; Chen, W.; Liang, H.; Liu, H.; Liang, C.; Zhi, X.; Hu, L.Q.; Yu, X.Z.; Wei, T.; Ma, T.; et al. Inhibition of mTORC2 Induces Cell-Cycle Arrest and Enhances the Cytotoxicity of Doxorubicin by Suppressing MDR1 Expression in HCC Cells. *Mol. Cancer Ther.* **2015**, *14*, 1805–1815. [CrossRef] [PubMed]

23. Albert, V.; Svensson, K.; Shimobayashi, M.; Colombi, M.; Munoz, S.; Jimenez, V.; Handschin, C.; Bosch, F.; Hall, M.N. mTORC2 sustains thermogenesis via Akt-induced glucose uptake and glycolysis in brown adipose tissue. *EMBO Mol. Med.* **2016**, *8*, 232–246. [CrossRef]

24. Liu, P.; Gan, W.; Chin, Y.R.; Ogura, K.; Guo, J.; Zhang, J.; Wang, B.; Blenis, J.; Cantley, L.C.; Toker, A.; et al. PtdIns(3,4,5)P3-Dependent Activation of the mTORC2 Kinase Complex. *Cancer Discov.* **2015**, *5*, 1194–1209. [CrossRef] [PubMed]

25. Sarbassov, D.D.; Guertin, D.A.; Ali, S.M.; Sabatini, D.M. Phosphorylation and regulation of Akt/PKB by the rictor-mTOR complex. *Science* **2005**, *307*, 1098–1101. [CrossRef] [PubMed]

26. Yang, G.; Murashige, D.S.; Humphrey, S.J.; James, D.E. A Positive Feedback Loop between Akt and mTORC2 via SIN1 Phosphorylation. *Cell Rep.* **2015**, *12*, 937–943. [CrossRef] [PubMed]

27. Humphrey, S.J.; Yang, G.; Yang, P.; Fazakerley, D.J.; Stockli, J.; Yang, J.Y.; James, D.E. Dynamic adipocyte phosphoproteome reveals that Akt directly regulates mTORC2. *Cell Metab.* **2013**, *17*, 1009–1020. [CrossRef]

28. Dibble, C.C.; Cantley, L.C. Regulation of mTORC1 by PI3K signaling. *Trends Cell Biol.* **2015**, *25*, 545–555. [CrossRef]

29. Mabuchi, S.; Kuroda, H.; Takahashi, R.; Sasano, T. The PI3K/AKT/mTOR pathway as a therapeutic target in ovarian cancer. *Gynecol. Oncol.* **2015**, *137*, 173–179. [CrossRef]

30. Inoki, K.; Li, Y.; Zhu, T.; Wu, J.; Guan, K.L. TSC2 is phosphorylated and inhibited by Akt and suppresses mTOR signalling. *Nat. Cell Biol.* **2002**, *4*, 648–657. [CrossRef]

31. Brunn, G.J.; Hudson, C.C.; Sekulić, A.; Williams, J.M.; Hosoi, H.; Houghton, P.J.; Lawrence, J.C.; Abraham, R.T. Phosphorylation of the Translational Repressor PHAS-I by the Mammalian Target of Rapamycin. *Science* **1997**, *277*, 99–101. [CrossRef] [PubMed]

32. Burnett, P.E.; Barrow, R.K.; Cohen, N.A.; Snyder, S.H.; Sabatini, D.M. RAFT1 phosphorylation of the translational regulators p70 S6 kinase and 4E-BP1. *Proc. Natl. Acad. Sci. USA* **1998**, *95*, 1432–1437. [CrossRef] [PubMed]

33. Levy, J.M.M.; Towers, C.G.; Thorburn, A. Targeting autophagy in cancer. *Nat. Rev. Cancer* **2017**, *17*, 528–542. [CrossRef] [PubMed]

34. Arias, E.; Cuervo, A.M. Chaperone-mediated autophagy in protein quality control. *Curr. Opin. Cell Biol.* **2011**, *23*, 184–189. [CrossRef] [PubMed]

35. Huber, L.A.; Teis, D. Lysosomal signaling in control of degradation pathways. *Curr. Opin. Cell Biol.* **2016**, *39*, 8–14. [CrossRef] [PubMed]

36. Jung, C.H.; Jun, C.B.; Ro, S.H.; Kim, Y.M.; Otto, N.M.; Cao, J.; Kundu, M.; Kim, D.H. ULK-Atg13-FIP200 complexes mediate mTOR signaling to the autophagy machinery. *Mol. Biol. Cell* **2009**, *20*, 1992–2003. [CrossRef] [PubMed]

37. Hosokawa, N.; Sasaki, T.; Iemura, S.; Natsume, T.; Hara, T.; Mizushima, N. Atg101, a novel mammalian autophagy protein interacting with Atg13. *Autophagy* **2009**, *5*, 973–979. [CrossRef]

38. Hurley, J.H.; Young, L.N. Mechanisms of Autophagy Initiation. *Annu. Rev. Biochem.* **2017**, *86*, 225–244. [CrossRef]

39. Kim, J.; Kundu, M.; Viollet, B.; Guan, K.L. AMPK and mTOR regulate autophagy through direct phosphorylation of Ulk1. *Nat. Cell Biol.* **2011**, *13*, 132–141. [CrossRef]

40. Shang, L.; Chen, S.; Du, F.; Li, S.; Zhao, L.; Wang, X. Nutrient starvation elicits an acute autophagic response mediated by Ulk1 dephosphorylation and its subsequent dissociation from AMPK. *Proc. Natl. Acad. Sci. USA* **2011**, *108*, 4788–4793. [CrossRef]

41. Lin, M.G.; Hurley, J.H. Structure and function of the ULK1 complex in autophagy. *Curr. Opin. Cell Biol.* **2016**, *39*, 61–68. [CrossRef] [PubMed]

42. Puente, C.; Hendrickson, R.C.; Jiang, X. Nutrient-regulated Phosphorylation of ATG13 Inhibits Starvation-induced Autophagy. *J. Biol. Chem.* **2016**, *291*, 6026–6035. [CrossRef] [PubMed]

43. Egan, D.F.; Chun, M.G.; Vamos, M.; Zou, H.; Rong, J.; Miller, C.J.; Lou, H.J.; Raveendra-Panickar, D.; Yang, C.C.; Sheffler, D.J.; et al. Small Molecule Inhibition of the Autophagy Kinase ULK1 and Identification of ULK1 Substrates. *Mol. Cell* **2015**, *59*, 285–297. [CrossRef] [PubMed]

44. Backer, J.M. The intricate regulation and complex functions of the Class III phosphoinositide 3-kinase Vps34. *Biochem. J.* **2016**, *473*, 2251–2271. [CrossRef] [PubMed]

45. Matsunaga, K.; Morita, E.; Saitoh, T.; Akira, S.; Ktistakis, N.T.; Izumi, T.; Noda, T.; Yoshimori, T. Autophagy requires endoplasmic reticulum targeting of the PI3-kinase complex via Atg14L. *J. Cell Biol.* **2010**, *190*, 511–521. [CrossRef] [PubMed]

46. Tan, X.; Thapa, N.; Liao, Y.; Choi, S.; Anderson, R.A. PtdIns(4,5)P2 signaling regulates ATG14 and autophagy. *Proc. Natl. Acad. Sci. USA* **2016**, *113*, 10896–10901. [CrossRef] [PubMed]

47. Ma, B.; Cao, W.; Li, W.; Gao, C.; Qi, Z.; Zhao, Y.; Du, J.; Xue, H.; Peng, J.; Wen, J.; et al. Dapper1 promotes autophagy by enhancing the Beclin1-Vps34-Atg14L complex formation. *Cell Res.* **2014**, *24*, 912–924. [CrossRef]

48. Byfield, M.P.; Murray, J.T.; Backer, J.M. hVps34 is a nutrient-regulated lipid kinase required for activation of p70 S6 kinase. *J. Biol. Chem.* **2005**, *280*, 33076–33082. [CrossRef]

49. Nobukuni, T.; Joaquin, M.; Roccio, M.; Dann, S.G.; Kim, S.Y.; Gulati, P.; Byfield, M.P.; Backer, J.M.; Natt, F.; Bos, J.L.; et al. Amino acids mediate mTOR/raptor signaling through activation of class 3 phosphatidylinositol 3OH-kinase. *Proc. Natl. Acad. Sci. USA* **2005**, *102*, 14238–14243. [CrossRef]

50. Yuan, H.-X.; Russell, R.C.; Guan, K.-L. Regulation of PIK3C3/VPS34 complexes by MTOR in nutrient stress-induced autophagy. *Autophagy* **2014**, *9*, 1983–1995. [CrossRef]

51. Ohashi, Y.; Soler, N.; Garcia Ortegon, M.; Zhang, L.; Kirsten, M.L.; Perisic, O.; Masson, G.R.; Burke, J.E.; Jakobi, A.J.; Apostolakis, A.A.; et al. Characterization of Atg38 and NRBF2, a fifth subunit of the autophagic Vps34/PIK3C3 complex. *Autophagy* **2016**, *12*, 2129–2144. [CrossRef] [PubMed]

52. Ma, X.; Zhang, S.; He, L.; Rong, Y.; Brier, L.W.; Sun, Q.; Liu, R.; Fan, W.; Chen, S.; Yue, Z.; et al. MTORC1-mediated NRBF2 phosphorylation functions as a switch for the class III PtdIns3K and autophagy. *Autophagy* **2017**, *13*, 592–607. [CrossRef] [PubMed]

53. Araki, Y.; Ku, W.C.; Akioka, M.; May, A.I.; Hayashi, Y.; Arisaka, F.; Ishihama, Y.; Ohsumi, Y. Atg38 is required for autophagy-specific phosphatidylinositol 3-kinase complex integrity. *J. Cell Biol.* **2013**, *203*, 299–313. [CrossRef] [PubMed]

54. Lu, J.; He, L.; Behrends, C.; Araki, M.; Araki, K.; Jun Wang, Q.; Catanzaro, J.M.; Friedman, S.L.; Zong, W.X.; Fiel, M.I.; et al. NRBF2 regulates autophagy and prevents liver injury by modulating Atg14L-linked phosphatidylinositol-3 kinase III activity. *Nat. Commun.* **2014**, *5*, 3920. [CrossRef] [PubMed]

55. Yang, C.; Cai, C.Z.; Song, J.X.; Tan, J.Q.; Durairajan, S.S.K.; Iyaswamy, A.; Wu, M.Y.; Chen, L.L.; Yue, Z.; Li, M.; et al. NRBF2 is involved in the autophagic degradation process of APP-CTFs in Alzheimer disease models. *Autophagy* **2017**, *13*, 2028–2040. [CrossRef] [PubMed]

56. Puertollano, R.; Ferguson, S.M.; Brugarolas, J.; Ballabio, A. The complex relationship between TFEB transcription factor phosphorylation and subcellular localization. *EMBO J.* **2018**, *37*. [CrossRef] [PubMed]

57. Sardiello, M.; Palmieri, M.; di Ronza, A.; Medina, D.L.; Valenza, M.; Gennarino, V.A.; Di Malta, C.; Donaudy, F.; Embrione, V.; Polishchuk, R.S.; et al. A gene network regulating lysosomal biogenesis and function. *Science* **2009**, *325*, 473–477. [CrossRef]

58. Martina, J.A.; Diab, H.I.; Lishu, L.; Jeong, A.L.; Patange, S.; Raben, N.; Puertollano, R. The nutrient-responsive transcription factor TFE3 promotes autophagy, lysosomal biogenesis, and clearance of cellular debris. *Sci. Signal.* **2014**, *7*, ra9. [CrossRef]

59. Raben, N.; Puertollano, R. TFEB and TFE3: Linking Lysosomes to Cellular Adaptation to Stress. *Annu. Rev. Cell Dev. Biol.* **2016**, *32*, 255–278. [CrossRef]

60. Napolitano, G.; Esposito, A.; Choi, H.; Matarese, M.; Benedetti, V.; Di Malta, C.; Monfregola, J.; Medina, D.L.; Lippincott-Schwartz, J.; Ballabio, A. mTOR-dependent phosphorylation controls TFEB nuclear export. *Nat. Commun.* **2018**, *9*, 3312. [CrossRef]

61. Chen, Y.; Yu, L. Scissors for autolysosome tubules. *EMBO J.* **2015**, *34*, 2217–2218. [CrossRef] [PubMed]

62. Munson, M.J.; Allen, G.F.; Toth, R.; Campbell, D.G.; Lucocq, J.M.; Ganley, I.G. mTOR activates the VPS34-UVRAG complex to regulate autolysosomal tubulation and cell survival. *EMBO J.* **2015**, *34*, 2272–2290. [CrossRef] [PubMed]

63. Yu, L.; McPhee, C.K.; Zheng, L.; Mardones, G.A.; Rong, Y.; Peng, J.; Mi, N.; Zhao, Y.; Liu, Z.; Wan, F.; et al. Termination of autophagy and reformation of lysosomes regulated by mTOR. *Nature* **2010**, *465*, 942–946. [CrossRef] [PubMed]

64. Zhang, J.; Zhou, W.; Lin, J.; Wei, P.; Zhang, Y.; Jin, P.; Chen, M.; Man, N.; Wen, L. Autophagic lysosomal reformation depends on mTOR reactivation in H2O2-induced autophagy. *Int. J. Biochem. Cell Biol.* **2016**, *70*, 76–81. [CrossRef] [PubMed]

65. Liu, J.; Liu, W.; Lu, Y.; Tian, H.; Duan, C.; Lu, L.; Gao, G.; Wu, X.; Wang, X.; Yang, H. Piperlongumine restores the balance of autophagy and apoptosis by increasing BCL2 phosphorylation in rotenone-induced Parkinson disease models. *Autophagy* **2018**, *14*, 845–861. [CrossRef] [PubMed]

66. Langston, J.W.; Ballard, P.; Tetrud, J.W.; Irwin, I. Chronic Parkinsonism in humans due to a product of meperidine-analog synthesis. *Science* **1983**, *219*, 979–980. [CrossRef] [PubMed]

67. Heikkila, R.E.; Manzino, L.; Cabbat, F.S.; Duvoisin, R.C. Protection against the dopaminergic neurotoxicity of 1-methyl-4-phenyl-1,2,5,6-tetrahydropyridine by monoamine oxidase inhibitors. *Nature* **1984**, *311*, 467–469. [CrossRef]

68. Recasens, A.; Dehay, B.; Bove, J.; Carballo-Carbajal, I.; Dovero, S.; Perez-Villalba, A.; Fernagut, P.O.; Blesa, J.; Parent, A.; Perier, C.; et al. Lewy body extracts from Parkinson disease brains trigger alpha-synuclein pathology and neurodegeneration in mice and monkeys. *Ann. Neurol.* **2014**, *75*, 351–362. [CrossRef] [PubMed]

69. Wong, Y.C.; Krainc, D. alpha-synuclein toxicity in neurodegeneration: Mechanism and therapeutic strategies. *Nat. Med.* **2017**, *23*, 1–13. [CrossRef]

70. Crews, L.; Spencer, B.; Desplats, P.; Patrick, C.; Paulino, A.; Rockenstein, E.; Hansen, L.; Adame, A.; Galasko, D.; Masliah, E. Selective molecular alterations in the autophagy pathway in patients with Lewy body disease and in models of alpha-synucleinopathy. *PLoS ONE* **2010**, *5*, e9313. [CrossRef] [PubMed]

71. Gao, S.; Duan, C.; Gao, G.; Wang, X.; Yang, H. Alpha-synuclein overexpression negatively regulates insulin receptor substrate 1 by activating mTORC1/S6K1 signaling. *Int. J. Biochem. Cell Biol.* **2015**, *64*, 25–33. [CrossRef] [PubMed]

72. Jiang, T.F.; Zhang, Y.J.; Zhou, H.Y.; Wang, H.M.; Tian, L.P.; Liu, J.; Ding, J.Q.; Chen, S.D. Curcumin ameliorates the neurodegenerative pathology in A53T alpha-synuclein cell model of Parkinson's disease through the downregulation of mTOR/p70S6K signaling and the recovery of macroautophagy. *J. Neuroimmune Pharmacol.* **2013**, *8*, 356–369. [CrossRef] [PubMed]

73. Malagelada, C.; Ryu, E.J.; Biswas, S.C.; Jackson-Lewis, V.; Greene, L.A. RTP801 is elevated in Parkinson brain substantia nigral neurons and mediates death in cellular models of Parkinson's disease by a mechanism involving mammalian target of rapamycin inactivation. *J. Neurosci.* **2006**, *26*, 9996–10005. [CrossRef] [PubMed]

74. Corradetti, M.N.; Inoki, K.; Guan, K.L. The stress-inducted proteins RTP801 and RTP801L are negative regulators of the mammalian target of rapamycin pathway. *J. Biol. Chem.* **2005**, *280*, 9769–9772. [CrossRef] [PubMed]

75. Brugarolas, J.; Lei, K.; Hurley, R.L.; Manning, B.D.; Reiling, J.H.; Hafen, E.; Witters, L.A.; Ellisen, L.W.; Kaelin, W.G., Jr. Regulation of mTOR function in response to hypoxia by REDD1 and the TSC1/TSC2 tumor suppressor complex. *Genes Dev.* **2004**, *18*, 2893–2904. [CrossRef] [PubMed]

76. Selvaraj, S.; Sun, Y.; Watt, J.A.; Wang, S.; Lei, S.; Birnbaumer, L.; Singh, B.B. Neurotoxin-induced ER stress in mouse dopaminergic neurons involves downregulation of TRPC1 and inhibition of AKT/mTOR signaling. *J. Clin. Investig.* **2012**, *122*, 1354–1367. [CrossRef] [PubMed]

77. Xu, Y.; Liu, C.; Chen, S.; Ye, Y.; Guo, M.; Ren, Q.; Liu, L.; Zhang, H.; Xu, C.; Zhou, Q.; et al. Activation of AMPK and inactivation of Akt result in suppression of mTOR-mediated S6K1 and 4E-BP1 pathways leading to neuronal cell death in in vitro models of Parkinson's disease. *Cell Signal.* **2014**, *26*, 1680–1689. [CrossRef]

78. Rajput, A.H. Factors predictive of the development of levodopa-induced dyskinesia and Wearing-Off in Parkinson's disease. *Mov. Disord.* **2014**, *29*, 429. [CrossRef]

79. Huot, P.; Johnston, T.H.; Koprich, J.B.; Fox, S.H.; Brotchie, J.M. The pharmacology of L-DOPA-induced dyskinesia in Parkinson's disease. *Pharmacol. Rev.* **2013**, *65*, 171–222. [CrossRef]

80. Urs, N.M.; Bido, S.; Peterson, S.M.; Daigle, T.L.; Bass, C.E.; Gainetdinov, R.R.; Bezard, E.; Caron, M.G. Targeting beta-arrestin2 in the treatment of L-DOPA-induced dyskinesia in Parkinson's disease. *Proc. Natl. Acad. Sci. USA* **2015**, *112*, E2517–E2526. [CrossRef]

81. Martin-Flores, N.; Fernandez-Santiago, R.; Antonelli, F.; Cerquera, C.; Moreno, V.; Marti, M.J.; Ezquerra, M.; Malagelada, C. MTOR Pathway-Based Discovery of Genetic Susceptibility to L-DOPA-Induced Dyskinesia in Parkinson's Disease Patients. *Mol. Neurobiol.* **2018**. [CrossRef] [PubMed]

82. Santini, E.; Heiman, M.; Greengard, P.; Valjent, E.; Fisone, G. Inhibition of mTOR signaling in Parkinson's disease prevents L-DOPA-induced dyskinesia. *Sci. Signal.* **2009**, *2*, ra36. [CrossRef] [PubMed]

83. Subramaniam, S.; Napolitano, F.; Mealer, R.G.; Kim, S.; Errico, F.; Barrow, R.; Shahani, N.; Tyagi, R.; Snyder, S.H.; Usiello, A. Rhes, a striatal-enriched small G protein, mediates mTOR signaling and L-DOPA-induced dyskinesia. *Nat. Neurosci.* **2011**, *15*, 191–193. [CrossRef] [PubMed]

84. Brugnoli, A.; Napolitano, F.; Usiello, A.; Morari, M. Genetic deletion of Rhes or pharmacological blockade of mTORC1 prevent striato-nigral neurons activation in levodopa-induced dyskinesia. *Neurobiol. Dis.* **2016**, *85*, 155–163. [CrossRef] [PubMed]

85. Moors, T.E.; Hoozemans, J.J.; Ingrassia, A.; Beccari, T.; Parnetti, L.; Chartier-Harlin, M.C.; van de Berg, W.D. Therapeutic potential of autophagy-enhancing agents in Parkinson's disease. *Mol. Neurodegener.* **2017**, *12*, 11. [CrossRef] [PubMed]

86. Verstraeten, A.; Theuns, J.; Van Broeckhoven, C. Progress in unraveling the genetic etiology of Parkinson disease in a genomic era. *Trends Genet.* **2015**, *31*, 140–149. [CrossRef] [PubMed]

87. Przedborski, S. The two-century journey of Parkinson disease research. *Nat. Rev. Neurosci.* **2017**, *18*, 251–259. [CrossRef] [PubMed]

88. Gan-Or, Z.; Dion, P.A.; Rouleau, G.A. Genetic perspective on the role of the autophagy-lysosome pathway in Parkinson disease. *Autophagy* **2015**, *11*, 1443–1457. [CrossRef]

89. Rocha, E.M.; Smith, G.A.; Park, E.; Cao, H.; Brown, E.; Hallett, P.; Isacson, O. Progressive decline of glucocerebrosidase in aging and Parkinson's disease. *Ann. Clin. Transl. Neurol.* **2015**, *2*, 433–438. [CrossRef]

90. Decressac, M.; Mattsson, B.; Weikop, P.; Lundblad, M.; Jakobsson, J.; Björklund, A. TFEB-mediated autophagy rescues midbrain dopamine neurons from α-synuclein toxicity. *Proc. Natl. Acad. Sci. USA* **2013**, E1817–E1826. [CrossRef] [PubMed]

91. Boland, B.; Yu, W.H.; Corti, O.; Mollereau, B.; Henriques, A.; Bezard, E.; Pastores, G.M.; Rubinsztein, D.C.; Nixon, R.A.; Duchen, M.R.; et al. Promoting the clearance of neurotoxic proteins in neurodegenerative disorders of ageing. *Nat. Rev. Drug Discov.* **2018**, *17*, 660–688. [CrossRef]

92. Dehay, B.; Bove, J.; Rodriguez-Muela, N.; Perier, C.; Recasens, A.; Boya, P.; Vila, M. Pathogenic lysosomal depletion in Parkinson's disease. *J. Neurosci.* **2010**, *30*, 12535–12544. [CrossRef] [PubMed]

93. Malagelada, C.; Jin, Z.H.; Jackson-Lewis, V.; Przedborski, S.; Greene, L.A. Rapamycin protects against neuron death in in vitro and in vivo models of Parkinson's disease. *J. Neurosci.* **2010**, *30*, 1166–1175. [CrossRef] [PubMed]

94. Bove, J.; Martinez-Vicente, M.; Vila, M. Fighting neurodegeneration with rapamycin: Mechanistic insights. *Nat. Rev. Neurosci.* **2011**, *12*, 437–452. [CrossRef]

95. Liu, J.; Chen, M.; Wang, X.; Wang, Y.; Duan, C.; Gao, G.; Lu, L.; Wu, X.; Wang, X.; Yang, H. Piperine induces autophagy by enhancing protein phosphotase 2A activity in a rotenone-induced Parkinson's disease model. *Oncotarget* **2016**, *7*, 60823–60843. [CrossRef] [PubMed]

96. Bekinschtein, P.; Katche, C.; Slipczuk, L.N.; Igaz, L.M.; Cammarota, M.; Izquierdo, I.; Medina, J.H. mTOR signaling in the hippocampus is necessary for memory formation. *Neurobiol. Learn. Mem.* **2007**, *87*, 303–307. [CrossRef] [PubMed]

97. Hoeffer, C.A.; Klann, E. mTOR signaling: At the crossroads of plasticity, memory and disease. *Trends Neurosci.* **2010**, *33*, 67–75. [CrossRef]

98. Sarkar, S.; Floto, R.A.; Berger, Z.; Imarisio, S.; Cordenier, A.; Pasco, M.; Cook, L.J.; Rubinsztein, D.C. Lithium induces autophagy by inhibiting inositol monophosphatase. *J. Cell Biol.* **2005**, *170*, 1101–1111. [CrossRef]

99. Sarkar, S.; Davies, J.E.; Huang, Z.; Tunnacliffe, A.; Rubinsztein, D.C. Trehalose, a novel mTOR-independent autophagy enhancer, accelerates the clearance of mutant huntingtin and alpha-synuclein. *J. Biol. Chem.* **2007**, *282*, 5641–5652. [CrossRef]

100. Song, J.X.; Lu, J.H.; Liu, L.F.; Chen, L.L.; Durairajan, S.S.; Yue, Z.; Zhang, H.Q.; Li, M. HMGB1 is involved in autophagy inhibition caused by SNCA/alpha-synuclein overexpression: A process modulated by the natural autophagy inducer corynoxine B. *Autophagy* **2014**, *10*, 144–154. [CrossRef]

101. Song, J.X.; Sun, Y.R.; Peluso, I.; Zeng, Y.; Yu, X.; Lu, J.H.; Xu, Z.; Wang, M.Z.; Liu, L.F.; Huang, Y.Y.; et al. A novel curcumin analog binds to and activates TFEB in vitro and in vivo independent of MTOR inhibition. *Autophagy* **2016**, *12*, 1372–1389. [CrossRef]

102. Sarkar, S.; Ravikumar, B.; Floto, R.A.; Rubinsztein, D.C. Rapamycin and mTOR-independent autophagy inducers ameliorate toxicity of polyglutamine-expanded huntingtin and related proteinopathies. *Cell Death Differ.* **2009**, *16*, 46–56. [CrossRef]

103. Dauer, W.; Przedborski, S. Parkinson's disease: Mechanisms and models. *Neuron* **2003**, *39*, 889–909. [CrossRef]

104. Domanskyi, A.; Geissler, C.; Vinnikov, I.A.; Alter, H.; Schober, A.; Vogt, M.A.; Gass, P.; Parlato, R.; Schutz, G. Pten ablation in adult dopaminergic neurons is neuroprotective in Parkinson's disease models. *FASEB J.* **2011**, *25*, 2898–2910. [CrossRef]

105. Long, X.; Lin, Y.; Ortiz-Vega, S.; Yonezawa, K.; Avruch, J. Rheb binds and regulates the mTOR kinase. *Curr. Biol.* **2005**, *15*, 702–713. [CrossRef]

106. Inoki, K.; Li, Y.; Xu, T.; Guan, K.L. Rheb GTPase is a direct target of TSC2 GAP activity and regulates mTOR signaling. *Genes Dev.* **2003**, *17*, 1829–1834. [CrossRef]

107. Aspuria, P.J.; Tamanoi, F. The Rheb family of GTP-binding proteins. *Cell Signal.* **2004**, *16*, 1105–1112. [CrossRef]

108. Potter, C.J.; Pedraza, L.G.; Xu, T. Akt regulates growth by directly phosphorylating Tsc2. *Nat. Cell Biol.* **2002**, *4*, 658. [CrossRef]

109. Kim, S.R.; Chen, X.; Oo, T.F.; Kareva, T.; Yarygina, O.; Wang, C.; During, M.; Kholodilov, N.; Burke, R.E. Dopaminergic pathway reconstruction by Akt/Rheb-induced axon regeneration. *Ann. Neurol.* **2011**, *70*, 110–120. [CrossRef]

110. Iwakawa, H.O.; Tomari, Y. The Functions of MicroRNAs: mRNA Decay and Translational Repression. *Trends Cell Biol.* **2015**, *25*, 651–665. [CrossRef]

111. Wilczynska, A.; Bushell, M. The complexity of miRNA-mediated repression. *Cell Death Differ.* **2015**, *22*, 22–33. [CrossRef]

112. Ma, L.; Wei, L.; Wu, F.; Hu, Z.; Liu, Z.; Yuan, W. Advances with microRNAs in Parkinson's disease research. *Drug Des. Dev.Ther.* **2013**, *7*, 1103–1113. [CrossRef]

113. Fragkouli, A.; Doxakis, E. miR-7 and miR-153 protect neurons against MPP(+)-induced cell death via upregulation of mTOR pathway. *Front. Cell. Neurosci.* **2014**, *8*, 182. [CrossRef]

114. Bee, J.; Fuller, S.; Miller, S.; Johnson, S.R. Lung function response and side effects to rapamycin for lymphangioleiomyomatosis: A prospective national cohort study. *Thorax* **2018**, *73*, 369–375. [CrossRef]

115. Lamming, D.W.; Ye, L.; Sabatini, D.M.; Baur, J.A. Rapalogs and mTOR inhibitors as anti-aging therapeutics. *J. Clin. Investig.* **2013**, *123*, 980–989. [CrossRef]

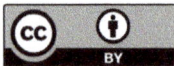

International Journal of
Molecular Sciences

MDPI

Review

Physical Activity Alleviates Cognitive Dysfunction of Alzheimer's Disease through Regulating the mTOR Signaling Pathway

Xianjuan Kou [1], Dandan Chen [2] and Ning Chen [1,*]

[1] Tianjiu Research and Development Center for Exercise Nutrition and Foods, Hubei Key Laboratory of Exercise Training and Monitoring, College of Health Science, Wuhan Sports University, Wuhan 430079, China; kouxianjuan@126.com

[2] Graduate School, Wuhan Sports University, Wuhan 430079, China; chendandan950310@163.com

* Correspondence: nchen510@gmail.com; Tel./Fax: +86-27-6784-6140

Received: 26 February 2019; Accepted: 27 March 2019; Published: 29 March 2019

Abstract: Alzheimer's disease (AD) is one of the most common aging-related progressive neurodegenerative disorders, and can result in great suffering for a large portion of the aged population. Although the pathogenesis of AD is being elucidated, the exact mechanisms are still unclear, thereby impeding the development of effective drugs, supplements, and other interventional strategies for AD. In recent years, impaired autophagy associated with microRNA (miRNA) dysfunction has been reported to be involved in aging and aging-related neurodegenerative diseases. Therefore, miRNA-mediated regulation for the functional status of autophagy may become one of the potent interventional strategies for AD. Mounting evidence from in vivo AD models has demonstrated that physical activity can exert a neuroprotective role in AD. In addition, autophagy is strictly regulated by the mTOR signaling pathway. In this article, the regulation of the functional status of autophagy through the mTOR signaling pathway during physical activity is systematically discussed for the prevention and treatment of AD. This concept will be beneficial to developing novel and effective targets that can create a direct link between pharmacological intervention and AD in the future.

Keywords: Alzheimer's disease; autophagy; mTOR signal pathway; physical activity; microRNA

1. Introduction

Alzheimer's disease (AD) is an insidious, age-dependent progressive neurodegenerative disorder characterized by deficits in cognitive function. The pathological changes of AD are diffuse atrophy of the cerebral cortex, deepening of cortical sulci, and narrowing of cerebral gyri, in which the loss of neurons, the extracellular deposition of amyloid-beta (Aβ) peptide as senile plaques (SPs), and the formation of neurofibrillary tangles (NFTs) are characteristic [1,2]. Up to now, a series of studies on the pathogenesis of AD have been conducted, and several hypotheses including Aβ cascade [3], abnormal tau phosphorylation [4], increased apolipoprotein E (APOE) [5], and neuroinflammation [6] have been widely recognized. However, no hypothesis has been completely elucidated on the complex pathological changes of AD.

Autophagy as an evolutionary-conserved process can maintain normal physiological events or regulate the progression of a series of diseases through sequestering mis-folded/toxic proteins in autophagosomes, thus executing its cytoprotective role [7,8]. Growing evidence demonstrates that autophagic capacity to degrade harmful proteins in cells declines with increasing age [9,10]. Moreover, dysfunctional autophagy has also been linked to several aging-related neurodegenerative diseases including AD [11–19]. Previous studies have documented the critical role of autophagy in the pathogenesis of AD, including Aβ production or deposition, Aβ precursor protein (APP) metabolism, and neuronal death [20,21]. Furthermore, insufficient or reduced autophagic activity can lead to the formation of harmful protein aggregates, which results in increased reactive oxygen species (ROS), cell death, and neurodegeneration [22]. As a result, autophagy has a crucial role in the regulation of longevity.

Mammalian target of rapamycin (mTOR) regulates a series of physiological processes. On the one hand, mTOR plays an important role in different cellular processes including cell survival, protein synthesis, mitochondrial biogenesis, proliferation, and cell death [23,24]. On the other hand, the mTOR signaling pathway can execute an important role in memory reconsolidation and maintaining synaptic plasticity for memory formation, due to its regulatory function for protein synthesis in neurons [25]. Moreover, mTOR also can interact with upstream signal components, such as growth factors, insulin, PI3K/Akt, 5'-adenosine monophosphate-activated protein kinase (AMPK), and glycogen synthase kinase 3 (GSK-3) [26,27]. Currently, although the molecular mechanisms responsible for AD remain unclear, more and more studies have confirmed the involvement of dys-regulated mTOR signaling in AD [28,29]. Activated mTOR signaling is a contributor to the progression of AD and is coordinated with both the pathological and clinical manifestations of AD [30]. Furthermore, there is a close relationship between mTOR signaling and the presence of Aβ plaques, NFTs, and cognitive impairment in clinical presentation [31–33]. Therefore, the development of mTOR inhibitors may be useful for the prevention and treatment of AD.

It has been reported that regular physical activity can improve brain health and provide cognitive and psychological benefits [34]. Mechanically, regular exercise training is related to the inhibition of oxidative stress and apoptotic signaling, thus effectively executing neuroprotection [35]. Previous studies have demonstrated that treadmill or voluntary wheel running is beneficial for the improvement of behavioral capacity, and can promote the dynamic recycling of mitochondria, thereby improving the health status of mitochondria in brain tissues [36]. Moreover, other studies have demonstrated that regular exercise has a beneficial effect on the structure, metabolism, and function of human and rodent brains [37,38]. Interestingly, our recent study has also documented that the brain aging of D-gal-induced aging rats can be noticeably attenuated by eight-week swimming training, due to the rescuing of impaired autophagy and abnormal mitochondrial dynamics in the presence of miR-34a mediation [39]. Therefore, physical activity is regarded as an effective approach against AD. The aim of this article is to overview the potential of physical activity as a preventive or therapeutic strategy for AD through regulating the mTOR signaling pathway. In this article, we summarize the main features of AD pathogenesis, the regulatory roles of mTOR in AD, and the preventive or therapeutic implications of targeting the mTOR signaling pathway with physical activity or exercise intervention.

2. The mTOR Signaling Pathway

2.1. The mTOR Signaling Pathway and Autophagy

mTOR can be divided into two different functional complexes: mTOR complex 1 (mTORC1) and mTOR complex 2 (mTORC2). These mTOR complexes are localized in the center of complex signaling pathways that are activated by growth factor signals or intracellular stress. mTOR can undergo self-phosphorylation via its own serine/threonine kinases, and can regulate the synthesis of other proteins by activating p70-S6K phosphorylation [40]. Similarly, as the first downstream substrate of mTOR, 4E-BP1 is a translational repressor that inhibits the translation initiation associated with eukaryotic translation initiation factor 4E (eIF4E). Under normal conditions, 4E-BP1 presents in a de-phosphorylation state in combination with eIF4E to form a complex. Under the stimulation of growth signals, 4E-BP1 can be inactivated due to the phosphorylation of mTOR, and p-4E-BP1 can be detached from eIF4E, thereby losing the inhibition of eIF4E [41]. When mTOR is activated, it can phosphorylate its key downstream molecules such as 4EBP1 and S6K1 to promote protein synthesis [42]. Furthermore, mTOR is also involved in the regulation of autophagy. Previous studies have demonstrated that the hyperactivation of mTOR can reduce autophagy and directly contribute to hyperphosphorylation and aggregation of tau protein [43,44].

Two mTOR complexes have different sensitivity to rapamycin. The mTORC1 is a rapamycin-sensitive complex and the mTORC2 is a rapamycin-independent complex. The mTORC1 can inhibit autophagy under the condition of sufficient nutrients and energy through phosphorylating Unc51-like kinase 1 (ULK1) and autophagy-related gene 13 (Atg13), which is essential for the formation of pre-autophagosomal structures [45]. Usually, mTOR regulates autophagy [46]. The inhibition of mTORC1 induces autophagy while its activation suppresses autophagy. Consistent with a previous study, the treatment with rapamycin in Alzheimer's transgenic mice (P301S mice) activates autophagy and suppresses tau hyperphosphorylation to prevent the aggregation of tau protein [47]. Therefore, mTOR inhibitors may have a protective role against AD. In addition, prolonged rapamycin treatment can inhibit Akt activity in many types of cells by suppressing mTORC2 assembly [48]. Since Akt positively regulates mTORC1, the phosphorylation of Akt by mTORC2 can stimulate the function of mTORC1, thereby inhibiting autophagy. In addition, mTOR also regulates protein synthesis in neurons at the translational level by phosphorylating several intracellular targets. One finding in invertebrates indicates that mTOR-dependent translational control is critical for synaptic plasticity and learning and memory reconsolidation [25]. The studies using various models have also confirmed mTOR as a critical signaling pathway for synaptic plasticity [49]. Considering its regulatory roles, mTOR could be a promising target for suppressing the neurodegenerative process and rescuing the adult brain from pathological changes.

A series of studies have demonstrated that the activation of autophagy can exert a neuroprotective function; in contrast, deficient autophagy or impaired autophagic flux can result in neurological damage in most neurological disorders [21,50,51]. For example, the deficiency of autophagy-related gene *Beclin1* in cultured neurons and transgenic mice provokes the deposition of Aβ, whereas its overexpression attenuates accumulation of Aβ [18]. Growing evidence has shown that lysosomal system defects are the key pathogenic factors in AD; thus, selectively restoring lysosomal function in mouse AD models can alleviate deficient cognitive capacity and synaptic function [52,53]. It has been reported that autophagic flux is altered in patients with AD, and the administration of autophagy enhancer rapamycin may alleviate cognitive impairment and Aβ neuropathology in APP/PS1 mouse models [54]. Consistent with these opinions, one recent report [55] has demonstrated that autophagic sequestration is stimulated in patients at the early stage of AD, while lysosomal clearance is progressively declining and autophagic flux is gradually hindered due to the lack of the substrate clearance. Previous studies have shown that rapamycin, a selective inhibitor of TORC1, can attenuate Aβ accumulation and inhibit tau phosphorylation in AD mouse models [56]. On the contrary, mTORC2 seems to indirectly suppress autophagy through phosphorylating Akt, thereby resulting in the activation of Akt/mTORC1 signaling [57]. Recent studies have also demonstrated that chronic intervention using rapamycin can retard the progression of AD-like deficits and decrease Aβ level by inducing autophagy in the mouse model with overexpression of human APP [58].

2.2. Activated mTOR Signaling Triggers Aβ Generation and Induces the Failure of Aβ Clearance

AD is a progressive neurodegenerative disease caused by the accumulation of toxic proteins that leads to neural damage and cell death [51]. A large number of studies have shown that the activation of mTOR is an enhancer of Aβ generation and deposition [31,59]. Under normal conditions, Aβ is degraded by the autophagic-lysosomal pathway, thus participating in protein quality control and the removal of aberrant forms of protein. mTOR also modulates the metabolism of APP by regulating β- and γ-secretases. Different animal and cell models have also provided evidence that excessive mTOR activity increases the activity of β- and γ-secretases, thus leading to the generation of Aβ plaques and the activation of mTOR related to the malfunction of Aβ elimination from the brain, since mTOR-mediated inhibition of autophagy could lead to the accumulation of Aβ [33,54,60]. The role of mTOR dependent autophagy dysfunction has been previously reported in a variety of neurological and neuropsychiatric disorders [61–65]. Increasing studies have proven that mTOR activation leads to the failure of Aβ removal from the brain, since the dysfunction of autophagy triggered by mTOR facilitates the process of Aβ generation and weakens its clearance [33,54,60]. In the 3xTg mouse model with AD, autophagy induced by rapamycin has been reported to ameliorate cognitive deficits through inhibiting mTOR signaling [66]. Chronic treatment with rapamycin reduces the progression of AD by inducing autophagy, which, in turn, reduces Aβ level in the mouse model with human APP [58]. Apart from this, the relationship between the immaturity of autophagolysosomes and the accumulation of autophagic vacuoles (AVs) that can contribute to the generation of Aβ has also been confirmed. In this case, the activation of mTOR signaling alters the autophagic process, thus leading to the accumulation of immature forms of AVs [67].

2.3. mTOR Activation Induces Hyperphosphorylation of Tau Protein

Tau is a microtubule-binding protein that promotes microtubule assembly and stabilization to form a stable cytoskeletal system. In contrast, the ability of hyperphosphorylated tau protein (pathological tau protein) to bind to microtubules is significantly reduced, thereby losing the ability to promote microtubule assembly and maintain microtubule stability, disrupting the cytoskeletal system, and impairing the normal function of neurons [4]. Wild-type tau in vivo can result in synaptic loss, whereas the deletion of tau can rescue Aβ-induced neurotoxicity at the synapse [68–70]. The chronic stress and mTOR-dependent inhibition of autophagy can lead to the accumulation of tau aggregates in P301L-tau-expressing mice and cells, which is validated by molecular, pharmacological, and behavioral analysis [71], suggesting that dys-regulated generation, phosphorylation, and aggregation of tau might be the key events for triggering neuronal degeneration in AD. Currently, little is known about the upstream intracellular effectors accounting for these molecular events in the process of tau deposition, but mTOR has been proposed. The signaling pathway mediated by mTOR kinase regulates protein homeostasis via facilitating protein translation [47]. The abnormal mTOR signaling can be observed in an AD brain [72]. Recent evidence indicates that tau can mediate learning and memory deficits in animal models with AD [68], suggesting that reducing tau level may represent a valid therapeutic approach. mTOR and its downstream p70S6K have been reported to be higher in human AD brains [73].

Growing evidence has shown that mTOR links to aging from lower organisms to mammals. For example, genetically increasing mTOR signaling can upregulate tau level and promote tau phosphorylation, but reducing mTOR signaling with rapamycin can ameliorate tau pathology and rescue motor deficits in a mouse model of tauopathy [74,75]. Consistent with in vivo experiment, in vitro results suggest that mTOR signaling regulates tau phosphorylation [43] and the activation of mTOR enhances tau-induced neurodegeneration in a Drosophila model of tauopathy [76]. Tau phosphorylation is dynamically regulated by mTOR. Numerous scientific data support the key role of mTOR in the tau-related pathological progress, thus implying that the activity of mTOR determines the abnormal hyperphosphorylation of tau and the formation of NFTs [47,56]. mTOR signaling activation increases abnormal phosphorylation of tau, while inhibiting mTOR attenuates abnormal phosphorylation of tau. Consistent with the above reports, a transgenic mouse model subjected to treatment with rapamycin revealed alleviated cognitive impairment and reduced accumulation of Aβ plaques and NFTs due to the induction of autophagy [77,78]. Therefore, mTOR is an effective preventive or therapeutic target for AD by regulating tau phosphorylation and controlling the autophagic signal pathway.

3. The Alteration of miRNAs in AD and Aging-Related Diseases

MicroRNAs (miRNAs), small non-coding RNAs with a length of 18–25 nucleotides, usually downregulate the expression of mRNA and protein upon targeting specific mRNAs, and are involved in complex post-transcriptional regulatory networks and the maintenance of healthy cellular functions [79–82]. Approximately 70% of known miRNAs enriched in the brain are involved in critical roles, including neuronal development and differentiation, synaptic plasticity, and the pathogenesis of neurodegenerative disorders [83]. The expression of some miRNAs is dynamically regulated during brain development, neurogenesis, and neuronal maturation [84]. In recent years, growing evidence has demonstrated that abnormal patterns of miRNAs are linked with most aging or aging-related neurodegenerative diseases [83,85]. In APP/PS1 mice, miR-99b-5p and miR-100-5p are reported to be decreased and increased at early and late disease stages compared with age-matched wild-type mice, respectively [86]. In addition, miR-99b-5p and miR-100-5p are reported to affect neuron survival by targeting mTOR, which is consistent with previous studies in cancer [87–89]. The defensive effect of miR-200b or miR-200c on Aβ-induced toxicity in AD models are observed, which is evidenced by the relieving of impaired spatial learning and memory induced by intracerebroventricular injection of oligomeric Aβ after the treatment of miR-200b or miR-200c [90]. Mechanically, the miR-200b/c could suppress the downstream effector of mTOR, S6K1. Chronic cerebral hypoperfusion (CCH) is a high-risk factor for vascular dementia and AD. Similar to a previous study, some miRNAs have also been validated to regulate autophagy-related signal pathways [39]. It is reported that the level of miR-96 is significantly increased in a CCH rat model established by two-vessel occlusion (2VO), and the inhibition of miR-96 can attenuate the cognitive impairment. Furthermore, miR-96 antagomir injection can attenuate the number of LC3 and Beclin1-positive autophagosomes in 2VO rats. In contrast, the overexpressed miR-96 can downregulate mTOR protein levels in 2VO rats and primary culture cells [91]. These findings suggest that miR-96 may play a key role in autophagy under CCH by regulating mTOR signaling. Since pathological changes occurring in AD and Parkinson's diseases (PD) brains are reflected in cerebrospinal fluid (CSF) composition, CSF represents an optimal biomarker source of neurodegenerative diseases. One study [92] related to CSF miRNAs has reported that 74 miRNAs are downregulated and 74 miRNAs are upregulated in AD patients when compared with controls based on a 1.5-fold change threshold. The study identified a set of genes involved in the regulation of tau and Aβ signal pathways in AD, with mTOR and BACE1 being targeted by the CSF miRNAs. Another study [93] has demonstrated that miR-153, miR-409-3p, miR-10a-5p, and let-7g-3p are significantly overexpressed in CSF exosomes from PD and AD patients. Bioinformatic analysis has demonstrated that mTOR signaling, ubiquitin-mediated proteolysis, dopaminergic synapses, and glutamatergic synapses are the most prominent pathways, with differential exosomal miRNA patterns associated with the development of PD and AD. These results have demonstrated that CSF miRNA molecules are reliable biomarkers with fair robustness in regard to specificity and sensitivity in differentiating PD and AD patients from healthy controls. Among these processes, the mTOR signaling pathway is an important target.

The roles of miRNAs in APP and Aβ production, synaptic remodeling, neuron survival, and glia cell activation have also been identified [94,95]. miRNAs, including miR-130a, miR-20a, miR-29a, miR-106b, miR-128a, miR-125b, and miR-let-7c, have been reported to be downregulated in aged individuals and in different human and animal cell aging models [85,96,97]. In the brain, miR-29 is reported to target BACE1, and the deregulation of miR-29b results in an increase of apoptosis in AD. The overexpression of miR-29 in humans and transgenic mice could decrease endogenous BACE1 levels and increase Aβ production [79]. MiR-107 also targets BACE1, and can induce cell cycle arrest, because cell cycle re-entry is an early event in AD pathogenesis [98]. Of course, there are some brain-specific miRNAs that participate in tau hyperphosphorylation, the physiological regulation of APP expression, and the generation and deposit of Aβ. The expression of extracellular signal-regulated kinase 1 (ERK1) is a direct tau kinase. Some miR-15 family members can target ERK1 to be involved in tau hyperphosphorylation [79]. For example, as a neuron-specific miRNA, the expression of mature miR-124 is reduced in a subset of AD patients [99]. Downregulation of miR-124 can result in the altered splicing of APP and promote the conversion of APP to Aβ. Similarly, the downregulation of miR-17, miR-101, and miR-16a also promotes accumulation of APP [33,37]. Previous studies have documented that the abnormally low expression of miR-16 could potentially lead to the accumulation of APP protein in the embryo of SAMP8 mice and BALb/c mice, suggesting APP as a target of miR-16 [100]. The miR-101 and miR-106 can also target APP, in turn, resulting in an elevated generation and accumulation of Aβ [101]. miR-455-3p is found to be significantly upregulated in serum samples, postmortem brains, mouse models, and cell lines of AD [102]. Recent evidence has shown that circulating miR-455-3p is upregulated in AD postmortem brains when compared with healthy control samples [81], suggesting that miR-455-3p may be a potential biomarker for AD. The miR-206 regulating brain-derived neurotrophic factor (BDNF) is markedly increased in AD model mice [103]. Because changes in gene expression and splicing of APP are associated with the generation and deposition of Aβ, specific neuronal miRNAs can regulate APP splicing. Therefore, the scanning and identification of miRNAs in the future could provide an important new insight and elucidation in the initiation and progression of AD. Nevertheless, the roles of far more miRNAs still remain enigmatic in AD etiology.

4. The Role of Physical Activity in AD

Physical activity not only affects skeletal muscle, but also has an important effect on the phenotype of the brain. The brain has high sensitivity to exercise, so that exercise in rodent models is easy to drive the neurogenesis within hippocampal and dentate gyrus (DG) areas, thus leading to enhanced learning and memory capabilities. Defining the optimal preventive strategy according to type, duration, and intensity of physical activity is a key practical question. In this article, the roles of physical activity as a potential preventive intervention against AD are summarized, which will be beneficial to exploring optimal exercise prescriptions for the prevention and treatment of AD, and providing references for developing novel and effective targets for the prevention and treatments of AD in the future.

4.1. Physical Activity is Beneficial for the Improvement of Learning and Memory Capacity

Cognitive decline has increasingly been reported in correlation with human aging [104]. This age-related decline of cognitive capacity also occurs in mice [105]. Some animal studies [106–108] demonstrate that cognitive impairment can occur in the absence of Aβ deposition and NFTs. However, several researchers have shown that a physically active lifestyle can modify cognitive decline in both humans and mice [109,110]. Moreover, regular physical activity can improve brain health and provide cognitive and psychological benefits. Physical activity has been shown to improve mental health and cognition, including in patients with AD [34]. Regular exercise may also improve different cognitive domains, such as memory and executive function, in older-age individuals with dementia and AD [111]. Different animal models with AD have displayed encouraging results from voluntary exercise training. It has been found that voluntary wheel running for 16 weeks could result in an improved capacity for exploring novel objects in a recognition memory paradigm when compared with forced exercise and sedentary controls in a Tg2576 mouse model [112]. In a transgenic APOE4 animal model aged 10–12 months, voluntary wheel running for six weeks promotes the more-noticeable recovery of cognitive impairment when compared to sedentary counterparts [113]. In addition, five-month voluntary wheel running has been demonstrated to decrease Aβ plaques in hippocampal tissue and improve learning capacity [114]. Tg2576 mice at the age of 17–19 months used as a mouse model of AD reveal a significant cognitive impairment and neuropathology consistent with AD; Kathryn [115] has found that wheel running intervention for three consecutive weeks effectively improved memory, thereby making the mouse models indistinguishable from wild-type mice on all tasks. A previous study using a TgCRND8 mouse model with AD also demonstrated that five-month voluntary wheel running begun at the age of one month improved cognitive performance when compared to the sedentary control group, which supports the hypothesis that an exercise-induced improvement in cognitive capacity if exercise is begun at the young age, prior to the AD pathogenesis. Furthermore, voluntary wheel running for 10 weeks can significantly delay cognitive decline in APPswe/PS1ΔE9 mouse models when compared with the sedentary controls [116]. Similarly, physical activity has been shown to produce positive effects on brain plasticity and regional gray matter volume [117].

4.2. Physical Activity Increases Neurogenesis

Reduced neurogenesis has been reported in different transgenic or knock-in mice with Swedish mutation of the APP or PS1 gene, or in double-transgenic mice with APP and PS1 genes. Exercise is beneficial for multiple pathways and can increase neurogenesis. Clinical exercise trials in normal aging populations have shown increased brain volume [118] following exercise. A previous study reported that voluntary wheel running for 10 weeks presented an enhanced level of hippocampal neurogenesis in APPswe-PS1ΔE9 mice [116]. Interestingly, an age-dependent promoting effect from voluntary wheel running on neurogenesis in hippocampal tissues of 18-month-old APP23 AD mouse model has been confirmed, but no promoting effect on neurogenesis in six-month-old control mice [119], suggesting that voluntary physical activity has the ability to upregulate cell proliferation and neuronal differentiation in AD brain.

4.3. Physical Activity Enhances Structural and Synaptic Plasticity in Hippocampus

Synaptic plasticity is the biological process of neurons with specific characteristics of changing their synaptic strength to communicate with others for the purpose of learning and memory capacity. Usually, two forms of synaptic plasticity can be measured in the hippocampus. Long-term potentiation (LTP) [120] is in charge of memory formation, depending on protein synthesis and kinase activation, which can be regarded as the major biological mechanisms for understanding the learning and memory processes. In contrast, long-term depression (LTD) is associated with memory clearance or forgetting. At a cellular level, the impairment of learning and memory in AD is associated with a decrease in LTP and an increase in LTD.

Currently, LTP is recognized as a valuable tool for evaluating therapeutic interventions for disorders of the central nervous system due to its close correlation with learning and memory. Previous findings have shown that Aβ oligomers can inhibit LTP in various hippocampal areas involved in learning and memory processes [114,121,122]. It is well documented that regular exercise can produce a positive effect on cognition and synaptic plasticity. Treadmill exercise can increase expression of LTP as the field excitatory postsynaptic potential (fEPSP) slope increases; it can also spike amplitude in DG both in vivo and in vitro, and enhance synaptic plasticity through lowering the LTP threshold [123,124]. In agreement with previous findings, long-term voluntary wheel running for two to four months has been confirmed to significantly increase the process of neuronal survival in female adult C57BL/6 mice, while concurrently enhancing synaptic plasticity and learning and memory performance, as demonstrated through a Morris water maze (MWM) test [125]. However, LTP could not be produced by a six-month voluntary wheel running treatment in 3xTg-AD animals, and regular exercise only reveals the weak protection from the impairment of LTP induction at the CA1-medial prefrontal cortex synapse [126]. More recently, studies on the effects of exercise on bidirectional plasticity have emerged, and it is reported that forced exercise has an evident effect on LTP in the CA1 region of hippocampus in the rats with sleep deprivation and aging and neurodegenerative diseases, but not in healthy rats [127,128].

4.4. Physical Activity Regulates Abnormal miRNAs

Currently, it is still difficult to predict whether the observed abnormal miRNA levels in humans are the cause or consequence of AD progression. Studies of miRNA-expression profiles in AD mouse models may be helpful to address these questions. Previous studies have shown that regular exercise can regulate the expression of miRNAs; however, the underlying mechanisms are still unclear [129]. Our recent findings have demonstrated that miR-34a is significantly increased in AD models when compared with the control; however, eight-week swimming training alleviates the abnormal expression of miR-34a in an AD rat model [39]. Neuroinflammation is a high risk of AD, and Toll-like receptor 4 (TLR4) participates in inflammatory responses. Aerobic exercise can significantly alter the expression of inflammatory cytokines and reduce vascular TLR4 levels in APOE-null mice through upregulating miR-146a and miR-126 and downregulating miR-155 [130]. Similarly, aerobic exercise can downregulate miR-143 level in cardiac tissue [131]. In addition, miRNAs such as miR-22, miR-101a, miR-720, and miR-721 have also been identified in murine brains during the aging process [132]. These findings suggest that miRNAs regulated by aerobic exercise may play an important role in AD. Therefore, aerobic exercise may regulate the expression of the above miRNAs, which should be helpful to prevent the progression of AD. Although studies on exercise to improve AD by regulating miRNAs are still at the stage of infancy, and numerous questions remain unanswered, whether or not miRNAs can be used for the diagnosis of AD depends on an elucidation of the precise characterization, specific distribution, and accurate regulation of miRNAs during the progression of AD. Therefore, further exploration of targets, regulatory networks, and functions is highly desired. Moreover, the scanning and identification of miRNAs during exercise intervention of AD will open a novel avenue for the diagnosis, prevention, and therapy of AD.

5. Clinical Studies of Physical Activity in AD

In addition to animal studies, a large prospective study has concluded that regular exercise in AD patients delays the onset of dementia and AD [133]. Human APOE maintains synaptic integrity in the CNS, and its allele APOE4 is associated with an early age of onset and increased risk of AD. Several human studies have shown the interactive effects of exercise and the APOE genotype on cognitive decline. Most studies have confirmed that the protective effects of exercise are more robust in carriers of the ε4 allele [134–137]. In particular, the impact of low activity is stronger in individuals carrying the APOE4 allele. For example, individuals participating at least twice a week in a leisure-time physical activity have 50% lower odds of dementia when compared with sedentary persons. However, there are inconsistent results about the effects of physical activity in patients with AD, and some studies claim that there is a negative correlation between physical activity and cognitive decline [136,138], while other studies report no relationship [139]. According to previous reports, leisure-time physical activity at midlife twice a week can delay the occurrence of AD for two decades in APOE4 carriers [136], whereas physical activity at the late stage of aging has shorter-term beneficial effects in APOE4 non-carriers [140]. Consistent with the above findings, previous studies on patients with mild cognitive impairment or neurological symptoms suggest that physical activity may still have some benefits in the prodromal or early stage of AD. Moreover, physical activity has a greater protective effect against AD and dementia in women than in men [138].

6. mTOR as a New Target for the Prevention and Treatment of AD During Physical Activity?

As reported above, mTOR seems to be an interesting candidate target for the regulation of AD, and the role of physical activity as a neuroprotective agent is well recognized. Some literature has also reported that mTOR is a regulatory target of AD during physical activity.

mTOR signaling is dynamically regulated by upstream components including PI3K/Akt, AMPK, mitogen-activated protein kinase (MAPK), p53, liver kinase B1 (LKB1), erb-b2 receptor tyrosine kinase 2 (ERBB2), insulin receptor substrate 1 (IRS-1), phosphatase and tensin homolog (PTEN), GSK-3, and insulin/insulin-like growth factor 1 (IGF-1). PI3K/Akt, AMPK, GSK-3, insulin/IGF-1, and AMPK play a critical role in regulating the generation of Aβ and the aberrant phosphorylation of tau [27,50,141,142]. PI3K-Akt can activate mTOR-mediated biosynthetic processes, whereas it also can also simultaneously repress autophagic degradation. Previous findings have demonstrated that aberrant activation of neuronal PI3K/Akt/mTOR signaling is an early pathogenesis in the brain of AD individuals and a major candidate for pathophysiological change of Aβ. In addition, the abnormal PI3K/Akt/mTOR signaling pathway has been shown to contribute to the development of AD [27]. Based on the relationship between upstream components of mTOR signaling and autophagy, physical activity should be beneficial to the prevention and alleviation of AD through regulating PI3K/Akt and AMPK signaling.

According to previous reports, the hyperactivation of mTOR can suppress autophagy, which directly contributes to hyperphosphorylation and the aggregation of tau protein [43,44]. Thus, the inhibition of mTOR represents one of the major mechanisms benefitting the pathogenesis of AD in the presence of physical activity. Of course, the effect of exercise on mTOR activity depends on the type and intensity of exercise. Jeong et al. [143] have reported abnormal mTOR phosphorylation and impaired autophagy, such as decreased Beclin1 and LC3B, and increased p62 in the cerebral cortex of NSE/htau23 transgenic mice. Interestingly, 12-week treadmill exercise intervention significantly improves learning and cognitive capacity of NSE/htau23 transgenic mice. Mechanically, abnormal mTOR, impaired autophagy, and the hyperphosphorylation and aggregation (Ser199/202, Ser404, Thr231, PHF-1) of tau protein are improved upon exercise intervention. Meanwhile, Antonella has observed a strong activation of the mTOR signaling pathway, and an increase in two mTOR downstream targets, p70S6K and 4EBP1, in both amnestic mild cognitive impairment (MCI) and AD patients when compared with that of the controls [144]. Interestingly, p70S6K and 4EBP1 are dramatically increased in AD, and are also positively correlated with tau phosphorylation [145,146], thus the activation of p70S6K and 4EBP1 has been identified as a contributor to hyperphosphorylated tau. In contrast, the significant autophagy impairment has also been found. These findings suggest that the alteration of mTOR signaling and autophagy occurs at the early stage of AD. Consistent with previous findings, one study has established a relationship between mTOR signal activation and AD, and a possible correlation of mTOR activation with the degree of cognitive impairment in AD [147]. Besides regulating autophagy and mTOR, 12-week treadmill exercise from the age of 24 months has been reported to markedly suppress Aβ-dependent neuronal cell death and upregulate the expression of NGF, BDNF, and phosphor-CREB in the hippocampal tissue of Tg mice [148]. Furthermore, treadmill exercise may specifically repress GSK-3α/β activity via elevated PI3K and Akt phosphorylation in hippocampal tissue. In a 20-week high-fat diet (HFD) rat model, eight-week treadmill exercise significantly decreased tau hyperphosphorylation and aggregation, while increasing insulin signaling-related protein activity [149]. The above findings suggest that treadmill exercise can provide a therapeutic potential to inhibit tau, Aβ-42, and neuronal-death signal pathways. Therefore, treadmill exercise may be beneficial in prevention or treatment of AD.

AMPK, as a key enzyme for energy metabolism, regulates cellular metabolism to maintain energy homeostasis in response to the reduction of intracellular ATP levels. AMPK is activated when cellular ADP level is increased with the accompanying changes in cellular energy status [150]. AMPK has been implicated in aging and neurodegenerative diseases [151,152]. In addition, AMPK also participates in the regulation of Aβ level and limits the generation of Aβ by inducing autophagy [141,153]. Increasing data have demonstrated the close relationship between AMPK signaling and major hallmarks of AD [154–157]. T2MD is a risk factor for AD, and diabetic populations at the midlife stage carry a 1.5-times higher risk for developing AD than those diagnosed with T2DM at a late stage in life [158]. Impaired insulin sensing in the brain, diabetes, and metabolic syndrome (MetS) are associated with the pathogenesis of AD, MCI, and other neurological disorders [159]. One recent study [160] demonstrated that mixed intervention, such as nutritional ketosis combined with high-intensity interval training (HIIT) (in order to inhibit mTOR signaling) for 10 weeks, can significantly reduce HgA1c, fasting insulin, and insulin resistance, as well as restore memory function, improve neuroplasticity, and normalize MetS biomarkers of patients via activating the AMPK signaling pathway. This finding suggests that mTOR suppression and AMPK induction may functionally halt neurological disease progression and restore early-stage memory loss. In addition, previous studies have reported mTOR as a target of physical activity in triple-negative breast cancer (TNBC), and physical activity at moderate to vigorous intensity induces the inhibition of PI3K-Akt-mTOR signaling and slows the growth of TNBC cells [161–163].

Up to now, the underlying mechanisms of physical activity for mediating these benefits have remained unclear. The neurophysiological effects of physical activity and regular exercise are thought to be mediated by various molecular mechanisms, including the upregulation of BDNF, IGF-1, and related molecules such as Ca^{2+}/calmodulin-dependent protein kinase II (CaMKII) and calcineurin, which are associated with learning and memory functions and can, in turn, enhance brain plasticity and improve performance of memory tasks. Forced treadmill running for five days can induce an increase of BDNF protein level within the brain tissues of animals by 70%, which is associated with the increased activation of BDNF receptors and subsequent mTORC1 signaling in hippocampal tissue [144]. Another study has also explored the effect of regular exercise on the upregulation of BDNF, the phosphorylation of BDNF receptors such as tropomyosin-related-kinase (Trk), and the activation of PI3K/Akt [145]. Reelin is an extracellular, secreted glycoprotein that is essential for neuronal migration, synaptic plasticity, and brain development. During the development of the brain, regular exercise increases the production of reelin [146]. In addition, regular exercise can shift the redox state of the brain. Previous studies have also confirmed the minimal change of lipid peroxidation in hippocampal tissue after regular exercise training [37]. Interestingly, BDNF also possesses metabotropic properties besides its neurotrophic effect. BDNF can upregulate expression of AMPK, ubiquitous mitochondrial creatine kinase (uMtCK), and uncoupling protein 2 (UCP2) [164]. Thus, it is reasonable to suggest that low expression or activity of BDNF can significantly lead to the alteration of these metabolic factors, thus eventually disrupting learning and memory functions. Meanwhile, AMPK, as an activator of autophagy, can slow down the progression of AD [153]. According to the data that the Aβ level in an AD brain is determined by the overall functional status of autophagy, AMPK activation can facilitate the triggering of autophagy and promote lysosomal degradation of Aβ through suppressing mTOR signaling.

In this review, we have reported that physical activity not only can attenuate cognitive impairment, but also inhibit the generation of Aβ in different AD models. What is more important, physical activity can induce autophagy in AD rats and mice. Furthermore, physical activity can significantly decrease expression of PI3K, p-Akt, and mTOR at the protein level, respectively. Taken together, AMPK/mTOR signaling may improve insufficient energy metabolism and execute the clearance of Aβ and NFTs via the autophagy signal pathway. Physical activity can inhibit Aβ generation and induce autophagy by downregulating the PI3K/Akt/mTOR signaling pathway, and further can reveal a neuroprotective effect. It seems that physical activity might be a candidate as a neuroprotective agent for AD treatment by inducing autophagy.

7. Conclusions and Future Perspectives

AD is one of the leading aging-related diseases worldwide due to its high rate of mortality and disability. Taking into account the scarcity of effective therapy for AD, developing novel and effective preventive or therapeutic exercise-based strategies based on these novel biological targets is highly desirable. Not all of these studies on regular exercise or physical activity have clearly elucidated a beneficial effect on AD, but regular exercise or physical activity should still be a potent preventive or treatment strategy of AD. Physical activity can alleviate cognitive dysfunction of AD through suppressing mTOR signaling pathways and rescuing abnormal expression of miRNAs, thereby regulating the dysfunctional status of autophagy, tau hyperphosphorylation, and the accumulation of Aβ and NFTs, and ultimately mitigating AD. However, the relationship among regular exercise or physical activity, mTOR suppression, neurogenesis and synaptic plasticity, and rescuing abnormal microRNAs still needs to be further explored in brain tissues, as summarized in Figure 1. Meanwhile, mTOR could be considered as the preventive and therapeutic target to develop novel and effective intervention strategies for AD and other neurodegenerative diseases.

How does regular exercise or physical activity initiate these neuroprotective effects in the CNS? Up to date, this is an intriguing question with no definitive answers. Now, the challenge is to address the cause-consequence relationship between miRNA dys-regulation and AD pathogenesis, and whether the changes in miRNA expression can contribute to AD pathogenesis. Therefore, future works for establishing the link with certainty are highly desired. Meanwhile, the following aspects should be conducted: (1) optimal exercise intervention should be screened according to behavioral results;

(2) target miRNAs in serum and hippocampal tissue during exercise intervention of AD should be screened and identified; (3) the manner in which physical activity regulates target miRNAs and autophagy for regulating AD should be further explored and elucidated.

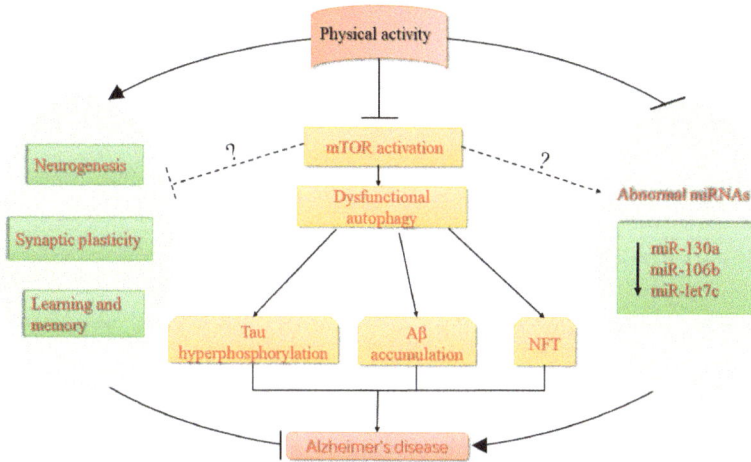

Figure 1. Physical activity as an mTOR suppressor can alleviate cognitive dysfunction and rescue abnormal miRNAs in AD for regulating functional status of autophagy, tau hyperphosphorylation, and the accumulation of Aβ and NFTs, thus accomplishing the mitigation of AD. Meanwhile, mTOR could be considered as the preventive and therapeutic target to develop novel and effective intervention strategies for AD and other neurodegenerative diseases. The solid arrows present the activation and the dotted arrows present the suppression, as well as question symbols presents the uncertainty.

Author Contributions: N.C. designed the outline of the manuscript. X.K., D.C. and N.C. collected the literatures. N.C. and X.K. wrote the manuscript, and N.C. reviewed and polished the manuscript, as well as X.K., D.C. and N.C. finally reviewed and approved the manuscript.

Funding: This work was financially supported by the National Natural Science Foundation of China (No. 81601228), National Science and Technology Program (2018YFF0300601-1), and Donghu Scholar Program from Wuhan Sports University to X.K., as well as the National Natural Science Foundation of China (No. 81571228), Hubei Superior Discipline Group of Physical Education and Health Promotion, and Outstanding Youth Scientific and Research Team (No. T201624) from Hubei Provincial Department of Education and Chutian Scholar Program and Innovative Start-Up Foundation from Wuhan Sports University to N.C.

Conflicts of Interest: These authors have declared no conflict of interest.

References

1. Hyman, B.T.; Phelps, C.H.; Beach, T.G.; Bigio, E.H.; Cairns, N.J.; Carrillo, M.C.; Dickson, D.W.; Duyckaerts, C.; Frosch, M.P.; Masliah, E.; et al. National Institute on Aging-Alzheimer's Association guidelines for the neuropathologic assessment of Alzheimer's disease. *Alzheimers Dement.* **2012**, *8*, 1–13. [CrossRef]

2. Montine, T.J.; Phelps, C.H.; Beach, T.G.; Bigio, E.H.; Cairns, N.J.; Dickson, D.W.; Duyckaerts, C.; Frosch, M.P.; Masliah, E.; Mirra, S.S.; et al. National Institute on Aging-Alzheimer's Association guidelines for the neuropathologic assessment of Alzheimer's disease: A practical approach. *Acta Neuropathol.* **2012**, *123*, 1–11. [CrossRef]

3. Karran, E.; De Strooper, B. The amyloid cascade hypothesis: Are we poised for success or failure? *J. Neurochem.* **2016**, *139*, 237–252. [CrossRef]

4. Krishnamurthy, P.K.; Johnson, G.V. Mutant (R406W) human tau is hyperphosphorylated and does not efficiently bind microtubules in a neuronal cortical cell model. *J. Biol. Chem.* **2004**, *279*, 7893–7900. [CrossRef]

5. Leoni, V. The effect of apolipoprotein E (ApoE) genotype on biomarkers of amyloidogenesis, tau pathology and neurodegeneration in Alzheimer's disease. *Clin. Chem. Lab. Med.* **2011**, *49*, 375–383. [CrossRef] [PubMed]

6. Ferretti, M.T.; Bruno, M.A.; Ducatenzeiler, A.; Klein, W.L.; Cuello, A.C. Intracellular Abeta-oligomers and early inflammation in a model of Alzheimer's disease. *Neurobiol. Aging* **2012**, *33*, 1329–1342. [CrossRef]

7. Chen, N.; Karantza-Wadsworth, V. Role and regulation of autophagy in cancer. *Biochim. Biophys. Acta* **2009**, *1793*, 1516–1523. [CrossRef]

8. Cuervo, A.M.; Bergamini, E.; Brunk, U.T.; Droge, W.; Ffrench, M.; Terman, A. Autophagy and aging: The importance of maintaining "clean" cells. *Autophagy* **2005**, *1*, 131–140. [CrossRef]

9. Salminen, A.; Kaarniranta, K. Regulation of the aging process by autophagy. *Trends Mol. Med.* **2009**, *15*, 217–224. [CrossRef] [PubMed]

10. Rubinsztein, D.C.; Marino, G.; Kroemer, G. Autophagy and aging. *Cell* **2011**, *146*, 682–695. [CrossRef] [PubMed]

11. Li, L.; Zhang, X.; Le, W. Autophagy dysfunction in Alzheimer's disease. *Neurodegener. Dis.* **2010**, *7*, 265–271. [CrossRef] [PubMed]

12. Wong, E.; Cuervo, A.M. Autophagy gone awry in neurodegenerative diseases. *Nat. Neurosci.* **2010**, *13*, 805–811. [CrossRef]

13. Kumar, A.; Dhawan, A.; Kadam, A.; Shinde, A. Autophagy and Mitochondria: Targets in Neurodegenerative Disorders. *CNS Neurol. Disord. Drug Targets* **2018**, *17*, 696–705. [CrossRef] [PubMed]

14. Limanaqi, F.; Biagioni, F.; Gambardella, S.; Ryskalin, L.; Fornai, F. Interdependency Between Autophagy and Synaptic Vesicle Trafficking: Implications for Dopamine Release. *Front. Mol. Neurosci.* **2018**, *11*, 299. [CrossRef] [PubMed]

15. Ferrucci, M.; Biagioni, F.; Ryskalin, L.; Limanaqi, F.; Gambardella, S.; Frati, A.; Fornai, F. Ambiguous Effects of Autophagy Activation Following Hypoperfusion/Ischemia. *Int. J. Mol. Sci.* **2018**, *19*, 2765. [CrossRef]

16. Martin, D.D.; Ladha, S.; Ehrnhoefer, D.E.; Hayden, M.R. Autophagy in Huntington disease and huntingtin in autophagy. *Trends Neurosci.* **2015**, *38*, 26–35. [CrossRef] [PubMed]

17. Natale, G.; Lenzi, P.; Lazzeri, G.; Falleni, A.; Biagioni, F.; Ryskalin, L.; Fornai, F. Compartment-dependent mitochondrial alterations in experimental ALS, the effects of mitophagy and mitochondriogenesis. *Front. Cell Neurosci.* **2015**, *9*, 434. [CrossRef] [PubMed]

18. Salminen, A.; Kaarniranta, K.; Kauppinen, A.; Ojala, J.; Haapasalo, A.; Soininen, H.; Hiltunen, M. Impaired autophagy and APP processing in Alzheimer's disease: The potential role of Beclin 1 interactome. *Prog. Neurobiol.* **2013**, *106–107*, 33–54. [CrossRef] [PubMed]

19. Pan, T.; Kondo, S.; Le, W.; Jankovic, J. The role of autophagy-lysosome pathway in neurodegeneration associated with Parkinson's disease. *Brain* **2008**, *131*, 1969–1978. [CrossRef]

20. Kou, X.; Chen, N. Resveratrol as a natural autophagy regulator for prevention and treatment of Alzheimer's disease. *Nutrients* **2017**, *9*, 927.

21. Yu, W.H.; Cuervo, A.M.; Kumar, A.; Peterhoff, C.M.; Schmidt, S.D.; Lee, J.H.; Mohan, P.S.; Mercken, M.; Farmery, M.R.; Tjernberg, L.O.; et al. Macroautophagy–a novel Beta-amyloid peptide-generating pathway activated in Alzheimer's disease. *J. Cell Biol.* **2005**, *171*, 87–98. [CrossRef] [PubMed]

22. Chen, N.; Karantza, V. Autophagy as a therapeutic target in cancer. *Cancer Biol. Ther.* **2011**, *11*, 157–168. [CrossRef]

23. Laplante, M.; Sabatini, D.M. mTOR signaling in growth control and disease. *Cell* **2012**, *149*, 274–293. [CrossRef]

24. Hung, C.M.; Garcia-Haro, L.; Sparks, C.A.; Guertin, D.A. mTOR-dependent cell survival mechanisms. *Cold Spring Harb. Perspect. Biol.* **2012**, *4*, a008771. [CrossRef]

25. Parsons, R.G.; Gafford, G.M.; Helmstetter, F.J. Translational control via the mammalian target of rapamycin pathway is critical for the formation and stability of long-term fear memory in amygdala neurons. *J. Neurosci.* **2006**, *26*, 12977–12983. [CrossRef]

26. Gouras, G.K. mTOR: At the crossroads of aging, chaperones, and Alzheimer's disease. *J. Neurochem.* **2013**, *124*, 747–748. [CrossRef] [PubMed]

27. O'neill, C. PI3-kinase/Akt/mTOR signaling: Impaired on/off switches in aging, cognitive decline and Alzheimer's disease. *Exp. Gerontol.* **2013**, *48*, 647–653. [CrossRef]

28. Gharibi, B.; Farzadi, S.; Ghuman, M.; Hughes, F.J. Inhibition of Akt/mTOR attenuates age-related changes in mesenchymal stem cells. *Stem Cells* **2014**, *32*, 2256–2266. [CrossRef] [PubMed]

29. Yang, F.; Chu, X.; Yin, M.; Liu, X.; Yuan, H.; Niu, Y.; Fu, L. mTOR and autophagy in normal brain aging and caloric restriction ameliorating age-related cognition deficits. *Behav. Brain Res.* **2014**, *264*, 82–90. [CrossRef] [PubMed]

30. Paccalin, M.; Pain-Barc, S.; Pluchon, C.; Paul, C.; Besson, M.N.; Carret-Rebillat, A.S.; Rioux-Bilan, A.; Gil, R.; Hugon, J. Activated mTOR and PKR kinases in lymphocytes correlate with memory and cognitive decline in Alzheimer's disease. *Dement. Geriatr. Cogn. Disord.* **2006**, *22*, 320–326. [CrossRef]

31. Cai, Z.; Zhao, B.; Li, K.; Zhang, L.; Li, C.; Quazi, S.H.; Tan, Y. Mammalian target of rapamycin: A valid therapeutic target through the autophagy pathway for Alzheimer's disease? *J. Neurosci. Res.* **2012**, *90*, 1105–1118. [CrossRef]

32. Pozueta, J.; Lefort, R.; Shelanski, M.L. Synaptic changes in Alzheimer's disease and its models. *Neuroscience* **2013**, *251*, 51–65. [CrossRef]

33. Lafay-Chebassier, C.; Paccalin, M.; Page, G.; Barc-Pain, S.; Perault-Pochat, M.C.; Gil, R.; Pradier, L.; Hugon, J. mTOR/p70S6k signalling alteration by Abeta exposure as well as in APP-PS1 transgenic models and in patients with Alzheimer's disease. *J. Neurochem.* **2005**, *94*, 215–225. [CrossRef]

34. Kaliman, P.; Parrizas, M.; Lalanza, J.F.; Camins, A.; Escorihuela, R.M.; Pallas, M. Neurophysiological and epigenetic effects of physical exercise on the aging process. *Ageing Res. Rev.* **2011**, *10*, 475–486. [CrossRef]

35. Marques-Aleixo, I.; Santos-Alves, E.; Balca, M.M.; Moreira, P.I.; Oliveira, P.J.; Magalhaes, J.; Ascensao, A. Physical exercise mitigates doxorubicin-induced brain cortex and cerebellum mitochondrial alterations and cellular quality control signaling. *Mitochondrion* **2016**, *26*, 43–57. [CrossRef] [PubMed]

36. Rees, P.S.; Davidson, S.M.; Harding, S.E.; McGregor, C.; Elliot, P.M.; Yellon, D.M.; Hausenloy, D.J. The mitochondrial permeability transition pore as a target for cardioprotection in hypertrophic cardiomyopathy. *Cardiovasc. Drugs Ther.* **2013**, *27*, 235–237. [CrossRef] [PubMed]

37. Radak, Z.; Ihasz, F.; Koltai, E.; Goto, S.; Taylor, A.W.; Boldogh, I. The redox-associated adaptive response of brain to physical exercise. *Free Radic. Res.* **2014**, *48*, 84–92. [CrossRef] [PubMed]

38. van Praag, H.; Fleshner, M.; Schwartz, M.W.; Mattson, M.P. Exercise, energy intake, glucose homeostasis, and the brain. *J. Neurosci.* **2014**, *34*, 15139–15149. [CrossRef] [PubMed]

39. Kou, X.; Li, J.; Liu, X.; Chang, J.; Zhao, Q.; Jia, S.; Fan, J.; Chen, N. Swimming attenuates d-galactose-induced brain aging via suppressing miR-34a-mediated autophagy impairment and abnormal mitochondrial dynamics. *J. Appl. Physiol.* **2017**, *122*, 1462–1469. [CrossRef]

40. Burnett, P.E.; Barrow, R.K.; Cohen, N.A.; Snyder, S.H.; Sabatini, D.M. RAFT1 phosphorylation of the translational regulators p70 S6 kinase and 4E-BP1. *Proc. Natl. Acad. Sci. USA* **1998**, *95*, 1432–1437. [CrossRef]

41. Hay, N.; Sonenberg, N. Upstream and downstream of mTOR. *Genes Dev.* **2004**, *18*, 1926–1945. [CrossRef]

42. Connolly, E.; Braunstein, S.; Formenti, S.; Schneider, R.J. Hypoxia inhibits protein synthesis through a 4E-BP1 and elongation factor 2 kinase pathway controlled by mTOR and uncoupled in breast cancer cells. *Mol. Cell. Biol.* **2006**, *26*, 3955–3965. [CrossRef] [PubMed]

43. Meske, V.; Albert, F.; Ohm, T.G. Coupling of mammalian target of rapamycin with phosphoinositide 3-kinase signaling pathway regulates protein phosphatase 2A- and glycogen synthase kinase-3 -dependent phosphorylation of tau. *J. Biol. Chem.* **2008**, *283*, 100–109. [CrossRef] [PubMed]

44. Caccamo, A.; Maldonado, M.A.; Majumder, S.; Medina, D.X.; Holbein, W.; Magri, A.; Oddo, S. Naturally secreted amyloid-beta increases mammalian target of rapamycin (mTOR) activity via a PRAS40-mediated mechanism. *J. Biol. Chem.* **2011**, *286*, 8924–8932. [CrossRef]

45. Mizushima, N. The role of the Atg1/ULK1 complex in autophagy regulation. *Curr. Opin. Cell Biol.* **2010**, *22*, 132–139. [CrossRef]

46. Shirooie, S.; Nabavi, S.F.; Dehpour, A.R.; Belwal, T.; Habtemariam, S.; Arguelles, S.; Sureda, A.; Daglia, M.; Tomczyk, M.; Sobarzo-Sanchez, E.; et al. Targeting mTORs by omega-3 fatty acids: A possible novel therapeutic strategy for neurodegeneration? *Pharmacol. Res.* **2018**, *135*, 37–48. [CrossRef]

47. Caccamo, A.; Magri, A.; Medina, D.X.; Wisely, E.V.; Lopez-Aranda, M.F.; Silva, A.J.; Oddo, S. mTOR regulates tau phosphorylation and degradation: Implications for Alzheimer's disease and other tauopathies. *Aging Cell* **2013**, *12*, 370–380. [CrossRef]

48. Sarbassov, D.D.; Ali, S.M.; Sengupta, S.; Sheen, J.H.; Hsu, P.P.; Bagley, A.F.; Markhard, A.L.; Sabatini, D.M. Prolonged rapamycin treatment inhibits mTORC2 assembly and Akt/PKB. *Mol. Cell* **2006**, *22*, 159–168. [CrossRef] [PubMed]

49. Cammalleri, M.; Lutjens, R.; Berton, F.; King, A.R.; Simpson, C.; Francesconi, W.; Sanna, P.P. Time-restricted role for dendritic activation of the mTOR-p70S6K pathway in the induction of late-phase long-term potentiation in the CA1. *Proc. Natl. Acad. Sci. USA* **2003**, *100*, 14368–14373. [CrossRef] [PubMed]

50. Maiese, K.; Chong, Z.Z.; Shang, Y.C.; Wang, S. mTOR: On target for novel therapeutic strategies in the nervous system. *Trends Mol. Med.* **2013**, *19*, 51–60. [CrossRef] [PubMed]

51. Zemke, D.; Azhar, S.; Majid, A. The mTOR pathway as a potential target for the development of therapies against neurological disease. *Drug News Perspect.* **2007**, *20*, 495–499. [CrossRef]

52. Lee, J.H.; McBrayer, M.K.; Wolfe, D.M.; Haslett, L.J.; Kumar, A.; Sato, Y.; Lie, P.P.; Mohan, P.; Coffey, E.E.; Kompella, U.; Mitchell, C.H.; et al. Presenilin 1 Maintains Lysosomal Ca(2+) Homeostasis via TRPML1 by Regulating vATPase-Mediated Lysosome Acidification. *Cell Rep.* **2015**, *12*, 1430–1444. [CrossRef] [PubMed]

53. Yang, D.S.; Stavrides, P.; Mohan, P.S.; Kaushik, S.; Kumar, A.; Ohno, M.; Schmidt, S.D.; Wesson, D.W.; Bandyopadhyay, U.; Jiang, Y.; et al. Therapeutic effects of remediating autophagy failure in a mouse model of Alzheimer disease by enhancing lysosomal proteolysis. *Autophagy* **2011**, *7*, 788–789. [CrossRef] [PubMed]

54. Li, L.; Zhang, S.; Zhang, X.; Li, T.; Tang, Y.; Liu, H.; Yang, W.; Le, W. Autophagy enhancer carbamazepine alleviates memory deficits and cerebral amyloid-beta pathology in a mouse model of Alzheimer's disease. *Curr. Alzheimer Res.* **2013**, *10*, 433–441. [CrossRef] [PubMed]

55. Bordi, M.; Berg, M.J.; Mohan, P.S.; Peterhoff, C.M.; Alldred, M.J.; Che, S.; Ginsberg, S.D.; Nixon, R.A. Autophagy flux in CA1 neurons of Alzheimer hippocampus: Increased induction overburdens failing lysosomes to propel neuritic dystrophy. *Autophagy* **2016**, *12*, 2467–2483. [CrossRef]

56. Caccamo, A.; Majumder, S.; Richardson, A.; Strong, R.; Oddo, S. Molecular interplay between mammalian target of rapamycin (mTOR), amyloid-beta, and tau: Effects on cognitive impairments. *J. Biol. Chem.* **2010**, *285*, 13107–13120. [CrossRef] [PubMed]

57. Oh, W.J.; Jacinto, E. mTOR complex 2 signaling and functions. *Cell Cycle* **2011**, *10*, 2305–2316. [CrossRef]

58. Pierce, A.; Podlutskaya, N.; Halloran, J.J.; Hussong, S.A.; Lin, P.Y.; Burbank, R.; Hart, M.J.; Galvan, V. Over-expression of heat shock factor 1 phenocopies the effect of chronic inhibition of TOR by rapamycin and is sufficient to ameliorate Alzheimer's-like deficits in mice modeling the disease. *J. Neurochem.* **2013**, *124*, 880–893. [CrossRef] [PubMed]

59. Chen, T.J.; Wang, D.C.; Chen, S.S. Amyloid-beta interrupts the PI3K-Akt-mTOR signaling pathway that could be involved in brain-derived neurotrophic factor-induced Arc expression in rat cortical neurons. *J. Neurosci. Res.* **2009**, *87*, 2297–2307. [CrossRef] [PubMed]

60. Son, S.M.; Song, H.; Byun, J.; Park, K.S.; Jang, H.C.; Park, Y.J.; Mook-Jung, I. Altered APP processing in insulin-resistant conditions is mediated by autophagosome accumulation via the inhibition of mammalian target of rapamycin pathway. *Diabetes* **2012**, *61*, 3126–3138. [CrossRef] [PubMed]

61. Ryskalin, L.; Limanaqi, F.; Frati, A.; Busceti, C.L.; Fornai, F. mTOR-Related Brain Dysfunctions in Neuropsychiatric Disorders. *Int. J. Mol. Sci.* **2018**, *19*, 2226. [CrossRef]

62. Costa-Mattioli, M.; Monteggia, L.M. mTOR complexes in neurodevelopmental and neuropsychiatric disorders. *Nat. Neurosci.* **2013**, *16*, 1537–1543. [CrossRef]

63. Fan, Q.W.; Weiss, W.A. Inhibition of PI3K-Akt-mTOR signaling in glioblastoma by mTORC1/2 inhibitors. *Methods Mol. Biol.* **2012**, *821*, 349–359. [PubMed]

64. Ryskalin, L.; Lazzeri, G.; Flaibani, M.; Biagioni, F.; Gambardella, S.; Frati, A.; Fornai, F. mTOR-Dependent Cell Proliferation in the Brain. *BioMed Res. Int.* **2017**, *2017*, 7082696. [CrossRef] [PubMed]

65. Wong, M. Mammalian target of rapamycin (mTOR) pathways in neurological diseases. *Biomed. J.* **2013**, *36*, 40–50. [CrossRef] [PubMed]

66. Majumder, S.; Richardson, A.; Strong, R.; Oddo, S. Inducing autophagy by rapamycin before, but not after, the formation of plaques and tangles ameliorates cognitive deficits. *PLoS ONE* **2011**, *6*, e25416. [CrossRef] [PubMed]

67. Boland, B.; Kumar, A.; Lee, S.; Platt, F.M.; Wegiel, J.; Yu, W.H.; Nixon, R.A. Autophagy induction and autophagosome clearance in neurons: Relationship to autophagic pathology in Alzheimer's disease. *J. Neurosci.* **2008**, *28*, 6926–6937. [CrossRef]

68. Roberson, E.D.; Scearce-Levie, K.; Palop, J.J.; Yan, F.; Cheng, I.H.; Wu, T.; Gerstein, H.; Yu, G.Q.; Mucke, L. Reducing endogenous tau ameliorates amyloid beta-induced deficits in an Alzheimer's disease mouse model. *Science* **2007**, *316*, 750–754. [CrossRef]

69. Rapoport, M.; Dawson, H.N.; Binder, L.I.; Vitek, M.P.; Ferreira, A. tau is essential to beta -amyloid-induced neurotoxicity. *Proc. Natl. Acad. Sci. USA* **2002**, *99*, 6364–6369. [CrossRef] [PubMed]

70. Ittner, L.M.; Gotz, J. Amyloid-beta and tau–a toxic pas de deux in Alzheimer's disease. *Nat. Rev. Neurosci.* **2011**, *12*, 65–72. [CrossRef] [PubMed]

71. Silva, J.M.; Rodrigues, S.; Sampaio-Marques, B.; Gomes, P.; Neves-Carvalho, A.; Dioli, C.; Soares-Cunha, C.; Mazuik, B.F.; Takashima, A.; Ludovico, P.; et al. Dysregulation of autophagy and stress granule-related proteins in stress-driven tau pathology. *Cell Death Differ.* **2018**. [CrossRef] [PubMed]

72. Griffin, R.J.; Moloney, A.; Kelliher, M.; Johnston, J.A.; Ravid, R.; Dockery, P.; O'Connor, R.; O'Neill, C. Activation of Akt/PKB, increased phosphorylation of Akt substrates and loss and altered distribution of Akt and PTEN are features of Alzheimer's disease pathology. *J. Neurochem.* **2005**, *93*, 105–117. [CrossRef] [PubMed]

73. Pei, J.J.; Bjorkdahl, C.; Zhang, H.; Zhou, X.; Winblad, B. p70 S6 kinase and tau in Alzheimer's disease. *J. Alzheimers Dis.* **2008**, *14*, 385–392. [CrossRef]

74. Harrison, D.E.; Strong, R.; Sharp, Z.D.; Nelson, J.F.; Astle, C.M.; Flurkey, K.; Nadon, N.L.; Wilkinson, J.E.; Frenkel, K.; Carter, C.S.; et al. Rapamycin fed late in life extends lifespan in genetically heterogeneous mice. *Nature* **2009**, *460*, 392–395. [CrossRef]

75. Selman, C.; Tullet, J.M.; Wieser, D.; Irvine, E.; Lingard, S.J.; Choudhury, A.I.; Claret, M.; Al-Qassab, H.; Carmignac, D.; Ramadani, F.; et al. Ribosomal protein S6 kinase 1 signaling regulates mammalian life span. *Science* **2009**, *326*, 140–144. [CrossRef]

76. Khurana, V.; Lu, Y.; Steinhilb, M.L.; Oldham, S.; Shulman, J.M.; Feany, M.B. TOR-mediated cell-cycle activation causes neurodegeneration in a Drosophila tauopathy model. *Curr. Biol.* **2006**, *16*, 230–241. [CrossRef] [PubMed]

77. Cai, Z.; Chen, G.; He, W.; Xiao, M.; Yan, L.J. Activation of mTOR: A culprit of Alzheimer's disease? *Neuropsychiatr. Dis. Treat.* **2015**, *11*, 1015–1030. [CrossRef]

78. Spilman, P.; Podlutskaya, N.; Hart, M.J.; Debnath, J.; Gorostiza, O.; Bredesen, D.; Richardson, A.; Strong, R.; Galvan, V. Inhibition of mTOR by rapamycin abolishes cognitive deficits and reduces amyloid-beta levels in a mouse model of Alzheimer's disease. *PLoS ONE* **2010**, *5*, e9979. [CrossRef]

79. Delay, C.; Mandemakers, W.; Hebert, S.S. MicroRNAs in Alzheimer's disease. *Neurobiol. Dis.* **2012**, *46*, 285–290. [CrossRef]

80. Fan, J.; Kou, X.; Yang, Y.; Chen, N. MicroRNA-regulated proinflammatory cytokines in sarcopenia. *Med. Inflamm.* **2016**, *2016*, 1438686. [CrossRef]

81. Kumar, S.; Reddy, P.H. MicroRNA-455-3p as a Potential Biomarker for Alzheimer's Disease: An Update. *Front. Aging Neurosci.* **2018**, *11*, 41. [CrossRef]

82. Zhang, S.; Chen, N. Regulatory role of microRNAs in muscle atrophy during exercise intervention. *Int. J. Mol. Sci.* **2018**, *19*, 405. [CrossRef]

83. Müller, M.; Perrone, G.; Kuiperij, H.B.; Verbeek, M.M. Expression of five miRNA targets in hippocampus and cerebrospinal fluid in Alzheimer's disease. *Alzheimers Dement. J. Alzheimers Assoc.* **2012**, *8*, P273. [CrossRef]

84. Kapsimali, M.; Kloosterman, W.P.; de Bruijn, E.; Rosa, F.; Plasterk, R.H.; Wilson, S.W. MicroRNAs show a wide diversity of expression profiles in the developing and mature central nervous system. *Genome Biol.* **2007**, *8*, R173. [CrossRef] [PubMed]

85. Hackl, M.; Brunner, S.; Fortschegger, K.; Schreiner, C.; Micutkova, L.; Muck, C.; Laschober, G.T.; Lepperdinger, G.; Sampson, N.; Berger, P.; et al. miR-17, miR-19b, miR-20a, and miR-106a are downregulated in human aging. *Aging Cell* **2010**, *9*, 291–296. [CrossRef] [PubMed]

86. Ye, X.; Luo, H.; Chen, Y.; Wu, Q.; Xiong, Y.; Zhu, J.; Diao, Y.; Wu, Z.; Miao, J.; Wan, J. MicroRNAs 99b-5p/100-5p Regulated by Endoplasmic Reticulum Stress are Involved in Abeta-Induced Pathologies. *Front. Aging Neurosci.* **2015**, *7*, 210. [CrossRef] [PubMed]

87. Sun, D.; Lee, Y.S.; Malhotra, A.; Kim, H.K.; Matecic, M.; Evans, C.; Jensen, R.V.; Moskaluk, C.A.; Dutta, A. miR-99 family of MicroRNAs suppresses the expression of prostate-specific antigen and prostate cancer cell proliferation. *Cancer Res.* **2011**, *71*, 1313–1324. [CrossRef] [PubMed]

88. Li, X.J.; Luo, X.Q.; Han, B.W.; Duan, F.T.; Wei, P.P.; Chen, Y.Q. MicroRNA-100/99a, deregulated in acute lymphoblastic leukaemia, suppress proliferation and promote apoptosis by regulating the FKBP51 and IGF1R/mTOR signalling pathways. *Br. J. Cancer* **2013**, *109*, 2189–2198. [CrossRef] [PubMed]

89. Xu, C.; Zeng, Q.; Xu, W.; Jiao, L.; Chen, Y.; Zhang, Z.; Wu, C.; Jin, T.; Pan, A.; Wei, R.; et al. miRNA-100 inhibits human bladder urothelial carcinogenesis by directly targeting mTOR. *Mol. Cancer Ther.* **2013**, *12*, 207–219. [CrossRef]

90. Higaki, S.; Muramatsu, M.; Matsuda, A.; Matsumoto, K.; Satoh, J.I.; Michikawa, M.; Niida, S. Defensive effect of microRNA-200b/c against amyloid-beta peptide-induced toxicity in Alzheimer's disease models. *PLoS ONE* **2018**, *13*, e0196929. [CrossRef] [PubMed]

91. Liu, P.; Liu, P.; Wang, Z.; Fang, S.; Liu, Y.; Wang, J.; Liu, W.; Wang, N.; Chen, L.; Wang, J.; Zhang, H.; Wang, L. Inhibition of MicroRNA-96 Ameliorates Cognitive Impairment and Inactivation Autophagy Following Chronic Cerebral Hypoperfusion in the Rat. *Cell Physiol. Biochem.* **2018**, *49*, 78–86. [CrossRef] [PubMed]

92. Denk, J.; Boelmans, K.; Siegismund, C.; Lassner, D.; Arlt, S.; Jahn, H. MicroRNA Profiling of CSF Reveals Potential Biomarkers to Detect Alzheimer's Disease. *PLoS ONE* **2015**, *10*, e0126423. [CrossRef] [PubMed]

93. Gui, Y.; Liu, H.; Zhang, L.; Lv, W.; Hu, X. Altered microRNA profiles in cerebrospinal fluid exosome in Parkinson disease and Alzheimer disease. *Oncotarget* **2015**, *6*, 37043–37053. [CrossRef] [PubMed]

94. Kocerha, J.; Kauppinen, S.; Wahlestedt, C. microRNAs in CNS disorders. *Neuromol. Med.* **2009**, *11*, 162–172. [CrossRef] [PubMed]

95. Schratt, G. microRNAs at the synapse. *Nat. Rev. Neurosci.* **2009**, *10*, 842–849. [CrossRef] [PubMed]

96. Noren Hooten, N.; Abdelmohsen, K.; Gorospe, M.; Ejiogu, N.; Zonderman, A.B.; Evans, M.K. microRNA expression patterns reveal differential expression of target genes with age. *PLoS ONE* **2010**, *5*, e10724. [CrossRef]

97. Zhang, H.; Yang, H.; Zhang, C.; Jing, Y.; Wang, C.; Liu, C.; Zhang, R.; Wang, J.; Zhang, J.; Zen, K.; et al. Investigation of microRNA expression in human serum during the aging process. *J. Gerontol. A Biol. Sci. Med. Sci.* **2015**, *70*, 102–109. [CrossRef]

98. Wang, W.X.; Rajeev, B.W.; Stromberg, A.J.; Ren, N.; Tang, G.; Huang, Q.; Rigoutsos, I.; Nelson, P.T. The expression of microRNA miR-107 decreases early in Alzheimer's disease and may accelerate disease progression through regulation of beta-site amyloid precursor protein-cleaving enzyme 1. *J. Neurosci.* **2008**, *28*, 1213–1223. [CrossRef] [PubMed]

99. Smith, P.; Al Hashimi, A.; Girard, J.; Delay, C.; Hebert, S.S. In vivo regulation of amyloid precursor protein neuronal splicing by microRNAs. *J. Neurochem.* **2011**, *116*, 240–247. [CrossRef]

100. Liu, W.; Liu, C.; Zhu, J.; Shu, P.; Yin, B.; Gong, Y.; Qiang, B.; Yuan, J.; Peng, X. MicroRNA-16 targets amyloid precursor protein to potentially modulate Alzheimer's-associated pathogenesis in SAMP8 mice. *Neurobiol. Aging* **2012**, *33*, 522–534. [CrossRef]

101. Hebert, S.S.; Horre, K.; Nicolai, L.; Bergmans, B.; Papadopoulou, A.S.; Delacourte, A.; De Strooper, B. MicroRNA regulation of Alzheimer's Amyloid precursor protein expression. *Neurobiol. Dis.* **2009**, *33*, 422–428. [CrossRef]

102. Kumar, S.; Vijayan, M.; Reddy, P.H. MicroRNA-455-3p as a potential peripheral biomarker for Alzheimer's disease. *Hum. Mol. Genet.* **2017**, *26*, 3808–3822. [CrossRef]

103. Lee, S.T.; Chu, K.; Jung, K.H.; Kim, J.H.; Huh, J.Y.; Yoon, H.; Park, D.K.; Lim, J.Y.; Kim, J.M.; Jeon, D.; et al. miR-206 regulates brain-derived neurotrophic factor in Alzheimer disease model. *Ann. Neurol.* **2012**, *72*, 269–277. [CrossRef]

104. Schafer, D. No old man ever forgot where he buried his treasure: Concepts of cognitive impairment in old age circa 1700. *J. Am. Geriatr. Soc.* **2005**, *53*, 2023–2027. [CrossRef]

105. Williams, A.F.; Gagnon, J. Neuronal cell Thy-1 glycoprotein: Homology with immunoglobulin. *Science* **1982**, *216*, 696–703. [CrossRef]

106. Mucke, L.; Masliah, E.; Yu, G.Q.; Mallory, M.; Rockenstein, E.M.; Tatsuno, G.; Hu, K.; Kholodenko, D.; Johnson-Wood, K.; McConlogue, L. High-level neuronal expression of abeta 1-42 in wild-type human amyloid protein precursor transgenic mice: Synaptotoxicity without plaque formation. *J. Neurosci.* **2000**, *20*, 4050–4058. [CrossRef] [PubMed]

107. Buttini, M.; Yu, G.Q.; Shockley, K.; Huang, Y.; Jones, B.; Masliah, E.; Mallory, M.; Yeo, T.; Longo, F.M.; Mucke, L. Modulation of Alzheimer-like synaptic and cholinergic deficits in transgenic mice by human apolipoprotein E depends on isoform, aging, and overexpression of amyloid beta peptides but not on plaque formation. *J. Neurosci.* **2002**, *22*, 10539–10548. [CrossRef] [PubMed]

108. Raber, J.; Wong, D.; Yu, G.Q.; Buttini, M.; Mahley, R.W.; Pitas, R.E.; Mucke, L. Apolipoprotein E and cognitive performance. *Nature* **2000**, *404*, 352–354. [CrossRef] [PubMed]

109. Churchill, J.D.; Galvez, R.; Colcombe, S.; Swain, R.A.; Kramer, A.F.; Greenough, W.T. Exercise, experience and the aging brain. *Neurobiol. Aging* **2002**, *23*, 941–955. [CrossRef]

110. Heyn, P.; Abreu, B.C.; Ottenbacher, K.J. The effects of exercise training on elderly persons with cognitive impairment and dementia: A meta-analysis. *Arch. Phys. Med. Rehabil.* **2004**, *85*, 1694–1704. [CrossRef]

111. Groot, C.; Hooghiemstra, A.M.; Raijmakers, P.G.; van Berckel, B.N.; Scheltens, P.; Scherder, E.J.; van der Flier, W.M.; Ossenkoppele, R. The effect of physical activity on cognitive function in patients with dementia: A meta-analysis of randomized control trials. *Ageing Res. Rev.* **2016**, *25*, 13–23. [CrossRef]

112. Yuede, C.M.; Zimmerman, S.D.; Dong, H.; Kling, M.J.; Bero, A.W.; Holtzman, D.M.; Timson, B.F.; Csernansky, J.G. Effects of voluntary and forced exercise on plaque deposition, hippocampal volume, and behavior in the Tg2576 mouse model of Alzheimer's disease. *Neurobiol. Dis.* **2009**, *35*, 426–432. [CrossRef] [PubMed]

113. Nichol, K.; Deeny, S.P.; Seif, J.; Camaclang, K.; Cotman, C.W. Exercise improves cognition and hippocampal plasticity in APOE epsilon4 mice. *Alzheimers Dement.* **2009**, *5*, 287–294. [CrossRef]

114. Adlard, P.A.; Perreau, V.M.; Pop, V.; Cotman, C.W. Voluntary exercise decreases amyloid load in a transgenic model of Alzheimer's disease. *J. Neurosci.* **2005**, *25*, 4217–4221. [CrossRef]

115. Nichol, K.E.; Parachikova, A.I.; Cotman, C.W. Three weeks of running wheel exposure improves cognitive performance in the aged Tg2576 mouse. *Behav. Brain Res.* **2007**, *184*, 124–132. [CrossRef]

116. Tapia-Rojas, C.; Aranguiz, F.; Varela-Nallar, L.; Inestrosa, N.C. Voluntary Running Attenuates Memory Loss, Decreases Neuropathological Changes and Induces Neurogenesis in a Mouse Model of Alzheimer's Disease. *Brain Pathol.* **2016**, *26*, 62–74. [CrossRef]

117. Erickson, K.I.; Gildengers, A.G.; Butters, M.A. Physical activity and brain plasticity in late adulthood. *Dialogues Clin. Neurosci.* **2013**, *15*, 99–108.

118. Colcombe, S.; Kramer, A.F. Fitness effects on the cognitive function of older adults: A meta-analytic study. *Psychol. Sci.* **2003**, *14*, 125–130. [CrossRef] [PubMed]

119. Mirochnic, S.; Wolf, S.; Staufenbiel, M.; Kempermann, G. Age effects on the regulation of adult hippocampal neurogenesis by physical activity and environmental enrichment in the APP23 mouse model of Alzheimer disease. *Hippocampus* **2009**, *19*, 1008–1018. [CrossRef] [PubMed]

120. Patten, A.R.; Yau, S.Y.; Fontaine, C.J.; Meconi, A.; Wortman, R.C.; Christie, B.R. The Benefits of Exercise on Structural and Functional Plasticity in the Rodent Hippocampus of Different Disease Models. *Brain Plast.* **2015**, *1*, 97–127. [CrossRef] [PubMed]

121. Barry, A.E.; Klyubin, I.; Mc Donald, J.M.; Mably, A.J.; Farrell, M.A.; Scott, M.; Walsh, D.M.; Rowan, M.J. Alzheimer's disease brain-derived amyloid-beta-mediated inhibition of LTP in vivo is prevented by immunotargeting cellular prion protein. *J. Neurosci.* **2011**, *31*, 7259–7263. [CrossRef] [PubMed]

122. Jo, J.; Whitcomb, D.J.; Olsen, K.M.; Kerrigan, T.L.; Lo, S.C.; Bru-Mercier, G.; Dickinson, B.; Scullion, S.; Sheng, M.; Collingridge, G.; et al. Abeta(1-42) inhibition of LTP is mediated by a signaling pathway involving caspase-3, Akt1 and GSK-3beta. *Nat. Neurosci.* **2011**, *14*, 545–547. [CrossRef] [PubMed]

123. O'Callaghan, R.M.; Ohle, R.; Kelly, A.M. The effects of forced exercise on hippocampal plasticity in the rat: A comparison of LTP, spatial- and non-spatial learning. *Behav. Brain Res.* **2007**, *176*, 362–366. [CrossRef]

124. Farmer, J.; Zhao, X.; van Praag, H.; Wodtke, K.; Gage, F.H.; Christie, B.R. Effects of voluntary exercise on synaptic plasticity and gene expression in the dentate gyrus of adult male Sprague-Dawley rats in vivo. *Neuroscience* **2004**, *124*, 71–79. [CrossRef] [PubMed]

125. van Praag, H.; Christie, B.R.; Sejnowski, T.J.; Gage, F.H. Running enhances neurogenesis, learning, and long-term potentiation in mice. *Proc. Natl. Acad. Sci. USA* **1999**, *96*, 13427–13431. [CrossRef]

126. Garcia-Mesa, Y.; Lopez-Ramos, J.C.; Gimenez-Llort, L.; Revilla, S.; Guerra, R.; Gruart, A.; Laferla, F.M.; Cristofol, R.; Delgado-Garcia, J.M.; Sanfeliu, C. Physical exercise protects against Alzheimer's disease in 3xTg-AD mice. *J. Alzheimers Dis.* **2011**, *24*, 421–454. [CrossRef]

127. Kumar, A.; Rani, A.; Tchigranova, O.; Lee, W.H.; Foster, T.C. Influence of late-life exposure to environmental enrichment or exercise on hippocampal function and CA1 senescent physiology. *Neurobiol. Aging* **2012**, *33*, 828.e1–828.e17. [CrossRef]

128. Dao, A.T.; Zagaar, M.A.; Levine, A.T.; Salim, S.; Eriksen, J.L.; Alkadhi, K.A. Treadmill exercise prevents learning and memory impairment in Alzheimer's disease-like pathology. *Curr. Alzheimer Res.* **2013**, *10*, 507–515. [CrossRef]

129. Nielsen, S.; Akerstrom, T.; Rinnov, A.; Yfanti, C.; Scheele, C.; Pedersen, B.K.; Laye, M.J. The miRNA plasma signature in response to acute aerobic exercise and endurance training. *PLoS ONE* **2014**, *9*, e87308. [CrossRef] [PubMed]

130. Wu, X.D.; Zeng, K.; Liu, W.L.; Gao, Y.G.; Gong, C.S.; Zhang, C.X.; Chen, Y.Q. Effect of aerobic exercise on miRNA-TLR4 signaling in atherosclerosis. *Int. J. Sports Med.* **2014**, *35*, 344–350. [CrossRef]

131. Fernandes, T.; Hashimoto, N.Y.; Magalhaes, F.C.; Fernandes, F.B.; Casarini, D.E.; Carmona, A.K.; Krieger, J.E.; Phillips, M.I.; Oliveira, E.M. Aerobic exercise training-induced left ventricular hypertrophy involves regulatory MicroRNAs, decreased angiotensin-converting enzyme-angiotensin ii, and synergistic regulation of angiotensin-converting enzyme 2-angiotensin (1-7). *Hypertension* **2011**, *58*, 182–189. [CrossRef] [PubMed]

132. Li, N.; Bates, D.J.; An, J.; Terry, D.A.; Wang, E. Upregulation of key microRNAs, and inverse downregulation of their predicted oxidative phosphorylation target genes, during aging in mouse brain. *Neurobiol. Aging* **2011**, *32*, 944–955. [CrossRef]

133. Larson, E.B.; Wang, L.; Bowen, J.D.; McCormick, W.C.; Teri, L.; Crane, P.; Kukull, W. Exercise is associated with reduced risk for incident dementia among persons 65 years of age and older. *Ann. Intern. Med.* **2006**, *144*, 73–81. [CrossRef] [PubMed]

134. Deeny, S.P.; Poeppel, D.; Zimmerman, J.B.; Roth, S.M.; Brandauer, J.; Witkowski, S.; Hearn, J.W.; Ludlow, A.T.; Contreras-Vidal, J.L.; Brandt, J.; et al. Exercise, APOE, and working memory: MEG and behavioral evidence for benefit of exercise in epsilon4 carriers. *Biol. Psychol.* **2008**, *78*, 179–187. [CrossRef]

135. Etnier, J.L.; Caselli, R.J.; Reiman, E.M.; Alexander, G.E.; Sibley, B.A.; Tessier, D.; McLemore, E.C. Cognitive performance in older women relative to ApoE-epsilon4 genotype and aerobic fitness. *Med. Sci. Sports Exerc.* **2007**, *39*, 199–207. [CrossRef]

136. Rovio, S.; Kareholt, I.; Helkala, E.L.; Viitanen, M.; Winblad, B.; Tuomilehto, J.; Soininen, H.; Nissinen, A.; Kivipelto, M. Leisure-time physical activity at midlife and the risk of dementia and Alzheimer's disease. *Lancet Neurol.* **2005**, *4*, 705–711. [CrossRef]

137. Schuit, A.J.; Feskens, E.J.; Launer, L.J.; Kromhout, D. Physical activity and cognitive decline, the role of the apolipoprotein e4 allele. *Med. Sci. Sports Exerc.* **2001**, *33*, 772–777. [CrossRef] [PubMed]

138. Laurin, D.; Verreault, R.; Lindsay, J.; MacPherson, K.; Rockwood, K. Physical activity and risk of cognitive impairment and dementia in elderly persons. *Arch. Neurol.* **2001**, *58*, 498–504. [CrossRef] [PubMed]

139. Verghese, J.; Lipton, R.B.; Katz, M.J.; Hall, C.B.; Derby, C.A.; Kuslansky, G.; Ambrose, A.F.; Sliwinski, M.; Buschke, H. Leisure activities and the risk of dementia in the elderly. *N. Engl. J. Med.* **2003**, *348*, 2508–2516. [CrossRef]

140. Akbaraly, T.N.; Portet, F.; Fustinoni, S.; Dartigues, J.F.; Artero, S.; Rouaud, O.; Touchon, J.; Ritchie, K.; Berr, C. Leisure activities and the risk of dementia in the elderly: Results from the Three-City Study. *Neurology* **2009**, *73*, 854–861. [CrossRef]

141. Cai, Z.; Yan, L.J.; Li, K.; Quazi, S.H.; Zhao, B. Roles of AMP-activated protein kinase in Alzheimer's disease. *Neuromol. Med.* **2012**, *14*, 1–14. [CrossRef] [PubMed]

142. O'Neill, C.; Kiely, A.P.; Coakley, M.F.; Manning, S.; Long-Smith, C.M. Insulin and IGF-1 signalling: Longevity, protein homoeostasis and Alzheimer's disease. *Biochem. Soc. Trans.* **2012**, *40*, 721–727. [CrossRef] [PubMed]

143. Kang, E.B.; Cho, J.Y. Effect of treadmill exercise on PI3K/AKT/mTOR, autophagy, and tau hyperphosphorylation in the cerebral cortex of NSE/htau23 transgenic mice. *J. Exerc. Nutr. Biochem.* **2015**, *19*, 199–209. [CrossRef]

144. Tramutola, A.; Triplett, J.C.; Di Domenico, F.; Niedowicz, D.M.; Murphy, M.P.; Coccia, R.; Perluigi, M.; Butterfield, D.A. Alteration of mTOR signaling occurs early in the progression of Alzheimer disease (AD): Analysis of brain from subjects with pre-clinical AD, amnestic mild cognitive impairment and late-stage AD. *J. Neurochem.* **2015**, *133*, 739–749. [CrossRef] [PubMed]

145. Li, S.Y.; Fang, C.X.; Aberle, N.S.; Ren, B.H.; Ceylan-Isik, A.F.; Ren, J. Inhibition of PI-3 kinase/Akt/mTOR, but not calcineurin signaling, reverses insulin-like growth factor I-induced protection against glucose toxicity in cardiomyocyte contractile function. *J. Endocrinol.* **2005**, *186*, 491–503. [CrossRef] [PubMed]

146. Li, X.; Alafuzoff, I.; Soininen, H.; Winblad, B.; Pei, J.J. Levels of mTOR and its downstream targets 4E-BP1, eEF2, and eEF2 kinase in relationships with tau in Alzheimer's disease brain. *FEBS J.* **2005**, *272*, 4211–4220. [CrossRef] [PubMed]

147. Yates, S.C.; Zafar, A.; Hubbard, P.; Nagy, S.; Durant, S.; Bicknell, R.; Wilcock, G.; Christie, S.; Esiri, M.M.; Smith, A.D.; Nagy, Z. Dysfunction of the mTOR pathway is a risk factor for Alzheimer's disease. *Acta Neuropathol. Commun.* **2013**, *1*, 3. [CrossRef] [PubMed]

148. Um, H.S.; Kang, E.B.; Koo, J.H.; Kim, H.T.; Jin, L.; Kim, E.J.; Yang, C.H.; An, G.Y.; Cho, I.H.; Cho, J.Y. Treadmill exercise represses neuronal cell death in an aged transgenic mouse model of Alzheimer's disease. *Neurosci. Res.* **2011**, *69*, 161–173. [CrossRef]

149. Jeong, J.H.; Kang, E.B. Effects of treadmill exercise on PI3K/AKT/GSK-3beta pathway and tau protein in high-fat diet-fed rats. *J. Exerc. Nutr. Biochem.* **2018**, *22*, 9–14. [CrossRef]

150. Jin, X.; Townley, R.; Shapiro, L. Structural insight into AMPK regulation: ADP comes into play. *Structure* **2007**, *15*, 1285–1295. [CrossRef]

151. Vingtdeux, V.; Davies, P.; Dickson, D.W.; Marambaud, P. AMPK is abnormally activated in tangle- and pre-tangle-bearing neurons in Alzheimer's disease and other tauopathies. *Acta Neuropathol.* **2011**, *121*, 337–349. [CrossRef]

152. Ju, T.C.; Chen, H.M.; Lin, J.T.; Chang, C.P.; Chang, W.C.; Kang, J.J.; Sun, C.P.; Tao, M.H.; Tu, P.H.; Chang, C.; et al. Nuclear translocation of AMPK-alpha1 potentiates striatal neurodegeneration in Huntington's disease. *J. Cell Biol.* **2011**, *194*, 209–227. [CrossRef] [PubMed]

153. Vingtdeux, V.; Chandakkar, P.; Zhao, H.; d'Abramo, C.; Davies, P.; Marambaud, P. Novel synthetic small-molecule activators of AMPK as enhancers of autophagy and amyloid-beta peptide degradation. *FASEB J.* **2011**, *25*, 219–231. [CrossRef] [PubMed]

154. Greco, S.J.; Sarkar, S.; Johnston, J.M.; Tezapsidis, N. Leptin regulates tau phosphorylation and amyloid through AMPK in neuronal cells. *Biochem. Biophys. Res. Commun.* **2009**, *380*, 98–104. [CrossRef]

155. Won, J.S.; Im, Y.B.; Kim, J.; Singh, A.K.; Singh, I. Involvement of AMP-activated-protein-kinase (AMPK) in neuronal amyloidogenesis. *Biochem. Biophys. Res. Commun.* **2010**, *399*, 487–491. [CrossRef] [PubMed]

156. Thornton, C.; Bright, N.J.; Sastre, M.; Muckett, P.J.; Carling, D. AMP-activated protein kinase (AMPK) is a tau kinase, activated in response to amyloid beta-peptide exposure. *Biochem. J.* **2011**, *434*, 503–512. [CrossRef] [PubMed]

157. Yoshida, H.; Goedert, M. Phosphorylation of microtubule-associated protein tau by AMPK-related kinases. *J. Neurochem.* **2012**, *120*, 165–176. [CrossRef] [PubMed]

158. Rönnemaa, E.; Zethelius, B.; Sundelöf, J.; Sundström, J.; Degerman-Gunnarsson, M.; Berne, C.; Lannfelt, L.; Kilander, L. Impaired insulin secretion increases the risk of Alzheimer disease. *Neurology* **2008**, *71*, 1065–1071. [CrossRef] [PubMed]

159. Gibas, M.K.; Gibas, K.J. Induced and controlled dietary ketosis as a regulator of obesity and metabolic syndrome pathologies. *Diabetes Metab. Syndr.* **2017**, *11*, S385–S390. [CrossRef]

160. Halikas, A.; Gibas, K.J. AMPK induced memory improvements in the diabetic population: A Case Study. *Diabetes Metab. Syndr.* **2018**, *12*, 1141–1146. [CrossRef]

161. Thompson, H.J.; Jiang, W.; Zhu, Z. Candidate mechanisms accounting for effects of physical activity on breast carcinogenesis. *IUBMB Life* **2009**, *61*, 895–901. [CrossRef] [PubMed]

162. Petersen, A.M.; Pedersen, B.K. The anti-inflammatory effect of exercise. *J. Appl. Physiol.* **2005**, *98*, 1154–1162. [CrossRef]

163. Dethlefsen, C.; Lillelund, C.; Midtgaard, J.; Andersen, C.; Pedersen, B.K.; Christensen, J.F.; Hojman, P. Exercise regulates breast cancer cell viability: Systemic training adaptations versus acute exercise responses. *Breast Cancer Res. Treat.* **2016**, *159*, 469–479. [CrossRef] [PubMed]

164. Gomez-Pinilla, F.; Vaynman, S.; Ying, Z. Brain-derived neurotrophic factor functions as a metabotrophin to mediate the effects of exercise on cognition. *Eur. J. Neurosci.* **2008**, *28*, 2278–2287. [CrossRef] [PubMed]

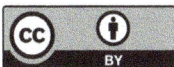

International Journal of
Molecular Sciences

MDPI

Review

mTORC Inhibitors as Broad-Spectrum Therapeutics for Age-Related Diseases

Hannah E. Walters and Lynne S. Cox *

Department of Biochemistry, University of Oxford, South Parks Road, Oxford OX1 3QU, UK;
hannah.walters@trinity.ox.ac.uk
* Correspondence: lynne.cox@bioch.ox.ac.uk

Received: 4 June 2018; Accepted: 30 July 2018; Published: 8 August 2018

Abstract: Chronological age represents the greatest risk factor for many life-threatening diseases, including neurodegeneration, cancer, and cardiovascular disease; ageing also increases susceptibility to infectious disease. Current efforts to tackle individual diseases may have little impact on the overall healthspan of older individuals, who would still be vulnerable to other age-related pathologies. However, recent progress in ageing research has highlighted the accumulation of senescent cells with chronological age as a probable underlying cause of pathological ageing. Cellular senescence is an essentially irreversible proliferation arrest mechanism that has important roles in development, wound healing, and preventing cancer, but it may limit tissue function and cause widespread inflammation with age. The serine/threonine kinase mTOR (mechanistic target of rapamycin) is a regulatory nexus that is heavily implicated in both ageing and senescence. Excitingly, a growing body of research has highlighted rapamycin and other mTOR inhibitors as promising treatments for a broad spectrum of age-related pathologies, including neurodegeneration, cancer, immunosenescence, osteoporosis, rheumatoid arthritis, age-related blindness, diabetic nephropathy, muscular dystrophy, and cardiovascular disease. In this review, we assess the use of mTOR inhibitors to treat age-related pathologies, discuss possible molecular mechanisms of action where evidence is available, and consider strategies to minimize undesirable side effects. We also emphasize the urgent need for reliable, non-invasive biomarkers of senescence and biological ageing to better monitor the efficacy of any healthy ageing therapy.

Keywords: mTOR; mTORC1; mTORC2; rapamycin; rapalogues; rapalogs; mTOR inhibitors; senescence; ageing; aging; cancer; neurodegeneration; immunosenescence; senolytics; biomarkers

1. Introduction

The greatest risk factor for all major life-threatening diseases, including cancer, neurodegeneration, and cardiovascular disease is age. Current therapies that target each of these age-related diseases (ARD) individually have had limited success, and a cure for one specific ARD may not greatly extend healthy lifespan, as elderly patients would still be vulnerable to other ARDs. However, mounting evidence suggests that it may be possible to develop broad-spectrum treatments for the diseases of old age by targeting the underlying biological mechanisms driving ageing and its associated pathologies. Indeed, several consistent hallmarks of ageing have been identified, including telomere attrition, epigenetic dysregulation, altered proteostasis, decreased autophagy, mitochondrial dysfunction, and increased DNA damage [1]. All of these processes contribute to the onset of cell senescence, a core driver of ageing, as demonstrated by improved health and extended lifespan of middle-aged mice upon the removal of senescent cells [2]. Furthermore, it is also possible that other hallmarks of ageing, including stem cell depletion and remodelling of the extracellular matrix [1], are in fact consequences of cell senescence.

1.1. Senescence

Cellular senescence is a programme of essentially permanent proliferative arrest, induced by stresses including replicative exhaustion, DNA damage, oncogene signalling, ER stress, and imbalances in ribosome biogenesis [3]. At least in vitro, senescent cells show greatly enlarged cell size, altered morphology, accumulation of lipid droplets and lipofuscin-type pigments [4], and prominent actin stress fibres. Mitochondrial load increases in senescence, possibly to compensate for chronically damaged mitochondria, and lysosomal stress is evident with dyes such as senescence-associated β-galactosidase (SA-β-gal) [5]. Senescent cells exhibit chronically elevated levels of DNA damage response proteins including 53BP1 and γH2AX indicating poor DNA repair capacity, while there is also marked restructuring of the epigenome, such that CpG methylation patterns can be used as an epigenetic clock to determine biological age [6]. At the biochemical level, activation of tumour suppressor proteins p53 and/or p16^{CDKN2}, together with cyclin-dependent kinase inhibitor p21^{CDKN1}, leads to cell cycle arrest and the cessation of proliferation that is characteristic of senescent cells, together with resistance to apoptosis.

While the original evolutionary role of senescence may lie in development [7], wound healing [8], or as a barrier to viral infection [9], it also provides a failsafe mechanism against proliferation of tumorigenic or aged cells [10]. However, this can be detrimental to tissue integrity, as such cells can no longer contribute to wound healing or the cell turnover necessary for tissue maintenance. Moreover, senescent cells do not simply exist as passive but ineffective components of a tissue: instead, they actively alter their microenvironment through a secretory programme termed the SASP (senescence-associated secretory phenotype) [11]. This pro-inflammatory programme comprising cytokines, chemokines, growth factors, and matrix-remodelling enzymes alerts immune cells to the presence of senescent cells, which in younger organisms is thought to promote immune clearance [12]. However, with increasing age comes both an increasingly unbalanced and dysfunctional immune system, and an increased rate of senescence onset via chronic exposure to extrinsic and intrinsic damaging agents, gradual loss of homeostasis, and progressive telomere erosion. Together, these cause the accumulation of senescent cells, observed in various tissues with chronological age [5,13,14]. Pleiotropic SASP signalling also induces paracrine senescence in neighbouring cells, amplifying the senescent cell burden, and possibly driving the chronic and sterile inflammation observed in old age—a contributing factor to the development of many ARDs. Components of the SASP also participate in paracrine pro-tumorigenic signalling (e.g., IL-6, IL-8, MMP-3), promoting tumour formation and progression [11]. Several notable experiments have provided evidence for the causative role of cellular senescence in organismal ageing and age-related pathology; most convincingly, the clearance of p16-expressing senescent cells in vivo rejuvenates naturally aged mice, improving health, and extending lifespan [2].

1.2. mTOR Signalling in Senescence and Ageing

The serine/threonine kinase mTOR is a major regulatory nexus that integrates signals, including levels of glucose, amino acids, oxygen, growth factors, and hormones to direct cell growth and proliferation under suitable conditions. mTOR is the functional enzyme within two distinct complexes—mTORC1 and mTORC2—where it associates with several other proteins that are either distinct to each complex (e.g., Raptor/Rictor) or present in both (e.g., Deptor, mLST8 (mammalian lethal with SEC13 protein 8), see Table 1). A novel mTOR complex containing GIT1 (GPCR kinase-interacting protein 1), but lacking Raptor and Rictor, has been identified by proteomic analysis of neural stem cells and astrocytes [15], highlighting the possible variation in mTOR complex composition between somatic tissues.

mTORC1 regulates pathways central to cell growth, proliferation, survival, motility, autophagy, and protein synthesis, whilst mTORC2 has a role in regulating actin organization as well as metabolic control [16]. mTORC1 is activated by recruitment to the lysosome through the action of Rag GTPases and regulators, such as the late endosomal/lysosomal adaptor and MAPK and mTOR activator (LAMTOR/Ragulator), whereas mTORC2 is ribosomally-associated on activation by insulin-signalling, mediated through IGFR (insulin-like growth factor receptor) and IRS1/2 (insulin receptor substrate) [16], though localisation at mitochondria, the plasma membrane, ER, and lysosomes has also been reported [17] (Table 2). There is significant cross-talk between the two complexes through various positive and negative feedback loops (particularly through the kinase Akt/PKB (protein kinase B)) [16], and possibly also through competition for FKBP (FK506 binding protein) subunits [18]. Recent research using unbiased phosphoproteomics has expanded the list of known direct mTOR substrates [19–21] and the mTOR signalling network has been reviewed extensively elsewhere [16,22,23]. Examples of key regulators, phosphorylation targets, and biochemical and biological outcomes for each complex are summarized in Table 2.

Table 1. mTOR complex subunits.

Contribution to Complex	mTORC1	mTORC2
core	mTOR mLST8/Gβ3 Deptor Tti1/Tel2	mTOR mLST8/Gβ3 Deptor Tti1/Tel2
complex-specific	Raptor PRAS40	Rictor mSIN1 Protor1/2

Table 2. Activities and localization of mTORC1 and mTORC2. Note that only a small subset of targets and modulators is shown. Proteins are named using standard nomenclature; for full gene names, please refer to the list of abbreviations.

	mTORC1	mTORC2
localization when active	lysosome	ribosome, plasma membrane, mitochondria, endoplasmic reticulum, lysosome
targets activated	S6K^{T389}, HIF 1α, GSK3, SOD1, Grb10, eIF4G, Acinus L, eEF2, IMP2	SGK1, PKC, paxillin, Rho GTPases, Akt^{S473}, IGFR, PDK1
targets inhibited	4EBP1/2, Maf1, Lipin-1, ULK1, ATG13, TFEB, DAP1, LARP1	FBW8
activated by	insulin, growth factors, Rheb, Rag, Akt, amino acids, high O$_2$, cytokines, TNFα, IkkB	PI3K, growth factors including IGFR, Akt (on mSIN1), membrane tension, ROS, ATM/ATR
inhibited by	AMPK, TSC1/2 (via Rheb inactivation), low O$_2$, low ATP, low amino acids	S6K on both Rictor and mSIN1 TSC1/2 (via Rheb inactivation)
biochemical outcomes of activation	protein, nucleotide, lipid and mitochondrial biosynthesis; inhibition of autophagy	actin reorganization, lipid biosynthesis
overall outcomes of activation	cell growth (increase in volume and biomass) cell proliferation suppression of oxidative damage	cell size (surface area increase) cell shape (cytoskeletal changes) survival under oxidative stresscell cycle progression metabolic control

The involvement of mTORC signalling in ageing is supported by a large body of experimental evidence. Mutations in TOR have been shown to increase the lifespan of yeast [24], *C. elegans* [25–27], and Drosophila [28]. Furthermore, deletion of S6K1 (ribosomal S6 protein kinase 1), which is a downstream target of mTOR, increases lifespan in female mice. Further, reduced mTOR signalling increases lifespan and reduces age-related pathologies, including motor dysfunction and loss of insulin sensitivity [29]. Notably, such findings contrast with other reports that chronic mTORC inhibition induces diabetes [30]. This finding has been attributed to differential effects on mTORC1 versus mTORC2, though in some instances loss of mTORC2 signalling also increases lifespan and improves health. For instance, in the nematode worm, reduction in mTORC2 signalling by RNAi depletion of Rictor can increase the lifespan under conditions of stress (high temperature) or high-quality food, whereas the opposite is seen at lower temperatures and on a less rich food source [31].

mTOR signalling is highly significant in senescence as well as in ageing. Notably, the proliferative arrest that characterizes cellular senescence is not accompanied by a down-regulation of growth signalling. In fact, mTOR signalling is constitutively active in senescence, resulting from replicative exhaustion, oncogene activation, and other stresses [32], and it may drive the process of geroconversion [33] i.e., the shift from proliferation to senescence without inhibition of growth. Inhibition of mTOR in cells approaching senescence reverses many of the characteristic senescence phenotypes [34] supporting a role for mTOR in driving senescence. Rather than being dramatically increased, however, mTOR signalling may instead be dysregulated in senescence; mTORC1 activity persists despite the removal of serum and amino acids in senescent but not proliferating fibroblasts, indicating constitutive activation that may be attributable to depolarization of the senescent cell plasma membrane [32].

Both the molecular mechanisms behind healthspan and lifespan extension afforded by mTOR inhibition, and the roles of mTOR signalling in senescence are likely to be multi-factorial, as mTOR regulates a multitude of downstream signalling events (Table 2 and Figure 1). Below, we consider major biochemical pathways that are important in ageing and cell senescence that are regulated by mTORC signalling, and that may therefore be amenable to modulation by mTORC inhibitors.

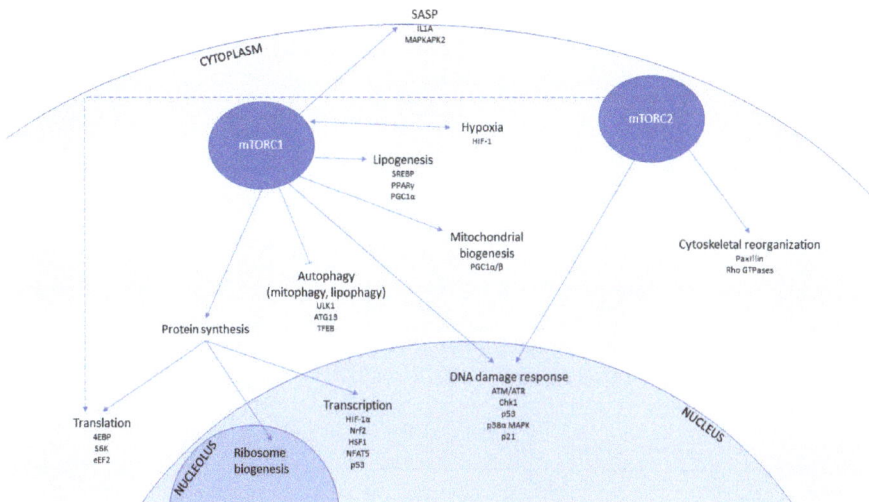

Figure 1. Summary of pathways targeted by mTOR signalling which are implicated in modulation of senescence and ageing. Arrows indicate that mTORC activity positively regulates the process, while bars indicate inhibition.

1.3. mTOR-Associated Pathways That Contribute to Senescence and Ageing

1.3.1. Transcription

mTOR signalling from both complexes can influence gene expression through interaction with a variety of transcription factors, including many involved in stress responses. For example, mTORC1 can modulate both the translational and the transcriptional activity of the hypoxia response factor HIF-1α during normoxia and hypoxia, respectively [35,36]. Furthermore, mTORC1 regulates the ROS-responsive transcription factor Nrf2 [37], as well as the heat-shock transcription factor HSF1 [38] and the osmotic stress transcription factor NFAT5 [39]. The effects of mTOR in modulating p53-dependent transcription are described in Section 1.3.7 (DNA damage response), below.

1.3.2. Protein Translation

Protein translation occurs within the ribosome, a large molecular factory that is composed of functional RNAs and proteins. Ribosomal biogenesis (and hence subsequent protein synthesis) requires the coordination of transcription of ribosomal RNAs (rRNA) within the nucleolus by RNA polymerase I, protein-encoding messenger RNAs (mRNA) by RNA polymerase II and transfer RNAs (tRNA) and a further 5S ribosomal RNA by RNA polymerase III, and is positively regulated by mTORC1 signalling at multiple stages [40]. Assembly of the ribosome from ribosomal RNAs and proteins also occurs within the nucleolus. Interestingly, nucleoli are enlarged in premature ageing [41], while small nucleoli are associated with longevity [42], suggesting that enhanced ribosomal production may be associated with ageing, either as a response to imbalances in ribosomal components or as a driver through increased protein synthesis.

Protein synthesis requires not only functional ribosomes but also coordinated activity of a number of translation initiation and elongation factors. Two well-established phosphorylation targets of mTORC1 signalling are 4EBP1 and S6K, which act as regulators of translation initiation. Unphosphorylated 4EBP1 binds to and inhibits eIF4E, which is a DEAD-box helicase necessary for unwinding secondary structures at the 5′ ends of transcripts, and that serves as a critical factor in recruiting 40S ribosomal subunits to mRNAs for cap-dependent translation initiation (thought to be the rate-limiting step in protein synthesis); this inhibition is relieved by mTORC1-mediated phosphorylation of 4EBP1 [43]. S6K is activated by phosphorylation by mTORC1 [16], and S6K then phosphorylates the S6 protein, a structural component of the 40S ribosomal subunit. S6K is also involved in ribosome biogenesis and in regulating the translation of 5′TOP (terminal oligopyrimidine tract) mRNAs; rapamycin and similar rapalogues attenuate translation of mRNAs with complex 5′ UTRs especially those encoding HIF1α and VEGF [44]. The impact of mTOR signalling on 4EBP1 and S6K does vary according to cell type [45], presumably allowing for the tailoring of translational responses to a cell's needs. Furthermore, mTOR also regulates translation elongation through activation of eEF2, which promotes the translocation of the ribosome along the mRNA. While regulation of protein synthesis has largely been attributed to mTORC1, recent evidence suggests a role for mTORC2 in co-translational processing of nascent polypeptides [46,47]. Direct activation of mTORC2 by association with the ribosome also suggests a strong link between translation and mTORC2, possibly ensuring that mTORC2 is only active in growing cells [46].

Mutations in 4EBP1, S6K, and several other components of the translational machinery can confer increased longevity, and mild restriction of protein synthesis by low dose cycloheximide can prevent induction of senescence [48]. It is possible that attenuating protein translation may prevent the production of damaged proteins by enhancing quality control to prevent translational errors, co-translational misfolding, or ER-stress, and that mTORC inhibitors, by reducing rates of protein synthesis, may prevent the formation of potentially toxic aggregates in the cell. mTOR is regulated by chaperone availability to link translation with quality control [49], suggesting that constitutively active mTOR signalling with elevated levels of translation may be detrimental to cell health. Notably, the dysregulation of protein synthesis and accumulation of protein aggregates are implicated in many age-related diseases, including diabetes and neurodegenerative Alzheimer's, Parkinson's and Huntington's diseases; such dysregulation is likely to occur through a combination of high levels of translation, poor post-translational quality control, and a failure of protein breakdown through autophagy.

1.3.3. Autophagy

Autophagy is a selective homoeostatic degradation pathway for cellular components, which are directed via double-membrane vesicles (autophagosomes) to lysosomes for degradation. Autophagy is activated in response to nutrient limitation and is suppressed by mTOR activity, through the inhibitory phosphorylation of the autophagy-initiating kinase ULK1 (ATG1) [50], ATG13, and lysosomally-located TFEB (reviewed in [51]).

The published literature contains some discrepancies about the association between autophagy and ageing. In acutely triggered oncogene-induced senescence, autophagy activation has been observed [52], possibly to rebalance the proteome for transition into a senescent state. However, in almost every other model described, decreased autophagy is linked to ageing. For instance, several proteins that are required for autophagy (Atg5, Atg7 and Beclin 1) are downregulated in normal human brain ageing [53] and in osteoarthritis (ULK1, Beclin 1 and LC3) [54], while knock-in of an activated form of Beclin 1 delays the onset of cardiac and renal fibrosis in normally ageing C57/BL6 mice, and even rescues the short lifespan of Klotho mutant mice [55]. Reduced autophagy has also been observed alongside mTOR activation in senescence resulting from treatment with the genotoxin adriamycin, and co-treatment with the autophagy inhibitor Bafilomycin A1 further increased the proportion of cells that are positively stained for SA-β-gal, a marker of senescence [56]. Increased autophagy has been suggested to mediate the pro-longevity effects of caloric restriction (CR), as inhibition of autophagy prevents CR-mediated anti-ageing effects [57]. Activation of autophagy by spermidine decreases immunosenescence and improves the response to influenza vaccination in mice [58]. Decreased autophagy in ageing may limit the removal of dysfunctional organelles, such as mitochondria, and lead to the accumulation of protein aggregates in neurodegenerative disorders. Autophagy has also been implicated as a mechanism for the antagonistic effects of SIRT6 expression on senescence in rat nucleus pulposus (NP) cells in a model of invertebral disc degeneration (IDD); SIRT6 expression declines in senescent NP cells, but when overexpressed, it attenuates senescence, with this effect being dependent on activation of autophagy and mTOR inhibition [59]. Furthermore, an acetylcholine esterase inhibitor designed as a potential Alzheimer's treatment was shown to induce senescence in MCF-7 breast cancer cells, while simultaneously inducing the onset of autophagy but blocking autophagic flux, leading to the production of single-membrane autolysosomes with non-degraded cargo [60]. Hence, initiation of autophagy with failure of autophagosome fusion with lysosomes for complete protein and organelle recycling may contribute to cell stress and senescence. These results taken in combination underline the complex role of mTOR signalling in regulating autophagy in senescence, and additionally highlight the inadequacy of usual markers of autophagy (autophagosome number or LC3-II/LC3-I ratio) as readouts for activation of such a complex pathway that is subject to further downstream regulation. On balance, we suggest that reactivation of autophagy through mTORC1 inhibition is likely to be beneficial in many different diseases that are associated with ageing, as discussed in Section 2 below.

1.3.4. Mitochondrial Function and Biogenesis

The progressive decline of mitochondrial efficiency in senescence represents a key hallmark of ageing [1]. Senescent cells accumulate dysfunctional mitochondria, with both reduced oxidative phosphorylation efficiency and increased ROS production [61,62]. Mitochondrial dysfunction is itself a driver of cell senescence, with senescent cells exhibiting an increased mitochondrial load and increased oxygen consumption [63]. The relationship between mitochondrial dysfunction and senescence may be inter-dependent, as the chronic DNA damage response of senescent cells also promotes mitochondrial dysfunction [64]. Furthermore, mitochondrial fission and fusion events are altered in senescence, resulting in increased connectivity of the mitochondrial network [65]. As well as the oxidative stress that is caused by dysfunctional mitochondria, mitochondrial nitrosative stress (excess S-nitrosylation) is implicated in senescence, through enhanced S-nitrosylation of proteins regulating mitophagy and mitochondrial dynamics [66].

mTOR provides a critical link between the energy balance of the cell and mitochondrial load, regulating both mitochondrial biogenesis and mitophagy. Biogenesis is controlled through several mechanisms, including PGC-1-β-dependent mitochondrial biogenesis and preferential translation of nuclear-encoded mitochondrial-related mRNAs via the relief of 4EBP inhibition [67], with mitochondrial oxidative function controlled through the YY1-PGC-1α transcriptional complex [68].

1.3.5. Hypoxia

The transcription factor HIF-1, active under hypoxic conditions, has been linked to ageing in *C. elegans*, with increased and reduced activity both causing lifespan extension, dependent on context. mTORC1 signalling is inhibited on HIF-1 activation, through transcription of REDD1, which activates the TSC1/TSC2 complex, resulting in mTORC1 inhibition. Conversely, high oxygen tensions lead to mTORC1 activation, while reactive oxygen species (ROS) may specifically activate mTORC2 [69,70] to promote survival under oxidative stress. However, high Rheb activity in many cancers leads to hyperactive mTOR signalling and increased HIF1 activity, resulting in the upregulation of VEGF and high vascularisation of the tumour [71]. Hence inhibition of mTORC through rapalogues or second-generation mTOR inhibitor ATP mimetics may have a beneficial impact on cancer through blocking this pathway. Whether this has direct relevance to ageing remains to be determined, though it has been suggested that ageing induces an mTOR-dependent pseudo-hypoxic state with high HIF1 and lactate production under normoxic conditions [72,73], which may be amenable to modulation by mTORC inhibition.

1.3.6. Immunomodulatory Signalling

A common feature of age-related pathologies is chronic sterile inflammation. The secretory phenotype (SASP) of senescent cells, through which pro-inflammatory mediators are released to stimulate clearance by immune cells, may be the source of such inflammation. The SASP has pleiotropic signalling effects, exhibiting not only paracrine immunomodulatory signalling, but also autocrine and paracrine pro-senescence, and paracrine pro-tumorigenic signalling. Therefore, the SASP may amplify the senescent cell burden of an elderly individual, exacerbate tissue dysfunction, and stimulate age-related tumorigenesis. The SASP is at least partially regulated by mTOR, possibly through feedback loops of IL1A translation or MAPKAPK2 signalling, and it can be suppressed while using rapamycin or Torin [74,75], or MAP kinase inhibitors [76]. These findings conflict with earlier studies showing the central importance of mTOR in innate immunity, specifically in the production of anti-inflammatory IL-10 and the suppression of pro-inflammatory cytokines IL-21 and IL1β. Rapamycin and Torin are also reported to suppress the anti-inflammatory effects of circulating glucocorticoids [77]. Furthermore, transplant patients receiving mTORC inhibitors showed more than double the expected rate of non-infectious fever [78], suggesting excess inflammation. It is possible that these important and marked discrepancies relate to dosage, with pro-inflammatory effects of mTORC inhibition being caused by high dosage, while anti-inflammatory suppression of the SASP may be achievable at much lower doses.

1.3.7. DNA Damage Response

Following DNA damage, cell cycle progression is halted through the activation of multiple checkpoints and cyclin-dependent kinase inhibitors. The damage-responsive ATM/ATR kinases phosphorylate and activate mTORC, which can then phosphorylate Chk1, leading to proliferative arrest at either S phase or G2/M; mTORC2 is specifically implicated in this arrest, at least in breast cancer cells [79]. In addition to Chk1, components of the mTOR/S6K axis are also phosphorylated by p38α MAPK following DNA damage. While mTOR activity can itself be modulated by the tumour suppressor protein p53 (e.g., through p53 transcriptional targets such as TSC2, AMPK, and REDD1 [80]), p53 activity is sensitive to mTOR signalling; mTORC1 can enhance the translation rate of p53 [81,82] or activate p53 through S6K1-dependent phosphorylation of and binding to MDM2, which releases p53 from inhibition [83] so that it can act as a transcription factor for repair factors, such as Gadd45 or pro-apoptotic factors Bax and PUMA (reviewed in [84,85]). Moreover, mTOR activity enhances p53-dependent transcription of p21^{CDKN1} and induction of senescence [86], a possible molecular explanation for the importance of mTOR in geroconversion.

The importance of mTORC in DNA damage responses suggests that mTORC inhibitors may be beneficial in cancer by sensitizing cells to genotoxic agents, though conflicting results have also been reported [21]. Very recent work suggests that the DNA damage response is defective in cells with hyper-activated mTORC1 signalling that lack the LKB1 tumour suppressor [87]. Chronic persistent DNA damage—and constitutively active mTOR—are also features of senescent cells. Hence, mTOR inhibitors may alleviate the burden of DNA damage on ageing, though their impact on cell cycle control should be closely monitored.

1.3.8. Lipid Metabolism

As a central regulator of cellular growth, mTOR also regulates lipid metabolism, through affecting lipogenesis as well as lipolysis and lipophagy. mTORC1 signalling activates SREBP transcription factors that drive fatty acid (FA) biosynthesis for lipogenesis [88] through an indirect mechanism, whereby mTORC1-phosphorylated Lipin-1 is no longer translocated to the nucleus [89,90]. (Lipin-1 is itself a phosphatidic acid phosphatase that is involved in triacylglycerol synthesis). Furthermore, PPARγ is a SREBP transcriptional target and mTORC1 may also regulate PPARγ activity [91], as well as inhibiting PPARα and PGC1α, which further regulate fatty acid oxidation [92]. PPARα activity is reduced in aged mice (alongside increased mTORC1 activity), but the inhibition of mTORC1 is sufficient to prevent the loss of PPARα activity [93]. The autophagic recycling of lipid droplets for degradation (lipophagy) is suppressed by mTORC1 signalling. Furthermore, decreased lipolysis and triacylglycerol accumulation are observed following the knockdown of 4EBP1 and 4EBP2, suggesting a role for mTORC1 signalling in lipolysis [94].

Senescent cells exhibit dysregulated lipid metabolism, characterized by increased uptake and accumulation of lipids, with coincident increase in oxidative damage to lipids. Notably, the addition of specific lipids such as triglycerides and cholesterol to delipidized media can induce senescence in vitro. This finding suggests altered lipid metabolism as a possible driver of senescence [95], potentially through adding to the ROS burden via β-oxidation of fats, and through lipid peroxidation producing aldehyde end-products, which can cause DNA and protein adducts [95]. Treatment with mTOR inhibitors in vitro has been shown to reduce lipid droplet accumulation in senescent cells [33].

1.4. Rapamycin and Other mTOR Inhibitors

Rapamycin is the natural macrolide antibiotic lactone that is produced by *Streptomyces hygroscopius*, discovered in soil samples from Easter Island, and initially noted for inhibiting the proliferation of yeast [96]. At high doses (e.g., 5 mg/day), rapamycin has immunosuppressive effects and it is FDA-approved for prevention of transplant rejection [97]. It is also in clinical use or in trials for a large number of cancers where mTORC signalling appears to be a key factor in promoting and/or sustaining oncogenic transformation (see Section 2.8 below). Reported side-effects of chronic administration include ulceration of mucosal tissues, haematological abnormalities, induction of insulin insensitivity, obesity, and diabetes, though these adverse effects may be largely dose-dependent.

As discovered through *S. cerevisiae* genetic screens [98], rapamycin mechanistically acts by binding the protein FKBP12, producing a complex that can bind the FRB region of mTOR and partially occlude the active site of mTOR kinase in the mTORC1 complex [99]. This induces cellular effects, including a decrease in protein synthesis, increase in autophagy, and inhibition of cellular growth [100]. Rapamycin does not inhibit the phosphorylation of all mTORC1 substrates equally—it completely inhibits S6K1 phosphorylation, while only partially blocking 4EBP1 phosphorylation [45]. A crystal structure of mTOR, rapamycin, and FKBP12 [101] suggests that this may be due to differential substrate access to the kinase active site, controlled by the mTOR FRB domain, though differential substrate quality (i.e., degree of divergence from the consensus sequence of the phosphorylation site) could also be important.

Structural and functional analogues of rapamycin (known as rapalogues) that also act by allosterically modulating the enzyme have been developed to improve bioavailability and pharmacokinetics, including drugs such as everolimus (RAD001). These agents also act by recruiting the immunophilin/prolyly isomerase FKBP12 to mTORC1.

By contrast to mTORC1, mTORC2 is not particularly sensitive to inhibition by rapamycin or rapalogues, though chronic administration does impact mTORC2 signalling [102], either through feedback via the insulin signalling pathway, and/or through competition for key subunits FKBP12, 51 and 52, which may set different thresholds for rapamycin sensitivity between the two complexes [18]. In human cells in culture, the 'chronic' effect on mTORC2 is observed as little as 24 h after drug treatment, though metabolic effects in animals and human patients require more prolonged treatment (over weeks or months). mTORC2 inhibition is implicated in impaired glucose homeostasis, insulin insensitivity, and diabetes, though studies on worms with tissue-specific RNAi have suggested that it is loss of mTORC2 activity, specifically in the intestine that results in the dysregulation of glucose metabolism [31]. It is important to note that such studies often rely on phosphorylation of mTORC2 target Akt on S473 as a readout of mTORC2 activity, but this site on Akt may also be targeted by kinases IKKε, TBK1 [103], and DNA-PK [104], potentially skewing the interpretation of mTORC2-specific effects.

Second-generation mTOR inhibitors have been developed, primarily as anti-cancer agents to target the hyperactive mTOR observed in many cancers [105]. These drugs compete with ATP for the active site of the mTOR kinase, and hence are effective in inhibiting both mTORC1 and mTORC2. Some agents have extremely high specificity and selectivity for the mTORC kinase. For example, AZD8055 has 1000-fold greater inhibitory effect on mTORC than on other PI3 kinases [106], whereas others (e.g., BEZ235) have dual inhibitory effects on both mTORC and PI3K [107], with a 3–5 fold higher K_d for damage response kinase ATR [108]. While these ATP-competitive inhibitors exhibit more potent apoptotic effects in vitro compared with rapalogues, and a number of such agents have been tested in clinical trials for safety, larger scale trials have not yet demonstrated greater efficacy than current best treatment regimens [105]. Therefore, drugs such as AZD8055, AZD2014, and WYE354 have not yet received FDA approval. The differential specificities of rapalogues and second generation mTORC inhibitors have proven useful in primary research to dissect the effect in senescence of mTORC1 inhibition (rapalogues) versus dual mTORC1/2 inhibition (competitive ATP mimetics) [34]. The major classes of mTOR inhibitors and other pathway modulators are listed in Table 3.

Table 3. Classes of mTOR pathway modulators with examples of each class.

Drug Class	Mode of Action	Drug Name	K_I or IC_{50}	Status
mTORC1 inhibitor	Binds FKBP12 which then associates with mTORC1 and partially occludes kinase active site; mTORC2 inhibited on chronic treatment (possibly through feedback loops)	Rapamycin (sirolimus)	mTORC1 IC_{50} 0.1 nM (in HEK293 cells)	FDA-approved for cancer and as immunosuppressant to prevent rejection in renal transplant; eluting stents in cardiovascular disease Delays senescence in cell culture [109]; extends lifespan and health in lab animals and improves cardiovascular health in companion dogs (see text)
		Everolimus (RAD001)	mTORC1 IC_{50} 1.6–2.4 nM (cell-free assay)	FDA-approved for cancer (e.g., monotherapy against advanced renal cell carcinoma, neuroendocrine tumours of pancreatic, gastrointestinal or lung origin, and SEGA associated with TSC, and as combination therapy with exemestane for HER2-negative breast cancer). Clinical trials show immune system rejuvenation [110,111]
		Temsirolimus; (CCI-779, NSC 683864)	IC_{50} 0.3–0.5 nM in cell culture	FDA approved, used at 10 mg/kg/day in acute lymphocytic leukaemia

Table 3. *Cont.*

Drug Class	Mode of Action	Drug Name	K$_i$ or IC$_{50}$	Status
Pan-mTOR inhibitor (inhibits both mTORC1 and mTORC2)	ATP-competitive mTORC1/2 inhibitor	AZD8055	mTOR IC$_{50}$ 0.8 nM (MDA-MB-468 cells); 1000-fold selectivity against PI3K isoforms and ATM/DNA-PK	Acceptable safety profile for treatment of advanced solid tumours and lymphoma in phase I trial [112]; reverses phenotypes of senescence in cell culture [34]
		Sapanisertib (AK-228, INK 128, MLN0128)	mTORC1 and mTORC2 1 nM (PI3K isoforms ~200 nM)	Phase 1 trials (cancer)
		OSI-027	22 nM mTORC1, 65 nM mTORC2 (>100× selectivity over PI3K)	Phase 1 trials; in experimental colorectal xenograft, OSI-027 (65 mg/kg) more effective than rapamycin [113], reviewed [114]
mTORC2-specific inhibitor	Prevents interaction of Rictor with mTOR hence blocking mTORC2	JR-AB2		Experimental, xenograft tumour models [115]
Dual PI3K and mTOR inhibitor	ATP-competitive dual PI3K and mTORC1/2 inhibitor	Apitolisib (GDC-0980, RG7422)	Dual PI3K/mTOR 5–14 nM Ki, 17 nM mTOR	Phase 2 trials (cancer)
		Dactolisib (NVP-BEZ235, BEZ235)	mTOR IC$_{50}$ 6 nM, PI3K p110α/γ/δ IC$_{50}$ 4/5/7 nM respectively; IC$_{50}$ ATR 21 nM (cell-free assays)	Passed phase I initial dose discovery trial [116]; modest efficacy in advanced or metastatic carcinoma in phase II [117] but poorly tolerated in advanced pancreatic neuroendocrine tumour patient phase II study [118]; beneficial outcomes in trial with everolimus for reversal of immune senescence [110]
		PF-04691502	PI3K(α/β/δ/γ)/mTOR dual inhibitor with K$_i$ of 1.8/2.1/1.6/1.9 and 16 nM (respectively)	Phase 1 clinical trials
PI3K, DNAPK and mTOR	ATP binding site competitor	PI-103	PI3K 2–15 nM, mTOR and DNAPK 30 nM	Experimental [119]
Other components of signalling pathway	PI3K and BRD bromodomain proteins	SF2523	DNAPK 9, 34–158 nM; BRD4 241 nM, mTOR 280 nM	Blocks Brd4; blocks Brd2 to overcome insulin resistance—may be useful as adjunct to prevent diabetic complications of mTOR inhibitors [120]
	Highly selective GSK3 inhibitor; ATP binding competitor	CHIR-98014	GSK3α 0.65 nM GSK3β 0.58 nM	Experimental [121,122]
mTOR activator	FKBP1A	3BDO	N/A	Experimental; inhibits autophagy; provides vascular protection [123]; improves neuronal function in App and Psen1 transgenic mice [124]

IC$_{50}$ and K$_i$ data derived from [125].

2. Ageing and Age-Related Pathologies Amenable to Treatment by mTOR Inhibition

2.1. Ageing

A landmark study from 2009 in which rapamycin was fed to middle aged mice provided the first evidence that any small molecule drug, taken orally, could significantly extend both the mean and maximum lifespan in mammals [126]. In this multi-centre, large cohort study of genetically heterogeneous (UM-HET3) mice, rapamycin delayed the ageing of 20-month old male and female mice. Further studies have not only validated these results, but have demonstrated that rapamycin improves health, in terms of lower incidence or decreased severity of age-related disease, as well as prolonging life [127]. Below, we assess the impact of mTOR inhibition on a number of age-associated diseases and pathologies, collating findings from model systems and human clinical trials.

2.2. Immunosenescence

The immune system undergoes a functional decline with age that both contributes to organismal ageing through decreased senescent cell clearance, and also compromises its ability to fight infection. The term immunosenescence is specifically associated with a decline in the haematopoietic stem cell proliferation compartment, a higher proportion of exhausted, PD-1$^+$ lymphocytes, an inverted CD4/CD8 ratio (<1), a low number of B cells, and seropositivity for cytomegalovirus (CMV) [128]. Age is associated with a high mortality rate from infectious disease, thought to be a direct consequence of loss of immune function. Activation of autophagy has been shown to rejuvenate the immune system in mice [58]; since mTOR activity inhibits autophagy, it follows that mild inhibition of mTOR could be beneficial for immune function with increasing age. Deriving an appropriate dose is critical, as at high doses rapamycin is immunosuppressive, blocking both the protein synthesis and cell division that are required to mount an adaptive immune response.

In mouse models, increased immune activity against both viral and bacterial pathogens has been observed on mild mTOR inhibition [129], suggesting that it is possible to improve at least some aspects of the ageing immune system with low dose mTOR inhibitors. Furthermore, a placebo-controlled, randomized, double-blind human clinical trial of over 200 elderly volunteers has shown similar results [110]. Volunteers were assigned to one of three regimes of the mTORC1 inhibitor RAD001 (everolimus—low: 0.5 mg daily or 5 mg weekly; high: 20 mg weekly) for a six-week period, followed by a two-week drug-free interval. These volunteers were then challenged with the seasonal influenza vaccine. Though the relatively small size of the study impeded powerful statistical analysis, the two low-dose RAD001 regimens improved immune function without causing serious side effects. Patients produced a broader and more powerful immune response, with improved HSC function and a decreased proportion of PD-1$^+$ lymphocytes. The increased breadth of the immune response was particularly promising; older individuals are more likely to die from influenza than younger people, but they generally produce a narrow, weak response to vaccination. Despite the lack of a young control population in the study, the improved response is thought to correspond to a rejuvenated immune system. In a subsequent follow-up study using combined BEZ235 and RAD001 treatment, again for just six weeks, better infection control was reported in older adults for a year after treatment ended [111]. Given the important role of the immune system in cancer surveillance and senescent cell clearance, it would be very interesting to test whether such a rejuvenated immune system is better equipped to clear senescent or tumorigenic cells in vivo.

2.3. Age-Related Neurodegeneration

mTOR hyperactivation is associated with cognitive deficit and brain dysfunction, as seen in Tuberous Sclerosis (TS), where the loss of TSC1/2 prevents negative regulation of mTOR. Hence, mTOR inhibition is being trialled for TS treatment, with beneficial results being reported (reviewed in [130]). Lifelong rapamycin administration to mice prevents the usual age-related decline in cognitive function, thought to be through suppression of IL1β [131]. Neurodegenerative diseases that are characterized by accumulation of abnormal protein aggregates (Alzheimer's disease, Parkinson's disease, and Huntington's disease) are further candidates for treatment with mTOR inhibitors. Not only does mTORC1 exert tight control over protein synthesis and degradation (autophagy) through 4EBP1/S6K, ULK1, and SCF/FBW8, but the mTOR pathway is involved in regulating the inflammatory responses that are known to be involved in the progression of neurodegeneration; it may also contribute to an energetic deficiency observed in such diseases. Conversely, however, the mTOR pathway has been proposed to regulate synaptic plasticity and memory consolidation, through the control of actin reorganization by mTORC2 [132], and neuronal Rictor knock-out mice do indeed show cognitive effects due to alterations in actin reorganisation needed for dendritic spine growth and formation of memories [133]. However, human trial data suggest that pharmacological inhibition, which is not equivalent to total loss of mTORC2, is if anything supportive of brain function since patients taking everolimus for immunosuppression after heart transplantation actually showed improvements in memory and concentration in comparison to those on calcineurin inhibitors [134].

2.3.1. Alzheimer's Disease

Alzheimer's disease (AD) is the most prevalent neurodegenerative disease, which is characterized by accumulation of aggregated extracellular amyloid β (Aβ) plaques and intracellular neurofibrillary tangles composed of tau protein. Neuronal loss and brain atrophy worsen with disease progression. mTOR signalling has been implicated in AD pathogenesis: evidence from human post-mortem exams suggests that mTOR activity is upregulated in AD brains compared to age-matched controls, as levels of phosphorylated mTOR, p70S6K and eIF4E are all increased in AD [135]. This upregulation of mTOR signalling could be mediated via Aβ accumulation, which may activate the PI3K/AKT pathway, and in turn, increased mTOR signalling has been linked to the development of tau pathology [136]. Aβ upregulates mTOR and mTOR is thought to increase levels of Aβ (reviewed in [137]), potentially generating a positive feedback loop in disease progression.

Rapamycin has been shown to prevent cognitive decline in the AD-Tg mouse model of Alzheimer's disease [138–140], and even to reverse already established memory deficits [141], though these effects were limited to mild cognitive decline before widespread plaques and tangles were observable. Improvements in memory and cognition with rapamycin or tersolimus treatment correlated with improvements in the three major hallmarks of AD (Aβ plaques, tau tangles, and microglia activation) [139–141]. A genetic mouse model lacking one mTOR gene copy in the brain exhibited reduced Aβ deposits and rescued memory deficits [142], hence reduced mTOR activity associates with cognitive improvement. It is likely that treatment must happen prior to major amyloid or tau deposition, as cognitive improvements are seen in mice on whole-life but not late-life administration of rapamycin—i.e., a therapeutic window exists, though it is not yet known what constitutes the point of no return.

Though the mechanism of improvement is still unclear, it is possible that decreased protein synthesis may avoid the build-up of toxic Aβ, or that the induction of autophagy through mTORC1 inhibition may result in the removal of protein aggregates. Healthy neurons have highly efficient and active autophagy, but this decreases with age (reviewed in [143]). In the mouse models where rapamycin was shown to decrease levels of Aβ, autophagy induction was necessary [138]. Further, in rapamycin-treated AD-Tg mice brains, increased localization of Aβ into lysosomes was detected, suggesting a more active degradation of these peptides [138], and the decrease in Aβ levels induced by rapamycin could be prevented by blocking autophagy. Hence, mTOR inhibition leading to increased autophagy may be beneficial in treating neuropathies that are associated with protein aggregation. Other components of the mTOR signalling cascade are also implicated in neurodegeneration, including GSK3, overactivity of which results in decreased lysosomal acidification. Hence, GSK3 inhibitors (such as peptide L803-mts) present a novel alternative to mTORC inhibition in AD, and appear to be active in the 5xFAD mouse model of AD [144].

2.3.2. Huntington's Disease

Huntington's disease (HD) is a neurodegenerative disorder where a genetic mutation causes an expansion of the polyglutamine tract within the Huntingtin protein (HTT), resulting in protein aggregation. As mTORC1 signalling suppresses autophagy, which is responsible for recycling protein aggregates, it has been implicated in HD pathology. Counter-intuitively, however, mTORC1 activation may actually be beneficial: in HD mouse models with increased mTOR activity, motor performance was improved relative to controls, coincident with improved mitochondrial function, cholesterol synthesis, and decreased HTT abundance. Further, phosphorylation of S6 was actually decreased in human HD patients as compared to controls, further suggesting a complicated association between mTOR signalling and HD [145].

2.3.3. Parkinson's Disease

Parkinson's disease (PD) is a progressive age-associated neurodegenerative disorder associated with the death of neurons in the substatia nigra. It manifests as loss of motor coordination, often associated with mood disturbance and in many cases followed by dementia. Current treatment is symptomatic, using L-DOPA to reinforce failing dopaminergic signalling. Though a number of genes are associated with PD, there is little overall understanding of the etiology, but lysosomal dysfunction (allowing for a build-up of intracellular α-synuclein as Lewy bodies) is implicated.

Failure of mitophagy, through defects in PINK1/Parkin, may also be important, and defective mitochondria are observed in PD [146].

mTORC1 has been suggested to be neuroprotective in PD, and consistent with this, suppression of mTORC1 signalling by several routes (AMPK, PTEN, or REDD1 activation, or rotenone treatment) results in neuronal cell death in models of PD [147,148]. Moreover, L-DOPA, the current symptomatic treatment of PD, activates mTORC1, supporting the idea that mTORC1 activity is beneficial. However, the opposite has also been reported: elevated mTORC signalling (by deletion of the gene Engrailed, or exposure to paraquat) leads to neuronal apoptosis, suggesting that a balance of mTORC activity is required for neuronal health.

To achieve this balance, mTORC inhibition is being explored as a possible treatment route for PD. Rapamycin has been shown to overcome dyskinesia in mice, which is a major side effect of treatment with L-DOPA, without interfering with the therapeutic effects of L-DOPA [149], while a number of other studies have also demonstrated benefits of rapamycin use in PD (reviewed in [150]). As in AD, other mTOR pathway factors, such as GSK3, might present therapeutic targets, particularly as lysosomal function appears important. It will be interesting to determine if mTORC inhibition promotes autophagic clearance of aggregated α-synuclein and/or dysfunctional mitochondria, and whether this is enhanced by co-treatment with GSK3-inhibiting peptides. However, it has been argued that specific pro-autophagic interventions may provide an even better therapeutic outcomes than global autophagy stimulation [151].

2.4. Age-Related Blindness: AMD

Age-related macular degeneration (AMD) is the most common cause of blindness in the Western world, whereby retinal damage leads to loss of vision in the centre of the visual field (macula). In senescence-accelerated OXYS rats, rapamycin administration in food decreased the incidence and severity of AMD-like retinopathy and prevented the destruction of ganglionar neurons in the retina [152]. These promising results accelerated rapamycin as an AMD therapeutic through to clinical trials, however conflicting results have since been produced, potentially because of dosing issues. For example, one small phase II clinical trial administered 440 μg rapamycin to one eye every three months for 24 months to eleven patients with an advanced form of dry AMD, but it was terminated early after finding that treatment may be detrimental to visual acuity [153]. High dose rapamycin is known to elicit unwanted side effects, so it is unfortunate that such high dosage trials have been designed and conducted, with negative outcomes, as they are likely to reinforce clinical prejudice against use of mTOR inhibitors for non-life-threatening illness. Full dose-response trials to obtain maximal benefit with minimal side effects are still needed, particularly as AMD treatment options are limited and pharmacological therapies should provide a cheaper and more accessible option to the successful stem cell treatments recently reported [154].

2.5. Musculoskeletal Disorders

2.5.1. Sarcopenia and Muscle Wasting

Structural and functional remodelling of skeletal muscle throughout ageing causes sarcopenia, a muscle-wasting syndrome that results in frailty. Muscle loss is consistently observed in premature ageing syndromes and associated with mTOR signalling. For example, muscle-derived stem/progenitor cells (MDSPCs) from the premature ageing Ercc1$^{-/\Delta}$ mouse show upregulated mTOR signalling and are defective in differentiation. Treatment with rapamycin improved myogenic differentiation, with increased levels of autophagy being detected in the isolated cells [155]. Hutchinson-Gilford progeria syndrome (HGPS), which is a human early onset premature ageing syndrome, is also associated with musculoskeletal abnormalities. HGPS results from a splice site mutation in the lamin A (LMNA) gene, leading to the production of an aberrant lamin protein termed progerin, though even in normal individuals, progerin accumulates during ageing, and is associated with vascular pathology. Rapamycin treatment can induce autophagy and reduce phenotypes of senescence induced by progerin in cell culture models of HGPS [156]. Based on such studies, everolimus has now been included in a clinical trial for 17 children with HGPS [157].

The muscle loss in premature ageing HGPS is highly similar to that seen in various other laminopathies, including Emery-Dreifuss muscular dystrophy, Limb-girdle muscular dystrophy, and dilated cardiomyopathy. mTORC1 is implicated in these LMNA-related dystrophies: both $Lmna^{H222P/H222P}$ and $Lmna^{-/-}$ mice show aberrant mTORC1 signalling [158]; $Lmna^{-/-}$ mice specifically showed increased mTORC1 signalling in cardiac and skeletal muscle, with impaired cardiac autophagy, while rapamycin treatment enhanced cardiac and skeletal muscle function and survival in the mutant mice [159].

Targeting mTORC1 signalling is the only therapeutic avenue yet explored for laminopathies that has promise against both dystrophic and progeroid laminopathies [160], but it has yet to be tested in sarcopenia. However, as a note of caution, patients taking rapamycin for more than six months for the treatment of renal cell carcinoma or paracrine neuroendocrine tumours demonstrated an increase in sarcopenia [161], a worrying finding as sarcopenia is predictive of outcomes in cancer patients. Longitudinal rapamycin studies in healthy subjects, such as those that are ongoing in companion dogs [162], are needed to inform on whether low dose mTOR inhibition may be able to delay or even prevent the onset of sarcopenia.

2.5.2. Osteoporosis

Osteoporosis is a common ARD that is characterized by loss of bone density, causing fragility. Falls, as a consequence of co-morbid sarcopenia and age-associated changes to vision and balance perception, often result in hip fractures, and a high number of elderly fracture patients die within six months of pneumonia (exacerbated by co-morbid immunosenescence) [163,164]. Increased activity of osteoclasts, which mediate bone resorption, together with decreased osteoblast activity, is frequently seen in multiple forms of bone loss (osteoporosis, rheumatoid arthritis, and cancer-induced bone loss). mTOR signalling regulates osteoclast differentiation by altering ratios of the LIP/LAP isoforms of transcription factor C/EBPβ [165], which enhances osteoclastogenesis. In mouse models and human cells, inhibition of mTORC1 signalling lowers the activity of the translation initiation factor eIF4E, in turn diminishing expression of the LIP isoform by inhibiting translation re-initiation. This increases the LAP to LIP ratio and inhibits osteoclastogenesis, hence rapamycin treatment limits bone resorption [166,167]. Furthermore, the mTORC1 inhibitor everolimus inhibits bone loss in an experimental rat model of osteoporosis induced by ovariectomy [168].

2.5.3. Rheumatoid Arthritis

Rheumatoid arthritis (RA) is a chronic autoimmune disease characterized by inflammation in joints. Highly effective treatments for RA include methotrexate and infliximab, but these have limited utility in elderly patients because of underlying renal insufficiency; factors such as transport/mobility difficulties also limit attendance at treatment centres for regular antibody infusion. Hence, a safer therapy is required in this patient cohort, which may be provided by mTOR inhibitors. Active mTOR signalling has been detected in synovial tissue from RA patients, and is crucial for joint destruction in experimental arthritis [169]. Such results appear to be relevant to human joints: in a recent proof-of-concept study (a multi-centre, randomized, double-blind study of 121 patients with RA), 6 mg everolimus daily for six months, in combination with methotrexate, showed improved clinical efficacy when compared with methotrexate alone, as well as causing few side effects [170].

Osteoarthritis (OA) is another ARD also characterized by joint inflammation but is thought to be caused by mechanical stress. Senescent cells have been detected in OA joints (Clinicaltrials.gov identifier NCT03100799), and SASP secretion of collagenase and other metalloproteases is likely to impact significantly on joint integrity. Hence, mTOR inhibition could also be beneficial in OA, by targeting constitutively active mTOR in senescent cells. Intraperitoneal administration of rapamycin reduced cartilage destruction and synovitis in experimentally-induced osteoarthritis in mice [171], this may occur at least in part through increased ULK1-mediated autophagy and through the suppression of MMP secretion by chondrocytes (reviewed in [172]). OA presents an ideal opportunity for intervention as intra-articular drug administration should avoid potential side-effects associated with systemic mTORC inhibitor treatment.

2.5.4. Diabetic Bone Fragility

Increased bone fragility is also seen in Type 1 and Type 2 diabetes mellitus (T1DM and T2DM), with increased cortical porosity and decreased cortical area in T2DM. Unlike other age-related bone pathologies, such as osteoporosis, diabetic bone fragility is not associated with decreased bone mineral density, nor does it impact on the balance between bone formation and bone resorption, but instead both bone remodelling and turnover are compromised (reviewed in [173]). This appears to arise from a combination of factors, including alterations in stem cell differentiation, glycation of collagen leading to decreased bone toughness [174], calcification of vascular smooth muscle cells though a RAGE-mediated MAPK-TGFβ-NFκB axis that increases fracture risk (at least in T1DM) through defective bone microvasculature [175], and deficits in muscle-dependent production of IL-6 on exercise that usually allow for bone to adapt to mechanical loading [176]. The decrease in bone turnover is likely to diminish capacity for microfracture repair, leading to a higher incidence of overt fractures. Notably, it has been suggested that the anti-diabetic drug metformin is protective of bone in diabetes by inhibiting adipogenesis that would otherwise be driven by mTOR/S6K signalling [177] and by lowering RAGE signalling [178]. Hence, metformin may support bone strength by acting as an mTOR pathway inhibitor, albeit indirectly.

2.6. Cardiovascular Disease

Cardiovascular disease is the leading cause of death in developed nations and its incidence increases with age. A number of studies have shown beneficial effects of rapamycin on cardiovascular disease in mice: for example, rapamycin has been shown to attenuate pressure overload-induced cardiac hypertrophy [179], to regress established cardiac hypertrophy and improve cardiac function [180], and to suppress experimental aortic aneurysm growth [181]. Recent studies have elaborated on this research. In female 24 month-old C57BL/6J mice fed rapamycin for three months, the greatest benefit measured was in cardiac health, with reversal or attenuation of age-related cardiac decline. Specifically, rapamycin appeared to slow or reverse the progression of age-related hypertrophy, and ventricular function of the ageing heart was also improved [182]. Through RNA-seq analysis, validated at the protein level and with bioinformatics analysis, it appeared that rapamycin reduced age-related sterile inflammation in the heart, while promoting the expression of RAD (Ras associated with diabetes), which mediates anti-hypertrophic signalling and enhances cardiomyocyte excitation-contraction coupling [183]. Caloric restriction and rapamycin treatment (both for 10 weeks) were also shown to rejuvenate the ageing mouse heart [184], with quantitative comparative proteomics revealing an age-dependent decrease in proteins that are involved in mitochondrial function, together with an increase in glycolytic enzymes, which could be reversed by either CR or rapamycin treatment. Improvements in mitochondrial function were implicated in the mechanism, as the mitochondrial proteome was rejuvenated [184], which is consistent with the known action of mTORC1 in mitochondrial biogenesis, and the contribution of mitochondrial accumulation to senescence. Hence, rapamycin could act both to suppress excessive mitochondrial biogenesis and to activate mitophagy. The authors did not observe any increase in autophagy by rapamycin or CR; instead, they observed a reduction in protein oxidative damage, alongside reduced protein turnover. Better preserved protein quality and slower turnover following CR or rapamycin treatment may therefore re-balance the oxidative phosphorylation to glycolysis shift usually seen in aged mice, though the impact of either treatment on cardiomyocyte senescence has not been analysed. It is of note that improved cardiovascular function was also the most marked outcome of the first year of a trial feeding rapamycin to companion dogs [162], thus reinforcing the potential for rapamycin to treat cardiovascular disease. It is possible that the mechanism here is through induction of autophagy by ULK1 upregulation on mTORC inhibition, as cardiac fibrosis is also decreased in older mice on the activation of autophagy by disrupting the Beclin 1-Bcl2 interaction [55]—alternatively or in addition, decreased inflammation by suppression of the SASP is also a potential mechanism.

mTOR inhibitors are also promising treatments for myocardial ischaemia/reperfusion (I/R) injury, for which diabetic patients are at especially severe risk. While the dosage and timing of administration may be critical for beneficial effects, rapamycin treatment has been shown to reduce infarct size after I/R injury in diabetic mice, through facilitating opening of mitochondrial ATP-sensitive potassium channels [185] with the effect also being dependent on STAT3 (signal transducer and activator of transcription 3) [186,187]. Improvements in oxidative stress, cytoskeleton organization, and glucose metabolism on rapamycin treatment have also been implicated in the mechanism [188].

Furthermore, rapamycin-eluting stents are now in widespread clinical use in coronary angioplasty to treat cardiovascular disease, after being approved in Europe in 2002 on the basis of very promising clinical trial results [189]. In this context, rapamycin may benefit coronary function by restricting cell proliferation and thus preventing fibrosis that could block the artery; everolimus is now also in clinical trials for this use. To date, therefore, mTOR inhibition appears to be a safe and effective intervention to improve cardiovascular function during ageing.

2.7. Kidney Disease

2.7.1. Adult Polycystic Kidney Disease

Age-related incontinence is a common cause of depression and isolation in the elderly. A possible heritable disease model for this condition, adult polycystic kidney disease, which is also known as autosomal-dominant polycystic kidney disease (ADPKD), is the most common heritable kidney disorder, with a prevalence of between 1/400 and 1/1000. Mutations in two genes are responsible for the condition: PKD1 (85% of cases—severe, early onset) and PKD2. PKD1 codes for polycystin-1, a membrane receptor protein, while PKD2 codes for polycystin-2, a Ca^{2+}-permeable channel that binds PKD1. Polycystins are involved in maintaining a differentiated epithelium in the kidney, liver and pancreas, but when mutated, excessive epithelial proliferation results in renal cysts. Mechanistically, they play a role in signalling—there are direct physical interactions between the cytoplasmic tail of polycystin-1 and tuberin, the product of the TSC2 gene, which regulates mTOR [190]. As mTOR signalling is therefore regulated by polycystin-1, and mTOR signalling is increased in murine models and in human ADPKD, mTOR activation may contribute to renal cyst expansion through excessive tubular epithelial cell proliferation. Hence, mTOR inhibition may be beneficial, and rapamycin has been shown to decrease proliferation in cystic and non-cystic tubules, to inhibit renal enlargement and to prevent the loss of kidney function in the Han:SPRD rat model of ADPKD [191–193]. While this model results from mutations in genes other than PKD1 and PKD2, rapamycin treatment was also effective in a more human-orthologous mouse model of conditional inactivation of PKD1 [194]. Still, both models exhibit early-onset, rapidly progressive disease, whereas human ADPKD is characterized by complex, slow, and heterogeneous progression. Therefore, retrospective analyses of human ADPKD patients after renal transplantations have been very informative. Using MRI-determined increases in kidney volume as a marker of disease progression, rapamycin-based regimens showed significantly reduced cystic kidney volumes when compared to alternative treatments [190,195,196]. Clinical trials using rapamycin to treat ADPKD have however produced varied results [197–199], though they may have been impeded by small sample size, reliance on poor markers of clinical progression, short follow up time for such a slow-progressing disease, and insufficient rapamycin doses [200].

2.7.2. Diabetic Nephropathy

High doses of rapamycin used for immunosuppression in renal transplantation and cancer are associated with type II diabetes [30]. However, there is some evidence that low doses of rapamycin may have therapeutic benefit in the treatment of diabetic nephropathy (DN), which is one of the major complications of both type I and II diabetes [201] that currently has very limited treatment options.

In diabetes, hyperglycaemia increases mTOR activity through activation of Akt and inhibition of AMPK, which has consequences for the development of podocytes, critical in production of the renal filtration barrier. Experimentally increasing mTORC1 activity in mouse podocytes induces DN phenotypes, podocyte loss, and mis-localization of Nephrin, a cell surface protein that is important in production of the renal filtration barrier [202], while reduced mTORC1 activity prevents DN progression [202]. Rapamycin and everolimus treatment has also shown therapeutic benefit for DN in other models, including rats with STZ-induced diabetes [203–207]. Some caution is required, however, as mTORC1 activity appears to protect diabetic livers from steatosis [208], though active mTORC2 promotes steatosis through induction of fatty acid and lipid synthesis [209], hence any treatment with mTORC inhibitors in diabetic patients must include close monitoring of a number of biomarkers for liver and kidney function as well as glucose homeostasis.

2.8. Age-Related Cancer

Consistent with its role as a central regulator of cell growth, proliferation, and angiogenesis, many oncogenic mutations activate mTOR signalling [210], meaning that the pathway is a key target in anti-cancer therapy. Elderly patients are particularly vulnerable to tumorigenesis; their inflamed tissue microenvironment and the paracrine pro-tumorigenic signalling in the SASP of accumulating senescent cells can drive progression of age-related cancer. In parallel, DNA-damaging chemotherapies given to cancer patients of any age can induce senescence (and the resulting SASP) in both cancerous and healthy collateral cells. This is thought to underlie the increased occurrence of secondary tumours as a side effect of chemotherapy [11,211,212]. Since the SASP is under the control of the mTOR pathway, treating senescent cells with mTOR inhibitors can suppress the secretion of inflammatory cytokines [74,75]. Notably, rapamycin treatment can prevent the stimulation of prostate tumour growth by senescent fibroblasts in mice [74]. Thus, rapamycin may be useful not only as an anti-cancer treatment but also as a preventative therapeutic against age-related cancers or those arising after genotoxic chemo- or radio-therapy.

Despite promising early findings, mTOR inhibitors have not fulfilled their potential as monotherapies against cancer. Combination regimens of mTOR inhibitors together with current best-in class chemotherapeutics do however show efficacy against a range of cancers. For example, combination treatment with rapamycin and resveratrol may be effective in inducing cell death in bladder cancer cells [213], with resveratrol blocking the Akt activation as induced by rapamycin. Similarly, rapamycin has been shown to enhance mitomycin C-induced apoptosis in peritoneal carcinomatosis [214]. In combination with anti-cancer agents, such as trastuzumab or exemestane, mTOR inhibitors exhibit promising anti-tumour activity, even against aromatase inhibitor-resistant breast tumours [215]. Rapamycin may also be beneficial in combination with radiotherapy treatment, for example inducing a significant decrease in tumour metabolic activity of rectal cancers before surgical resection, as assessed by positron emission tomography (PET)-scanning [216].

Currently (June 2018), 461 clinical trials are listed on Clinicaltrials.gov involving the use of mTOR inhibitors in cancer, in a range of tissue types, including breast, cervix, prostate, ovary, pancreas, lung and colon carcinomas, various sarcomas, and lymphomas, while PubMed lists 601 publications for the search terms "mTOR inhibitor cancer clinical trial". The reported outcomes are highly variable, with some suggesting markedly better outcomes (e.g., Hodgkin's lymphoma on mTOR inhibition [217,218]), while others showed no improvement or even faster disease progression. It is likely that the variability represents both the stage and grade of cancer, and mTOR status, which should be assessed by 'personalised medicine' prior to the use of mTOR inhibitors in cancer treatment, as not all will be driven by hyperactive mTOR, and even those that are may not be sensitive to rapalogue inhibition (e.g., if mutated in the FKBP12 binding site). For those tumours with activated drug-sensitive mTOR, however, mTOR inhibition can give remarkably good outcomes; with the complete response to therapy being reported in one patient during a Phase I trial of everolimus in combination with pazopanib [219]. Use of specific mTORC2 inhibitors has been suggested as route to overcoming the pro-survival effect of PI3K/PDK1/Akt feedback loops [220], though pan-mTOR inhibitors may be equally valuable in this context. The choice to test any drug in aggressive and treatment-refractory or relapsing tumours would present significant challenges, as the cancers by this stage will be genetically heterogeneous and hard to treat; the use of mTOR inhibitors in many such late-stage/refractory cancer trials may therefore not reveal their true potential. It is possible that earlier intervention with mTOR inhibitors, and in combination therapies, may provide more reliable anti-cancer activity. However, a major goal would instead be prevention. In this context, mTOR inhibitors used to intervene in other age-related disease may, in fact, serve a preventative role in cancer, possibly by blocking the deleterious SASP.

3. Perspectives

3.1. Balancing Efficacy Against Side Effects

Treating otherwise healthy ageing individuals with mTOR inhibitors to treat or prevent progression of age-related disease is only viable if the treatment does not induce unacceptable or undesirable side effects. The studies of immunosenescence from Mannick et al. [110,111] may provide critical insights into side effect profiles of low-dose mTOR inhibition in ageing humans. These studies showed that everolimus and BEZ235 were generally well tolerated, although with an increased incidence of mouth ulceration. Particularly promising is the finding that the two lowest dose regimens of everolimus (0.5 mg daily or 5 mg weekly [111]) proved both the most effective and the best tolerated, with the fewest overall adverse events per cohort. Hence, using as low dose as possible whilst retaining efficacy is critical in minimising side effects.

High dose rapamycin (~20 ng/mL blood) that is used for immunosuppression after transplant or cancer treatment is associated with deleterious side effects, such as the development of type II diabetes [30], though evidence from experimental models produces conflicting results. For example, two short-term studies in mice found that chronic rapamycin treatment induced deleterious metabolic side effects such as weight gain, glucose intolerance [221], and progression of type II diabetes [222], while a longer study showed that these effects could be transient [182]. The dose of rapamycin used may be of critical importance in determining the side effect profile; far lower doses are required for anti-ageing effects than for cancer treatment or immunosuppression and as doses decrease, so do serious adverse events. Disruption of mTORC2 may be behind the metabolic side effects of rapamycin treatment, since it is widely considered that mTORC2 primarily drives the response to insulin signalling and causes lipid biosynthesis (though note the caveats above concerning Akt^{S473} phosphorylation as a sole readout of mTORC2 activity). Carefully considered intermittent treatment regimens may minimize the undesirable effects of rapamycin treatment, such as impaired glucose tolerance [223]. A further alternative strategy to circumvent high dose rapalogue-induced glucose intolerance is to use mTOR inhibitors in combination with anti-diabetes medicines, such as metformin—another promising longevity therapeutic in its own right. Indeed, this strategy has been shown to be highly effective in HET3 female mice treated with both rapamycin and metformin, where glucose tolerance readings were indistinguishable from control mice, though the protective effect was not seen in males [224]. Hence complex-specific mTORC inhibitors, with additional agents to counteract adverse side effects, could retain treatment efficacy over the long-term, a necessary requirement for anti-ageing medicines.

An alternative approach to minimising side effects would be to use a topical application of mTOR inhibitors. This is possible in age-related diseases that occur in discrete compartments, such as OA and AMD, where injection into the affected site is possible. However, as ageing affects the entire body, systemic therapies should be more effective at treating aging per se, and hence in minimising the onset of multiple age-related diseases. mTOR inhibitors currently provide a promising avenue for further research and development, and may promote healthy ageing by modulating the harmful aspects of senescent cells, but they should be considered in combination with other treatment approaches.

In this context, alternative anti-ageing therapies are also being developed—notably the growing field of senolytic drugs that are designed to selectively target and kill senescent cells. These agents exploit the reliance of senescent cells on survival pathways, and they can induce apoptosis specifically in senescent cells, for example, by inducing p53 or disrupting Bcl2. Treatment of aged mice with senolytic agents has been shown to rejuvenate tissues and reverse several age-related pathologies (e.g., [225,226]) and a human clinical trial for senolytic treatment of OA is currently recruiting (Clinicaltrials.gov identifier NCT03513016). However, while senolytics are indisputably exciting, it is well established that senescent cells are beneficial in various instances, such as in wound healing and regeneration. Furthermore, a recent study investigating the senescent cell burden of several tissues of old mice found that up to 14% of cells were senescent [13], with estimates of 20–60% senescent cells in aged primate skin [14,227]. It is therefore important to investigate whether killing a significant proportion of cells in the tissues of elderly patients is safe, whether stem cells are able to refill this empty niche to restore structural and functional tissue integrity, and to assess whether wound healing and regeneration are compromised by senolytic agents. Furthermore, senescent cells from different tissues and in different contexts rely on different survival pathways to avoid apoptosis and are therefore only vulnerable to specific senolytic agents, meaning that a range of senolytics will be required to treat different ARDs. Modulation of the antagonistically pleiotropic and highly heterogeneous state that is cell senescence undoubtedly requires careful and context-dependent consideration.

3.2. Monitoring Therapeutic Outcomes: The Need for Ageing Biomarkers

There is an urgent need for reliable, non-invasive, and quantitative biomarkers of senescence and ageing to both measure disease susceptibility or progression, and promptly monitor the outcome of any intervention. It is highly likely that single factors will not be able to adequately reflect the panoply of changes that is associated with ageing and that instead a panel of biomarkers will be required to account for the multi-factorial and complex nature of pathological ageing. Molecular markers that are currently in use include telomere length analysis, DNA methylation patterns, and SAβGAL staining, while functional and morphological markers are also available. The choice of marker may depend on the trial to be conducted—for example, PET scanning for amyloid deposition may be necessary in AD trials, though a recently described blood test for amyloid could substitute [228]. Notably, a number of simple biochemical biomarkers (e.g., glycated haemoglobin) that are selected for inclusion in UK Biobank appear to be valid for assessment of age-related changes, while functional readouts including hand grip strength produce reliable measures of frailty. Clinical trials and any licensed treatments may thus require the development and validation of a panel of biomarkers that could be analysed in a low cost, straightforward, and quick in-house procedure from readily available patient material e.g., urine or blood.

In conclusion, ageing and age-related diseases that arise from hyperactive mTORC signalling may benefit from the use of mTORC inhibitors. However, any such treatment strategy must consider both of the beneficial effects, such as those that are afforded by activation of autophagy and improved quality control of protein synthesis, as well as potential detrimental effects from modifying cellular or organismal metabolism. We believe that mTORC inhibitors hold much promise in the field of anti-ageing medicine, and that clinical prejudice against their use needs to be overcome by careful dosage trials. To obtain maximal therapeutic benefit, whilst minimising side-effects, combinatorial therapies may prove useful. Overall outcomes on ageing and age-related diseases require the use of a panel of robust biomarkers that should provide rapid readouts of age-associated factors in a minimally invasive and cost-effective format. Biochemical pathways that intersect with mTORC signalling may also provide fruitful avenues for anti-ageing drug discovery.

Int. J. Mol. Sci. **2018**, *19*, 2325

Author Contributions: H.E.W. and L.S.C. both researched and wrote the article.

Acknowledgments: H.E.W. is funded by a generous donation from an anonymous donor through the University of Oxford Development Office; L.S.C. is supported by the Higher Education Funding Council of England (HEFCE). The work in L.S.C.'s lab is also supported by the Biotechnology and Biological Sciences Research Council (BBSRC grant number [BB/M006727/1]) and Amway. L.S.C. is grateful to the Glenn Foundation for Medical Research for a Glenn Award. No specific funds have been provided for publishing open access. We thank the reviewers for their useful contributions and are grateful to Ronald Pearson for critical reading of the manuscript.

Conflicts of Interest: L.S.C. is co-I on an Open Innovation research agreement with Astra Zeneca to study mTOR inhibitor AZD8055. The authors declare no other conflict of interest.

Abbreviations

4EBP1	eIF4E binding protein
53BP1	p53 binding protein 1
Aβ	amyloid beta
AD	Alzheimer's disease
ADPKD	adult polycystic kidney disease
Akt/PKB	protein kinase B
AMD	age-related macular degeneration
AMPK	AMP-activated protein kinase
ARD	age-related disease
ATG13	autophagy related protein 13
ATM	ataxia telangiectasia mutated
ATR	ATM-related
ATP	adenosine triphosphate
CMV	cytomegalovirus
CpG	5'-C-p-G-3'
CR	caloric restriction
DAP1	death associated protein 1
DN	diabetic neuropathy
eEF2	eukaryotic elongation factor 2
eIF	eukaryotic translation initiation factor
ER	endoplasmic reticulum
FA	fatty acid
FBW8	F-Box And WD Repeat Domain Containing 8
FDA	Food and Drug Administration
FKBP	FK506 binding protein
FK506	Tacrolimus
FRB	FKBP12-Rapamycin Binding (FRB) domain of mTOR
GIT1	GPCR-kinase interacting protein 1
GSK3	glycogen synthase kinase 3
HD	Huntington's disease
HGPS	Hutchinson Gilford progeroid syndrome
HIF1	hypoxia inducible factor 1
HTT	huntingtin protein
IC$_{50}$	half maximal inhibitory concentration
IKK	IkB kinase
IL	Interleukin
IGFR	insulin-like growth factor receptor
IMP2	insulin-like growth factor 2 mRNA binding protein 2
IRS	insulin receptor substrate
Ki	inhibitory constant
LAMTOR	late endosomal/lysosomal adaptor and MAPK and MTOR activator
LAP	liver-enriched activator protein
LARP1	La related protein

LIP	liver-enriched inhibitory protein
LKB1	liver kinase B1
LMNA	lamin A
L-DOPA	L-dopamine
MAPKAPK2	mitogen-activated protein kinase-activated protein kinase 2
MCF-7	Michigan Cancer Foundation-7 (breast cancer cell line)
mLST8	mammalian lethal with SEC13 protein 8
MMP	matrix metalloproteinase
mTOR	mammalian/mechanistic target of rapamycin
mTORC1/2	mTOR complex 1 or 2
NFAT5	nuclear factor of activated T cells 5
OA	osteoarthritis
PD	Parkinson's disease
PD-1	programmed death 1
PDK1/2	pyruvate dehydrogenase kinase 1/2
PGC-1-β	peroxisome proliferator-activated receptor gamma coactivator 1-β
PKC	protein kinase C
PPAR	Peroxisome Proliferator Activated Receptor
RA	rheumatoid arthritis
RAD	Ras associated with diabetes
RAGE	receptor for advanced glycation end products
REDD1	regulated in development and DNA damage 1
RNAi	RNA interference
ROS	reactive oxygen species
S6K	protein kinase that phosphorylates S6 ribosomal protein
SAβGAL	senescence associated beta galactosidase
SASP	senescence-associated secretory phenotype
SGK1	serine/threonine protein kinase
SIRT	sirtuin
SOD1	superoxide dismutase 1
SREBP	sterol regulatory element-binding protein
STAT3	signal transducer and activator of transcription 3
T1DM	type 1 diabetes mellitus
T2DM	type 2 diabetes mellitus
TFEB	transcription factor EB
TNFα	tumour necrosis factor α
TSC1/2	tuberous sclerosis complex 1 or 2
ULK1	Unc-51 like autophagy activating kinase
UTR	untranslated region
VEGF	vascular endothelial growth factor
γH2AX	Ser-139 phosphorylated histone 2A variant X

References

1. Lopez-Otin, C.; Blasco, M.A.; Partridge, L.; Serrano, M.; Kroemer, G. The hallmarks of aging. *Cell* **2013**, *153*, 1194–1217. [CrossRef] [PubMed]
2. Baker, D.J.; Childs, B.G.; Durik, M.; Wijers, M.E.; Sieben, C.J.; Zhong, J.; Saltness, R.A.; Jeganathan, K.B.; Verzosa, G.C.; Pezeshki, A.; et al. Naturally occurring p16[Ink4a]-positive cells shorten healthy lifespan. *Nature* **2016**, *530*, 184–189. [CrossRef] [PubMed]
3. Munoz-Espin, D.; Serrano, M. Cellular senescence: From physiology to pathology. *Nat. Rev. Mol. Cell Biol.* **2014**, *15*, 482–496. [CrossRef] [PubMed]

4. Georgakopoulou, E.A.; Tsimaratou, K.; Evangelou, K.; Fernandez Marcos, P.J.; Zoumpourlis, V.; Trougakos, I.P.; Kletsas, D.; Bartek, J.; Serrano, M.; Gorgoulis, V.G. Specific lipofuscin staining as a novel biomarker to detect replicative and stress-induced senescence. A method applicable in cryo-preserved and archival tissues. *Aging* **2013**, *5*, 37–50. [CrossRef] [PubMed]

5. Dimri, G.P.; Lee, X.; Basile, G.; Acosta, M.; Scott, G.; Roskelley, C.; Medrano, E.E.; Linskens, M.; Rubelj, I.; Pereira-Smith, O.; et al. A biomarker that identifies senescent human cells in culture and in aging skin in vivo. *Proc. Natl. Acad. Sci. USA* **1995**, *92*, 9363–9367. [CrossRef] [PubMed]

6. Horvath, S. DNA methylation age of human tissues and cell types. *Genome Biol.* **2013**, *14*, R115. [CrossRef] [PubMed]

7. Munoz-Espin, D.; Canamero, M.; Maraver, A.; Gomez-Lopez, G.; Contreras, J.; Murillo-Cuesta, S.; Rodriguez-Baeza, A.; Varela-Nieto, I.; Ruberte, J.; Collado, M.; et al. Programmed cell senescence during mammalian embryonic development. *Cell* **2013**, *155*, 1104–1118. [CrossRef] [PubMed]

8. Demaria, M.; Ohtani, N.; Youssef, S.A.; Rodier, F.; Toussaint, W.; Mitchell, J.R.; Laberge, R.M.; Vijg, J.; Van Steeg, H.; Dolle, M.E.; et al. An essential role for senescent cells in optimal wound healing through secretion of PDGF-AA. *Dev. Cell* **2014**, *31*, 722–733. [CrossRef] [PubMed]

9. Chuprin, A.; Gal, H.; Biron-Shental, T.; Biran, A.; Amiel, A.; Rozenblatt, S.; Krizhanovsky, V. Cell fusion induced by ERVWE1 or measles virus causes cellular senescence. *Genes Dev.* **2013**, *27*, 2356–2366. [CrossRef] [PubMed]

10. Serrano, M.; Lin, A.W.; McCurrach, M.E.; Beach, D.; Lowe, S.W. Oncogenic ras provokes premature cell senescence associated with accumulation of p53 and p16INK4a. *Cell* **1997**, *88*, 593–602. [CrossRef]

11. Coppe, J.P.; Patil, C.K.; Rodier, F.; Sun, Y.; Munoz, D.P.; Goldstein, J.; Nelson, P.S.; Desprez, P.Y.; Campisi, J. Senescence-associated secretory phenotypes reveal cell-nonautonomous functions of oncogenic RAS and the p53 tumor suppressor. *PLoS Biol.* **2008**, *6*, 2853–2868. [CrossRef] [PubMed]

12. Van Deursen, J.M. The role of senescent cells in ageing. *Nature* **2014**, *509*, 439–446. [CrossRef] [PubMed]

13. Biran, A.; Zada, L.; Abou Karam, P.; Vadai, E.; Roitman, L.; Ovadya, Y.; Porat, Z.; Krizhanovsky, V. Quantitative identification of senescent cells in aging and disease. *Aging Cell* **2017**, *16*, 661–671. [CrossRef] [PubMed]

14. Herbig, U.; Ferreira, M.; Condel, L.; Carey, D.; Sedivy, J.M. Cellular senescence in aging primates. *Science* **2006**, *311*, 1257. [CrossRef] [PubMed]

15. Smithson, L.J.; Gutmann, D.H. Proteomic analysis reveals GIT1 as a novel mTOR complex component critical for mediating astrocyte survival. *Genes Dev.* **2016**, *30*, 1383–1388. [CrossRef] [PubMed]

16. Huang, K.; Fingar, D.C. Growing knowledge of the mTOR signaling network. *Semin. Cell Dev. Biol.* **2014**, *36*, 79–90. [CrossRef] [PubMed]

17. Ebner, M.; Sinkovics, B.; Szczygiel, M.; Ribeiro, D.W.; Yudushkin, I. Localization of mTORC2 activity inside cells. *J. Cell Biol.* **2017**, *216*, 343–353. [CrossRef] [PubMed]

18. Schreiber, K.H.; Ortiz, D.; Academia, E.C.; Anies, A.C.; Liao, C.Y.; Kennedy, B.K. Rapamycin-mediated mTORC2 inhibition is determined by the relative expression of FK506-binding proteins. *Aging Cell* **2015**, *14*, 265–273. [CrossRef] [PubMed]

19. Hsu, P.P.; Kang, S.A.; Rameseder, J.; Zhang, Y.; Ottina, K.A.; Lim, D.; Peterson, T.R.; Choi, Y.; Gray, N.S.; Yaffe, M.B.; et al. The mTOR-regulated phosphoproteome reveals a mechanism of mTORC1-mediated inhibition of growth factor signaling. *Science* **2011**, *332*, 1317–1322. [CrossRef] [PubMed]

20. Schwarz, J.J.; Wiese, H.; Tolle, R.C.; Zarei, M.; Dengjel, J.; Warscheid, B.; Thedieck, K. Functional Proteomics Identifies Acinus L as a Direct Insulin- and Amino Acid-Dependent Mammalian Target of Rapamycin Complex 1 (mTORC1) Substrate. *Mol. Cell. Proteom.* **2015**, *14*, 2042–2055. [CrossRef] [PubMed]

21. Bandhakavi, S.; Kim, Y.M.; Ro, S.H.; Xie, H.; Onsongo, G.; Jun, C.B.; Kim, D.H.; Griffin, T.J. Quantitative nuclear proteomics identifies mTOR regulation of DNA damage response. *Mol. Cell. Proteom.* **2010**, *9*, 403–414. [CrossRef] [PubMed]

22. Fonseca, B.D.; Smith, E.M.; Yelle, N.; Alain, T.; Bushell, M.; Pause, A. The ever-evolving role of mTOR in translation. *Semin. Cell Dev. Biol.* **2014**, *36*, 102–112. [CrossRef] [PubMed]

23. Laplante, M.; Sabatini, D.M. mTOR signaling in growth control and disease. *Cell* **2012**, *149*, 274–293. [CrossRef] [PubMed]

24. Kaeberlein, M.; Powers, R.W., 3rd; Steffen, K.K.; Westman, E.A.; Hu, D.; Dang, N.; Kerr, E.O.; Kirkland, K.T.; Fields, S.; Kennedy, B.K. Regulation of yeast replicative life span by TOR and Sch9 in response to nutrients. *Science* **2005**, *310*, 1193–1196. [CrossRef] [PubMed]

25. Vellai, T.; Takacs-Vellai, K.; Zhang, Y.; Kovacs, A.L.; Orosz, L.; Muller, F. Genetics: Influence of TOR kinase on lifespan in *C. elegans*. *Nature* **2003**, *426*, 620. [CrossRef] [PubMed]

26. Jia, K.; Levine, B. Autophagy is required for dietary restriction-mediated life span extension in *C. elegans*. *Autophagy* **2007**, *3*, 597–599. [CrossRef] [PubMed]

27. Hansen, M.; Taubert, S.; Crawford, D.; Libina, N.; Lee, S.J.; Kenyon, C. Lifespan extension by conditions that inhibit translation in *Caenorhabditis elegans*. *Aging Cell* **2007**, *6*, 95–110. [CrossRef] [PubMed]

28. Kapahi, P.; Zid, B.M.; Harper, T.; Koslover, D.; Sapin, V.; Benzer, S. Regulation of lifespan in Drosophila by modulation of genes in the TOR signaling pathway. *Curr. Biol.* **2004**, *14*, 885–890. [CrossRef] [PubMed]

29. Selman, C.; Tullet, J.M.; Wieser, D.; Irvine, E.; Lingard, S.J.; Choudhury, A.I.; Claret, M.; Al-Qassab, H.; Carmignac, D.; Ramadani, F.; et al. Ribosomal protein S6 kinase 1 signaling regulates mammalian life span. *Science* **2009**, *326*, 140–144. [CrossRef] [PubMed]

30. Gyurus, E.; Kaposztas, Z.; Kahan, B.D. Sirolimus therapy predisposes to new-onset diabetes mellitus after renal transplantation: A long-term analysis of various treatment regimens. *Transpl. Proc.* **2011**, *43*, 1583–1592. [CrossRef] [PubMed]

31. Mizunuma, M.; Neumann-Haefelin, E.; Moroz, N.; Li, Y.; Blackwell, T.K. mTORC2-SGK-1 acts in two environmentally responsive pathways with opposing effects on longevity. *Aging Cell* **2014**, *13*, 869–878. [CrossRef] [PubMed]

32. Carroll, B.; Nelson, G.; Rabanal-Ruiz, Y.; Kucheryavenko, O.; Dunhill-Turner, N.A.; Chesterman, C.C.; Zahari, Q.; Zhang, T.; Conduit, S.E.; Mitchell, C.A.; et al. Persistent mTORC1 signaling in cell senescence results from defects in amino acid and growth factor sensing. *J. Cell Biol.* **2017**, *216*, 1949–1957. [CrossRef] [PubMed]

33. Leontieva, O.V.; Blagosklonny, M.V. Gerosuppression by pan-mTOR inhibitors. *Aging* **2016**, *8*, 3535–3551. [CrossRef] [PubMed]

34. Walters, H.E.; Deneka-Hannemann, S.; Cox, L.S. Reversal of phenotypes of cellular senescence by pan-mTOR inhibition. *Aging* **2016**, *8*, 231–244. [CrossRef] [PubMed]

35. Majumder, P.K.; Febbo, P.G.; Bikoff, R.; Berger, R.; Xue, Q.; McMahon, L.M.; Manola, J.; Brugarolas, J.; McDonnell, T.J.; Golub, T.R.; et al. mTOR inhibition reverses Akt-dependent prostate intraepithelial neoplasia through regulation of apoptotic and HIF-1-dependent pathways. *Nat. Med.* **2004**, *10*, 594–601. [CrossRef] [PubMed]

36. Nakamura, H.; Makino, Y.; Okamoto, K.; Poellinger, L.; Ohnuma, K.; Morimoto, C.; Tanaka, H. TCR engagement increases hypoxia-inducible factor-1α protein synthesis via rapamycin-sensitive pathway under hypoxic conditions in human peripheral T cells. *J. Immunol.* **2005**, *174*, 7592–7599. [CrossRef] [PubMed]

37. Lerner, C.; Bitto, A.; Pulliam, D.; Nacarelli, T.; Konigsberg, M.; Van Remmen, H.; Torres, C.; Sell, C. Reduced mammalian target of rapamycin activity facilitates mitochondrial retrograde signaling and increases life span in normal human fibroblasts. *Aging Cell* **2013**, *12*, 966–977. [CrossRef] [PubMed]

38. Santagata, S.; Mendillo, M.L.; Tang, Y.C.; Subramanian, A.; Perley, C.C.; Roche, S.P.; Wong, B.; Narayan, R.; Kwon, H.; Koeva, M.; et al. Tight coordination of protein translation and HSF1 activation supports the anabolic malignant state. *Science* **2013**, *341*, 1238303. [CrossRef] [PubMed]

39. Ortells, M.C.; Morancho, B.; Drews-Elger, K.; Viollet, B.; Laderoute, K.R.; Lopez-Rodriguez, C.; Aramburu, J. Transcriptional regulation of gene expression during osmotic stress responses by the mammalian target of rapamycin. *Nucleic Acids Res.* **2012**, *40*, 4368–4384. [CrossRef] [PubMed]

40. Iadevaia, V.; Liu, R.; Proud, C.G. mTORC1 signaling controls multiple steps in ribosome biogenesis. *Semin. Cell Dev. Biol.* **2014**, *36*, 113–120. [CrossRef] [PubMed]

41. Buchwalter, A.; Hetzer, M.W. Nucleolar expansion and elevated protein translation in premature aging. *Nat. Commun.* **2017**, *8*, 328. [CrossRef] [PubMed]

42. Tiku, V.; Jain, C.; Raz, Y.; Nakamura, S.; Heestand, B.; Liu, W.; Spath, M.; Suchiman, H.E.D.; Muller, R.U.; Slagboom, P.E.; et al. Small nucleoli are a cellular hallmark of longevity. *Nat. Commun.* **2016**, *8*, 16083. [CrossRef] [PubMed]

43. Gingras, A.-C.; Gygi, S.P.; Raught, B.; Polakiewicz, R.D.; Abraham, R.T.; Hoekstra, M.F.; Aebersold, R.; Sonenberg, N. Regulation of 4E-BP1 phosphorylation: A novel two-step mechanism. *Genes Dev.* **1999**, *13*, 1422–1437. [CrossRef] [PubMed]

44. Opdenaker, L.M.; Farach-Carson, M.C. Rapamycin selectively reduces the association of transcripts containing complex 5′ UTRs with ribosomes in C4-2B prostate cancer cells. *J. Cell. Biochem.* **2009**, *107*, 473–481. [CrossRef] [PubMed]

45. Choo, A.Y.; Yoon, S.O.; Kim, S.G.; Roux, P.P.; Blenis, J. Rapamycin differentially inhibits S6Ks and 4E-BP1 to mediate cell-type-specific repression of mRNA translation. *Proc. Natl. Acad. Sci. USA* **2008**, *105*, 17414–17419. [CrossRef] [PubMed]

46. Zinzalla, V.; Stracka, D.; Oppliger, W.; Hall, M.N. Activation of mTORC2 by association with the ribosome. *Cell* **2011**, *144*, 757–768. [CrossRef] [PubMed]

47. Oh, W.J.; Wu, C.C.; Kim, S.J.; Facchinetti, V.; Julien, L.A.; Finlan, M.; Roux, P.P.; Su, B.; Jacinto, E. mTORC2 can associate with ribosomes to promote cotranslational phosphorylation and stability of nascent Akt polypeptide. *EMBO J.* **2010**, *29*, 3939–3951. [CrossRef] [PubMed]

48. Takauji, Y.; Wada, T.; Takeda, A.; Kudo, I.; Miki, K.; Fujii, M.; Ayusawa, D. Restriction of protein synthesis abolishes senescence features at cellular and organismal levels. *Sci. Rep.* **2016**, *6*, 18722. [CrossRef] [PubMed]

49. Qian, S.B.; Zhang, X.; Sun, J.; Bennink, J.R.; Yewdell, J.W.; Patterson, C. mTORC1 links protein quality and quantity control by sensing chaperone availability. *J. Biol. Chem.* **2010**, *285*, 27385–27395. [CrossRef] [PubMed]

50. Kim, J.; Kundu, M.; Viollet, B.; Guan, K.L. AMPK and mTOR regulate autophagy through direct phosphorylation of Ulk1. *Nat. Cell Biol.* **2011**, *13*, 132–141. [CrossRef] [PubMed]

51. Kennedy, B.K.; Lamming, D.W. The Mechanistic Target of Rapamycin: The Grand ConducTOR of Metabolism and Aging. *Cell Metab.* **2016**, *23*, 990–1003. [CrossRef] [PubMed]

52. Young, A.R.; Narita, M.; Ferreira, M.; Kirschner, K.; Sadaie, M.; Darot, J.F.; Tavare, S.; Arakawa, S.; Shimizu, S.; Watt, F.M.; et al. Autophagy mediates the mitotic senescence transition. *Genes Dev.* **2009**, *23*, 798–803. [CrossRef] [PubMed]

53. Lipinski, M.M.; Zheng, B.; Lu, T.; Yan, Z.; Py, B.F.; Ng, A.; Xavier, R.J.; Li, C.; Yankner, B.A.; Scherzer, C.R.; et al. Genome-wide analysis reveals mechanisms modulating autophagy in normal brain aging and in Alzheimer's disease. *Proc. Natl. Acad. Sci. USA* **2010**, *107*, 14164–14169. [CrossRef] [PubMed]

54. Carames, B.; Taniguchi, N.; Otsuki, S.; Blanco, F.J.; Lotz, M. Autophagy is a protective mechanism in normal cartilage, and its aging-related loss is linked with cell death and osteoarthritis. *Arthritis Rheum.* **2010**, *62*, 791–801. [CrossRef] [PubMed]

55. Fernandez, A.F.; Sebti, S.; Wei, Y.; Zou, Z.; Shi, M.; McMillan, K.L.; He, C.; Ting, T.; Liu, Y.; Chiang, W.C.; et al. Disruption of the beclin 1-BCL2 autophagy regulatory complex promotes longevity in mice. *Nature* **2018**. [CrossRef] [PubMed]

56. Sung, J.Y.; Lee, K.Y.; Kim, J.R.; Choi, H.C. Interaction between mTOR pathway inhibition and autophagy induction attenuates adriamycin-induced vascular smooth muscle cell senescence through decreased expressions of p53/p21/p16. *Exp. Gerontol.* **2017**. [CrossRef] [PubMed]

57. Rubinsztein, D.C.; Marino, G.; Kroemer, G. Autophagy and aging. *Cell* **2011**, *146*, 682–695. [CrossRef] [PubMed]

58. Puleston, D.J.; Zhang, H.; Powell, T.J.; Lipina, E.; Sims, S.; Panse, I.; Watson, A.S.; Cerundolo, V.; Townsend, A.R.; Klenerman, P.; et al. Autophagy is a critical regulator of memory CD8$^+$ T cell formation. *eLife* **2014**, *3*. [CrossRef] [PubMed]

59. Chen, J.; Xie, J.J.; Jin, M.Y.; Gu, Y.T.; Wu, C.C.; Guo, W.J.; Yan, Y.Z.; Zhang, Z.J.; Wang, J.L.; Zhang, X.L.; et al. Sirt6 overexpression suppresses senescence and apoptosis of nucleus pulposus cells by inducing autophagy in a model of intervertebral disc degeneration. *Cell Death Dis.* **2018**, *9*, 56. [CrossRef] [PubMed]

60. Kucharewicz, K.; Dudkowska, M.; Zawadzka, A.; Ogrodnik, M.; Szczepankiewicz, A.A.; Czarnocki, Z.; Sikora, E. Simultaneous induction and blockade of autophagy by a single agent. *Cell Death Dis.* **2018**, *9*, 353. [CrossRef] [PubMed]

61. Passos, J.F.; Saretzki, G.; Ahmed, S.; Nelson, G.; Richter, T.; Peters, H.; Wappler, I.; Birket, M.J.; Harold, G.; Schaeuble, K.; et al. Mitochondrial dysfunction accounts for the stochastic heterogeneity in telomere-dependent senescence. *PLoS Biol.* **2007**, *5*, e110. [CrossRef] [PubMed]

62. Korolchuk, V.I.; Miwa, S.; Carroll, B.; von Zglinicki, T. Mitochondria in Cell Senescence: Is Mitophagy the Weakest Link? *EBioMedicine* **2017**, *21*, 7–13. [CrossRef] [PubMed]

63. Correia-Melo, C.; Marques, F.D.; Anderson, R.; Hewitt, G.; Hewitt, R.; Cole, J.; Carroll, B.M.; Miwa, S.; Birch, J.; Merz, A.; et al. Mitochondria are required for pro-ageing features of the senescent phenotype. *EMBO J.* **2016**, *35*, 724–742. [CrossRef] [PubMed]

64. Passos, J.F.; Nelson, G.; Wang, C.; Richter, T.; Simillion, C.; Proctor, C.J.; Miwa, S.; Olijslagers, S.; Hallinan, J.; Wipat, A.; et al. Feedback between p21 and reactive oxygen production is necessary for cell senescence. *Mol. Syst. Biol.* **2010**, *6*, 347. [CrossRef] [PubMed]

65. Mai, S.; Klinkenberg, M.; Auburger, G.; Bereiter-Hahn, J.; Jendrach, M. Decreased expression of Drp1 and Fis1 mediates mitochondrial elongation in senescent cells and enhances resistance to oxidative stress through PINK1. *J. Cell Sci.* **2010**, *123 Pt 6*, 917–926. [CrossRef]

66. Rizza, S.; Cardaci, S.; Montagna, C.; Di Giacomo, G.; De Zio, D.; Bordi, M.; Maiani, E.; Campello, S.; Borreca, A.; Puca, A.A.; et al. S-nitrosylation drives cell senescence and aging in mammals by controlling mitochondrial dynamics and mitophagy. *Proc. Natl. Acad. Sci. USA* **2018**, *115*, E3388–E3397. [CrossRef] [PubMed]

67. Morita, M.; Gravel, S.P.; Chenard, V.; Sikstrom, K.; Zheng, L.; Alain, T.; Gandin, V.; Avizonis, D.; Arguello, M.; Zakaria, C.; et al. mTORC1 controls mitochondrial activity and biogenesis through 4E-BP-dependent translational regulation. *Cell Metab.* **2013**, *18*, 698–711. [CrossRef] [PubMed]

68. Cunningham, J.T.; Rodgers, J.T.; Arlow, D.H.; Vazquez, F.; Mootha, V.K.; Puigserver, P. mTOR controls mitochondrial oxidative function through a YY1-PGC-1α transcriptional complex. *Nature* **2007**, *450*, 736–740. [CrossRef] [PubMed]

69. Niles, B.J.; Joslin, A.C.; Fresques, T.; Powers, T. TOR complex 2-Ypk1 signaling maintains sphingolipid homeostasis by sensing and regulating ROS accumulation. *Cell Rep.* **2014**, *6*, 541–552. [CrossRef] [PubMed]

70. Cai, W.; Andres, D.A. mTORC2 is required for rit-mediated oxidative stress resistance. *PLoS ONE* **2014**, *9*, e115602. [CrossRef] [PubMed]

71. Land, S.C.; Tee, A.R. Hypoxia-inducible factor 1α is regulated by the mammalian target of rapamycin (mTOR) via an mTOR signaling motif. *J. Biol. Chem.* **2007**, *282*, 20534–20543. [CrossRef] [PubMed]

72. Gomes, A.P.; Price, N.L.; Ling, A.J.; Moslehi, J.J.; Montgomery, M.K.; Rajman, L.; White, J.P.; Teodoro, J.S.; Wrann, C.D.; Hubbard, B.P.; et al. Declining NAD$^+$ induces a pseudohypoxic state disrupting nuclear-mitochondrial communication during aging. *Cell* **2013**, *155*, 1624–1638. [CrossRef] [PubMed]

73. Leontieva, O.V.; Blagosklonny, M.V. M(o)TOR of pseudo-hypoxic state in aging: Rapamycin to the rescue. *Cell Cycle* **2014**, *13*, 509–515. [CrossRef] [PubMed]

74. Laberge, R.M.; Sun, Y.; Orjalo, A.V.; Patil, C.K.; Freund, A.; Zhou, L.; Curran, S.C.; Davalos, A.R.; Wilson-Edell, K.A.; Liu, S.; et al. MTOR regulates the pro-tumorigenic senescence-associated secretory phenotype by promoting IL1A translation. *Nat. Cell Biol.* **2015**, *17*, 1049–1061. [CrossRef] [PubMed]

75. Herranz, N.; Gallage, S.; Mellone, M.; Wuestefeld, T.; Klotz, S.; Hanley, C.J.; Raguz, S.; Acosta, J.C.; Innes, A.J.; Banito, A.; et al. mTOR regulates MAPKAPK2 translation to control the senescence-associated secretory phenotype. *Nat. Cell Biol.* **2015**, *17*, 1205–1217. [CrossRef] [PubMed]

76. Alimbetov, D.; Davis, T.; Brook, A.J.; Cox, L.S.; Faragher, R.G.; Nurgozhin, T.; Zhumadilov, Z.; Kipling, D. Suppression of the senescence-associated secretory phenotype (SASP) in human fibroblasts using small molecule inhibitors of p38 MAP kinase and MK2. *Biogerontology* **2016**, *17*, 305–315. [CrossRef] [PubMed]

77. Weichhart, T.; Haidinger, M.; Katholnig, K.; Kopecky, C.; Poglitsch, M.; Lassnig, C.; Rosner, M.; Zlabinger, G.J.; Hengstschlager, M.; Muller, M.; et al. Inhibition of mTOR blocks the anti-inflammatory effects of glucocorticoids in myeloid immune cells. *Blood* **2011**, *117*, 4273–4283. [CrossRef] [PubMed]

78. Saemann, M.D.; Haidinger, M.; Hecking, M.; Horl, W.H.; Weichhart, T. The multifunctional role of mTOR in innate immunity: Implications for transplant immunity. *Am. J. Transpl.* **2009**, *9*, 2655–2661. [CrossRef] [PubMed]

79. Selvarajah, J.; Elia, A.; Carroll, V.A.; Moumen, A. DNA damage-induced S and G2/M cell cycle arrest requires mTORC2-dependent regulation of Chk1. *Oncotarget* **2015**, *6*, 427–440. [CrossRef] [PubMed]

80. Feng, Z.; Hu, W.; de Stanchina, E.; Teresky, A.K.; Jin, S.; Lowe, S.; Levine, A.J. The regulation of AMPK β1, TSC2, and PTEN expression by p53: Stress, cell and tissue specificity, and the role of these gene products in modulating the IGF-1-AKT-mTOR pathways. *Cancer Res.* **2007**, *67*, 3043–3053. [CrossRef] [PubMed]

81. Lee, C.H.; Inoki, K.; Karbowniczek, M.; Petroulakis, E.; Sonenberg, N.; Henske, E.P.; Guan, K.L. Constitutive mTOR activation in TSC mutants sensitizes cells to energy starvation and genomic damage via p53. *EMBO J.* **2007**, *26*, 4812–4823. [CrossRef] [PubMed]

82. Vadysirisack, D.D.; Ellisen, L.W. mTOR activity under hypoxia. *Methods Mol. Biol.* **2012**, *821*, 45–58. [CrossRef] [PubMed]

83. Lai, K.P.; Leong, W.F.; Chau, J.F.; Jia, D.; Zeng, L.; Liu, H.; He, L.; Hao, A.; Zhang, H.; Meek, D.; et al. S6K1 is a multifaceted regulator of Mdm2 that connects nutrient status and DNA damage response. *EMBO J.* **2010**, *29*, 2994–3006. [CrossRef] [PubMed]

84. Cox, L.S.; Lane, D.P. Tumour suppressors, kinases and clamps: How p53 regulates the cell cycle in response to DNA damage. *Bioessays* **1995**, *17*, 501–508. [CrossRef] [PubMed]

85. Shen, Y.; White, E. p53-dependent apoptosis pathways. *Adv. Cancer Res.* **2001**, *82*, 55–84. [PubMed]

86. Astle, M.V.; Hannan, K.M.; Ng, P.Y.; Lee, R.S.; George, A.J.; Hsu, A.K.; Haupt, Y.; Hannan, R.D.; Pearson, R.B. AKT induces senescence in human cells via mTORC1 and p53 in the absence of DNA damage: Implications for targeting mTOR during malignancy. *Oncogene* **2012**, *31*, 1949–1962. [CrossRef] [PubMed]

87. Xie, X.; Hu, H.; Tong, X.; Li, L.; Liu, X.; Chen, M.; Yuan, H.; Xie, X.; Li, Q.; Zhang, Y.; et al. The mTOR-S6K pathway links growth signalling to DNA damage response by targeting RNF168. *Nat. Cell Biol.* **2018**, *20*, 320–331. [CrossRef] [PubMed]

88. Yokoyama, C.; Wang, X.; Briggs, M.R.; Admon, A.; Wu, J.; Hua, X.; Goldstein, J.L.; Brown, M.S. SREBP-1, a basic-helix-loop-helix-leucine zipper protein that controls transcription of the low density lipoprotein receptor gene. *Cell* **1993**, *75*, 187–197. [CrossRef]

89. Porstmann, T.; Santos, C.R.; Griffiths, B.; Cully, M.; Wu, M.; Leevers, S.; Griffiths, J.R.; Chung, Y.L.; Schulze, A. SREBP activity is regulated by mTORC1 and contributes to Akt-dependent cell growth. *Cell Metab.* **2008**, *8*, 224–236. [CrossRef] [PubMed]

90. Peterson, T.R.; Sengupta, S.S.; Harris, T.E.; Carmack, A.E.; Kang, S.A.; Balderas, E.; Guertin, D.A.; Madden, K.L.; Carpenter, A.E.; Finck, B.N.; et al. mTOR complex 1 regulates lipin 1 localization to control the SREBP pathway. *Cell* **2011**, *146*, 408–420. [CrossRef] [PubMed]

91. Blanchard, P.G.; Festuccia, W.T.; Houde, V.P.; St-Pierre, P.; Brule, S.; Turcotte, V.; Cote, M.; Bellmann, K.; Marette, A.; Deshaies, Y. Major involvement of mTOR in the PPARγ-induced stimulation of adipose tissue lipid uptake and fat accretion. *J. Lipid Res.* **2012**, *53*, 1117–1125. [CrossRef] [PubMed]

92. Lefebvre, P.; Chinetti, G.; Fruchart, J.C.; Staels, B. Sorting out the roles of PPARα in energy metabolism and vascular homeostasis. *J. Clin. Investig.* **2006**, *116*, 571–580. [CrossRef] [PubMed]

93. Sengupta, S.; Peterson, T.R.; Laplante, M.; Oh, S.; Sabatini, D.M. mTORC1 controls fasting-induced ketogenesis and its modulation by ageing. *Nature* **2010**, *468*, 1100–1104. [CrossRef] [PubMed]

94. Le Bacquer, O.; Petroulakis, E.; Paglialunga, S.; Poulin, F.; Richard, D.; Cianflone, K.; Sonenberg, N. Elevated sensitivity to diet-induced obesity and insulin resistance in mice lacking 4E-BP1 and 4E-BP2. *J. Clin. Investig.* **2007**, *117*, 387–396. [CrossRef] [PubMed]

95. Flor, A.C.; Wolfgeher, D.; Wu, D.; Kron, S.J. A signature of enhanced lipid metabolism, lipid peroxidation and aldehyde stress in therapy-induced senescence. *Cell Death Discov.* **2017**, *3*, 17075. [CrossRef] [PubMed]

96. Vezina, C.; Kudelski, A.; Sehgal, S.N. Rapamycin (AY-22,989), a new antifungal antibiotic. I. Taxonomy of the producing streptomycete and isolation of the active principle. *J. Antibiot.* **1975**, *28*, 721–726. [CrossRef] [PubMed]

97. Dominguez, J.; Mahalati, K.; Kiberd, B.; McAlister, V.C.; MacDonald, A.S. Conversion to rapamycin immunosuppression in renal transplant recipients: Report of an initial experience. *Transplantation* **2000**, *70*, 1244–1247. [CrossRef] [PubMed]

98. Heitman, J.; Movva, N.R.; Hall, M.N. Targets for cell cycle arrest by the immunosuppressant rapamycin in yeast. *Science* **1991**, *253*, 905–909. [CrossRef] [PubMed]

99. Caron, E.; Ghosh, S.; Matsuoka, Y.; Ashton-Beaucage, D.; Therrien, M.; Lemieux, S.; Perreault, C.; Roux, P.P.; Kitano, H. A comprehensive map of the mTOR signaling network. *Mol. Syst. Biol.* **2010**, *6*, 453. [CrossRef] [PubMed]

100. Stanfel, M.N.; Shamieh, L.S.; Kaeberlein, M.; Kennedy, B.K. The TOR pathway comes of age. *Biochim. Biophys. Acta* **2009**, *1790*, 1067–1074. [CrossRef] [PubMed]

101. Yang, H.; Rudge, D.G.; Koos, J.D.; Vaidialingam, B.; Yang, H.J.; Pavletich, N.P. mTOR kinase structure, mechanism and regulation. *Nature* **2013**, *497*, 217–223. [CrossRef] [PubMed]

102. Sarbassov, D.D.; Ali, S.M.; Sengupta, S.; Sheen, J.H.; Hsu, P.P.; Bagley, A.F.; Markhard, A.L.; Sabatini, D.M. Prolonged rapamycin treatment inhibits mTORC2 assembly and Akt/PKB. *Mol. Cell* **2006**, *22*, 159–168. [CrossRef] [PubMed]

103. Joung, S.M.; Park, Z.Y.; Rani, S.; Takeuchi, O.; Akira, S.; Lee, J.Y. Akt contributes to activation of the TRIF-dependent signaling pathways of TLRs by interacting with TANK-binding kinase 1. *J. Immunol.* **2011**, *186*, 499–507. [CrossRef] [PubMed]

104. Toulany, M.; Schickfluss, T.A.; Fattah, K.R.; Lee, K.J.; Chen, B.P.; Fehrenbacher, B.; Schaller, M.; Chen, D.J.; Rodemann, H.P. Function of erbB receptors and DNA-PKcs on phosphorylation of cytoplasmic and nuclear Akt at S473 induced by erbB1 ligand and ionizing radiation. *Radiother. Oncol.* **2011**, *101*, 140–146. [CrossRef] [PubMed]

105. Kim, L.C.; Cook, R.S.; Chen, J. mTORC1 and mTORC2 in cancer and the tumor microenvironment. *Oncogene* **2017**, *36*, 2191–2201. [CrossRef] [PubMed]

106. Chresta, C.M.; Davies, B.R.; Hickson, I.; Harding, T.; Cosulich, S.; Critchlow, S.E.; Vincent, J.P.; Ellston, R.; Jones, D.; Sini, P.; et al. AZD8055 is a potent, selective, and orally bioavailable ATP-competitive mammalian target of rapamycin kinase inhibitor with in vitro and in vivo antitumor activity. *Cancer Res.* **2010**, *70*, 288–298. [CrossRef] [PubMed]

107. Maira, S.M.; Stauffer, F.; Brueggen, J.; Furet, P.; Schnell, C.; Fritsch, C.; Brachmann, S.; Chene, P.; De Pover, A.; Schoemaker, K.; et al. Identification and characterization of NVP-BEZ235, a new orally available dual phosphatidylinositol 3-kinase/mammalian target of rapamycin inhibitor with potent in vivo antitumor activity. *Mol. Cancer Ther.* **2008**, *7*, 1851–1863. [CrossRef] [PubMed]

108. Toledo, L.I.; Murga, M.; Zur, R.; Soria, R.; Rodriguez, A.; Martinez, S.; Oyarzabal, J.; Pastor, J.; Bischoff, J.R.; Fernandez-Capetillo, O. A cell-based screen identifies ATR inhibitors with synthetic lethal properties for cancer-associated mutations. *Nat. Struct. Mol. Biol.* **2011**, *18*, 721–727. [CrossRef] [PubMed]

109. Demidenko, Z.N.; Zubova, S.G.; Bukreeva, E.I.; Pospelov, V.A.; Pospelova, T.V.; Blagosklonny, M.V. Rapamycin decelerates cellular senescence. *Cell Cycle* **2009**, *8*, 1888–1895. [CrossRef] [PubMed]

110. Mannick, J.B.; Morris, M.; Hockey, H.-U.P.; Roma, G.; Beibel, M.; Kulmatycki, K.; Watkins, M.; Shavlakadze, T.; Zhou, W.; Quinn, D.; et al. TORC1 inhibition enhances immune function and reduces infections in the elderly. *Sci. Transl. Med.* **2018**, *10*. [CrossRef] [PubMed]

111. Mannick, J.B.; Del Giudice, G.; Lattanzi, M.; Valiante, N.M.; Praestgaard, J.; Huang, B.; Lonetto, M.A.; Maecker, H.T.; Kovarik, J.; Carson, S.; et al. mTOR inhibition improves immune function in the elderly. *Sci. Transl. Med.* **2014**, *6*, 268ra179. [CrossRef] [PubMed]

112. Naing, A.; Aghajanian, C.; Raymond, E.; Olmos, D.; Schwartz, G.; Oelmann, E.; Grinsted, L.; Burke, W.; Taylor, R.; Kaye, S.; et al. Safety, tolerability, pharmacokinetics and pharmacodynamics of AZD8055 in advanced solid tumours and lymphoma. *Br. J. Cancer* **2012**, *107*, 1093–1099. [CrossRef] [PubMed]

113. Bhagwat, S.V.; Gokhale, P.C.; Crew, A.P.; Cooke, A.; Yao, Y.; Mantis, C.; Kahler, J.; Workman, J.; Bittner, M.; Dudkin, L.; et al. Preclinical characterization of OSI-027, a potent and selective inhibitor of mTORC1 and mTORC2: Distinct from rapamycin. *Mol. Cancer Ther.* **2011**, *10*, 1394–1406. [CrossRef] [PubMed]

114. Bahrami, A.; Khazaei, M.; Hasanzadeh, M.; ShahidSales, S.; Joudi Mashhad, M.; Farazestanian, M.; Sadeghnia, H.R.; Rezayi, M.; Maftouh, M.; Hassanian, S.M.; et al. Therapeutic Potential of Targeting PI3K/AKT Pathway in Treatment of Colorectal Cancer: Rational and Progress. *J. Cell. Biochem.* **2018**, *119*, 2460–2469. [CrossRef] [PubMed]

115. Benavides-Serrato, A.; Lee, J.; Holmes, B.; Landon, K.A.; Bashir, T.; Jung, M.E.; Lichtenstein, A.; Gera, J. Specific blockade of Rictor-mTOR association inhibits mTORC2 activity and is cytotoxic in glioblastoma. *PLoS ONE* **2017**, *12*, e0176599. [CrossRef] [PubMed]

116. Bendell, J.C.; Kurkjian, C.; Infante, J.R.; Bauer, T.M.; Burris, H.A., 3rd; Greco, F.A.; Shih, K.C.; Thompson, D.S.; Lane, C.M.; Finney, L.H.; et al. A phase 1 study of the sachet formulation of the oral dual PI3K/mTOR inhibitor BEZ235 given twice daily (BID) in patients with advanced solid tumors. *Investig. New Drugs* **2015**, *33*, 463–471. [CrossRef] [PubMed]

117. Seront, E.; Rottey, S.; Filleul, B.; Glorieux, P.; Goeminne, J.C.; Verschaeve, V.; Vandenbulcke, J.M.; Sautois, B.; Boegner, P.; Gillain, A.; et al. Phase II study of dual phosphoinositol-3-kinase (PI3K) and mammalian target of rapamycin (mTOR) inhibitor BEZ235 in patients with locally advanced or metastatic transitional cell carcinoma. *BJU Int.* **2016**, *118*, 408–415. [CrossRef] [PubMed]

118. Fazio, N.; Buzzoni, R.; Baudin, E.; Antonuzzo, L.; Hubner, R.A.; Lahner, H.; WW, D.E.H.; Raderer, M.; Teule, A.; Capdevila, J.; et al. A Phase II Study of BEZ235 in Patients with Everolimus-resistant, Advanced Pancreatic Neuroendocrine Tumours. *Anticancer Res.* **2016**, *36*, 713–719. [PubMed]

119. Fan, Q.W.; Knight, Z.A.; Goldenberg, D.D.; Yu, W.; Mostov, K.E.; Stokoe, D.; Shokat, K.M.; Weiss, W.A. A dual PI3 kinase/mTOR inhibitor reveals emergent efficacy in glioma. *Cancer Cell* **2006**, *9*, 341–349. [CrossRef] [PubMed]

120. Sun, R.; Wu, Y.; Hou, W.; Sun, Z.; Wang, Y.; Wei, H.; Mo, W.; Yu, M. Bromodomain-containing protein 2 induces insulin resistance via the mTOR/Akt signaling pathway and an inflammatory response in adipose tissue. *Cell. Signal.* **2017**, *30*, 92–103. [CrossRef] [PubMed]

121. Ring, D.B.; Johnson, K.W.; Henriksen, E.J.; Nuss, J.M.; Goff, D.; Kinnick, T.R.; Ma, S.T.; Reeder, J.W.; Samuels, I.; Slabiak, T.; et al. Selective glycogen synthase kinase 3 inhibitors potentiate insulin activation of glucose transport and utilization in vitro and in vivo. *Diabetes* **2003**, *52*, 588–595. [CrossRef] [PubMed]

122. Qiu, Y.S.; Jiang, N.N.; Zhou, Y.; Yu, K.Y.; Gong, H.Y.; Liao, G.J. LMO3 promotes gastric cancer cell invasion and proliferation through Akt-mTOR and Akt-GSK3β signaling. *Int. J. Mol. Med.* **2018**, *41*, 2755–2763. [CrossRef] [PubMed]

123. Peng, N.; Meng, N.; Wang, S.; Zhao, F.; Zhao, J.; Su, L.; Zhang, S.; Zhang, Y.; Zhao, B.; Miao, J. An activator of mTOR inhibits oxLDL-induced autophagy and apoptosis in vascular endothelial cells and restricts atherosclerosis in apolipoprotein E$^{-/-}$ mice. *Sci. Rep.* **2014**, *4*, 5519. [CrossRef] [PubMed]

124. Ge, D.; Han, L.; Huang, S.; Peng, N.; Wang, P.; Jiang, Z.; Zhao, J.; Su, L.; Zhang, S.; Zhang, Y.; et al. Identification of a novel MTOR activator and discovery of a competing endogenous RNA regulating autophagy in vascular endothelial cells. *Autophagy* **2014**, *10*, 957–971. [CrossRef] [PubMed]

125. Selleckchem.com. Available online: http://www.selleckchem.com/ (accessed on 3 June 2018).

126. Harrison, D.E.; Strong, R.; Sharp, Z.D.; Nelson, J.F.; Astle, C.M.; Flurkey, K.; Nadon, N.L.; Wilkinson, J.E.; Frenkel, K.; Carter, C.S.; et al. Rapamycin fed late in life extends lifespan in genetically heterogeneous mice. *Nature* **2009**, *460*, 392–395. [CrossRef] [PubMed]

127. Wilkinson, J.E.; Burmeister, L.; Brooks, S.V.; Chan, C.C.; Friedline, S.; Harrison, D.E.; Hejtmancik, J.F.; Nadon, N.; Strong, R.; Wood, L.K.; et al. Rapamycin slows aging in mice. *Aging Cell* **2002**, *11*, 675–682. [CrossRef] [PubMed]

128. Pera, A.; Campos, C.; Lopez, N.; Hassouneh, F.; Alonso, C.; Tarazona, R.; Solana, R. Immunosenescence: Implications for response to infection and vaccination in older people. *Maturitas* **2015**, *82*, 50–55. [CrossRef] [PubMed]

129. Hurez, V.; Dao, V.; Liu, A.; Pandeswara, S.; Gelfond, J.; Sun, L.; Bergman, M.; Orihuela, C.J.; Galvan, V.; Padron, A.; et al. Chronic mTOR inhibition in mice with rapamycin alters T, B, myeloid, and innate lymphoid cells and gut flora and prolongs life of immune-deficient mice. *Aging Cell* **2015**, *14*, 945–956. [CrossRef] [PubMed]

130. Capal, J.K.; Franz, D.N. Profile of everolimus in the treatment of tuberous sclerosis complex: An evidence-based review of its place in therapy. *Neuropsychiatr. Dis. Treat.* **2016**, *12*, 2165–2172. [CrossRef] [PubMed]

131. Majumder, S.; Caccamo, A.; Medina, D.X.; Benavides, A.D.; Javors, M.A.; Kraig, E.; Strong, R.; Richardson, A.; Oddo, S. Lifelong rapamycin administration ameliorates age-dependent cognitive deficits by reducing IL-1β and enhancing NMDA signaling. *Aging Cell* **2012**, *11*, 326–335. [CrossRef] [PubMed]

132. Josselyn, S.A.; Frankland, P.W. mTORC2: Actin on your memory. *Nat. Neurosci.* **2013**, *16*, 379–380. [CrossRef] [PubMed]

133. Thomanetz, V.; Angliker, N.; Cloetta, D.; Lustenberger, R.M.; Schweighauser, M.; Oliveri, F.; Suzuki, N.; Ruegg, M.A. Ablation of the mTORC2 component rictor in brain or Purkinje cells affects size and neuron morphology. *J. Cell Biol.* **2013**, *201*, 293–308. [CrossRef] [PubMed]

134. Lang, U.E.; Heger, J.; Willbring, M.; Domula, M.; Matschke, K.; Tugtekin, S.M. Immunosuppression using the mammalian target of rapamycin (mTOR) inhibitor everolimus: Pilot study shows significant cognitive and affective improvement. *Transpl. Proc.* **2009**, *41*, 4285–4288. [CrossRef] [PubMed]

135. An, W.L.; Cowburn, R.F.; Li, L.; Braak, H.; Alafuzoff, I.; Iqbal, K.; Iqbal, I.G.; Winblad, B.; Pei, J.J. Up-regulation of phosphorylated/activated p70 S6 kinase and its relationship to neurofibrillary pathology in Alzheimer's disease. *Am. J. Pathol.* **2003**, *163*, 591–607. [CrossRef]

136. Pei, J.J.; Hugon, J. mTOR-dependent signalling in Alzheimer's disease. *J. Cell. Mol. Med.* **2008**, *12*, 2525–2532. [CrossRef] [PubMed]

137. Oddo, S. The role of mTOR signaling in Alzheimer disease. *Front. Biosci.* **2012**, *4*, 941–952. [CrossRef]

138. Caccamo, A.; Majumder, S.; Richardson, A.; Strong, R.; Oddo, S. Molecular interplay between mammalian target of rapamycin (mTOR), amyloid-β, and Tau: Effects on cognitive impairments. *J. Biol. Chem.* **2010**, *285*, 13107–13120. [CrossRef] [PubMed]

139. Spilman, P.; Podlutskaya, N.; Hart, M.J.; Debnath, J.; Gorostiza, O.; Bredesen, D.; Richardson, A.; Strong, R.; Galvan, V. Inhibition of mTOR by rapamycin abolishes cognitive deficits and reduces amyloid-β levels in a mouse model of Alzheimer's disease. *PLoS ONE* **2010**, *5*, e9979. [CrossRef] [PubMed]

140. Majumder, S.; Richardson, A.; Strong, R.; Oddo, S. Inducing autophagy by rapamycin before, but not after, the formation of plaques and tangles ameliorates cognitive deficits. *PLoS ONE* **2011**, *6*, e25416. [CrossRef] [PubMed]

141. Lin, A.L.; Zheng, W.; Halloran, J.J.; Burbank, R.R.; Hussong, S.A.; Hart, M.J.; Javors, M.; Shih, Y.Y.; Muir, E.; Solano Fonseca, R.; et al. Chronic rapamycin restores brain vascular integrity and function through NO synthase activation and improves memory in symptomatic mice modeling Alzheimer's disease. *J. Cereb. Blood Flow Metab.* **2013**, *33*, 1412–1421. [CrossRef] [PubMed]

142. Caccamo, A.; De Pinto, V.; Messina, A.; Branca, C.; Oddo, S. Genetic reduction of mammalian target of rapamycin ameliorates Alzheimer's disease-like cognitive and pathological deficits by restoring hippocampal gene expression signature. *J. Neurosci.* **2014**, *34*, 7988–7998. [CrossRef] [PubMed]

143. Cuervo, A.M. Autophagy and aging: Keeping that old broom working. *Trends Genet.* **2008**, *24*, 604–612. [CrossRef] [PubMed]

144. Avrahami, L.; Farfara, D.; Shaham-Kol, M.; Vassar, R.; Frenkel, D.; Eldar-Finkelman, H. Inhibition of glycogen synthase kinase-3 ameliorates beta-amyloid pathology and restores lysosomal acidification and mammalian target of rapamycin activity in the Alzheimer disease mouse model: In vivo and in vitro studies. *J. Biol. Chem.* **2013**, *288*, 1295–1306. [CrossRef] [PubMed]

145. Lee, J.H.; Tecedor, L.; Chen, Y.H.; Monteys, A.M.; Sowada, M.J.; Thompson, L.M.; Davidson, B.L. Reinstating aberrant mTORC1 activity in Huntington's disease mice improves disease phenotypes. *Neuron* **2015**, *85*, 303–315. [CrossRef] [PubMed]

146. Winklhofer, K.F.; Haass, C. Mitochondrial dysfunction in Parkinson's disease. *Biochim. Biophys. Acta* **2010**, *1802*, 29–44. [CrossRef] [PubMed]

147. Xu, Y.; Liu, C.; Chen, S.; Ye, Y.; Guo, M.; Ren, Q.; Liu, L.; Zhang, H.; Xu, C.; Zhou, Q.; et al. Activation of AMPK and inactivation of Akt result in suppression of mTOR-mediated S6K1 and 4E-BP1 pathways leading to neuronal cell death in in vitro models of Parkinson's disease. *Cell. Signal.* **2014**, *26*, 1680–1689. [CrossRef] [PubMed]

148. Zhou, Q.; Liu, C.; Liu, W.; Zhang, H.; Zhang, R.; Liu, J.; Zhang, J.; Xu, C.; Liu, L.; Huang, S.; et al. Rotenone induction of hydrogen peroxide inhibits mTOR-mediated S6K1 and 4E-BP1/eIF4E pathways, leading to neuronal apoptosis. *Toxicol. Sci.* **2015**, *143*, 81–96. [CrossRef] [PubMed]

149. Santini, E.; Heiman, M.; Greengard, P.; Valjent, E.; Fisone, G. Inhibition of mTOR signaling in Parkinson's disease prevents L-DOPA-induced dyskinesia. *Sci. Signal.* **2009**, *2*, ra36. [CrossRef] [PubMed]

150. Lan, A.P.; Chen, J.; Zhao, Y.; Chai, Z.; Hu, Y. mTOR Signaling in Parkinson's Disease. *Neuromol. Med.* **2017**, *19*, 1–10. [CrossRef] [PubMed]

151. Moors, T.E.; Hoozemans, J.J.; Ingrassia, A.; Beccari, T.; Parnetti, L.; Chartier-Harlin, M.C.; van de Berg, W.D. Therapeutic potential of autophagy-enhancing agents in Parkinson's disease. *Mol. Neurodegener.* **2017**, *12*, 11. [CrossRef] [PubMed]

152. Kolosova, N.G.; Muraleva, N.A.; Zhdankina, A.A.; Stefanova, N.A.; Fursova, A.Z.; Blagosklonny, M.V. Prevention of age-related macular degeneration-like retinopathy by rapamycin in rats. *Am. J. Pathol.* **2012**, *181*, 472–477. [CrossRef] [PubMed]

153. Wong, W.T.; Dresner, S.; Forooghian, F.; Glaser, T.; Doss, L.; Zhou, M.; Cunningham, D.; Shimel, K.; Harrington, M.; Hammel, K.; et al. Treatment of geographic atrophy with subconjunctival sirolimus: Results of a phase I/II clinical trial. *Investig. Ophthalmol. Vis. Sci.* **2013**, *54*, 2941–2950. [CrossRef] [PubMed]

154. Da Cruz, L.; Fynes, K.; Georgiadis, O.; Kerby, J.; Luo, Y.H.; Ahmado, A.; Vernon, A.; Daniels, J.T.; Nommiste, B.; Hasan, S.M.; et al. Phase 1 clinical study of an embryonic stem cell-derived retinal pigment epithelium patch in age-related macular degeneration. *Nat. Biotechnol.* **2018**, *36*, 328–337. [CrossRef] [PubMed]

155. Takayama, K.; Kawakami, Y.; Lavasani, M.; Mu, X.; Cummins, J.H.; Yurube, T.; Kuroda, R.; Kurosaka, M.; Fu, F.H.; Robbins, P.D.; et al. mTOR signaling plays a critical role in the defects observed in muscle-derived stem/progenitor cells isolated from a murine model of accelerated aging. *J. Orthop. Res.* **2017**, *35*, 1375–1382. [CrossRef] [PubMed]

156. Cao, K.; Graziotto, J.J.; Blair, C.D.; Mazzulli, J.R.; Erdos, M.R.; Krainc, D.; Collins, F.S. Rapamycin reverses cellular phenotypes and enhances mutant protein clearance in Hutchinson-Gilford progeria syndrome cells. *Sci. Transl. Med.* **2011**, *3*, 89ra58. [CrossRef] [PubMed]

157. Progeria Research Foundation (PRF). Available online: https://www.progeriaresearch.org/clinical-trials/ (accessed on 3 June 2018).

158. Choi, J.C.; Wu, W.; Muchir, A.; Iwata, S.; Homma, S.; Worman, H.J. Dual specificity phosphatase 4 mediates cardiomyopathy caused by lamin A/C (LMNA) gene mutation. *J. Biol. Chem.* **2012**, *287*, 40513–40524. [CrossRef] [PubMed]

159. Ramos, F.J.; Chen, S.C.; Garelick, M.G.; Dai, D.F.; Liao, C.Y.; Schreiber, K.H.; MacKay, V.L.; An, E.H.; Strong, R.; Ladiges, W.C.; et al. Rapamycin reverses elevated mTORC1 signaling in lamin A/C-deficient mice, rescues cardiac and skeletal muscle function, and extends survival. *Sci. Transl. Med.* **2012**, *4*, 144ra103. [CrossRef] [PubMed]

160. Schreiber, K.H.; Kennedy, B.K. When lamins go bad: Nuclear structure and disease. *Cell* **2013**, *152*, 1365–1375. [CrossRef] [PubMed]

161. Gyawali, B.; Shimokata, T.; Honda, K.; Kondoh, C.; Hayashi, N.; Yoshino, Y.; Sassa, N.; Nakano, Y.; Gotoh, M.; Ando, Y. Muscle wasting associated with the long-term use of mTOR inhibitors. *Mol. Clin. Oncol.* **2016**, *5*, 641–646. [CrossRef] [PubMed]

162. Urfer, S.R.; Kaeberlein, T.L.; Mailheau, S.; Bergman, P.J.; Creevy, K.E.; Promislow, D.E.L.; Kaeberlein, M. A randomized controlled trial to establish effects of short-term rapamycin treatment in 24 middle-aged companion dogs. *Geroscience* **2017**, *39*, 117–127. [CrossRef] [PubMed]

163. Hazeldine, J.; Naumann, D.N.; Toman, E.; Davies, D.; Bishop, J.R.B.; Su, Z.; Hampson, P.; Dinsdale, R.J.; Crombie, N.; Duggal, N.A.; et al. Prehospital immune responses and development of multiple organ dysfunction syndrome following traumatic injury: A prospective cohort study. *PLoS Med.* **2017**, *14*, e1002338. [CrossRef] [PubMed]

164. Wilson, D.; Jackson, T.; Sapey, E.; Lord, J.M. Frailty and sarcopenia: The potential role of an aged immune system. *Ageing Res. Rev.* **2017**, *36*, 1–10. [CrossRef] [PubMed]

165. Smink, J.J.; Begay, V.; Schoenmaker, T.; Sterneck, E.; de Vries, T.J.; Leutz, A. Transcription factor C/EBPβ isoform ratio regulates osteoclastogenesis through MafB. *EMBO J.* **2009**, *28*, 1769–1781. [CrossRef] [PubMed]

166. Smink, J.J.; Leutz, A. Rapamycin and the transcription factor C/EBPβ as a switch in osteoclast differentiation: Implications for lytic bone diseases. *J. Mol. Med.* **2010**, *88*, 227–233. [CrossRef] [PubMed]

167. Glantschnig, H.; Fisher, J.E.; Wesolowski, G.; Rodan, G.A.; Reszka, A.A. M-CSF, TNFα and RANK ligand promote osteoclast survival by signaling through mTOR/S6 kinase. *Cell Death Differ.* **2003**, *10*, 1165–1177. [CrossRef] [PubMed]

168. Kneissel, M.; Luong-Nguyen, N.H.; Baptist, M.; Cortesi, R.; Zumstein-Mecker, S.; Kossida, S.; O'Reilly, T.; Lane, H.; Susa, M. Everolimus suppresses cancellous bone loss, bone resorption, and cathepsin K expression by osteoclasts. *Bone* **2004**, *35*, 1144–1156. [CrossRef] [PubMed]

169. Cejka, D.; Hayer, S.; Niederreiter, B.; Sieghart, W.; Fuereder, T.; Zwerina, J.; Schett, G. Mammalian target of rapamycin signaling is crucial for joint destruction in experimental arthritis and is activated in osteoclasts from patients with rheumatoid arthritis. *Arthritis Rheum.* **2010**, *62*, 2294–2302. [CrossRef] [PubMed]

170. Bruyn, G.A.; Tate, G.; Caeiro, F.; Maldonado-Cocco, J.; Westhovens, R.; Tannenbaum, H.; Bell, M.; Forre, O.; Bjorneboe, O.; Tak, P.P.; et al. Everolimus in patients with rheumatoid arthritis receiving concomitant methotrexate: A 3-month, double-blind, randomised, placebo-controlled, parallel-group, proof-of-concept study. *Ann. Rheum. Dis.* **2008**, *67*, 1090–1095. [CrossRef] [PubMed]

171. Carames, B.; Hasegawa, A.; Taniguchi, N.; Miyaki, S.; Blanco, F.J.; Lotz, M. Autophagy activation by rapamycin reduces severity of experimental osteoarthritis. *Ann. Rheum. Dis.* **2012**, *71*, 575–581. [CrossRef] [PubMed]

172. Pal, B.; Endisha, H.; Zhang, Y.; Kapoor, M. mTOR: A potential therapeutic target in osteoarthritis? *Drugs R&D* **2015**, *15*, 27–36. [CrossRef]

173. Lecka-Czernik, B. Diabetes, bone and glucose-lowering agents: Basic biology. *Diabetologia* **2017**, *60*, 1163–1169. [CrossRef] [PubMed]

174. Creecy, A.; Uppuganti, S.; Merkel, A.R.; O'Neal, D.; Makowski, A.J.; Granke, M.; Voziyan, P.; Nyman, J.S. Changes in the Fracture Resistance of Bone with the Progression of Type 2 Diabetes in the ZDSD Rat. *Calcif. Tissue Int.* **2016**, *99*, 289–301. [CrossRef] [PubMed]

175. Tanikawa, T.; Okada, Y.; Tanikawa, R.; Tanaka, Y. Advanced glycation end products induce calcification of vascular smooth muscle cells through RAGE/p38 MAPK. *J. Vasc. Res.* **2009**, *46*, 572–580. [CrossRef] [PubMed]

176. Mera, P.; Laue, K.; Ferron, M.; Confavreux, C.; Wei, J.; Galan-Diez, M.; Lacampagne, A.; Mitchell, S.J.; Mattison, J.A.; Chen, Y.; et al. Osteocalcin Signaling in Myofibers Is Necessary and Sufficient for Optimum Adaptation to Exercise. *Cell Metab.* **2016**, *23*, 1078–1092. [CrossRef] [PubMed]

177. Chen, S.C.; Brooks, R.; Houskeeper, J.; Bremner, S.K.; Dunlop, J.; Viollet, B.; Logan, P.J.; Salt, I.P.; Ahmed, S.F.; Yarwood, S.J. Corrigendum to "Metformin suppresses adipogenesis through both AMP-activated protein kinase (AMPK)-dependent and AMPK-independent mechanisms" [Mol. Cell. Endocrinol. 440 15 January 2017 57–68]. *Mol. Cell. Endocrinol.* **2017**, *443*, 176. [CrossRef] [PubMed]

178. Zhou, Z.; Tang, Y.; Jin, X.; Chen, C.; Lu, Y.; Liu, L.; Shen, C. Metformin Inhibits Advanced Glycation End Products-Induced Inflammatory Response in Murine Macrophages Partly through AMPK Activation and RAGE/NFkappaB Pathway Suppression. *J. Diabetes Res.* **2016**, *2016*, 4847812. [CrossRef] [PubMed]

179. Shioi, T.; McMullen, J.R.; Tarnavski, O.; Converso, K.; Sherwood, M.C.; Manning, W.J.; Izumo, S. Rapamycin attenuates load-induced cardiac hypertrophy in mice. *Circulation* **2003**, *107*, 1664–1670. [CrossRef] [PubMed]

180. McMullen, J.R.; Sherwood, M.C.; Tarnavski, O.; Zhang, L.; Dorfman, A.L.; Shioi, T.; Izumo, S. Inhibition of mTOR signaling with rapamycin regresses established cardiac hypertrophy induced by pressure overload. *Circulation* **2004**, *109*, 3050–3055. [CrossRef] [PubMed]

181. Lawrence, D.M.; Singh, R.S.; Franklin, D.P.; Carey, D.J.; Elmore, J.R. Rapamycin suppresses experimental aortic aneurysm growth. *J. Vasc. Surg.* **2004**, *40*, 334–338. [CrossRef] [PubMed]

182. Flynn, J.M.; O'Leary, M.N.; Zambataro, C.A.; Academia, E.C.; Presley, M.P.; Garrett, B.J.; Zykovich, A.; Mooney, S.D.; Strong, R.; Rosen, C.J.; et al. Late-life rapamycin treatment reverses age-related heart dysfunction. *Aging Cell* **2013**, *12*, 851–862. [CrossRef] [PubMed]

183. Wang, G.; Zhu, X.; Xie, W.; Han, P.; Li, K.; Sun, Z.; Wang, Y.; Chen, C.; Song, R.; Cao, C.; et al. Rad as a novel regulator of excitation-contraction coupling and β-adrenergic signaling in heart. *Circ. Res.* **2010**, *106*, 317–327. [CrossRef] [PubMed]

184. Dai, D.F.; Karunadharma, P.P.; Chiao, Y.A.; Basisty, N.; Crispin, D.; Hsieh, E.J.; Chen, T.; Gu, H.; Djukovic, D.; Raftery, D.; et al. Altered proteome turnover and remodeling by short-term caloric restriction or rapamycin rejuvenate the aging heart. *Aging Cell* **2014**, *13*, 529–539. [CrossRef] [PubMed]

185. Khan, S.; Salloum, F.; Das, A.; Xi, L.; Vetrovec, G.W.; Kukreja, R.C. Rapamycin confers preconditioning-like protection against ischemia-reperfusion injury in isolated mouse heart and cardiomyocytes. *J. Mol. Cell. Cardiol.* **2006**, *41*, 256–264. [CrossRef] [PubMed]

186. Das, A.; Salloum, F.N.; Durrant, D.; Ockaili, R.; Kukreja, R.C. Rapamycin protects against myocardial ischemia-reperfusion injury through JAK2-STAT3 signaling pathway. *J. Mol. Cell. Cardiol.* **2012**, *53*, 858–869. [CrossRef] [PubMed]

187. Das, A.; Salloum, F.N.; Filippone, S.M.; Durrant, D.E.; Rokosh, G.; Bolli, R.; Kukreja, R.C. Inhibition of mammalian target of rapamycin protects against reperfusion injury in diabetic heart through STAT3 signaling. *Basic Res. Cardiol.* **2015**, *110*, 31. [CrossRef] [PubMed]

188. Das, A.; Durrant, D.; Koka, S.; Salloum, F.N.; Xi, L.; Kukreja, R.C. Mammalian target of rapamycin (mTOR) inhibition with rapamycin improves cardiac function in type 2 diabetic mice: Potential role of attenuated oxidative stress and altered contractile protein expression. *J. Biol. Chem.* **2014**, *289*, 4145–4160. [CrossRef] [PubMed]

189. Morice, M.C.; Serruys, P.W.; Sousa, J.E.; Fajadet, J.; Ban Hayashi, E.; Perin, M.; Colombo, A.; Schuler, G.; Barragan, P.; Guagliumi, G.; et al. A randomized comparison of a sirolimus-eluting stent with a standard stent for coronary revascularization. *N. Engl. J. Med.* **2002**, *346*, 1773–1780. [CrossRef] [PubMed]

190. Shillingford, J.M.; Murcia, N.S.; Larson, C.H.; Low, S.H.; Hedgepeth, R.; Brown, N.; Flask, C.A.; Novick, A.C.; Goldfarb, D.A.; Kramer-Zucker, A.; et al. The mTOR pathway is regulated by polycystin-1, and its inhibition reverses renal cystogenesis in polycystic kidney disease. *Proc. Natl. Acad. Sci. USA* **2006**, *103*, 5466–5471. [CrossRef] [PubMed]

191. Tao, Y.; Kim, J.; Schrier, R.W.; Edelstein, C.L. Rapamycin markedly slows disease progression in a rat model of polycystic kidney disease. *J. Am. Soc. Nephrol.* **2005**, *16*, 46–51. [CrossRef] [PubMed]

192. Wahl, P.R.; Serra, A.L.; Le Hir, M.; Molle, K.D.; Hall, M.N.; Wuthrich, R.P. Inhibition of mTOR with sirolimus slows disease progression in Han:SPRD rats with autosomal dominant polycystic kidney disease (ADPKD). *Nephrol. Dial. Transpl.* **2006**, *21*, 598–604. [CrossRef] [PubMed]

193. Zafar, I.; Belibi, F.A.; He, Z.; Edelstein, C.L. Long-term rapamycin therapy in the Han:SPRD rat model of polycystic kidney disease (PKD). *Nephrol Dial. Transpl.* **2009**, *24*, 2349–2353. [CrossRef] [PubMed]

194. Shillingford, J.M.; Piontek, K.B.; Germino, G.G.; Weimbs, T. Rapamycin ameliorates PKD resulting from conditional inactivation of Pkd1. *J. Am. Soc. Nephrol.* **2010**, *21*, 489–497. [CrossRef] [PubMed]

195. Peces, R.; Peces, C.; Perez-Duenas, V.; Cuesta-Lopez, E.; Azorin, S.; Selgas, R. Rapamycin reduces kidney volume and delays the loss of renal function in a patient with autosomal-dominant polycystic kidney disease. *NDT Plus* **2009**, *2*, 133–135. [CrossRef] [PubMed]

196. Qian, Q.; Du, H.; King, B.F.; Kumar, S.; Dean, P.G.; Cosio, F.G.; Torres, V.E. Sirolimus reduces polycystic liver volume in ADPKD patients. *J. Am. Soc. Nephrol.* **2008**, *19*, 631–638. [CrossRef] [PubMed]

197. Liu, Y.M.; Shao, Y.Q.; He, Q. Sirolimus for treatment of autosomal-dominant polycystic kidney disease: A meta-analysis of randomized controlled trials. *Transpl. Proc.* **2014**, *46*, 66–74. [CrossRef] [PubMed]

198. Myint, T.M.; Rangan, G.K.; Webster, A.C. Treatments to slow progression of autosomal dominant polycystic kidney disease: Systematic review and meta-analysis of randomized trials. *Nephrology* **2014**, *19*, 217–226. [CrossRef] [PubMed]

199. Bolignano, D.; Palmer, S.C.; Ruospo, M.; Zoccali, C.; Craig, J.C.; Strippoli, G.F. Interventions for preventing the progression of autosomal dominant polycystic kidney disease. *Cochrane Database Syst. Rev.* **2015**, CD010294. [CrossRef] [PubMed]

200. Jardine, M.J.; Liyanage, T.; Buxton, E.; Perkovic, V. mTOR inhibition in autosomal-dominant polycystic kidney disease (ADPKD): The question remains open. *Nephrol. Dial. Transpl.* **2013**, *28*, 242–244. [CrossRef] [PubMed]

201. Remuzzi, G.; Schieppati, A.; Ruggenenti, P. Clinical practice. Nephropathy in patients with type 2 diabetes. *N. Engl. J. Med.* **2002**, *346*, 1145–1151. [CrossRef] [PubMed]

202. Inoki, K.; Mori, H.; Wang, J.; Suzuki, T.; Hong, S.; Yoshida, S.; Blattner, S.M.; Ikenoue, T.; Ruegg, M.A.; Hall, M.N.; et al. mTORC1 activation in podocytes is a critical step in the development of diabetic nephropathy in mice. *J. Clin. Investig.* **2011**, *121*, 2181–2196. [CrossRef] [PubMed]

203. Lloberas, N.; Cruzado, J.M.; Franquesa, M.; Herrero-Fresneda, I.; Torras, J.; Alperovich, G.; Rama, I.; Vidal, A.; Grinyo, J.M. Mammalian target of rapamycin pathway blockade slows progression of diabetic kidney disease in rats. *J. Am. Soc. Nephrol.* **2006**, *17*, 1395–1404. [CrossRef] [PubMed]

204. Yang, Y.; Wang, J.; Qin, L.; Shou, Z.; Zhao, J.; Wang, H.; Chen, Y.; Chen, J. Rapamycin prevents early steps of the development of diabetic nephropathy in rats. *Am. J. Nephrol.* **2007**, *27*, 495–502. [CrossRef] [PubMed]

205. Sakaguchi, M.; Isono, M.; Isshiki, K.; Sugimoto, T.; Koya, D.; Kashiwagi, A. Inhibition of mTOR signaling with rapamycin attenuates renal hypertrophy in the early diabetic mice. *Biochem. Biophys. Res. Commun.* **2006**, *340*, 296–301. [CrossRef] [PubMed]

206. Mori, H.; Inoki, K.; Masutani, K.; Wakabayashi, Y.; Komai, K.; Nakagawa, R.; Guan, K.L.; Yoshimura, A. The mTOR pathway is highly activated in diabetic nephropathy and rapamycin has a strong therapeutic potential. *Biochem. Biophys. Res. Commun.* **2009**, *384*, 471–475. [CrossRef] [PubMed]

207. Cheng, L.; Chen, J.; Mao, X. Everolimus vs. rapamycin for treating diabetic nephropathy in diabetic mouse model. *J. Huazhong Univ. Sci. Technol. Med. Sci.* **2011**, *31*, 457–462. [CrossRef] [PubMed]

208. Kenerson, H.L.; Subramanian, S.; McIntyre, R.; Kazami, M.; Yeung, R.S. Livers with constitutive mTORC1 activity resist steatosis independent of feedback suppression of Akt. *PLoS ONE* **2015**, *10*, e0117000. [CrossRef] [PubMed]

209. Guri, Y.; Colombi, M.; Dazert, E.; Hindupur, S.K.; Roszik, J.; Moes, S.; Jenoe, P.; Heim, M.H.; Riezman, I.; Riezman, H.; et al. mTORC2 Promotes Tumorigenesis via Lipid Synthesis. *Cancer Cell* **2017**, *32*, 807–823. [CrossRef] [PubMed]

210. Grabiner, B.C.; Nardi, V.; Birsoy, K.; Possemato, R.; Shen, K.; Sinha, S.; Jordan, A.; Beck, A.H.; Sabatini, D.M. A diverse array of cancer-associated MTOR mutations are hyperactivating and can predict rapamycin sensitivity. *Cancer Discov.* **2014**, *4*, 554–563. [CrossRef] [PubMed]

211. Krtolica, A.; Parrinello, S.; Lockett, S.; Desprez, P.Y.; Campisi, J. Senescent fibroblasts promote epithelial cell growth and tumorigenesis: A link between cancer and aging. *Proc. Natl. Acad. Sci. USA* **2001**, *98*, 12072–12077. [CrossRef] [PubMed]

212. Liu, D.; Hornsby, P.J. Senescent human fibroblasts increase the early growth of xenograft tumors via matrix metalloproteinase secretion. *Cancer Res.* **2007**, *67*, 3117–3126. [CrossRef] [PubMed]

213. Alayev, A.; Salamon, R.S.; Schwartz, N.S.; Berman, A.Y.; Wiener, S.L.; Holz, M.K. Combination of Rapamycin and Resveratrol for Treatment of Bladder Cancer. *J. Cell. Physiol.* **2017**, *232*, 436–446. [CrossRef] [PubMed]

214. Song, X.; Dilly, A.K.; Kim, S.Y.; Choudry, H.A.; Lee, Y.J. Rapamycin-enhanced mitomycin C-induced apoptotic death is mediated through the S6K1-Bad-Bak pathway in peritoneal carcinomatosis. *Cell Death Dis.* **2014**, *5*, e1281. [CrossRef] [PubMed]

215. Sendur, M.A.; Zengin, N.; Aksoy, S.; Altundag, K. Everolimus: A new hope for patients with breast cancer. *Curr. Med. Res. Opin.* **2014**, *30*, 75–87. [CrossRef] [PubMed]

216. Buijsen, J.; van den Bogaard, J.; Jutten, B.; Belgers, E.; Sosef, M.; Leijtens, J.W.; Beets, G.L.; Jansen, R.L.; Riedl, R.G.; Clarijs, R.; et al. A phase I-II study on the combination of rapamycin and short course radiotherapy in rectal cancer. *Radiother. Oncol.* **2015**, *116*, 214–220. [CrossRef] [PubMed]

217. Bennani, N.N.; LaPlant, B.R.; Ansell, S.M.; Habermann, T.M.; Inwards, D.J.; Micallef, I.N.; Johnston, P.B.; Porrata, L.F.; Colgan, J.P.; Markovic, S.N.; et al. Efficacy of the oral mTORC1 inhibitor everolimus in relapsed or refractory indolent lymphoma. *Am. J. Hematol.* **2017**, *92*, 448–453. [CrossRef] [PubMed]

218. Johnston, P.B.; Pinter-Brown, L.C.; Warsi, G.; White, K.; Ramchandren, R. Phase 2 study of everolimus for relapsed or refractory classical Hodgkin lymphoma. *Exp. Hematol. Oncol.* **2018**, *7*, 12. [CrossRef] [PubMed]

219. Wagle, N.; Grabiner, B.C.; Van Allen, E.M.; Hodis, E.; Jacobus, S.; Supko, J.G.; Stewart, M.; Choueiri, T.K.; Gandhi, L.; Cleary, J.M.; et al. Activating mTOR mutations in a patient with an extraordinary response on a phase I trial of everolimus and pazopanib. *Cancer Discov.* **2014**, *4*, 546–553. [CrossRef] [PubMed]

220. Yang, G.; Murashige, D.S.; Humphrey, S.J.; James, D.E. A Positive Feedback Loop between Akt and mTORC2 via SIN1 Phosphorylation. *Cell Rep.* **2015**, *12*, 937–943. [CrossRef] [PubMed]

221. Yang, S.B.; Lee, H.Y.; Young, D.M.; Tien, A.C.; Rowson-Baldwin, A.; Shu, Y.Y.; Jan, Y.N.; Jan, L.Y. Rapamycin induces glucose intolerance in mice by reducing islet mass, insulin content, and insulin sensitivity. *J. Mol. Med.* **2012**, *90*, 575–585. [CrossRef] [PubMed]

222. Fraenkel, M.; Ketzinel-Gilad, M.; Ariav, Y.; Pappo, O.; Karaca, M.; Castel, J.; Berthault, M.F.; Magnan, C.; Cerasi, E.; Kaiser, N.; et al. mTOR inhibition by rapamycin prevents β-cell adaptation to hyperglycemia and exacerbates the metabolic state in type 2 diabetes. *Diabetes* **2008**, *57*, 945–957. [CrossRef] [PubMed]

223. Arriola Apelo, S.I.; Neuman, J.C.; Baar, E.L.; Syed, F.A.; Cummings, N.E.; Brar, H.K.; Pumper, C.P.; Kimple, M.E.; Lamming, D.W. Alternative rapamycin treatment regimens mitigate the impact of rapamycin on glucose homeostasis and the immune system. *Aging Cell* **2016**, *15*, 28–38. [CrossRef] [PubMed]

224. Weiss, R.; Fernandez, E.; Liu, Y.; Strong, R.; Salmon, A.B. Metformin reduces glucose intolerance caused by rapamycin treatment in genetically heterogeneous female mice. *Aging* **2018**. [CrossRef] [PubMed]

225. Ogrodnik, M.; Miwa, S.; Tchkonia, T.; Tiniakos, D.; Wilson, C.L.; Lahat, A.; Day, C.P.; Burt, A.; Palmer, A.; Anstee, Q.M.; et al. Cellular senescence drives age-dependent hepatic steatosis. *Nat. Commun.* **2017**, *8*, 15691. [CrossRef] [PubMed]

226. Jeon, O.H.; Kim, C.; Laberge, R.M.; Demaria, M.; Rathod, S.; Vasserot, A.P.; Chung, J.W.; Kim, D.H.; Poon, Y.; David, N.; et al. Local clearance of senescent cells attenuates the development of post-traumatic osteoarthritis and creates a pro-regenerative environment. *Nat. Med.* **2017**, *23*, 775–781. [CrossRef] [PubMed]

227. Lewis, D.A.; Travers, J.B.; Machado, C.; Somani, A.K.; Spandau, D.F. Reversing the aging stromal phenotype prevents carcinoma initiation. *Aging* **2011**, *3*, 407–416. [CrossRef] [PubMed]

228. Nakamura, A.; Kaneko, N.; Villemagne, V.L.; Kato, T.; Doecke, J.; Dore, V.; Fowler, C.; Li, Q.X.; Martins, R.; Rowe, C.; et al. High performance plasma amyloid-β biomarkers for Alzheimer's disease. *Nature* **2018**, *554*, 249–254. [CrossRef] [PubMed]

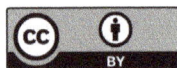

International Journal of
Molecular Sciences

MDPI

Review

The Cutting Edge: The Role of mTOR Signaling in Laminopathies

Francesca Chiarini [1,2,*], Camilla Evangelisti [1,2], Vittoria Cenni [1,2], Antonietta Fazio [3], Francesca Paganelli [3], Alberto M. Martelli [3] and Giovanna Lattanzi [1,2,*]

1   CNR National Research Council of Italy, Institute of Molecular Genetics, Unit of Bologna, 40136 Bologna, Italy; camilla.evangelisti@cnr.it (C.E.); vittoria.cenni@cnr.it (V.C.)
2   IRCCS Istituto Ortopedico Rizzoli, 40136 Bologna, Italy
3   Department of Biomedical and Neuromotor Sciences, University of Bologna, 40126 Bologna, Italy; antonietta.fazio@studio.unibo.it (A.F.); francesca.paganell15@studio.unibo.it (F.P.); alberto.martelli@unibo.it (A.M.M.)
*   Correspondence: francesca.chiarini@cnr.it (F.C.); giovanna.lattanzi@cnr.it (G.L.); Tel.: +39-051-209-1582 (F.C.); +39-051-636-6857 (G.L.); Fax: +39 051-209-1695 (F.C.); +39-051-468-9922 (G.L.)

Received: 21 January 2019; Accepted: 12 February 2019; Published: 15 February 2019

Abstract: The mechanistic target of rapamycin (mTOR) is a ubiquitous serine/threonine kinase that regulates anabolic and catabolic processes, in response to environmental inputs. The existence of mTOR in numerous cell compartments explains its specific ability to sense stress, execute growth signals, and regulate autophagy. mTOR signaling deregulation is closely related to aging and age-related disorders, among which progeroid laminopathies represent genetically characterized clinical entities with well-defined phenotypes. These diseases are caused by *LMNA* mutations and feature altered bone turnover, metabolic dysregulation, and mild to severe segmental progeria. Different *LMNA* mutations cause muscular, adipose tissue and nerve pathologies in the absence of major systemic involvement. This review explores recent advances on mTOR involvement in progeroid and tissue-specific laminopathies. Indeed, hyper-activation of protein kinase B (AKT)/mTOR signaling has been demonstrated in muscular laminopathies, and rescue of mTOR-regulated pathways increases lifespan in animal models of Emery-Dreifuss muscular dystrophy. Further, rapamycin, the best known mTOR inhibitor, has been used to elicit autophagy and degradation of mutated lamin A or progerin in progeroid cells. This review focuses on mTOR-dependent pathogenetic events identified in Emery-Dreifuss muscular dystrophy, *LMNA*-related cardiomyopathies, Hutchinson-Gilford Progeria, mandibuloacral dysplasia, and type 2 familial partial lipodystrophy. Pharmacological application of mTOR inhibitors in view of therapeutic strategies is also discussed.

Keywords: mTOR; laminopathies; lamin A/C; Emery-Dreifuss muscular dystrophy (EDMD); Hutchinson-Gilford progeria syndrome (HGPS); autophagy; cellular signaling; metabolism; bone remodeling; ageing

1. Introduction

1.1. Lamin A and Lamin C

Lamin A and lamin C are the two major splicing products of the *LMNA* gene, which also encodes lamin A delta 10 and lamin C2 [1]. Lamin A/C forms polymers of around 3.5 nm in diameter [2], which are interconnected in a meshwork underneath the nuclear envelope. Further, lamin A and C are also found in the nucleoplasm, bound to chromatin-related proteins as LAP2 alpha [3] and BAF (barrier to autointegration factor) [4]. Lamin A is transcribed and translated as a precursor protein known as prelamin A, which is subjected to a complex post-translational processing yielding mature lamin A [1,5]. Prelamin A C-terminal CaaX box, which is typical of farnesylated proteins, undergoes farnesylation by farnesyl transferase, cleavage of the last three aminoacids by the zinc metallopeptidase STE24 (ZMPSTE24) and carboxymethylation by the isoprenylcysteine carboxyl methyltransferase (ICMT). Thereafter, further cleavage by ZMPSTE24 eliminates the last 15 aminoacids, thus producing a short peptide and mature lamin A [5]. Prelamin A and its processing pathway have been implicated in both physiological and pathogenetic mechanisms [6,7]. Thus, prelamin A plays a physiological role during myogenic differentiation in recruiting inner nuclear membrane proteins SUN1, SUN2 (Sad1 and UNC-84) [8], and Samp1 [9], required for proper myonuclear positioning. Moreover, prelamin A modulation during stress response is a physiological mechanism related to import of DNA repair factors [10] or activation of chromatin remodeling enzymes (Mattioli et al., in preparation). On the other hand, prelamin A accumulation in cells causes toxicity leading to cellular senescence [11] as well as organism ageing [1]. Mature lamin A and lamin C are usually considered as participating in the same cellular mechanisms, although some lamin C-specific pathways have recently emerged [12,13] and lamin C has been shown to form homodimers [14]. Lamin A/C has been implicated in nuclear structure, mechanosignaling, chromatin and genome organization, and cellular response to stress and cellular differentiation [1,5]. All these mechanisms are related to the occurrence of a high number of lamin post-translational modifications, such as phosphorylation, sumoylation, and acetylation, which influence lamin polymerization and lamin interactions with partner proteins [15]. Among the most relevant lamin partners are nuclear envelope proteins emerin, SUN1, SUN2, and nesprins, which form the so-called LINC complex, connecting the nucleus to the cytoskeleton [8,16]. Moreover, lamins bind and regulate translocation of some transcription factors, including SREBP1 [7], Oct-1 [17], Sp-1 [18], NRF2 [19], and mechanoresponsive myocardin-related transcription factor A (MRTFA) [20], and bind and stabilize pRb [21,22] in an Erk1/2-dependent mechanism [23]. Lamin A/C also influences chromatin organization through binding to chromatin-associated proteins such as BAF [4] and histone deacetylases [24]. Further, association of lamins with specific chromatin domains called lamina-associated domains (LADs) has been widely studied in recent years and shown to affect the transcriptional landscape in a cell-type-specific way [25,26].

A role for lamins in cellular signaling has been mostly described in models of muscle differentiation and in muscular laminopathies [15]. In particular, the phosphoinositide 3-kinase (PI3K)/ AKT and Erk 1/2 pathway has been extensively investigated in mouse models of EDMD [27–29]. In the same context, a major player appears to be TGFβ 2 signaling. TGFβ 2 levels are increased both in EDMD patient serum [30] and in mouse models of muscular laminopathies [31] and in both cases TGFβ 2 elicits upregulation of fibrogenic molecules. TGFβ 2 signals through the mechanistic target of the rapamycin (mTOR) pathway, although different involvement of AKT, mTOR itself, or p70 ribosomal S6 kinase 1 (S6K1) occur depending on cell types [30]. Of note, it has been demonstrated that lamin A mutations causing MADA or other progeroid laminopathies are also able to trigger TGFβ 2 signaling with downstream effects on mTOR pathway and osteoclastogenic activity [32]. On the other hand, AKT is a lamin A and prelamin A kinase, which phosphorylates Serine 404 in the protein rod domain [33] and targets prelamin A to lysosomal degradation [34]. It is tempting to speculate that feedback mechanisms aimed at the maintenance of proper lamin A levels [34] could involve activation of mTOR under both normal and pathological conditions. This review is aimed at providing an overview of available data to stimulate a new interpretation and suggest new experimental approaches to the issue of an mTOR-lamin A relationship.

1.2. Laminopathies

Laminopathies are rare diseases caused by mutations in *LMNA* or other nuclear envelope genes or in genes structurally or functionally related to the nuclear envelope (Figure 1).

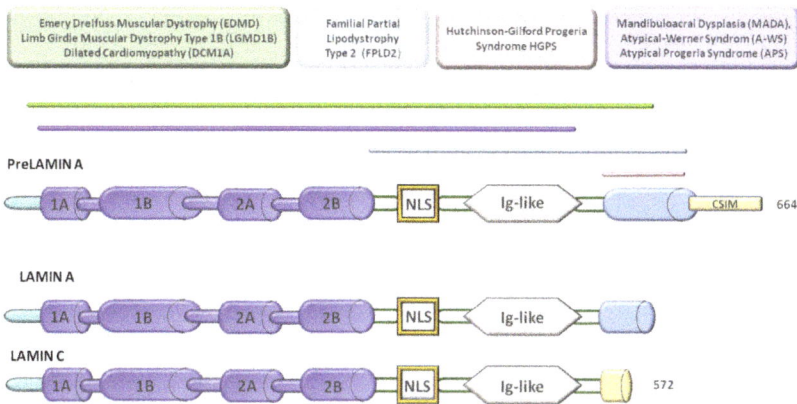

Figure 1. Diagram of prelamin A, lamin A, and lamin C structures with domains mutated in laminopathies. Laminopathies are grouped in the upper boxes referring to muscular laminopathies, lipodystrophy, Hutchinson-Gilford progeria syndrome (HGPS), and other progeroid laminopathies. Under physiological conditions and in muscular laminopathies, prelamin A is hardly detectable due to rapid maturation to lamin A. Most cases of laminopathies carry *LMNA* missense mutations. In progeroid laminopathies, prelamin A levels increase. In HGPS, truncated prelamin A (progerin) is accumulated due to a splicing defect. The pink bar spans the prelamin A domain missing in progerin. For bar colors, refer to the disease boxes.

Most laminopathies are rare to very rare diseases and feature an autosomal dominant inheritance, although recessive inheritance can also occur, as in mandibuloacral dysplasia (MADA), Charcot–Marie tooth neuropathy (CMT2B1), and restrictive dermopathy (RD). Muscular laminopathies include muscular dystrophies characterized by joint contractures, muscle weakness and wasting, and cardiomyopathy—*LMNA*-linked congenital muscular dystrophy (L-CMD) and isolated cardiomyopathies with conduction defects [30,35]. Among muscular dystrophies, EDMD1 is linked to emerin mutations (*EMD* gene), EDMD2 and limb -girdle muscular dystrophy type 1B are caused by dominant lamin A/C mutations (*LMNA* gene), other forms of EDMD are caused by nesprin (*SYNE1* and *SYNE2* genes), FHL1, SUN1, or SUN2 mutations (Table 1) [1,30]. Cardiomyopathies occurring in the absence of muscular dystrophy have been so far mostly linked to *LMNA* mutations, although cases related to nesprin gene defects have also been reported, and an association of *LMNA* with modifier gene variants has been suggested [36–38].

Table 1. The most representative laminopathies are listed. * nomenclature for these forms is provisional; ** potential hotspot; *** cardiomyopathy with conduction defect type 1A (DCM1A).

Disease	Gene	Protein	Hotspot	Inheritance	Phenotype	Ref.
Muscular Laminopathies						
EDMD2	*LMNA*	Lamin A/C	R453	AD	Joint contractures, muscle weakness and wasting, cardiomyopathy	[39,40]
EDMD1	*EMD*	Emerin		X-linked	Joint contractures, muscle weakness and wasting, cardiomyopathy	[39,40]
EDMD3	*LMNA*	Lamin A/C		AR	Joint contractures, muscle weakness and wasting, cardiomyopathy	[39,40]
EDMD4	*SYNE1*	Nesprin 1		AD	Joint contractures, muscle weakness and wasting, cardiomyopathy	[39,41]
EDMD5	*SYNE2*	Nesprin 2		AD	Joint contractures, muscle weakness and wasting, cardiomyopathy	[39,41]

Table 1. *Cont.*

Disease	Gene	Protein	Hotspot	Inheritance	Phenotype	Ref.
Muscular Laminopathies						
EDMD6	*FHL1*	FHL1		X-linked	Joint contractures, muscle weakness and wasting, cardiomyopathy, vocal cord involvement	[40,42]
EDMD7	*TMEM43*	LUMA		AD	Muscle weakness, cardiomyopathy with cardiac conduction defects	[40,43]
LGMD1B	*LMNA*	Lamin A/C		AD	Joint contractures, muscle weakness and wasting, cardiomyopathy	[39,40]
L-CMD	*LMNA*	Lamin A/C		AD	Severe and early onset muscle weakness and wasting, contractures, delayed/absent motor milestones, dropped head, cardiomyopathy	[39,40]
MD*	*SUN1, SUN2*	SUN1, SUN2		AD	Cardiomyopathy, skeletal muscle weakness and wasting	[37,44]
Cardiomyopathies						
DCM1A***	*LMNA*	Lamin A/C		AD	Dilated cardiomyopathy and conduction defects	[35,45]
DCM	*SYNE1*	Nesprin 1		AD	Dilated cardiomyopathy	[46,47]
DCM-CD	*TMPO*	Lap2 α			Dilated cardiomyopathy joint contractures	[48,49]
Lipodystrophies						
FPLD2	*LMNA*	Lamin A/C	R482	AD	Loss of subcutaneous fat, accumulation of fat in the neck, diabetes, polycystic ovary syndrome	[50,51]
APL	*LMNB2*	Lamin B2		AR	Symmetrical loss of subcutaneous fat from the face, neck, upper extremities, thorax, and abdomen, sparing the lower extremities	[52,53]
Progeroid Laminopathies						
HGPS	*LMNA*	Lamin A/C	G608		Premature and accelerated aging, growth arrest, lipodystrophy mandible, clavicle, phalanges osteolysis, osteoporosis, atherosclerosis	[54,55]
APS	*LMNA*	Lamin A/C			Premature aging, lipodystrophy, cardiovascular disease, short stature, diabetes and alopecia	[24,56]
A-WS	*LMNA*	Lamin A/C		AD	Late onset premature aging, atherosclerosis, lipodystrophy, diabetes	[1,57]
MADA	*LMNA*	Lamin A/C	R527	AR AD	Mandible, clavicle, phalanges osteolysis, osteoporosis, partial lipodystrophy, short stature, metabolic abnormalities, mildly accelerated aging	[1,58]
MADB	*ZMPSTE24*	ZMPSTE24	1085dupT **	AR AD	Accelerated aging, mandible, clavicle, phalanges osteolysis, osteoporosis, generalized lipodystrophy, short stature, metabolic abnormalities	[1,59]

Laminopathies featuring a lipodystrophy phenotype acquire partial lipodystrophy due to *LMNB2* gene mutations, type 2 familial partial lipodystrophy (FPLD2), type A and B mandiboloacral dysplasia (MADA and MADB) associated with mutations in *LMNA*, or the prelamin A endoprotease ZMPSTE24 gene, respectively. Lipodystrophy can be partial, causing loss of specific fat depots and fat accumulation in other districts, or generalized, as in MADB. MADA and MADB are also considered progeroid laminopathies since patient experience mildly accelerated ageing and bone and skin defects typical of aged individuals [1,58]. The latter symptoms are present with increased severity in HGPS, a premature aging syndrome with very early onset also causing cardiovascular disorders and premature death [58] (Table 1).

2. mTOR Complexes and Signaling Regulation

2.1. mTOR Complexes

mTOR is a Ser/Thr kinase in the phosphoinositide kinase-related family of protein kinases (PIKK) [60]. Other members of the PIKK family include ataxia telangiectasia mutated (ATM), ataxia telangiectasia gene product- and RAD3-related (ATR), human suppressor of morphogenesis in genitalia-1 (hSMG-1), and the catalytic subunit of DNA-dependent protein kinase (DNA-PK) (Figure 2) [61].

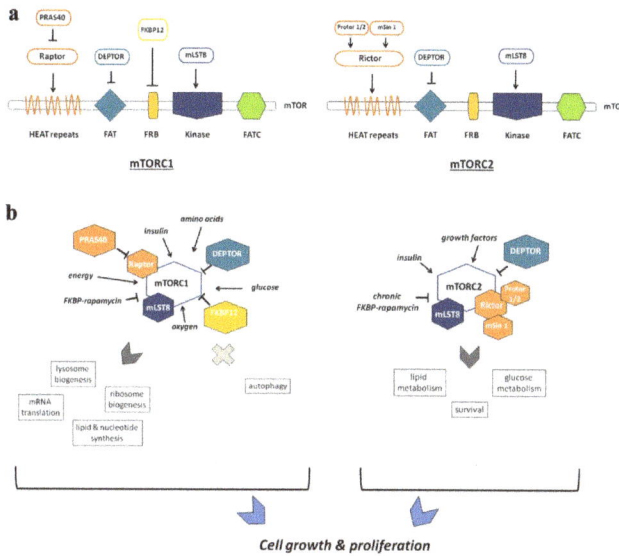

Figure 2. mTORC1 and mTORC2 domains and interactors. (**a**) Deptor, DEP domain-containing mTOR-interacting protein; FAT, FKBP/ATM/TRRAP; FATC, FRAP/ATM/TRRAP/Carboxy terminal; FKBP-12, FK506-binding protein-12; FRB, FKBP, rapamycin-binding; HEAT, Huntingtin/Elongation factor 3/A subunit of protein phosphatase-2A/ TOR1; mLST8, mammalian lethal with SEC13 protein 8; mSin1, mammalian stress-activated protein kinase interacting protein 1; mTOR, mechanistic target of rapamycin; mTORC1, mTOR complex 1; mTORC2: mTOR complex 2; PRAS40, proline-rich AKT substrate 1 40 kDa; Protor 1/2, protein observed with Rictor; Raptor, regulatory-associated protein of TOR; Rictor, rapamycin-insensitive companion of TOR. (**b**) mTORC1 and mTORC2 complexes and their role in cell growth and proliferation.

mTOR works as a crucial integrator of growth factor-activated and nutrient sensing pathways to coordinate several cellular functions, and linking nutrient availability with metabolic control [62]. mTOR is the catalytic subunit of two functionally and structurally distinct protein complexes known as mTORC1 and mTORC2 (Figure 2a,b) [60].

2.1.1. mTORC1

mTORC1 is composed of mTOR, RAPTOR (regulatory-associated protein of mTOR), which is important for the subcellular localization of mTORC1, mLST8 (mammalian lethal with Sec13 protein 8), PRAS40 (proline rich AKT substrate 40 kDa), and DEPTOR (DEP-domain containing mTOR interacting protein), the latter two having an inhibitory function on mTORC1 (Figure 2).

Multiple inputs converge on mTORC1: growth factors, chemokines, nutrients (glucose, amino acids), and the cell energy status (i.e., a high ATP/AMP ratio) [63]. Growth factors and cytokines stimulate mTORC1 mostly through the PI3K/AKT signaling pathway. However, growth factors and chemokines signal to mTORC1 also occur through the Ras/Raf/MEK/ Erk 1/2 network. Moreover, recent studies have shown that mTORC1 and mTORC2 also respond to inputs via the Wnt and liver kinase 1 (LKB1)/AMP-activated protein kinase (AMPK) signaling pathways (Figure 3) [62].

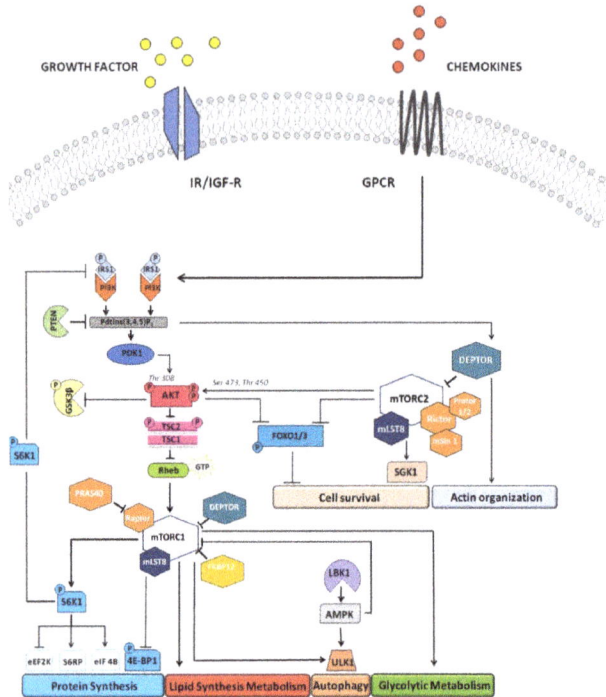

Figure 3. mTOR signaling network. The serine/threonine kinase mTOR is found in two multiprotein complexes: mTORC1 is composed of RAPTOR, PRAS40, mLST8, and DEPTOR, which has an inhibitory function on mTORC1. The mTORC1 is activated by growth factors, chemokines, nutrients (glucose, amino acids), and the cell energy status (i.e., a high ATP/AMP ratio). mTORC1 stimulation is activated by growth factors through the phosphoinositide 3-kinase (PI3K)-AKT signaling pathway. AKT phosphorylates tuberous sclerosis complex 2 (TSC2 or hamartin) at multiple sites. TSC2 is a GTPase-activating protein (GAP) that associates with tuberous sclerosis 1 (TSC1 or tuberin) for inactivating the small G protein Rheb (Ras homolog enriched in brain). Once AKT phosphorylates TSC2, the GAP activity of the TSC1/TSC2 complex is repressed, allowing Rheb to accumulate in a GTP-bound state. Therefore, Rheb-GTP upregulates mTORC1 protein kinase activity. AKT also phosphorylates PRAS40 (at Thr246), which dissociates from mTORC1 in response to growth factors, or glucose and nutrients, thereby releasing the inhibitory function of PRAS40 on mTORC1. mTORC1 activates S6K1 through phosphorylation, and S6K1 in turn phosphorylates or binds proteins such as eukaryotic elongation factor 2 kinase (eEF2K), which targets eEF2 and regulates the elongation step of protein translation, ribosomal protein S6 (S6RP), and eukaryotic initiation factor 4B (eIF4B), ultimately promoting translation initiation and elongation. mTORC1 also phosphorylayes and inactivates the translation inhibitor 4E-BP1, which has a role in inhibiting cap-dependent translation through the binding of the translation initiation factor eIF4E. mTORC1 is a repressor of autophagy, through phosphorylation of Unc-51 like autophagy activating kinase 1 (ULK1), and positively controls lipid synthesis and glycolytic metabolism.

Upon activation, mTORC1 regulates ribosomal and lysosomal biogenesis, cap-dependent translation, autophagy, mitochondrial biogenesis, lipid synthesis, and thermogenesis, acting through direct phosphorylation of many substrates. mTORC1 can also sustain nucleotide biogenesis promoting the expression of genes involved in the pentose phosphate pathway and pirimidine biosynthesis (Figure 3) [64].

It has been demonstrated that reducing mTOR activity increases autophagic flux, reducing reactive oxygen species within the cell and increasing replicative lifespan. At the same time, it has been established that impaired mitochondrial function is associated with aging and age-related diseases, in which decreased mitochondrial function can have a significant impact on ATP production, maintenance of NAD/NADH ratios, and reactive oxygen species (ROS) production [65]. In the case of laminopathies, defective mitochondrial activity has been documented in FPLD2 [66], models of DCM [67], and HGPS cells [68].

Activation of mTORC1 relieves the inhibitory effect of 4E-BP1 on eIF4E and stimulates the translation of nuclear-encoded mRNAs of mitochondrial proteins, including the mitochondrial transcription factor A (TFAM) and mitochondrial ribosomal proteins and components of complex I and V. In addition, mTORC1 regulates mitochondrial function by modulating transcription of mitochondrial nuclear-encoded genes via Yin Yang 1 (YY1) and peroxisome proliferator-activated receptor-gamma coactivator 1 α (PGC-1α) [69]. Hence, it is likely that mTORC1 stimulates mitochondrial function by orchestrating translation and transcription of distinct mitochondria-related genes [70].

It has been demonstrated in models of senescence and Hutchinson–Gilford progeria that senescence is accompanied by elevated glycolysis and increased oxidative phosphorylation, which are both reduced by rapamycin or rapalogs [68].

Concerning protein synthesis, mTOR is able to control the balance between anabolism and catabolism in response to environmental cues [71] and to act through phosphorylation of the effectors of the protein synthesis machinery, including S6K1 and the translation inhibitor, eukaryotic translation initiation factor 4E-binding protein 1 (4E-BP1) [72,73]. S6K1 is phosphorylated by mTORC1 in Th389, enabling its complete phosphorylation and activation by PDK1. S6K1 phosphorylates ribosomal protein S6 (RPS6), leading to active translation of mRNAs involved in ribosome biogenesis. S6K1 has also several substrates, including insulin receptor substrate-1 (IRS1), which is upstream of mTORC1. Importantly, IRS1 phosphorylation by S6K1 is fundamental for its proteasomal degradation and impairs growth factors (insulin, insulin-like growth factor-1) signaling downstream of receptor tyrosine kinases (RTKs) [60]. The consequence is a negative feedback loop, in which PI3K/AKT axis is inhibited and mTORC1 activity is regulated. In addition, also Grb10 acts as a negative regulator of mTORC1 through phosphorylation-dependent feedback mechanisms. Regarding 4E-BP1, its phosphorylation by mTORC1 triggers its dissociation to the cap-binding protein eukaryotic initiation factor 4E (eIF4E), enabling it to constitute the eIF4F complex, necessary for the initiation of cap-dependent mRNA translation (Figure 3) [60,72].

Further, mTORC1 acts increasing the glycolytic flux, promoting a shift in glucose metabolism, by activating the transcription and the translation of hypoxia inducible factor 1α (HIF1α), a positive regulator of many glycolytic genes, and facilitating cell growth [60].

mTORC1 also controls de novo lipid synthesis, necessary for proliferating cells to generate membranes, acting mainly through the sterol regulatory element-binding proteins 1 (SREBP1), which are transcription factors of lipogenic genes, as well as through peroxisome proliferator-activated receptor gamma (PPARγ), the master regulator of adipogenesis [60].

In addition to various anabolic roles, mTORC1 is a negative regulator of autophagic processes, required to eliminate damaged organelles and recycle molecules as well as for cellular adaptation to nutrient starvation [74]. When mTORC1 is inhibited, autophagosomes sequester cytoplasmic components and then fuse with lysosomes, leading to degradation of cell components and recycling of cellular building blocks.

mTORC1 directly phosphorylates and suppresses ULK1/Atg13/FIP200 (unc-51-like kinase 1/mammalian autophagy-related gene 13/focal adhesion kinase family-interacting protein of 200 kDa), a kinase complex which is required to drive autophagosome formation [75]. mTORC2 is composed of RICTOR, SIN1, mLST8, PROTOR, and DEPTOR. It regulates cell survival through serum and glucocorticoid activated kinase 1 (SGK1) and AKT. mTORC2 phosphorylates AKT on Ser473, priming AKT for further phosphorylation by PDK1 at the Thr308 residue. Loss of phosphorylation at Ser 473 site, however, only affects some of AKT substrates, such as FOXO transcription factors, but not TSC2, in response to growth factor signaling. mTORC2 associates with actively translating ribosome to co-translationally phosphorylate AKT (at Thr450), which prevents ubiquitinylation and degradation of AKT. mTORC2 is involved in the spatial control of cell growth via cytoskeleton regulation. Arrows indicate activating events, while perpendicular lines indicate inhibitory events. GPCR: G protein-coupled receptor; IGF-R, insulin-like growth factor receptor; IR: insulin receptor.

On the contrary, during nutrient deprivation, lysosomal mTORC1 is inactivated, partially due to lack of amino acids. Under energy starvation conditions, an increase in AMP levels stimulates the activity of AMPK, and inhibits mTORC1. It is observed that the relative activity of mTORC1 and AMPK in different contexts may determinate the level of autophagy induction. AMPK, which is activated by LKB1 under metabolic stress conditions, phosphorylates ULK1 at multiple sites, thus upregulating ULK1 activity, and activates tuberous sclerosis complex 2 (TSC2), which is an indirect inhibitor of mTORC1 activity. Following mTORC1 inhibition, derepressed ULK1, by binding to ATG14L (ATG—autophagy related-14 Like), is recruited to a molecular platform composed of vacuolar protein sorting 34 (Vps34) and beclin-1. This leads to the phosphorylation of beclin-1 on Ser 14, and activation of Vps34, which has an important role in regulating membrane trafficking and autophagy, releasing PI3-phosphate at the nascent autophagosome [76]. In this condition, microtubule-associated protein 1 light chain 3 (LC3), a structural protein found in the cytoplasm in its precursor form (LC3I), is cleaved, coupled to phosphatidylethanolamine and converted into its active autophagosomal, membrane-bound form, LC3II [76].

Protein turnover is controlled by the ubiquitin proteasome system (UPS), through which proteins are targeted for degradation by the proteasome after ubiquitination. mTORC1 was recently found involved in the control of proteasome-dependent proteolysis. Acute mTORC1 inhibition seems to increase proteasome-dependent proteolysis likely to restore aminoacid pools. Prolonged hyperactivation of mTORC1 signaling increases proteasome activity through elevated expression of proteasome subunits downstream of Nrf1, as a compensatory mechanism to balance the increase in protein turnover and protein synthesis [77].

2.1.2. mTORC2

mTORC2 is composed of RICTOR (rapamycin-insensible companion of mTOR), SIN1 (stress activated protein kinase-interacting 1), PROTOR1/2 (protein observed with Rictor), mLST8, and DEPTOR (Figure 2b) [60]. Unlike mTORC1, mTORC2 is not sensitive to nutrients, but it responds to growth factors via the PI3K signaling pathway. In fact, the most relevant role of mTORC2 is AKT phosphorylation in Ser473 and its activation, which is required for the phosphorylation of Forkhead box O 1/3a (FoxO1/3a) transcription factors. This phosphorylation allows AKT to promote cell growth and survival via PI3K/AKT signaling. AKT also phosphorylates and inhibits GSK3beta and the mTORC1 inhibitor TSC2. Thus, mTORC2 acts as an effector of insulin/PI3K signaling. The mTORC2 protein mSin1 contains a PH domain, essential for the insulin-dependent regulation of mTORC2 activity. mSin1 inhibits the catalytic activity of mTORC2 in the absence of insulin, and this autoinhibition is relieved upon binding to PIP3 generated by the PI3K at the plasma membrane (Figure 3). Localization at the plasma membrane is a key aspect of mTORC2 regulation. mSin1 can also be phosphorylated by AKT, with a positive feedback loop, while the partial activation of AKT promotes mTORC2 activation, which causes in turn AKT phosphorylation (and activation) at Ser473 [78].

mTORC2 controls cell survival/metabolism also through serum and glucocorticoid activated kinase 1 (SGK1), and it is involved in the spatial control of cell growth via cytoskeleton remodeling, through actin fibers, paxilin, RhoA, Rac1, and protein kinase C (PKC) family phosphorylation, all of which regulate several aspects of cytoskeleton remodeling and cell migration [60].

mTORC2 signaling is also regulated by mTORC1, due to the negative feedback loop between insulin/PI3K and mTORC1. In fact, mTORC1 can phosphorylate and activate Grb10, a negative regulator of insulin/IGF1receptor signaling, upstream of AKT and mTORC2, while S6K1 also suppresses mTORC2 activation through the phosphorylation dependent degradation of IRS1, as has been mentioned [78].

3. mTOR Signaling in Physiological Conditions

3.1. mTOR Signaling in Muscular Tissue

As in all the other tissues of the organism, in normal skeletal and cardiac muscle, the mTOR pathway plays a pivotal role in cell growth, proliferation, and survival. In particular, in skeletal muscle cells, mTOR controls both the anabolic and catabolic signaling resulting in the modulation of muscle hypertrophy and muscle wasting [79]. mTOR functions as a positive regulator of muscle hypertrophy, being downregulated by muscle atrophy-inducing signals, such as myostatin [80] and glucocorticoids [81] as well as by sarcopenia, an age-related decline in muscle mass due to a reduction of circulatory IGF1 levels. On the other hand, mTOR is strongly activated by anabolic stimuli such as muscle contraction, insulin, IGF1, and nutrients, and triggers an increase of protein synthesis and as such of muscle hypertrophy. In the cardiovascular system, mTOR activity is involved in the regulation of embryonic cardiovascular development and in the control of vital cellular processes necessary for postnatal growth and maintenance of cardiac function. Ablation of cardiac mTOR in murine models is in fact associated with a high rate of embryonic lethality [82], and cardiac disruption of mTORC1 activity is associated with cardiac dilation, dysfunction, apoptosis, mitochondrial and metabolic derangements, heart failure, and ultimately mortality in the postnatal stage [83]. In addition, complete genetic disruption of mTORC1 impairs the ability of the heart to respond to pressure overload and to undergo compensatory hypertrophy, resulting in the development of dilated cardiomyopathy [83]. On the other hand, mTOR inhibition triggers autophagy, protects cardiomyocytes during energy deprivation [84], extends lifespan, and reduces cardiac hyperthrophy in aged mouse models [85]. All these data suggest a complex and multifaceted role of mTOR signaling in the heart [86].

3.2. mTOR Signaling in Adipose Tissue

mTOR signaling plays a critical role in the regulation of adipogenesis, lipid metabolism, thermogenesis, and adipokine synthesis/secretion. However, a complex picture emerges from literature data, which suggests a condition highly dependent on environmental stimuli, adipose tissue depot, developmental stage, and the type of adipocyte precursors involved. White and brown adipose tissue have diverse morphology and functions [87]. Whereas white adipocytes are formed by large lipid droplets deputed to store energy in the form of triglycerides, brown adipocytes present small droplets and convert lipid-derived chemical energy into heat for thermogenesis [87]. mTORC1 is indispensable for adipose tissue homeostasis, as indicated by the occurrence of lipodystrophy, defects in dietary lipid intake and metabolic disorders in mice lacking mTORC1 in all mature adipocytes [88]. However, knocking out all adipocyte AKT activity by simultaneously deleting AKT1 and AKT2 in adipocytes, elicits an even more severe lipodystrophy phenotype, showing that AKT also regulates mTOR-independent adipocyte activities and that mTORC1-AKT interplay contributes to adipose tissue maintenance [88]. On the other hand, mTOR inhibition leading to the activation of autophagy contributes to white adipose tissue formation. Consistently, partial knockdown of mTOR increases adipogenesis, although complete inhibition of activity as well as inactivation of pS6K1 impairs adipocyte differentiation [89]. Several genes including PPARγ, a master regulator of adipogenesis, are upregulated by mTOR inhibition [89]. However, the best-known effect of mTOR downregulation, i.e., autophagy induction, plays a major role. In fact, autophagy is required for white adipogenesis [90], while inhibition of autophagy has been shown to convert white adipocytes into brown-like cells called brite or beige adipocytes [91]. Autophagy triggers degradation of PPARγ 2 proteases, thus contributing to PPARγ 2 increase. Further, autophagy promotes vesicle fusion, thus triggering a formation of large lipid droplets in white adipocytes [92]. Nevertheless, a recent paper shows that the thyroid hormone triiodothyronine (T3) stimulates autophagy in brown adipose tissue by reducing mTOR activity, and this elicits mitophagy and a more efficient mitochondrial respiratory chain [93].

3.3. mTOR in Bone Turnover

Mammalian bones are formed through two different mechanisms, endochondral or intramembranous ossification. During intramembranous ossification, mesenchymal progenitors directly differentiate into osteoblasts, while, in endochondral bone formation, a first stage of cartilage production is followed by remodeling of hypertrophic cartilage by osteoclasts and the production of bone matrix by osteoblasts [94]. mTORC1 has been studied in models of cartilage formation and chondrocyte differentiation, and diverse mechanisms have been proposed and partially validated by experimental evidence [95]. Further, mTORC1 and mTORC2 have been implicated in regulating osteoblast differentiation and function. Bone marrow stromal cells lacking Rictor gene exhibited reduced osteogenic potential and an increased tendency to undergo adipogenic differentiation, suggesting that mTOR signaling may regulate cellular fate, thus affecting bone homeostasis [95]. mTORC1 is required for the transition of preosteoblasts to mature osteoblasts and both mTORC1 and mTORC2 dysregulation have been linked to osteoarthritis and osteoporosis [95]. Moreover, mTOR activity affects osteoclasts and bone resorption, although effectors are not fully elucidated [95].

4. EDMD, DCM and Other Muscular Laminopathies

4.1. Muscular Laminopathies

LMNA-associated muscular laminopathies include EDMD2 and EDMD3 [96], DCM [97,98], LGMD1B [99], *LMNA*-related congenital muscular dystrophy (L-CMD) [100], and "heart-hand" syndrome (HHS) [101].

To date, there are multiple hypotheses regarding the onset of muscular dystrophies due to genetic mutations on *LMNA* or genes encoding for lamin A/C-associated proteins. The first one is the "structural hypothesis," which suggests that a loss of structural integrity of the nuclear lamina leads to nuclear structural weakness, which ultimately results in a decrease in the ability of the nucleus to resist to the high mechanical strain typical of skeletal muscles [102]. This theory is validated by the fact that lamin A/C interacts with structural proteins including emerin SUN1 [8], nesprins, LAP2α [103], and Ankrd2 [104]. The interaction of lamin A/C with SUN proteins and nesprins is particularly relevant for nuclear positioning in muscle [8], and mutations in lamins affect LINC complex-lamin A/C interplay, thus leading to myonuclear clustering, a further determinant of *LMNA* pathogenetic mechanisms [8,9]. The "gene-expression" hypothesis suggests that some lamin A/C mutations may alter gene expression during muscle differentiation. Supporting this hypothesis, A-type lamins and some of their binding partners (e.g., LAP2 or emerin) interact with muscle specific transcription factors such as MyoD [105]. Moreover, myoblasts with altered lamin A/C or emerin are characterized by low levels of proteins involved in cell cycle regulation and muscle differentiation, such as MyoD, desmin, pRb, and M-cadherin [106]. Furthermore, the microRNA profile in skeletal muscles of patients affected by muscular laminopathies has revealed a significant alteration of proteins involved in muscle repair pathways, such as MAPK, TGF-β, and Wnt, as well as in differentiation and regenerative processes [107]. These pathogenetic hypotheses are not mutually exclusive and most likely concur to the onset of the pathology.

mTOR Signaling in Muscular Laminopathies

Several studies indicate that the molecular pathway ruled by mTOR is deeply affected in muscular laminopathies. As a consequence of the sustained mechanical strain to which they are constantly subjected, cardiac and skeletal muscle cells feature a particularly high amount of waste material, including mitochondrial-derived ROS (reactive oxygen species) and toxic molecules [108]. In normal conditions, ROSs block mTORC1 activity through the already described AMPK/mTOR pathway, triggering the activation of autophagy, that results in a prompt degradation of toxic molecules and dysfunctional organelles (for a review of autophagy regulation by ROSs, please read Filomeni et al. [109].

In muscle cells from laminopathic patients, there is an overall increase in the amount of ROS, due to both the reduction of nuclear plasticity [104] and the loss of the properties of "ROS acceptor" of the altered nuclear lamina unable to neutralize cellular ROSs [110]. In spite of this, the significant drop of autophagic activity has been described in models of muscular laminopathies. In 2012, the group of B. Kennedy demonstrated that, in the heart of $Lmna^{-/-}$ mice suffering of muscular dystrophy and cardiomyopathy, the increased levels of LC3-BII, Atg7, and beclin 1 proteins, generally indicating an ongoing autophagic pathway, were not followed by a decrease in p62/SQSTM1 [111], which is a marker of an active autophagic flux. Almost simultaneously, the group of H. Worman demonstrated that cardiac cells from a mouse model carrying the p.H222P lamin A/C mutation causing EDMD2 in humans exhibited defective autophagy in response to starvation [97,112]. Interestingly, in this study the authors also found a clear correlation between the expression level of mutated lamin A/C and the hyperactivation of both AKT and Erk 1/2 [97,112], which results in the activation of mTORC1. Finally, the confirmation that the mTORC1/autophagy axis plays a central role in the pathophysiology of cardio-muscular laminopathies, came from the evidences that rapamycin or its analog temsirolimus improve cardiac and muscle functions, and extend the lifespan in both laminopathic mouse models [97,111]. In serum from patients affected by muscular laminopathies, a wide study conducted by the Italian Network for Laminopathies demonstrated a significant increase in TGFβ 2 levels [30]. This was associated with hyperactivation of mTOR in cultured myoblasts and AKT and pS6K1 in fibroblasts [30]. Intriguingly, in both cell types, neutralization by a TGFβ 2 antibody rescued mTOR or AKT hyperactivation, thus showing a major role of TGFβ 2 in the signaling pathway in EDMD2 [30]. Downstream events in that experimental context reduced myoblast differentiation and fibrogenic conversion of myoblasts ad tenocytes [30], the latter being a poorly investigated cell type with potential involvement in joint contractures typical of EDMD. The relevance of TGFβ 2 signaling in pathogenetic events, mostly leading to fibrogenic conversion of myoblasts, has also shown in the H222P/H222P *Lmna* mouse model of EDMD2 [31].

The group of B. Kennedy also wondered if mTOR was involved in the activation of pathways promoting metabolic response via phosphorylation of S6K1 and 4E-BP1 [113]. The authors reported that heterozygosity for S6K1 (S6K1$^{+/-}$) extended lifespan of $Lmna^{-/-}$ mice exactly as rapamycin treatment did. Intriguingly, life extension of $Lmna^{-/-}$ S6K1$^{+/-}$ mice was not due to improvement in cardiac function (as seen for rapamycin treatment) or to the rescue of metabolic alterations, but to the amelioration of skeletal muscle deficits. In contrast, whole-body overexpression of 4E-BP1 shortened the survival of $Lmna^{-/-}$ mice, likely by accelerating lipolysis, pointing to the conclusion that rapamycin possibly extends survival of $Lmna^{-/-}$ mice through the mTORC1-S6K1 branch, but not the mTORC1/4E-BP1 one of the mTOR signaling pathway [113].

Altered autophagic activity has been also observed in hearts of transgenic *Drosophila* expressing mutated LamC (the genetic counterpart of human *LMNA*) and affected by cardiomyopathy [114]. In this model, mutant Lamin C accumulated in the cytosol, resulting in upregulation and accumulation of p62/SQSTM1. These events caused inactivation of AMPK, activation of mTOR, and ultimately inhibition of autophagy [114]. Interestingly, similar evidence had been previously obtained in heart and muscle from other transgenic *Drosophila* models carrying other EDMD2-causative mutations in LamC [115]. In support to mTOR signaling pathway alteration in laminopathic muscle cells, cardiac cells from transgenic flies also featured metabolic alterations, including an age-dependent increase in size of fat bodies and enhanced triglyceride amount [114]. Overexpression of *Atg1* (a kinase promoting autophagy) suppressed cardiac defects associated with mutant LamC and restored cardiac function and lifespan. At the molecular level, the reactivation of autophagy induced by *Atg1* overexpression elicited clearance of cytoplasmic LamC aggregates, reduction of p62 accumulation, reactivation of AMPK pathway, and ultimately restoration of mTOR activity [114].

Finally, in support of the involvement of mTORC1 signaling in the pathophysiology of muscular laminopathies, it is important to emphasize some results obtained from muscular models with a phenotype very similar to the dystrophic one, that is aged non-pathological muscle. Aged muscle cells have in fact several traits in common with dystrophic cells, such as reduced regenerative and differentiative potential and high levels of basal ROSs. In 2015, the group of E. Volpi reported that, despite a basal level of hyperphosphorylated mTORC1, aged muscle cells presented a poor protein synthesis, suggesting that, in these model, mTORC1 phosphorylation was not sufficient per se to activate protein synthesis pathway as usually did [116]. In another study, performed in aged muscles of a TSC1 KO mice, it was observed that chronic mTORC1 activation, obtained by the lack of TSC1, did not lead to muscle hypertrophy, mainly because of the inability to induce autophagy [117]. Similar to that reported regarding cardio-laminopathic mice [97,111], in aged and stressed heart, mTORC1 inhibition, obtained by the use of selective mTOR inhibitors, resulted in cardioprotection and extended lifespan [118], reducing cardiac hypertrophy and improving cardiac function in the presence of pressure overload [119].

These findings independently obtained from different models of laminopathic and aged muscles perfectly support each other, and corroborate the relevance of altered autophagic processes in muscular laminopathies (Figure 4).

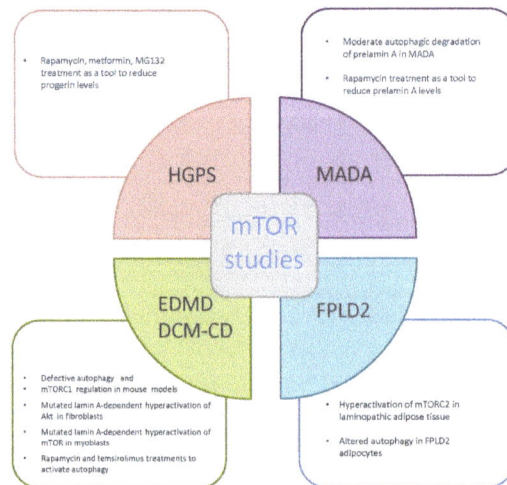

Figure 4. mTOR studies in laminopathies. Schematic representation of mTOR studies in EDMD, HGPS, MADA, and FPLD2. For EDMD see refs: [97,112]; for HGPS see refs: [120]; for MADA see refs: [5]; for FPLD2 see refs: [121] (Pellegrini et al., in preparation).

5. FPLD2

5.1. Laminopathic Lipodystrophies

Monogenic causes of lipodystrophies mostly converge in primary alterations of the adipose tissue, such as impaired defects in the formation, maintenance, and regulation of the adipocyte lipid droplets, leading to a loss of fat in specific district or in the whole body and secondary metabolic dysfunction [53].

As said above, mutations in lamin A/C, lamin B2, or ZMPSTE24 gene or alterations of prelamin A maturation are the cause of laminopathies featuring lipodystrophy.

From a clinical point of view, FPLD2 and MADA feature type A lipodystrophy, i.e., a loss of fat from the limbs and trunk and accumulation in the neck, while MADB presents with a generalized loss of adipose tissue (type B lipodystrophy) [122]. Metabolic alterations such as insulin resistance, diabetes, dyslipidemia, and nonalcoholic fatty liver diseases are found in laminopathic lipodystrophies with some variability among individuals [51]. The onset of lipodystrophy is at puberty, while up to that age most mutation carriers appear unaffected [122]. Of note, fat loss is much more evident in females and some male patients remain asymptomatic for several years [122]. A main clinical phenotype in MADA and MADB is accelerated ageing with onset in the second decade [1].

FPLD2

FPLD2 is typical partial lipodystrophy caused by mutations in the *LMNA* gene. More than 85% of FPLD2 mutations affect arginine 482 (p.Arg482Trp, p.Arg482Gln, p.Arg482Leu), located in exon 8, which encodes the globular portion of the protein. Different *LMNA* missense mutations have been reported in patients with FPLD2, most of them occurring in lamin A/C C-terminal domains [123,124].

FPLD2 is characterized by a loss of fat from the limbs, buttocks, and trunk, with cushingoid appearance, due to fat accumulation in the neck, face, and axillary regions [51,53,122]. In addition, patients may present muscular hypertrophy. FPLD2 patients also show early-onset atherosclerosis leading in some cases to cardiovascular pathologies and premature coronary heart disease, peripheral arteritis, and stroke [125].

Adipose tissue endocrine functions are also affected, with decrease in adiponectin- and leptin-circulating levels, leading to a worse prognosis in female patients, thus indicating that steroids could be involved in lipodystrophic phenotypes, resulting from *LMNA* mutations [124].

At the molecular level, FPLD2, MADA, and MADB are also characterized by accumulation of prelamin A at the nuclear periphery [66,126]. In FPLD2 and MADA, prelamin A accumulation is associated with recruitment of BAF to the nuclear periphery [127] and interferes with import and transactivation activity of the adipocyte transcription factor SREBP1 [7]. With a similar mechanism, accumulation of prelamin A by treatment of cells with anti-retroviral protease inhibitors, drugs that caused a lipodystrophy phenotype in patients subjected to therapy, has been shown to affect Sp1 import in nuclei of mesenchymal stem cells and Sp1-dependent regulation of genes related to lipid metabolism [18].

In FPLD2, it was observed that lamin A connection with chromatin at the nuclear periphery and in the nuclear interior could be affected and associated with tridimensional rearrangements of chromatin [128]. 3D genome models of fibroblasts from FPLD2 patients have shown a repositioning in the nuclear center of the T/Brachyury gene, a key regulator of mesodermal differentiation, an event favoring gene transcription [129].

To address FPLD2 pathogenesis, the particular clinical condition must be considered. Patients lose subcutaneous fat, while they accumulate adipose tissue in the neck and in some instances in visceral depots [122]. In a study aimed at evaluating different fat districts, it was shown that prelamin A accumulation in lipoatrophic fat is associated with altered expression of cyclin D3, pRB, and PPARγ genes, involved in adipocyte differentiation and proliferation [130]. On the other hand, fibrosis, altered expression of adipogenic factors, a mitochondrion number increase, and enhanced levels of uncoupling protein 1 (UCP1, a marker of brown adipocytes) have been reported in the neck adipose tissue from FPLD2 patients, suggesting that the hypertrophic adipose tissue found in that particular district is of brown origin [126,130]. It is plausible that *LMNA* defects might affect a group of adipogenic genes or differentiation mechanisms depending on the type of adipogenic precursors [5]. Our recent work has demonstrated that impaired autophagy due to hyperphosphorylation of pS6K1 contributes to downregulation of white adipose tissue genes in cells from FPLD2 patients, while aberrant activation of autophagy in brown preadipocytes from the neck of FPLD2 patients contributes to direct cell differentiation towards a white adipocyte phenotype (Pellegrini et al., in preparation). As a consequence of impaired autophagic signaling, lipid droplet formation is impaired in FPLD2, as observed in an in vitro model of *LMNA*-lipodystrophy (Pellegrini et al., in preparation).

Aberrant differentiation or even determination of adipocyte precursors might play a major role in FPLD2 pathogenesis. Along this line, the Collas group showed that altered lamin A association with the RNA-binding protein Fragile X syndrome-related protein 1 (FXR1P) and upregulation of FXR1P in FPLD2 adipogenic precursors leads to conversion to the myogenic lineage [131]. However, a complex pathogenetic picture is emerging from FPLD2 studies, also involving the anti-adipogenic factors. For instance, the p.R482W mutation impairs differentiation-dependent lamin A binding to the MIR335 locus and overexpression of the MIR355 gene after adipogenic induction [25]. Moreover, tissue and depot specific effects might be related to lamin A tissue-specific interactions, such as the one with the adipocyte nuclear envelope protein TMEM120 [132].

Involvement of mTOR signaling in laminopathic adipose tissue defects has been also explored in $Lmna^{-/-}$ mice [111] used to study cardiomyopathy and muscle dystrophy. In that mouse model, mTORC2 inactivation specifically in adipose tissue elicited weight gain and improved the whole body metabolism [111]. Importantly, high energy expenditure was observed in this mouse model, while rapamycin reversed this condition, indicating that mTOR-dependent signaling affected the rate of energy expenditure [121]. The reduction in adiposity in $Lmna^{-/-}$ mice seems to be linked to lipolysis, which is decreased after rapamycin treatment. Very interestingly, mTOR was found to be aberrantly activated in adipose tissue, while rapamycin suppressed hyperactivated mTOR signaling, rescuing the phenotype. These results suggest a link between A-type lamin functions and mTOR signaling in adipose tissue and imply that not only adipose tissue homeostasis and differentiation, but also metabolic regulation may be related to altered mTOR regulation in the absence of a functional lamina (Figure 4) [121].

6. Progeroid Laminopathies

6.1. HGPS

Progeroid laminopathies include several forms linked to *LMNA* mutations and a few forms associated with *ZMPSTE24* gene variants or the *POLD1* gene [1]. Among *LMNA*-linked progeroid syndromes are HGPS, MADA, atypical-Werner syndrome, and atypical progeria syndrome [1]. MADB is linked to ZMPSTE24 mutations, while a form of mandibuloacral dysplasia also featuring hearing loss is associated with *POLD1* mutations [1].

HGPS is a rare genetic disorder characterized by very early onset accelerated ageing with hair loss, short stature, skin tightness, joint contractures, progressive cardiovascular disease resembling atherosclerosis, osteolysis of clavicles, mandible and terminal phalanges, osteoporosis, and death due to cardiovascular problems at an average age of 14.6 years [133]. Children with HGPS are healthy at birth but rapidly develop a progeroid phenotype [133]. HGPS is due to a sporadic mutation in the *LMNA* gene (c.1824C<T) [134,135], resulting in a silent polymorphism at codon 608 (G608G) that activates a cryptic splice site. This leads to a deletion of 50 amino acids near the C-terminus of prelamin A. The abnormal protein produced, called progerin, lacks the second site for endoproteolytic cleavage, and thus remains permanently farnesylated. Accumulation of progerin exerts toxic effects disrupting the integrity of nuclear envelope and leading to nuclear architecture abnormalities [136]. Even though G608G is the most frequent mutation in HGPS patients (at least 90% of all progeria cases), other mutations in the gene cause progeroid phenotypes classified as atypical progeria syndrome, with onset in the first decade, variable bone phenotype and lipodystrophy, or atypical-Werner syndrome, with onset of accelerated ageing in the second decade [137–139].

6.2. mTOR Signaling in HGPS

AKT-mTOR signaling has been analyzed in HGPS fibroblasts. AKT phosphorylation was reduced in HGPS cells [140], and mTOR phosphorylation, possibly leading to autophagy activation, was reduced in HGPS fibroblasts [141]. Moreover, in a mouse model of progeria, the Zmpste24 null mouse, which accumulates toxic levels of prelamin A, AKT, and S6 kinase phosphorylation were significantly reduced in liver and skeletal muscle, [140], suggesting activation of the autophagic signaling. Unexpectedly, in the same mouse model, genetic ablation of the prelamin A methyltransferase Icmt caused a significant activation of AKT and its downstream effectors in the mTOR pathway, leading to phosphorylation and degradation of p21 and reduced cellular senescence [140]. Thus, mTOR inactivation seems to play a dual role in progeroid cells, modulating both the autophagic signaling and p21-dependent cellular senescence [140]. Although autophagy is considered an anti-aging mechanism, increased levels of p21 are associated with senescence. Moreover, we did not observe any degradation of progerin in HGPS cells unless rapamycin was used to further inhibit the mTOR activity [141,142]. More recently, autophagy has been proposed as a mechanism to recycle nutrients in *Lmna* G609G progeroid mice [143], which were affected by severe weight loss and cachexia. In these mice subjected to high fat diet, LC3 II levels were reduced compared to individual under normal diet regimen [143]. The authors did not explore mTOR signaling but suggest that elevated energy intake by high fat diet could downregulate autophagy in progeroid mice. This complex picture needs further investigation, mostly to understand to which extent the HGPS phenotype could be improved by treatment with rapamycin or other rapalogs.

6.3. mTOR in Ageing Models

Several mouse models have been developed to better understand the effects of mTOR signaling in promoting aging and age-related phenotypes. Mice lacking S6K1 [144] and mice bearing heterozygous deletions of mTOR and mLST8 [145] show extended longevity. Moreover, mTOR hypomorphic mice display increased median lifespan, and they are healthier and seem to be protected from many age-related diseases [118].

Interestingly, many other studies support the effects of the mTOR signaling pathway on aging through a pharmacological approach [146–150]. Several evidences suggest that rapamycin could modulate a number of aging-related mechanisms and could be a potential anti-aging therapy, extending average and maximum lifespan in mice and delaying several age-related pathologies [148,151–153]. Rapamycin may also reverse features of ageing in mice, such as cardiac hypertrophy, liver degeneration, adrenal glands and endometrium decline, and tendon elasticity [137].

Besides to limit the set of problems caused by prolonged exposure to rapalogs, different approaches have been carried out, reporting that an intermittent rapamycin treatment schedule is associated with fewer side effects on the immune system and on glucose metabolism, and with a lifespan extension in mouse models [154–156]. Another possible dosing regimen for delaying the aging phenotype and minimizing the side effects has been suggested by Mannick and colleagues, proposing low-dose and short-time everolimus administration [157]. Finally, a very recent paper has demonstrated that a methionine restriction diet extended lifespan in *LmnaG609G/G609G* and *Zmpste24−/−* HGPS mouse models, rescuing the pathologic phenotype, by reversing the transcriptome alterations in inflammation and DNA-damage response genes, improving the lipid profile and changing bile acid levels and conjugation. Methionine restriction also induced downregulation of the mTOR pathway, suggesting the existence of a metabolic signaling involved in the longevity extension achieved by the methionine restriction diet [158].

6.4. mTOR Inhibitors in HGPS

Rapamycin reduces progerin levels in HGPS cells, avoids farnesylated prelamin A accumulation, and rescues physiological chromatin dynamics [142]. Temsirolimus, another rapalog, has been tested in

HGPS cells [68]. Nevertheless, mitochondrial dysfunction [159] and elevated DNA damage observed in HGPS cells are not rescued by the drug [68]. Combination of drugs is currently considered the most promising approach to HGPS therapy, not only because of the complex clinical condition but also to take advantage of the synergistic effects of drugs that allow for the use of a low dosage, thus limiting toxicity. In a study we performed in HGPS cells, all-trans retinoid acid (ATRA) and rapamycin were shown to synergistically improve the lamin A to progerin ratio. The beneficial effect leading to reduction of DNA damage and improvement of BAF and chromatin dynamics was elicited through a transcriptional effect, possibly due to ATRA, and through rapamycin-dependent activation of progerin autophagic degradation (Figure 4) [160]. The combined treatment is currently being tested in animal models. The administration of rapalogs with the anti-diabetes drug metformin, able to minimize adverse effects, may represent a further strategy for the use of mTOR inhibitors [160]. Metformin is a regulator of the mTORC1-dependent translation process, activating the AMP-activated protein kinase (AMPK) axis [161] and directly inhibiting mTOR [162]. This drug shows anti-aging effects in many models [163], and an observational and retrospective study in diabetic patients revealed that metformin treatment leads to a strong decrease in all-cause death and in the onset of age-related diseases [164]. Recently, it has reported in a mouse model that a combination of rapamycin and metformin reduces the strong metabolic deficits caused by rapamycin treatment [120]. Interestingly, in HGPS fibroblasts and *Lmna* G609G/G609G mouse fibroblasts, metformin diminishes progerin expression [165], suggesting a possible therapeutic potential of metformin for HGPS.

A recent approach to HGPS treatment involves lonafarnib (a prelamin A and progerin farnesylation inhibitor [166] combined with everolimus (an analogue of rapamycin that has a more favorable pharmacokinetic profile) and an ongoing phase I/II trial has been launched by the Progeria Research Foundation [NCT02579044].

Another strategy to modulate autophagy and decrease the progerin levels in HGPS patients' cells employed proteasome inhibitor MG132 as an activator of lysosomal degradation in response to proteasome inhibition. Moreover, progerin degradation, following MG132 treatment, was observed in HGPS IPSC-derived cell lines as well as in vivo in an *Lmna* G609G/G609G mouse model, showing an amelioration of cellular HGPS phenotype (Figure 4) [167]. Finally, various nanoparticles (NPs) have demonstrated an ability to modulate mTOR activity and proliferation. This approach to mTOR modulation warrants further investigation [168,169].

6.5. MADA and MADB

MAD is a rare laminopathy characterized by progeroid features, including growth retardation, fat distribution, and metabolic abnormalities (diabetes, glucose intolerance, and insulin resistance) and severe osteolysis and osteoporosis [1,141]. MADA fibroblasts show nuclear blebbing and reduced proliferation. Patients with MADA have a less severe phenotype as compared to MADB harboring *ZMPSTE24* mutations, consistent with the accumulation of a higher amount of prelamin A in MADB. Several therapeutic approaches have been reported to rescue the cellular abnormalities, such as farnesyl transferase inhibitors, statins, and bisphosphonate [16].

Interestingly, some activation of autophagy in MADA has been suggested by studies performed with chloroquine. In MADA fibroblasts subjected to chloroquine treatment, prelamin A level is increased, while, as expected, the autophagic process is impaired (Figure 3) [170]. Thus, it appears that an autophagic mechanism of removal of mutated prelamin A (MADA cells carry homozygous *LMNA* mutations and are devoid of wild-type lamin A/C) is activated in those cells [170]. Consistent with this observation, inhibition of mTOR by rapamycin triggers lysosomal degradation of farnesylated prelamin A in MADA fibroblasts and rescues markers of cellular senescence as well as chromatin epigenetic mechanisms [5,170]. In contrast to what observed in MADA fibroblasts, osteoblast-like cells overexpressing lamin A R527H showed activation of the mTOR pathway, although mTOR itself was not phosphorylated. Inhibition of this pathway by everolimus treatment significantly improved the mutant phenotype and its pathogenetic pathways, including the ability of R527H *LMNA* osteoblasts to stimulate osteoclastogenesis, suggesting that everolimus can be explored as a therapeutic approach for MADA [32].

Rapamycin treatment may be a therapeutic strategy for MADB as well. Indeed, it has been demonstrated that inhibition of the mTOR signaling pathway induces improvement of nuclear aberrations and ameliorates the overall phenotype of fibroblasts from MADB patients, even if changes in the phosphorylation status of mTOR have not been determined (Figure 4) [171].

7. Perspectives

From a basic point of view, the main finding of mTOR studies conducted in models of laminopathies is that functional lamin A/C is required for mTOR-dependent pathways that regulate autophagy and fibrogenic processes. The link between a functional lamina and autophagy is consistent with the observed involvement of autophagy in lamina homeostasis through degradation of defective or excess A or B type lamins [142,160,170,172]. Thus, a feedback mechanism could be hypothesized, whereby proteins of the nuclear lamina inhibit mTOR activity and trigger autophagy to maintain their physiological levels. This hypothesis has been widely proven for lamin B [172]. Mutated lamins, including the R527H-mutated lamin A/C and prelamin A found in many cases of MADA and progerin, likely fail to trigger efficient mTOR-dependent autophagic signaling, thus causing protein accumulation. However, while EDMD2 and FPLD2 appear to be characterized by activation of the AKT/mTOR pathway either through mTOR itself or through direct phosphorylation of p70S6 kinase, ultimately impairing the autophagic activity [30,32,111,121,173], HGPS and MADA cells show some activation of the autophagic pathway. Nevertheless, despite this relevant difference in mTOR signaling, in experimental models of all these laminopathies, rapamycin, everolimus, and temsirolimus have been demonstrated to efficiently degrade toxic molecules and/or rescue the phenotype. Despite the known side effects of rapamycin and rapalogs, those results suggest that therapeutic approaches based on mTOR inhibition and activation of autophagy be explored. However, recent findings showing that other mTOR dependent mechanisms such as nutrient intake and energy expenditure are affected in laminopathies suggest a more complex therapeutic strategy aimed at rescuing good metabolic conditions while reducing levels of mutated lamins.

Author Contributions: All of the authors contributed to the writing and editing of the article.

Funding: The authors' work was supported by grants from MIUR PRIN 2015FBNB5Y to G.L.

Acknowledgments: The authors thank Aurelio Valmori for the technical assistance. The authors also thank Associazione Italiana Progeria Sammy Basso (AIProSaB) and Associazione Italiana Distrofia di Emery-Dreifuss (AIDMED). G.L. is a partner of the E-RARE 2017 project "TREAT-HGPS".

Conflicts of Interest: The authors declare no conflict of interest.

Abbreviations

4E-BP1	Eukariotic translation initiation factor 4E-binding protein 1
AMPK	AMP-activated protein kinase
ATG14L	ATG autophagy related-14 like
ATM	Atacsia telangectasia-mutated
ATR	Atacsia telangectasia- and RAD3-related
ATRA	All-trans retinoid acid
BAF	Barrier to autointegration factor
CMT2B1	Charcot–Marie tooth neuropathy
DEPTOR	DEP domain-containing mTOR-interacting protein
DNA-PK	DNA-dependent protein kinase
EDMD	Emery-Dreifuss muscular dystrophy
eEF2K	Eukaryotic elongation factor 2 kinase
eIF-4E	Eukaryotic initiation factor-4E
FAT	FKBP/ATM/TRRAP

FATC	FRAP/ATM/TRRAP/carboxy terminal
FKBP-12	FK506-binding protein-12
FoxO	Forkhead box O
FPLD2	Familial partial lipodistrphy 2
FRB	FKBP, rapamycin-binding
FXR1P	Fragile X syndrome-related protein 1
GAP	PTPase activating protein
HEAT	Huntingtin/elongation factor 3/A subunit of protein phosphatase-2A/TOR1
HGPS	Hutchinson–Gilford progeria syndrome
HHS	"Heart hand" syndrome
HIF1 alpha	Hypoxia inducible factor 1
hSMG-1	Human suppressor of morphogenesis in genitalia-1
IGFR	Insulin-like growth factor receptor
IR	Insulin receptor
IRS1	Insulin receptor substrate 1
LAD	Lamina-associated domain
LC3	Microtubule-associated protein 1 light chain 3
L-CMD	Cardiomyopathy-lmna-linked congenital muscular distrophy
LKB1	Liver kinase 1
MADA	Mandibuloacral dysplasia
mLST8	Mammalian sethal with SEC13 protein 8
MRTFA	Mechanoresponsive myocardin-related transcription factor A
mSin	Mammalian stress-activated protein kinase Interacting protein 1
mTOR	Mechanistic target of rapamycin
PI3K	Phosphoinositide 3-kinase
PIKK	Phosphoinositide kinase-related family of protein kinases
PKC	Protein kinase C
PPARgamma	Peroxisome proliferatio-activated receptor gamma
PRAS40	Proline-rich AKT substrate 1 40 kDa
PROTOR 1/2	Protein observed with Rictor
RAPTOR	Regulatory-associated protein of TOR
RD	Restrictive dermopathy
RHEB	Ras homolog enriched in brain
RICTOR	Rapamycin-insensitive companion of TOR
RPS6	Ribosomal protein S6
RTK	Receptor tyrosine kinase
S6K1	P70 ribosomal S6 kinase 1
SGK1	Serum and glucocorticoid-activated kinase 1
SREBP1	Sterol regulatory element-binding protein 1
TSC2	Tuberous sclerosis complex 2
UCP1	Uncoupling protein 1
UPS	Ubiquitin proteasome system
Vps34	Vacuolar protein sorting 34

References

1. Cenni, V.; D'Apice, M.R.; Garagnani, P.; Columbaro, M.; Novelli, G.; Franceschi, C.; Lattanzi, G. Mandibuloacral dysplasia: A premature ageing disease with aspects of physiological ageing. *Ageing Res. Rev.* **2018**, *42*, 1–13. [CrossRef] [PubMed]
2. Turgay, Y.; Medalia, O. The structure of lamin filaments in somatic cells as revealed by cryo-electron tomography. *Nucleus* **2017**, *8*, 475–481. [CrossRef] [PubMed]
3. Vidak, S.; Georgiou, K.; Fichtinger, P.; Naetar, N.; Dechat, T.; Foisner, R. Nucleoplasmic lamins define growth-regulating functions of lamina-associated polypeptide 2alpha in progeria cells. *J. Cell Sci.* **2018**, *131*. [CrossRef] [PubMed]

4. Loi, M.; Cenni, V.; Duchi, S.; Squarzoni, S.; Lopez-Otin, C.; Foisner, R.; Lattanzi, G.; Capanni, C. Barrier-to-autointegration factor (BAF) involvement in prelamin A-related chromatin organization changes. *Oncotarget* **2016**, *7*, 15662–15677. [CrossRef] [PubMed]

5. Camozzi, D.; Capanni, C.; Cenni, V.; Mattioli, E.; Columbaro, M.; Squarzoni, S.; Lattanzi, G. Diverse lamin-dependent mechanisms interact to control chromatin dynamics. Focus on laminopathies. *Nucleus* **2014**, *5*, 427–440. [CrossRef] [PubMed]

6. Navarro, C.L.; De Sandre-Giovannoli, A.; Bernard, R.; Boccaccio, I.; Boyer, A.; Genevieve, D.; Hadj-Rabia, S.; Gaudy-Marqueste, C.; Smitt, H.S.; Vabres, P.; et al. Lamin A and ZMPSTE24 (FACE-1) defects cause nuclear disorganization and identify restrictive dermopathy as a lethal neonatal laminopathy. *Hum. Mol. Genet.* **2004**, *13*, 2493–2503. [CrossRef] [PubMed]

7. Capanni, C.; Mattioli, E.; Columbaro, M.; Lucarelli, E.; Parnaik, V.K.; Novelli, G.; Wehnert, M.; Cenni, V.; Maraldi, N.M.; Squarzoni, S.; et al. Altered pre-lamin A processing is a common mechanism leading to lipodystrophy. *Hum. Mol. Genet.* **2005**, *14*, 1489–1502. [CrossRef]

8. Mattioli, E.; Columbaro, M.; Capanni, C.; Maraldi, N.M.; Cenni, V.; Scotlandi, K.; Marino, M.T.; Merlini, L.; Squarzoni, S.; Lattanzi, G. Prelamin A-mediated recruitment of SUN1 to the nuclear envelope directs nuclear positioning in human muscle. *Cell Death Differ.* 2011. [CrossRef]

9. Mattioli, E.; Columbaro, M.; Jafferali, M.H.; Schena, E.; Hallberg, E.; Lattanzi, G. Samp1 Mislocalization in Emery–Dreifuss Muscular Dystrophy. *Cells* **2018**, *7*. [CrossRef]

10. Lattanzi, G.; Ortolani, M.; Columbaro, M.; Prencipe, S.; Mattioli, E.; Lanzarini, C.; Maraldi, N.M.; Cenni, V.; Garagnani, P.; Salvioli, S.; et al. Lamins are rapamycin targets that impact human longevity: A study in centenarians. *J. Cell Sci.* **2014**, *127*, 147–157. [CrossRef]

11. Liu, Y.; Drozdov, I.; Shroff, R.; Beltran, L.E.; Shanahan, C.M. Prelamin A accelerates vascular calcification via activation of the DNA damage response and senescence-associated secretory phenotype in vascular smooth muscle cells. *Circ. Res.* **2013**, *112*, e99–e109. [CrossRef] [PubMed]

12. Gonzalez-Cruz, R.D.; Dahl, K.N.; Darling, E.M. The Emerging Role of Lamin C as an Important LMNA Isoform in Mechanophenotype. *Front. Cell Dev. Biol.* **2018**, *6*, 151. [CrossRef] [PubMed]

13. Patni, N.; Xing, C.; Agarwal, A.K.; Garg, A. Juvenile-onset generalized lipodystrophy due to a novel heterozygous missense LMNA mutation affecting lamin C. *Am. J. Med. Genet. A* **2017**, *173*, 2517–2521. [CrossRef] [PubMed]

14. Kolb, T.; Maass, K.; Hergt, M.; Aebi, U.; Herrmann, H. Lamin A and lamin C form homodimers and coexist in higher complex forms both in the nucleoplasmic fraction and in the lamina of cultured human cells. *Nucleus* **2011**, *2*, 425–433. [CrossRef] [PubMed]

15. Maraldi, N.M.; Capanni, C.; Cenni, V.; Fini, M.; Lattanzi, G. Laminopathies and lamin-associated signaling pathways. *J. Cell. Biochem.* **2011**, *112*, 979–992. [CrossRef] [PubMed]

16. Camozzi, D.; D'Apice, M.R.; Schena, E.; Cenni, V.; Columbaro, M.; Capanni, C.; Maraldi, N.M.; Squarzoni, S.; Ortolani, M.; Novelli, G.; et al. Altered chromatin organization and SUN2 localization in mandibuloacral dysplasia are rescued by drug treatment. *Histochem. Cell Biol.* **2012**, *138*, 643–651. [CrossRef] [PubMed]

17. Infante, A.; Gago, A.; de Eguino, G.R.; Calvo-Fernandez, T.; Gomez-Vallejo, V.; Llop, J.; Schlangen, K.; Fullaondo, A.; Aransay, A.M.; Martin, A.; et al. Prelamin A accumulation and stress conditions induce impaired Oct-1 activity and autophagy in prematurely aged human mesenchymal stem cell. *Aging* **2014**, *6*, 264–280. [CrossRef]

18. Ruiz de Eguino, G.; Infante, A.; Schlangen, K.; Aransay, A.M.; Fullaondo, A.; Soriano, M.; Garcia-Verdugo, J.M.; Martin, A.G.; Rodriguez, C.I. Sp1 transcription factor interaction with accumulated prelamin a impairs adipose lineage differentiation in human mesenchymal stem cells: Essential role of sp1 in the integrity of lipid vesicles. *Stem Cells Transl. Med.* **2012**, *1*, 309–321. [CrossRef]

19. Kubben, N.; Zhang, W.; Wang, L.; Voss, T.C.; Yang, J.; Qu, J.; Liu, G.H.; Misteli, T. Repression of the Antioxidant NRF2 Pathway in Premature Aging. *Cell* **2016**, *165*, 1361–1374. [CrossRef]

20. Osmanagic-Myers, S.; Kiss, A.; Manakanatas, C.; Hamza, O.; Sedlmayer, F.; Szabo, P.L.; Fischer, I.; Fichtinger, P.; Podesser, B.K.; Eriksson, M.; et al. Endothelial progerin expression causes cardiovascular pathology through an impaired mechanoresponse. *J. Clin. Investig.* 2018. [CrossRef]

21. Nitta, R.T.; Jameson, S.A.; Kudlow, B.A.; Conlan, L.A.; Kennedy, B.K. Stabilization of the retinoblastoma protein by A-type nuclear lamins is required for INK4A-mediated cell cycle arrest. *Mol. Cell. Biol.* **2006**, *26*, 5360–5372. [CrossRef] [PubMed]

22. Nitta, R.T.; Smith, C.L.; Kennedy, B.K. Evidence that proteasome-dependent degradation of the retinoblastoma protein in cells lacking A-type lamins occurs independently of gankyrin and MDM2. *PLoS ONE* **2007**, *2*, e963. [CrossRef] [PubMed]

23. Rodriguez, J.; Calvo, F.; Gonzalez, J.M.; Casar, B.; Andres, V.; Crespo, P. ERK1/2 MAP kinases promote cell cycle entry by rapid, kinase-independent disruption of retinoblastoma-lamin A complexes. *J. Cell Biol.* **2010**, *191*, 967–979. [CrossRef] [PubMed]

24. Mattioli, E.; Andrenacci, D.; Garofalo, C.; Prencipe, S.; Scotlandi, K.; Remondini, D.; Gentilini, D.; Di Blasio, A.M.; Valente, S.; Scarano, E.; et al. Altered modulation of lamin A/C-HDAC2 interaction and p21 expression during oxidative stress response in HGPS. *Aging Cell* **2018**, *17*, e12824. [CrossRef] [PubMed]

25. Oldenburg, A.; Briand, N.; Sorensen, A.L.; Cahyani, I.; Shah, A.; Moskaug, J.O.; Collas, P. A lipodystrophy-causing lamin A mutant alters conformation and epigenetic regulation of the anti-adipogenic MIR335 locus. *J. Cell Biol.* **2017**, *216*, 2731–2743. [CrossRef] [PubMed]

26. Briand, N.; Collas, P. Laminopathy-causing lamin A mutations reconfigure lamina-associated domains and local spatial chromatin conformation. *Nucleus* **2018**, *9*, 216–226. [CrossRef]

27. Chatzifrangkeskou, M.; Yadin, D.; Marais, T.; Chardonnet, S.; Cohen-Tannoudji, M.; Mougenot, N.; Schmitt, A.; Crasto, S.; Di Pasquale, E.; Macquart, C.; et al. Cofilin-1 phosphorylation catalyzed by ERK1/2 alters cardiac actin dynamics in dilated cardiomyopathy caused by lamin A/C gene mutation. *Hum. Mol. Genet.* **2018**, *27*, 3060–3078. [CrossRef]

28. Choi, J.C.; Wu, W.; Phillips, E.; Plevin, R.; Sera, F.; Homma, S.; Worman, H.J. Elevated dual specificity protein phosphatase 4 in cardiomyopathy caused by lamin A/C gene mutation is primarily ERK1/2-dependent and its depletion improves cardiac function and survival. *Hum. Mol. Genet.* **2018**, *27*, 2290–2305. [CrossRef]

29. Gerbino, A.; Procino, G.; Svelto, M.; Carmosino, M. Role of Lamin A/C Gene Mutations in the Signaling Defects Leading to Cardiomyopathies. *Front. Physiol.* **2018**, *9*, 1356. [CrossRef]

30. Bernasconi, P.; Carboni, N.; Ricci, G.; Siciliano, G.; Politano, L.; Maggi, L.; Mongini, T.; Vercelli, L.; Rodolico, C.; Biagini, E.; et al. Elevated TGF beta2 serum levels in Emery–Dreifuss Muscular Dystrophy: Implications for myocyte and tenocyte differentiation and fibrogenic processes. *Nucleus* **2018**, *9*, 292–304. [CrossRef]

31. Chatzifrangkeskou, M.; Le Dour, C.; Wu, W.; Morrow, J.P.; Joseph, L.C.; Beuvin, M.; Sera, F.; Homma, S.; Vignier, N.; Mougenot, N.; et al. ERK1/2 directly acts on CTGF/CCN2 expression to mediate myocardial fibrosis in cardiomyopathy caused by mutations in the lamin A/C gene. *Hum. Mol. Genet.* **2016**, *25*, 2220–2233. [CrossRef] [PubMed]

32. Evangelisti, C.; Bernasconi, P.; Cavalcante, P.; Cappelletti, C.; D'Apice, M.R.; Sbraccia, P.; Novelli, G.; Prencipe, S.; Lemma, S.; Baldini, N.; et al. Modulation of TGFβ 2 levels by lamin A in U2-OS osteoblast-like cells: Understanding the osteolytic process triggered by altered lamins. *Oncotarget* **2015**, *6*, 7424–7437. [CrossRef] [PubMed]

33. Cenni, V.; Bertacchini, J.; Beretti, F.; Lattanzi, G.; Bavelloni, A.; Riccio, M.; Ruzzene, M.; Marin, O.; Arrigoni, G.; Parnaik, V.; et al. Lamin A Ser404 is a nuclear target of Akt phosphorylation in C2C12 cells. *J. Proteome Res.* **2008**, *7*, 4727–4735. [CrossRef] [PubMed]

34. Bertacchini, J.; Beretti, F.; Cenni, V.; Guida, M.; Gibellini, F.; Mediani, L.; Marin, O.; Maraldi, N.M.; de Pol, A.; Lattanzi, G.; et al. The protein kinase Akt/PKB regulates both prelamin A degradation and Lmna gene expression. *FASEB J.* **2013**, *27*, 2145–2155. [CrossRef] [PubMed]

35. Boriani, G.; Biagini, E.; Ziacchi, M.; Malavasi, V.L.; Vitolo, M.; Talarico, M.; Mauro, E.; Gorlato, G.; Lattanzi, G. Cardiolaminopathies from bench to bedside: Challenges in clinical decision-making with focus on arrhythmia-related outcomes. *Nucleus* **2018**, *9*, 442–459. [CrossRef] [PubMed]

36. Roncarati, R.; Viviani Anselmi, C.; Krawitz, P.; Lattanzi, G.; von Kodolitsch, Y.; Perrot, A.; di Pasquale, E.; Papa, L.; Portararo, P.; Columbaro, M.; et al. Doubly heterozygous LMNA and TTN mutations revealed by exome sequencing in a severe form of dilated cardiomyopathy. *Eur. J. Hum. Genet.* **2013**, *21*, 1105–1111. [CrossRef] [PubMed]

37. Meinke, P.; Mattioli, E.; Haque, F.; Antoku, S.; Columbaro, M.; Straatman, K.R.; Worman, H.J.; Gundersen, G.G.; Lattanzi, G.; Wehnert, M.; et al. Muscular dystrophy-associated SUN1 and SUN2 variants disrupt nuclear-cytoskeletal connections and myonuclear organization. *PLoS Genet.* **2014**, *10*, e1004605. [CrossRef] [PubMed]

38. van Tintelen, J.P.; Pinto, Y.M. Additional Genetic Variants in Inherited Dilated Cardiomyopathy: Just Another Brick in the Wall? *Circ. Genom. Precis. Med.* **2018**, *11*, e002249. [CrossRef]

39. Brull, A.; Morales Rodriguez, B.; Bonne, G.; Muchir, A.; Bertrand, A.T. The Pathogenesis and Therapies of Striated Muscle Laminopathies. *Front. Physiol.* **2018**, *9*, 1533. [CrossRef]

40. Madej-Pilarczyk, A. Clinical aspects of Emery–Dreifuss muscular dystrophy. *Nucleus* **2018**, *9*, 268–274. [CrossRef]

41. Rajgor, D.; Shanahan, C.M. Nesprins: From the nuclear envelope and beyond. *Expert Rev. Mol. Med.* **2013**, *15*, e5. [CrossRef] [PubMed]

42. Gueneau, L.; Bertrand, A.T.; Jais, J.P.; Salih, M.A.; Stojkovic, T.; Wehnert, M.; Hoeltzenbein, M.; Spuler, S.; Saitoh, S.; Verschueren, A.; et al. Mutations of the FHL1 gene cause Emery–Dreifuss muscular dystrophy. *Am. J. Hum. Genet.* **2009**, *85*, 338–353. [CrossRef] [PubMed]

43. Liang, W.C.; Mitsuhashi, H.; Keduka, E.; Nonaka, I.; Noguchi, S.; Nishino, I.; Hayashi, Y.K. TMEM43 mutations in Emery–Dreifuss muscular dystrophy-related myopathy. *Ann. Neurol.* **2011**, *69*, 1005–1013. [CrossRef] [PubMed]

44. Stroud, M.J. Linker of nucleoskeleton and cytoskeleton complex proteins in cardiomyopathy. *Biophys. Rev.* **2018**, *10*, 1033–1051. [CrossRef] [PubMed]

45. Captur, G.; Arbustini, E.; Bonne, G.; Syrris, P.; Mills, K.; Wahbi, K.; Mohiddin, S.A.; McKenna, W.J.; Pettit, S.; Ho, C.Y.; et al. Lamin and the heart. *Heart* **2018**, *104*, 468–479. [CrossRef] [PubMed]

46. Zhou, C.; Li, C.; Zhou, B.; Sun, H.; Koullourou, V.; Holt, I.; Puckelwartz, M.J.; Warren, D.T.; Hayward, R.; Lin, Z.; et al. Novel nesprin-1 mutations associated with dilated cardiomyopathy cause nuclear envelope disruption and defects in myogenesis. *Hum. Mol. Genet.* **2017**, *26*, 2258–2276. [CrossRef] [PubMed]

47. Gimpel, P.; Lee, Y.L.; Sobota, R.M.; Calvi, A.; Koullourou, V.; Patel, R.; Mamchaoui, K.; Nedelec, F.; Shackleton, S.; Schmoranzer, J.; et al. Nesprin-1alpha-Dependent Microtubule Nucleation from the Nuclear Envelope via Akap450 Is Necessary for Nuclear Positioning in Muscle Cells. *Curr. Biol.* **2017**, *27*, 2999–3009. [CrossRef]

48. Taylor, M.R.; Slavov, D.; Gajewski, A.; Vlcek, S.; Ku, L.; Fain, P.R.; Carniel, E.; Di Lenarda, A.; Sinagra, G.; Boucek, M.M.; et al. Thymopoietin (lamina-associated polypeptide 2) gene mutation associated with dilated cardiomyopathy. *Hum. Mutat.* **2005**, *26*, 566–574. [CrossRef]

49. Gesson, K.; Vidak, S.; Foisner, R. Lamina-associated polypeptide (LAP)2alpha and nucleoplasmic lamins in adult stem cell regulation and disease. *Semin. Cell Dev. Biol.* **2014**, *29*, 116–124. [CrossRef]

50. Lattanzi, G.; Maggi, L.; Araujo-Vilar, D. Laminopathies. *Nucleus* **2018**, *9*, 543–544. [CrossRef]

51. Vigouroux, C.; Guenantin, A.C.; Vatier, C.; Capel, E.; Le Dour, C.; Afonso, P.; Bidault, G.; Bereziat, V.; Lascols, O.; Capeau, J.; et al. Lipodystrophic syndromes due to LMNA mutations: Recent developments on biomolecular aspects, pathophysiological hypotheses and therapeutic perspectives. *Nucleus* **2018**, *9*, 235–248. [CrossRef] [PubMed]

52. Hegele, R.A.; Cao, H.; Liu, D.M.; Costain, G.A.; Charlton-Menys, V.; Rodger, N.W.; Durrington, P.N. Sequencing of the reannotated LMNB2 gene reveals novel mutations in patients with acquired partial lipodystrophy. *Am. J. Hum. Genet.* **2006**, *79*, 383–389. [CrossRef]

53. Araujo-Vilar, D.; Santini, F. Diagnosis and treatment of lipodystrophy: A step-by-step approach. *J. Endocrinol. Investig.* **2019**, *42*, 61–73. [CrossRef] [PubMed]

54. Harhouri, K.; Frankel, D.; Bartoli, C.; Roll, P.; De Sandre-Giovannoli, A.; Levy, N. An overview of treatment strategies for Hutchinson–Gilford Progeria syndrome. *Nucleus* **2018**, *9*, 246–257. [CrossRef]

55. Gonzalo, S.; Kreienkamp, R.; Askjaer, P. Hutchinson–Gilford Progeria Syndrome: A premature aging disease caused by LMNA gene mutations. *Ageing Res. Rev.* **2017**, *33*, 18–29. [CrossRef]

56. Garg, A.; Subramanyam, L.; Agarwal, A.K.; Simha, V.; Levine, B.; D'Apice, M.R.; Novelli, G.; Crow, Y. Atypical progeroid syndrome due to heterozygous missense LMNA mutations. *J. Clin. Endocrinol. Metab.* **2009**, *94*, 4971–4983. [CrossRef]

57. Renard, D.; Fourcade, G.; Milhaud, D.; Bessis, D.; Esteves-Vieira, V.; Boyer, A.; Roll, P.; Bourgeois, P.; Levy, N.; De Sandre-Giovannoli, A. Novel LMNA mutation in atypical Werner syndrome presenting with ischemic disease. *Stroke* **2009**, *40*, e11–e14. [CrossRef] [PubMed]

58. Gargiuli, C.; Schena, E.; Mattioli, E.; Columbaro, M.; D'Apice, M.R.; Novelli, G.; Greggi, T.; Lattanzi, G. Lamins and bone disorders: Current understanding and perspectives. *Oncotarget* **2018**, *9*, 22817–22831. [CrossRef]

59. Ben Yaou, R.; Navarro, C.; Quijano-Roy, S.; Bertrand, A.T.; Massart, C.; De Sandre-Giovannoli, A.; Cadinanos, J.; Mamchaoui, K.; Butler-Browne, G.; Estournet, B.; et al. Type B mandibuloacral dysplasia with congenital myopathy due to homozygous ZMPSTE24 missense mutation. *Eur. J. Hum. Genet.* **2011**, *19*, 647–654. [CrossRef]

60. Laplante, M.; Sabatini, D.M. mTOR signaling in growth control and disease. *Cell* **2012**, *149*, 274–293. [CrossRef]

61. Abraham, R.T. PI 3-kinase related kinases: 'big' players in stress-induced signaling pathways. *DNA Repair.* **2004**, *3*, 883–887. [CrossRef] [PubMed]

62. Shimobayashi, M.; Hall, M.N. Making new contacts: The mTOR network in metabolism and signalling crosstalk. *Nat. Rev. Mol. Cell. Biol.* **2014**, *15*, 155–162. [CrossRef] [PubMed]

63. Lee, P.L.; Jung, S.M.; Guertin, D.A. The Complex Roles of Mechanistic Target of Rapamycin in Adipocytes and Beyond. *Trends Endocrinol. Metab.* **2017**, *28*, 319–339. [CrossRef]

64. Cai, H.; Dong, L.Q.; Liu, F. Recent Advances in Adipose mTOR Signaling and Function: Therapeutic Prospects. *Trends Pharmacol. Sci.* **2016**, *37*, 303–317. [CrossRef]

65. Nacarelli, T.; Azar, A.; Altinok, O.; Orynbayeva, Z.; Sell, C. Rapamycin increases oxidative metabolism and enhances metabolic flexibility in human cardiac fibroblasts. *Geroscience* 2018. [CrossRef] [PubMed]

66. Caron, M.; Auclair, M.; Donadille, B.; Bereziat, V.; Guerci, B.; Laville, M.; Narbonne, H.; Bodemer, C.; Lascols, O.; Capeau, J.; et al. Human lipodystrophies linked to mutations in A-type lamins and to HIV protease inhibitor therapy are both associated with prelamin A accumulation, oxidative stress and premature cellular senescence. *Cell Death Differ.* **2007**, *14*, 1759–1767. [CrossRef] [PubMed]

67. Galata, Z.; Kloukina, I.; Kostavasili, I.; Varela, A.; Davos, C.H.; Makridakis, M.; Bonne, G.; Capetanaki, Y. Amelioration of desmin network defects by alphaB-crystallin overexpression confers cardioprotection in a mouse model of dilated cardiomyopathy caused by LMNA gene mutation. *J. Mol. Cell. Cardiol.* **2018**, *125*, 73–86. [CrossRef] [PubMed]

68. Gabriel, D.; Gordon, L.B.; Djabali, K. Temsirolimus Partially Rescues the Hutchinson–Gilford Progeria Cellular Phenotype. *PLoS ONE* **2016**, *11*, e0168988. [CrossRef] [PubMed]

69. Morita, M.; Gravel, S.P.; Chenard, V.; Sikstrom, K.; Zheng, L.; Alain, T.; Gandin, V.; Avizonis, D.; Arguello, M.; Zakaria, C.; et al. mTORC1 controls mitochondrial activity and biogenesis through 4E-BP-dependent translational regulation. *Cell Metab.* **2013**, *18*, 698–711. [CrossRef]

70. Liu, X.; Zhang, Y.; Ni, M.; Cao, H.; Signer, R.A.J.; Li, D.; Li, M.; Gu, Z.; Hu, Z.; Dickerson, K.E.; et al. Regulation of mitochondrial biogenesis in erythropoiesis by mTORC1-mediated protein translation. *Nat. Cell Biol.* **2017**, *19*, 626–638. [CrossRef]

71. Sengupta, S.; Peterson, T.R.; Sabatini, D.M. Regulation of the mTOR complex 1 pathway by nutrients, growth factors, and stress. *Mol. Cell* **2010**, *40*, 310–322. [CrossRef] [PubMed]

72. Thoreen, C.C.; Chantranupong, L.; Keys, H.R.; Wang, T.; Gray, N.S.; Sabatini, D.M. A unifying model for mTORC1-mediated regulation of mRNA translation. *Nature* **2012**, *485*, 109–113. [CrossRef] [PubMed]

73. Yuan, H.X.; Xiong, Y.; Guan, K.L. Nutrient sensing, metabolism, and cell growth control. *Mol. Cell* **2013**, *49*, 379–387. [CrossRef] [PubMed]

74. Dunlop, E.A.; Tee, A.R. mTOR and autophagy: A dynamic relationship governed by nutrients and energy. *Semin. Cell Dev. Biol.* 2014. [CrossRef] [PubMed]

75. Alers, S.; Loffler, A.S.; Wesselborg, S.; Stork, B. The incredible ULKs. *Cell Commun. Signal.* **2012**, *10*, 7. [CrossRef] [PubMed]

76. Evangelisti, C.; Chiarini, F.; McCubrey, J.A.; Martelli, A.M. Therapeutic Targeting of mTOR in T-Cell Acute Lymphoblastic Leukemia: An Update. *Int. J. Mol. Sci.* **2018**, *19*. [CrossRef] [PubMed]

77. Zhao, J.; Zhai, B.; Gygi, S.P.; Goldberg, A.L. mTOR inhibition activates overall protein degradation by the ubiquitin proteasome system as well as by autophagy. *Proc. Natl. Acad. Sci. USA* **2015**, *112*, 15790–15797. [CrossRef]

78. Saxton, R.A.; Sabatini, D.M. mTOR Signaling in Growth, Metabolism, and Disease. *Cell* **2017**, *169*, 361–371. [CrossRef]

79. Yoon, M.-S. mTOR as a Key Regulator in Maintaining Skeletal Muscle Mass. *Front. Physiol.* **2017**, *8*, 788. [CrossRef]

80. McPherron, A.C.; Lawler, A.M.; Lee, S.-J. Regulation of skeletal muscle mass in mice by a new TGF-p superfamily member. *Nature* **1997**, *387*, 83. [CrossRef]

81. Shimizu, N.; Yoshikawa, N.; Ito, N.; Maruyama, T.; Suzuki, Y.; Takeda, S.; Nakae, J.; Tagata, Y.; Nishitani, S.; Takehana, K.; et al. Crosstalk between Glucocorticoid Receptor and Nutritional Sensor mTOR in Skeletal Muscle. *Cell Metab.* **2011**, *13*, 170–182. [CrossRef] [PubMed]

82. Zhu, Y.; Pires, K.M.P.; Whitehead, K.J.; Olsen, C.D.; Wayment, B.; Zhang, Y.C.; Bugger, H.; Ilkun, O.; Litwin, S.E.; Thomas, G.; et al. Mechanistic target of rapamycin (Mtor) is essential for murine embryonic heart development and growth. *PLoS ONE* **2013**, *8*, e54221. [CrossRef] [PubMed]

83. Zhang, D.; Contu, R.; Latronico, M.V.G.; Zhang, J.; Rizzi, R.; Catalucci, D.; Miyamoto, S.; Huang, K.; Ceci, M.; Gu, Y.; et al. MTORC1 regulates cardiac function and myocyte survival through 4E-BP1 inhibition in mice. *J. Clin. Investig.* **2010**, *120*, 2805–2816. [CrossRef] [PubMed]

84. Sciarretta, S.; Zhai, P.; Shao, D.; Maejima, Y.; Robbins, J.; Volpe, M.; Condorelli, G.; Sadoshima, J. Rheb is a critical regulator of autophagy during myocardial ischemia: Pathophysiological implications in obesity and metabolic syndrome. *Circulation* **2012**, *125*, 1134–1146. [CrossRef] [PubMed]

85. Sciarretta, S.; Volpe, M.; Sadoshima, J. Mammalian target of rapamycin signaling in cardiac physiology and disease. *Circ. Rese.* **2014**, *114*, 549–564. [CrossRef] [PubMed]

86. Sciarretta, S.; Yee, D.; Shenoy, V.; Nagarajan, N.; Sadoshima, J. The importance of autophagy in cardioprotection. *High. Blood Press. Cardiovasc. Prev.* **2014**, *21*, 21–28. [CrossRef] [PubMed]

87. Cinti, S. The adipose organ at a glance. *Dis. Model. Mech.* **2012**, *5*, 588–594. [CrossRef] [PubMed]

88. Lee, P.L.; Tang, Y.; Li, H.; Guertin, D.A. Raptor/mTORC1 loss in adipocytes causes progressive lipodystrophy and fatty liver disease. *Mol. Metab.* **2016**, *5*, 422–432. [CrossRef]

89. Yoon, M.S.; Zhang, C.; Sun, Y.; Schoenherr, C.J.; Chen, J. Mechanistic target of rapamycin controls homeostasis of adipogenesis. *J. Lipid Res.* **2013**, *54*, 2166–2173. [CrossRef]

90. Zhang, Y.; Goldman, S.; Baerga, R.; Zhao, Y.; Komatsu, M.; Jin, S. Adipose-specific deletion of autophagy-related gene 7 (atg7) in mice reveals a role in adipogenesis. *Proc. Natl. Acad. Sci. USA* **2009**, *106*, 19860–19865. [CrossRef]

91. Armani, A.; Cinti, F.; Marzolla, V.; Morgan, J.; Cranston, G.A.; Antelmi, A.; Carpinelli, G.; Canese, R.; Pagotto, U.; Quarta, C.; et al. Mineralocorticoid receptor antagonism induces browning of white adipose tissue through impairment of autophagy and prevents adipocyte dysfunction in high-fat-diet-fed mice. *FASEB J.* **2014**, *28*, 3745–3757. [CrossRef] [PubMed]

92. Zhang, C.; He, Y.; Okutsu, M.; Ong, L.C.; Jin, Y.; Zheng, L.; Chow, P.; Yu, S.; Zhang, M.; Yan, Z. Autophagy is involved in adipogenic differentiation by repressesing proteasome-dependent PPARgamma2 degradation. *Am. J. Physiol. Endocrinol. Metab.* **2013**, *305*, E530–E539. [CrossRef] [PubMed]

93. Yau, W.W.; Singh, B.K.; Lesmana, R.; Zhou, J.; Sinha, R.A.; Wong, K.A.; Wu, Y.; Bay, B.H.; Sugii, S.; Sun, L.; et al. Thyroid hormone (T3) stimulates brown adipose tissue activation via mitochondrial biogenesis and MTOR-mediated mitophagy. *Autophagy* **2019**, *15*, 131–150. [CrossRef] [PubMed]

94. Long, F.; Ornitz, D.M. Development of the endochondral skeleton. *Cold Spring Harb. Perspect. Biol.* **2013**, *5*, a008334. [CrossRef] [PubMed]

95. Chen, J.; Long, F. mTOR signaling in skeletal development and disease. *Bone Res.* **2018**, *6*, 1. [CrossRef] [PubMed]

96. Bonne, G.; Mercuri, E.; Muchir, A.; Urtizberea, A.; Bécane, H.M.; Recan, D.; Merlini, L.; Wehnert, M.; Boor, R.; Reuner, U.; et al. Clinical and molecular genetic spectrum of autosomal dominant Emery–Dreifuss muscular dystrophy due to mutations of the lamin A/C gene. *Ann. Neurol.* **2000**, *48*, 170–180. [CrossRef]

97. Choi, J.C.; Muchir, A.; Wu, W.; Iwata, S.; Homma, S.; Morrow, J.P.; Worman, H.J. Temsirolimus activates autophagy and ameliorates cardiomyopathy caused by lamin A/C gene mutation. *Sci. Transl. Med.* **2012**, *4*, 144ra102. [CrossRef]

98. Fatkin, D.; MacRae, C.; Sasaki, T.; Wolff, M.R.; Porcu, M.; Frenneaux, M.; Atherton, J.; Vidaillet, H.J., Jr.; Spudich, S.; De Girolami, U.; et al. Missense mutations in the rod domain of the lamin A/C gene as causes of dilated cardiomyopathy and conduction-system disease. *N. Engl. J. Med.* **1999**, *341*, 1715–1724. [CrossRef]

99. van der Kooi, A.J.; van Meegen, M.; Ledderhof, T.M.; McNally, E.M.; de Visser, M.; Bolhuis, P.A. Genetic localization of a newly recognized autosomal dominant limb-girdle muscular dystrophy with cardiac involvement (LGMD1B) to chromosome 1q11-21. *Am. J. Hum. Genet.* **1997**, *60*, 891–895.

100. Quijano-Roy, S.; Mbieleu, B.; Bönnemann, C.G.; Jeannet, P.-Y.; Colomer, J.; Clarke, N.F.; Cuisset, J.-M.; Roper, H.; De Meirleir, L.; D'Amico, A.; et al. De novo LMNA mutations cause a new form of congenital muscular dystrophy. *Ann. Neurol.* **2008**, *64*, 177–186. [CrossRef]

101. Renou, L.; Stora, S.; Yaou, R.B.; Volk, M.; Šinkovec, M.; Demay, L.; Richard, P.; Peterlin, B.; Bonne, G. Heart–hand syndrome of Slovenian type: A new kind of laminopathy. *J. Med. Genet.* **2008**, *45*, 666. [CrossRef] [PubMed]

102. Brosig, M.; Ferralli, J.; Gelman, L.; Chiquet, M.; Chiquet-Ehrismann, R. Interfering with the connection between the nucleus and the cytoskeleton affects nuclear rotation, mechanotransduction and myogenesis. *Int. J. Biochem. Cell Biol.* **2010**, *42*, 1717–1728. [CrossRef] [PubMed]

103. Dechat, T.; Korbei, B.; Vaughan, O.A.; Vlcek, S.; Hutchison, C.J.; Foisner, R. Lamina-associated polypeptide 2alpha binds intranuclear A-type lamins. *J. Cell Sci.* **2000**, *113*, 3473. [PubMed]

104. Angori, S.; Capanni, C.; Faulkner, G.; Bean, C.; Boriani, G.; Lattanzi, G.; Cenni, V. Emery–Dreifuss Muscular Dystrophy-Associated Mutant Forms of Lamin A Recruit the Stress Responsive Protein Ankrd2 into the Nucleus, Affecting the Cellular Response to Oxidative Stress. *Cell. Physiol. Biochem.* **2017**, *42*, 169–184. [CrossRef] [PubMed]

105. Markiewicz, E.; Ledran, M.; Hutchison, C.J. Remodelling of the nuclear lamina and nucleoskeleton is required for skeletal muscle differentiation in vitro. *J. Cell Sci.* **2005**, *118*, 409. [CrossRef] [PubMed]

106. Frock, R.L.; Kudlow, B.A.; Evans, A.M.; Jameson, S.A.; Hauschka, S.D.; Kennedy, B.K. Lamin A/C and emerin are critical for skeletal muscle satellite cell differentiation. *Genes Dev.* **2006**, *20*, 486–500. [CrossRef] [PubMed]

107. Sylvius, N.; Bonne, G.; Straatman, K.; Reddy, T.; Gant, T.W.; Shackleton, S. MicroRNA expression profiling in patients with lamin A/C-associated muscular dystrophy. *FASEB J.* **2011**, *25*, 3966–3978. [CrossRef]

108. Rahman, M.; Mofarrahi, M.; Kristof, A.S.; Nkengfac, B.; Harel, S.; Hussain, S.N.A. Reactive Oxygen Species Regulation of Autophagy in Skeletal Muscles. *Antioxid. Redox Signal.* **2013**, *20*, 443–459. [CrossRef]

109. Filomeni, G.; De Zio, D.; Cecconi, F. Oxidative stress and autophagy: The clash between damage and metabolic needs. *Cell Death Differ.* **2015**, *22*, 377–388. [CrossRef]

110. Pekovic, V.; Gibbs-Seymour, I.; Markiewicz, E.; Alzoghaibi, F.; Benham, A.M.; Edwards, R.; Wenhert, M.; von Zglinicki, T.; Hutchison, C.J. Conserved cysteine residues in the mammalian lamin A tail are essential for cellular responses to ROS generation. *Aging Cell* **2011**, *10*, 1067–1079. [CrossRef]

111. Ramos, F.J.; Chen, S.C.; Garelick, M.G.; Dai, D.F.; Liao, C.Y.; Schreiber, K.H.; MacKay, V.L.; An, E.H.; Strong, R.; Ladiges, W.C.; et al. Rapamycin reverses elevated mTORC1 signaling in lamin A/C-deficient mice, rescues cardiac and skeletal muscle function, and extends survival. *Sci. Transl. Med.* **2012**, *4*, 144ra103. [CrossRef] [PubMed]

112. Choi, J.C.; Worman, H.J. Reactivation of autophagy ameliorates LMNA cardiomyopathy. *Autophagy* **2013**, *9*, 110–111. [CrossRef] [PubMed]

113. Liao, C.-Y.; Anderson, S.S.; Chicoine, N.H.; Mayfield, J.R.; Garrett, B.J.; Kwok, C.S.; Academia, E.C.; Hsu, Y.-M.; Miller, D.M.; Bair, A.M.; et al. Evidence that S6K1, but not 4E-BP1, mediates skeletal muscle pathology associated with loss of A-type lamins. *Cell Discov.* **2017**, *3*, 17039. [CrossRef]

114. Bhide, S.; Trujillo, A.S.; O'Connor, M.T.; Young, G.H.; Cryderman, D.E.; Chandran, S.; Nikravesh, M.; Wallrath, L.L.; Melkani, G.C. Increasing autophagy and blocking Nrf2 suppress laminopathy-induced age-dependent cardiac dysfunction and shortened lifespan. *Aging Cell* **2018**, *17*, e12747. [CrossRef]

115. Dialynas, G.; Shrestha, O.K.; Ponce, J.M.; Zwerger, M.; Thiemann, D.A.; Young, G.H.; Moore, S.A.; Yu, L.; Lammerding, J.; Wallrath, L.L. Myopathic lamin mutations cause reductive stress and activate the nrf2/keap-1 pathway. *PLoS Genet.* **2015**, *11*, e1005231. [CrossRef]

116. Markofski, M.M.; Dickinson, J.M.; Drummond, M.J.; Fry, C.S.; Fujita, S.; Gundermann, D.M.; Glynn, E.L.; Jennings, K.; Paddon-Jones, D.; Reidy, P.T.; et al. Effect of age on basal muscle protein synthesis and mTORC1 signaling in a large cohort of young and older men and women. *Exp. Gerontol.* **2015**, *65*, 1–7. [CrossRef] [PubMed]

117. Castets, P.; Lin, S.; Rion, N.; Di Fulvio, S.; Romanino, K.; Guridi, M.; Frank, S.; Tintignac, L.A.; Sinnreich, M.; Rüegg, M.A. Sustained Activation of mTORC1 in Skeletal Muscle Inhibits Constitutive and Starvation-Induced Autophagy and Causes a Severe, Late-Onset Myopathy. *Cell Metab.* **2013**, *17*, 731–744. [CrossRef] [PubMed]

118. Wu, J.J.; Liu, J.; Chen, E.B.; Wang, J.J.; Cao, L.; Narayan, N.; Fergusson, M.M.; Rovira, I.I.; Allen, M.; Springer, D.A.; et al. Increased Mammalian Lifespan and a Segmental and Tissue-Specific Slowing of Aging after Genetic Reduction of mTOR Expression. *Cell Rep.* **2013**, *4*, 913–920. [CrossRef] [PubMed]

119. Wu, X.; Cao, Y.; Nie, J.; Liu, H.; Lu, S.; Hu, X.; Zhu, J.; Zhao, X.; Chen, J.; Chen, X.; et al. Genetic and Pharmacological Inhibition of Rheb1-mTORC1 Signaling Exerts Cardioprotection against Adverse Cardiac Remodeling in Mice. *Am. J. Pathol.* **2013**, *182*, 2005–2014. [CrossRef] [PubMed]

120. Weiss, R.; Fernandez, E.; Liu, Y.; Strong, R.; Salmon, A.B. Metformin reduces glucose intolerance caused by rapamycin treatment in genetically heterogeneous female mice. *Aging* **2018**. [CrossRef]

121. Liao, C.Y.; Anderson, S.S.; Chicoine, N.H.; Mayfield, J.R.; Academia, E.C.; Wilson, J.A.; Pongkietisak, C.; Thompson, M.A.; Lagmay, E.P.; Miller, D.M.; et al. Rapamycin Reverses Metabolic Deficits in Lamin A/C-Deficient Mice. *Cell Rep.* **2016**, *17*, 2542–2552. [CrossRef] [PubMed]

122. Guillin-Amarelle, C.; Fernandez-Pombo, A.; Sanchez-Iglesias, S.; Araujo-Vilar, D. Lipodystrophic laminopathies: Diagnostic clues. *Nucleus* **2018**, *9*, 249–260. [CrossRef] [PubMed]

123. Cao, H.; Hegele, R.A. Nuclear lamin A/C R482Q mutation in canadian kindreds with Dunnigan-type familial partial lipodystrophy. *Hum. Mol. Genet.* **2000**, *9*, 109–112. [CrossRef] [PubMed]

124. Guenantin, A.C.; Briand, N.; Bidault, G.; Afonso, P.; Bereziat, V.; Vatier, C.; Lascols, O.; Caron-Debarle, M.; Capeau, J.; Vigouroux, C. Nuclear envelope-related lipodystrophies. *Semin. Cell Dev. Biol.* **2014**, *29*, 148–157. [CrossRef] [PubMed]

125. Bidault, G.; Garcia, M.; Vantyghem, M.C.; Ducluzeau, P.H.; Morichon, R.; Thiyagarajah, K.; Moritz, S.; Capeau, J.; Vigouroux, C.; Bereziat, V. Lipodystrophy-linked LMNA p.R482W mutation induces clinical early atherosclerosis and in vitro endothelial dysfunction. *Arterioscler. Thromb. Vasc. Biol.* **2013**, *33*, 2162–2171. [CrossRef] [PubMed]

126. Bereziat, V.; Cervera, P.; Le Dour, C.; Verpont, M.C.; Dumont, S.; Vantyghem, M.C.; Capeau, J.; Vigouroux, C.; Lipodystrophy Study, G. LMNA mutations induce a non-inflammatory fibrosis and a brown fat-like dystrophy of enlarged cervical adipose tissue. *Am. J. Pathol.* **2011**, *179*, 2443–2453. [CrossRef]

127. Capanni, C.; Squarzoni, S.; Cenni, V.; D'Apice, M.R.; Gambineri, A.; Novelli, G.; Wehnert, M.; Pasquali, R.; Maraldi, N.M.; Lattanzi, G. Familial partial lipodystrophy, mandibuloacral dysplasia and restrictive dermopathy feature barrier-to-autointegration factor (BAF) nuclear redistribution. *Cell Cycle* **2012**, *11*, 3568–3577. [CrossRef]

128. Briand, N.; Cahyani, I.; Madsen-Osterbye, J.; Paulsen, J.; Ronningen, T.; Sorensen, A.L.; Collas, P. Lamin A, Chromatin and FPLD2: Not Just a Peripheral Menage-a-Trois. *Front. Cell Dev. Biol.* **2018**, *6*, 73. [CrossRef]

129. Briand, N.; Guenantin, A.C.; Jeziorowska, D.; Shah, A.; Mantecon, M.; Capel, E.; Garcia, M.; Oldenburg, A.; Paulsen, J.; Hulot, J.S.; et al. The lipodystrophic hotspot lamin A p.R482W mutation deregulates the mesodermal inducer T/Brachyury and early vascular differentiation gene networks. *Hum. Mol. Genet.* **2018**, *27*, 1447–1459. [CrossRef]

130. Araujo-Vilar, D.; Lattanzi, G.; Gonzalez-Mendez, B.; Costa-Freitas, A.T.; Prieto, D.; Columbaro, M.; Mattioli, E.; Victoria, B.; Martinez-Sanchez, N.; Ramazanova, A.; et al. Site-dependent differences in both prelamin A and adipogenic genes in subcutaneous adipose tissue of patients with type 2 familial partial lipodystrophy. *J. Med. Genet.* **2009**, *46*, 40–48. [CrossRef]

131. Oldenburg, A.R.; Delbarre, E.; Thiede, B.; Vigouroux, C.; Collas, P. Deregulation of Fragile X-related protein 1 by the lipodystrophic lamin A p.R482W mutation elicits a myogenic gene expression program in preadipocytes. *Hum. Mol. Genet.* **2014**, *23*, 1151–1162. [CrossRef] [PubMed]

132. Batrakou, D.G.; de Las Heras, J.I.; Czapiewski, R.; Mouras, R.; Schirmer, E.C. TMEM120A and B: Nuclear Envelope Transmembrane Proteins Important for Adipocyte Differentiation. *PLoS ONE* **2015**, *10*, e0127712. [CrossRef] [PubMed]

133. Gordon, L.B.; Rothman, F.G.; Lopez-Otin, C.; Misteli, T. Progeria: A paradigm for translational medicine. *Cell* **2014**, *156*, 400–407. [CrossRef] [PubMed]

134. De Sandre-Giovannoli, A.; Bernard, R.; Cau, P.; Navarro, C.; Amiel, J.; Boccaccio, I.; Lyonnet, S.; Stewart, C.L.; Munnich, A.; Le Merrer, M.; et al. Lamin a truncation in Hutchinson–Gilford progeria. *Science* **2003**, *300*, 2055. [CrossRef] [PubMed]

135. Eriksson, M.; Brown, W.T.; Gordon, L.B.; Glynn, M.W.; Singer, J.; Scott, L.; Erdos, M.R.; Robbins, C.M.; Moses, T.Y.; Berglund, P.; et al. Recurrent de novo point mutations in lamin A cause Hutchinson–Gilford progeria syndrome. *Nature* **2003**, *423*, 293–298. [CrossRef] [PubMed]

136. Goldman, R.D.; Shumaker, D.K.; Erdos, M.R.; Eriksson, M.; Goldman, A.E.; Gordon, L.B.; Gruenbaum, Y.; Khuon, S.; Mendez, M.; Varga, R.; et al. Accumulation of mutant lamin A causes progressive changes in nuclear architecture in Hutchinson–Gilford progeria syndrome. *Proc. Natl. Acad. Sci. USA* **2004**, *101*, 8963–8968. [CrossRef] [PubMed]

137. Barthelemy, F.; Navarro, C.; Fayek, R.; Da Silva, N.; Roll, P.; Sigaudy, S.; Oshima, J.; Bonne, G.; Papadopoulou-Legbelou, K.; Evangeliou, A.E.; et al. Truncated prelamin A expression in HGPS-like patients: A transcriptional study. *Eur. J. Hum. Genet.* **2015**, *23*, 1051–1061. [CrossRef]

138. Moulson, C.L.; Fong, L.G.; Gardner, J.M.; Farber, E.A.; Go, G.; Passariello, A.; Grange, D.K.; Young, S.G.; Miner, J.H. Increased progerin expression associated with unusual LMNA mutations causes severe progeroid syndromes. *Hum. Mutat.* **2007**, *28*, 882–889. [CrossRef]

139. Kang, S.M.; Yoon, M.H.; Park, B.J. Laminopathies; Mutations on single gene and various human genetic diseases. *BMB Rep.* **2018**, *51*, 327–337. [CrossRef]

140. Ibrahim, M.X.; Sayin, V.I.; Akula, M.K.; Liu, M.; Fong, L.G.; Young, S.G.; Bergo, M.O. Targeting isoprenylcysteine methylation ameliorates disease in a mouse model of progeria. *Science* **2013**, *340*, 1330–1333. [CrossRef]

141. Evangelisti, C.; Cenni, V.; Lattanzi, G. Potential therapeutic effects of the MTOR inhibitors for preventing ageing and progeria-related disorders. *Br. J. Clin. Pharmacol.* **2016**, *82*, 1229–1244. [CrossRef] [PubMed]

142. Cenni, V.; Capanni, C.; Columbaro, M.; Ortolani, M.; D'Apice, M.R.; Novelli, G.; Fini, M.; Marmiroli, S.; Scarano, E.; Maraldi, N.M.; et al. Autophagic degradation of farnesylated prelamin A as a therapeutic approach to lamin-linked progeria. *Eur. J. Histochem.* **2011**, *55*, e36. [CrossRef] [PubMed]

143. Kreienkamp, R.; Billon, C.; Bedia-Diaz, G.; Albert, C.J.; Toth, Z.; Butler, A.A.; McBride-Gagyi, S.; Ford, D.A.; Baldan, A.; Burris, T.P.; et al. Doubled lifespan and patient-like pathologies in progeria mice fed high-fat diet. *Aging Cell* **2018**, e12852. [CrossRef]

144. Selman, C.; Tullet, J.M.; Wieser, D.; Irvine, E.; Lingard, S.J.; Choudhury, A.I.; Claret, M.; Al-Qassab, H.; Carmignac, D.; Ramadani, F.; et al. Ribosomal protein S6 kinase 1 signaling regulates mammalian lifespan. *Science* **2009**, *326*, 140–144. [CrossRef]

145. Lamming, D.W.; Ye, L.; Katajisto, P.; Goncalves, M.D.; Saitoh, M.; Stevens, D.M.; Davis, J.G.; Salmon, A.B.; Richardson, A.; Ahima, R.S.; et al. Rapamycin-induced insulin resistance is mediated by mTORC2 loss and uncoupled from longevity. *Science* **2012**, *335*, 1638–1643. [CrossRef]

146. Chen, C.; Liu, Y.; Zheng, P. mTOR regulation and therapeutic rejuvenation of aging hematopoietic stem cells. *Sci. Signal.* **2009**, *2*, ra75. [CrossRef]

147. Dai, D.F.; Karunadharma, P.P.; Chiao, Y.A.; Basisty, N.; Crispin, D.; Hsieh, E.J.; Chen, T.; Gu, H.; Djukovic, D.; Raftery, D.; et al. Altered proteome turnover and remodeling by short-term caloric restriction or rapamycin rejuvenate the aging heart. *Aging Cell* **2014**, *13*, 529–539. [CrossRef]

148. Harrison, D.E.; Strong, R.; Sharp, Z.D.; Nelson, J.F.; Astle, C.M.; Flurkey, K.; Nadon, N.L.; Wilkinson, J.E.; Frenkel, K.; Carter, C.S.; et al. Rapamycin fed late in life extends lifespan in genetically heterogeneous mice. *Nature* **2009**, *460*, 392–395. [CrossRef]

149. Spilman, P.; Podlutskaya, N.; Hart, M.J.; Debnath, J.; Gorostiza, O.; Bredesen, D.; Richardson, A.; Strong, R.; Galvan, V. Inhibition of mTOR by rapamycin abolishes cognitive deficits and reduces amyloid-beta levels in a mouse model of Alzheimer's disease. *PLoS ONE* **2010**, *5*, e9979. [CrossRef]

150. Wilkinson, J.E.; Burmeister, L.; Brooks, S.V.; Chan, C.C.; Friedline, S.; Harrison, D.E.; Hejtmancik, J.F.; Nadon, N.; Strong, R.; Wood, L.K.; et al. Rapamycin slows aging in mice. *Aging Cell* **2012**, *11*, 675–682. [CrossRef]

151. Miller, R.A.; Harrison, D.E.; Astle, C.M.; Baur, J.A.; Boyd, A.R.; de Cabo, R.; Fernandez, E.; Flurkey, K.; Javors, M.A.; Nelson, J.F.; et al. Rapamycin, but not resveratrol or simvastatin, extends lifespan of genetically heterogeneous mice. *J. Gerontol. A Biol. Sci. Med. Sci.* **2011**, *66*, 191–201. [CrossRef] [PubMed]

152. Miller, R.A.; Harrison, D.E.; Astle, C.M.; Fernandez, E.; Flurkey, K.; Han, M.; Javors, M.A.; Li, X.; Nadon, N.L.; Nelson, J.F.; et al. Rapamycin-mediated lifespan increase in mice is dose and sex dependent and metabolically distinct from dietary restriction. *Aging Cell* **2014**, *13*, 468–477. [CrossRef] [PubMed]

153. Zhang, Y.; Bokov, A.; Gelfond, J.; Soto, V.; Ikeno, Y.; Hubbard, G.; Diaz, V.; Sloane, L.; Maslin, K.; Treaster, S.; et al. Rapamycin extends life and health in C57BL/6 mice. *J. Gerontol. A Biol. Sci. Med. Sci.* **2014**, *69*, 119–130. [CrossRef] [PubMed]

154. Arriola Apelo, S.I.; Neuman, J.C.; Baar, E.L.; Syed, F.A.; Cummings, N.E.; Brar, H.K.; Pumper, C.P.; Kimple, M.E.; Lamming, D.W. Alternative rapamycin treatment regimens mitigate the impact of rapamycin on glucose homeostasis and the immune system. *Aging Cell* **2016**, *15*, 28–38. [CrossRef] [PubMed]

155. Carter, C.S.; Khamiss, D.; Matheny, M.; Toklu, H.Z.; Kirichenko, N.; Strehler, K.Y.; Tumer, N.; Scarpace, P.J.; Morgan, D. Rapamycin Versus Intermittent Feeding: Dissociable Effects on Physiological and Behavioral Outcomes When Initiated Early and Late in Life. *J. Gerontol. A Biol. Sci. Med. Sci.* **2016**, *71*, 866–875. [CrossRef] [PubMed]

156. Longo, V.D.; Fontana, L. Intermittent supplementation with rapamycin as a dietary restriction mimetic. *Aging* **2011**, *3*, 1039–1040. [CrossRef] [PubMed]

157. Mannick, J.B.; Del Giudice, G.; Lattanzi, M.; Valiante, N.M.; Praestgaard, J.; Huang, B.; Lonetto, M.A.; Maecker, H.T.; Kovarik, J.; Carson, S.; et al. mTOR inhibition improves immune function in the elderly. *Sci. Transl. Med.* **2014**, *6*, 268ra179. [CrossRef] [PubMed]

158. Barcena, C.; Quiros, P.M.; Durand, S.; Mayoral, P.; Rodriguez, F.; Caravia, X.M.; Marino, G.; Garabaya, C.; Fernandez-Garcia, M.T.; Kroemer, G.; et al. Methionine Restriction Extends Lifespan in Progeroid Mice and Alters Lipid and Bile Acid Metabolism. *Cell Rep.* **2018**, *24*, 2392–2403. [CrossRef] [PubMed]

159. Rivera-Torres, J.; Acin-Perez, R.; Cabezas-Sanchez, P.; Osorio, F.G.; Gonzalez-Gomez, C.; Megias, D.; Camara, C.; Lopez-Otin, C.; Enriquez, J.A.; Luque-Garcia, J.L.; et al. Identification of mitochondrial dysfunction in Hutchinson–Gilford progeria syndrome through use of stable isotope labeling with amino acids in cell culture. *J. Proteomics* **2013**, *91*, 466–477. [CrossRef] [PubMed]

160. Pellegrini, C.; Columbaro, M.; Capanni, C.; D'Apice, M.R.; Cavallo, C.; Murdocca, M.; Lattanzi, G.; Squarzoni, S. All-trans retinoic acid and rapamycin normalize Hutchinson Gilford progeria fibroblast phenotype. *Oncotarget* **2015**, *6*, 29914–29928. [CrossRef] [PubMed]

161. Cho, K.; Chung, J.Y.; Cho, S.K.; Shin, H.W.; Jang, I.J.; Park, J.W.; Yu, K.S.; Cho, J.Y. Antihyperglycemic mechanism of metformin occurs via the AMPK/LXRalpha/POMC pathway. *Sci. Rep.* **2015**, *5*, 8145. [CrossRef] [PubMed]

162. Nair, V.; Sreevalsan, S.; Basha, R.; Abdelrahim, M.; Abudayyeh, A.; Rodrigues Hoffman, A.; Safe, S. Mechanism of metformin-dependent inhibition of mammalian target of rapamycin (mTOR) and Ras activity in pancreatic cancer: Role of specificity protein (Sp) transcription factors. *J. Biol. Chem.* **2014**, *289*, 27692–27701. [CrossRef] [PubMed]

163. Barzilai, N.; Crandall, J.P.; Kritchevsky, S.B.; Espeland, M.A. Metformin as a Tool to Target Aging. *Cell Metab.* **2016**, *23*, 1060–1065. [CrossRef] [PubMed]

164. Campbell, J.M.; Bellman, S.M.; Stephenson, M.D.; Lisy, K. Metformin reduces all-cause mortality and diseases of ageing independent of its effect on diabetes control: A systematic review and meta-analysis. *Ageing Res. Rev.* **2017**, *40*, 31–44. [CrossRef] [PubMed]

165. Egesipe, A.L.; Blondel, S.; Cicero, A.L.; Jaskowiak, A.L.; Navarro, C.; Sandre-Giovannoli, A.; Levy, N.; Peschanski, M.; Nissan, X. Metformin decreases progerin expression and alleviates pathological defects of Hutchinson–Gilford progeria syndrome cells. *NPJ Aging Mech. Dis.* **2016**, *2*, 16026. [CrossRef] [PubMed]

166. Gordon, L.B.; Kleinman, M.E.; Miller, D.T.; Neuberg, D.S.; Giobbie-Hurder, A.; Gerhard-Herman, M.; Smoot, L.B.; Gordon, C.M.; Cleveland, R.; Snyder, B.D.; et al. Clinical trial of a farnesyltransferase inhibitor in children with Hutchinson–Gilford progeria syndrome. *Proc. Natl. Acad. Sci. USA* **2012**, *109*, 16666–16671. [CrossRef]

167. Harhouri, K.; Navarro, C.; Depetris, D.; Mattei, M.G.; Nissan, X.; Cau, P.; De Sandre-Giovannoli, A.; Levy, N. MG132-induced progerin clearance is mediated by autophagy activation and splicing regulation. *EMBO Mol. Med.* **2017**, *9*, 1294–1313. [CrossRef]

168. Lunova, M.; Smolkova, B.; Lynnyk, A.; Uzhytchak, M.; Jirsa, M.; Kubinova, S.; Dejneka, A.; Lunov, O. Targeting the mTOR Signaling Pathway Utilizing Nanoparticles: A Critical Overview. *Cancers* **2019**, *11*. [CrossRef]

169. Lunova, M.; Prokhorov, A.; Jirsa, M.; Hof, M.; Olzynska, A.; Jurkiewicz, P.; Kubinova, S.; Lunov, O.; Dejneka, A. Nanoparticle core stability and surface functionalization drive the mTOR signaling pathway in hepatocellular cell lines. *Sci. Rep.* **2017**, *7*, 16049. [CrossRef]

170. Cenni, V.; Capanni, C.; Mattioli, E.; Columbaro, M.; Wehnert, M.; Ortolani, M.; Fini, M.; Novelli, G.; Bertacchini, J.; Maraldi, N.M.; et al. Rapamycin treatment of Mandibuloacral dysplasia cells rescues localization of chromatin-associated proteins and cell cycle dynamics. *Aging* **2014**, *6*, 755–770. [CrossRef]

Int. J. Mol. Sci. **2019**, *20*, 847

171. Akinci, B.; Sankella, S.; Gilpin, C.; Ozono, K.; Garg, A.; Agarwal, A.K. Progeroid syndrome patients with ZMPSTE24 deficiency could benefit when treated with rapamycin and dimethylsulfoxide. *Cold Spring Harb. Mol. Case Stud.* **2017**, *3*, a001339. [CrossRef] [PubMed]

172. Dou, Z.; Xu, C.; Donahue, G.; Shimi, T.; Pan, J.A.; Zhu, J.; Ivanov, A.; Capell, B.C.; Drake, A.M.; Shah, P.P.; et al. Autophagy mediates degradation of nuclear lamina. *Nature* **2015**, *527*, 105–109. [CrossRef] [PubMed]

173. Muchir, A.; Reilly, S.A.; Wu, W.; Iwata, S.; Homma, S.; Bonne, G.; Worman, H.J. Treatment with selumetinib preserves cardiac function and improves survival in cardiomyopathy caused by mutation in the lamin A/C gene. *Cardiovasc. Res.* **2012**, *93*, 311–319. [CrossRef] [PubMed]

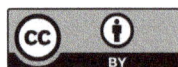

International Journal of
Molecular Sciences

MDPI

Article

In Vitro Identification of New Transcriptomic and miRNomic Profiles Associated with Pulmonary Fibrosis Induced by High Doses Everolimus: Looking for New Pathogenetic Markers and Therapeutic Targets

Simona Granata [1], Gloria Santoro [1], Valentina Masola [1], Paola Tomei [1], Fabio Sallustio [2,3], Paola Pontrelli [2], Matteo Accetturo [2], Nadia Antonucci [1], Pierluigi Carratù [4], Antonio Lupo [1] and Gianluigi Zaza [1,*]

[1] Renal Unit, Department of Medicine, University of Verona, Piazzale Stefani 1, 37126 Verona, Italy; simona.granata@univr.it (S.G.); gloria.santoro@univr.it (G.S.); valentina.masola@unipd.it (V.M.); paola.tomei@univr.it (P.T.); nadia.antonucci@univr.it (N.A.); antonio.lupo@univr.it (A.L.)
[2] Department of Emergency and Organ Transplantation, University of Bari "Aldo Moro", Piazza Giulio Cesare 11, 70124 Bari, Italy; fabio.sallustio@uniba.it (F.S.); paola.pontrelli@uniba.it (P.P.); accetturo.m@gmail.com (M.A.)
[3] Department of Basic Medical Sciences, Neuroscience and Sense Organs, University of Bari "Aldo Moro", Piazza Giulio Cesare 11, 70124 Bari, Italy
[4] Department of Respiratory Diseases, University of Bari "Aldo Moro", Piazza Giulio Cesare 11, 70124 Bari, Italy; pierluigi.carratu@uniba.it
* Correspondence: gianluigi.zaza@univr.it; Tel.: +39-045-812-2521

Received: 23 March 2018; Accepted: 17 April 2018; Published: 20 April 2018

Abstract: The administration of Everolimus (EVE), a mTOR inhibitor used in transplantation and cancer, is often associated with adverse effects including pulmonary fibrosis. Although the underlying mechanism is not fully clarified, this condition could be in part caused by epithelial to mesenchymal transition (EMT) of airway cells. To improve our knowledge, primary bronchial epithelial cells (BE63/3) were treated with EVE (5 and 100 nM) for 24 h. EMT markers (α-SMA, vimentin, fibronectin) were measured by RT-PCR. Transepithelial resistance was measured by Millicell-ERS ohmmeter. mRNA and microRNA profiling were performed by Illumina and Agilent kit, respectively. Only high dose EVE increased EMT markers and reduced the transepithelial resistance of BE63/3. Bioinformatics showed 125 de-regulated genes that, according to enrichment analysis, were implicated in collagen synthesis/metabolism. Connective tissue growth factor (*CTGF*) was one of the higher up-regulated mRNA. Five nM EVE was ineffective on the pro-fibrotic machinery. Additionally, 3 miRNAs resulted hyper-expressed after 100 nM EVE and able to regulate 31 of the genes selected by the transcriptomic analysis (including *CTGF*). RT-PCR and western blot for *MMP12* and *CTGF* validated high-throughput results. Our results revealed a complex biological network implicated in EVE-related pulmonary fibrosis and underlined new potential disease biomarkers and therapeutic targets.

Keywords: epithelial to mesenchymal transition; mTOR inhibitor; pulmonary fibrosis; transcriptomics; miRNome; everolimus

1. Introduction

Everolimus (EVE), marketed as Certican, is a pharmacological agent widely used in the anti-rejection therapy of solid organ transplantation and in the treatment of certain tumors (e.g., in advanced renal cell carcinoma, subependymal giant cell astrocytoma associated with tuberous sclerosis, pancreatic neuroendocrine tumors, breast cancer) [1]. Similar to Sirolimus and Tamsilorimus, it exerts its immunosuppressive activity by inhibiting mammalian target of rapamycin (mTOR), a phosphoinositide 3-kinase-related protein that controls cell cycle, protein synthesis, angiogenesis and autophagy [2]. These important multi-factorial biological/cellular effects allow this drug to avoid/minimize the onset of acute rejection episodes and to slow down the progression of chronic allograft lesions [3,4].

However, some authors have reported a high rate of discontinuation secondary to side effects after the introduction of this drug [5–7]. Among them, pneumonitis or interstitial lung disease with a range of pulmonary histopathologic changes (including alveolar hemorrhage, pulmonary alveolar proteinosis, focal fibrosis, bronchiolitis obliterans organizing pneumonia) have been largely reported in clinical records and they have been associated with worsened patients' clinical outcomes and drug discontinuation [8–16]. The incidence of this complications is 2–11%, frequently reported between 1 and 51 months after the beginning of mTOR inhibitor therapy [17–19].

The pathogenic mechanism underlying lung toxicity is multi-factorial and epithelial to mesenchymal transition (EMT) of airway cells seems to have a pivotal role [20–23]. Our group has recently demonstrated that high doses of EVE are associated with a reprogramming of gene expression in several epithelial cell lines (airway, renal epithelial proximal tubular and hepatic cells) with a consequent loss of their phenotype (junctions and apical-basal polarity) and the acquisition of mesenchymal traits increasing the motility and enabling the development of an invasive and pro-fibrotic phenotype [24–26].

High dosage of EVE eliminating negative crosstalk from mTORC1/S6K, leads to activation of mTORC2 that enhances AKT phosphorylation at Ser473 and stimulates PI3K-AKT signaling that induces renal fibrosis [26–30].

The pro-fibrotic attitude of EVE has also been confirmed in vivo in renal transplant patients through the estimation of an arbitrary pulmonary fibrosis index score in renal transplant patients chronically treated with this drug. In this patients' subset, high blood trough level of EVE was associated with a high rate of pulmonary signs of fibrosis [24].

However, although the aforementioned studies and the large clinical evidences, the complete biological machinery involved in this condition has not been completely clarified.

Therefore, we employed, for the first time, a highthroughput approach combining a transcriptomic with a miRNome analysis to study the capability of EVE to induce pro-fibrotic changes in primary bronchial epithelial cells.

All together our results could represent a step forward in the comprehension of the mTOR-I associated biological machinery and in the identification of new targets for therapeutic interventions.

2. Results

2.1. High Dosage Everolimus (EVE) Induced Epithelial to Mesenchymal Transition (EMT) of BE63/3 (Primary Bronchial Epithelial Cells)

To confirm our previous results obtained in immortalized bronchial and pulmonary cell lines [24], we decided to measure by Real Time-PCR the expression level of alpha smooth muscle actin (*α-SMA*), vimentin (*VIM*), and fibronectin (*FN*) in BE63/3 treated for 24 h with 2 different dosages of EVE (5 and 100 nM) chosen according to literature evidences [31–34] and previous experiments performed by our research group in different cell lines [24–26].

Only high dose of EVE (100 nM), similarly to TGF-β (20 ng/mL), increased the mRNA level of the EMT-related markers (Figure 1A–C). Moreover E-cadherin resulted downregulated although it did not reach a statistically significant level (Figure S1). Contrarily, 5 nM EVE was ineffective (Figure 1A–C).

Additionally, high dosage of EVE was also able to reduce the transepithelial resistance (TER) evaluated by a Millicell-ERS ohmmeter indicating dysfunctional tight junctions (Figure 1D).

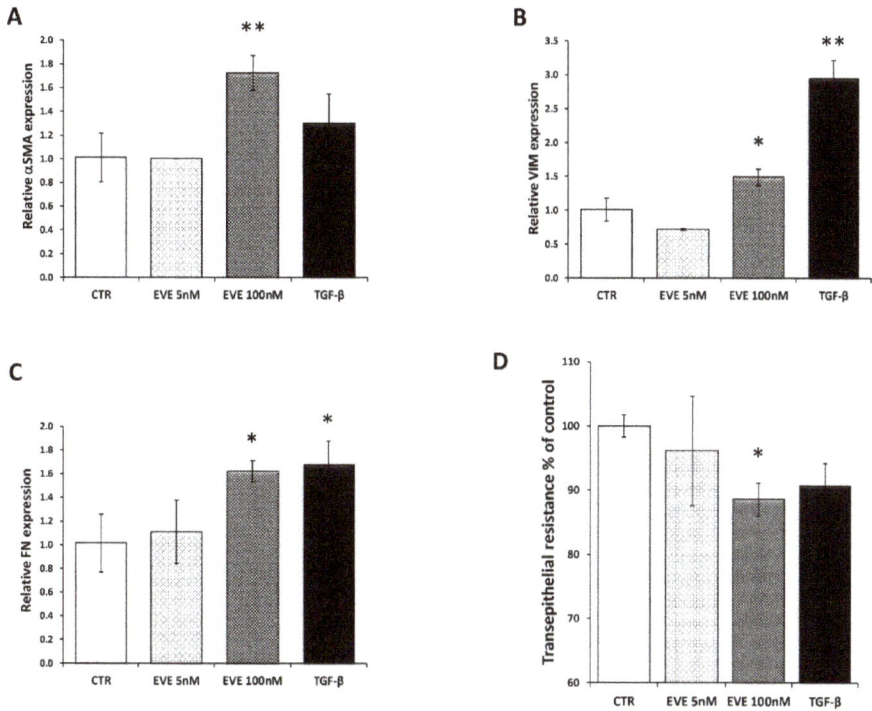

Figure 1. Gene expression of epithelial to mesenchymal transition (EMT) related markers. Relative (**A**) alpha smooth muscle actin (*α-SMA*), (**B**) fibronectin (*FN*) and (**C**) vimentin (*VIM*) expression evaluated by Real-time PCR in BE 63/3 cells treated or untreated with Everolimus (EVE) (5 and 100 nM) or TGF-β (20 ng/mL); expression values were normalized to glyceraldehyde-3-phosphate dehydrogenase (GAPDH). Mean ± S.D. (error bars) of three separate experiments performed in triplicate. * $p < 0.05$, ** $p < 0.01$ vs. control (CTR). (**D**) Histogram represents transepithelial resistance as percentage change with respect to control cells. * $p < 0.05$ vs. CTR.

2.2. Transcriptomic Analysis Revealed That High Dosage of EVE Up-Regulated Genes Involved in Collagen Synthesis and Metabolism

Gene expression profiling evaluated by transcriptomic analysis revealed that in vitro treatment of BE63/3 cells with 100 nM EVE for 24 h deregulated 147 probe sets (corresponding to 125 genes): 60/147 probe sets (47 genes) resulted up-regulated while 87/147 probe sets (corresponding to 78 genes) were down-regulated ($\geq$1.5-fold change) in EVE-treated cells compared with control (CTR) (Table 1). According to enrichment analysis, selected genes belonged to 44 pathways (Table 2) and 5 of them were involved in collagen synthesis/metabolism and regulation of stress fiber assembly. Interestingly, connective tissue growth factor (*CTGF*) was a representative gene in all these pro-fibrotic pathways.

Instead, low dosage EVE (5 nM) was able to change the expression level of only 33 probe sets (24 genes): 25/33 probe sets (20 genes) were hyper-expressed and 4 probe sets (4 genes) down-regulated after treatment (Table 3). None of the selected pathways was associated with the pro-fibrotic cellular machinery (Table 4).

Principal component analysis (PCA) and volcano plot showed the degree of separation of untreated versus treated cells at both EVE dosages (Figure 2).

Table 1. List of the differentially expressed probe sets after treatment with 100 nM EVE.

Probe ID	Fold Change	Regulation	Symbol	Entrez Gene ID	Definition
4760626	2.275	Up	MMP12	4321	matrix metallopeptidase 12 (macrophage elastase), mRNA.
4780209	2.218	Up	MMP12	4321	matrix metallopeptidase 12 (macrophage elastase) mRNA.
670041	1.925	Up	AKAP12	9590	A kinase (PRKA) anchor protein (gravin) 12, transcript variant 2, mRNA.
6770746	1.903	Up	LOC728715	728715	similar to hCG38149 (LOC728715), mRNA.
4640086	1.814	Up	FOXQ1	94234	forkhead box Q1, mRNA.
2810246	1.808	Up	LBH	81606	limb bud and heart development homolog (mouse) (LBH), mRNA.
6330270	1.804	Up	GPC4	2239	glypican 4, mRNA.
6620201	1.789	Up	KLHL24	54800	kelch-like 24 (Drosophila), mRNA.
5690687	1.783	Up	CTGF	1490	connective tissue growth factor, mRNA.
5420577	1.775	Up	CLCA4	22802	chloride channel, calcium activated, family member 4, mRNA.
2640292	1.769	Up	CTGF	1490	connective tissue growth factor, mRNA.
1070477	1.753	Up	ALDH1A1	216	aldehyde dehydrogenase 1 family, member A1, mRNA.
3130301	1.729	Up	PIM1	5292	pim-1 oncogene, mRNA.
6620008	1.705	up	KAL1	3730	Kallmann syndrome 1 sequence, mRNA.
4040576	1.704	up	IL6	3569	interleukin 6 (interferon, beta 2), mRNA.
1820315	1.677	up	C4orf26	152816	chromosome 4 open reading frame 26 (C4orf26), mRNA.
1990142	1.671	up	C20orf114	92747	chromosome 20 open reading frame 114 (C20orf114), mRNA.
1940647	1.668	up	HBP1	26959	HMG-box transcription factor 1, mRNA.
2640324	1.665	up	SLC46A3	283537	solute carrier family 46, member 3, mRNA.
3800241	1.651	up	CDH6	1004	cadherin 6, type 2, K-cadherin (fetal kidney), mRNA.
6110736	1.646	up	IRS2	8660	insulin receptor substrate 2, mRNA.
4610056	1.641	up	FLRT2	23768	fibronectin leucine rich transmembrane protein 2, mRNA.
6420687	1.638	up	PLUNC	51297	palate, lung and nasal epithelium carcinoma associated, transcript variant 2, mRNA.
6420465	1.625	up	GABARAPL1	23710	GABA(A) receptor-associated protein like 1, mRNA.
4780128	1.625	up	ATF3	467	activating transcription factor 3, transcript variant 4, mRNA.
160242	1.622	up	C13orf15	28984	chromosome 13 open reading frame 15 (C13orf15), mRNA.
2650709	1.620	up	CDH11	1009	cadherin 11, type 2, OB-cadherin (osteoblast), mRNA.
2230767	1.615	up	LOC387825	387825	misc_RNA (LOC387825), miscRNA.
6860228	1.610	up	C5orf41	153222	chromosome 5 open reading frame 41 (C5orf41), mRNA.
6510754	1.609	up	ALDH1A1	216	aldehyde dehydrogenase 1 family, member A1, mRNA.
1980255	1.605	up	RNF39	80352	ring finger protein 39, transcript variant 2, mRNA.
6840491	1.604	up	C5orf41	153222	chromosome 5 open reading frame 41 (C5orf41), mRNA.
4280228	1.595	up	IVNS1ABP	10625	influenza virus NS1A binding protein, mRNA.
5080021	1.593	up	BIRC3	330	baculoviral IAP repeat-containing 3, transcript variant 1, mRNA.
6400131	1.589	up	CYP24A1	1591	cytochrome P450, family 24, subfamily A, polypeptide 1, nuclear gene encoding mitochondrial protein, mRNA.
7160239	1.580	up	FOSB	2354	FBJ murine osteosarcoma viral oncogene homolog B, mRNA.
380689	1.578	up	TSC22D1	8848	TSC22 domain family, member 1, transcript variant 1, mRNA.
3060095	1.574	up	COL12A1	1303	collagen, type XII, alpha 1, transcript variant short, mRNA.
1410209	1.571	up	SGK1	6446	serum/glucocorticoid regulated kinase 1, transcript variant 1, mRNA.
2190553	1.556	up	FZD6	8323	frizzled homolog 6 (Drosophila), mRNA.
4570075	1.544	up	KIAA1641	57730	KIAA1641, transcript variant 7, mRNA.
5090626	1.540	up	FAP	2191	fibroblast activation protein, alpha, mRNA.
6620538	1.540	up	UBL3	5412	ubiquitin-like 3, mRNA.

Table 1. *Cont.*

Probe ID	Fold Change	Regulation	Symbol	Entrez Gene ID	Definition
5960398	1.537	up	NT5E	4907	5′-nucleotidase, ecto (CD73), mRNA.
5570731	1.533	up	C8orf4	56892	chromosome 8 open reading frame 4 (C8orf4), mRNA.
830639	1.531	up	LOC653778	653778	similar to solute carrier family 25, member 37 (LOC653778), mRNA.
3290187	1.529	up	PCMTD1	115294	protein-L-isoaspartate (D-aspartate) O-methyltransferase domain containing 1 (PCMTD1), mRNA.
3440670	1.517	up	LOC402251	402251	similar to eukaryotic translation elongation factor 1 alpha 2 (LOC402251), mRNA.
630315	1.514	up	DHRS9	10170	dehydrogenase/reductase (SDR family) member 9, transcript variant 1, mRNA.
1410161	1.513	up	KLHL5	51088	kelch-like 5 (Drosophila), transcript variant 3, mRNA.
4150575	1.513	up	LETMD1	25875	LETM1 domain containing 1, transcript variant 2, mRNA.
7210497	1.513	up	NUAK1	9891	NUAK family, SNF1-like kinase, 1, mRNA.
1240440	1.511	up	TXNIP	10628	thioredoxin interacting protein, mRNA.
4760747	1.509	up	TPST1	8460	tyrosylprotein sulfotransferase 1, mRNA.
2360220	1.508	up	MATR3	9782	matrin 3, transcript variant 1, mRNA.
3800431	1.508	up	RCOR3	55758	REST corepressor 3, mRNA.
4390450	1.504	up	SGK	6446	serum/glucocorticoid regulated kinase, mRNA.
2450465	1.503	up	CYBRD1	79901	cytochrome b reductase 1, mRNA.
6110053	1.501	up	ZNF32	7580	zinc finger protein 32, transcript variant 2, mRNA.
4570398	1.501	up	F2R	2149	coagulation factor II (thrombin) receptor, mRNA.
3800050	−1.503	down	ADCY3	109	adenylate cyclase 3, mRNA.
5900008	−1.504	down	KLK11	11012	kallikrein-related peptidase 11, transcript variant 2, mRNA.
5080605	−1.504	down	SNRPA1	6627	small nuclear ribonucleoprotein polypeptide A′, mRNA.
4560541	−1.521	down	MLKL	197259	mixed lineage kinase domain-like, mRNA.
520682	−1.523	down	CPA4	51200	carboxypeptidase A4, mRNA.
4010296	−1.527	down	RNASE1	6035	ribonuclease, RNase A family, 1 (pancreatic), transcript variant 1, mRNA.
6350161	−1.530	down	LCP1	3936	lymphocyte cytosolic protein 1 (L-plastin), mRNA.
4730605	−1.532	down	AURKA	6790	aurora kinase A, transcript variant 5, mRNA.
6840075	−1.532	down	NP	4860	nucleoside phosphorylase, mRNA.
6770187	−1.533	down	SPRR2A	6700	small proline-rich protein 2A, mRNA.
870131	−1.533	down	HSPA5	3309	heat shock 70 kDa protein 5 (glucose-regulated protein, 78 kDa), mRNA.
1570193	−1.535	down	ARHGDIB	397	Rho GDP dissociation inhibitor (GDI) beta, mRNA.
2450167	−1.537	down	RPL29	6159	ribosomal protein L29, mRNA.
7510709	−1.540	down	CEP55	55165	centrosomal protein 55 kDa, mRNA.
2350465	−1.544	down	RPL29	6159	ribosomal protein L29, mRNA.
160097	−1.546	down	MELK	9833	maternal embryonic leucine zipper kinase, mRNA.
3930703	−1.547	down	WDR4	10785	WD repeat domain 4, transcript variant 2, mRNA.
1170066	−1.554	down	SULT2B1	6820	sulfotransferase family, cytosolic, 2B, member 1, transcript variant 1, mRNA.
2070520	−1.556	down	CDCA7	83879	cell division cycle associated 7, transcript variant 1, mRNA.
6550048	−1.559	down	DHCR7	1717	7-dehydrocholesterol reductase, mRNA.
5310634	−1.566	down	FASN	2194	fatty acid synthase, mRNA.
6560494	−1.566	down	ARTN	9048	artemin, transcript variant 2, mRNA.
5860348	−1.568	down	SC4MOL	6307	sterol-C4-methyl oxidase-like, transcript variant 2, mRNA.
5270112	−1.570	down	HMGCS1	3157	3-hydroxy-3-methylglutaryl-Coenzyme A synthase 1 (soluble), transcript variant 2, mRNA.
5690274	−1.571	down	MCM6	4175	minichromosome maintenance complex component 6, mRNA.

Table 1. *Cont.*

Probe ID	Fold Change	Regulation	Symbol	Entrez Gene ID	Definition
940487	−1.573	down	FUT3	2525	fucosyltransferase 3 (galactoside 3(4)-L-fucosyltransferase, Lewis blood group), transcript variant 4, mRNA.
5810154	−1.580	down	ALOX15B	247	arachidonate 15-lipoxygenase, type B, transcript variant b, mRNA.
870546	−1.581	down	MAD2L1	4085	MAD2 mitotic arrest deficient-like 1 (yeast), mRNA.
6020139	−1.588	down	KLK7	5650	kallikrein-related peptidase 7, transcript variant 1, mRNA.
4250156	−1.589	down	LBP	10682	emopamil binding protein (sterol isomerase), mRNA.
10341	−1.599	down	SHMT2	6472	serine hydroxymethyltransferase 2 (mitochondrial), nuclear gene encoding mitochondrial protein, mRNA.
5360678	−1.602	down	DHCR7	1717	7-dehydrocholesterol reductase, transcript variant 1, mRNA.
6580059	−1.610	down	UCP2	7351	uncoupling protein 2 (mitochondrial, proton carrier), nuclear gene encoding mitochondrial protein, mRNA.
5090278	−1.610	down	GPX2	2877	glutathione peroxidase 2 (gastrointestinal), mRNA.
3940673	−1.617	down	LOC728285	728285	similar to keratin associated protein 2-4 (LOC728285), mRNA.
2650564	−1.623	down	RARRES3	5920	retinoic acid receptor responder (tazarotene induced) 3, mRNA.
360367	−1.625	down	PCDH7	5099	protocadherin 7, transcript variant a, mRNA.
7560364	−1.635	down	LOC729779	729779	misc_RNA (LOC729779), miscRNA.
780528	−1.635	down	CKS2	1164	CDC28 protein kinase regulatory subunit 2, mRNA.
5960224	−1.636	down	PTTG3P	26255	pituitary tumor-transforming 3 (pseudogene), non-coding RNA.
4730196	−1.653	down	TK1	7083	thymidine kinase 1, soluble, mRNA.
1510296	−1.656	down	ASNS	440	asparagine synthetase, transcript variant 1, mRNA.
1190142	−1.657	down	EMILIN2	84034	elastin microfibril interfacer 2, mRNA.
1170170	−1.662	down	STC2	8614	stanniocalcin 2, mRNA.
2140128	−1.670	down	SCD	6319	stearoyl-CoA desaturase (delta-9-desaturase), mRNA.
5360070	−1.674	down	CCNB2	9133	cyclin B2, mRNA.
3990619	−1.675	down	TOP2A	7153	topoisomerase (DNA) II alpha 170 kDa, mRNA.
3780047	−1.679	down	GBP6	163351	guanylate binding protein family, member 6, mRNA.
2000148	−1.683	down	IFIT1	3434	interferon-induced protein with tetratricopeptide repeats 1, transcript variant 2, mRNA.
2070494	−1.700	down	PRC1	9055	protein regulator of cytokinesis 1, transcript variant 2, mRNA.
10414	−1.704	down	PTTG1	9232	pituitary tumor-transforming 1, mRNA.
2940110	−1.720	down	UHRF1	29128	ubiquitin-like with PHD and ring finger domains 1, transcript variant 1, mRNA.
1510291	−1.733	down	PTTG1	9232	pituitary tumor-transforming 1, mRNA.
1780446	−1.739	down	PCK2	5106	phosphoenolpyruvate carboxykinase 2 (mitochondrial), nuclear gene encoding mitochondrial protein, transcript variant 1, mRNA.
1660521	−1.745	down	SPRR2D	6703	small proline-rich protein 2D, mRNA.
730689	−1.763	down	LOC652595	652595	similar to U2 small nuclear ribonucleoprotein A (U2 snRNP-A) (LOC652595), mRNA.
5090754	−1.766	down	KIAA0101	9768	KIAA0101, transcript variant 1, mRNA.
5080139	−1.789	down	PRSS3	5646	protease, serine, 3 (mesotrypsin), mRNA.
3800452	−1.805	down	EMP3	2014	epithelial membrane protein 3, mRNA.
1230047	−1.810	down	CBS	875	cystathionine-beta-synthase, mRNA.
6370615	−1.858	down	TGM1	7051	transglutaminase 1 (K polypeptide epidermal type I, protein-glutamine-gamma-glutamyltransferase), mRNA.
5310471	−1.894	down	UBE2C	11065	ubiquitin-conjugating enzyme E2C, transcript variant 6, mRNA.
7380719	−1.897	down	IGFBP6	3489	insulin-like growth factor binding protein 6, mRNA.

Table 1. *Cont.*

Probe ID	Fold Change	Regulation	Symbol	Entrez Gene ID	Definition
940327	−1.907	down	KLK13	26085	kallikrein-related peptidase 13, mRNA.
520195	−1.914	down	TMEM79	84283	transmembrane protein 79, mRNA.
4040398	−1.954	down	MAL	4118	mal, T-cell differentiation protein, transcript variant d, mRNA.
1990630	−1.979	down	TRIB3	57761	tribbles homolog 3 (Drosophila), mRNA.
430446	−1.996	down	KRT81	3887	keratin 81, mRNA.
4260368	−2.022	down	UBE2C	11065	ubiquitin-conjugating enzyme E2C, transcript variant 3, mRNA.
290767	−2.038	down	KRTDAP	388533	keratinocyte differentiation-associated protein, mRNA.
6520139	−2.046	down	FGFR3	2261	fibroblast growth factor receptor 3 (achondroplasia, thanatophoric dwarfism), transcript variant 2, mRNA.
620102	−2.046	down	MALL	7851	mal, T-cell differentiation protein-like, mRNA.
5870653	−2.050	down	LOC651397	651397	misc_RNA (LOC651397), miscRNA.
4050398	−2.071	down	KLK12	43849	kallikrein-related peptidase 12, transcript variant 1, mRNA.
7330753	−2.102	down	ACAT2	39	acetyl-Coenzyme A acetyltransferase 2, mRNA.
4900458	−2.147	down	KRT14	3861	keratin 14 (epidermolysis bullosa simplex, Dowling-Meara, Koebner), mRNA.
540546	−2.283	down	KRT4	3851	keratin 4, mRNA.
1500010	−2.322	down	CDC20	991	cell division cycle 20 homolog (*S. cerevisiae*), mRNA.
6550356	−2.430	down	SPRR2C	6702	small proline-rich protein 2C (pseudogene), non-coding RNA.
4850674	−2.452	down	PSAT1	29968	phosphoserine aminotransferase 1, transcript variant 2, mRNA.
5890400	−2.577	down	SPRR2E	6704	small proline-rich protein 2E, mRNA.
240086	−2.608	down	PHGDH	26227	phosphoglycerate dehydrogenase, mRNA.
7650441	−2.696	down	FGFBP1	9982	fibroblast growth factor binding protein 1, mRNA.
5810546	−2.894	down	SPRR2E	6704	small proline-rich protein 2E, mRNA.
7330184	−2.933	down	SPRR1A	6698	small proline-rich protein 1A, mRNA.
2230035	−2.936	down	KRT13	3860	keratin 13, transcript variant 2, mRNA.
4610131	−3.284	down	SPRR3	6707	small proline-rich protein 3, transcript variant 1, mRNA.

In red up-regulated and in green down-regulated genes in BE63/3 cells treated with 100 nM EVE compared to CTR.

Table 2. List of pathways differentially regulated after 100 nM EVE.

Pathways	Adj. *p* Value	Associated Genes
Epidermis development	1.24×10^{-6}	ALOX15B, CTGF, FOXQ1, FZD6, KLK7, KRT14, RNASE1, SPRR1A, SPRR2A, SPRR2D, SPRR2E, SPRR3, TGM1, TMEM79, TXNIP
Keratinization	5.22×10^{-6}	SPRR1A, SPRR2A, SPRR2D, SPRR2E, SPRR3, TGM1, TMEM79
Negative regulation of cell division	2.58×10^{-5}	CDC20, FGFR3, MAD1L1, PTTG1, PTTG3P, RGCC, TXNIP, UBE2C
Negative regulation of mitotic nuclear division	2.81×10^{-5}	CDC20, FGFR3, MAD1L1, PTTG1, PTTG3P, RGCC, UBE2C
Keratinocyte differentiation	3.05×10^{-5}	ALOX15B, SPRR1A, SPRR2A, SPRR2D, SPRR2E, SPRR3, TGM1, TMEM79, TXNIP
L-serine metabolic process	3.54×10^{-5}	CBS, PHGDH, PSAT1, SHMT2
Epidermal cell differentiation	9.21×10^{-5}	ALOX15B, RNASE1, SPRR1A, SPRR2A, SPRR2D, SPRR2E, SPRR3, TGM1, TMEM79, TXNIP
L-serine biosynthetic process	9.75×10^{-5}	PHGDH, PSAT1, SHMT2

Table 2. *Cont.*

Pathways	Adj. *p* Value	Associated Genes
Negative regulation of nuclear division	1.10×10^{-4}	CDC20, FGFR3, MAD2L1, PTTG1, PTTG3P, RGCC, UBE2C
Skin development	1.82×10^{-4}	ALOX15B, FOXQ1, FZD6, SPRR1A, SPRR2A, SPRR2D, SPRR2E, SPRR3, TGM1, TMEM79, TXNIP
Peptide cross-linking	2.05×10^{-4}	SPRR1A, SPRR2A, SPRR2D, SPRR2E, SPRR3, TGM1
Serine family amino acid biosynthetic process	3.55×10^{-4}	CBS, PHGDH, PSAT1, SHMT2
Regulation of collagen metabolic process	5.84×10^{-4}	CTGF, F2R, FAP, IL6, RGCC
Regulation of multicellular organismal metabolic process	6.51×10^{-4}	CTGF, F2R, FAP, IL6, RGCC
Steroid biosynthesis	6.77×10^{-4}	CYP24A1, DHCR7, EBP, MSMO1
Chromosome separation	0.00192	CDC20, MAD2L1, PTTG1, PTTG3P, TOP2A, UBE2C
Negative regulation of mitotic sister chromatid separation	0.00199	CDC20, MAD2L1, PTTG1, PTTG3P, UBE2C
Collagen metabolic process	0.00200	COL12A1, CTGF, F2R, FAP, IL6, MMP12, RGCC
Negative regulation of mitotic sister chromatid segregation	0.00231	CDC20, MAD2L1, PTTG1, PTTG3P, UBE2C
Multicellular organismal macromolecule metabolic process	0.00248	COL12A1, CTGF, F2R, FAP, IL6, MMP12, RGCC
Negative regulation of sister chromatid segregation	0.00267	CDC20, MAD2L1, PTTG1, PTTG3P, UBE2C
Negative regulation of chromosome segregation	0.00267	CDC20, MAD2L1, PTTG1, PTTG3P, UBE2C
Regulation of nuclear division	0.00302	AURKA, CDC20, FGFR3, MAD2L1, PTTG1, PTTG3P, RGCC, UBE2C
Multicellular organismal metabolic process	0.00456	COL12A1, CTGF, F2R, FAP, IL6, MMP12, RGCC
Regulation of collagen biosynthetic process	0.00457	CTGF, F2R, IL6, RGCC
Mitotic sister chromatid separation	0.00664	CDC20, MAD2L1, PTTG1, PTTG3P, UBE2C
Regulation of mitotic sister chromatid segregation	0.00834	CDC20, MAD2L1, PTTG1, PTTG3P, UBE2C
Sister chromatid segregation	0.00851	CDC20, CEP55, MAD2L1, PTTG1, PTTG3P, TOP2A, UBE2C
Glycine, serine and threonine metabolism	0.00873	CBS, PHGDH, PSAT1, SHMT2
Collagen biosynthetic process	0.00873	CTGF, F2R, IL6, RGCC
Oocyte meiosis	0.01153	ADCY3, AURKA, CCNB2, CDC20, MAD2L1, PTTG1
Regulation of sister chromatid segregation	0.01277	CDC20, MAD2L1, PTTG1, PTTG3P, UBE2C
Negative regulation of chromosome organization	0.01396	ARTN, CDC20, MAD2L1, PTTG1, PTTG3P, UBE2C
PERK-mediated unfolded protein response	0.01404	ASNS, ATF3, HSPA5
Regulation of stress fiber assembly	0.01630	CTGF, RGCC, RNASE1
FoxO signaling pathway	0.01634	CCNB2, GABARAPL1, IL6, IRS2, PCK2, SGK1
Anaphase-promoting complex-dependent proteasomal ubiquitin-dependent protein catabolic process	0.01664	AURKA, CDC20, MAD2L1, PTTG1, UBE2C
Alpha-amino acid biosynthetic process	0.01664	ASNS, CBS, PHGDH, PSAT1, SHMT2
Positive regulation of collagen biosynthetic process	0.02234	CTGF, F2R, RGCC
Regulation of systemic arterial blood pressure by circulatory renin-angiotensin	0.02412	CPA4, F2R, MMP12
Positive regulation of multicellular organismal metabolic process	0.02412	CTGF, F2R, RGCC
Secondary alcohol biosynthetic process	0.02578	DHCR7, EBP, HMGCS1, MSMO1
Regulation of chromosome segregation	0.02590	CDC20, MAD2L1, PTTG1, PTTG3P, UBE2C
Negative regulation of proteasomal ubiquitin-dependent protein catabolic process	0.03145	CDC20, MAD2L1, UBE2C

In red up-regulated and in green down-regulated genes in BE63/3 cells treated with 100 nM EVE compared to CTR.

Table 3. List of probe sets differentially expressed after treatment with 5 nM EVE.

Probe ID	Fold Change	Regulation	Symbol	Entrez Gene ID	Definition
2230035	7.508	up	KRT13	3860	keratin 13, transcript variant 2, mRNA.
6510754	3.841	up	ALDH1A1	216	aldehyde dehydrogenase 1 family, member A1, mRNA.
1070477	3.395	up	ALDH1A1	216	aldehyde dehydrogenase 1 family, member A1, mRNA.
540546	2.749	up	KRT4	3851	keratin 4, mRNA.
1990142	2.644	up	C20orf114	92747	chromosome 20 open reading frame 114, mRNA.
5900368	2.385	up	MSMB	4477	microseminoprotein, beta-, transcript variant PSP94, mRNA.
4610131	2.358	up	SPRR3	6707	small proline-rich protein 3, transcript variant 1, mRNA.
3190110	2.194	up	MSMB	4477	microseminoprotein, beta-, transcript variant PSP94, mRNA.
630315	2.151	up	DHRS9	10170	dehydrogenase/reductase (SDR family) member 9, transcript variant 1, mRNA.
5420577	2.149	up	CLCA4	22802	chloride channel, calcium activated, family member 4, mRNA.
5560369	2.107	up	ALDH3A1	218	aldehyde dehydrogenase 3 family, memberA1, mRNA.
4150598	1.990	up	MSMB	4477	microseminoprotein, beta-, transcript variant PSP57, mRNA.
1820414	1.897	up	ATP12A	479	ATPase, H$^+$/K$^+$ transporting, nongastric, alpha polypeptide, mRNA.
3520709	1.888	up	ADH7	131	alcohol dehydrogenase 7 (class IV), mu or sigma polypeptide, mRNA.
7160468	1.807	up	DHRS9	10170	dehydrogenase/reductase (SDR family) member 9, transcript variant 1, mRNA.
5310646	1.795	up	AKR1B10	57016	aldo-keto reductase family 1, member B10 (aldose reductase), mRNA.
4250092	1.749	up	C10orf99	387695	chromosome 10 open reading frame 99, mRNA.
110372	1.748	up	CSTA	1475	cystatin A (stefin A), mRNA.
3710671	1.712	up	KRT15	3866	keratin 15, mRNA.
1770603	1.705	up	TCN1	6947	transcobalamin I (vitamin B12 binding protein, R binder family), mRNA.
6100537	1.655	up	FAM3D	131177	family with sequence similarity 3, member D, mRNA.
4540400	1.623	up	CYP4B1	1580	cytochrome P450, family 4, subfamily B, polypeptide 1, transcript variant 2, mRNA.
2900050	1.611	up	GSTA1	2938	glutathione S-transferase alpha 1, mRNA.
1510170	1.565	up	NLRP2	55655	NLR family, pyrin domain containing 2, mRNA.
5820400	1.526	up	CYP4B1	1580	cytochrome P450, family 4, subfamily B, polypeptide 1, mRNA.
130561	1.525	up	GSTA4	2941	glutathione S-transferase A4, mRNA.
3850246	1.513	up	HOPX	84525	HOP homeobox, transcript variant 3, mRNA.
7200612	−1.522	down	LOC730417	730417	hypothetical protein LOC730417, mRNA.
1510296	−1.556	down	ASNS	440	asparagine synthetase, transcript variant 1, mRNA.
3290390	−1.563	down	LOC729841	729841	misc_RNA, miscRNA.
7380193	−1.574	down	ARPC3	10094	actin related protein 2/3 complex, subunit 3, 21 kDa, mRNA.
130717	−1.610	down	ARPC1B	10095	actin related protein 2/3 complex, subunit 1B, 41 kDa, mRNA.
430446	−1.689	down	KRT81	3887	keratin 81, mRNA.

In red up-regulated and in green down-regulated genes in BE63/3 cells treated with 5 nM EVE compared to CTR.

Table 4. List of pathways differentially regulated after treatment with 5 nM EVE.

PATHWAYS	Adj. *p* Value	Associated Genes Found
Retinol metabolism	8.58×10^{-5}	ADH7, ALDH1A1, DHRS9
Metabolism of xenobiotics by cytochrome P450	1.48×10^{-5}	ADH7, ALDH3A1, GSTA1, GSTA4
Drug metabolism	1.37×10^{-5}	ADH7, ALDH3A1, GSTA1, GSTA4
Retinoid metabolic process	1.41×10^{-5}	ADH7, AKR1B10, ALDH1A1, DHRS9
Chemical carcinogenesis	1.96×10^{-5}	ADH7, ALDH3A1, GSTA1, GSTA4
Cellular aldehyde metabolic process	2.60×10^{-5}	ADH7, AKR1B10, ALDH1A1, ALDH3A1
Primary alcohol metabolic process	3.30×10^{-6}	ADH7, AKR1B10, ALDH1A1, DHRS9
Retinol metabolic process	1.99×10^{-5}	ADH7, ALDH1A1, DHRS9

In red up-regulated genes in BE63/3 cells treated with 5 nM EVE compared to CTR.

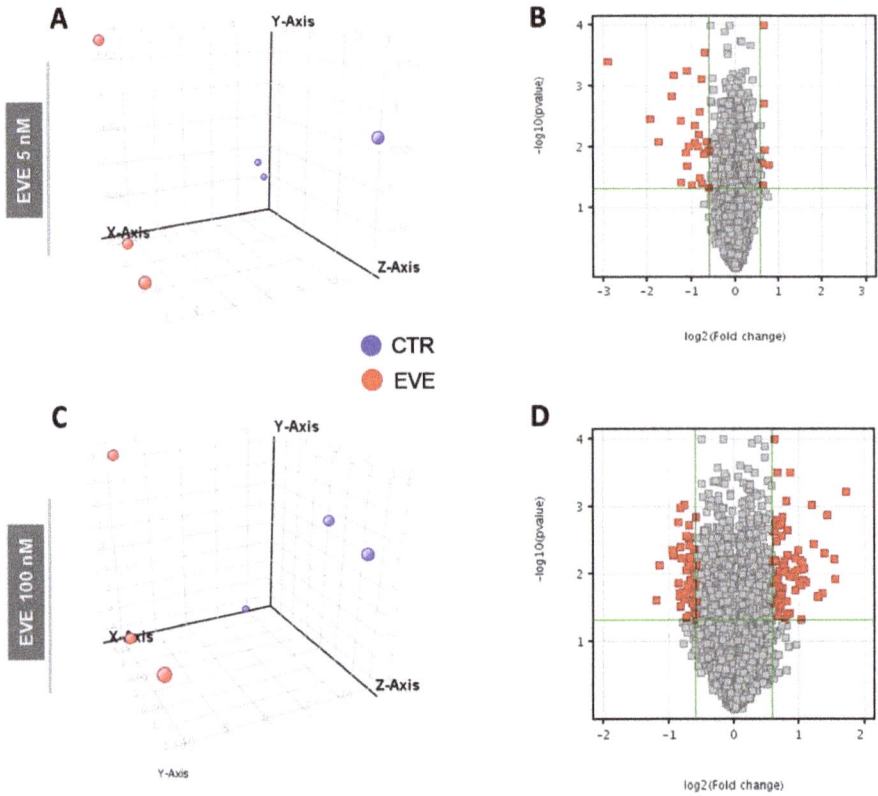

Figure 2. Principal Component Analysis (PCA) and Volcano Plot discriminating BE63/3 CTR from EVE treated cells. PCA plots were built using the expression level of all differentially expressed genes obtained from mRNA expression profiling after treatment with (**A**) 5 nM and (**C**) 100 nM EVE. Volcano Plot based on fold change (Log2) and p value (−Log10) of all genes identified in BE63/3 after treatment with (**B**) 5 nM and (**D**) 100 nM EVE. In both graphs red circles indicate the genes that showed statistically significant change.

2.3. MiRNome Analysis Identified Specific MicroRNAs Deregulated by EVE

To gain insights into the mechanism leading to EMT induced by EVE and to discover possible regulatory miRNAs of this effect, we performed a miRNome analysis by miRNA Complete Labeling and Hybridization kit. Statistical analysis identified three miRNAs up-regulated after high dosage (100 nM) (Table 5) and four after treatment with EVE at low dosage (5 nM) (Table 6). Among these, miR-8485 was the most up-regulated miRNA (more than 4-fold changes in both treatments).

Table 5. List of microRNAs differentially regulated after treatment with 100 nM EVE.

Systematic Name	Regulation	Fold Change
hsa-miR-8485	up	5.372
hsa-miR-937-5p	up	1.787
hsa-miR-5194	up	1.694

Table 6. List of microRNAs differentially regulated after treatment with 5 nM EVE.

Systematic Name	Regulation	Fold Change
hsa-miR-8485	up	9.183
hsa-miR-4730	up	2.900
hsa-miR-5194	up	2.732
hsa-miR-6716-3p	up	2.561

By matching mRNA and miRNA expression data, we found that 31 genes were specific target of the three identified miRNAs (Table 7).

Table 7. miRNA/mRNA pairs matched on the basis of mRNA and miRNA profiling results.

Cell Treatments	miRNA	Fold Change	mRNA Target	Gene Name
EVE 5 nM	miR-8485	9.183	CYP4B1	cytochrome P450, family 4, subfamily B, polypeptide 1
	miR-5194	2.732	ARPC3	actin related protein 2/3 complex, subunit 3, 21 kDa
EVE 100 nM	miR-8485	5.372	CYP24A1	cytochrome P450, family 24, subfamily A, polypeptide 1
			KAL1	Kallmann syndrome 1 sequence
			UBL3	ubiquitin-like 3
			IRS2	insulin receptor substrate 2
			CTGF	connective tissue growth factor
			LBH	limb bud and heart development
			FLRT2	fibronectin leucine rich transmembrane protein 2
			CDH6	cadherin 6, type 2, K-cadherin (fetal kidney)
			CYBRD1	cytochrome b reductase 1
			LETMD1	LETM1 domain containing 1
			FGFR3	fibroblast growth factor receptor 3
			CPA4	carboxypeptidase A4
			AURKA	aurora kinase A
			CBS	cystathionine-beta-synthase
			MAD2L1	MAD2 mitotic arrest deficient-like 1 (yeast)
			ADCY3	adenylate cyclase 3
			TMEM79	transmembrane protein 79
			IFIT1	interferon-induced protein with tetratricopeptide repeats 1
			PTTG1	pituitary tumor-transforming 1
			PCDH7	protocadherin 7
	miR-937-5p	1.787	CDH6	cadherin 6, type 2, K-cadherin (fetal kidney)
			KIAA0101	KIAA0101
			EMILIN2	elastin microfibril interfacer 2
	miR-5194	1.694	KLHL24	kelch-like family member 24
			FAP	fibroblast activation protein, alpha
			LBH	limb bud and heart development
			PIM1	pim-1 oncogene
			FLRT2	fibronectin leucine rich transmembrane protein 2
			LETMD1	LETM1 domain containing 1
			FGFR3	fibroblast growth factor receptor 3
			KIAA0101	KIAA0101
			RARRES3	retinoic acid receptor responder (tazarotene induced) 3
			ARTN	artemin
			IGFBP6	insulin-like growth factor binding protein 6
			LCP1	lymphocyte cytosolic protein 1 (L-plastin)
			MALL	small integral membrane protein 5
			SCD	LSM14B, SCD6 homolog B (*S. cerevisiae*)
			IFIT1	interferon-induced protein with tetratricopeptide repeats 1

In red up-regulated and in green down-regulated genes in BE63/3 cells treated with EVE (5 or 100 nM) compared to CTR.

2.4. Gene Expression and Protein Analysis for Matrix Metalloproteinase 12 (MMP12) and Connective Tissue Growth Factor (CTGF) Validated High-Throughput Results

In order to validate microarray results, we measured by Real-Time PCR the level of mRNA expression of *MMP12* and *CTGF*. Both transcripts were up-regulated after treatment with 100 nM EVE.

Contrarily 5 nM EVE had no effect (Figure 3A,B). In addition, western blot analysis of *CTGF* confirmed gene expression results at protein level (Figure 3C,D).

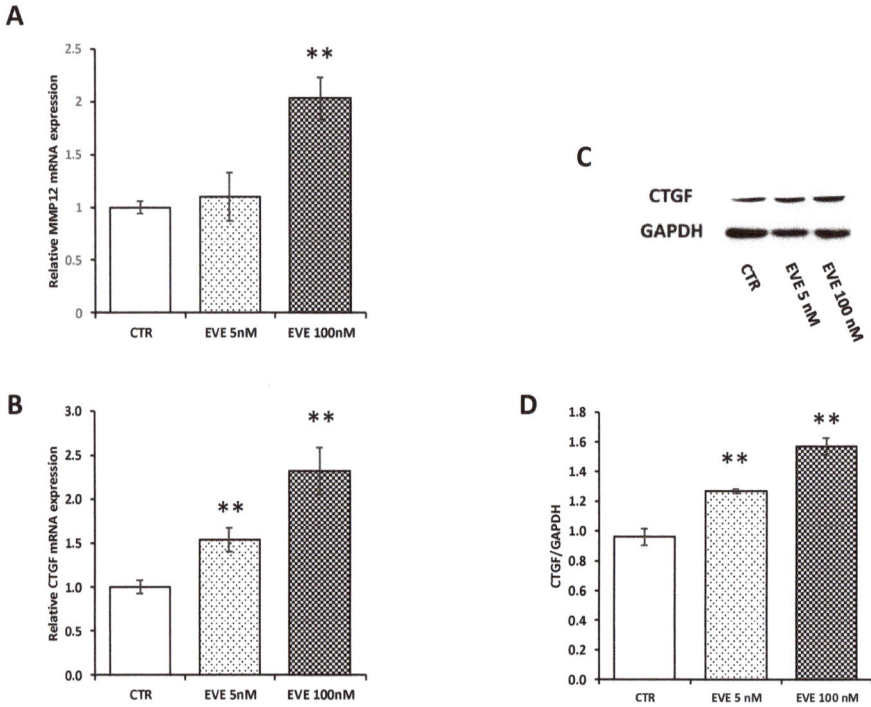

Figure 3. Gene expression of *MMP12* and connective tissue growth factor (*CTGF*). mRNA level of (**A**) *MMP12* and (**B**) *CTGF* evaluated by real-time PCR in BE63/3 cells treated or not with EVE (5 and 100 nM). Data were normalized to GAPDH expression. Mean ± SD (error bars) of two separate experiments performed in triplicate. ** $p < 0.001$, * $p < 0.05$ vs. CTR. (**C**) Representative western blotting experiments for *CTGF*. (**D**) Histogram represents the mean ± SD of *CTGF* protein level. *GAPDH* was included as loading control. ** $p < 0.001$ vs. CTR.

2.5. Validation of Transcriptomic Results in an Additional Primary Cell Line (BE121/3)

To confirm transcriptomic results, we decided to measure the expression level of 8 selected genes (involved in EMT) up-regulated after high dosage EVE in a new primary bronchial epithelial cell line. As showed in Figure 4, results were in line with those obtained in BE63/3 (Figure 4).

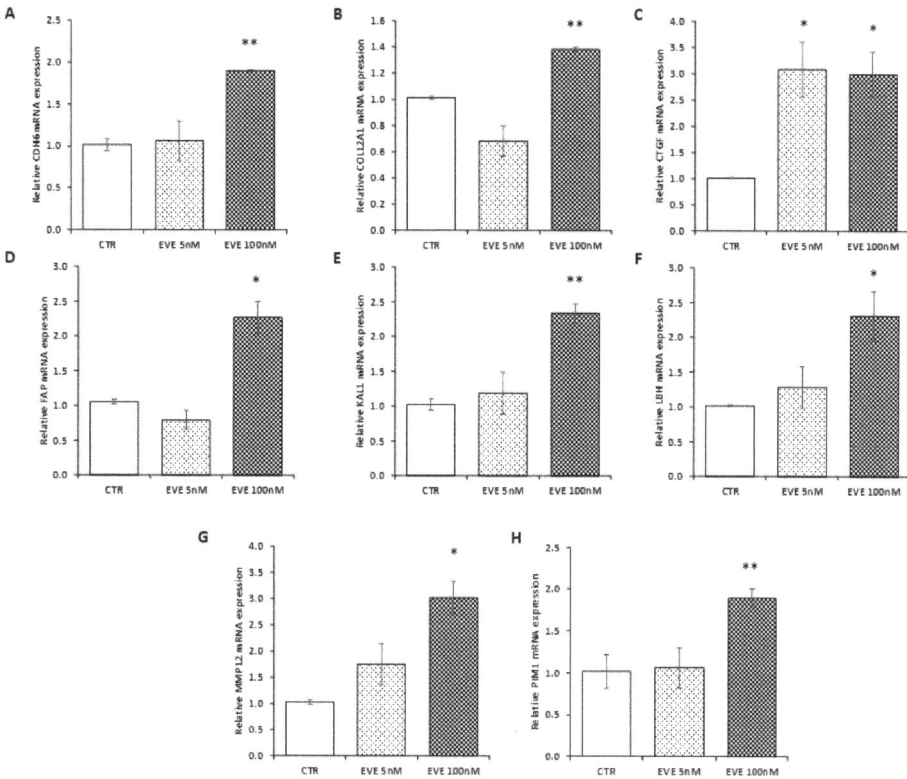

Figure 4. Gene expression in BE121/3. mRNA level of (**A**) *CDH6*, (**B**) *COL12A1*, (**C**) *CTGF*, (**D**) *FAP*, (**E**) *KAL1*, (**F**) *LBH*, (**G**) *MMP12*, (**H**) *PIM1* evaluated by real-time PCR in BE121/3 cells treated or not with EVE (5 and 100 nM). Data were normalized to *GAPDH* expression. Mean ± SD (error bars) of two separate experiments performed in triplicate. ** $p < 0.001$, * $p < 0.05$ vs. CTR.

2.6. High Dosage EVE Up-Regulated CTGF and Collagen1 in Fibroblasts and Hepatic Stellate Cells

To validate the pro-fibrotic effect of high dosage EVE we measured the expression level of collagen1 and CTGF in NIH/3T3 (mouse embryo fibroblast cell line) treated with EVE.

Interestingly, also in fibroblasts high dosage EVE up-regulated the protein levels of collagen1 and CTGF (Figure 5).

Also, in hepatic stellate cells high dosage EVE induced the up-regulation of CTGF and collagen1 (Figure S2).

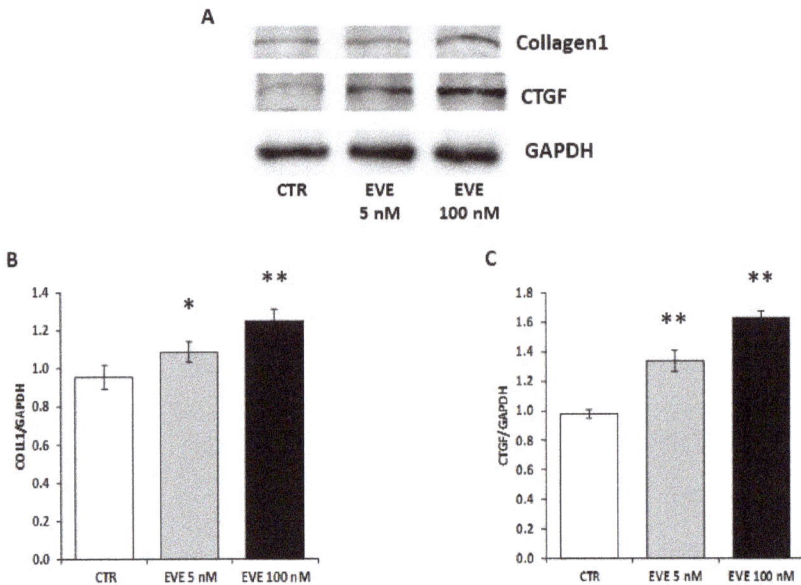

Figure 5. Protein levels of collagen1 and CTGF in NIH/3T3 cells. (**A**) Representative western blotting experiments for collagen1 and CTGF. Histograms represent the mean ± SD of (**B**) collagen1 and (**C**) CTGF protein levels. GAPDH was included as loading control. ** $p < 0.001$, * $p < 0.05$ vs. CTR.

3. Discussion

Pulmonary fibrosis is a potential serious adverse effect following administration of mTOR-I in patients undergoing solid organ transplantation or receiving anti-cancer therapies. It is generally accepted that pulmonary disease is related to mTOR-I therapy, whether the following conditions are present: (1). The symptoms of pulmonary disease occur after initiation of mTOR-I therapy; (2). Infection, other pulmonary diseases or toxicity associated with other drugs are excluded; (3). mTOR-I minimization or discontinuation lead to resolution of the symptoms. In fact, the dose-dependent effect was proved by the observation of this disease particularly in patients receiving high doses of mTOR-I.

Pulmonary manifestations in these patients are numerous and include several clinical/histological phenotypes (e.g., focal pulmonary fibrosis, bronchiolitis obliterans with organizing pneumonia) [8,9,35,36].

This multi-factorial and heterogeneous clinical condition is often responsible for drug discontinuation and it requires long and expensive clinical evaluations and treatments (e.g., antibiotics, corticosteroids, immunosuppressive drugs) [14] with the involvement of a multidisciplinary team of experts (e.g., pulmonologists, infectivologists, nephrologists).

The etiopathogenic mechanism of pulmonary toxicity associated with mTOR-I therapy is not known and several in vivo and in vitro studies have tried to define the underlying mechanisms. It has been proposed a T cell-mediated autoimmune response induced when pulmonary cryptic antigens are exposed, leading to lymphocytic alveolitis and interstitial pneumonitis [15]. Other possible pathogenic mechanisms could be a delayed-type hypersensitivity reaction [9] or pulmonary inflammation as a direct effect of mTOR-I to stimulate cells of the innate immune system to produce proinflammatory cytokines [37,38].

Additionally, Ussavarungsi et al. have reported that sirolimus may induce granulomatous interstitial inflammation and proposed a mechanism of T-cell mediated hypersensitivity reaction triggered by circulating antigens or immune complexes in the lungs [39].

Moreover, several authors have emphasized the pathogenetic role of the EMT of bronchial epithelial cells in these important Everolimus (EVE)-related adverse events [20–23].

To obtain more insights, we decided to employ, for the first time, innovative high throughput technologies, to identify new elements involved in the biological/cellular reprogramming induced by high dose of mTOR-I and leading to fibrosis.

In vitro experiments using classical bio-molecular strategies, confirmed, in primary bronchial epithelial cell lines, our previous results demonstrating the ability of high dosages EVE to induce EMT. In particular, 100 nM EVE caused the up-regulation of EMT-related genes (*α-SMA*, *VIM*, *FN*) and reduced the trans-epithelial resistance to the same levels induced by TGF-β. Then, high doses of this drug significantly changed the expression level of 125 genes (47 up- and 78 down-regulated).

Several of the selected genes were target of miR-8485, the top significant and up-regulated microRNA (miRNA) by EVE 100 nM. Other 2 miRNAs were identified after the same treatment: miR-937-5p and miR-5194. Except for miR-8485, at our knowledge, none of them has been previously associated with fibrosis or supposed to be regulatory of genes implicated in this process. It's unquestionable that further studies are warranted to confirm the involvement of these miRNAs in EVE induced EMT since all identified miRNAs were up-regulated demonstrating their possible role as enhancer of fibrotic machinery. This could be in line with recent findings suggesting that miRNA-mediated down-regulation is not a one-way process and some miRNAs could up-regulate gene expression in specific cell types and conditions with distinct transcripts and proteins [40,41]. It is noteworthy that these miRNAs are up-regulated also after treatment with 5 nM EVE. Many reasons could be responsible of this effect. In particular, the expression of these miRNAs could be regulated by several factors and networks (some of them also unrelated to mTOR-I treatment). Additional studies are needed to clarify the role of miRNA in EVE-mediated pro-fibrotic effect.

Moreover, analyzing the results of the transcriptomic analysis and the hypothetic targets of miR-8485, we found that connective tissue growth factor (*CTGF*), a protein secreted into the extracellular environment where it interacts with distinct cell surface receptors, growth factors and extra-cellular matrix [42,43] was one of the top scored genes. Gene expression by RT-PCR and protein analysis by western blotting confirmed the result obtained by microarray.

It is well known that CTGF modulates the activities of TGF-β or vascular endothelial growth factor (*VEGF*), with consequent pro-fibrotic and angiogenetic effects [44–47]. However, the overexpression of CTGF in fibroblast of mice caused tissue fibrosis in vivo [48] without involving the canonical TGF-β pathway. This is in line with several reports that demonstrated a mTOR-I dose-related induction of CTGF at gene and protein levels in vitro and in vivo [49–52].

Moreover, Xu et al. have demonstrated that rapamycin, an analogue of EVE, exerted a profibrotic effect in lung epithelial cells as well as in lung fibroblasts via up-regulation of CTGF expression and PI3K/AKT pathway [50,51]. Similarly, Mikaelian et al. using a combination of RNAi and pharmacological approaches showed that inhibition of mTOR triggers EMT in mammalian epithelial cells by a mechanism TGF-β independent [53]. In the transplant context it has been described a synergistic fibrotic effect of sirolimus with cyclosporine in kidney also mediated by the up-regulation of CTGF [54,55].

Another interested gene up-regulated by EVE, selected by microarray and validated by RT-PCR, was metalloproteinase 12 (*MMP12*), a member of the zinc-dependent endopeptidases family able to proteolyze all components of the extracellular matrix [56,57] by degrading collagen, other extracellular filaments, cytokines, growth factors and their receptors. *MMP12* has a pivotal role in TGF-β mediated pulmonary fibrosis [58,59].

Interestingly, other identified genes by transcriptomic analysis and target of miR-8485 (Table 7) were Kallmann syndrome-1 gene (*KAL1*, fold change: 1.705), Limb-bud and heart (*LBH*, fold change: 1.808) and insulin receptor substrates 2 (*IRS2*, fold change: 1.646) that resulted up-regulated after 100 nM EVE treatment and Protocadherin 7 (*PCDH7*, fold change: −1.625) down-regulated by similar treatment. All of them have been described in literature as directly or indirectly involved in the EMT.

KAL1, codes for anosmin-1, a cell adhesion protein in extracellular matrix induced by TGF-β [60,61]. *IRS2* expression appears to repress the expression of E-cadherin [62], marker of epithelial cells deregulated during EMT.

LBH is a transcription cofactor with both transcriptional activator and corepressor functions. *LBH* is a direct Wnt/β-catenin target gene and is induced by TGF-β [63,64]. Wnt/β-catenin signaling activation occurs in cells during EMT [65] and treated with mTOR-I.

Protocadherin 7 is an integral membrane protein having a role in cell–cell recognition and adhesion. Down-regulation of *PCDH7* gene was correlated with E-cadherin inhibition [66].

All these findings, although speculatively interesting, need to be validated in vivo. Our study is an hypothesis generating study that should be considered a starting point for bio-molecular study involving transplanted patients or animal models.

Nevertheless, after 21 days in culture, most of the cells were not ciliated and we cannot exclude that differentiation state may have affected the response to EVE (Figure S3).

However, our results suggested that high concentrations of EVE, through the activation of a multi-factorial biological/cellular machinery, may lead to pulmonary fibrosis and underlined potential pathogenetic, diagnostic biomarkers and targets for future pharmacological interventions to introduce in the "day by day" clinical practice. Finally, at a clinical point of view, we confirm that, whenever possible, the dose of EVE should be the minimized in patients with early signs of lung toxicity.

4. Materials and Methods

4.1. Cell Culture Treatment

Primary wild-type bronchial epithelial cells (BE63/3 and BE121/3) were obtained from "Servizio Colture Primarie" of the Italian Cystic Fibrosis Research Foundation (ICFRF) and cultured following the supplier instructions [67]. The protocols to isolate, culture, store, and study bronchial epithelial cells from patients undergoing lung transplant was approved by the Ethical Committee of Gaslini Institute (ethical approval number IGG:192 date of approval: 9/24/2010) under the supervision of the Italian Ministry of Health. Cells were grown on rat tail collagen-coated tissue culture plates in serum-free LHC9/RPMI 1640 medium at 37 °C and 5% CO_2.

After 4–5 passages, cells were seeded on Transwell porous inserts. After 24 h from seeding, the medium was switched to DMEM/F12 supplemented with 2% Ultroser G, 2 mM L-glutammine, 100 U/mL penicillin, 100 µg/mL streptomycin.

Exchange of culture medium is repeated every day on both sides of permeable supports up to 5 days. Then the apical culture medium was removed, and the medium was added only in the basolateral side (air-liquid interface) favoring a differentiation of the epithelium (Figure S3). After 11 days the epithelium was treated with EVE (5 nM and 100 nM) and TGF-β (20 ng/mL), an EMT inducer, for 24 h. "The timing of cell culture for gene expression and western blot experiments (17 days) was based on clear instructions supplied by the "Servizio Colture Primarie" of the ICFRF in order to reach the differentiation of epithelium". Although the in vitro model cannot completely represent the in vivo pharmacokinetic/effect of this drug, we can postulate that 5 nM EVE corresponds to a trough level of approximately 5 ng/mL (drug level frequently reached in the immunosuppressive maintenance therapy of solid organ transplantation), while 100 nM may correspond to very high dosages (trough level more than 50 ng/mL) that patients could reach in anticancer therapy.

NIH/3T3 fibroblasts, purchased from American Type Culture Collection (Manassas, VA, USA) were maintained at 37 °C in DMEM supplemented with 10% FCS, 100 U/mL penicillin, 100 µg/mL streptomycin, and 2 mM L-glutamine. Cells were treated with or without 5 and 100 nM Everolimus for 24 h.

4.2. RNA Extraction and Gene Expression Profiling

Trizol reagent (Invitrogen) was used to extract total RNA and then, yield and purity were checked using a Nanodrop spectrophotometer.

Gene expression data were produced using the HumanHT-12 v3 Expression BeadChip (Release 38, Illumina, San Diego, CA, USA). Five hundred ng total RNA from BE63/3 was used to synthesize biotin-labeled cRNA using the Illumina®TotalPrep™ RNA amplification kit (Applied Biosystems, Foster City, CA, USA). Quality of labelled cRNA was assessed by NanoDrop® ND-100 spectrophotometer and the Agilent 2100 Bioanalyzer. Then, 750 ng biotinylated cRNA was used for hybridization to illumina microarrays that were then scanned with the HiScanSQ.

4.3. Pathway Analysis

The Ingenuity Pathway Analysis software (IPA, Ingenuity System, Redwood City, CA, USA) was used to assess biological relationships among differentially regulated genes. The reference gene selection was performed by own software written in Java program language. The canonical pathways generated by IPA are the most significant for the uploaded data set. Fischer's exact test with false discovery rate (FDR) option was used to calculate the significance of the canonical pathway.

4.4. MicroRNA Expression Profiling

Fluorescently-labeled miRNAs were generated using the miRNA Complete Labeling and Hybridization kit (Agilent Technologies, Santa Clara, CA, USA), with a sample input of 100 ng of total RNA from BE63/3 and hybridized for 20 h at 55 °C on the Agilent 8 × 60 K Human miRNA Microarray slide (Agilent Technologies), based on miRBase database (Release 21.0). Following hybridization, the slides were washed and scanned using the High-Resolution Microarray C Scanner (Agilent Technologies). The image files were processed using the Agilent Feature Extraction software (v10.7.3): the microarray grid was correctly placed; inlier pixels were identified, and outlier pixels were rejected.

4.5. Real-Time PCR

Five hundred ng total RNA from each sample was reverse transcribed into cDNA using the High Capacity cDNA Reverse Transcription Kit (Applied Biosystems). Real-time PCR amplification reactions were performed in duplicate via SYBR Green chemistry on CFX-connect (Bio-Rad, Hercules, CA, USA) and SsoAdvanced™ Universal SYBR® Green Supermix (Bio-Rad). Primers for α-SMA, VIM, FN, MMP12, CTGF, CDH6, COL12A1, FAP, KAL1, LBH, PIM1 and glyceraldehyde-3-phosphate dehydrogenase (GAPDH) were obtained from Qiagen (QuantiTect Primer Assay, Hilden, Germany).

The comparative C_t method ($\Delta\Delta C_t$) was used to quantify gene expression and the relative quantification was calculated as $2^{-\Delta\Delta Ct}$. Melting curve analysis was employed to exclude non-specific amplification products.

4.6. Western Blot

Equal amounts of proteins were resolved in 10% SDS-PAGE and electrotransferred to nitrocellulose membranes. Non-specific binding was blocked for 1 h at room temperature with non-fat milk (5%) in TBST buffer (50 mM Tris-HCl, pH 7.4, 150 mM NaCl, 0.1% Tween 20). Membranes were exposed to primary antibodies directed against GAPDH (Santa Cruz sc-25778), CTGF (NovusBio, Littleton, CO, USA) and collagen1 (ORIGENE TA309096) (overnight at 4 °C) and incubated with a secondary peroxidase-conjugated antibody for 1 h at room temperature. The signal was detected with SuperSignals West Pico Chemiluminescent substrate solution (Pierce) according to the manufacturer's instructions.

4.7. Transepithelial Resistance (TER)

Millicell-ERS ohmmeter with electrodes (Millipore) was used to measure TER (alternating current applied between the electrodes: ± 20 µA and frequency: 12.5 Hz). The resistance of the monolayer multiplied by the effective surface area was used to obtain the electrical resistance of the monolayer (Ω cm^2). Once stable resistances were obtained, different culture media (control, EVE 5 nM, EVE 100 nM, TGF-β 20 ng/mL) were tested. After the addition of test solutions, measurements were taken at 24 h.

4.8. Statistical Analysis

For transcriptomics statistical analyses were carried out by Genespring GX 11.0 software (Agilent Technologies). Gene probe sets were filtered based on the FDR method of Benjamini–Hochberg and fold-change. Only genes that were significantly (adjusted-p value < 0.05 and fold-change > 1.5) modulated were considered for further analysis.

In the miRNome analysis, after normalization (Quantile method), unpaired t-test (p-value cut-off: 0.05 and fold-change cut-off: 2.0, after Benjamini–Hochberg multiple testing correction) was employed to identify most differentially expressed probes.

For the statistical analysis of RT-PCR and western-blot, differences between control and treated cell were compared using Student's t-test. A p-value < 0.05 was set as statistically significant.

Supplementary Materials: Supplementary materials can be found at http://www.mdpi.com/1422-0067/19/4/1250/s1.

Acknowledgments: This study was funded by grants from the Italian Cystic Fibrosis (CF) Research Foundation (FFC#28/2014, Delegazione FFC di Torino, Lodi/Latina, Italy) and from the Fondazione Cariverona 2015. This study was performed in the LURM (Laboratorio Universitario di Ricerca Medica) Research Center, University of Verona, Verona, Italy.

Author Contributions: Gianluigi Zaza, Simona Granata, Valentina Masola conceived and designed the experiments; Simona Granata, Valentina Masola, Gloria Santoro, Nadia Antonucci, Fabio Sallustio, Paola Pontrelli, Matteo Accetturo, Paola Tomei performed the experiments; Gianluigi Zaza, Simona Granata, Antonio Lupo, Pierluigi Carratù analyzed the data; Gianluigi Zaza and Simona Granata wrote the manuscript. All co-authors revised and approved the final manuscript.

Conflicts of Interest: The authors declare no conflict of interest.

References

1. Fasolo, A.; Sessa, C. Targeting mTOR pathways in human malignancies. *Curr. Pharm. Des.* **2012**, *18*, 2766–2777. [CrossRef] [PubMed]
2. Sarbassov, D.D.; Ali, S.M.; Sabatini, D.M. Growing roles for the mTOR pathway. *Curr. Opin. Cell Biol.* **2005**, *17*, 596–603. [CrossRef] [PubMed]
3. Chan, L.; Hartmann, E.; Cibrik, D.; Cooper, M.; Shaw, L.M. Optimal everolimus concentration is associated with risk reduction for acute rejection in de novo renal transplant recipients. *Transplantation* **2010**, *90*, 31–37. [CrossRef] [PubMed]
4. Romagnoli, J.; Citterio, F.; Favi, E.; Salerno, M.P.; Tondolo, V.; Spagnoletti, G.; Renna, R.; Castagneto, M. Higher incidence of acute rejection in renal transplant recipients with low everolimus exposure. *Transplant. Proc.* **2007**, *39*, 1823–1826. [CrossRef] [PubMed]
5. Zaza, G.; Tomei, P.; Ria, P.; Granata, S.; Boschiero, L.; Lupo, A. Systemic and nonrenal adverse effects occurring in renal transplant patients treated with mTOR inhibitors. *Clin. Dev. Immunol.* **2013**, *2013*, 403280. [CrossRef] [PubMed]
6. Kaplan, B.; Qazi, Y.; Wellen, J.R. Strategies for the management of adverse events associated with mTOR inhibitors. *Transplant. Rev.* **2014**, *28*, 126–133. [CrossRef] [PubMed]
7. Engelen, M.A.; Welp, H.A.; Gunia, S.; Amler, S.; Klarner, M.P.; Dell'aquila, A.M.; Stypmann, J. Prospective study of everolimus with calcineurin inhibitor-free immunosuppression after heart transplantation: Results at four years. *Ann. Thorac. Surg.* **2014**, *97*, 888–893. [CrossRef] [PubMed]

8. Champion, L.; Stern, M.; Israël-Biet, D.; Mamzer-Bruneel, M.-F.; Peraldi, M.-N.; Kreis, H.; Porcher, R.; Morelon, E. Sirolimus-associated pneumonitis: 24 cases in renal transplant recipients. *Ann. Intern. Med.* **2006**, *144*, 505–509. [CrossRef] [PubMed]

9. Pham, P.T.; Pham, P.C.; Danovitch, G.M.; Ross, D.J.; Gritsch, H.A.; Kendrick, E.A.; Singer, J.; Shah, T.; Wilkinson, A.H. Sirolimus-associated pulmonary toxicity. *Transplantation* **2004**, *77*, 1215–1220. [CrossRef] [PubMed]

10. Weiner, S.M.; Sellin, L.; Vonend, O.; Schenker, P.; Buchner, N.J.; Flecken, M.; Viebahn, R.; Rump, L.C. Pneumonitis associated with sirolimus: Clinical characteristics, risk factors and outcome—A single-centre experience and review of the literature. *Nephrol. Dial. Transplant.* **2007**, *22*, 3631–3637. [CrossRef] [PubMed]

11. West, M.L. Bronchiolitis obliterans and organizing pneumonia in renal transplant recipients. *Transplantation* **2000**, *69*, 1531. [CrossRef]

12. Feagans, J.; Victor, D.; Moehlen, M.; Florman, S.S.; Regenstein, F.; Balart, L.A.; Joshi, S.; Killackey, M.T.; Slakey, D.P.; Paramesh, A.S. Interstitial pneumonitis in the transplant patient: Consider sirolimus-associated pulmonary toxicity. *J. La. State Med. Soc.* **2009**, *161*, 166–172. [PubMed]

13. Molas-Ferrer, G.; Soy-Muner, D.; Anglada-Martínez, H.; Riu-Viladoms, G.; Estefanell-Tejero, A.; Ribas-Sala, J. Interstitial pneumonitis as an adverse reaction to mTOR inhibitors. *Nefrologia* **2013**, *33*, 297–300. [PubMed]

14. Lopez, P.; Kohler, S.; Dimri, S. Interstitial lung disease associated with mTOR inhibitors in solid organ transplant recipients: Results from a large phase III clinical trial program of everolimus and review of the literature. *J. Transplant.* **2014**, *2014*, 305931. [CrossRef] [PubMed]

15. Morelon, E.; Stern, M.; Israël-Biet, D.; Correas, J.M.; Danel, C.; Mamzer-Bruneel, M.F.; Peraldi, M.N.; Kreis, H. Characteristics of sirolimus-associated interstitial pneumonitis in renal transplant patients. *Transplantation* **2001**, *72*, 787–790. [CrossRef] [PubMed]

16. Hasni, K.; Slusher, J.; Siddiqui, W.; Matsumura, D.; Malek, B.; Heifets, M.; Ahmed, Z. Bronchiolitis obliterans organizing pneumonia in renal transplant patients. *Dial. Transplant.* **2010**, *39*, 449–451. [CrossRef]

17. Errasti, P.; Izquierdo, D.; Martín, P.; Errasti, M.; Slon, F.; Romero, A.; Lavilla, F.J. Pneumonitis associated with mammalian target of rapamycin inhibitors in renal transplant recipients: A single-center experience. *Transplant. Proc.* **2010**, *42*, 3053–3054. [CrossRef] [PubMed]

18. Alexandru, S.; Ortiz, A.; Baldovi, S.; Milicua, J.M.; Ruíz-Escribano, E.; Egido, J.; Plaza, J.J. Severe everolimus-associated pneumonitis in a renal transplant recipient. *Nephrol. Dial. Transplant.* **2008**, *23*, 3353–3355. [CrossRef] [PubMed]

19. Rodríguez-Moreno, A.; Ridao, N.; García-Ledesma, P.; Calvo, N.; Pérez-Flores, I.; Marques, M.; Barrientos, A.; Sánchez-Fructuoso, A.I. Sirolimus and everolimus induced pneumonitis in adult renal allograft recipients: Experience in a center. *Transplant. Proc.* **2009**, *41*, 2163–2165. [CrossRef] [PubMed]

20. Kage, H.; Borok, Z. EMT and interstitial lung disease: A mysterious relationship. *Curr. Opin. Pulm. Med.* **2012**, *18*, 517–523. [CrossRef] [PubMed]

21. Horowitz, J.C.; Thannickal, V.J. Epithelial-mesenchymal interactions in pulmonary fibrosis. *Semin. Respir. Crit. Care Med.* **2006**, *27*, 600–612. [CrossRef] [PubMed]

22. Strieter, R.M.; Mehrad, B. New mechanisms of pulmonary fibrosis. *Chest* **2009**, *136*, 1364–1370. [CrossRef] [PubMed]

23. Felton, V.M.; Inge, L.J.; Willis, B.C.; Bremner, R.M.; Smith, M.A. Immunosuppression-induced bronchial epithelial-mesenchymal transition: A potential contributor to obliterative bronchiolitis. *J. Thorac. Cardiovasc. Surg.* **2011**, *141*, 523–530. [CrossRef] [PubMed]

24. Tomei, P.; Masola, V.; Granata, S.; Bellin, G.; Carratù, P.; Ficial, M.; Ventura, V.A.; Onisto, M.; Resta, O.; Gambaro, G.; et al. Everolimus-induced epithelial to mesenchymal transition (EMT) in bronchial/pulmonary cells: When the dosage does matter in transplantation. *J. Nephrol.* **2016**, *29*, 881–891. [CrossRef] [PubMed]

25. Masola, V.; Carraro, A.; Zaza, G.; Bellin, G.; Montin, U.; Violi, P.; Lupo, A.; Tedeschi, U. Epithelial to mesenchymal transition in the liver field: The double face of Everolimus in vitro. *BMC Gastroenterol.* **2015**, *15*, 118. [CrossRef] [PubMed]

26. Masola, V.; Zaza, G.; Granata, S.; Gambaro, G.; Onisto, M.; Lupo, A. Everolimus-induced epithelial to mesenchymal transition in immortalized human renal proximal tubular epithelial cells: Key role of heparanase. *J. Transl. Med.* **2013**, *11*, 292. [CrossRef] [PubMed]

27. Breuleux, M.; Klopfenstein, M.; Stephan, C.; Doughty, C.A.; Barys, L.; Maira, S.M.; Kwiatkowski, D.; Lane, H.A. Increased AKT S473 phosphorylation after mTORC1 inhibition is rictor dependent and does not predict tumor cell response to PI3 K/mTOR inhibition. *Mol. Cancer Ther.* **2009**, *8*, 742–753. [CrossRef] [PubMed]

28. Wan, X.; Harkavy, B.; Shen, N.; Grohar, P.; Helman, L.J. Rapamycin induces feedback activation of Akt signaling through an IGF-1R-dependent mechanism. *Oncogene* **2007**, *26*, 1932–1940. [CrossRef] [PubMed]

29. Bhaskar, P.T.; Hay, N. The two TORCs and Akt. *Dev. Cell* **2007**, *12*, 487–502. [CrossRef] [PubMed]

30. Carracedo, A.; Ma, L.; Teruya-Feldstein, J.; Rojo, F.; Salmena, L.; Alimonti, A.; Egia, A.; Sasaki, A.T.; Thomas, G.; Kozma, S.C.; et al. Inhibition of mTORC1 leads to MAPK pathway activation through a PI3K-dependent feedback loop in human cancer. *J. Clin. Investig.* **2008**, *118*, 3065–3074. [CrossRef] [PubMed]

31. Witzig, T.E.; Reeder, C.; Han, J.J.; LaPlant, B.; Stenson, M.; Tun, H.W.; Macon, W.; Ansell, S.M.; Habermann, T.M.; Inwards, D.J.; et al. The mTORC1 inhibitor everolimus has antitumor activity in vitro and produces tumor responses in patients with relapsed T-cell lymphoma. *Blood* **2015**, *126*, 328–335. [CrossRef] [PubMed]

32. Guo, H.; Zhong, Y.; Jackson, A.L.; Clark, L.H.; Kilgore, J.; Zhang, L.; Han, J.; Sheng, X.; Gilliam, T.P.; Gehrig, P.A.; et al. Everolimus exhibits anti-tumorigenic activity in obesity-induced ovarian cancer. *Oncotarget* **2016**, *7*, 20338–20356. [CrossRef] [PubMed]

33. Yunokawa, M.; Koizumi, F.; Kitamura, Y.; Katanasaka, Y.; Okamoto, N.; Kodaira, M.; Yonemori, K.; Shimizu, C.; Ando, M.; Masutomi, K.; et al. Efficacy of everolimus, a novel mTOR inhibitor, against basal-like triple-negative breast cancer cells. *Cancer Sci.* **2012**, *103*, 1665–1671. [CrossRef] [PubMed]

34. Browne, A.J.; Kubasch, M.L.; Göbel, A.; Hadji, P.; Chen, D.; Rauner, M.; Stölzel, F.; Hofbauer, L.C.; Rachner, T.D. Concurrent antitumor and bone-protective effects of everolimus in osteotropic breast cancer. *Breast Cancer Res.* **2017**, *19*, 92. [CrossRef] [PubMed]

35. Vandewiele, B.; Vandecasteele, S.J.; Vanwalleghem, L.; De Vriese, A.S. Diffuse alveolar hemorrhage induced by everolimus. *Chest* **2010**, *137*, 456–459. [CrossRef] [PubMed]

36. Vlahakis, N.E.; Rickman, O.B.; Morgenthaler, T. Sirolimus-associated diffuse alveolar hemorrhage. *Mayo Clin. Proc.* **2004**, *79*, 541–545. [CrossRef] [PubMed]

37. Cravedi, P.; Ruggenenti, P.; Remuzzi, G. Sirolimus for calcineurin inhibitors in organ transplantation: Contra. *Kidney Int.* **2010**, *78*, 1068–1074. [CrossRef] [PubMed]

38. Schmitz, F.; Heit, A.; Dreher, S.; Eisenächer, K.; Mages, J.; Haas, T.; Krug, A.; Janssen, K.P.; Kirschning, C.J.; Wagner, H. Mammalian target of rapamycin (mTOR) orchestrates the defense program of innate immune cells. *Eur. J. Immunol.* **2008**, *38*, 2981–2992. [CrossRef] [PubMed]

39. Ussavarungsi, K.; Elsanjak, A.; Laski, M.; Raj, R.; Nugent, K. Sirolimus induced granulomatous interstitial pneumonitis. *Respir. Med. Case Rep.* **2012**, *7*, 8–11. [CrossRef] [PubMed]

40. Vasudevan, S.; Steitz, J.A. AU-rich-element-mediated upregulation of translation by FXR1 and Argonaute 2. *Cell* **2007**, *128*, 1105–1118. [CrossRef] [PubMed]

41. Valinezhad Orang, A.; Safaralizadeh, R.; Kazemzadeh-Bavili, M. Mechanisms of miRNA-mediated gene regulation from common downregulation to mRNA-specific upregulation. *Int. J. Genom.* **2014**, *2014*, 970607. [CrossRef] [PubMed]

42. Duncan, M.R.; Frazier, K.S.; Abramson, S.; Williams, S.; Klapper, H.; Huang, X.; Grotendorst, G.R. Connective tissue growth factor mediates transforming growth factor β-induced collagen synthesis: Down-regulation by cAMP. *FASEB J.* **1999**, *13*, 1774–1786. [CrossRef] [PubMed]

43. Cicha, I.; Goppelt-Struebe, M. Connective tissue growth factor: Context-dependent functions and mechanisms of regulation. *Biofactors* **2009**, *35*, 200–208. [CrossRef] [PubMed]

44. Pan, L.H.; Yamauchi, K.; Uzuki, M.; Nakanishi, T.; Takigawa, M.; Inoue, H.; Sawai, T. Type II alveolar epithelial cells and interstitial fibroblasts express connective tissue growth factor in IPF. *Eur. Respir. J.* **2001**, *17*, 1220–1227. [CrossRef] [PubMed]

45. Lipson, K.E.; Wong, C.; Teng, Y.; Spong, S. CTGF is a central mediator of tissue remodeling and fibrosis and its inhibition can reverse the process of fibrosis. *Fibrogenes. Tissue Repair* **2012**, *5*, S24. [CrossRef] [PubMed]

46. Grotendorst, G.R. Connective tissue growth factor: A mediator of TGF-beta action on fibroblasts. *Cytokine Growth Factor Rev.* **1997**, *8*, 171–179. [CrossRef]

47. Nishida, T.; Kondo, S.; Maeda, A.; Kubota, S.; Lyons, K.M.; Takigawa, M. CCN family 2/connective tissue growth factor (CCN2/CTGF) regulates the expression of Vegf through Hif-1α expression in a chondrocytic cell line, HCS-2/8, under hypoxic condition. *Bone* **2009**, *44*, 24–31. [CrossRef] [PubMed]

48. Sonnylal, S.; Shi-Wen, X.; Leoni, P.; Naff, K.; van Pelt, C.S.; Nakamura, H.; Leask, A.; Abraham, D.; Bou-Gharios, G.; de Crombrugghe, B. Selective expression of connective tissue growth factor in fibroblasts in vivo promotes systemic tissue fibrosis. *Arthritis Rheumatol.* **2010**, *62*, 1523–1532. [CrossRef] [PubMed]

49. Balah, A.; Ezzate, O. The mTOR inhibitor rapamycin induces CTGF and TIMP-1 expression in rat kidney: Implication of TGF-β/SMAD signaling cascade. *Eur. J. Pharm. Med. Res.* **2017**, *4*, 49–56.

50. Xu, X.; Dai, H.; Geng, J.; Wan, X.; Huang, X.; Li, F.; Jiang, D.; Wang, C. Rapamycin increases CCN2 expression of lung fibroblasts via phosphoinositide 3-kinase. *Lab. Investig.* **2015**, *95*, 846–859. [CrossRef] [PubMed]

51. Xu, X.; Wan, X.; Geng, J.; Li, F.; Yang, T.; Dai, H. Rapamycin regulates connective tissue growth factor expression of lung epithelial cells via phosphoinositide 3-kinase. *Exp. Biol. Med.* **2013**, *238*, 1082–1094. [CrossRef] [PubMed]

52. Finckenberg, P.; Inkinen, K.; Ahonen, J.; Merasto, S.; Louhelainen, M.; Vapaatalo, H.; Müller, D.; Ganten, D.; Luft, F.; Mervaala, E. Angiotensin II induces connective tissue growth factor gene expression via calcineurin-dependent pathways. *Am. J. Pathol.* **2003**, *163*, 355–366. [CrossRef]

53. Mikaelian, I.; Malek, M.; Gadet, R.; Viallet, J.; Garcia, A.; Girard-Gagnepain, A.; Hesling, C.; Gillet, G.; Gonzalo, P.; Rimokh, R.; et al. Genetic and pharmacologic inhibition of mTORC1 promotes EMT by a TGF-β-independent mechanism. *Cancer Res.* **2013**, *73*, 6621–6631. [CrossRef] [PubMed]

54. Shihab, F.S.; Bennett, W.M.; Yi, H.; Andoh, T.F. Effect of cyclosporine and sirolimus on the expression of connective tissue growth factor in rat experimental chronic nephrotoxicity. *Am. J. Nephrol.* **2006**, *26*, 400–407. [CrossRef] [PubMed]

55. O'Connell, S.; Slattery, C.; Ryan, M.P.; McMorrow, T. Sirolimus enhances cyclosporine a-induced cytotoxicity in human renal glomerular mesangial cells. *J. Transplant.* **2012**, *2012*, 980910. [CrossRef] [PubMed]

56. Catania, J.M.; Chen, G.; Parrish, A.R. Role of matrix metalloproteinases in renal pathophysiologies. *Am. J. Physiol. Renal. Physiol.* **2007**, *292*, F905–F911. [CrossRef] [PubMed]

57. Parks, W.C.; Wilson, C.L.; López-Boado, Y.S. Matrix metalloproteinases as modulators of inflammation and innate immunity. *Nat. Rev. Immunol.* **2004**, *4*, 617–629. [CrossRef] [PubMed]

58. Matute-Bello, G.; Wurfel, M.M.; Lee, J.S.; Park, D.R.; Frevert, C.W.; Madtes, D.K.; Shapiro, S.D.; Martin, T.R. Essential role of MMP-12 in Fas-induced lung fibrosis. *Am. J. Respir. Cell Mol. Biol.* **2007**, *37*, 210–221. [CrossRef] [PubMed]

59. Kang, H.R.; Cho, S.J.; Lee, C.G.; Homer, R.J.; Elias, J.A. Transforming growth factor (TGF)-β1 stimulates pulmonary fibrosis and inflammation via a Bax-dependent, Bid-activated pathway that involves matrix metalloproteinase-12. *J. Biol. Chem.* **2007**, *282*, 7723–7732. [CrossRef] [PubMed]

60. Tanaka, Y.; Kanda, M.; Sugimoto, H.; Shimizu, D.; Sueoka, S.; Takami, H.; Ezaka, K.; Hashimoto, R.; Okamura, Y.; Iwata, N.; et al. Translational implication of Kallmann syndrome-1 gene expression in hepatocellular carcinoma. *Int. J. Oncol.* **2015**, *46*, 2546–2554. [CrossRef] [PubMed]

61. Raju, R.; Jian, B.; Hooks, J.J.; Nagineni, C.N. Transforming growth factor-β regulates the expression of anosmin (KAL-1) in human retinal pigment epithelial cells. *Cytokine* **2013**, *61*, 724–727. [CrossRef] [PubMed]

62. Carew, R.M.; Browne, M.B.; Hickey, F.B.; Brazil, D.P. Insulin receptor substrate 2 and FoxO3a signalling are involved in E-cadherin expression and transforming growth factor-β1-induced repression in kidney epithelial cells. *FEBS J.* **2011**, *278*, 3370–3380. [CrossRef] [PubMed]

63. Rieger, M.E.; Sims, A.H.; Coats, E.R.; Clarke, R.B.; Briegel, K.J. The embryonic transcription cofactor LBH is a direct target of the Wnt signaling pathway in epithelial development and in aggressive basal subtype breast cancers. *Mol. Cell Biol.* **2010**, *30*, 4267–4279. [CrossRef] [PubMed]

64. Liu, Q.; Guan, X.; Lv, J.; Li, X.; Wang, Y.; Li, L. Limb-bud and Heart (LBH) functions as a tumor suppressor of nasopharyngeal carcinoma by inducing G1/S cell cycle arrest. *Sci. Rep.* **2015**, *5*, 7626. [CrossRef] [PubMed]

65. Lam, A.P.; Flozak, A.S.; Russell, S.; Wei, J.; Jain, M.; Mutlu, G.M.; Budinger, G.R.; Feghali-Bostwick, C.A.; Varga, J.; Gottardi, C.J. Nuclear β-catenin is increased in systemic sclerosis pulmonary fibrosis and promotes lung fibroblast migration and proliferation. *Am. J. Respir. Cell Mol. Biol.* **2011**, *45*, 915–922. [CrossRef] [PubMed]

66. Chen, H.F.; Ma, R.R.; He, J.Y.; Zhang, H.; Liu, X.L.; Guo, X.Y.; Gao, P. Protocadherin 7 inhibits cell migration and invasion through E-cadherin in gastric cancer. *Tumour Biol.* **2017**, *39*, 1010428317697551. [CrossRef] [PubMed]

67. Galietta, L.J.; Lantero, S.; Gazzolo, A.; Sacco, O.; Romano, L.; Rossi, G.A.; Zegarra-Moran, O. An improved method to obtain highly differentiated monolayers of human bronchial epithelial cells. *In Vitro Cell. Dev. Biol. Anim.* **1998**, *34*, 478–481. [CrossRef] [PubMed]

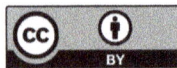

International Journal of
Molecular Sciences

MDPI

Review

Molecular Mechanisms Controlled by mTOR in Male Reproductive System

Bruno P. Moreira [1], Pedro F. Oliveira [1,2,3] and Marco G. Alves [1,*]

[1] Department of Microscopy, Laboratory of Cell Biology, Institute of Biomedical Sciences Abel Salazar (ICBAS) and Unit for Multidisciplinary Research in Biomedicine (UMIB), University of Porto, 4050-313 Porto, Portugal; brunommoreira9@gmail.com (B.P.M.); pfobox@gmail.com (P.F.O.)
[2] i3S-Instituto de Investigação e Inovação em Saúde, University of Porto, 4200-135 Porto, Portugal
[3] Department of Genetics, Faculty of Medicine, University of Porto, 4200-450 Porto, Portugal
*   Correspondence: alvesmarc@gmail.com; Tel.: +351-967245248

Received: 12 March 2019; Accepted: 28 March 2019; Published: 2 April 2019

Abstract: In recent years, the mammalian target of rapamycin (mTOR) has emerged as a master integrator of upstream inputs, such as amino acids, growth factors and insulin availability, energy status and many others. The integration of these signals promotes a response through several downstream effectors that regulate protein synthesis, glucose metabolism and cytoskeleton organization, among others. All these biological processes are essential for male fertility, thus it is not surprising that novel molecular mechanisms controlled by mTOR in the male reproductive tract have been described. Indeed, since the first clinical evidence showed that men taking rapamycin were infertile, several studies have evidenced distinct roles for mTOR in spermatogenesis. However, there is a lack of consensus whether mTOR inhibition, which remains the experimental approach that originates the majority of available data, has a negative or positive impact on male reproductive health. Herein we discuss the latest findings concerning mTOR activity in testes, particularly its role on spermatogonial stem cell (SSC) maintenance and differentiation, as well as in the physiology of Sertoli cells (SCs), responsible for blood–testis barrier maintenance/restructuring and the nutritional support of spermatogenesis. Taken together, these recent advances highlight a crucial role for mTOR in determining the male reproductive potential.

Keywords: mTOR; spermatogenesis; male fertility; Sertoli cells

1. Introduction

Homeostasis, a term coined by Walter Bradford Cannon [1], represents the state of internal conditions of an organism where the equilibrium for optimal functioning is achieved. This equilibrium is constantly being threatened by internal and external stimuli which can compromise key processes including cell growth, proliferation and apoptosis, therefore compromising biological homeostasis. These processes are regulated by several factors including nutrients and hormones, which trigger complex signaling pathways. One of these pathways, involving the mammalian target of rapamycin (mTOR), has emerged in the last decade as a central regulator of biological homeostasis, being associated with protein synthesis, glucose metabolism and cytoskeleton organization among other functions [2,3]. mTOR is a well conserved Ser/Thr protein kinase of approximately 290 kDa, which was originally identified in yeast but is present in all mammalian and non-mammalian cells integrating cellular energy status, thus regulating cellular metabolism [3]. This kinase exists in two functionally and structurally distinct forms depending on the proteins that associate with the core component: The mTOR complex 1 (mTORC1) and the mTOR complex 2 (mTORC2) [4–6]. Interestingly, both complexes present different sensitivities to mTOR inhibitors [7,8]. As a consequence of being so versatile, the study of mTOR has a high degree of complexity.

In recent years, mTOR has been associated with spermatogenesis. Studies have demonstrated that mTOR controls glucose consumption and redox balance in Sertoli cells (SCs), highlighting a direct involvement for this pathway in the nutritional support of spermatogenesis [9]. Furthermore, mTOR is also involved in the maintenance and restructuring of the blood–testis barrier (BTB), a key event in the seminiferous epithelium cycle [10–12].

Notably, mTOR is intimately linked with eukaryotic cell growth and metabolism, regulating these processes according to several environmental inputs [3]. Metabolism is known to be pivotal to spermatogenesis [13] as it is responsible for the formation of spermatozoa and thus is directly associated with the fertility potential of an individual. This is highlighted in the seminiferous tubule epithelium across the different stages that are classified according to the development stage of germ cells and their association with SCs [14]. The somatic SCs have key roles for the success of spermatogenesis as they are responsible for the physical and nutritional support of germ cells. The metabolic cooperation established between Sertoli and germ cells is essential, since germ cells cannot use glucose and rely on SCs production of lactate to satisfy their metabolic needs [15,16]. Adjacent SCs establish the BTB, an immune-privileged environment, where germ cells safely develop from the attack of immune system cells [17]. During spermatogenesis, BTB is reorganized to allow the transport of germ cells to the lumen of the seminiferous tubules, where one of the last steps of spermatogenesis occurs. This complex network of steps and checkpoints is tightly coordinated to ensure that no disruption occurs, which could lead to infertility. In the last decade, several studies were focused on these two steps and how mTOR regulates them, which revealed new clues into the molecular and biochemical mechanisms behind mTOR pathway and male fertility [9–12,18,19]. Herein, we do a follow up concerning the most recent studies focused on mTOR and male reproduction, which revealed new clues in the everlasting puzzle of mTOR as a central regulator of spermatogenesis, and hence male fertility.

2. mTOR Signaling and Cell Physiology: Brief Overview

Life began billions of years ago with the appearance of unicellular organisms [20]. These simple life forms satisfy their metabolic needs according to the availability of nutrients [21]. Fast-forwarding in time, these organisms evolved into pluricellular organisms, which are composed of millions of cells, each one with a specific purpose [22]. These organisms react accordingly to external stimuli, that is, they have the ability to adapt their metabolic needs to the situation [21]. This is only possibly due to the existence of metabolic pathways that can integrate the information and react accordingly. mTOR plays a central role in the signaling network that balances the metabolic signals of growth factors, energy status, oxygen, stress and amino acids, and outputs the correct cascade of events resulting in protein and lipids synthesis or autophagy, accordingly to the stimuli [3].

mTOR can form two functionally and structurally distinct forms, depending on the associated proteins. mTORC1 is formed by mTOR, regulatory associated protein of mTOR (raptor), proline-rich Akt substrate 40 kDa (pras40), DEP (Dishevelled, Egl-10 and Pleckstrin) domain-containing mTOR-interacting protein (deptor), mammalian lethal with sec-13 protein 8 (mLST8) and the Tti1/Tel2 complex (Figure 1) [5,23–27]. Although mTORC2 shares several protein components with mTORC1 including mTOR, deptor, mLST8 and the Tti1/Tel2 complex; it is composed by rapamycin insensitive companion of mTOR (rictor), mammalian stress-activated protein kinase interacting protein (mSIN1) and protein observed with rictor 1 and 2 (protor1/2) (Figure 1) [6,28,29]. Thus, mTORC1 or mTORC2 are formed depending on whether raptor or rictor associate with the core component. Nonetheless, there is still much to be discovered concerning mTOR complex proteins and how they interact with mTOR structure and signaling.

Int. J. Mol. Sci. **2019**, *20*, 1633

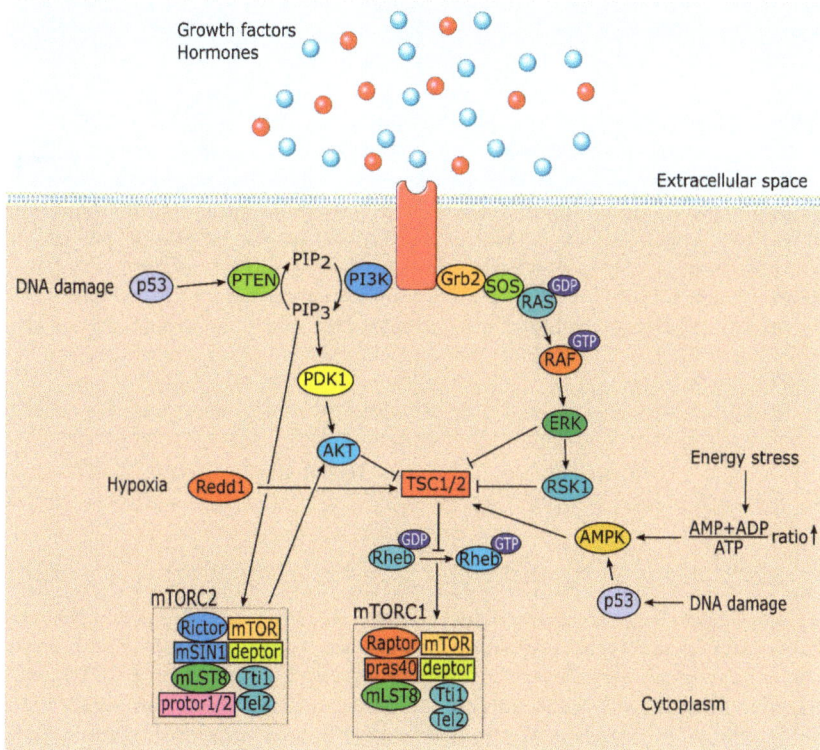

Figure 1. Schematic illustration of rapamycin (mTOR) signaling pathway. mTOR forms two functional complexes, mTORC1 and mTORC2 which are involved in different physiological processes. mTORC1 is regulated by growth factors/hormones, DNA damage, energy status and oxygen levels. mTORC2 is also regulated by growth factors and is involved in AKT phosphorylation. Abbreviations: AKT: protein kinase B; AMPK: AMP-activated protein kinase; deptor: DEP (Dishevelled, Egl-10 and Pleckstrin) domain-containing mTOR-interacting protein; ERK: Extracellular signal regulated kinase; Grb2: Growth factor receptor bound protein 2; mLST8: Mammalian lethal with sec-13 protein 8; mSIN1: Mammalian stress-activated protein kinase interacting protein; p53: Cellular tumor antigen p53; PDK1: 3-phosphoinositide-dependent protein kinase-1; PI3K: Phosphoinositide 3-kinase; pras40: Proline-rich Akt substrate 40 kDa; protor1/2: Protein observed with rictor 1 and 2; PTEN: Phosphatase and tensin homolog; raptor: Regulatory associated protein of mTOR; Redd1: Protein regulated in development and DNA damage response 1; Rheb: Ras homolog enriched in brain GTPase; rictor: rapamycin insensitive companion of mTOR; RSK1: p90 ribosomal S6 kinase 1; SOS: Ras-guanine exchange factor; TSC1/2: Tuberous sclerosis 1/2. → stimulation. ⊣ inhibition.

mTORC1 is considered the rapamycin-sensitive complex [8] while mTORC2 was usually known as the rapamycin-insensitive complex [7]. This concept has changed since mTORC2 assembly was shown to be inhibited by long term rapamycin treatment in some cell types [30]. This probably occurs due to the inability of mTOR bounded to rapamycin to associate with rictor, therefore impairing the formation of new mTORC2 complexes. Thus, as the name easily suggests, mTOR is referred as the mammalian target of rapamycin, a 31-membered macrocyclic natural product produced by several actinomycetes. Interestingly, rapamycin was found in a screening for anti-fungal agents [31]. Besides antifungal properties, rapamycin also has immunosuppressive, antitumoral and lifespan extension properties, which turned this molecule into a desired tool to study cell growth, and lately to be used as a potential tool to fight metabolic diseases [32–34]. Rapamycin inhibits mTORC1 by associating with its intracellular receptor FK506-binding protein 12 (FKBP12) forming a gain of function complex which interacts with the corresponding FKBP12–rapamycin binding domain located in mTOR, inhibiting mTOR activity by occluding substrates from the active site [8].

Tuberous sclerosis complex (TSC1/2), formed by TSC1 and TSC2, a GTPase-activating protein, functions as an upstream regulator of mTORC1, converting the Ras homolog enriched in brain GTPase (Rheb) into its inactive GDP bound state (Figure 1) [35,36]. This conversion blocks Rheb from stimulating mTORC1 kinase activity. mTORC1 kinase activity can be triggered by several stimuli such as: Growth factors via the IRS-PI3K and MAPK/ERK pathways; the energy status of the cell (ATP/AMP ratio) and DNA damage via AMP-activated protein kinase (AMPK) pathway; certain stresses including oxygen levels; and nutrient status via amino acids that function as sensors (Figure 1). Nutrient level detection by mTOR is the least described mechanism, although progress has been made in recent years [37,38]. These inputs, excluding nutrient level detection, exert their action on mTOR through modulation of TSC1/2 activity (Figure 1) [39]. As their name suggests, mutations on TSC1/2 originate tuberous sclerosis, a disease characterized by the development of hamartomas (mostly benign malformations) in multiple organ systems [40]. Stimulation by growth factors (e.g., insulin and IGF-1) activates PI3K and MAPK pathways, which results in the phosphorylation of TSC1/2 by protein kinase B (Akt), by p90 ribosomal S6 kinase 1 (RSK1) and by extracellular signal regulated kinase (ERK) (Figure 1) [41–45]. This phosphorylation inactivates TSC1/2, which results in mTORC1 activation.

mTORC1 is also involved in the response to stress signals such as low energy levels. AMPK, a vital enzyme that functions as an intracellular energy sensor, phosphorylates TSC1/2 in these cases increasing TSC1/2 activity culminating in the reduction of mTORC1 kinase activity (Figure 1) [46]. DNA damage signals are also regulated by mTORC1 activity. In these cases, p53 dependent transcription activates AMPK resulting in mTOR inhibition (Figure 1) [47,48]. Another mechanism involved in the response to stress signals is phosphatase and tensin homolog (PTEN) activation mediated by p53, which downregulates the entire PI3K-Akt-mTORC1 axis culminating in autophagy (Figure 1) [47,49]. TSC1/2 can also be directly activated by protein regulated in development and DNA damage response 1 (Redd1) in hypoxia situations which inhibits mTOR (Figure 1) [50,51].

Concerning mTORC2, less information is known about this complex signaling pathways and its upstream and downstream regulators. Nonetheless, studies have shown mSIN1 is required for mTORC2 assembly and kinase activity [52], which in turn activates Akt (Figure 1), and serum and glucocorticoid-regulated kinase 1 [53,54]. Moreover, under non-stimulated conditions, pleckstrin homology (PH) domain of mSIN1 interacts with mTOR kinase domain to suppress mTORC2 activity. However, upon stimulation by insulin, activated PI3K forms PtdIns(3,4,5)P$_3$, which interacts with PH-mSIN1 to release its inhibition on mTOR kinase domain, leading to mTORC2 activation (Figure 1) [55]. This activation results in phosphorylation of Akt at the hydrophobic motif of Ser^{473} setting in motion a cascade of phosphorylation by other proteins until Akt is fully activated creating a positive feedback loop between Akt and mTORC2 [56]. Interestingly, while TSC1/2 inhibits mTORC1, it can activate and associate with mTORC2 [57]. Another mechanism suggests that mTORC2 associates with ribosomes in a growth factor sensitive manner and these ribosomes are necessary for mTORC2 kinase activity [58]. Furthermore, the rapamycin insensitive complex also modulates the phosphorylation of several members of the protein kinase C (PKC) involved in the regulation of the actin cytoskeleton and cell migration [6,7].

As referred above, mTOR complexes are different per se. Besides structural differences, they also have different sensitivities to rapamycin and different upstream and downstream outputs. mTORC1 integrates signals from several sources, including growth factors, stress signals and amino acids status, and responds accordingly, regulating cell growth by promoting protein and lipids synthesis, ribosomes biogenesis, cell metabolism and ATP production. mTORC1 also has a key role in inhibiting autophagy. Concerning mTORC2, it is involved in cell proliferation, surveillance, metabolism and cytoskeleton organization, mainly through Akt, which phosphorylates downstream targets positively regulating these processes.

3. mTOR and Male Fertility: Evidence from Testis Signaling

mTOR is regarded as the central integrator of several signals, as listed above, regulating metabolism, cellular growth and proliferation. However, little information concerning mTOR and its functions was known just a couple of decades ago. This paradigm has shifted and mTOR has been a target of great scientific interest in recent years. This outburst of information occurred due to the use of mTOR inhibitors in several works with clinical intentions [59–62]. Currently, mTOR inhibitors are still a target of several studies with the aim to be used as pharmacological agents in the treatment of diseases, including cancer and diabetes [63–65]. These studies paved the way to outline mTOR signaling pathway and functions, although there is still much to be done. Thus, most of the information gathered concerning mTOR is due to the use of rapamycin. As mentioned before, rapamycin, also known as sirolimus, is an allosteric inhibitor of mTOR, approved in 1999 by the Food and Drug Administration under the commercial name of ®Rapamune to be used as an immunosuppressant preventing organ rejection in transplants [66]. Although rapamycin fulfilled its purpose, several side effects emerged from its use. Male infertility was one of the most striking side effects described in patients after few years of rapamycin use [67]. Specifically, the most relevant reported effects were low sperm count, decreased motility and decreased sperm vitality as well as negative impact on sexual hormone levels and lower rate of fathered pregnancies when compared with individuals treated with other immunosuppressants (Figure 2) [68–70]. These were the first studies that provided evidence for a negative effect of prolonged rapamycin use on male fertility. Subsequent studies were more focused on the root responsible for the impaired fertility parameters reported and, using mice models, revealed that mTOR inhibitors, particularly rapamycin, induced major histological changes in testicular structure followed by impairment of testicular development and of spermatogenesis (Figure 2) [71,72]. Overall, rapamycin was clearly demonstrated to be capable of inducing testicular toxicity. However, those effects mediated by rapamycin were shown to be reversible. Switching from a rapamycin-based therapy to another immunosuppressant recovered normal fertility parameters and sexual hormone levels, thus restoring the fertility of men previously treated with rapamycin [72,73]. Nevertheless, the mechanisms through which mTOR inhibitors induce infertility remain largely unknown.

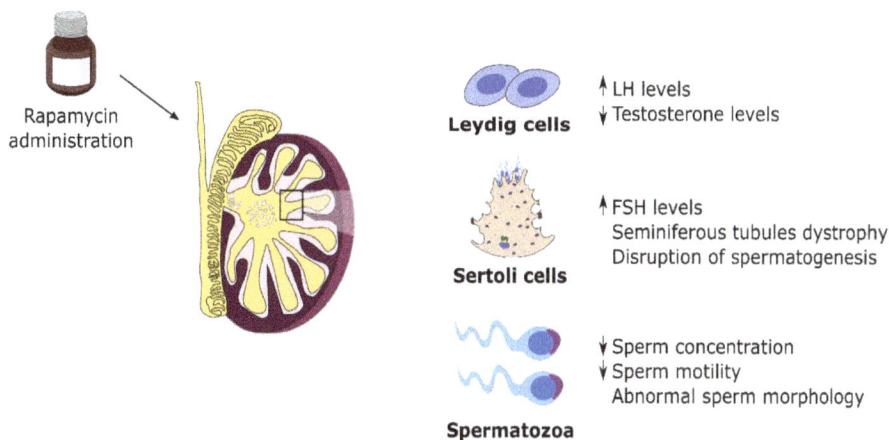

Figure 2. Effects of mTORC1 inhibitor (rapamycin) administration on the testicular function and sperm production. The figure depicts the outcomes of several clinical studies where rapamycin was used as an immunosuppressant which resulted in male infertility. Posterior studies using mice models exposed to rapamycin revealed the deleterious effects of this compound to testicular morphology, gonadotropins and testosterone levels, and overall for spermatogenesis.

In 2010, Hobbs et al., showed that mTOR plays an important role in spermatogonial stem cell (SSC) maintenance [74]. For clarification, in this review, SSCs will be used to define undifferentiated germline cells that can self-renewal. It was shown that mice lacking promyelocytic leukaemia zinc finger (Plzf) ($Plzf^{-/-}$), a transcription factor essential for SSCs maintenance (Figure 3) [75,76], presented aberrant mTORC1 activity which inhibited SSC response to glial cell-derived neurotrophic factor (GNDF), a known growth factor required for SSC self-renewal, through negative feedback. $Plzf^{-/-}$ mice mTORC1 hyperactivity was due to lack of Plzf-mediated Redd1 transcriptional activity which inhibits mTORC1 (Figure 3) [74]. Interestingly, a recent study by Daguia Zambe et al., suggested that Plzf inhibition of mTOR was regulated by micro-RNAs, specifically miR-19b-3p, opening new exciting possibilities to further understand mTOR's role in SSC maintenance [77]. Other study has suggested that conditional knockout of *FOXO* (forkhead box protein O) *1*, *FOXO3* and *FOXO4*, Akt-regulated factors involved in stem-cell renewal [78], within the germ line-specific Vasa-Cre blocks SSCs self-renewal and differentiation [79]. Conditional knockout of *PTEN* also phenocopied FOXOs conditional inactivation phenotype suggesting that PI3K-Akt signaling and Akt inhibition of FOXOs are involved in the homeostasis of SSCs proliferation and differentiation (Figure 3) [79]. Interestingly, similar results were obtained with conditional knockout of *PTEN* in hematopoietic stem cells, a phenotype that could be partially rescued by rapamycin [80]. *PTEN* conditional inactivation should result in mTOR activation which would explain why rapamycin treatment restored hematopoietic stem cells self-renewal ability. Logically, conditional inactivation of PTEN in germ cells should result in Akt-stimulated mTOR activation further corroborating the results described by Hobbs et al., evidencing the role of mTOR in SSCs maintenance and differentiation. Nevertheless, this remains to be confirmed.

p53, the well-recognized tumor suppressor agent, seems to be another agent involved in suppressing mTOR activity to allow for SSC self-renewal. Under genotoxic conditions, p53 induces cell-cycle arrest through inhibition of mTOR [81]. Although many studies were focused on p53 functions under these conditions, mounting evidence has suggested the involvement of p53 in the regulation of stem cell processes under normal physiological conditions [82]. Recently, *p53* knockout mice testes were shown to augment mTORC1 activity during early spermatogonial differentiation which induced exhaustion of the SSC pool, driving them out of the undifferentiated state, indicating that the p53-mTORC1 pathway is also involved in regulating the SSC differentiation process (Figure 3) [83]. Furthermore, recent studies in mice, where germ cell conditional knockouts were created for *TSC1* and *TSC2*, resulted in mTOR aberrant activity which induced spermatogonial differentiation depleting the SSC pool (Figure 3) [84,85]. Both studies reported lower testis weight and a higher percentage of degenerated seminiferous tubules when compared with controls which clearly highlights a role for mTOR in spermatogenesis. Interestingly, in those studies, mTOR activation was shown to be stage-dependent concerning spermatogonial development. Self-renewing stem cells had mTORC1 activity suppressed while progenitors committed to differentiation had mTORC1 activity induced, in both conditional knockout mice models [84,85]. Those findings clearly suggest a role for mTORC1 supervising and deciding stem cells fate.

Glucocorticoid-induced leucine zipper (GILZ), an essential factor for spermatogenesis [86,87], was also demonstrated to be an essential modulator of growth factor signaling in SCCs. Indeed, adult mice knockout for *GILZ* are characterized by SCCs exhaustion and germline degeneration [88]. *GILZ* knockout mice present aberrant mTORC1 activation, which was a downstream effect of aberrant activation of ERK/MAPK pathways (Figure 3) [88]. Treatment of these mice with Torin1, an mTOR inhibitor, rescued SSC depletion. Interestingly, expression of the spermatogonial deubiquitinase probable ubiquitin carboxyl-terminal hydrolase FAF-X (USP9X), an essential factor for a proper spermatogenesis [89], was also downregulated in *GILZ* knockout mice (Figure 3) [88]. Altogether, these data pinpoint exact mechanisms that help to explain how the decisions for the fate of SSCs are chosen. mTORC1 seems to be inhibited by GILZ through USP9X expression. GILZ also modulates mTORC1 through inhibition of upstream signals, including MAPK/ERK pathways which indicates that GILZ operates as an essential rheostat for growth factor signaling. In fact, Wang et al., demonstrated that mTORC1 balance between phosphorylated and inhibited states seems to be a key factor modulating SSCs fate. In that study, Wang and colleagues used an interesting approach to detect phosphorylated protein and phosphorylated sites after stimulation by GDNF, a growth factor required for SSC self-renewal [90,91]. This revealed that SSC proliferation is dependent on the GDNF/ERK modulation since the inhibition of this pathway impaired proliferation [92]. Interestingly, this process was dependent on mTORC1 phosphorylation, specifically in the Ser[863] of mTORC1 component, raptor [92]. In vitro overexpression of this component resulted in an accelerated growth of SSCs while inhibition of raptor by deletion in mouse germline cells resulted in SSC depletion and impaired spermatogenesis. Taken together, these data validated previous studies and further expanded the knowledge on mTORC1 relevance in deciding the fate of SSCs. It seems that a specific raptor phosphorylation is required to decide the future of SSCs, and ERK pathway is involved. Indeed, two recent studies from Serra et al. focused on these issues and gave new insights on mTOR's involvement in the fate of SSCs. Using two different germ cell knockout mice models of *mTOR* and *raptor* component respectively, these studies produced very interesting and surprising results. In the first study, germ cell knockout of *mTOR* core component (not the mTORC1 complex as a whole) resulted in no sperm production due to impairment of spermatogonial differentiation [93]. Interestingly, a small subset of SSCs remained in adult testes, indicating that mTOR is not required for the survival and maintenance of SSCs but rather for their proliferation and differentiation [93]. This phenotype clearly resembles the one reported by Busada et al., where inhibition of mTORC1 by rapamycin lead to impairment of spermatogonial differentiation [94]. This similarity suggests that mTOR effects on spermatogonial differentiation and proliferation are primarily mediated by mTORC1 and not mTORC2. In the second study, germ cell knockout of *raptor*, mTORC1's core component, also resulted in no sperm production. However, interesting differences were observed comparatively to the first study. Spermatogonia from germ cell *raptor* knockout mice entered meiosis but were unable to complete it [95]. Interestingly, adult testes seminiferous tubules only had SCs due to SSC depletion [95]. These results clearly suggest that raptor is essential in the completion of meiosis and for the formation and maintenance of a fully functional pool of SSCs (Figure 3). Furthermore, unlike other studies where mTORC1 hyperactivation resulted in SSC differentiation but not a total depletion, the reported total depletion of the SSC pool could be attributed to inhibition of FOXOs, important factors in self-renewal of SSCs [79]. This could be due to a higher number of mTORC2 complexes being formed in response to the knockout of raptor. One of the well-known functions of mTORC2 is activation of Akt [54] which, as referred to above, is involved in the inhibition of FOXOs [79]. Nevertheless, this hypothesis remains to be fully tested and demonstrated.

Several other studies also showed that mTOR is heavily involved in spermatogenesis [96–98]. For instance, conditional knockout of *Rheb* in male germline resulted in oligoasthenoteratozoospermia and male infertility [96]. The authors could observe multiple defects in meiotic and post-meiotic stages of spermatogenesis, which resulted in an increase of sperm defects and overall severe reduction on epididymal sperm numbers (Figure 3) [96]. In addition, spermatid and spermatocytes production decreased with age while undifferentiated spermatogonia maintained the normal numbers, reflecting a delay in meiotic progression. Interestingly, Hobbs et al. previously observed that Rheb was not required for SSC self-renewal [74], but it seems that Rheb is crucial for meiotic progression. This is also a subject that deserves attention in years to come regarding mTOR and SSCs self-renewal and progression.

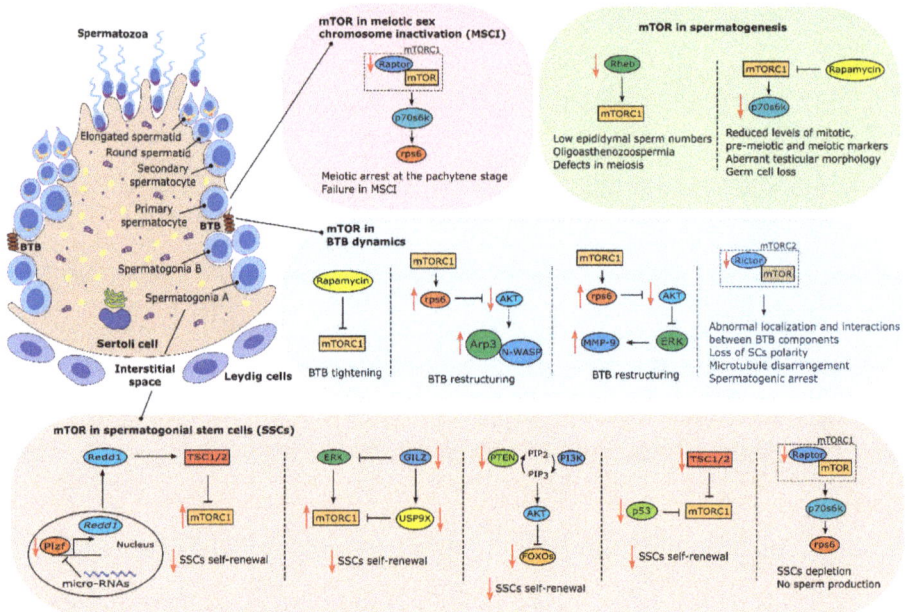

Figure 3. Involvement of mTOR in several processes linked with male fertility. mTORC1 is required for a correct meiotic sex chromosome inactivation. Furthermore, mTOR inhibition of mTORC1 or knockdown of Rheb results in germ cell loss, reduced epididymal sperm numbers, defects in testicular morphology and impairment of meiosis. mTOR is also directly involved in BTB dynamics, with mTORC1 promoting BTB restructuring and mTORC2 promoting BTB maintenance. mTOR inhibition is also required for spermatogonial stem cell (SSC) self-renewal. However, knockdown of raptor impairs spermatogenesis which shows that mTORC1 presence is required for SSCs self-renewal and a balance must occur between mTOR inhibition and mTOR activation for a correct SSCs proliferation and differentiation. Abbreviations: BTB: Blood–testis barrier; AKT: Protein kinase B; ERK: Extracellular signal regulated kinase; FOXOs: Forkhead box proteins; GILZ: Glucocorticoid-induced leucine zipper; MMP-9: Matrix metallopeptidase 9; MSCI: Meiotic sex chromosome inactivation; mTOR: Mammalian target of rapamycin; N-WASP: Neuronal Wiskott–Aldrich syndrome protein; p53: Cellular tumor antigen p53; p70s6k: p70S6 kinase; PI3K: Phosphoinositide 3-kinase; Plzf: Promyelocytic leukaemia zinc finger; PTEN: Phosphatase and tensin homolog; raptor: Regulatory associated protein of mTOR; Redd1: Protein regulated in development and DNA damage response 1; Rheb: Ras homolog enriched in brain GTPase; rictor: Rapamycin insensitive companion of mTOR; rps6: Ribosomal protein S6; TSC1/2: Tuberous sclerosis complex; USP9X: Spermatogonial deubiquitinase probable ubiquitin carboxyl-terminal hydrolase FAF-X. → stimulation. ⊣ inhibition. ↓ downregulation/knockout. ↑ upregulation.

Retinoic acid is a key regulator of spermatogenesis, regulating spermatogonial differentiation via retinoic acid stimulated gene 8 (*STRA8*), a gene expressed in SSCs and preleptotene spermatocytes [99,100]. *STRA8* was shown to be necessary for differentiating spermatogonia to undergo morphological changes that define meiotic prophase and for these cells to exhibit the molecular hallmarks of meiotic chromosome cohesion, synapsis and recombination. In fact, male mice lacking *STRA8* gene function fail to enter meiotic prophase [101]. Sahin et al. confirmed that SSCs and preleptotene spermatocytes express several downstream effectors of the mTOR pathway including mTOR, p-mTOR, p70s6k, phosphorylated p70S6 kinase (p-p70s6k) and phosphorylated eukaryotic initiation factor 4E binding protein 1 (p-4E-BP1) [102]. Interestingly, inhibition of mTOR by rapamycin using cultured seminiferous tubules decreased the levels of p-p70s6k and p-4E-BP1, and also decreased the levels of proliferating cell nuclear antigen (PCNA) and STRA8, markers for proliferation and differentiation, respectively [102]. This clearly indicates that mTOR signaling is involved in the differentiation and stimulation of meiotic initiation of undifferentiated spermatogonia. A further study by this team aimed to unveil mTOR's role in meiotic initiation and progression during post-natal development, specifically in the first wave of spermatogenesis, and in the adult mice. Administration of rapamycin in post-natal testes decreased p-p70s6k and STRA8 levels while STRA8 levels were increased after administration of retinoic acid, as expected [97]. Interestingly, administration of rapamycin during four weeks in adult testes induced germ cell loss, disorganization of testicular morphology and vacuolization (Figure 3). Furthermore, the levels of STRA8 and DNA meiotic recombinase 1 (Dmc1), a meiotic marker, were decreased [97]. Overall, mTOR signaling seems to be involved in the meiotic progression of spermatogenesis during not only the first wave of spermatogenesis but also in adult testes. Recently, Xu et al. demonstrated that mTOR and its downstream effectors are positively correlated with spermatogenesis at different development stages [98]. Interestingly, phosphorylated levels of p70s6k, ribosomal protein S6 (rps6) and 4E-BP1 were also gradually downregulated with age which could explain the decrease in male fertility potential that occurs as a consequence of aging. Inhibition of mTOR signaling by rapamycin decreased sperm number and downregulated protein levels of the phosphorylated effectors of mTOR referred above, except 4E-BP1 [98]. Interestingly, treatment with a PI3K inhibitor downregulated phosphorylated levels of 4E-BP1 suggesting that PI3K regulates this protein [98]. Overall, we can conclude that mTOR plays an important role in spermatogenesis by regulating this process through p70s6k activation.

In recent years, mTOR is also being closely related with meiotic sex chromosome inactivation (MSCI). MSCI is a process that, as the name suggests, occurs during the meiotic phase of spermatogenesis. In short, at the pachytene stage, transcriptional silencing of the male X and Y chromosomes occurs after autosomal chromosomes have completed pairing [103]. X and Y chromosomes are compartmentalized into a peripheral nuclear subdomain known as the XY body. Following meiosis II, when haploid daughter cells are formed, X and Y chromosomes are thought to be repressed until the end of spermatogenesis, although this is still a matter of debate [103]. Thus, MSCI is crucial for male fertility, as mutant mice with defects in MSCI are infertile due to meiotic arrest in prophase I [104,105]. A study by Xiong et al. revealed that raptor is an essential mTORC1 component for a correct MSCI and consequently, a correct meiosis. Mice with conditional knockout of *raptor* were sterile and had increased numbers of SSCs [106]. Furthermore, these mice exhibited meiotic arrest at the pachytene stage and XY chromosome were not repressed which suggests that mTORC1 is crucial for MSCI (Figure 3). MSCI failure was due to lower accumulation of ATR, a key mediator of meiotic silencing which is required to induce repressive epigenetic modifications on sex chromatin in pachytene spermatocytes [106]. On the contrary, another study has shown that meiotic progression and recruitment of silencing factors to sex chromosomes was normal in testes with conditional knockout of mTORC2 component *rictor* [107]. Overall, these reports suggest that rapamycin-mediated defects in meiosis and MSCI are mTORC1-dependent. In another study, inhibition of mTORC1 by chronic rapamycin treatment also caused defects in MSCI resulting in spermatogenic arrest. Recruitment of the essential silencing factor ATR to the chromatin was attenuated in the pachytene stage [108]. Interestingly, the rapamycin inhibitory effect was reversible following treatment withdrawal. Furthermore, rapamycin treated mice had a reduction in pachytene piRNA populations, suggesting that mTOR is involved in the homeostasis of noncoding RNA [108].

4. mTOR Pathway in Sertoli Cells and Male Fertility

SCs are unique polarized mesoepithelial cells responsible for the seminiferous tubules structure [109]. Extending from the basement membrane to the lumen of the seminiferous tubule, these cells are responsible for a panoply of functions, ranging from nourishment and structural support of developing germ cells, integration of upstream signals and secretion of factors and hormones accordingly, phagocytic activity of defective spermatogenic cells and the control of the microenvironment responsible for the correct development of germ cells [13,110]. SCs are known as "nurse cells" as they babysit germ cells through the different stages of spermatogenesis. In fact, SC extensions are in direct and permanent contact with germ cells to ensure their correct development. During spermatogenesis, germ cells must cross the seminiferous tubule to reach the border where spermiation is completed [111]. SC extensions and their microtubular network guide germ cells during this process. Finally, adjacent SCs establish the BTB, an immunoprivileged environment, restricting access by the immune system to these cells which could be identified as foreign agents by the immune system [17]. Structurally, BTB is composed by tight junctions, basal ectoplasmic specializations, desmosomes and gap junctions [17]. Those junctions are connected to the actin cytoskeleton and possess packed actin filament bundles that lie perpendicularly, connecting each adjacent SC through the plasma membrane [112]. These actin filament bundles are also enclosed by the endoplasmic reticulum cisternae giving BTB a remarkable strength and adaptability. In addition, BTB divides the seminiferous epithelium into two functionally and anatomically distinct compartments: 1) The basal compartment where SSCs and preleptotene spermatocytes reside not protected by the BTB; 2) the adluminal compartment where both meiosis and post-meiotic development occurs under the protection of the BTB [113]. Logically, this division suggests that developing spermatocytes must cross the BTB barrier to reach the lumen in order to fulfill the last steps of spermatogenesis. Preleptotene spermatocytes are the only germ cells transported across the BTB in different seminiferous epithelium stages according to the species (rat, mouse or human) [14,114]. Interestingly, this transport takes place quite rapidly, which suggests the existence of a tight and complex network regulating BTB modulation. The existence of a BTB, designated as old, which then gives origin to another BTB, designated as new, was initially pointed as the main mechanism. This was named as the intermediate compartment, in an attempt to explain this phenomenon [115]. This view has changed, and several important studies have shed new light on this topic.

Several studies have suggested that BTB remodeling is regulated, at least in part, by mTORC1 and mTORC2 (specifically by their particular subunits, raptor and rictor, respectively) [10–12,18]. This pathway targets several actin-regulating proteins which causes the cyclic reorganization of the F-actin network, remodeling the BTB. Several studies have shown a stage-specific expression of mTORC1 and mTORC2 subunits and downstream effectors (raptor/p-rps6 and rictor, respectively) during the epithelial cycle with the first being predominantly expressed at later stages of the seminiferous epithelium cycle and virtually undetectable in other stages while rictor expression is predominant in earlier stages of the epithelial cycle [10–12]. This expression pattern suggests that mTORC1 and mTORC2 have opposing effects in BTB dynamics and remodeling. In fact, it was reported that mTORC1 pathway promotes BTB remodeling, which causes this barrier to be "leaky". Several studies using in vitro and in vivo approaches reported that inhibiting mTORC1 signaling, either by knockdown of *rps6* using RNAi or by rapamycin administration, promoted SCs tight junction permeability barrier effectively turning BTB "tighter" (Figure 3) [19]. In those studies, stage-specific p-rps6 expression in the BTB was colocalized with several putative BTB proteins including zonula occludens-1 (ZO-1) (adaptor protein connecting tight junctions to actin cytoskeleton), N-cadherin (a basal endoplasmic specialization protein), Arp3 (a component of the Arp2/3 complex at the BTB involved in changing the conformation of the actin network) and F-actin suggesting an involvement of p-rps6 in BTB remodeling in order to facilitate preleptotene spermatocytes transit to the adluminal compartment [19]. Other studies in mice with a constitutively active quadruple phosphomimetic mutant p-rps6 reported that this turns the BTB "leaky", due to changes in F-actin bundle organization [10,11]. These studies also identified two pathways through which mTORC1 regulates BTB dynamics, the prpS6/Akt/Arp3/N-WASP and the p-rps6/Akt/MMP-9 pathways (Figure 3). In the first, alterations in the organization of actin microfilaments and in actin bundling activity destabilized BTB dynamics and SC tight junction barrier function [10]. These changes were caused by the rps6 mutant which through upregulation of p-rps6 downregulated p-Akt causing an increase in the association of Arp3 and its upstream activator N-WASP (neuronal Wiskott–Aldrich syndrome protein) [10]. This was further confirmed using a knockdown of p-Akt by RNAi in SCs which also led to reorganization of actin filaments and BTB restructuring [10]. In the second pathway, the constitutively active quadruple phosphomimetic mutant p-rps6 disrupted insulin/IGF-1 signaling, which inhibited Akt phosphorylation leading to expression of matrix metallopeptidase 9 (MMP-9), a proprotein involved in the proteolysis of tight junction proteins of the BTB contributing for a "leaky" barrier [11]. This was also confirmed using a MMP-9 inhibitor, which effectively blocked the SCs tight junction disruption induced by the active p-rps6 mutant [11]. Importantly, a knockdown of p-Akt using RNAi in SCs resulted in a phenotype identical to the induced by the active p-rps6 mutant causing the SCs tight junction disruption [11]. These findings were recently confirmed by an in vivo study. Using a constitutively active quadruple phosphomimetic mutant to overexpress p-rps6 in vivo, the authors observed a similar phenotype to the previously reported in vitro findings where p-rps6 caused disruption of the BTB, resulting in impaired spermatogenesis due to loss of spermatid polarity and failure in the transport of germ cells [116]. This was a result of p-rps6 induced changes in the spatiotemporal expression of actin and microtubule-based binding and regulatory proteins [116]. In sum, mTORC1 and rps6 signaling control BTB remodeling through changes in actin and microtubule-based binding regulating the transition of preleptotene spermatocytes to the adluminal compartment, and overall spermatogenesis itself.

Interestingly, a recent study by Xiong et al., has suggested a Rheb–mTORC1-independent pathway controlling cell polarity and cytoskeleton organization [117]. Using the Cre–LoxP system to generate two SC-specific mutants (*raptor* and *Rheb* knockout mice), the authors observed that adult *raptor* KO mice displayed azoospermia and disrupted cytoskeletal organization and cell polarity while adult *Rheb* KO mice had intact seminiferous tubules, sperm present in the epididymis and normal fertility [117]. Furthermore, activity of mTORC1 downstream molecules was similar in both models, which suggests that these phenotypic changes were caused by raptor and not by canonical mTOR signaling. In fact, *raptor* but not *Rheb* KO mice had reduced Rac1 activity [118], a GTPase which is part of the Rho family of GTPases, suggesting that this GTPase is involved in raptor-mediated cytoskeletal organization. Whole-transcriptome sequencing revealed that *cingulin*, a gene coding a protein involved in the mediation of interactions between actin and tight junction proteins, was downregulated and even disappeared in some tubules in adult *raptor* but not *Rheb* KO mice [117]. As Rac1 is a GTPase, downregulation could be caused by an increase in GTPase-activating protein (GAP) or a decrease in guanine-nucleotide exchange factors (GEFs). In this case, lower expression of rho guanine nucleotide exchange factor 4 (ARHGEF4), a GEF, was detected [117]. Taken together, these results indicate novel raptor/non-canonical mTORC1 signaling roles for cytoskeleton and cell polarity regulation through the modulation of Rac1 activity by *cingulin*.

Nonetheless, mTORC1 involvement in BTB remodeling is only half of the puzzle. Mounting evidence has shown that rictor, a key component of mTORC2, is also involved in BTB dynamics. Rictor expression is also stage dependent and it is downregulated in late stages, coinciding with BTB restructuring [12]. Studies have shown that *rictor* knockdown by RNAi turns the BTB "leaky" (Figure 3) [12]. In vivo, similar results were observed, as knockdown of *rictor* perturbed BTB integrity due to changes in F-actin organization and a loss of interaction between actin and proteins involved in BTB constitution (α-catenin and ZO-1) [12]. Furthermore, SC-specific amh–Cre-mediated ablation of rictor in mice caused infertility [18]. Loss of rictor also caused microtubule disarrangement and impaired actin organization, which disrupted SC polarity and overall BTB integrity (Figure 3) [18]. These mice had spermatogenic arrest, which supports that mTORC2 is required for BTB integrity. Interestingly, a recent study by Bai et al. explored the possibilities of a conditional germ-cell specific knockout of *rictor* using Ngn3–Cre technology. In this study, *rictor^cko* mice were also infertile due to impairment of spermatogonial differentiation, which reduced the number of germ cells entering meiosis [107]. Interestingly, loss of rictor also caused apoptosis of early spermatocytes, which further exacerbated this effect. BTB integrity of *rictor^cko* mice was also compromised due to abnormal localization of BTB components, including basal ectoplasmic specialization and gap junction proteins [107]. Microtubular interactions with actin were also abnormal which disrupted cell–cell junctions and Sertoli–germ cell adhesion [107]. Overall, this study further confirmed mTORC2 involvement in BTB maintenance and suggested new roles for mTORC2 in spermatogonial differentiation, indicating that mTORC1 and mTORC2 overlap, at least partially, in some functions but also have fundamental differences in others. Furthermore, mTORC2 signaling in germ cells seems to orchestrate with SCs to form the correct architecture for a successful spermatogenesis.

Another recent topic of study linking SCs with mTOR has been focused on the metabolic control of these cells by this serine/threonine protein kinase complex. As discussed, SCs are known as "nurse cells" due to their role in providing structural and nutritional support to germ cells [119]. Indeed, these cells also have unique metabolic features, exhibiting a 'Warburg-like' metabolism [120] since germ cell metabolism is entirely dependent on SCs that produce the lactate needed as substrate for germ cell development [13]. Thus, the control of SC metabolism is a key event for a correct spermatogenesis. Interestingly, a recent report demonstrated that human SCs exposed to rapamycin had several metabolic parameters altered, including glucose consumption and mitochondrial complex III protein levels [9]. Increased lipid peroxidation and a partial inhibition of mTOR phosphorylation at Ser2448 was also observed in SCs exposed to rapamycin [9]. Finally, phosphorylated 4E-BP1 levels remained unchanged after the treatment which led the authors to speculate regarding a rephosphorylation of this mTOR downstream effector during the treatment [9]. A recent study also reported no alterations in phosphorylated 4E-BP1 levels after rapamycin treatment. However, after exposure to a specific PI3K inhibitor, 4E-BP1 levels were downregulated [98]. These results suggest that rapamycin inhibition of mTOR is not sufficient to inhibit p-4E-BP1, which seems to be directly or indirectly regulated by PI3K. Nevertheless, the mechanisms through which mTOR modulates the SC metabolic state affecting the nutritional support of spermatogenesis remain undisclosed. mTOR dysregulation has also been associated with the establishment of metabolic diseases, including obesity [2]. Several studies have shown the importance of the metabolic state of the individual for a correct spermatogenesis [120–123]. In fact, subfertility or infertility associated with metabolic diseases has been linked with SC metabolic dysregulation. A recent study reported that treatment of human SCs with glucagon-like peptide-1 (GLP-1) increased p-mTOR levels at Ser244 [124]. GLP-1 analogues are used for the treatment of diabetes and obesity [125] promoting weight loss. Thus, that work suggests novel roles for mTOR in the restoration of fertility in individuals with subfertility or infertility induced by metabolic diseases. However, further studies are required to determine how mTOR signaling is involved and if mTOR is dysregulated in subfertility or infertility cases associated with metabolic diseases.

5. Concluding Remarks

Knowledge concerning mTOR indicates that it functions as a master integrator of several upstream signals (amino acids, growth factors, insulin and energy status, among others), which responds accordingly through several downstream effectors. This multiprotein complex is composed by two complexes that share components, mTORC1 and mTORC2, that carry and respond to upstream signals accordingly. Several advancements have been made trying to understand the assembly of mTOR complexes and protein–protein interactions resulting from that process. However, there is still much to be done, particularly in an in vivo environment, which could closely resemble physiological conditions. This subject is of particular importance as only with an exact view of each complex functions and the role of each component in the assembly of mTOR complexes can we fully understand mTOR functions. In fact, there are still components of mTOR complexes whose functions and role are yet to be defined.

mTOR inhibition by rapamycin has been extensively used to better understand mTOR functions. Furthermore, this inhibition has been pursued as a linchpin to better manage several metabolic diseases (including cancer) and the associated co-morbidities. Interestingly, male infertility derived from rapamycin treatment was the first sign of mTOR involvement in male reproduction. Nowadays, several studies have shown different ways of involvement for mTOR in spermatogenesis. However, there is a lack of consensus whether mTOR's role is positive or negative concerning male reproductive health. As discussed above, several studies in upstream and downstream mTOR effectors present both positive and negative effects concerning SSC maintenance, BTB maintenance/restructuring and overall male fertility. Several studies have also shown that mTOR inhibition is crucial for SSC maintenance. However, mounting evidence in models using knockout of upstream mTOR inhibitors shows that mTOR activation leads to exhaustion of the SSC pool. Different modulators of this mTOR inhibition are also starting to be discovered and some of these modulators are even suggested to be regulated by micro-RNAs. Interestingly, studies have started to show that mTOR activation is stage-dependent, being active in progenitors committed to differentiation. In fact, mTOR transition between active and inactive states also seems to be essential to decide the fate of an SSC. Retinoic acid treatment, a key regulator of spermatogenesis which is involved in spermatogonia differentiation, also resulted in mTOR phosphorylation, and thus also suggests an involvement of mTOR in this process. Taken together, these studies reinforce the deciding role of mTOR in controlling the fate of SSCs.

Another topic of interest is mTOR's involvement in BTB dynamics. Studies using in vitro and in vivo approaches have shown different actions of mTORC1 and mTORC2 in this barrier. The first is involved in BTB remodeling while the latter is involved in making the BTB "tighter". As before, mTOR complexes expression is also stage-dependent, which explains the transition of preleptotene spermatocytes to the adluminal compartment due to a timely upregulation of mTORC1 at later stages while mTORC2 is upregulated at earlier stages of the seminiferous epithelial cycle. The attention of the scientific community is now focused on identifying possible signaling pathways regulating this complex interaction and this focus already produced interesting results, identifying the prpS6/Akt/Arp3/N-WASP and the p-rps6/Akt/MMP-9 pathways as mediators of mTORC1 effects in BTB dynamics.

It seems that a small part of the puzzle is starting to be deciphered and that the answer is not what we expected. mTOR seems to be much more than a simple positive or negative trigger in male reproduction. In physiological conditions, it acts as a master integrator of several signals, which is also regulated by different factors in a joint effort to decide the outcome for several processes, including SSC differentiation or self-renewal and BTB restructuring. Nevertheless, these apparently conflicting roles of mTOR in male reproduction underline the complex web of interactions that these multiprotein complexes regulate, which makes the attempt to study them an uphill battle. Trying to translate in vitro results to physiological conditions is also difficult, highlighting the need for more integrative studies that can mimic physiological conditions in order to fully disclose mTOR's function in male reproductive health. There is no doubt that mTOR's involvement in male reproduction deserves special merit and attention in the years to come.

Author Contributions: Conceptualization by M.G.A. and P.F.O.; methodology by M.G.A.; investigation by B.P.M.; writing and draft preparation by B.P.M., supervised by P.F.O. and M.G.A.; revision and editing by P.F.O. and M.G.A.; funding acquisition by P.F.O. and M.G.A.

Funding: This work was supported by the Portuguese Foundation for Science and Technology: B.P.M. (PTDC/MEC-AND/28691/2017); M.G.A. (IFCT2015, PTDC/BIM-MET/4712/2014 and PTDC/MEC-AND/28691/2017); P.F.O. (IFCT2015 and PTDC/BBB-BQB/1368/2014) and Unit for Multidisciplinary Research in Biomedicine (UMIB) (Pest-OE/SAU/UI0215/2014); co-funded by FEDER funds through the POCI/COMPETE 2020.

Acknowledgments: The figures used elements from Servier Medical Art, provided by Servier, licensed under a Creative Commons Attribution 3.0 unported license (available at http://smart.servier.com).

Abbreviations

mTOR	Mammalian target of rapamycin
SSCs	Spermatogonial stem cells
SCs	Sertoli cells
mTORC1	Mammalian target of rapamycin 1
mTORC2	Mammalian target of rapamycin 2
BTB	Blood-testis barrier
raptor	Regulatory associated protein of mTOR
pras40	Proline-rich Akt substrate 40 kDa
deptor	DEP (Dishevelled, Egl-10 and Pleckstrin) domain-containing mTOR-interacting protein
mLST8	Mammalian lethal with sec-13 protein 8
rictor	Rapamycin insensitive companion of mTOR
mSIN1	Mammalian stress-activated protein kinase interacting protein
protor1/2	Protein observed with rictor 1 and 2
FKBP12	FK506-binding protein 12
TSC1/2	Tuberous sclerosis complex
Rheb	Ras homolog enriched in brain GTPase
Akt	Protein kinase B
RSK1	p90 ribosomal S6 kinase 1
ERK	Extracellular signal regulated kinase
PTEN	Phosphatase and tensin homolog
Redd1	Protein regulated in development and DNA damage response 1
PKC	Protein kinase C
Plzf	Promyelocytic leukaemia zinc finger
GNDF	Glial cell-derived neurotrophic factor
FOXOs	Forkhead box proteins
GILZ	Glucocorticoid-induced leucine zipper
USP9X	Spermatogonial deubiquitinase probable ubiquitin carboxyl-terminal hydrolase FAF-X
STRA8	Retinoic acid stimulated gene 8
p-p70s6k	Phosphorylated p70S6 kinase
p-4E-BP1	Phosphorylated eukaryotic initiation factor 4E binding protein 1
PCNA	Proliferating cell nuclear antigen
Dmc1	DNA meiotic recombinase 1
Rps6	Ribosomal protein S6
MSCI	Meiotic sex chromosome inactivation
ZO-1	Zonula occludens-1
N-WASP	Neuronal Wiskott-Aldrich syndrome protein
MMP-9	Matrix metallopeptidase 9
ARHGEF4	Rho guanine nucleotide exchange factor 4
GLP-1	Glucagon-like peptide-1
AMPK	AMP-activated protein kinase

References

1. Cannon, W.B. *Physiological Regulation of Normal States: Some Tentative Postulates Concerning Biological Homeostatics*; éditions Médicales: Paris, France, 1926.
2. Laplante, M.; Sabatini, D.M. Mtor signaling in growth control and disease. *Cell* **2012**, *149*, 274–293. [CrossRef]
3. Saxton, R.A.; Sabatini, D.M. Mtor signaling in growth, metabolism, and disease. *Cell* **2017**, *168*, 960–976. [CrossRef] [PubMed]
4. Kim, D.H.; Sarbassov, D.D.; Ali, S.M.; King, J.E.; Latek, R.R.; Erdjument-Bromage, H.; Tempst, P.; Sabatini, D.M. Mtor interacts with raptor to form a nutrient-sensitive complex that signals to the cell growth machinery. *Cell* **2002**, *110*, 163–175. [CrossRef]

5. Hara, K.; Maruki, Y.; Long, X.; Yoshino, K.; Oshiro, N.; Hidayat, S.; Tokunaga, C.; Avruch, J.; Yonezawa, K. Raptor, a binding partner of target of rapamycin (tor), mediates tor action. *Cell* **2002**, *110*, 177–189. [CrossRef]

6. Sarbassov, D.D.; Ali, S.M.; Kim, D.H.; Guertin, D.A.; Latek, R.R.; Erdjument-Bromage, H.; Tempst, P.; Sabatini, D.M. Rictor, a novel binding partner of mtor, defines a rapamycin-insensitive and raptor-independent pathway that regulates the cytoskeleton. *Curr. Biol.* **2004**, *14*, 1296–1302. [CrossRef] [PubMed]

7. Jacinto, E.; Loewith, R.; Schmidt, A.; Lin, S.; Ruegg, M.A.; Hall, A.; Hall, M.N. Mammalian tor complex 2 controls the actin cytoskeleton and is rapamycin insensitive. *Nat. Cell Biol.* **2004**, *6*, 1122–1128. [CrossRef]

8. Sabatini, D.M.; Erdjument-Bromage, H.; Lui, M.; Tempst, P.; Snyder, S.H. Raft1: A mammalian protein that binds to fkbp12 in a rapamycin-dependent fashion and is homologous to yeast tors. *Cell* **1994**, *78*, 35–43. [CrossRef]

9. Jesus, T.T.; Oliveira, P.F.; Silva, J.; Barros, A.; Ferreira, R.; Sousa, M.; Cheng, C.Y.; Silva, B.M.; Alves, M.G. Mammalian target of rapamycin controls glucose consumption and redox balance in human sertoli cells. *Fertil. Steril.* **2016**, *105*, 825–833. [CrossRef]

10. Mok, K.W.; Chen, H.; Lee, W.M.; Cheng, C.Y. Rps6 regulates blood-testis barrier dynamics through arp3-mediated actin microfilament organization in rat sertoli cells. An in vitro study. *Endocrinology* **2015**, *156*, 1900–1913. [CrossRef]

11. Mok, K.W.; Mruk, D.D.; Cheng, C.Y. Rps6 regulates blood-testis barrier dynamics through akt-mediated effects on mmp-9. *J. Cell Sci.* **2014**, *127*, 4870–4882. [CrossRef] [PubMed]

12. Mok, K.W.; Mruk, D.D.; Lee, W.M.; Cheng, C.Y. Rictor/mtorc2 regulates blood-testis barrier dynamics via its effects on gap junction communications and actin filament network. *FASEB J. Off. Publ. Fed. Am. Soc. Exp. Biol.* **2013**, *27*, 1137–1152. [CrossRef]

13. Rato, L.; Alves, M.G.; Socorro, S.; Duarte, A.I.; Cavaco, J.E.; Oliveira, P.F. Metabolic regulation is important for spermatogenesis. *Nat. Rev. Urol.* **2012**, *9*, 330–338. [CrossRef]

14. Hess, R.A.; Renato de Franca, L. Spermatogenesis and cycle of the seminiferous epithelium. *Adv. Exp. Med. Biol.* **2008**, *636*, 1–15.

15. Rato, L.; Meneses, M.J.; Silva, B.M.; Sousa, M.; Alves, M.G.; Oliveira, P.F. New insights on hormones and factors that modulate sertoli cell metabolism. *Histol. Histopathol.* **2016**, *31*, 499–513.

16. Boussouar, F.; Benahmed, M. Lactate and energy metabolism in male germ cells. *Trends Endocrinol. Metab.* **2004**, *15*, 345–350. [CrossRef]

17. Mruk, D.D.; Cheng, C.Y. The mammalian blood-testis barrier: Its biology and regulation. *Endocr. Rev.* **2015**, *36*, 564–591. [CrossRef]

18. Dong, H.; Chen, Z.; Wang, C.; Xiong, Z.; Zhao, W.; Jia, C.; Lin, J.; Lin, Y.; Yuan, W.; Zhao, A.Z.; et al. Rictor regulates spermatogenesis by controlling sertoli cell cytoskeletal organization and cell polarity in the mouse testis. *Endocrinology* **2015**, *156*, 4244–4256. [CrossRef]

19. Mok, K.W.; Mruk, D.D.; Silvestrini, B.; Cheng, C.Y. Rps6 regulates blood-testis barrier dynamics by affecting f-actin organization and protein recruitment. *Endocrinology* **2012**, *153*, 5036–5048. [CrossRef]

20. Libby, E.; Ratcliff, W.C. Evolution. Ratcheting the evolution of multicellularity. *Science* **2014**, *346*, 426–427. [CrossRef]

21. Dussutour, A.; Latty, T.; Beekman, M.; Simpson, S.J. Amoeboid organism solves complex nutritional challenges. *Proc. Natl. Acad. Sci. USA* **2010**, *107*, 4607–4611. [CrossRef]

22. Szathmáry, E.; Smith, J.M. The major evolutionary transitions. *Nature* **1995**, *374*, 227–232. [CrossRef] [PubMed]

23. Sancak, Y.; Thoreen, C.C.; Peterson, T.R.; Lindquist, R.A.; Kang, S.A.; Spooner, E.; Carr, S.A.; Sabatini, D.M. Pras40 is an insulin-regulated inhibitor of the mtorc1 protein kinase. *Mol. Cell* **2007**, *25*, 903–915. [CrossRef]

24. Thedieck, K.; Polak, P.; Kim, M.L.; Molle, K.D.; Cohen, A.; Jeno, P.; Arrieumerlou, C.; Hall, M.N. Pras40 and prr5-like protein are new mtor interactors that regulate apoptosis. *PLoS ONE* **2007**, *2*, e1217. [CrossRef] [PubMed]

25. Peterson, T.R.; Laplante, M.; Thoreen, C.C.; Sancak, Y.; Kang, S.A.; Kuehl, W.M.; Gray, N.S.; Sabatini, D.M. Deptor is an mtor inhibitor frequently overexpressed in multiple myeloma cells and required for their survival. *Cell* **2009**, *137*, 873–886. [CrossRef]

26. Aylett, C.H.; Sauer, E.; Imseng, S.; Boehringer, D.; Hall, M.N.; Ban, N.; Maier, T. Architecture of human mtor complex 1. *Science* **2016**, *351*, 48–52. [CrossRef]

27. Kaizuka, T.; Hara, T.; Oshiro, N.; Kikkawa, U.; Yonezawa, K.; Takehana, K.; Iemura, S.; Natsume, T.; Mizushima, N. Tti1 and tel2 are critical factors in mammalian target of rapamycin complex assembly. *J. Boil. Chem.* **2010**, *285*, 20109–20116. [CrossRef] [PubMed]

28. Frias, M.A.; Thoreen, C.C.; Jaffe, J.D.; Schroder, W.; Sculley, T.; Carr, S.A.; Sabatini, D.M. Msin1 is necessary for akt/pkb phosphorylation, and its isoforms define three distinct mtorc2s. *Curr. Biol.* **2006**, *16*, 1865–1870. [CrossRef]

29. Pearce, L.R.; Huang, X.; Boudeau, J.; Pawlowski, R.; Wullschleger, S.; Deak, M.; Ibrahim, A.F.; Gourlay, R.; Magnuson, M.A.; Alessi, D.R. Identification of protor as a novel rictor-binding component of mtor complex-2. *Biochem. J.* **2007**, *405*, 513–522. [CrossRef] [PubMed]

30. Sarbassov, D.D.; Ali, S.M.; Sengupta, S.; Sheen, J.H.; Hsu, P.P.; Bagley, A.F.; Markhard, A.L.; Sabatini, D.M. Prolonged rapamycin treatment inhibits mtorc2 assembly and akt/pkb. *Mol. Cell* **2006**, *22*, 159–168. [CrossRef]

31. Vezina, C.; Kudelski, A.; Sehgal, S.N. Rapamycin (ay-22,989), a new antifungal antibiotic. I. Taxonomy of the producing streptomycete and isolation of the active principle. *J. Antibiot.* **1975**, *28*, 721–726. [CrossRef]

32. Martel, R.R.; Klicius, J.; Galet, S. Inhibition of the immune response by rapamycin, a new antifungal antibiotic. *Can. J. Physiol. Pharmacol.* **1977**, *55*, 48–51. [CrossRef]

33. Eng, C.P.; Sehgal, S.N.; Vezina, C. Activity of rapamycin (ay-22,989) against transplanted tumors. *J. Antibiot.* **1984**, *37*, 1231–1237. [CrossRef] [PubMed]

34. Harrison, D.E.; Strong, R.; Sharp, Z.D.; Nelson, J.F.; Astle, C.M.; Flurkey, K.; Nadon, N.L.; Wilkinson, J.E.; Frenkel, K.; Carter, C.S.; et al. Rapamycin fed late in life extends lifespan in genetically heterogeneous mice. *Nature* **2009**, *460*, 392–395. [CrossRef] [PubMed]

35. Tee, A.R.; Manning, B.D.; Roux, P.P.; Cantley, L.C.; Blenis, J. Tuberous sclerosis complex gene products, tuberin and hamartin, control mtor signaling by acting as a gtpase-activating protein complex toward rheb. *Curr. Biol.* **2003**, *13*, 1259–1268. [CrossRef]

36. Long, X.; Lin, Y.; Ortiz-Vega, S.; Yonezawa, K.; Avruch, J. Rheb binds and regulates the mtor kinase. *Curr. Biol.* **2005**, *15*, 702–713. [CrossRef]

37. Wolfson, R.L.; Sabatini, D.M. The dawn of the age of amino acid sensors for the mtorc1 pathway. *Cell Metab.* **2017**, *26*, 301–309. [CrossRef]

38. Bröer, S.; Bröer, A. Amino acid homeostasis and signalling in mammalian cells and organisms. *Biochem. J.* **2017**, *474*, 1935–1963. [CrossRef] [PubMed]

39. Menon, S.; Dibble, C.C.; Talbott, G.; Hoxhaj, G.; Valvezan, A.J.; Takahashi, H.; Cantley, L.C.; Manning, B.D. Spatial control of the tsc complex integrates insulin and nutrient regulation of mtorc1 at the lysosome. *Cell* **2014**, *156*, 771–785. [CrossRef] [PubMed]

40. Randle, S.C. Tuberous sclerosis complex: A review. *Pediatr. Ann.* **2017**, *46*, e166–e171. [CrossRef]

41. Ma, L.; Chen, Z.; Erdjument-Bromage, H.; Tempst, P.; Pandolfi, P.P. Phosphorylation and functional inactivation of tsc2 by erk implications for tuberous sclerosis and cancer pathogenesis. *Cell* **2005**, *121*, 179–193. [CrossRef]

42. Inoki, K.; Li, Y.; Zhu, T.; Wu, J.; Guan, K.L. Tsc2 is phosphorylated and inhibited by akt and suppresses mtor signalling. *Nat. Cell Biol.* **2002**, *4*, 648–657. [CrossRef]

43. Manning, B.D.; Tee, A.R.; Logsdon, M.N.; Blenis, J.; Cantley, L.C. Identification of the tuberous sclerosis complex-2 tumor suppressor gene product tuberin as a target of the phosphoinositide 3-kinase/akt pathway. *Mol. Cell* **2002**, *10*, 151–162. [CrossRef]

44. Potter, C.J.; Pedraza, L.G.; Xu, T. Akt regulates growth by directly phosphorylating tsc2. *Nat. Cell Biol.* **2002**, *4*, 658–665. [CrossRef] [PubMed]

45. Roux, P.P.; Ballif, B.A.; Anjum, R.; Gygi, S.P.; Blenis, J. Tumor-promoting phorbol esters and activated ras inactivate the tuberous sclerosis tumor suppressor complex via p90 ribosomal s6 kinase. *Proc. Natl. Acad. Sci. USA* **2004**, *101*, 13489–13494. [CrossRef]

46. Gwinn, D.M.; Shackelford, D.B.; Egan, D.F.; Mihaylova, M.M.; Mery, A.; Vasquez, D.S.; Turk, B.E.; Shaw, R.J. Ampk phosphorylation of raptor mediates a metabolic checkpoint. *Mol. Cell* **2008**, *30*, 214–226. [CrossRef]

47. Feng, Z.; Hu, W.; de Stanchina, E.; Teresky, A.K.; Jin, S.; Lowe, S.; Levine, A.J. The regulation of ampk beta1, tsc2, and pten expression by p53: Stress, cell and tissue specificity, and the role of these gene products in modulating the igf-1-akt-mtor pathways. *Cancer Res.* **2007**, *67*, 3043–3053. [CrossRef]

48. Feng, Z.; Zhang, H.; Levine, A.J.; Jin, S. The coordinate regulation of the p53 and mtor pathways in cells. *Proc. Natl. Acad. Sci. USA* **2005**, *102*, 8204–8209. [CrossRef]

49. Stambolic, V.; MacPherson, D.; Sas, D.; Lin, Y.; Snow, B.; Jang, Y.; Benchimol, S.; Mak, T.W. Regulation of pten transcription by p53. *Mol. Cell* **2001**, *8*, 317–325. [CrossRef]

50. Brugarolas, J.; Lei, K.; Hurley, R.L.; Manning, B.D.; Reiling, J.H.; Hafen, E.; Witters, L.A.; Ellisen, L.W.; Kaelin, W.G., Jr. Regulation of mtor function in response to hypoxia by redd1 and the tsc1/tsc2 tumor suppressor complex. *Genes Dev.* **2004**, *18*, 2893–2904. [CrossRef]

51. DeYoung, M.P.; Horak, P.; Sofer, A.; Sgroi, D.; Ellisen, L.W. Hypoxia regulates tsc1/2-mtor signaling and tumor suppression through redd1-mediated 14-3-3 shuttling. *Genes Dev.* **2008**, *22*, 239–251. [CrossRef] [PubMed]

52. Yang, Q.; Inoki, K.; Ikenoue, T.; Guan, K.L. Identification of sin1 as an essential torc2 component required for complex formation and kinase activity. *Genes Dev.* **2006**, *20*, 2820–2832. [CrossRef] [PubMed]

53. Garcia-Martinez, J.M.; Alessi, D.R. Mtor complex 2 (mtorc2) controls hydrophobic motif phosphorylation and activation of serum- and glucocorticoid-induced protein kinase 1 (sgk1). *Biochem. J.* **2008**, *416*, 375–385. [CrossRef] [PubMed]

54. Sarbassov, D.D.; Guertin, D.A.; Ali, S.M.; Sabatini, D.M. Phosphorylation and regulation of akt/pkb by the rictor-mtor complex. *Science* **2005**, *307*, 1098–1101. [CrossRef] [PubMed]

55. Liu, P.; Gan, W.; Chin, Y.R.; Ogura, K.; Guo, J.; Zhang, J.; Wang, B.; Blenis, J.; Cantley, L.C.; Toker, A.; et al. Ptdins(3,4,5)p3-dependent activation of the mtorc2 kinase complex. *Cancer Discov.* **2015**, *5*, 1194–1209. [CrossRef] [PubMed]

56. Yang, G.; Murashige, D.S.; Humphrey, S.J.; James, D.E. A positive feedback loop between akt and mtorc2 via sin1 phosphorylation. *Cell Rep.* **2015**, *12*, 937–943. [CrossRef] [PubMed]

57. Huang, J.; Dibble, C.C.; Matsuzaki, M.; Manning, B.D. The tsc1-tsc2 complex is required for proper activation of mtor complex 2. *Mol. Cell. Biol.* **2008**, *28*, 4104–4115. [CrossRef]

58. Zinzalla, V.; Stracka, D.; Oppliger, W.; Hall, M.N. Activation of mtorc2 by association with the ribosome. *Cell* **2011**, *144*, 757–768. [CrossRef] [PubMed]

59. Huang, Z.; Wu, Y.; Zhou, X.; Qian, J.; Zhu, W.; Shu, Y.; Liu, P. Clinical efficacy of mtor inhibitors in solid tumors: A systematic review. *Future Oncol.* **2015**, *11*, 1687–1699. [CrossRef]

60. Fouque, A.; Jean, M.; Weghe, P.; Legembre, P. Review of pi3k/mtor inhibitors entering clinical trials to treat triple negative breast cancers. *Recent Patents Anti-Cancer Drug Discov.* **2016**, *11*, 283–296. [CrossRef]

61. Ortolani, S.; Ciccarese, C.; Cingarlini, S.; Tortora, G.; Massari, F. Suppression of mtor pathway in solid tumors: Lessons learned from clinical experience in renal cell carcinoma and neuroendocrine tumors and new perspectives. *Future Oncol.* **2015**, *11*, 1809–1828. [CrossRef]

62. Citraro, R.; Leo, A.; Constanti, A.; Russo, E.; De Sarro, G. Mtor pathway inhibition as a new therapeutic strategy in epilepsy and epileptogenesis. *Pharmacol. Res.* **2016**, *107*, 333–343. [CrossRef]

63. De Fijter, J.W. Cancer and mtor inhibitors in transplant recipients. *Transplantation* **2017**, *101*, 45–55. [CrossRef]

64. Ghidini, M.; Petrelli, F.; Ghidini, A.; Tomasello, G.; Hahne, J.C.; Passalacqua, R.; Barni, S. Clinical development of mtor inhibitors for renal cancer. *Expert Opin. Investig. Drugs* **2017**, *26*, 1229–1237. [CrossRef] [PubMed]

65. Verges, B.; Cariou, B. Mtor inhibitors and diabetes. *Diabetes Res. Clin. Pract.* **2015**, *110*, 101–108. [CrossRef]

66. Yoo, Y.J.; Kim, H.; Park, S.R.; Yoon, Y.J. An overview of rapamycin: From discovery to future persp ctives. *J. Ind. Microbiol. Biotechnol.* **2017**, *44*, 537–553. [CrossRef] [PubMed]

67. Huyghe, E.; Zairi, A.; Nohra, J.; Kamar, N.; Plante, P.; Rostaing, L. Gonadal impact of target of rapamycin inhibitors (sirolimus and everolimus) in male patients: An overview. *Transpl. Int. Off. J. Eur. Soc. Organ Transplant.* **2007**, *20*, 305–311. [CrossRef] [PubMed]

68. Bererhi, L.; Flamant, M.; Martinez, F.; Karras, A.; Thervet, E.; Legendre, C. Rapamycin-induced oligospermia. *Transplantation* **2003**, *76*, 885–886. [CrossRef] [PubMed]

69. Kaczmarek, I.; Groetzner, J.; Adamidis, I.; Landwehr, P.; Mueller, M.; Vogeser, M.; Gerstorfer, M.; Uberfuhr, P.; Meiser, B.; Reichart, B. Sirolimus impairs gonadal function in heart transplant recipients. *Am. J. Transplant. Off. J. Am. Soc. Transplant. Am. Soc. Transpl. Surg.* **2004**, *4*, 1084–1088. [CrossRef]

70. Zuber, J.; Anglicheau, D.; Elie, C.; Bererhi, L.; Timsit, M.O.; Mamzer-Bruneel, M.F.; Ciroldi, M.; Martinez, F.; Snanoudj, R.; Hiesse, C.; et al. Sirolimus may reduce fertility in male renal transplant recipients. *Am. J. Transplant. Off. J. Am. Soc. Transplant. Am. Soc. Transpl. Surg.* **2008**, *8*, 1471–1479. [CrossRef]

71. Chen, Y.; Zhang, Z.; Lin, Y.; Lin, H.; Li, M.; Nie, P.; Chen, L.; Qiu, J.; Lu, Y.; Chen, L.; et al. Long-term impact of immunosuppressants at therapeutic doses on male reproductive system in unilateral nephrectomized rats: A comparative study. *BioMed Res. Int.* **2013**, *2013*, 690382. [CrossRef]

72. Rovira, J.; Diekmann, F.; Ramirez-Bajo, M.J.; Banon-Maneus, E.; Moya-Rull, D.; Campistol, J.M. Sirolimus-associated testicular toxicity: Detrimental but reversible. *Transplantation* **2012**, *93*, 874–879. [CrossRef] [PubMed]

73. Skrzypek, J.; Krause, W. Azoospermia in a renal transplant recipient during sirolimus (rapamycin) treatment. *Andrologia* **2007**, *39*, 198–199. [CrossRef]

74. Hobbs, R.M.; Seandel, M.; Falciatori, I.; Rafii, S.; Pandolfi, P.P. Plzf regulates germline progenitor self-renewal by opposing mtorc1. *Cell* **2010**, *142*, 468–479. [CrossRef] [PubMed]

75. Costoya, J.A.; Hobbs, R.M.; Barna, M.; Cattoretti, G.; Manova, K.; Sukhwani, M.; Orwig, K.E.; Wolgemuth, D.J.; Pandolfi, P.P. Essential role of plzf in maintenance of spermatogonial stem cells. *Nat. Genet.* **2004**, *36*, 653–659. [CrossRef]

76. Buaas, F.W.; Kirsh, A.L.; Sharma, M.; McLean, D.J.; Morris, J.L.; Griswold, M.D.; de Rooij, D.G.; Braun, R.E. Plzf is required in adult male germ cells for stem cell self-renewal. *Nat. Genet.* **2004**, *36*, 647–652. [CrossRef]

77. Daguia Zambe, J.C.; Zhai, Y.; Zhou, Z.; Du, X.; Wei, Y.; Ma, F.; Hua, J. Mir-19b-3p induces cell proliferation and reduces heterochromatin-mediated senescence through plzf in goat male germline stem cells. *J. Cell. Physiol.* **2018**, *233*, 4652–4665. [CrossRef]

78. Tarnawa, E.D.; Baker, M.D.; Aloisio, G.M.; Carr, B.R.; Castrillon, D.H. Gonadal expression of foxo1, but not foxo3, is conserved in diverse mammalian species. *Biol. Reprod.* **2013**, *88*, 103. [CrossRef] [PubMed]

79. Goertz, M.J.; Wu, Z.; Gallardo, T.D.; Hamra, F.K.; Castrillon, D.H. Foxo1 is required in mouse spermatogonial stem cells for their maintenance and the initiation of spermatogenesis. *J. Clin. Investig.* **2011**, *121*, 3456–3466. [CrossRef] [PubMed]

80. Yilmaz, O.H.; Valdez, R.; Theisen, B.K.; Guo, W.; Ferguson, D.O.; Wu, H.; Morrison, S.J. Pten dependence distinguishes haematopoietic stem cells from leukaemia-initiating cells. *Nature* **2006**, *441*, 475–482. [CrossRef]

81. Feng, Z.; Levine, A.J. The regulation of energy metabolism and the igf-1/mtor pathways by the p53 protein. *Trends Cell Boil.* **2010**, *20*, 427–434. [CrossRef]

82. Solozobova, V.; Blattner, C. P53 in stem cells. *World J. Biol. Chem.* **2011**, *2*, 202–214. [CrossRef]

83. Xiong, M.; Ferder, I.C.; Ohguchi, Y.; Wang, N. Quantitative analysis of male germline stem cell differentiation reveals a role for the p53-mtorc1 pathway in spermatogonial maintenance. *Cell Cycle* **2015**, *14*, 2905–2913. [CrossRef] [PubMed]

84. Hobbs, R.M.; La, H.M.; Makela, J.A.; Kobayashi, T.; Noda, T.; Pandolfi, P.P. Distinct germline progenitor subsets defined through tsc2-mtorc1 signaling. *EMBO Rep.* **2015**, *16*, 467–480. [CrossRef] [PubMed]

85. Wang, C.; Wang, Z.; Xiong, Z.; Dai, H.; Zou, Z.; Jia, C.; Bai, X.; Chen, Z. Mtorc1 activation promotes spermatogonial differentiation and causes subfertility in mice. *Biol. Reprod.* **2016**, *95*, 97. [CrossRef] [PubMed]

86. Bruscoli, S.; Velardi, E.; Di Sante, M.; Bereshchenko, O.; Venanzi, A.; Coppo, M.; Berno, V.; Mameli, M.G.; Colella, R.; Cavaliere, A.; et al. Long glucocorticoid-induced leucine zipper (l-gilz) protein interacts with ras protein pathway and contributes to spermatogenesis control. *J. Biol. Chem.* **2012**, *287*, 1242–1251. [CrossRef]

87. Ngo, D.; Cheng, Q.; O'Connor, A.E.; DeBoer, K.D.; Lo, C.Y.; Beaulieu, E.; De Seram, M.; Hobbs, R.M.; O'Bryan, M.K.; Morand, E.F. Glucocorticoid-induced leucine zipper (gilz) regulates testicular foxo1 activity and spermatogonial stem cell (ssc) function. *PLoS ONE* **2013**, *8*, e59149. [CrossRef]

88. La, H.M.; Chan, A.L.; Legrand, J.M.D.; Rossello, F.J.; Gangemi, C.G.; Papa, A.; Cheng, Q.; Morand, E.F.; Hobbs, R.M. Gilz-dependent modulation of mtorc1 regulates spermatogonial maintenance. *Development* **2018**, *145*, dev165324. [CrossRef]

89. Kishi, K.; Uchida, A.; Takase, H.M.; Suzuki, H.; Kurohmaru, M.; Tsunekawa, N.; Kanai-Azuma, M.; Wood, S.A.; Kanai, Y. Spermatogonial deubiquitinase usp9x is essential for proper spermatogenesis in mice. *Reproduction* **2017**, *154*, 135–143. [CrossRef]

90. Meng, X.; Lindahl, M.; Hyvonen, M.E.; Parvinen, M.; de Rooij, D.G.; Hess, M.W.; Raatikainen-Ahokas, A.; Sainio, K.; Rauvala, H.; Lakso, M.; et al. Regulation of cell fate decision of undifferentiated spermatogonia by gdnf. *Science* **2000**, *287*, 1489–1493. [CrossRef] [PubMed]

91. Kubota, H.; Avarbock, M.R.; Brinster, R.L. Growth factors essential for self-renewal and expansion of mouse spermatogonial stem cells. *Proc. Natl. Acad. Sci. USA* **2004**, *101*, 16489–16494. [CrossRef]

92. Wang, M.; Guo, Y.; Wang, M.; Zhou, T.; Xue, Y.; Du, G.; Wei, X.; Wang, J.; Qi, L.; Zhang, H.; et al. The glial cell-derived neurotrophic factor (gdnf)-responsive phosphoprotein landscape identifies raptor phosphorylation required for spermatogonial progenitor cell proliferation. *Mol. Cell. Proteom.* **2017**, *16*, 982–997. [CrossRef] [PubMed]

93. Serra, N.D.; Velte, E.K.; Niedenberger, B.A.; Kirsanov, O.; Geyer, C.B. Cell-autonomous requirement for mammalian target of rapamycin (mtor) in spermatogonial proliferation and differentiation in the mousedagger. *Biol. Reprod.* **2017**, *96*, 816–828. [CrossRef] [PubMed]

94. Busada, J.T.; Niedenberger, B.A.; Velte, E.K.; Keiper, B.D.; Geyer, C.B. Mammalian target of rapamycin complex 1 (mtorc1) is required for mouse spermatogonial differentiation in vivo. *Dev. Biol.* **2015**, *407*, 90–102. [CrossRef]

95. Serra, N.; Velte, E.K.; Niedenberger, B.A.; Kirsanov, O.; Geyer, C.B. The mtorc1 component rptor is required for maintenance of the foundational spermatogonial stem cell pool in mice. *Biol. Reprod.* **2018**, *100*, 429–439. [CrossRef]

96. Baker, M.D.; Ezzati, M.; Aloisio, G.M.; Tarnawa, E.D.; Cuevas, I.; Nakada, Y.; Castrillon, D.H. The small gtpase rheb is required for spermatogenesis but not oogenesis. *Reproduction* **2014**, *147*, 615–625.

97. Sahin, P.; Gungor-Ordueri, N.E.; Celik-Ozenci, C. Inhibition of mtor pathway decreases the expression of pre-meiotic and meiotic markers throughout postnatal development and in adult testes in mice. *Andrologia* **2018**, *50*, e12811. [CrossRef]

98. Xu, H.; Shen, L.; Chen, X.; Ding, Y.; He, J.; Zhu, J.; Wang, Y.; Liu, X. Mtor/p70s6k promotes spermatogonia proliferation and spermatogenesis in sprague dawley rats. *Reprod. Biomed. Online* **2016**, *32*, 207–217. [CrossRef]

99. Koubova, J.; Menke, D.B.; Zhou, Q.; Capel, B.; Griswold, M.D.; Page, D.C. Retinoic acid regulates sex-specific timing of meiotic initiation in mice. *Proc. Natl. Acad. Sci. USA* **2006**, *103*, 2474–2479. [CrossRef] [PubMed]

100. Zhou, Q.; Nie, R.; Li, Y.; Friel, P.; Mitchell, D.; Hess, R.A.; Small, C.; Griswold, M.D. Expression of stimulated by retinoic acid gene 8 (stra8) in spermatogenic cells induced by retinoic acid: An in vivo study in vitamin a-sufficient postnatal murine testes. *Biol. Reprod.* **2008**, *79*, 35–42.

101. Anderson, E.L.; Baltus, A.E.; Roepers-Gajadien, H.L.; Hassold, T.J.; de Rooij, D.G.; van Pelt, A.M.; Page, D.C. Stra8 and its inducer, retinoic acid, regulate meiotic initiation in both spermatogenesis and oogenesis in mice. *Proc. Natl. Acad. Sci. USA* **2008**, *105*, 14976–14980. [CrossRef]

102. Sahin, P.; Sahin, Z.; Gungor-Ordueri, N.E.; Donmez, B.O.; Celik-Ozenci, C. Inhibition of mammalian target of rapamycin signaling pathway decreases retinoic acid stimulated gene 8 expression in adult mouse testis. *Fertil. Steril.* **2014**, *102*, 1482–1490. [CrossRef]

103. Turner, J.M. Meiotic sex chromosome inactivation. *Development* **2007**, *134*, 1823–1831. [PubMed]

104. Fernandez-Capetillo, O.; Mahadevaiah, S.K.; Celeste, A.; Romanienko, P.J.; Camerini-Otero, R.D.; Bonner, W.M.; Manova, K.; Burgoyne, P.; Nussenzweig, A. H2ax is required for chromatin remodeling and inactivation of sex chromosomes in male mouse meiosis. *Dev. Cell* **2003**, *4*, 497–508. [CrossRef]

105. Turner, J.M.; Mahadevaiah, S.K.; Ellis, P.J.; Mitchell, M.J.; Burgoyne, P.S. Pachytene asynapsis drives meiotic sex chromosome inactivation and leads to substantial postmeiotic repression in spermatids. *Dev. Cell* **2006**, *10*, 521–529. [CrossRef] [PubMed]

106. Xiong, M.; Zhu, Z.; Tian, S.; Zhu, R.; Bai, S.; Fu, K.; Davis, J.G.; Sun, Z.; Baur, J.A.; Zheng, K.; et al. Conditional ablation of raptor in the male germline causes infertility due to meiotic arrest and impaired inactivation of sex chromosomes. *FASEB J. Off. Publ. Fed. Am. Soc. Exp. Biol.* **2017**, *31*, 3934–3949. [CrossRef]

107. Bai, S.; Cheng, L.; Zhang, Y.; Zhu, C.; Zhu, Z.; Zhu, R.; Cheng, C.Y.; Ye, L.; Zheng, K. A germline-specific role for the mtorc2 component rictor in maintaining spermatogonial differentiation and intercellular adhesion in mouse testis. *Mol. Hum. Reprod.* **2018**, *24*, 244–259. [CrossRef]

108. Zhu, Z.; Yue, Q.; Xie, J.; Zhang, S.; He, W.; Bai, S.; Tian, S.; Zhang, Y.; Xiong, M.; Sun, Z.; et al. Rapamycin-mediated mtor inhibition impairs silencing of sex chromosomes and the pachytene pirna pathway in the mouse testis. *Aging* **2019**, *11*, 185–208.

109. Weber, J.E.; Russell, L.D.; Wong, V.; Peterson, R.N. Three-dimensional reconstruction of a rat stage v sertoli cell: Ii. Morphometry of sertoli–sertoli and sertoli–germ-cell relationships. *Am. J. Anat.* **1983**, *167*, 163–179. [CrossRef]

110. Kaur, G.; Thompson, L.A.; Dufour, J.M. Sertoli cells–immunological sentinels of spermatogenesis. *Semin. Cell Dev. Boil.* **2014**, *30*, 36–44. [CrossRef]

111. O'Donnell, L. Mechanisms of spermiogenesis and spermiation and how they are disturbed. *Spermatogenesis* **2014**, *4*, e979623. [CrossRef]

112. Li, N.; Mruk, D.D.; Cheng, C.Y. Actin binding proteins in blood-testis barrier function. *Curr. Opin. Endocrinol. Diabetes Obes.* **2015**, *22*, 238–247. [CrossRef]

113. Yan, H.H.; Mruk, D.D.; Lee, W.M.; Cheng, C.Y. Cross-talk between tight and anchoring junctions-lesson from the testis. *Adv. Exp. Med. Biol.* **2008**, *636*, 234–254. [PubMed]

114. Xiao, X.; Mruk, D.D.; Wong, C.K.; Cheng, C.Y. Germ cell transport across the seminiferous epithelium during spermatogenesis. *Physiology* **2014**, *29*, 286–298. [PubMed]

115. Russell, L. Movement of spermatocytes from the basal to the adluminal compartment of the rat testis. *Am. J. Anat.* **1977**, *148*, 313–328. [CrossRef]

116. Li, S.Y.T.; Yan, M.; Chen, H.; Jesus, T.; Lee, W.M.; Xiao, X.; Cheng, C.Y. Mtorc1/rps6 regulates blood-testis barrier dynamics and spermatogenetic function in the testis in vivo. *Am. J. Physiol. Endocrinol. Metab.* **2018**, *314*, E174–E190.

117. Xiong, Z.; Wang, C.; Wang, Z.; Dai, H.; Song, Q.; Zou, Z.; Xiao, B.; Zhao, A.Z.; Bai, X.; Chen, Z. Raptor directs sertoli cell cytoskeletal organization and polarity in the mouse testis. *Biol. Reprod.* **2018**, *99*, 1289–1302. [PubMed]

118. Saci, A.; Cantley, L.C.; Carpenter, C.L. Rac1 regulates the activity of mtorc1 and mtorc2 and controls cellular size. *Mol. Cell* **2011**, *42*, 50–61. [CrossRef]

119. Alves, M.G.; Rato, L.; Carvalho, R.A.; Moreira, P.I.; Socorro, S.; Oliveira, P.F. Hormonal control of sertoli cell metabolism regulates spermatogenesis. *Cell. Mol. Life Sci.* **2013**, *70*, 777–793. [CrossRef]

120. Oliveira, P.F.; Martins, A.D.; Moreira, A.C.; Cheng, C.Y.; Alves, M.G. The warburg effect revisited–lesson from the sertoli cell. *Med. Res. Rev.* **2015**, *35*, 126–151. [CrossRef]

121. Martins, A.D.; Moreira, A.C.; Sa, R.; Monteiro, M.P.; Sousa, M.; Carvalho, R.A.; Silva, B.M.; Oliveira, P.F.; Alves, M.G. Leptin modulates human sertoli cells acetate production and glycolytic profile: A novel mechanism of obesity-induced male infertility? *Biochim. Biophys. Acta* **2015**, *1852*, 1824–1832. [CrossRef]

122. Martins, A.D.; Sá, R.; Monteiro, M.P.; Barros, A.; Sousa, M.; Carvalho, R.A.; Silva, B.M.; Oliveira, P.F.; Alves, M.G. Ghrelin acts as energy status sensor of male reproduction by modulating sertoli cells glycolytic metabolism and mitochondrial bioenergetics. *Mol. Cell. Endocrinol.* **2016**, *434*, 199–209. [CrossRef] [PubMed]

123. Alves, M.G.; Jesus, T.T.; Sousa, M.; Goldberg, E.; Silva, B.M.; Oliveira, P.F. Male fertility and obesity: Are ghrelin, leptin and glucagon-like peptide-1 pharmacologically relevant? *Curr. Pharm. Des.* **2016**, *22*, 783–791. [CrossRef] [PubMed]

124. Martins, A.D.; Monteiro, M.P.; Silva, B.M.; Barros, A.; Sousa, M.; Carvalho, R.A.; Oliveira, P.F.; Alves, M.G. Metabolic dynamics of human sertoli cells are differentially modulated by physiological and pharmacological concentrations of glp-1. *Toxicol. Appl. Pharmacol.* **2019**, *362*, 1–8. [CrossRef] [PubMed]

125. Crane, J.; McGowan, B. The glp-1 agonist, liraglutide, as a pharmacotherapy for obesity. *Ther. Adv. Chronic Dis.* **2016**, *7*, 92–107. [CrossRef] [PubMed]

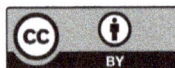

International Journal of
Molecular Sciences

MDPI

Article

Early Developmental Exposure to General Anesthetic Agents in Primary Neuron Culture Disrupts Synapse Formation via Actions on the mTOR Pathway

Jing Xu [1], R. Paige Mathena [1], Michael Xu [1], YuChia Wang [1], CheJui Chang [2], Yiwen Fang [2], Pengbo Zhang [1] and C. David Mintz [1],*

[1] Department of Anesthesiology and Critical Care Medicine, The Johns Hopkins University School of Medicine, Baltimore, MD 21205, USA; jxu72@jhmi.edu (J.X.); rmathen1@jhmi.edu (R.P.M.); michael.xu@downstate.edu (M.X.); yw3af@virginia.edu (Y.W.); zhpbo@mail.xjtu.edu.cn (P.Z.)
[2] Chang Gung Memorial Hospital, Taoyuan City 33305, Taiwan; jeff83831@gmail.com (C.C.); gs1606890220@gmail.com (Y.F.)
* Correspondence: cmintz2@jhmi.edu; Tel.: +1-917-733-0422

Received: 7 June 2018; Accepted: 20 July 2018; Published: 26 July 2018

Abstract: Human epidemiologic studies and laboratory investigations in animal models suggest that exposure to general anesthetic agents (GAs) have harmful effects on brain development. The mechanism underlying this putative iatrogenic condition is not clear and there are currently no accepted strategies for prophylaxis or treatment. Recent evidence suggests that anesthetics might cause persistent deficits in synaptogenesis by disrupting key events in neurodevelopment. Using an in vitro model consisting of dissociated primary cultured mouse neurons, we demonstrate abnormal pre- and post-synaptic marker expression after a clinically-relevant isoflurane anesthesia exposure is conducted during neuron development. We find that pharmacologic inhibition of the mechanistic target of rapamycin (mTOR) pathway can reverse the observed changes. Isoflurane exposure increases expression of phospho-S6, a marker of mTOR pathway activity, in a concentration-dependent fashion and this effect occurs throughout neuronal development. The mTOR 1 complex (mTORC1) and the mTOR 2 complex (mTORC2) branches of the pathway are both activated by isoflurane exposure and this is reversible with branch-specific inhibitors. Upregulation of mTOR is also seen with sevoflurane and propofol exposure, suggesting that this mechanism of developmental anesthetic neurotoxicity may occur with all the commonly used GAs in pediatric practice. We conclude that GAs disrupt the development of neurons during development by activating a well-defined neurodevelopmental disease pathway and that this phenotype can be reversed by pharmacologic inhibition.

Keywords: anesthesia; neurotoxicity; synapse; mTOR; neurodevelopment

---

1. Introduction

The United States Food and Drug Administration has recently required that 12 commonly used anesthetic and sedative agents with mechanisms of action on NMDA and GABA receptors carry labels warning that repeated or lengthy exposure to these drugs between the third trimester and the first three years of life may result in adverse consequences for brain development (FDA Drug Safety Communication). An estimated 115,000 children each year are anesthetized for surgery and other procedures in the U.S. alone, suggesting that millions of children are exposed to anesthesia each year worldwide [1]. It is not yet clear which patients are potentially at risk of cognitive dysfunction related to this exposure, but early results from the only two clinical trials that have reached endpoints give reassurance that short, single exposures in healthy children do not have deleterious effects [2,3].

This finding is consistent with data from large epidemiologic studies showing no effect of short, single early life exposures to surgery and anesthesia, but a correlation between long or multiple exposures and reduced scores on cognitive testing, worsened scores in educational testing assessments, and increased billing codes indicates developmental or behavioral disorders [4–6]. Numerous studies have found that early postnatal exposure to GA in rodents results in deficits in performance on tests of learning and memory [7–15], but rodent anesthesia models introduce a confound of physiologic perturbation that is difficult to measure and also the short timeline of rodent brain development might exaggerate the consequences of a toxic developmental exposure. However, recent data in non-human primates have provided definitive evidence that early postnatal GA exposure can have lasting effects on cognition, including deficits in socioemotional and learning function [16–19].

The mechanism by which a transient exposure to GA could have lasting consequences on brain development has been the subject of considerable investigation, but no clear conclusion has been reached [20,21]. We have found evidences in an in vivo mouse model that early postnatal exposure to isoflurane causes a lasting increase in activity in the mTOR pathway in the hippocampal dentate gyrus. Inhibition of mTOR upregulation with rapamycin reversed a loss of neuronal spines in dentate gyrus granule neurons and also restored performance on hippocampal-dependent learning tests that are impaired by isoflurane exposure [8]. The mTOR pathway is a complex and heterogeneous signaling system that integrates intra- and extracellular cue sensing and links to numerous other signaling pathways in order to regulate metabolism, growth, and homeostasis [22]. A lasting anesthetic action on mTOR function is an intriguing potential mechanism of developmental anesthetic neurotoxicity. The mTOR system is critical for neuronal development [23] and a causative role of mTOR system dysfunction has been proposed for better understood neurodevelopmental disorders, such as Fragile X, autism, schizophrenia, and drug addiction [24]. However, mTOR has not been extensively studied in this context, and the evidence linking it to anesthetic toxicity is mixed [25].

Here we use an in vitro primary rat neuron culture system to further explore the hypothesis that GAs disrupt neuron development via an upregulation of mTOR signaling. To this end we employ quantitative immunohistochemistry to examine the effects of anesthetic-induced mTOR changes on synapse development. We also test for contributions of the mTOR1 and mTOR2 complexes, which represent a divergence in the pathway. Finally, we ask whether the effects on the mTOR pathway generalize to multiple anesthetic agents.

2. Results and Discussion

2.1. Effects of Isoflurane Exposure for 6 h on Apoptosis

In order to exclude the possible effects of isoflurane on the health of the primary neurons, we first tested the difference in apoptosis in the 1.8% and 2.4% isoflurane exposure group compared to the control group. A small number of cells stained positive in the TUNEL assay following a 6 h exposure both when the cells were harvested immediately after exposure and when they were harvested 24 h after exposure (Figure 1B). There was no significant difference between the control group ($7.95 \pm 7.86\%$) and the isoflurane 1.8% ($13.85 \pm 7.69\%$) and 2.4% ($14.14 \pm 7.67\%$) groups when harvested directly after exposure using one-way ANOVA with Dunnett's multiple comparisons (Figure 1C). The same results were found when the cells were harvested 24 h following exposure ((control group ($3.83 \pm 5.47\%$), isoflurane 1.8% ($6.81 \pm 5.77\%$), and 2.4% ($10.91 \pm 6.25\%$) groups)) (Figure 1D). These results indicate that 1.8% and 2.4% isoflurane exposure on seven days in vitro (DIV) for 6 h does not affect normal baseline levels of cell apoptosis.

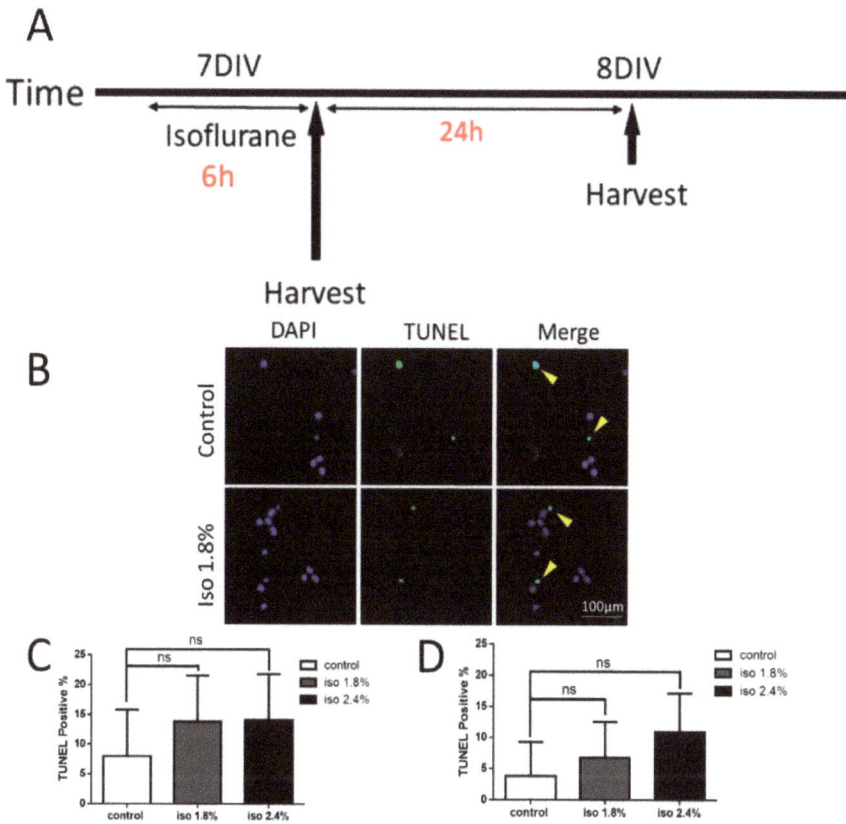

Figure 1. Isoflurane exposure at different doses did not show any significant apoptosis in our exposure paradigms. (**A**) The TUNEL experiment timeline in vitro. The neurons were exposed to either carrier gas or 1.8%/2.4% isoflurane for 6 h on their 7 DIV, and the cells were harvested immediately after exposure or 24 h after the exposure; (**B**). Representative images of DAPI (blue) and TUNEL (green) immunofluorescence in the dissociated neurons at 8 DIV; (**C,D**) 6 h of isoflurane treatment on 7 DIV did not show a significant apoptosis difference among all the DAPI/TUNEL neurons compared to the control groups immediately after the exposure (**C**) or 24 h after the exposure (**D**) (n = 15 fields that were measured per group, n.s. indicates no significant difference, one-way ANOVA with Dunnett's multiple comparisons test).

2.2. Effects of 1.8% Isoflurane Exposure for 6 h on Synaptogenesis

Our previous work in newborn dentate gyrus granule neurons in the intact mouse showed that isoflurane could act via an mTOR-mediated mechanism to cause a lasting reduction in the numbers of dendritic spines, which represent a morphological marker for excitatory post-synaptic elements. To determine whether this effect is an acute one that occurs during neuron synapse development and to test whether it generalizes to multiple neuronal types, we explored the effects of isoflurane administered during the period of ongoing synaptogenesis in cultured neocortical neurons, a population that is both heterogeneous and distinctly different from dentate gyrus neurons. Exposures consisting of 1.8% isoflurane for 6 h were performed at 7 DIV when synaptogenesis is ongoing, and results were assayed at 10 DIV when it is largely complete [26] (Figure 2). Double immunofluorescence staining was performed using MAP-2 as a dendritic marker to define the area over which synaptic markers were measured, and either Synapsin-1 to identify pre-synaptic elements or Homer-1 to identify excitatory post-synaptic elements. The locations of the images taken for analysis were 50 μm from the nucleus, representative images are shown in Figure 3A (scale bar: 50 μm) and Figure 3B (scale bar: 2 μm).

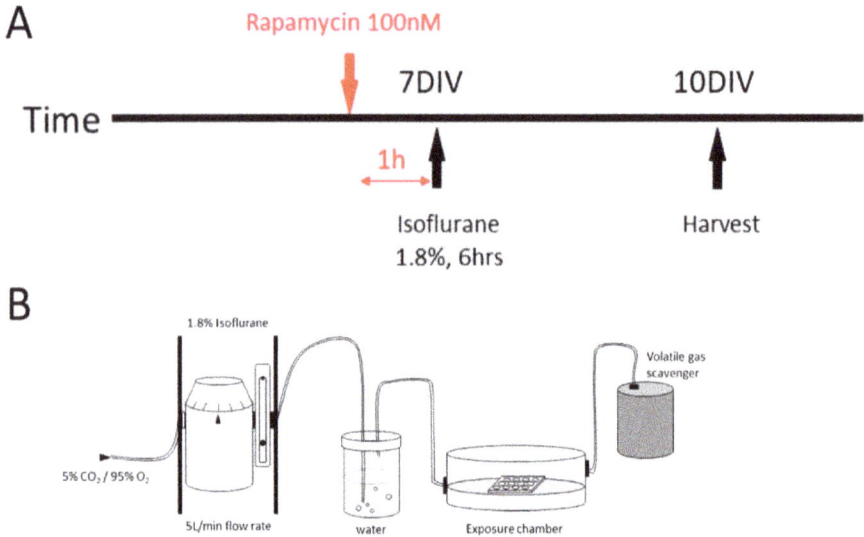

Figure 2. Schematic representation of the experimental timeline and exposure induction diagram in vitro. (**A**) The general experiment timeline in vitro. The neurons were exposed to 1.8% isoflurane for 6 h on their 7 DIV, and 100 nM rapamycin was added into the media 1 h before the exposure according to the experiment design. The fresh media change was done regularly. The cells were fixed for immunohistochemistry on 10 DIV; (**B**) Coverslips in 12-well plates were placed in identical air-tight, humidified chambers. Isoflurane was delivered using an agent-specific, calibrated inline and was diluted in 5% CO_2/95% O_2 carrier gas. Controls for these experiments received 5% CO_2/95% O_2 carrier gas only. After a 15-min equilibration period, the sealed chambers were placed in an incubator to maintain a temperature at 37 °C for the duration of the anesthesia exposure.

We found that 6 h of isoflurane treatment at a concentration of 1.8% resulted in a significant decrease in the intensity of Synapsin-1 immunoreactivity ($20.46 \pm 7.33\%$) compared to the control group ($48.95 \pm 19.02\%$, $p < 0.001$) (Figure 3C). Rapamycin treatment results in Synapsin-1 intensity levels ($32.11 \pm 9.10\%$) that are not significantly different from the control plus rapamycin treatment group ($36.13 \pm 11.70\%$), while there was a significant interaction of isoflurane treatment and rapamycin using two-way ANOVA with Bonferroni's multiple comparisons test, suggesting a rescue effect of rapamycin (Figure 3D). Carrier gas and isoflurane treatment were also used in the presence of the rapamycin diluent, dimethyl sulfoxide (DMSO), and the results did not differ from the same experiment performed without DMSO, indicating that the diluent has no independent effect. Isoflurane treatment at 1.8% for 6 h resulted in a significant reduction in intensity of Homer-1 immunoreactivity ($30.47 \pm 5.22\%$) compared to the control group ($68.46 \pm 11.18\%$, $p < 0.0001$) (Figure 3E). As was found with Synapsin-1, rapamycin treatment after isoflurane exposure prevented the effects of isoflurane. Homer-1 immunoreactivity after rapamycin treatment did not differ significantly between the isoflurane ($49.33 \pm 7.32\%$) and carrier gas groups ($56.14 \pm 8.91\%$) (Figure 3F). Taken together, these data indicate that isoflurane interferes with the formation of excitatory synapses in developing cultured neocortical neurons and that this effect may be due to actions on the mTOR pathway.

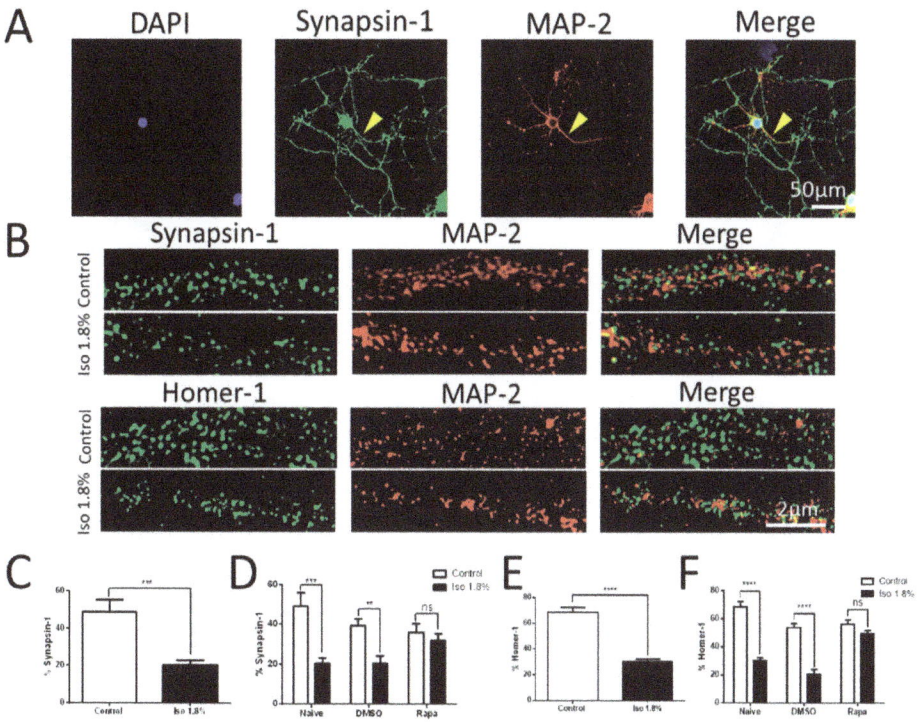

Figure 3. A 1.8% isoflurane exposure for 6 h decreases pre- and post-synaptic marker intensity in vitro. (**A,B**) Representative images of Synapsin-1/Homer-1 (green), MAP-2 (red), DAPI (blue) immunofluorescence in neurons in dissociated culture at 10 DIV are shown. The segment for the dendrite was picked according to MAP-2 staining from each neuron and the locations for images taken were defined as 20–30 μm from the nucleus according to DAPI (shown as the yellow arrow pointing in (**A**); (**C–F**) 6 h of isoflurane exposure on 7 DIV caused a significant difference in the intensity decrease of Synapsin-1 compared to the control group (**C**), while rapamycin treatment before the isoflurane exposure reversed the Synapsin-1 intensity to normal compared to the control with rapamycin treatment group (**D**). The intensity of Homer-1 also decreased compared to the control group (**E**), while rapamycin treatment before the isoflurane exposure reversed the Homer-1 intensity to normal compared to the control with rapamycin treatment group (**F**). (*n* = 30 neurons measured per group, ** $p < 0.01$, *** $p < 0.001$, **** $p < 0.0001$, n.s. indicates no significant difference, *t*-test for (**C,E**), two-way ANOVA with Bonferroni's multiple comparisons test for (**D,F**).

Our own work in vivo shows that newborn dentate gyrus neurons in mice exposed to GA with isoflurane are found to have reduced numbers of spines overall, and profoundly-reduced numbers of mushroom morphology spines over a month later [8]. As in our culture model, we found that this effect was reversible by treatment with rapamycin not acutely, but for a week after the exposure. While dendritic spines are generally the sites of excitatory post-synaptic elements, the correlation is imperfect, and our finding of reduced Homer-1 immunoreactivity in culture lends weight to our previous findings in vivo, particularly as we also found a decrease in expression of a pre-synaptic marker as well. However, our results in this manuscript differ in some important ways. Our anesthesia exposure occurred during synaptogenesis, rather than at the point of generation, and also the neurons observed in a cortical culture differ morphologically and functionally from dentate gyrus granule cells, which have many unusual features compared to other neurons. Thus, we predict, based on our findings, that mTOR-mediated effects on synapse formation are likely to generalize across a broad range of contexts. The current literature does not have any other studies of mTOR and anesthetic effects on synapses, but the preponderance of evidence suggests at least that GA exposure during development can disrupt synapse formation or maintenance. Two in vivo rodent studies using electron microscopy to identify synapses found decreased synaptic density in the hippocampus of young adult mice that had been exposed to GAs during the early postnatal phase [27,28]. Interestingly, when this phenomenon was studied in the rodent pre-frontal cortex using light microscopy to quantify spine numbers, it was found that a P5 exposure reduced spine number but a P15 exposure actually increased the spine number [29], suggesting that the state of the neuron at the time of exposure is critically important to determine the effect of GAs. Our findings in this manuscript support the conclusion that GA exposure prior to stabilization of synapses leads to a failure of synapse formation.

2.3. Parameters of Activation of mTOR by Isoflurane in Cultured Neurons

We have previously shown that isoflurane exposure causes a lasting increase in expression of phospho-S6 (pS6), a commonly used marker of activity in the mTOR pathway [8,25]. However, the constraints of in vivo experimentation are such that we were unable to determine at what stage of development neurons are subject to this phenomenon, and we were also unable to test the minimum time of exposure and exposure dose required. To address these questions, we stained for DAPI (grey) to define cell bodies and immunolabeled for βIII-tubulin (blue) to verify neuronal cell type. To measure the activity in the mTOR pathway, we co-labeled for unphosphorylated-S6 (red) and phosphorylated-S6 (green) to assess mTOR activation. A representative example of control and isoflurane 1.8% for 6 h treatment on 7 DIV with harvest on 10 DIV is shown (Figure 4A, scale bar: 50 μm).

We first tested the effects of varying the time of exposure to isoflurane on pS6 expression. We found that 6 h of 1.8% isoflurane treatment on 3 DIV caused a significant increase in the percentage of pS6 positive neurons (as the yellow arrows pointed out in Figure 4A) compared to the control group with harvest at 5 DIV ($64.25 \pm 15.95\%$ vs. $17.22 \pm 10.15\%$, $p < 0.0001$), 7 DIV ($54.33 \pm 37.69\%$ vs. $23.98 \pm 11.54\%$, $p < 0.0001$), 10 DIV ($65.53 \pm 15.26\%$ vs. $23.73 \pm 9.60\%$, $p < 0.0001$), and 14 DIV ($64.17 \pm 21.40\%$ vs. $28.01 \pm 11.92\%$, $p < 0.0001$) (Figure 4B). Isoflurane treatment at 5 DIV caused a significant increase in the percentage of pS6+ neurons compared to the control group at 7 DIV ($48.00 \pm 11.43\%$ vs. $23.60 \pm 11.33\%$, $p < 0.05$), 10 DIV ($36.65 \pm 14.74\%$ vs. $25.13 \pm 9.63\%$, $p < 0.05$), and 14 DIV ($44.36 \pm 15.36\%$ vs. $26.65 \pm 9.57\%$, $p < 0.05$) (Figure 4C). Exposure at 7 DIV caused a significant increase in pS6 positive neurons compared to the control group on 10 DIV ($79.21 \pm 16.54\%$ vs. $23.86 \pm 18.39\%$, $p < 0.0001$), but no difference was detected at the 14 DIV ($42.51 \pm 12.51\%$ vs. $32.74 \pm 7.70\%$) harvest time point (Figure 4D). These findings suggest that isoflurane exposure causes pS6 to increase at any early developmental time point, but that the effect is reduced as the neuron approaches maturity.

Next, we tested the effects of different concentrations of isoflurane delivered at 7 DIV and assayed for pS6 on 10 DIV. There was a significant difference between the 1.2% isoflurane group ($67.33 \pm 22.31\%$, ANOVA, $p < 0.01$), 1.8% isoflurane group ($79.20 \pm 16.53\%$, ANOVA, $p < 0.01$), and 2.4% isoflurane group ($71 \pm 32.31\%$, ANOVA, $p < 0.05$), compared to the control group ($23.86 \pm 18.39\%$), while there was no significant difference between the 0.6% isoflurane group ($37.80 \pm 11.13\%$), 0.9% isoflurane group ($29.65 \pm 13.18\%$), and the control group using one-way ANOVA with Dunnett's multiple comparisons (Figure 4E). This represents a clear inflection point at a value corresponding to one adult minimum alveolar concentration (MAC), which is a clinically-reasonable dose in pediatric settings.

We then sought to determine the minimum duration of exposure to isoflurane that is required to cause an increase in mTOR signaling. We exposed P7 neurons to 1.8% isoflurane with varying durations and measured pS6 levels on 10 DIV. There was a significant difference between the 0.5 h isoflurane group ($67.28 \pm 26.06\%$) compared to the control group ($21.40 \pm 10.43\%$, $p < 0.0001$), 1 h isoflurane group ($58.00 \pm 10.62\%$) compared to the control group ($35.07 \pm 19.39\%$, $p < 0.0001$), and 6 h isoflurane group ($79.20 \pm 16.53\%$) compared to the control group ($23.86 \pm 18.39\%$, $p < 0.0001$) (Figure 4F). Half an hour exposure is the shortest practical duration to measure in our model, and we conclude that even brief exposures have the potential to act on the mTOR pathway.

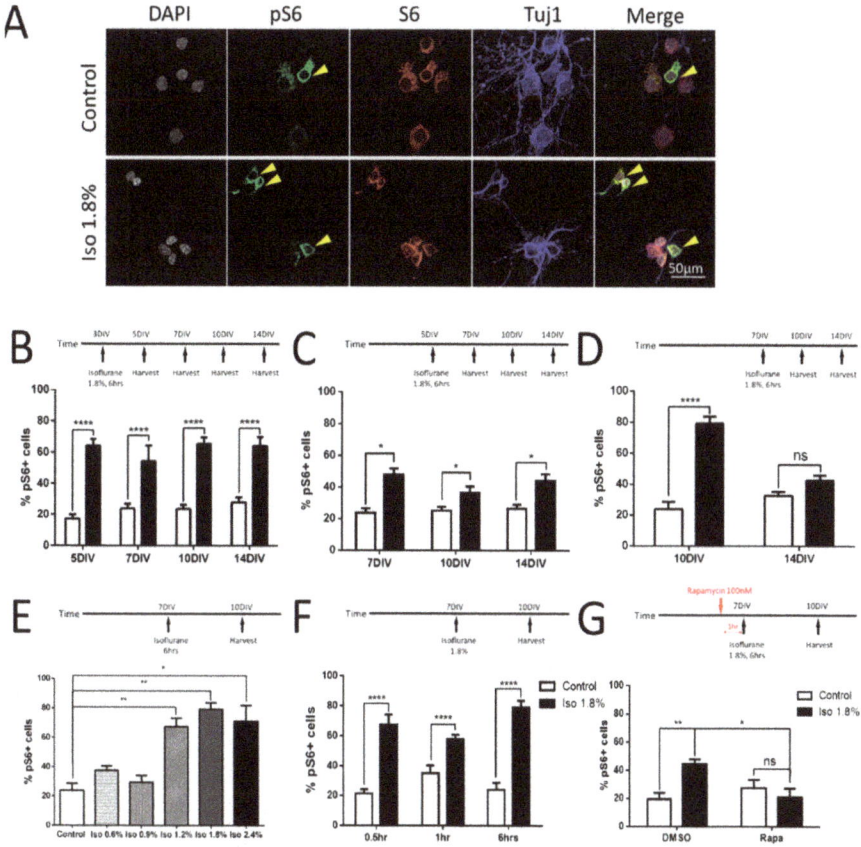

Figure 4. Isoflurane exposure at different time points showed effects on the downstream marker of mTOR pathway. (**A**) Representative images of DAPI (grey), pS6 (green), S6 (red), βIII Tubulin (blue) immunofluorescence in the dissociated neurons at 10 DIV. (**B–G**) 6 h of 1.8% isoflurane treatment on different early time points caused significant increases in the percentage of pS6 positive cells among all the DAPI/Tubulin neurons compared to the control group at late time points except the ones exposed on 7 DIV and tested on 14 DIV (**B–D**). The effect on pS6 levels at 10 DIV varied depending on the doses of isoflurane. There was a significant increase in immunoactivity starting from the 1.2% isoflurane group to the 2.4% isoflurane group, while lower doses (0.6% and 0.9%) remained at control levels of pS6 immunoactivity (**E**). Different exposure durations (0.5 h, 1 h and 6 h) of 1.8% isoflurane also resulted in increased pS6 immunoactivity at all exposure times compared to control (**F**). Adding rapamycin, an mTOR pathway inhibitor, reversed the increase of pS6 after isoflurane exposure on 7 DIV (**G**). (*n* = 15 fields that were measured per group, * *p* < 0.05, ** *p* < 0.01, **** *p* < 0.0001, n.s. indicates no significant difference, *t*-test for (**B–F**). one-way ANOVA with Dunnett's multiple comparisons test for (**E**), two-way ANOVA with Bonferroni's multiple comparisons test for (**G**).

In order to further confirm that the increase in pS6 labeling that we observe is, in fact, evidence of mTOR pathway activation, we treated the cultures with rapamycin as in Figure 1. With the significant interaction between isoflurane and rapamycin treatment using two-way ANOVA with Bonferroni's multiple comparisons test, we found that there was a significant increase in the percentage of pS6 positive cells among all the DAPI/Tubulin neurons between the isoflurane + vehicle (DMSO) group (44.49 ± 9.73%) compared to the control + vehicle (DMSO) group (19.44 ± 16.86%, $p < 0.01$). Rapamycin treatment prevented the increase of pS6 immunoactivity in the isoflurane group (21.00 ± 23.25%) compared to the isoflurane group without rapamycin (44.49 ± 9.73%, $p < 0.05$), and there was no significant difference between isoflurane + rapamycin group compared to the control+ rapamycin group (27.52 ± 23.06%) (Figure 4G).

The use of a dissociated culture model presents a substantial advantage for studying the pharmacology of anesthetic toxicity as compared to in vivo models, as the short timeline of experiments and the lesser requirements for resources allow for the study of a broad range of doses and exposure paradigms. The general consensus in the literature is that the period of synaptogenesis represents the peak window of vulnerability to developmental anesthetic neurotoxicity in vivo [30,31], but in vivo synaptogenesis is a heterogeneous process that occurs over long periods of time as different cohorts of neurons mature over widely variable timelines. Using the culture model, in which synaptogenesis is synchronous starting from 5 DIV and ending about 14 DIV [32], we asked which stages of synaptogenesis are vulnerable to a potentially harmful increase in the mTOR pathway in response to isoflurane exposure to gain a clearer understanding of the potential window of vulnerability. The only time point we studied at which pS6 up-regulation due to isoflurane exposure was at all abated was the P7 exposure with measurement of pS6 at 14 DIV. Synapses are highly dependent on filamentous actin for stability during the first week in culture, but during the second week there is a marked shift towards persistence of synapses even when actin is perturbed [33]. Several previous studies have suggested that isoflurane toxicity during development may be mediated in part via effects on the actin cytoskeleton [34,35], and our results are consistent with the period of actin-dependent synapse formation as the window of vulnerability to the mTOR-mediated effects on synaptogenesis. One of the principal concerns in the study of developmental anesthetic toxicity is that many reported phenomena may lack clinical relevance as they are reported by studies that use only supra-therapeutic doses, sometimes in excess of 2 adult MAC, or unrealistically long exposure times, which in some cases are as much as 24 h [36]. Our findings in cultured neurons show that the vulnerability of neurons to isoflurane-induced mTOR activation appears to have a threshold between 0.9% and 1.2% isoflurane, which is a dose that is clinically realistic as it represents less than 1 MAC for pediatric patients [37]. Furthermore, the duration of exposure required to generate a significant effect is strikingly short at 30 min, the briefest exposure that is practical in our system. This finding does call into question the clinical relevance of mTOR activation as the evidence from clinical trials suggests that anesthetic exposures under an hour do not have measurable effects on children [38,39]. However, it is reasonable to suppose that, in vivo, particularly in the setting of a complex brain with a long developmental timeline, there may be a high threshold for phenotypically detectable events, which exceeds the threshold for detectable change at the cellular and molecular levels. Nevertheless, the discrepancy between thresholds of toxicity in rodent models, humans, and non-human primates remains an unsolved problem in the field of anesthetic toxicity in neuro-development [40].

2.4. Effects of Isoflurane Exposure on the mTORC1 and mTORC2 Pathway

The mTOR pathway has two principal branches, which arise from mTORC1 and mTORC2. These pathways perform biologically distinct functions in some settings, but there is substantial communication between them [41]. We next sought to determine whether the effects of isoflurane are mediated through one branch of the pathway. This was accomplished via a series of experiments using mTOR pathway inhibitors with differential effects between mTORC1 and mTORC2, and by measuring levels of immunoreactivity of downstream phospho-proteins that are activated differentially between the pathway branches. Inhibitors were added into the media one hour before the 1.8% isoflurane/carrier gas exposure at 7 DIV for a harvest at 10 DIV (Figure 5A). The concentrations of the inhibitor were maintained after the exposure by media change with fresh inhibitor on 8 DIV and 9 DIV. The branch specific inhibitor and readout strategy (shown in Figure 4B) is as follows: PP242 was used as an inhibitor to block both mTORC1 and mTORC2 pathways simultaneously. Rapamycin was used as an mTORC1-specific pathway inhibitor. Ser473 phosphorylated Akt (pAkt, Ser473) was used as an mTORC2 downstream activity marker, while Thr389 phosphorylated 70S6 (p70S6, Thr389) was used as an activity marker downstream from mTORC1 (Figure 5B). The combination of these inhibitors and markers has been shown to be effective in differentiating activity in between the mTORC1 and mTORC2 branches [42].

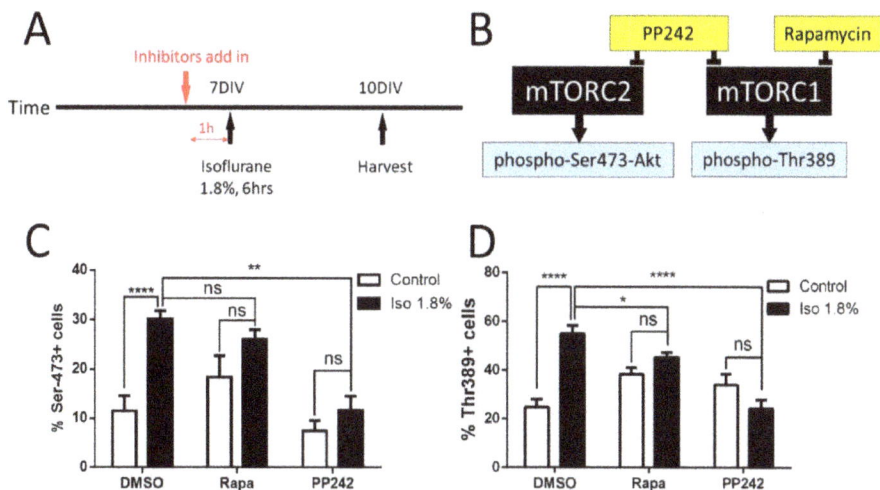

Figure 5. Effects of 1.8% isoflurane exposure for 6 h on the downstream marker of mTORC1 and mTORC2 pathway. (**A**) The timeline for adding mTORC1/mTORC2 inhibitors. The inhibitors were added to the media 1 h before the 1.8% isoflurane/carrier gas exposure on 7 DIV. The cells were fixed for immunohistochemistry on 10 DIV; (**B**). Visual diagram showing the inhibition of PP242 and rapamycin on mTORC1 and mTORC2 pathways, (**C,D**) For the mTORC2 downstream marker Ser473-Akt, there is a significant increase after 1.8% isoflurane exposure for 6 h on 7 DIV compared to the control group. Adding rapamycin did not fully reverse it back to normal, but adding PP242 made a significant difference between the isoflurane + PP242 and isoflurane + DMSO groups, while the positive Ser-473 cells returned back to normal compared to the control + PP242 group. This indicates that the mTORC2 pathway is involved in the isoflurane neurotoxicity changes (**C**). For the mTORC1 downstream marker Thr389, isoflurane exposure increased its immunoactivity significantly, while adding either rapamycin or PP242 reversed its immunoactivity back to normal. This indicates that mTORC1 pathway is also involved in the deficiency of neuron growth caused by isoflurane as well (**D**). ($n = 15$ fields that were measured per group, * $p < 0.05$, ** $p < 0.01$, **** $p < 0.0001$, n.s. indicates no significant difference, two-way ANOVA with Bonferroni's multiple comparisons test for (**C,D**).

We found a significant difference in the percentage of pAkt positive neurons between the isoflurane + vehicle (DMSO) group ($30.19 \pm 6.12\%$) and the control + vehicle (DMSO) group ($11.45 \pm 11.71\%$, $p < 0.0001$). As expected, with the significant interaction between isoflurane and inhibitor treatments using two-way ANOVA with Bonferroni's multiple comparisons test, rapamycin treatment did not change the pAkt levels which were shown in the isoflurane + rapamycin group ($26.09 \pm 7.04\%$) compared to the isoflurane + DMSO group, but there was a significant difference between the isoflurane + PP242 group ($14.60 \pm 14.50\%$) compared to the isoflurane + DMSO group ($p < 0.01$). A comparison between the isoflurane + PP242 group and the control + PP242 group ($4.16 \pm 5.27\%$) showed no significant difference (Figure 5C). Taken together, this data suggests that the mTORC2 pathway is involved in the toxic effect of isoflurane on neurons. There was a significant increase in the percentage of Thr-389 positive cells among all the DAPI/Tubulin neurons between the isoflurane + vehicle (DMSO) group (54.88 ± 10.56%) compared to those of the control + vehicle (DMSO) group (24.67 ± 10.19%, $p < 0.0001$) while there was a significant interaction between isoflurane and inhibitor treatments using two-way ANOVA with Bonferroni's multiple comparisons test (Figure 4D). Adding rapamycin before the exposure prevented the changes in Thr-389 levels (45.37 ± 6.09%) seen with the isoflurane + DMSO group ($p < 0.05$), and there was a significant difference between the isoflurane + PP242 group (24.22 ± 13.66%) compared to the isoflurane + DMSO group ($p < 0.0001$). Comparison between the isoflurane + PP242 group and the control + PP242 group (34.15 ± 16.55%) showed no significant difference (Figure 5D). Taken together, these data indicate that isoflurane acts on both the mTORC1 and mTORC2 branches. This is principally significant because it shows that therapeutic strategies cannot be designed around only one pathway branch or the other, unless it can be determined that the deleterious effects occur downstream of only one of the two branches.

2.5. Effects of Sevoflurane and Propofol on the Downstream Marker of the mTOR Pathway

A key question in developmental anesthesia toxicity is whether unwanted effects of anesthetic agents could be avoided through different choices of the primary anesthetic drug used. Thus, we asked what the effects of sevoflurane, the most commonly used volatile agent in pediatric anesthesia practice, and propofol, which is an intravenous agent that serves as the next likely alternative to isoflurane or sevoflurane, are on the mTOR pathway. Sevoflurane exposure in cultured neurons was accomplished using the same methods used for isoflurane exposure. Propofol exposure was accomplished by adding propofol in a carrier to the culture media, followed by media replacement at the appropriate time to terminate the exposure.

We measured the effect of a range of clinically relevant concentrations of sevoflurane and propofol delivered at 7 DIV on pS6 levels measures at 10 DIV. Using one-way ANOVA with Dunnett's multiple comparisons test, we found no significant difference in the percentage of neurons positive for pS6 between the 0.9% sevoflurane group (22.29 ± 14.86%) or the 1.8% sevoflurane group (26.03 ± 10.52%) and the control group (23.85 ± 18.39%) (Figure 6A). However, at 2.7% sevoflurane (59.00 ± 12.11%, $p < 0.0001$), 3.6% sevoflurane (71.35 ± 21.27%, $p < 0.0001$), and 4.5% sevoflurane group (42.39 ± 20.91%, $p < 0.05$), there was a significant increase in the percentage of pS6+ neurons over control (Figure 5A). With the significant interaction between isoflurane and rapamycin treatment using two-way ANOVA with Bonferroni's multiple comparisons test, rapamycin prevented the increase in pS6 labeling with 3.6% sevoflurane exposure (45.13 ± 8.77% for sevoflurane plus rapamycin compared to 39.42 ± 10.10% for rapamycin plus carrier gas, no significant difference) (Figure 6B). One adult MAC of sevoflurane is approximately 1.8% and, thus, compared to isoflurane, a higher dose of sevoflurane, which is at the high end of a clinically-reasonable concentration, is required to show an increase in pS6 expression.

Next, we tested the effects of propofol on pS6 expression. There was a significant increase in the percentage of pS6 positive cells measured in the 1nM propofol group (22.71 ± 5.46%, $p < 0.0001$), the 2 nM propofol group (23.96 ± 6.78%, $p < 0.0001$), and the 4 nM propofol group (29.02 ± 5.30%, $p < 0.0001$), compared to the control group (11.00 ± 6.52%) using one-way ANOVA with Dunnett's multiple comparisons test (Figure 6C). Adding rapamycin 1 h before the 2nM propofol exposure decreased the pS6 immunoactivity (15.02 ± 2.63%) compared to the ones without rapamycin treatment (28.96 ± 3.78%, $p < 0.01$), and there was no significant difference between the 2 nM propofol + rapamycin group and the control + rapamycin group (13.29 ± 4.50%) using two-way ANOVA with Bonferroni's multiple comparisons test, and there was a significant interaction between isoflurane and rapamycin treatment (Figure 6D). These data indicate that propofol may also mediate its effects though the mTOR pathway, although there is no clear way to draw equivalence in dosing between isoflurane or sevoflurane and propofol. One of the most practical strategies to potentially avoid anesthetic toxicity would be to choose drugs that do not activate pathways that result in toxic effects related to neural development. While numerous studies have identified mechanisms specific to either the potent volatile agents or to propofol [20], relatively few studies have conducted head-to-head comparisons between these two principal approaches to general anesthesia. Our data suggest to the extent that mTOR is a key mechanism in developmental anesthetic neurotoxicity, the choice of the agent may not be protective.

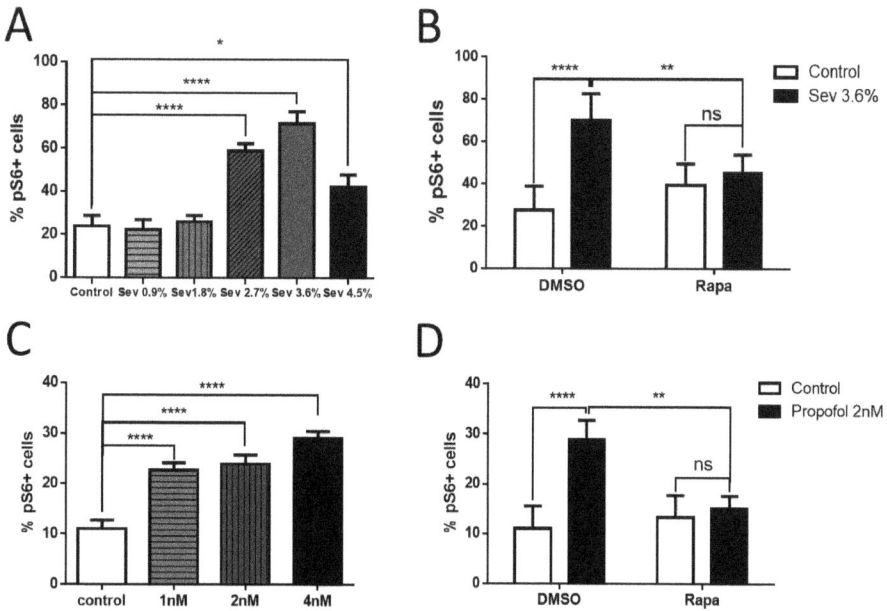

Figure 6. Effects of sevoflurane and propofol on the downstream marker of the mTOR pathway. (**A,B**) The effect on pS6 levels at 10 DIV varied depending on the doses of sevoflurane at 7 DIV. There was a significant increase in immunoactivity starting from the 2.7% sevoflurane group to the 4.5% sevoflurane group, while lower doses (0.9% and 1.8%) remained at control levels of pS6 (**A**). Rapamycin treatment prevented the increase in pS6 labeling with 3.6% sevoflurane exposure (**B**). (**C,D**) Different doses of propofol at 7 DIV had similar effects on pS6 levels at 10 DIV. There was a significant increase in pS6 immunoactivity starting from the 1 nM propofol group to the 4 nM propofol group (**C**). Rapamycin treatment prevented the increase in pS6 labeling with 2 nM propofol exposure (**D**). ($n = 15$ fields that were measured per group, * $p < 0.05$, ** $p < 0.01$, **** $p < 0.0001$, n.s. indicates no significant difference, one-way ANOVA with Dunnett's multiple comparisons test for (**A,C**), two-way ANOVA with Bonferroni's multiple comparisons test for (**B,D**).

3. Materials and Methods

3.1. Neuronal Cultures

Primary neuron cultures were obtained from BrainBits, LLC (Springfield, IL, USA). Cultures consisted of dissociated neurons obtained from neocortex dissected from E18 Sprague Dawley rat embryos according to the company protocols. Neurons were plated on 12 mm glass coverslips at 16,000 cells/cm^2 and maintained in NbActiv4 medium (BrainBits, Springfield, IL, USA) with half media changes conducted three times per week. Pilot experiments showed over 95% of cells from these cultures were immunopositive for β-tubulin, suggesting a high degree of purity. Experiments were performed on neurons between 3 and 14 DIV, and all experiments incorporated coverslips cultured from a minimum of three individual litters of pups.

3.2. Anesthetic Agent Exposure

Coverslips in 12-well plates were placed in identical air-tight, humidified chambers (Billups-Rothenberg, Del Mar, CA, USA) as previously described [43]. Isoflurane (Baxter Healthcare Cooperation, Deerfield, IL, USA) or sevoflurane (AbbVie Inc., North Chicago, IL, USA) were delivered using an agent-specific, calibrated inline vaporizer (SuperaVet, Vaporizer Sales and Services Inc., Rockmart, GA, USA), and were diluted in 5% CO_2/95% O_2 carrier gas. Controls for these experiments received 5% CO_2/95% O_2 carrier gas only. There was a 15-min equilibration period, which was required to achieve the correct concentration of isoflurane or sevoflurane as measured by a 5250 RGM gas analyzer (Datex-Ohmeda, Madison, WI, USA). Then the sealed chambers were placed in an incubator to maintain temperature at 37 °C for the duration of anesthesia exposure. Isoflurane/sevoflurane concentration was periodically measured at the end of the experimental period to verify that it was appropriately maintained throughout the exposure.

The propofol exposure was done by adding pure 2,6-diisopropylphenol (Sigma Aldrich, Saint Louis, MO, USA) (1 nM, 2 nM, 4 nM) into experiment wells, and incubated at 37 °C for the duration of anesthesia exposure. The exposure was terminated by removing all the media and by adding a combination of previously-removed media without propofol and fresh media.

3.3. The mTOR Pathway Inhibition

The mTOR inhibitors used in this study were as follows: PP242 at 1 µM (EMD Millipore, Billerica, MA, USA), and rapamycin at 100 nM (Sigma Aldrich, Saint Louis, MO, USA). They were used to inhibit mTORC1 or mTORC2, which are distinct functional pathways of the mTOR pathway. The same volume of the vehicle (DMSO) was added to the control groups. The neurons were pretreated with inhibitors 1 h before isoflurane or carrier gas exposure. The inhibitor concentration was maintained until the time of fixation by incorporating inhibitor in media changes.

3.4. TUNEL Assay

After isoflurane exposure, cells were harvested either immediately after the exposure or 24 h later. Neurons on coverslips were briefly fixed with 4% paraformaldehyde at room temperature for 10 min, then permeabilized and blocked for 1 h at room temperature in 5% donkey serum with 0.1% Triton X-100. Apoptosis was detected using an in situ cell death detection kit (Roche, Mannheim, Germany) and neurons were mounted on coverslips using 2.5% PVA/DABCO Mounting Media. An apoptotic index (AI) was defined as the number of TUNEL positive cells per field (400×) under a Leica SP8 confocal microscope (Leica, Wetzlar, Germany).

3.5. Immunocytochemistry

Fluorescent immunocytochemistry and labeling with fluorescently tagged F-actin was conducted as previously described [44]. Neurons on coverslips were briefly fixed with 4% paraformaldehyde at room temperature for 10 min, then permeabilized and blocked for 1 h at room temperature in 5% donkey serum with 0.1% Triton X-100. Neurons were incubated overnight at 4 °C in using the following antibodies: rabbit-anti-Synapsin-1 (1:200, EMD Millipore, Burlington, MA, USA), chicken-anti-Homer-1 (1:400, Synaptic Systems, Goettingen, Germany), mouse-anti-MAP-2 (1:200, Abcam, Cambridge, MA, USA), rabbit anti-human phospho-p70S6K (Thr-389, 1:1000, EMD Millipore, Billrecia, MA, USA), rabbit anti-human phospho-AKT (Ser-473,1:500, Cell Signaling Technologies, Danvers, MA, USA), rabbit anti-human S6 (1:100, Cell Signaling Technologies, Danvers, MA, USA), rabbit anti-human phospho-S6 (Ser-235/236, Cell Signaling Technologies, Danvers, MA, USA), and chicken-anti-human anti-β-III Tubulin (Tuj 1, 1:1000, EMD Millipore, Billrecia, MA, USA). All the antibodies were diluted in phosphate-buffered saline solution containing 0.1% Triton X-100. After rinsing, neurons were incubated for 2 h with a fluorescent secondary antibody and 4′,6-diamidino-2-phenylindole (DAPI) at the manufacturer's recommended concentration (Jackson Immuno Research Labs, West Grove, PA, USA). Subsequently, neurons were mounted on coverslips using 2.5% PVA/DABCO mounting medium.

3.6. Imaging and Microscopic Analysis

A Leica SP8 confocal microscope was used to capture all microscopic images. Cell counting analyses were conducted manually. Excluding the coverslips for TUNEL assay, the counting field for each coverslip was conducted by capturing five 63× fields that were selected to represent all four quadrants and the center of the coverslip. Neuronal cell bodies were identified as those positive for both β-III Tubulin and DAPI, and representative images were taken using a 63× 1.0 N.A. objective with an additional 1.0× magnification lens in line. For the synaptic marker analysis, five neurons from each sample were evenly distributed throughout the coverslip to represent all four quadrants and the center was randomly selected for analysis. Images were taken using a 63× 1.0 N.A. objective with an additional 5× magnification lens in line. One dendrite was picked according to MAP-2 staining from each neuron and the locations for image taken were defined as 20–30 μm from the nucleus according to DAPI. Synaptic puncta were quantified using ImageJ software (NIH, Bethesda, MD, USA). The dendrite segment outline was traced and the area quantification was done according to the MAP-2 channel, and the threshold was maintained the same for the synaptic marker channel. The intensity of Synapsin-1/Homer-1 puncta inside the dendrite outline was measured and recorded. For TUNEL assay, neuronal cell bodies were identified as those positive for DAPI, and representative images were taken using a 40× 1.0 N.A. objective with an additional 1.0× magnification lens in line. The counting field for each coverslip was conducted by capturing five 40× fields that were selected to represent all four quadrants and the center of the coverslip. Both imaging and analysis were conducted by an investigator blind to the conditions.

3.7. Statistical Analysis

Results are expressed as mean ± SEM. All statistical analysis was conducted using Prism 6.0 (GraphPad, San Diego, CA, USA). Student's *t*-test was used to determining statistical differences between each experiment group and the control-group data. One-way ANOVA with Dunnett's multiple comparisons was used for the data with group number over two. Two-way ANOVA with Bonferroni's multiple comparisons were used between groups that have the same exposure condition but different inhibitor treatments. All data examined with parametric tests were determined to be normally distributed and were conducted by an investigator blind to the conditions. Statistical significance for all tests were set a priori at $p < 0.05$.

4. Conclusions

In summary, we conclude that the potent volatile anesthetics and propofol, which are the mainstays of nearly all pediatric anesthetics, all have the capacity to up-regulate signaling in both branches of the mTOR pathway, mTOR1 and mTOR2, in neurons during synaptogenesis. Anesthetic exposure in this setting inhibits synaptogenesis, and this effect is reversible with the mTOR inhibitor, rapamycin. Our study has several limitations, principally related to the study of neural development in culture, where there is no patterned activity. In addition, because manipulation of mTOR via genetic means is problematic, only pharmacologic inhibition was used. Nevertheless, we believe that future studies of mTOR as a putative mechanism for developmental anesthetic neurotoxicity in dissociated culture will prove informative, and that questions about which types of neurons and synapses are at risk and what the effects on neural function are could be successfully addressed in this model system.

Author Contributions: Data curation: J.X., C.C. and Y.F.; formal analysis: J.X.; funding acquisition: J.X. and C.D.M.; methodology: J.X., R.P.M., M.X., C.C., Y.F., and C.D.M.; software: J.X. and R.P.M.; supervision: P.Z. and C.D.M.; writing—original draft: J.X. and C.D.M.; Writing—review and editing: R.P.M., M.X., Y.W., C.C., Y.F., P.Z., and C.D.M.

Funding: This research was funded by 1R01GM120519-01 to C.D.M., and a grant from the Chinese Scholarship Council (201606280280) to J.X.

Conflicts of Interest: The authors declare no conflict of interest. The funders had no role in the design of the study; in the collection, analyses, or interpretation of data; in the writing of the manuscript; or in the decision to publish the results.

Abbreviations

GA	General anesthetics
mTOR	Mechanistic target of rapamycin
mTORC1	mTOR 1 complex
mTORC2	mTOR 2 complex
DIV	Days in vitro
DAPI	4',6-diamidino-2-phenylindole
DMSO	Dimethyl sulfoxide
pS6	Phosphorylated S6
MAC	Minimum alveolar concentration
Ser473	Ser473 phosphorylated Akt
Thr389	Thr389 phosphorylated 70S6

References

1. Tzong, K.Y.; Han, S.; Roh, A.; Ing, C. Epidemiology of pediatric surgical admissions in US children: Data from the HCUP kids inpatient database. *J. Neurosurg. Anesthesiol.* **2012**, *24*, 391–395. [CrossRef] [PubMed]
2. Davidson, A.J.; Disma, N.; de Graaff, J.C.; Withington, D.E.; Dorris, L.; Bell, G.; Stargatt, R.; Bellinger, D.C.; Schuster, T.; Arnup, S.J.; et al. Neurodevelopmental outcome at 2 years of age after general anaesthesia and awake-regional anaesthesia in infancy (GAS): An international multicentre, randomised controlled trial. *Lancet* **2016**, *387*, 239–250. [CrossRef]
3. Sun, L.S.; Li, G.; Miller, T.L.; Salorio, C.; Byrne, M.W.; Bellinger, D.C.; Ing, C.; Park, R.; Radcliffe, J.; Hays, S.R.; et al. Association Between a Single General Anesthesia Exposure before Age 36 Months and Neurocognitive Outcomes in Later Childhood. *JAMA* **2016**, *315*, 2312–2320. [CrossRef] [PubMed]
4. DiMaggio, C.; Sun, L.S.; Li, G. Early childhood exposure to anesthesia and risk of developmental and behavioral disorders in a sibling birth cohort. *Anesthesia Analg.* **2011**, *113*, 1143–1151. [CrossRef] [PubMed]
5. Ing, C.; Dimaggio, C.; Whitehouse, A.; Hegarty, M.K.; Brady, J.; von Ungern-Sternberg, B.S.; Davidson, A.; Wood, A.J.; Li, G.; Sun, L.S. Long-term Differences in Language and Cognitive Function After Childhood Exposure to Anesthesia. *Pediatrics* **2012**, *130*, e476–e485. [CrossRef] [PubMed]
6. Wilder, R.T.; Flick, R.P.; Sprung, J.; Katusic, S.K.; Barbaresi, W.J.; Mickelson, C.; Gleich, S.J.; Schroeder, D.R.; Weaver, A.L.; Warner, D.O. Early exposure to anesthesia and learning disabilities in a population-based birth cohort. *Anesthesiology* **2009**, *110*, 796–804. [CrossRef] [PubMed]
7. Jevtovic-Todorovic, V.; Hartman, R.E.; Izumi, Y.; Benshoff, N.D.; Dikranian, K.; Zorumski, C.F.; Olney, J.W.; Wozniak, D.F. Early exposure to common anesthetic agents causes widespread neurodegeneration in the developing rat brain and persistent learning deficits. *J. Neurosci. Off. J. Soc. Neurosci.* **2003**, *23*, 876–882. [CrossRef]
8. Kang, E.; Jiang, D.; Ryu, Y.K.; Lim, S.; Kwak, M.; Gray, C.D.; Xu, M.; Choi, J.H.; Junn, S.; Kim, J.; et al. Early postnatal exposure to isoflurane causes cognitive deficits and disrupts development of newborn hippocampal neurons via activation of the mTOR pathway. *PLoS Biol.* **2017**, *15*, e2001246. [CrossRef] [PubMed]
9. Lee, B.H.; Chan, J.T.; Hazarika, O.; Vutskits, L.; Sall, J.W. Early exposure to volatile anesthetics impairs long-term associative learning and recognition memory. *PLoS ONE* **2014**, *9*, e105340. [CrossRef] [PubMed]
10. Levin, E.D.; Uemura, E.; Bowman, R.E. Neurobehavioral toxicology of halothane in rats. *Neurotoxicol. Teratol.* **1991**, *13*, 461–470. [CrossRef]
11. Sanders, R.D.; Xu, J.; Shu, Y.; Januszewski, A.; Halder, S.; Fidalgo, A.; Sun, P.; Hossain, M.; Ma, D.; Maze, M. Dexmedetomidine attenuates isoflurane-induced neurocognitive impairment in neonatal rats. *Anesthesiology* **2009**, *110*, 1077–1085. [CrossRef] [PubMed]

12. Satomoto, M.; Satoh, Y.; Terui, K.; Miyao, H.; Takishima, K.; Ito, M.; Imaki, J. Neonatal exposure to sevoflurane induces abnormal social behaviors and deficits in fear conditioning in mice. *Anesthesiology* **2009**, *110*, 628–637. [CrossRef] [PubMed]

13. Stratmann, G.; Sall, J.W.; May, L.D.; Bell, J.S.; Magnusson, K.R.; Rau, V.; Visrodia, K.H.; Alvi, R.S.; Ku, B.; Lee, M.T.; et al. Isoflurane differentially affects neurogenesis and long-term neurocognitive function in 60-day-old and 7-day-old rats. *Anesthesiology* **2009**, *110*, 834–848. [CrossRef] [PubMed]

14. Fang, F.; Xue, Z.; Cang, J. Sevoflurane exposure in 7-day-old rats affects neurogenesis, neurodegeneration and neurocognitive function. *Neurosci. Bull.* **2012**, *28*, 499–508. [CrossRef] [PubMed]

15. Gonzales, E.L.; Yang, S.M.; Choi, C.S.; Mabunga, D.F.; Kim, H.J.; Cheong, J.H.; Ryu, J.H.; Koo, B.N.; Shin, C.Y. Repeated neonatal propofol administration induces sex-dependent long-term impairments on spatial and recognition memory in rats. *Biomol. Ther.* **2015**, *23*, 251–260. [CrossRef] [PubMed]

16. Alvarado, M.C.; Murphy, K.L.; Baxter, M.G. Visual recognition memory is impaired in rhesus monkeys repeatedly exposed to sevoflurane in infancy. *Br. J. Anaesth.* **2017**, *119*, 517–523. [CrossRef] [PubMed]

17. Coleman, K.; Robertson, N.D.; Dissen, G.A.; Neuringer, M.D.; Martin, L.D.; Cuzon Carlson, V.C.; Kroenke, C.; Fair, D.; Brambrink, A.M. Isoflurane Anesthesia Has Long-term Consequences on Motor and Behavioral Development in Infant Rhesus Macaques. *Anesthesiology* **2017**, *126*, 74–84. [CrossRef] [PubMed]

18. Raper, J.; Alvarado, M.C.; Murphy, K.L.; Baxter, M.G. Multiple Anesthetic Exposure in Infant Monkeys Alters Emotional Reactivity to an Acute Stressor. *Anesthesiology* **2015**, *123*, 1084–1092. [CrossRef] [PubMed]

19. Raper, J.; De Biasio, J.C.; Murphy, K.L.; Alvarado, M.C.; Baxter, M.G. Persistent alteration in behavioural reactivity to a mild social stressor in rhesus monkeys repeatedly exposed to sevoflurane in infancy. *Br. J. Anaesth.* **2018**, *120*, 761–767. [CrossRef] [PubMed]

20. Vutskits, L.; Xie, Z. Lasting impact of general anaesthesia on the brain: Mechanisms and relevance. *Nat. Rev. Neurosci.* **2016**, *17*, 705–717. [CrossRef] [PubMed]

21. Yu, D.; Li, L.; Yuan, W. Neonatal anesthetic neurotoxicity: Insight into the molecular mechanisms of long-term neurocognitive deficits. *Biomed. Pharmacother. Biomedecine Pharmacother.* **2017**, *87*, 196–199. [CrossRef] [PubMed]

22. Laplante, M.; Sabatini, D.M. mTOR signaling in growth control and disease. *Cell* **2012**, *149*, 274–293. [CrossRef] [PubMed]

23. Takei, N.; Nawa, H. mTOR signaling and its roles in normal and abnormal brain development. *Front. Mol. Neurosci.* **2014**, *7*, 28. [CrossRef] [PubMed]

24. Costa-Mattioli, M.; Monteggia, L.M. mTOR complexes in neurodevelopmental and neuropsychiatric disorders. *Nat. Neurosci.* **2013**, *16*, 1537–1543. [CrossRef] [PubMed]

25. Xu, J.; Kang, E.; Mintz, C.D. Anesthetics disrupt brain development via actions on the mTOR pathway. *Commun. Integr. Boil.* **2018**, e1451719. [CrossRef]

26. Goslin, K.; Banker, G. Experimental observations on the development of polarity by hippocampal neurons in culture. *J. Cell Boil.* **1989**, *108*, 1507–1516. [CrossRef]

27. Amrock, L.G.; Starner, M.L.; Murphy, K.L.; Baxter, M.G. Long-term effects of single or multiple neonatal sevoflurane exposures on rat hippocampal ultrastructure. *Anesthesiology* **2015**, *122*, 87–95. [CrossRef] [PubMed]

28. Lunardi, N.; Ori, C.; Erisir, A.; Jevtovic-Todorovic, V. General anesthesia causes long-lasting disturbances in the ultrastructural properties of developing synapses in young rats. *Neurotox. Res.* **2010**, *17*, 179–188. [CrossRef] [PubMed]

29. Briner, A.; Nikonenko, I.; De Roo, M.; Dayer, A.; Muller, D.; Vutskits, L. Developmental Stage-dependent persistent impact of propofol anesthesia on dendritic spines in the rat medial prefrontal cortex. *Anesthesiology* **2011**, *115*, 282–293. [CrossRef] [PubMed]

30. Jevtovic-Todorovic, V. General Anesthetics and Neurotoxicity: How Much Do We Know? *Anesthesiol. Clin.* **2016**, *34*, 439–451. [CrossRef] [PubMed]

31. Lei, X.; Guo, Q.; Zhang, J. Mechanistic insights into neurotoxicity induced by anesthetics in the developing brain. *Int. J. Mol. Sci.* **2012**, *13*, 6772–6799. [CrossRef] [PubMed]

32. Banker, G.; Goslin, K. *Culturing Nerve Cells*, 2nd ed.; MIT Press: Cambridge, UK, 1998; 666p.

33. Zhang, W.; Benson, D.L. Stages of synapse development defined by dependence on F-actin. *J. Neurosci. Off. J. Soc. Neurosci.* **2001**, *21*, 5169–5181. [CrossRef]

34. Lemkuil, B.P.; Head, B.P.; Pearn, M.L.; Patel, H.H.; Drummond, J.C.; Patel, P.M. Isoflurane neurotoxicity is mediated by p75NTR-RhoA activation and actin depolymerization. *Anesthesiology* **2011**, *114*, 49–57. [CrossRef] [PubMed]

35. Lunardi, N.; Hucklenbruch, C.; Latham, J.R.; Scarpa, J.; Jevtovic-Todorovic, V. Isoflurane impairs immature astroglia development in vitro: The role of actin cytoskeleton. *J. Neuropathol. Exp. Neurol.* **2011**, *70*, 281–291. [CrossRef] [PubMed]

36. Brown, R.E., Jr. Safety considerations of anesthetic drugs in children. *Expert Opin. Drug Saf.* **2017**, *16*, 445–454. [CrossRef] [PubMed]

37. Murray, D.J.; Mehta, M.P.; Forbes, R.B. The additive contribution of nitrous oxide to isoflurane MAC in infants and children. *Anesthesiology* **1991**, *75*, 186–190. [CrossRef] [PubMed]

38. Sun, L. Early childhood general anaesthesia exposure and neurocognitive development. *Br. J. Anaesth.* **2010**, *105* (Suppl. 1), i61–i68. [CrossRef] [PubMed]

39. Sanders, R.D.; Hassell, J.; Davidson, A.J.; Robertson, N.J.; Ma, D. Impact of anaesthetics and surgery on neurodevelopment: An update. *Br. J. Anaesth.* **2013**, *110* (Suppl. 1), i53–i72. [CrossRef] [PubMed]

40. Rappaport, B.A.; Suresh, S.; Hertz, S.; Evers, A.S.; Orser, B.A. Anesthetic neurotoxicity—Clinical implications of animal models. *N. Engl. J. Med.* **2015**, *372*, 796–797. [CrossRef] [PubMed]

41. Dowling, R.J.; Topisirovic, I.; Fonseca, B.D.; Sonenberg, N. Dissecting the role of mTOR: Lessons from mTOR inhibitors. *Biochim. Biophys. Acta* **2010**, *1804*, 433–439. [CrossRef] [PubMed]

42. Warren, K.J.; Fang, X.; Gowda, N.M.; Thompson, J.J.; Heller, N.M. The TORC1-activated Proteins, p70S6K and GRB10, Regulate IL-4 Signaling and M2 Macrophage Polarization by Modulating Phosphorylation of Insulin Receptor Substrate-2. *J. Boil. Chem.* **2016**, *291*, 24922–24930. [CrossRef] [PubMed]

43. Mintz, C.D.; Barrett, K.M.; Smith, S.C.; Benson, D.L.; Harrison, N.L. Anesthetics interfere with axon guidance in developing mouse neocortical neurons in vitro via a gamma-aminobutyric acid type A receptor mechanism. *Anesthesiology* **2013**, *118*, 825–833. [CrossRef] [PubMed]

44. Mintz, C.D.; Smith, S.C.; Barrett, K.M.; Benson, D.L. Anesthetics interfere with the polarization of developing cortical neurons. *J. Neurosurg. Anesthesiol.* **2012**, *24*, 368–375. [CrossRef] [PubMed]

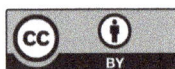

International Journal of
Molecular Sciences

MDPI

Review

Role of mTOR in Glucose and Lipid Metabolism

Zhuo Mao [1] and Weizhen Zhang [1,2,*]

[1]   Center for Diabetes, Obesity and Metabolism, Department of Physiology, Shenzhen University Health
      Science Center, Shenzhen 518060, China; maoz@szu.edu.cn
[2]   Department of Physiology and Pathophysiology, Peking University Health Science Center,
      Beijing 100191, China
*   Correspondence: weizhenzhang@bjmu.edu.cn; Tel.: +86-150-1090-9001

Received: 31 May 2018; Accepted: 11 July 2018; Published: 13 July 2018

Abstract: The mammalian target of rapamycin, mTOR is the master regulator of a cell's growth and metabolic state in response to nutrients, growth factors and many extracellular cues. Its dysregulation leads to a number of metabolic pathological conditions, including obesity and type 2 diabetes. Here, we review recent findings on the role of mTOR in major metabolic organs, such as adipose tissues, liver, muscle, pancreas and brain. And their potentials as the mTOR related pharmacological targets will be also discussed.

Keywords: mTOR; metabolic diseases; glucose and lipid metabolism

---

Multicellular organisms evolve essential mechanisms to sense and accommodate the ever-changing extracellular environments for their survival and growth. The mechanistic target of rapamycin (mTOR) signaling is the most important intracellular pathway that coordinates local nutrients and systemic energy status at the organismal and cellular level. Dysregulation in mTOR signaling is associated with various diseases such as obesity, type 2 diabetes, cancer, and neurological diseases [1]. Obesity and over-nutrition induce a chronic hyper-activation of mTOR activity in multiple tissues [2–4]. In turn, mTOR signaling dysregulation may facilitate the development of type 2 diabetes mellitus (T2DM) or insulin resistance. In this review, we provide a comprehensive summary on the mTOR signaling in the regulation of glucose and lipid metabolism. We will focus on the recent findings about the role of mTOR complex (mTORC) pathways in the regulation of energy balance and metabolism in key metabolic tissues, including adipose tissue, liver, skeletal muscle, pancreas and the brain. We will also briefly discuss the therapeutic potential of mTOR signaling for the metabolic disorders.

1. mTOR Signaling

mTOR is the conserved serine/threonine kinase which exists in two distinct multi-complexes with different protein components and downstream substrates: mTOR complex 1 (mTORC1) and mTOR complex 2 (mTORC2) (Figure 1). Both two complexes shared some common protein components: mTOR (a serine/threonine protein kinase), mLST8 (mammalian lethal with sec-13 protein 8) and DEPTOR (DEP-domain containing mTOR-interacting protein). The additional mTORC1 complex proteins include scaffold protein Raptor (regulatory-associated protein of TOR) and Akt substrate protein PRAS40 (proline-rich Akt substrate 40 kDa). The mTORC2 core components include scaffold protein Rictor (rapamycin insensitive companion of mTOR), mSIN1 (stress-activated protein kinase-interacting protein 1), and protein observed with rictor 1 and 2 (PROTOR1/2) [1,3].

mTORC1 mainly maintains a cellular balance between anabolism and catabolism in response to the environmental cues such as growth factors, amino acids, and stress. Growth factors such as insulin and insulin-like growth factor (IGF) regulate mTORC1 through phosphoinositide 3-kinase (PI3K)-AKT-Tuberous sclerosis (TSC)-RHEB signaling. PI3K-AKT signaling phosphorylates, and inhibits TSC1 which is the GTPase-activating protein (GAP) for the RHEB (the small GTPase

Ras homologue enriched in brain), thus activating RHEB. mTORC1 activity is strongly enhanced by active RHEB. Amino acids activate mTORC signaling by stimulating the Rag family of GTPases, which promotes mTORC1 translocation to the lysosome and is activated by RHEB [5,6]. Stress such as hypoxia, DNA damage also signals to mTORC with multiple mechanisms while in general through TSC1/2 [3,7].

Activation of mTORC1 induces protein synthesis by promoting ribosome biogenesis and mRNA translation. The major downstream effectors of mTORC1 are the ribosomal S6 kinase (S6K) and the inhibitory eIF4E-binding proteins (4E-BPs). Activation of S6K by mTORC1 phosphorylates its downstream substrates such as ribosomal protein S6, protein synthesis initiation factor 4B (eIF4B), and elongation factor 2 kinase (eEF2K), which subsequently promote translation initiation and elongation. Phosphorylation of 4E-BP by mTORC1 dissociates its binding with the eukaryotic translation initiation factor 4F (eIF4F), promoting 5′ cap-dependent translation [1,8].

In addition to protein synthesis, activation of mTORC1 is sufficient to stimulate other metabolic pathways. For example, mTORC1 enhances nucleotide synthesis by increasing ATF-dependent expression of MTHFD2, the key enzyme in mitochondrial tetrahydrofolate (mTHF) cycle, increasing the production of purine nucleotides [9]. mTORC1 promotes de novo lipogenesis in SREBP1 dependent pathway either through S6K1 phosphorylation [10] or by modulating the Lipin 1 localization and SREBP1 expression [11]. mTORC1 also stimulates glycolysis and glucose uptake through modulating the transcription factor hypoxia-inducible factor (HIF1α) [10].

The autophagy-lysosome and ubiquitin-proteasome are two major pathways for protein and organelle turnover. mTORC1 is implicated in these two routes to affect protein degradation. ULK1 is the mammalian autophagy-initiating kinase which drives autophagosome formation. Under nutrient sufficient condition, mTORC1 phosphorylates ULK1 and prevents its activation by adenosine 5′-monophosphate (AMP)-activated protein kinase (AMPK), blocking autophagy induction [12]. mTORC1 activation suppresses lysosome pathway through inhibiting the activity of the master regulator of lysosomal biogenesis, transcription factor EB (TFEB). Nutrient deprivation or inhibition of mTORC1 activates TFEB by promoting its nuclear translocation, thus initiating the expression of lysosomal and autophagic genes [13]. Recently, two reports have demonstrated that the ubiquitin proteasome system (UPS) in mammalian cells is increased when mTORC1 signaling pathway is inactivated [14,15]. Therefore, mTORC1 activation induces a coordinated response between lysosomal and proteasomal degradation in order to meet the rising needs of cells.

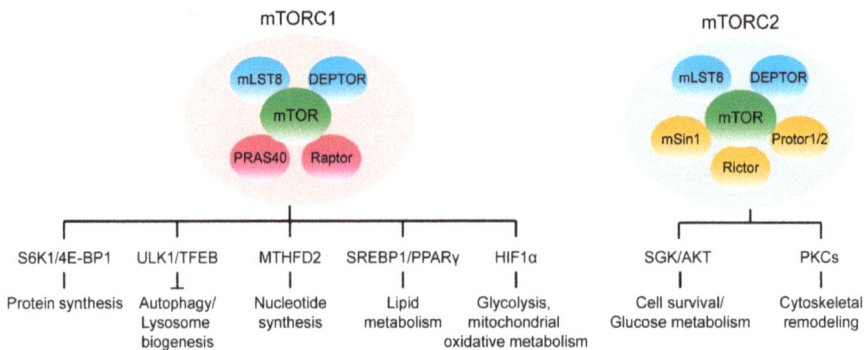

Figure 1. The protein components and the major downstream signaling pathway of mTORC1 and mTORC2. Simplified illustration of the protein components of mTORC1 and mTORC2 complex. Activation of mTORC1 promotes protein synthesis, nucleotide synthesis, lipogenesis, glycolysis, and inhibits autophagy and lysosome biogenesis. Alternatively, mTORC2 regulates cell survival/glucose metabolism and cytoskeletal remodeling.

Relative to mTORC1, the upstream signals and downstream substrates of mTORC2 are less known. mTORC2 can be activated by the growth factors such as insulin and IGF, but insensitive to the nutrients. Activated mTORC2 phosphorylates AGC kinase family, including AKT, SGK, and PKCα, to regulate cellular survival and metabolism, as well as cytoskeletal remodeling. The most well characterized substrate of mTORC2 is AKT which is phosphorylated at the serine 473. AKT could further phosphorylate TSC2, the upstream inhibitor of mTORC1. Therefore, activation of mTORC2 inactivates mTORC1. Vice versa, mTORC1-S6K axis could also directly phosphorylate mSIN1, the core component of mTORC2 and inactivate it. Therefore, mTORC1 and mTORC2 form a feedback loop regulating the complex activity.

2. mTOR Signaling in Adipose Tissue

Fat or adipose tissue is a critical organ in the development of obesity and insulin resistance. mTORC signaling has been involved in adipose tissue biology in multiple aspects. mTOR is critical for adipogenesis and maintenance of fat tissues. Adipocyte-specific mTOR knockout mice have reduced adipose tissue mass, insulin resistance and fatty liver, suggesting its critical role in adipogenesis and systemic energy metabolism [16]. The role of mTORC1 complex in adipose tissue has been examined using different transgenic mouse models, including genetic depletion of S6K, S6K1, and Raptor in systemic or adipose tissue specific manner. These models consistently showed that ablation of mTORC1 signaling induces reduced adipose tissue mass and resistance to diet-induced obesity. Recent finding has identified glutamylprolyl-tRNA synthetase (EPRS) as the downstream effector of mTORC1-S6K1 axis for adiposity. Activation of mTORC1-S6K1 phosphorylates EPRS at Ser999 and induces its release from the amino acyl tRNA multisynthetase complex. Phosphorylated EPRS interacts with fatty acid transport protein 1 (FATP1), promoting its translocation to the plasma membrane and importing fatty acid to the cells [17].

There are two major adipose tissues, white adipose tissue (WAT) and brown adipose tissue (BAT). WAT stores energy in the form of triglyceride droplets and BAT dissipates energy through uncoupled respiration and heat production. WAT is able to acquire brown fat characteristics, a process named browning or beigeing, which is an important physiological response to cold or stress. mTORC1 is involved in the conversion of these two adipose tissues. In 2015, Xiang et al. found that activation of mTORC1 in adipose tissue increases lipid accumulation in BAT which is associated with down-regulation of brown adipocyte markers and concurrent up-regulation of WAT markers. These observations indicate a phenotypic switch of BAT to WAT. Rapamycin treatment reverses this process in vivo and in cultured brown adipocytes [18]. Later, another study found that WAT browning stimulated by catecholamine also requires mTORC1 and Raptor. Catecholamine stimulates β3 adrenergic receptor mediated cAMP-PKA signaling. PKA phosphorylates mTOR and Raptor, thus initializes browning of WAT via mTORC1-S6K1 axis. Mice with genetic deletion of Raptor or treated with rapamycin are cold intolerant with decreased browning/beigeing ability [19,20].

The role of mTORC2 in adipose tissue has also been examined using adipose-specific deletion of mTORC2 core component Rictor in mice. These transgenic mice have increased body size and enlarged organs, such as pancreas and heart, indicating a role of adipose mTORC2 in controlling whole body growth [21]. In addition, Rictor-null adipose cells are unable to suppress lipolysis in response to insulin, leading to elevated circulating fatty acids and glycerol [22]. mTORC2 promotes the phosphorylation of the BSD domain containing signal transducer and Akt interactor (BSTA) and its interaction with Akt1. BSTA-Akt1 interaction suppresses the expression of FoxC2, the transcription factor critical for adipocyte differentiation [23]. Moreover, mTORC2 in adipose tissue promotes de novo lipogenesis and hepatic glucose metabolism through increasing the expression of the lipogenic transcription factor ChREBPβ [24]. The role of mTORC2 in BAT growth was examined using Myf5-Cre expressed BAT precursor cells. Rictor deficiency blocks the BAT differentiation and shifts BAT metabolism to a more oxidative and less lipogenic state and protects mice from obesity and metabolic disorders [25]. mTORC2 is also implicated in WAT browning process. β-adrenergic stimulation activates mTORC2 and stimulates Akt-mediated glucose uptake and glycolysis. Loss of mTORC2 in BAT leads to cold intolerance due to defective insulin stimulated glucose uptake [26].

In conclusion, mTORC1 participates in normal adipose tissue growth and BAT-WAT phenotypic switch. mTORC2 regulates fat cell and whole body organ size, systemic glucose and lipid metabolism and BAT differentiation.

3. mTOR Signaling in Liver

The liver is a critical organ for systemic metabolism. In the fasted state, the liver increases ketone body production (ketogenesis), providing energy sources for peripheral tissues. mTORC1 controls ketogenesis in mice in response to fasting. Hyperactivation of mTORC1 in liver leads to a pronounced defect in ketone body production and a fasting-resistant increase in liver size. PPARα (peroxisome proliferator activated receptor α) is the master transcriptional activator of ketongenic genes which is induced by fasting. Inhibition of mTOR is required for this process. Activation of mTORC1 suppresses PPARα activity and thus the ketone production [27].

In addition, activation of mTORC1 signaling stimulates de novo lipogenesis in hepatocytes [28]. mTORC1 regulates hepatic lipid metabolism mainly through SREBP1, the master regulator of lipid synthesis. It is initially synthesized as an inactive precursor and localized in the ER. In response to the insulin signaling, SREBP1 is cleaved and transported to the nucleus to induce lipogenic gene expression. Liver-specific inhibition of mTORC1 abrogates SREBP1 function and renders mice resistant to hepatic steatosis and hypercholesterolemia induced by the Western diet. In 2011, Peterson et al. found that mTORC1 regulates SREBP1 through controlling the nuclear entry of a phosphatidic acid phosphatase, Lipin 1. Normally, dephosphorylated Lipin1 traffics to the nucleus and inhibits SREBP transcriptional activity and SREBP protein abundance. mTORC1 could phosphorylate Lipin 1, preventing its translocation to nucleus and hence promoting SREBP1-mediated lipogenesis [11]. Later, Han et al. demonstrated that mTORC1 also regulates SREBP1's trafficking and maturation through CREB regulated transcription coactivator 2 (CRTC2). CRTC2 disrupts COPII dependent SREBP1 trafficking by competing with Sec23A for the interaction with Sec31A, and thus inhibits SREBP1's maturation and function. In the feeding state or under the insulin signaling, mTOR activation phosphorylates and attenuates its inhibitory effect on SREBP1 maturation, thus enhancing lipogenesis [29].

Raptor is the important component of mTORC1 signaling pathway. Raptor deficient mice or cellular models have been used to study the biological functions of mTORC1 inactivation. Recently, Kim et al. have found that there are two forms of Raptor in cells, the mTORC1-bound and the free state. Although mTORC1-Raptor promotes lipogenesis through SREBP1 as previously discussed, free Raptor could increase the Akt phosphatase PHLPP2 level and decrease hepatic Akt activity, thus suppressing lipogenesis. It is proposed that the balance between free and mTORC1-bound Raptor is an important modulation mechanism for hepatic lipid accumulation [30].

In addition, activation of mTORC1 regulates whole-body behavior and metabolism. Liver-specific Tsc1 knockout mice have reduced level of hepatic and plasma glutamine, leading to peroxisome proliferator—activated receptor γ coactivator-1α (PGC-1α)—dependent fibroblast growth factor 21 (FGF21) expression in the liver. FGF21 significantly impacts the locomotor activity, body temperature, and hepatic lipid content [31].

The Sestrins are a family of stress-inducible proteins which suppress mTORC1 signaling activity through activation of AMPK. There are three Sestrins, named Sestrin 1, Sestrin 2, and Sestrin 3 in mammals. Hepatic mTORC1 signaling is regulated by Sestrin2. Over-nutrition and obesity induces hepatic Sestrin 2 expression primarily through activation of ER stress signaling. Increased Sestrin 2 potentiates AMPK activation and suppresses mTORC1-S6K activity in the liver, alleviating insulin resistance and obesity associated nonalcoholic fatty liver disease (NAFLD) pathologies including steatohepatitis and hepatic fibrosis. Loss of Sestrin 2 in mice displayed hyperactivation of mTORC1-S6K signaling in the liver and leads to insulin resistance and glucose intolerance when fed with high fat diet [32,33]. In addition to Sestrin 2, metformin, the most widely used drug for T2DM patients, also regulates mTORC1 activity. Recently it is found that metformin robustly inhibits mTORC1 activity and protein synthesis in liver. This inhibition is dependent on AMPK and TSC complex [34].

Hepatic mTORC2 regulates glucose and lipid metabolism via AKT signaling. The role of hepatic mTORC2 has been examined in vivo using the mice lacking Rictor in liver. Deficient expression of mTORC2 in liver leads to defective insulin-stimulated AKT phosphorylation, resulting in constitutive gluconeogenesis, impaired glycolysis and lipogenesis by altering hepatic glucokinase and SREBP1c activity [35,36]. In addition, mTORC2 has been known to regulate gluconeogenesis and lipogenesis through a number of transcription factors including FOXO1, FOXA2, and PPARγ. Genomic and phosphoproteomic analyses have shown that hepatic mTORC2 regulates a complex genetic expression which affects intermediary metabolism, ribosomal biogenesis, and proteasomal biogenesis. These findings suggest that hepatic mTORC2 exerts broad biological effects under physiological conditions [37]. Similar to Sestrin 2, Sestrin 3 is an upstream regulator of mTORC2 activity. Sestrin 3 interacts with Rictor to activate mTORC2 and AKT. Therefore, deletion of Sestrin 3 in the liver results in insulin resistance and glucose intolerance and Sestrin 3 transgenic mice are protected against insulin resistance induced by a high-fat diet [38].

mTORC1 and mTORC2 can be regulated by an upstream regulator Reptin, an AAA + ATPase that is overexpressed in hepatocellular carcinoma. In normal adult liver, Reptin exerts opposite regulation on mTORC1 and mTORC2. It activates mTORC1 activity while inactivates mTORC2 activity, thus regulating global glucido-lipidic homeostasis. Liver-specific ablation of Reptin strongly inhibits hepatic mTORC1 activity, leading to significant decrease in *de novo* lipogenesis and cholesterol production. Meanwhile, mTORC2 activity is greatly enhanced and hepatic glucose production is inhibited [39].

4. mTOR Signaling in Muscle

Skeletal muscle tissues comprise 40% of the total body lean mass and contributes to the regulation of whole-body metabolism in various ways. It is the main organ responsible for insulin-induced glucose uptake. Insulin resistance in skeletal muscle is the primary defect during the development of type 2 diabetes. The complex role of mTOR activity in skeletal muscle has been examined, as in other organs, using genetic deletion mouse models.

Skeletal muscle specific deletion of Raptor causes a number of symptoms, including shorter life expectancy, progressively dystrophic muscle with impaired oxidative capacity and increased glycogen stores [40,41]. Activation of mTORC1 signaling in muscle has been examined using mice model with TSC1 deletion specifically in muscle (TSCmKO mice). Although these mice are lean, they develop glucose intolerance and insulin resistance characterized by reduced glucose uptake in the muscle and reduced glycogen and lipid deposition in the liver under high fat diet condition [42,43]. The mechanism of mTORC1 activation induced insulin sensitivity has been examined elaborately. When mTORC1 is activated, S6K1 could directly phosphorylate IRS1 (S307 and S636/S639) and promote its degradation, which subsequently blunts PI3K-AKT activation and its downstream effects such as glucose uptake, glycogen accumulation, etc. [2,3].

Interestingly, the other mTORC1 substrate 4E-BP1 in skeletal muscle has a more general effect on systemic metabolism. Overexpression of the mTORC1-nonresponsive form 4E-BP1 in skeletal muscle results in increased energy expenditure, with enhanced respiratory activity both in skeletal muscle and brown fat. Increased PGC-1α activity and the myokine FGF21 expression may partially responsible for the altered metabolic effects in these two tissues [44].

Regulated in development and DNA damage response 1 (REDD1) is an upstream inhibitor of mTORC1 pathway. REDD1 suppresses mTORC1 signaling pathway through de-phosphorylation of AKT and activation of TSC1/TSC2 complex [45]. In turn, mTORC1 activation could stabilize NEDD1 protein as a mTORC1-REDD1 feedback loop [46]. Under the obese or T2DM condition, both mTORC1 signaling and REDD1 protein level are elevated in the skeletal muscle [47,48]. It is proposed that hyper-activation of mTORC1 stabilizes REDD1 protein, which inhibits insulin-induced

AKT phosphorylation, attenuating glucose uptake in the skeletal muscle. This may also contribute to hyperglycemia and insulin resistance in T2DM and obese patients [48].

It should be noted that mTORC1 activity exerts a significant effect on muscle mass by affecting autophagy process. Sustained activation of mTORC1 in skeletal muscle reduces muscle mass and muscle fiber size in old mice, leading to a late-onset myopathy which is tightly associated with other metabolic pathways [49]. Furthermore, skeletal muscle mass and function are also regulated by motor innervation. mTORC1 is substantially increased in denervated muscle. Mice with mTORC1 activation exhibited increased sensitivity to denervation-induced atrophy. These data reveal that mTORC1 is central to the muscle catabolism and atrophy [50]. The cause and effect relation between glucose metabolism and muscle mass upon mTORC1 activation in skeletal muscle remains to be explored.

The role of mTORC2 in muscle has been evaluated using muscle specific Rictor knockout mice. Similar to mTORC1, mTORC2 regulates insulin-mediated glucose uptake and glucose tolerance. The insulin stimulated phosphorylatin of AKT at Ser473 is significantly reduced in Rictor knockout mice. This alteration is associated with a defect in insulin signaling and the defective glucose transport [51]. Recently Klieinert et al. also found that muscle mTORC2 activity negatively modulates whole body lipid metabolism and intramyocellular triglyceride content through regulating the lipid droplet binding protein Perilipin 3 via FoxO1 [52,53].

5. mTOR Signaling in Pancreas

mTORC1 has been regarded as a positive regulator of beta cell mass, due to enhancement of beta cell growth and proliferation. The loss-of-function studies of mTOR signaling in vivo have been examined in mice deficient for mTOR or Raptor specifically in beta cells or pancreatic endocrine progenitor cells (mating with PDX1- or Neurog3-cre mice). These mice consistently exhibit reduced beta cells mass, defective postnatal islet development, hypoinsulinemia, and glucose intolerance [54–58]. Conversely, activation of mTORC1 signaling by deletion of TSC1 leads to beta cell hypertrophy and hyperinsulinemia [59]. These observations suggest that mTORC1 is critical for the islet development and function, and consequent glucose homeostasis. mTOR also protects islets from apoptosis by inhibiting the expression of thioredoxin-interacting protein (TXNIP), a potent inducer of β cell death and oxidative stress. TXNIP can be transcriptionally activated by the carbohydrate-response element–binding protein (ChREBP). mTOR physically interacts with ChREBP–Max-like protein complex, consequently suppressing its transcriptional activity on TXNIP [55].

However, study of constitutive activation of mTOR reveals a biphasic role of mTOR in the glucose homeostasis. Young mice with beta cell-specific deletion of TSC2 display beta cell hypertrophy, hyperinsulinemia, and improved glucose tolerance. On the other hand, beta cell mass in aging mice is gradually lost due to increased apoptosis, which triggers hyperglycemia [60,61]. Moreover, mTORC1 is aberrantly activated in islets from T2DM patients and diabetic mouse islets, suggesting that sustained hyperactivation of mTORC1 contributes to impaired beta cell function and survival upon the metabolic stress [4]. Chronic hyper-activation of mTORC1 signaling also results in impaired autophagy/mitophagy process and ER stress, evidenced by an accumulation of p62 protein (an indication of impaired autophagic response) and ER stress markers in the older TSC2 knockout beta cells [60]. Consistently, mTOR inhibition protects lipid accumulation, ER stress and beta cell dysfunction under nutrient overload conditions [4,62]. Therefore, mTORC1 activation increases beta cell mass and improves glucose metabolism in the short term, while sustained mTORC1 activation ultimately deteriorates beta cell mass and function, which is reminiscent in type 2 diabetic beta cells.

The molecular mechanisms underlying the detrimental effects of hyper-activation of mTOR signaling in beta cells has been elaborately reviewed recently [63]. Several mechanisms have been proposed: (1) mTORC1 directly phosphorylates IRS1/2 and promotes its degradation, impairs insulin signaling pathway and induces insulin resistance. (2) mTORC1 can phosphorylate and activate Growth-Factor-Bound Protein 10 (Grb10), which disrupts the interaction between IR and IRS1/2, induces IRS2 proteasomal degradation, and ultimately leads to defective insulin signaling pathway [64,65]. (3) mTORC1 can also phosphorylate mTORC2 components, such as Rictor and Sin1, abrogate mTORC2 activity and AKT signaling [66,67].

In addition to beta cells, mTORC1 also regulates α cell mass and glucagon secretion. Mice lacking Raptor specifically in α cell have normal α cell mass, but defective α cell maturation and glucagon secretion. FoxA2 is the downstream transcription factor regulating the critical genes responsible for α cell function [68]. Type 2 diabetes patients have elevated glucagon. Glucagon stimulates hepatic digestion of proteins to amino acids. Increased amino acids induce alpha cell hyperplasia by an mTORC1-dependent mechanism [69–71].

Similar to mTORC1, mTORC2 is also critical for maintaining beta cell mass and glucose homeostasis. Rictor null mice exhibits glucose intolerance caused by a reduction in β-cell mass, beta-cell proliferation, pancreatic insulin content, and glucose-stimulated insulin secretion [72]. In contrast to mTORC1, mTORC2 activity is declined in beta cells under diabetogenic conditions and in human diabetic islets [4].

6. mTOR Signaling in Brain

mTOR pathway has been implicated in neural development and neurodegenerative disorders [73]. Hypothalamus is the main structure in the central nervous system (CNS) involved in the control of glucose homeostasis and systemic energy balance. The hypothalamic region comprises several nuclei with distinct functions and serves as a hub which integrates nutrient and hormones signals, regulating the systemic energy balance. Within hypothalamus, mTOR functions as a cellular signaling hub which integrates internal and external cues to control the central or peripheral tissue functions [74].

In the hypothalamus, there are two groups of neurons, orexigenic neuropeptide Y (NPY), and agouti-related protein (AgRP) co-expressing neurons, and anorexigenic proopiomelanocortin (POMC) and cocaine and amphetamine related transcript (CART) co-expressing neurons. mTORC1 activity in the hypothalamus is complex and varies by cell and stimulus type. S6K is expressed in orexigenic NPY and AgRP neurons, as well as POMC neurons, both of which are critically involved in the regulation of energy homeostasis. Increased S6K activity by adenoviral injection of constitutive active form of S6K in the mediobasal hypothalamus (MBH) decreases body weight, food intake, and hypothalamic leptin sensitivity, while increasing thermogenesis during cold challenge. Overexpression of S6K protects high fat feeding induced hyperphagia, fat accumulation and insulin resistance suggesting a critical role of MBH S6K activity in energy homeostasis [75]. Constitutive activation of mTORC1 signaling in the AgRP neurons modulates sympathetic tone to increase BAT thermogenesis and energy expenditure and protects against diet-induced obesity [76]. However, a recent study has shown that specific ablation of S6K1 in POMC or AgRP neurons causes no significant change in food intake and body weight. This discrepancy has been proposed to be possibly caused by high level of adenovirus-mediated gene expression, the local inflammation, the post-operative stress, and/or another group of neurons other than AgRP and POMC neurons involved. In their study, although S6K1 is not required for the hypothalamic regulation of food intake and body weight, it alters the hepatic glucose output (HGP), peripheral lipid metabolism and skeletal muscle insulin sensitivity, suggesting an important role of hypothalamic S6K1 in glucose and energy homeostasis [77]. However, studies using genetic or pharmcological manipulation of mTOR activation in mice demonstrated that mTORC1 hyperactivation in POMC neurons leads to increased body mass and defective neuron activation [78,79]. Therefore, the role of mTORC1 in hypothalamus is elusive and needs further investigation.

DEPTOR is the inhibitor protein of mTOR which is shared by mTORC1 and mTORC2. It is widely expressed in the brain and highly expressed in MBH neurons. Overexpression of DEPTOR specifically in the MBH neurons protects mice from HFD-induced obesity and improves systemic glucose homeostasis due to decreased food intake and elevated oxygen consumption [80]. Since DEPTOR co-localizes with POMC neurons, it is possible that the POMC neurons mediate the effects of hypothalamic DEPTOR overexpression. Unexpectedly, none of these phenotypes is reproduced in the mice with POMC–specific overexpression of mTORC1, suggesting that other neuronal populations in the MBH are responsible for the energy and glucose metabolism control [81]. It should be noted that the mTORC1 signaling is implicated in the neuronal growth/migration and synaptic plasticity. Brain somatic activating mutations in components of the PI3K-AKT-TSC1/2-mTOR pathway have also been identified in the epileptogenic neurodevelopmental disease, focal cortical dysplasia (FCD) type II [82–84]. The critical developmental defects may profoundly impact the systemic metabolism.

The implication of mTORC2 in central regulation of energy balance is much less well defined. Kocalis et al. found that mice lacking Rictor in nestin-positive neural cells exhibits increased fat mass and adiposity, as well as glucose intolerance. Moreover, they examined mice with Rictor deletion in POMC and AgRP neurons. Loss of Rictor in POMC neurons reproduces most of phenotypes such as hyperphagia, obesity, and glucose intolerance, while loss of Rictor in AgRP neurons has no significant effects on energy homeostasis [85]. Since mTORC2 signaling is also implicated in the neural development [86], it is possible that the energy dys-homeostasis is caused by defective neuron morphology and function.

7. Therapeutic Potential of Targeting mTOR Signaling Pathway

Since mTORC1 has been aberrantly increased in the diabetes or metabolic stressed conditions, targeting mTORC1 signaling pathway represents a potential treatment for metabolic dys-regulation. Rapamycin is the well-known, classical mTORC1 inhibitor. It forms a protein complex with FKBP12 or FKBP51 and inhibits mTORC1 function. Rapamycin treatment exerts significant effects on systemic metabolism affecting multiple organs [87]. Acute treatment of rapamycin enhances insulin secretion and prevents nutrient-induced insulin resistance. However, a number of studies have demonstrated that chronic rapamycin treatment induces detrimental effects on metabolic profiling, including reduced beta cell mass and function, increased hepatic gluconeogenesis, and impaired insulin sensitivity [37,88–91].

Recently, one interesting study has compared the effects of rapamycin treatment on different diabetic mouse models and unexpectedly demonstrated that rapamycin improves insulin sensitivity and reduces hyperinsulinemia better in mice with lower pancreatic insulin content. It has thus been proposed that the beneficial or detrimental effects of rapamycin treatment are determined by the pancreatic insulin contents and pancreas biology [92].

Another explanation for the detrimental effects of rapamycin is the "off-target" effect on mTORC2 disruption. Chronic administration of rapamycin also disrupts mTORC2 complex and impairs mTORC2 signaling, which is required for the insulin-mediated suppression of hepatic gluconeogenesis [37]. Rapamycin also causes mTORC2-dependent insulin resistance in C2C12 myotubes [93]. These findings prompt the development of specific inhibitors of mTORC1 which might provide beneficial effects on health and longevity avoiding of the detrimental effects on systemic metabolism.

In order to inhibit mTORC1 signaling pathway more specifically, an inhibitor of S6K1, PF-4708671 has been generated and used for delineating S6K1-specific roles downstream of mTOR [94]. Shum et al. have compared the effects of glucose metabolism using rapamycin and PF-4708671 in vitro and in vivo. In contrast to the adverse effects associated with chronic rapamycin treatment, S6K1 inhibition with PF-4708671 improves glucose tolerance with increased AKT phosphorylation in both cellular and high fat diet induced obese mouse models [95]. Therefore, specific S6K1 blockade is a promising pharmacological approach to improve metabolic homeostasis in obese or diabetic individuals.

8. Concluding Remarks

During the past few decades, our knowledge on mTOR regulatory mechanism in these key metabolic organs at the molecular, cellular, and organismal level has been emerging (Table 1). Rapamycin and several other mTOR targeting drugs have been used for cancers and immuno-suppressive therapies. However, their side effects leading to dys-regulated metabolic profiling limit their clinical use. More basic and clinical studies are required to better understand the beneficial and side effects of mTOR inhibiting strategy against metabolic disorders. In addition, a comprehensive understanding of mTORC2 pathway, identification of new mTOR signaling substrates and molecular mechanisms would pave the way for developing more specific treatment in the future.

Table 1. The effects of altered mTOR signaling on glucose and lipid metabolism in metabolic tissues.

	mTORC1	mTORC2
Adipose tissue	Normal adipose tissue growth [16]; BAT-WAT phenotypic switch [18–20]	Regulate fat and whole body organ size [21]; systemic glucose and lipid metabolism [22]; BAT differentiation [25]
Liver	Suppress ketogenesis in response to fasting [27]; promote lipogenesis [28,29]	Regulate constitutive gluconeogenesis, increase glycolysis and lipogenesis [35,36]
Muscle	Glucose intolerance and insulin resistance, hypertrophy [42,43]	Promote glucose uptake and improve insulin signaling [51]; negatively modualtes systemic lipid metabolism and intramyocellular triglycerid content [52,53]
Pancreas	Promote beta cell growth and proliferation [54–58]; improved glucose tolerance in short term, deteriorates beta cell mass and function in long term [60,61]; maintain α cell maturation and glucagon secretion [68]	Maintaining beta cell mass and glucose homeostasis [72]
Brain	Regulate the hepatic glucose output, peripheral lipid metabolism and skeletal muscle insulin sensitivity [75–77]	Regulate fat mass and adiposity, and glucose tolerance [85]

Funding: This work was funded by the National Natural Science Foundation of China (81500619, 81730020), the National Key R&D Program of China (2017YFC0908900), Natural Science Foundation of Guangdong Province (2016A030310040), Shenzhen Science and Technology Project (JCYJ20160422091658982, JCYJ20150324140036854) Shenzhen Peacocok Plan (KQTD20140630100746562, 827-000107) and Natural Science Foundation of SZU (201567).

Conflicts of Interest: The authors declare no conflict of interest.

References

1. Saxton, R.A.; Sabatini, D.M. mTOR Signaling in Growth, Metabolism, and Disease. *Cell* **2017**, *168*, 960–976. [CrossRef] [PubMed]

2. Um, S.H.; Frigerio, F.; Watanabe, M.; Picard, F.; Joaquin, M.; Sticker, M.; Fumagalli, S.; Allegrini, P.R.; Kozma, S.C.; Auwerx, J.; et al. Absence of S6K1 protects against age- and diet-induced obesity while enhancing insulin sensitivity. *Nature* **2004**, *431*, 200–205. [CrossRef] [PubMed]

3. Laplante, M.; Sabatini, D.M. mTOR signaling in growth control and disease. *Cell* **2012**, *149*, 274–293. [CrossRef] [PubMed]

4. Yuan, T.; Rafizadeh, S.; Gorrepati, K.D.D.; Lupse, B.; Oberholzer, J.; Maedler, K.; Ardestani, A. Reciprocal regulation of mTOR complexes in pancreatic islets from humans with type 2 diabetes. *Diabetologia* **2017**, *60*, 668–678. [CrossRef] [PubMed]

5. Sancak, Y.; Bar-Peled, L.; Zoncu, R.; Markhard, A.L.; Nada, S.; Sabatini, D.M. Ragulator-Rag Complex Targets mTORC1 to the Lysosomal Surface and Is Necessary for Its Activation by Amino Acids. *Cell* **2010**, *141*, 290–303. [CrossRef] [PubMed]

6. Kim, E.; Goraksha-Hicks, P.; Li, L.; Neufeld, T.P.; Guan, K.-L. Regulation of TORC1 by Rag GTPases in nutrient response. *Nat. Cell Biol.* **2008**, *10*, 935–945. [CrossRef] [PubMed]

7. Inoki, K.; Zhu, T.; Guan, K.L. TSC2 mediates cellular energy response to control cell growth and survival. *Cell* **2003**, *115*, 577–590. [CrossRef]

8. Cornu, M.; Albert, V.; Hall, M.N. mTOR in aging, metabolism, and cancer. *Curr. Opin. Genet. Dev.* **2013**, *23*, 53–62. [CrossRef] [PubMed]

9. Ben-Sahra, I.; Hoxhaj, G.; Ricoult, S.J.H.; Asara, J.M.; Manning, B.D. mTORC1 induces purine synthesis through control of the mitochondrial tetrahydrofolate cycle. *Science* **2016**, *351*, 728–733. [CrossRef] [PubMed]

10. Düvel, K.; Yecies, J.L.; Menon, S.; Raman, P.; Lipovsky, A.I.; Souza, A.L.; Triantafellow, E.; Ma, Q.; Gorski, R.; Cleaver, S.; et al. Activation of a Metabolic Gene Regulatory Network Downstream of mTOR Complex 1. *Mol. Cell* **2010**, *39*, 171–183. [CrossRef] [PubMed]

11. Peterson, T.R.; Sengupta, S.S.; Harris, T.E.; Carmack, A.E.; Kang, S.A.; Balderas, E.; Guertin, D.A.; Madden, K.L.; Carpenter, A.E.; Finck, B.N.; et al. mTOR Complex 1 Regulates Lipin 1 Localization to Control the SREBP Pathway. *Cell* **2011**, *146*, 408–420. [CrossRef] [PubMed]

12. Kim, J.; Kundu, M.; Viollet, B.; Guan, K.-L. AMPK and mTOR regulate autophagy through direct phosphorylation of Ulk1. *Nat. Cell Biol.* **2011**, *13*, 132. [CrossRef] [PubMed]

13. Settembre, C.; Zoncu, R.; Medina, D.L.; Vetrini, F.; Erdin, S.; Erdin, S.; Huynh, T.; Ferron, M.; Karsenty, G.; Vellard, M.C.; et al. A lysosome-to-nucleus signalling mechanism senses and regulates the lysosome via mTOR and TFEB. *EMBO J.* **2012**, *31*, 1095–1108. [CrossRef] [PubMed]

14. Zhao, J.; Zhai, B.; Gygi, S.P.; Goldberg, A.L. mTOR inhibition activates overall protein degradation by the ubiquitin proteasome system as well as by autophagy. *Proc. Natl. Acad. Sci. USA* **2015**, *112*, 15790–15797. [CrossRef] [PubMed]

15. Rousseau, A.; Bertolotti, A. An evolutionarily conserved pathway controls proteasome homeostasis. *Nature* **2016**, *536*, 184–189. [CrossRef] [PubMed]

16. Shan, T.; Zhang, P.; Jiang, Q.; Xiong, Y.; Wang, Y.; Kuang, S. Adipocyte-specific deletion of mTOR inhibits adipose tissue development and causes insulin resistance in mice. *Diabetologia* **2016**, *59*, 1995–2004. [CrossRef] [PubMed]

17. Arif, A.; Terenzi, F.; Potdar, A.A.; Jia, J.; Sacks, J.; China, A.; Halawani, D.; Vasu, K.; Li, X.X.; Brown, J.M.; et al. EPRS is a critical mTORC1-S6K1 effector that influences adiposity in mice. *Nature* **2017**, *542*, 357–361. [CrossRef] [PubMed]

18. Xiang, X.; Lan, H.; Tang, H.; Yuan, F.; Xu, Y.; Zhao, J.; Li, Y.; Zhang, W. Tuberous Sclerosis Complex 1–Mechanistic Target of Rapamycin Complex 1 Signaling Determines Brown-to-White Adipocyte Phenotypic Switch. *Diabetes* **2015**, *64*, 519–528. [CrossRef] [PubMed]

19. Liu, D.X.; Bordicchia, M.; Zhang, C.Y.; Fang, H.F.; Wei, W.; Li, J.L.; Guilherme, A.; Guntur, K.; Czech, M.P.; Collins, S. Activation of mTORC1 is essential for beta-adrenergic stimulation of adipose browning. *J. Clin. Investig.* **2016**, *126*, 1704–1716. [CrossRef] [PubMed]

20. Tran, C.M.; Mukherjee, S.; Ye, L.; Frederick, D.W.; Kissig, M.; Davis, J.G.; Lamming, D.W.; Seale, P.; Baur, J.A. Rapamycin Blocks Induction of the Thermogenic Program in White Adipose Tissue. *Diabetes* **2016**, *65*, 927–941. [CrossRef] [PubMed]

21. Cybulski, N.; Polak, P.; Auwerx, J.; Rüegg, M.A.; Hall, M.N. mTOR complex 2 in adipose tissue negatively controls whole-body growth. *Proc. Natl. Acad. Sci. USA* **2009**, *106*, 9902–9907. [CrossRef] [PubMed]

22. Kumar, A.; Lawrence, J.C., Jr.; Jung, D.Y.; Ko, H.J.; Keller, S.R.; Kim, J.K.; Magnuson, M.A.; Harris, T.E. Fat cell-specific ablation of rictor in mice impairs insulin-regulated fat cell and whole-body glucose and lipid metabolism. *Diabetes* **2010**, *59*, 1397–1406. [CrossRef] [PubMed]

23. Yao, Y.; Suraokar, M.; Darnay, B.G.; Hollier, B.G.; Shaiken, T.E.; Asano, T.; Chen, C.-H.; Chang, B.H.-J.; Lu, Y.; Mills, G.B.; et al. BSTA Promotes mTORC2-Mediated Phosphorylation of Akt1 to Suppress Expression of FoxC2 and Stimulate Adipocyte Differentiation. *Sci. Signal.* **2013**, *6*, ra2. [CrossRef] [PubMed]

24. Tang, Y.F.; Wallace, M.; Sanchez-Gurmaches, J.; Hsiao, W.Y.; Li, H.W.; Lee, P.L.; Vernia, S.; Metallo, C.M.; Guertin, D.A. Adipose tissue mTORC2 regulates ChREBP-driven de novo lipogenesis and hepatic glucose metabolism. *Nat. Commun.* **2016**, *7*, 14. [CrossRef] [PubMed]

25. Hung, C.-M.; Calejman, C.M.; Sanchez-Gurmaches, J.; Li, H.; Clish, C.B.; Hettmer, S.; Wagers, A.J.; Guertin, D.A. Rictor/mTORC2 loss in the Myf5 lineage reprograms brown fat metabolism and protects mice against obesity and metabolic disease. *Cell Rep.* **2014**, *8*, 256–271. [CrossRef] [PubMed]

26. Albert, V.; Svensson, K.; Shimobayashi, M.; Colombi, M.; Muñoz, S.; Jimenez, V.; Handschin, C.; Bosch, F.; Hall, M.N. mTORC2 sustains thermogenesis via Akt-induced glucose uptake and glycolysis in brown adipose tissue. *EMBO Mol. Med.* **2016**, *8*, 232–246. [CrossRef] [PubMed]

27. Sengupta, S.; Peterson, T.R.; Laplante, M.; Oh, S.; Sabatini, D.M. mTORC1 controls fasting-induced ketogenesis and its modulation by ageing. *Nature* **2010**, *468*, 1100. [CrossRef] [PubMed]

28. Li, Z.; Xu, G.; Qin, Y.; Zhang, C.; Tang, H.; Yin, Y.; Xiang, X.; Li, Y.; Zhao, J.; Mulholland, M.; et al. Ghrelin promotes hepatic lipogenesis by activation of mTOR-PPARγ signaling pathway. *Proc. Natl. Acad. Sci. USA* **2014**, *111*, 13163–13168. [CrossRef] [PubMed]

29. Han, J.B.; Li, E.W.; Chen, L.Q.; Zhang, Y.Y.; Wei, F.C.; Liu, J.Y.; Deng, H.T.; Wang, Y.G. The CREB coactivator CRTC2 controls hepatic lipid metabolism by regulating SREBP1. *Nature* **2015**, *524*, 243. [CrossRef] [PubMed]

30. Kim, K.; Qiang, L.; Hayden, M.S.; Sparling, D.P.; Purcell, N.H.; Pajvani, U.B. mTORC1-independent Raptor prevents hepatic steatosis by stabilizing PHLPP2. *Nat. Commun.* **2016**, *7*, 10. [CrossRef] [PubMed]

31. Cornu, M.; Oppliger, W.; Albert, V.; Robitaille, A.M.; Trapani, F.; Quagliata, L.; Fuhrer, T.; Sauer, U.; Terracciano, L.; Hall, M.N. Hepatic mTORC1 controls locomotor activity, body temperature, and lipid metabolism through FGF21. *Proc. Natl. Acad. Sci. USA* **2014**, *111*, 11592–11599. [PubMed]

32. Lee, J.H.; Budanov, A.V.; Talukdar, S.; Park, E.J.; Park, H.L.; Park, H.W.; Bandyopadhyay, G.; Li, N.; Aghajan, M.; Jang, I.; et al. Maintenance of metabolic homeostasis by Sestrin2 and Sestrin3. *Cell Metab.* **2012**, *16*, 311–321. [CrossRef] [PubMed]

33. Park, H.W.; Park, H.; Ro, S.H.; Jang, I.; Semple, I.A.; Kim, D.N.; Kim, M.; Nam, M.; Zhang, D.; Yin, L.; et al. Hepatoprotective role of Sestrin2 against chronic ER stress. *Nat. Commun.* **2014**, *5*, 4233. [CrossRef] [PubMed]

34. Howell, J.J.; Hellberg, K.; Turner, M.; Talbott, G.; Kolar, M.J.; Ross, D.S.; Hoxhaj, G.; Saghatelian, A.; Shaw, R.J.; Manning, B.D. Metformin Inhibits Hepatic mTORC1 Signaling via Dose-Dependent Mechanisms Involving AMPK and the TSC Complex. *Cell Metab.* **2017**, *25*, 463–471. [CrossRef] [PubMed]

35. Hagiwara, A.; Cornu, M.; Cybulski, N.; Polak, P.; Betz, C.; Trapani, F.; Terracciano, L.; Heim, M.H.; Rüegg, M.A.; Hall, M.N. Hepatic mTORC2 Activates Glycolysis and Lipogenesis through Akt, Glucokinase, and SREBP1c. *Cell Metab.* **2012**, *15*, 725–738. [CrossRef] [PubMed]

36. Yuan, M.; Pino, E.; Wu, L.; Kacergis, M.; Soukas, A.A. Identification of Akt-independent Regulation of Hepatic Lipogenesis by Mammalian Target of Rapamycin (mTOR) Complex 2. *J. Biol. Chem.* **2012**, *287*, 29579–29588. [CrossRef] [PubMed]

37. Lamming, D.W.; Ye, L.; Katajisto, P.; Goncalves, M.D.; Saitoh, M.; Stevens, D.M.; Davis, J.G.; Salmon, A.B.; Richardson, A.; Ahima, R.S.; et al. Rapamycin-Induced Insulin Resistance Is Mediated by mTORC2 Loss and Uncoupled from Longevity. *Science* **2012**, *335*, 1638–1643. [PubMed]

38. Tao, R.; Xiong, X.; Liangpunsakul, S.; Dong, X.C. Sestrin 3 Protein Enhances Hepatic Insulin Sensitivity by Direct Activation of the mTORC2-Akt Signaling. *Diabetes* **2015**, *64*, 1211–1223. [CrossRef] [PubMed]

39. Javary, J.; Allain-Courtois, N.; Saucisse, N.; Costet, P.; Heraud, C.; Benhamed, F.; Pierre, R.; Bure, C.; Pallares-Lupon, N.; Do Cruzeiro, M.; et al. Liver Reptin/RUVBL2 controls glucose and lipid metabolism with opposite actions on mTORC1 and mTORC2 signalling. *Gut* **2017**. [CrossRef] [PubMed]

40. Bentzinger, C.F.; Romanino, K.; Cloëtta, D.; Lin, S.; Mascarenhas, J.B.; Oliveri, F.; Xia, J.; Casanova, E.; Costa, C.F.; Brink, M.; et al. Skeletal Muscle-Specific Ablation of raptor, but Not of rictor, Causes Metabolic Changes and Results in Muscle Dystrophy. *Cell Metab.* **2008**, *8*, 411–424. [CrossRef] [PubMed]

41. Lopez, R.J.; Mosca, B.; Treves, S.; Maj, M.; Bergamelli, L.; Calderon, J.C.; Bentzinger, C.F.; Romanino, K.; Hall, M.N.; Ruegg, M.A.; et al. Raptor ablation in skeletal muscle decreases Cav1.1 expression and affects the function of the excitation-contraction coupling supramolecular complex. *Biochem. J.* **2015**, *466*, 123–135. [CrossRef] [PubMed]

42. Guridi, M.; Kupr, B.; Romanino, K.; Lin, S.; Falcetta, D.; Tintignac, L.; Rüegg, M.A. Alterations to mTORC1 signaling in the skeletal muscle differentially affect whole-body metabolism. *Skeletal Muscle* **2016**, *6*, 13. [CrossRef] [PubMed]

43. Guridi, M.; Tintignac, L.A.; Lin, S.; Kupr, B.; Castets, P.; Rüegg, M.A. Activation of mTORC1 in skeletal muscle regulates whole-body metabolism through FGF21. *Sci. Signal.* **2015**, *8*, ra113. [CrossRef] [PubMed]

44. Tsai, S.; Sitzmann, J.M.; Dastidar, S.G.; Rodriguez, A.A.; Vu, S.L.; McDonald, C.E.; Academia, E.C.; O'Leary, M.N.; Ashe, T.D.; La Spada, A.R.; et al. Muscle-specific 4E-BP1 signaling activation improves metabolic parameters during aging and obesity. *J. Clin. Investig.* **2015**, *125*, 2952–2964. [CrossRef] [PubMed]

45. Lipina, C.; Hundal, H.S. Is REDD1 a Metabolic Eminence Grise? *Trends Endocrinol. Metab. TEM* **2016**, *27*, 868–880. [CrossRef] [PubMed]

46. Tan, C.Y.; Hagen, T. mTORC1 dependent regulation of REDD1 protein stability. *PLoS ONE* **2013**, *8*, e63970. [CrossRef] [PubMed]

47. Williamson, D.L.; Li, Z.; Tuder, R.M.; Feinstein, E.; Kimball, S.R.; Dungan, C.M. Altered nutrient response of mTORC1 as a result of changes in REDD1 expression: Effect of obesity vs. REDD1 deficiency. *J. Appl. Physiol.* **2014**, *117*, 246–256. [CrossRef] [PubMed]

48. Williamson, D.L.; Dungan, C.M.; Mahmoud, A.M.; Mey, J.T.; Blackburn, B.K.; Haus, J.M. Aberrant REDD1-mTORC1 responses to insulin in skeletal muscle from Type 2 diabetics. *Am. J. Physiol. Regul. Integr. Comp. Physiol.* **2015**, *309*, R855–R863. [CrossRef] [PubMed]

49. Castets, P.; Lin, S.; Rion, N.; Di Fulvio, S.; Romanino, K.; Guridi, M.; Frank, S.; Tintignac, L.A.; Sinnreich, M.; Rüegg, M.A. Sustained Activation of mTORC1 in Skeletal Muscle Inhibits Constitutive and Starvation-Induced Autophagy and Causes a Severe, Late-Onset Myopathy. *Cell Metab.* **2013**, *17*, 731–744. [CrossRef] [PubMed]

50. Tang, H.; Inoki, K.; Lee, M.; Wright, E.; Khuong, A.; Khuong, A.; Sugiarto, S.; Garner, M.; Paik, J.; DePinho, R.A.; et al. mTORC1 Promotes Denervation-Induced Muscle Atrophy Through a Mechanism Involving the Activation of FoxO and E3 Ubiquitin Ligases. *Sci. Signal.* **2014**, *7*, ra18. [CrossRef] [PubMed]

51. Kumar, A.; Harris, T.E.; Keller, S.R.; Choi, K.M.; Magnuson, M.A.; Lawrence, J.C., Jr. Muscle-specific deletion of rictor impairs insulin-stimulated glucose transport and enhances Basal glycogen synthase activity. *Mol. Cell Biol.* **2008**, *28*, 61–70. [CrossRef] [PubMed]

52. Kleinert, M.; Sylow, L.; Fazakerley, D.J.; Krycer, J.R.; Thomas, K.C.; Oxboll, A.J.; Jordy, A.B.; Jensen, T.E.; Yang, G.; Schjerling, P.; et al. Acute mTOR inhibition induces insulin resistance and alters substrate utilization in vivo. *Mol. Metab.* **2014**, *3*, 630–641. [CrossRef] [PubMed]

53. Kleinert, M.; Parker, B.L.; Chaudhuri, R.; Fazakerley, D.J.; Serup, A.; Thomas, K.C.; Krycer, J.R.; Sylow, L.; Fritzen, A.M.; Hoffman, N.J.; et al. mTORC2 and AMPK differentially regulate muscle triglyceride content via Perilipin 3. *Mol. Metab.* **2016**, *5*, 646–655. [CrossRef] [PubMed]

54. Blandino-Rosano, M.; Barbaresso, R.; Jimenez-Palomares, M.; Bozadjieva, N.; Werneck-de-Castro, J.P.; Hatanaka, M.; Mirmira, R.G.; Sonenberg, N.; Liu, M.; Ruegg, M.A.; et al. Loss of mTORC1 signalling impairs beta-cell homeostasis and insulin processing. *Nat. Commun.* **2017**, *8*, 16014. [CrossRef] [PubMed]

55. Chau, G.C.; Im, D.U.; Kang, T.M.; Bae, J.M.; Kim, W.; Pyo, S.; Moon, E.-Y.; Um, S.H. mTOR controls ChREBP transcriptional activity and pancreatic β cell survival under diabetic stress. *J. Cell Biol.* **2017**. [CrossRef] [PubMed]

56. Elghazi, L.; Blandino-Rosano, M.; Alejandro, E.; Cras-Méneur, C.; Bernal-Mizrachi, E. Role of nutrients and mTOR signaling in the regulation of pancreatic progenitors development. *Mol. Metab.* **2017**, *6*, 560–573. [CrossRef] [PubMed]

57. Ni, Q.; Gu, Y.; Xie, Y.; Yin, Q.; Zhang, H.; Nie, A.; Li, W.; Wang, Y.; Ning, G.; Wang, W.; et al. Raptor regulates functional maturation of murine beta cells. *Nat. Commun.* **2017**, *8*, 15755. [CrossRef] [PubMed]

58. Sinagoga, K.L.; Stone, W.J.; Schiesser, J.V.; Schweitzer, J.I.; Sampson, L.; Zheng, Y.; Wells, J.M. Distinct roles for the mTOR pathway in postnatal morphogenesis, maturation and function of pancreatic islets. *Development* **2017**, *144*, 2402–2414. [CrossRef] [PubMed]

59. Ding, L.; Yin, Y.; Han, L.; Li, Y.; Zhao, J.; Zhang, W. TSC1-mTOR signaling determines the differentiation of islet cells. *J. Endocrinol.* **2017**, *232*, 59–70. [CrossRef] [PubMed]

60. Bartolome, A.; Kimura-Koyanagi, M.; Asahara, S.I.; Guillen, C.; Inoue, H.; Teruyama, K.; Shimizu, S.; Kanno, A.; Garcia-Aguilar, A.; Koike, M.; et al. Pancreatic beta-Cell Failure Mediated by mTORC1 Hyperactivity and Autophagic Impairment. *Diabetes* **2014**, *63*, 2996–3008. [CrossRef] [PubMed]

61. Rachdi, L.; Balcazar, N.; Osorio-Duque, F.; Elghazi, L.; Weiss, A.; Gould, A.; Chang-Chen, K.J.; Gambello, M.J.; Bernal-Mizrachi, E. Disruption of Tsc2 in pancreatic beta cells induces beta cell mass expansion and improved glucose tolerance in a TORC1-dependent manner. *Proc. Natl. Acad. Sci. USA* **2008**, *105*, 9250–9255. [CrossRef] [PubMed]

62. Varshney, R.; Varshney, R.; Mishra, R.; Roy, P. Kaempferol alleviates palmitic acid-induced lipid stores, endoplasmic reticulum stress and pancreatic β-cell dysfunction through AMPK/mTOR-mediated lipophagy. *J. Nutr. Biochem.* **2018**. [CrossRef] [PubMed]

63. Ardestani, A.; Lupse, B.; Kido, Y.; Leibowitz, G.; Maedler, K. mTORC1 Signaling: A Double-Edged Sword in Diabetic beta Cells. *Cell Metab.* **2018**, *27*, 314–331. [CrossRef] [PubMed]

64. Warren, K.J.; Fang, X.; Gowda, N.M.; Thompson, J.J.; Heller, N.M. The TORC1-activated Proteins, p70S6K and GRB10, Regulate IL-4 Signaling and M2 Macrophage Polarization by Modulating Phosphorylation of Insulin Receptor Substrate-2. *J. Biol. Chem.* **2016**, *291*, 24922–24930. [CrossRef] [PubMed]

65. Wick, K.R.; Werner, E.D.; Langlais, P.; Ramos, F.J.; Dong, L.Q.; Shoelson, S.E.; Liu, F. Grb10 Inhibits Insulin-stimulated Insulin Receptor Substrate (IRS)-Phosphatidylinositol 3-Kinase/Akt Signaling Pathway by Disrupting the Association of IRS-1/IRS-2 with the Insulin Receptor. *J. Biol. Chem.* **2003**, *278*, 8460–8467. [CrossRef] [PubMed]

66. Julien, L.-A.; Carriere, A.; Moreau, J.; Roux, P.P. mTORC1-activated S6K1 phosphorylates Rictor on threonine 1135 and regulates mTORC2 signaling. *Mol. Cell. Biol.* **2010**, *30*, 908–921. [CrossRef] [PubMed]

67. Liu, P.; Gan, W.; Inuzuka, H.; Lazorchak, A.S.; Gao, D.; Arojo, O.; Liu, D.; Wan, L.; Zhai, B.; Yu, Y.; et al. Sin1 phosphorylation impairs mTORC2 complex integrity and inhibits downstream Akt signalling to suppress tumorigenesis. *Nat. Cell Biol.* **2013**, *15*, 1340. [CrossRef] [PubMed]

68. Bozadjieva, N.; Blandino-Rosano, M.; Chase, J.; Dai, X.-Q.; Cummings, K.; Gimeno, J.; Dean, D.; Powers, A.C.; Gittes, G.K.; Rüegg, M.A.; et al. Loss of mTORC1 signaling alters pancreatic α cell mass and impairs glucagon secretion. *J. Clin. Investig.* **2017**, *127*, 4379–4393. [CrossRef] [PubMed]

69. Dean, E.D.; Li, M.; Prasad, N.; Wisniewski, S.N.; Von Deylen, A.; Spaeth, J.; Maddison, L.; Botros, A.; Sedgeman, L.R.; Bozadjieva, N.; et al. Interrupted Glucagon Signaling Reveals Hepatic α Cell Axis and Role for L-Glutamine in α Cell Proliferation. *Cell Metab.* **2017**, *25*, 1362–1373. [CrossRef] [PubMed]

70. Kim, J.; Okamoto, H.; Huang, Z.; Anguiano, G.; Chen, S.; Liu, Q.; Cavino, K.; Xin, Y.; Na, E.; Hamid, R.; et al. Amino Acid Transporter Slc38a5 Controls Glucagon Receptor Inhibition-Induced Pancreatic α Cell Hyperplasia in Mice. *Cell Metab.* **2017**, *25*, 1348–1361. [CrossRef] [PubMed]

71. Solloway, M.J.; Madjidi, A.; Gu, C.; Eastham-Anderson, J.; Clarke, H.J.; Kljavin, N.; Zavala-Solorio, J.; Kates, L.; Friedman, B.; Brauer, M.; et al. Glucagon Couples Hepatic Amino Acid Catabolism to mTOR-Dependent Regulation of α-Cell Mass. *Cell Rep.* **2015**, *12*, 495–510. [CrossRef] [PubMed]

72. Gu, Y.; Lindner, J.; Kumar, A.; Yuan, W.; Magnuson, M.A. Rictor/mTORC2 Is Essential for Maintaining a Balance Between β-Cell Proliferation and Cell Size. *Diabetes* **2011**, *60*, 827–837. [CrossRef] [PubMed]

73. Bockaert, J.; Marin, P. mTOR in Brain Physiology and Pathologies. *Physiol. Rev.* **2015**, *95*, 1157–1187. [CrossRef] [PubMed]

74. Hu, F.; Xu, Y.; Liu, F. Hypothalamic roles of mTOR complex I: Integration of nutrient and hormone signals to regulate energy homeostasis. *Am. J. Physiol.-Endocrinol. Metab.* **2016**, *310*, E994–E1002. [CrossRef] [PubMed]

75. Blouet, C.; Ono, H.; Schwartz, G.J. Mediobasal Hypothalamic p70 S6 Kinase 1 Modulates the Control of Energy Homeostasis. *Cell Metab.* **2008**, *8*, 459–467. [CrossRef] [PubMed]

76. Burke, L.K.; Darwish, T.; Cavanaugh, A.R.; Virtue, S.; Roth, E.; Morro, J.; Liu, S.M.; Xia, J.; Dalley, J.W.; Burling, K.; et al. mTORC1 in AGRP neurons integrates exteroceptive and interoceptive food-related cues in the modulation of adaptive energy expenditure in mice. *eLife* **2017**, *6*, 22. [CrossRef] [PubMed]

77. Smith, M.A.; Katsouri, L.; Irvine, E.E.; Hankir, M.K.; Pedroni, S.M.A.; Voshol, P.J.; Gordon, M.W.; Choudhury, A.I.; Woods, A.; Vidal-Puig, A.; et al. Ribosomal S6K1 in POMC and AgRP Neurons Regulates Glucose Homeostasis but Not Feeding Behavior in Mice. *Cell Rep.* **2015**, *11*, 335–343. [CrossRef] [PubMed]

78. Mori, H.; Inoki, K.; Munzberg, H.; Opland, D.; Faouzi, M.; Villanueva, E.C.; Ikenoue, T.; Kwiatkowski, D.; MacDougald, O.A.; Myers, M.G., Jr.; et al. Critical role for hypothalamic mTOR activity in energy balance. *Cell Metab.* **2009**, *9*, 362–374. [CrossRef] [PubMed]

79. Yang, S.B.; Tien, A.C.; Boddupalli, G.; Xu, A.W.; Jan, Y.N.; Jan, L.Y. Rapamycin ameliorates age-dependent obesity associated with increased mTOR signaling in hypothalamic POMC neurons. *Neuron* **2012**, *75*, 425–436. [CrossRef] [PubMed]

80. Caron, A.; Labbé, S.M.; Lanfray, D.; Blanchard, P.-G.; Villot, R.; Roy, C.; Sabatini, D.M.; Richard, D.; Laplante, M. Mediobasal hypothalamic overexpression of DEPTOR protects against high-fat diet-induced obesity. *Mol. Metab.* **2016**, *5*, 102–112. [CrossRef] [PubMed]

81. Caron, A.; Labbe, S.M.; Mouchiroud, M.; Huard, R.; Lanfray, D.; Richard, D.; Laplante, M. DEPTOR in POMC neurons affects liver metabolism but is dispensable for the regulation of energy balance. *Am. J. Physiol.-Regul. Integr. Comp. Physiol.* **2016**, *310*, R1322–R1331. [CrossRef] [PubMed]

82. Park, A.H.; Park, E.K.; Cho, Y.W.; Kim, S.; Kim, H.M.; Kim, J.A.; Kim, J.; Rhee, H.; Kang, S.G.; Kim, H.D.; et al. Brain somatic mutations in MTOR cause focal cortical dysplasia type II leading to intractable epilepsy. *Nat. Med.* **2015**, *21*, 395–400.

83. Lim, J.S.; Gopalappa, R.; Kim, S.H.; Ramakrishna, S.; Lee, M.; Kim, W.I.; Kim, J.; Park, S.M.; Lee, J.; Oh, J.H.; et al. Somatic Mutations in TSC1 and TSC2 Cause Focal Cortical Dysplasia. *Am. J. Hum. Genet.* **2017**, *100*, 454–472. [CrossRef] [PubMed]

84. Park, S.M.; Lim, J.S.; Ramakrishina, S.; Kim, S.H.; Kim, W.K.; Lee, J.; Kang, H.C.; Reiter, J.F.; Kim, D.S.; Kim, H.H.; et al. Brain Somatic Mutations in MTOR Disrupt Neuronal Ciliogenesis, Leading to Focal Cortical Dyslamination. *Neuron* **2018**. [CrossRef] [PubMed]

85. Kocalis, H.E.; Hagan, S.L.; George, L.; Turney, M.K.; Siuta, M.A.; Laryea, G.N.; Morris, L.C.; Muglia, L.J.; Printz, R.L.; Stanwood, G.D.; et al. Rictor/mTORC2 facilitates central regulation of energy and glucose homeostasis. *Mol. Metab.* **2014**, *3*, 394–407. [CrossRef] [PubMed]

86. Thomanetz, V.; Angliker, N.; Cloëtta, D.; Lustenberger, R.M.; Schweighauser, M.; Oliveri, F.; Suzuki, N.; Rüegg, M.A. Ablation of the mTORC2 component rictor in brain or Purkinje cells affects size and neuron morphology. *J. Cell Biol.* **2013**, *201*, 293–308. [CrossRef] [PubMed]

87. Harrison, D.E.; Strong, R.; Sharp, Z.D.; Nelson, J.F.; Astle, C.M.; Flurkey, K.; Nadon, N.L.; Wilkinson, J.E.; Frenkel, K.; Carter, C.S.; et al. Rapamycin fed late in life extends lifespan in genetically heterogeneous mice. *Nature* **2009**, *460*, 392–395. [CrossRef] [PubMed]

88. Barlow, A.D.; Nicholson, M.L.; Herbert, T.P. Evidence for Rapamycin Toxicity in Pancreatic β-Cells and a Review of the Underlying Molecular Mechanisms. *Diabetes* **2013**, *62*, 2674–2682. [CrossRef] [PubMed]

89. Deblon, N.; Bourgoin, L.; Veyrat-Durebex, C.; Peyrou, M.; Vinciguerra, M.; Caillon, A.; Maeder, C.; Fournier, M.; Montet, X.; Rohner-Jeanrenaud, F.; et al. Chronic mTOR inhibition by rapamycin induces muscle insulin resistance despite weight loss in rats. *Br. J. Pharmacol.* **2012**, *165*, 2325–2340. [CrossRef] [PubMed]

90. Houde, V.P.; Brule, S.; Festuccia, W.T.; Blanchard, P.G.; Bellmann, K.; Deshaies, Y.; Marette, A. Chronic Rapamycin Treatment Causes Glucose Intolerance and Hyperlipidemia by Upregulating Hepatic Gluconeogenesis and Impairing Lipid Deposition in Adipose Tissue. *Diabetes* **2010**, *59*, 1338–1348. [CrossRef] [PubMed]

91. Pereira, M.J.; Palming, J.; Rizell, M.; Aureliano, M.; Carvalho, E.; Svensson, M.K.; Eriksson, J.W. mTOR inhibition with rapamycin causes impaired insulin signalling and glucose uptake in human subcutaneous and omental adipocytes. *Mol. Cell. Endocrinol.* **2012**, *355*, 96–105. [CrossRef] [PubMed]

92. Reifsnyder, P.C.; Flurkey, K.; Te, A.; Harrison, D.E. Rapamycin treatment benefits glucose metabolism in mouse models of type 2 diabetes. *Aging* **2016**, *8*, 3120–3130. [CrossRef] [PubMed]

93. Ye, L.; Varamini, B.; Lamming, D.; Sabatini, D.; Baur, J. Rapamycin has a biphasic effect on insulin sensitivity in C2C12 myotubes due to sequential disruption of mTORC1 and mTORC2. *Front. Genet.* **2012**, *3*, 177. [CrossRef] [PubMed]

94. Pearce, L.R.; Alton, G.R.; Richter, D.T.; Kath, J.C.; Lingardo, L.; Chapman, J.; Hwang, C.; Alessi, D.R. Characterization of PF-4708671, a novel and highly specific inhibitor of p70 ribosomal S6 kinase (S6K1). *Biochem. J.* **2010**, *431*, 245–255. [CrossRef] [PubMed]

95. Shum, M.; Bellmann, K.; St-Pierre, P.; Marette, A. Pharmacological inhibition of S6K1 increases glucose metabolism and Akt signalling in vitro and in diet-induced obese mice. *Diabetologia* **2016**, *59*, 592–603. [CrossRef] [PubMed]

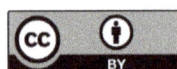

International Journal of
Molecular Sciences

MDPI

Review

mTOR is a Key Protein Involved in the Metabolic Effects of Simple Sugars

Gemma Sangüesa [1,2,†], **Núria Roglans** [1,2,3], **Miguel Baena** [1,2,‡], **Ana Magdalena Velázquez** [1], **Juan Carlos Laguna** [1,2,3] **and Marta Alegret** [1,2,3,*]

1   Department of Pharmacology, Toxicology and Therapeutic Chemistry, School of Pharmacy and Food Science, University of Barcelona, 08028 Barcelona, Spain; gemmasanguesa@gmail.com (G.S.); roglans@ub.edu (N.R.); mbaena@uic.es (M.B.); avelazquezpy@gmail.com (A.M.V.); jclagunae@ub.edu (J.C.L.)

2   Institute of Biomedicine, University of Barcelona, 08028 Barcelona, Spain

3   Centro de Investigación Biomédica en Red de Fisiopatología de la Obesidad y Nutrición (CIBERObn), 28029 Madrid, Spain

*   Correspondence: alegret@ub.edu; Tel.: +34-93-4024531

†   Current Address: Institut d'Investigacions Biomèdiques August Pi i Sunyer (IDIBAPS), Barcelona, Spain. Centro de Investigación Biomédica en Red Cardiovascular (CIBERCV), Spain.

‡   Current Address: Department of Basic Areas, Faculty of Medicine and Health Sciences, Universitat Internacional de Catalunya, Barcelona, Spain.

Received: 23 January 2019; Accepted: 28 February 2019; Published: 5 March 2019

Abstract: One of the most important threats to global human health is the increasing incidences of metabolic pathologies (including obesity, type 2 diabetes and non-alcoholic fatty liver disease), which is paralleled by increasing consumptions of hypercaloric diets enriched in simple sugars. The challenge is to identify the metabolic pathways affected by the excessive consumption of these dietary components when they are consumed in excess, to unravel the molecular mechanisms leading to metabolic pathologies and identify novel therapeutic targets to manage them. Mechanistic (mammalian) target of rapamycin (mTOR) has emerged as one of the key molecular nodes that integrate extracellular signals, such as energy status and nutrient availability, to trigger cell responses that could lead to the above-mentioned diseases through the regulation of lipid and glucose metabolism. By activating mTOR signalling, excessive consumption of simple sugars (such as fructose and glucose), could modulate hepatic gluconeogenesis, lipogenesis and fatty acid uptake and catabolism and thus lipid deposition in the liver. In the present review we will discuss some of the most recent studies showing the central role of mTOR in the metabolic effects of excessive simple sugar consumption.

Keywords: mTOR; fructose; glucose; liver; lipid metabolism; gluconeogenesis

1. Introduction

Mechanistic (formerly mammalian) target of rapamycin (mTOR) is a serine/threonine protein kinase that forms the catalytic centre of two multi-protein complexes termed mTORC1 and mTORC2, which have different compositions and responses to upstream signals [1,2]. As it is shown in Figure 1, both complexes share the core proteins mTOR and mammalian lethal with SEC13 protein 8 (mLST8), the Tti1/Tel2 complex and the inhibitory protein DEP domain-containing mTOR-interacting protein (DEPTOR). The mTORC1 complex contains regulatory-associated protein of mTOR (Raptor) and the inhibitory subunit proline-rich Akt substrate of 40 kDa (PRAS40), whereas mTORC2 contains rapamycin-insensitive companion of mTOR (Rictor) and the regulatory proteins Protor1/2 and mSin1. Both complexes are activated by insulin and related growth factors, such as insulin-like growth factors, while mTORC1 can also be activated by nutrients (amino acids, cholesterol and simple sugars), oxygen and the cellular energy status (sensed via ATP levels) [1,3].

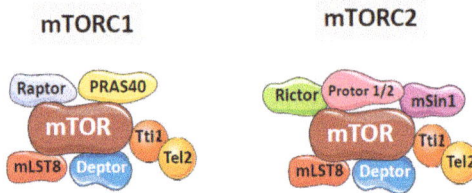

Figure 1. Components of mTORC1 and mTORC2 complexes. mTORC1 and mTORC2 share the core proteins mTOR and mammalian lethal with SEC13 protein 8 (mLST8), the Tti1/Tel2 complex and the inhibitory protein DEP domain-containing mTOR-interacting protein (DEPTOR). In addition, mTORC1 contains regulatory-associated protein of mTOR (Raptor) and the inhibitory subunit proline-rich Akt substrate of 40 kDa (PRAS40), whereas mTORC2 contains rapamycin-insensitive companion of mTOR (Rictor) and the regulatory proteins Protor1/2 and mSin1.

The downstream effects of mTORC1 and mTORC2 activity (reviewed in Reference [4]) are also different. Briefly, mTORC1 activation induces cellular growth through: (i) activation of mRNA translation, driven by the phosphorylation of the ribosomal protein S6 kinases (S6K1/2), which activate several substrates associated with the initiation of mRNA translation and the phosphorylation of eIF4E binding proteins (4EBP), which release factor eIF4E to enable the formation of the translation initiation complex; (ii) promotion of metabolic effects including increased de novo lipid synthesis via the activation of sterol response element-binding protein (SREBP) and a shift to glycolysis instead of oxidative phosphorylation; and (iii) inhibition of catabolic pathways such as autophagy, mainly by the phosphorylation of UNC-51-like kinase 1 (ULK-1). By contrast, mTORC2 activation promotes cell survival and proliferation through the phosphorylation of several kinases including Akt, which is one of the main transducers of insulin signalling.

In summary, the role of mTOR complexes is to coordinate cell responses to energy availability by promoting or repressing anabolic and catabolic molecular pathways in response to different stimuli, including nutrients and growth factors. This review focuses on mTOR regulation by a specific type of nutrients (simple sugars) and its consequences on lipid and carbohydrate metabolism, aiming to gain insight into the mechanisms by which an excessive intake of simple sugars causes metabolic diseases such as dyslipidaemia, diabetes and non-alcoholic fatty liver disease (NAFLD).

2. Regulation of mTORC1 Activity by Simple Sugars

Of the two mTOR complexes, only mTORC1 seems to be regulated by simple sugars (Figure 2). Direct regulation of mTORC1 activity by carbohydrates is less well known than that by amino acids. Activation of mTORC1 by amino acids is initiated by the stimulation of the Rag family of GTPases, which recruits mTORC1 to the outer lysosomal membrane [2]. Using mice that constitutively express an active form of RagA, Efeyan et al. showed that mTORC1 activation by carbohydrates also involves the Rag-GTPases [5,6]. This shared mechanism between amino acids and carbohydrates does not directly activate mTORC1 but causes its lysosomal localization, where the Ras-homolog enriched in brain (Rheb) GTPase resides and activates mTORC1 by promoting mTOR kinase activity. mTOR phosphorylates several substrates, including its autophosphorylation at Ser-2481, which indicates mTOR-specific catalytic activity [7].

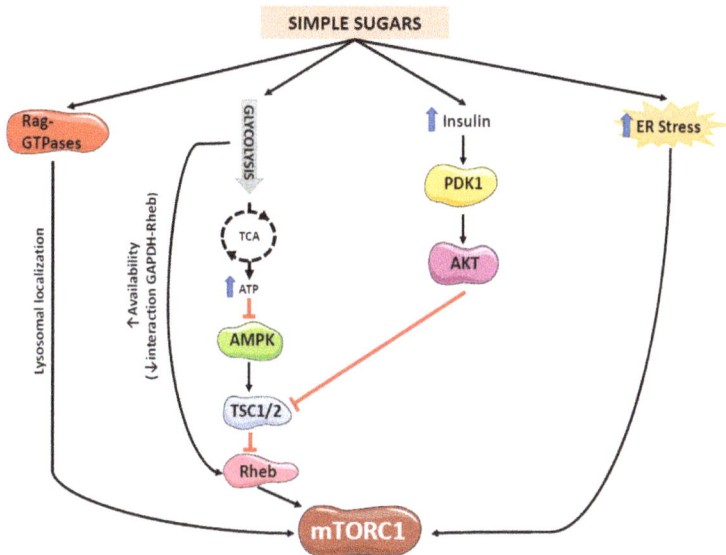

Figure 2. Proposed mechanisms of mTORC1 activity regulation by simple sugars. mTORC1 activation by simple sugars might be mediated by several mechanisms, including (i) Rag-GTPases activation, which cause mTORC1 lysosomal localization, (ii) increased glycolytic flux, which might increase Rheb availability and inhibit AMPK activity, (iii) increased plasma insulin levels and (iv) increased ER stress.

In studies conducted by our group in female rats supplemented with 10% (*w/v*) liquid fructose for different periods of time (two weeks, two months and seven months), we consistently showed a marked increase in hepatic mTOR phosphorylation at Ser-2481 [8–10]. As Rheb overexpression has been reported to promote the phosphorylation of mTOR at this position [11], we explored whether fructose induced mTOR phosphorylation by increasing Rheb expression. We did not detect a significant increase in the hepatic levels of Rheb protein in female rats supplemented with liquid fructose for two months [8]. A cell-based model of mTORC1 regulation by glucose proposed that high glucose levels increased glycolytic flux and reduced the interaction of Rheb with GAPDH, thus increasing the availability of Rheb to interact with and activate mTORC1 [12]. Our co-immunoprecipitation experiments showed that this was not the mechanism for fructose-induced mTORC1 activation, since Rheb-GAPDH and Rheb-mTOR interactions were not affected in the livers of fructose-supplemented rats [8].

Carbohydrates also regulate mTORC1 indirectly via adenosine monophosphate-activated protein kinase (AMPK), which senses the fluctuations in energy levels due to glucose availability. AMPK is another cellular energy sensor that is activated by increased AMP/ATP ratio caused by either reduced ATP production or excessive ATP consumption [13]. AMPK has the opposite role to that of the mTOR system. While mTOR is activated by high energy availability and promotes anabolic routes to use this energy in cell growth and proliferation, AMPK senses low energy statuses, for example glucose deprivation and promotes catabolic processes to obtain energy. Glucose deprivation activates AMPK not only by increasing the AMP/ATP ratio but also by depletion of the glucose metabolite fructose-1,6-biphosphate. Reduced levels of this metabolite facilitate the formation of an AMPK-containing protein complex in the lysosomal membrane, which stimulates the kinase LKB1 to phosphorylate and activate AMPK [14]. AMPK activation can inhibit the mTORC1 pathway through two main mechanisms: phosphorylation of tuberous sclerosis complex (TSC) 2 at Ser-1387, which activates the upstream mTOR inhibitor TSC1/TSC2 complex [15,16] or direct inhibition by phosphorylating Raptor [17]. It is not yet known which of these mechanisms predominate but it has been proposed that TSC2 phosphorylation may counteract growth factor-activated mTORC1, whereas Raptor phosphorylation has been reported to inhibit basal mTORC1 activity [18].

When glucose enters the glycolytic pathway to form pyruvate for the tricarboxylic acid (TCA) cycle, ATP is generated and AMPK is inhibited, which leads to mTORC1 activation. However, before entering the glycolytic pathway, carbohydrates are phosphorylated by hexokinases in an irreversible reaction that consumes ATP. Although this process is similar for all carbohydrates, there are some differences. For example, glucose is phosphorylated first by glucokinase and after isomerization the resulting molecule is phosphorylated by phosphofructokinase, whose activity is tightly controlled by end-product inhibition (ATP and citrate) [19]. By contrast, fructose is phosphorylated by fructokinase and enters the glycolytic pathway by skipping the negative feedback control system. Moreover, fructose up-regulates fructokinase expression, thus inducing its own metabolism. Therefore, despite both fructose and glucose phosphorylation consuming ATP, this consumption is more rapid and intense for fructose, which may deplete ATP [20]. Paradoxically, this mechanism could lead to AMPK activation and, consequently, mTORC1 inhibition. Results from our own studies in female rats supplemented with simple sugars in liquid form for seven months indicated that fructose does not activate hepatic AMPK [21], suggesting that if ATP depletion does occur it may be transient and not associated with chronic fructose intake. In a recent study, Hu et al. confirmed this transient inhibitory effect of fructose: in mice sacrificed 30 min after receiving a 10% fructose or glucose solution by gavage, mTORC1 activity was inhibited by fructose but this inhibitory effect was lost in mice receiving a diet containing 60% fructose for one week [22]. In contrast to fructose, our results in female rats showed that chronic consumption of an equicaloric glucose solution activated AMPK, as demonstrated by a modest but significant 30% increase in phospho-AMPK α (Thr172) levels [21]. We attributed this effect to the increased plasma adiponectin levels observed only in rats consuming glucose [9], as the liver has been described to be one of the main targets of circulating adiponectin, which activates hepatic AMPK by phosphorylation [23].

Carbohydrates can also regulate mTORC1 activity through endoplasmic reticulum (ER) stress. The ER has a key role in cellular homeostasis by controlling the synthesis, folding and posttranslational modification of proteins. Perturbations in the ER folding capacity cause ER stress and trigger the unfolded protein response (UPR), which involves the activation of specific transmembrane proteins acting as stress sensors (activating transcription factor 6 [ATF6], inositol-requiring enzyme 1 [IRE1] and protein kinase RNA-like ER kinase [PERK]) to restore cell homeostasis by proper protein folding and reduction of the ER protein load [24]. The UPR is activated not only by the accumulation of unfolded proteins but also by other stimuli, including nutrient availability. Both deprivation and excessive levels of carbohydrates can induce ER stress, which may influence mTORC activity. Thus, glucose starvation causes energy stress by reducing ATP levels, which at least in some cell types can induce calcium efflux from the ER and activate the PERK branch of the UPR [25]. In addition, protein glycosylation occurs in the ER and, therefore, alterations in this process due to glucose depletion could perturb ER homeostasis and elicit also ER stress [18]. On the other hand, high levels of glucose stimulate ER stress in hepatic cells, as shown by higher levels of PERK phosphorylation [26]. Interestingly, the glucose-induced ER stress response in these cells is mediated by mTORC1, as specific mTORC1 inhibition by rapamycin prevents the phosphorylation of PERK and its downstream effector eIF2α [26]. ER stress can also elicit mTORC1 activation through ATF6 and the induction of the phosphoinositide 3-kinase (PI3K)-Akt axis; however, Akt and mTORC1 are inhibited under conditions of chronic ER stress [27].

Results from our own studies in female rats showed that fructose consumption activated mTORC1 independently of ER stress [8,9]. As mentioned before, we observed that fructose induced hepatic mTOR phosphorylation at Ser-2481 but the only UPR marker that was increased was phosphorylated IRE1, whereas the PERK branch of the UPR remained unaffected [8,9]. In fact, mTOR activation in renal cells has been shown to selectively induce IRE1 without affecting PERK and ATF6 [28]. In contrast to PERK activation, which leads to CHOP induction and JNK-mediated apoptosis, selective IRE1 activation might protect cells by promoting the elimination of misfolded proteins without inducing cell death. Moreover, as it was shown in hepatocyte-specific IRE1-null mice, IRE1 is required to prevent hepatic steatosis [29] and when it is chronically activated it may cause the regression of pre-existing steatosis. Accordingly, the lack of hepatic steatosis observed in rats supplemented with fructose or glucose for seven months could be attributed to the selective and chronic activation of IRE1 in their livers [9].

Interestingly, when we compared the effects of glucose and fructose supplementation in female rats, we found that fructose induced hepatic mTOR Ser-2481 phosphorylation to a greater extent than glucose and that only fructose activated downstream effectors of mTORC1 such as phosphorylated 4EBP1 [9]. The fact that fructose had a greater effect on mTORC1 than glucose could not be attributed to the amount of energy provided by the sugar supplementation, as rats consumed equicaloric amounts of glucose and fructose. Instead, this could be due to an indirect mechanism involving changes in plasma insulin levels. Insulin, after binding to its receptor, activates the PI3K-phosphoinositide-dependent kinase 1 (PDK1)-Akt pathway, leading to the phosphorylation of TSC2 at multiple sites, which inactivates the TSC2/TSC1 complex and activates Rheb and mTORC1 [2]. Our results showed that only fructose-supplemented rats displayed significant hyperinsulinemia after seven months of treatment and therefore, the lower level of mTORC1 activation observed with the equicaloric glucose supplementation could be attributed, at least in part, to a lack of effect on plasma insulin levels [9]. Another factor contributing to this differential effect is that, as commented before, only glucose supplementation activates AMPK [9], which has an inhibitory effect on mTORC1.

3. The Effects of mTOR on Lipid Metabolism and Modulation by Carbohydrates

The mTOR system plays a key role in the response to nutrient abundance, in part by activating anabolic processes such as lipid synthesis. Both mTORC1 and mTORC2 can modulate lipogenesis but much more attention has been paid to mTORC1. Lipogenesis is activated by mTOR mainly through the master regulator of this process, the transcription factor SREBP1c, which belongs to the basic-helix loop-helix-leucine zipper family. SREBP1c is synthesized as a precursor that remains anchored to the ER membrane through its interaction with SREBP cleavage-activating protein (SCAP) [30]. Through a mechanism that remains unclear [31], the SCAP-SREBP1c heterodimer is transferred to the Golgi apparatus, where SREBP1c is processed by proteolytic enzymes into its mature form, that then translocates to the nucleus to induce the transcription of target genes, including those encoding the main lipogenic enzymes. The mTOR system can regulate SREBP1c activity at different levels, including transcription of its encoding gene Srebf1, processing of the precursor protein and nuclear transport of the mature protein (Figure 3) [2,31].

mTORC1 activates SREBP1c partly through S6K1 by mechanisms that have not been completely elucidated [2]. For example, a study in rat hepatocytes in which the transcriptional effects of insulin on the SREBP1c gene were eliminated showed that S6K1 is essential for SREBP1c processing but not for its transcription [32]. However, other studies have shown that S6K1 depletion in the liver of obese mice reduces the abundance of hepatic SREBP1c mRNA [33]. Moreover, a recent report showed that mTORC1-S6K1 activation may induce lipogenesis independently of SREBP1c by promoting the splicing of lipogenic mRNAs, that increases their stability [34]. In addition, mTORC1 may activate SREBP1c via S6K1-independent pathways such as by: (i) the phosphorylation of CREB-regulated transcription coactivator 2 (CRTC2), which increases the trafficking of SREBP1c to the Golgi apparatus where it is processed [35]; (ii) the phosphorylation and nuclear exclusion of lipin-1, which prevents its blocking effect on SREBP1c transcriptional activity [36]; and (iii) inducing ER stress, which may activate hepatic SREBP1c [2]. Furthermore, mTORC2 might also regulate SREBP1c, as mice with specific hepatic deletion of Rictor have been reported to show reduced SREBP1c activity and lipogenesis [37].

Thus, it could be hypothesized that simple sugars promote lipogenesis by activating the mTORC1-SREBP pathway. Our studies in rats supplemented with 10% liquid fructose (*w/v*) for two weeks or two months did not show increases in the nuclear active form of SREBP1c, despite higher levels of mTOR phosphorylation [8,10]. By contrast, nuclear SREBP1c levels were significantly increased in rats fed a 63% fructose in solid form for two weeks [38]. Similarly, in our chronic study in which 10% liquid sugars were supplemented for seven months, fructose but not glucose caused an increase in nuclear SREBP1c [9]. Therefore, it seems that the ability of fructose to activate SREBP1c depends on the burden of fructose to the organism, taking into account both the amount of fructose consumed and the duration of the supplementation. Moreover, the different effects of fructose and glucose on SREBP1c activity could be due to the greater effect of fructose on mTOR phosphorylation, combined with the hyperinsulinemia caused by fructose but not glucose supplementation.

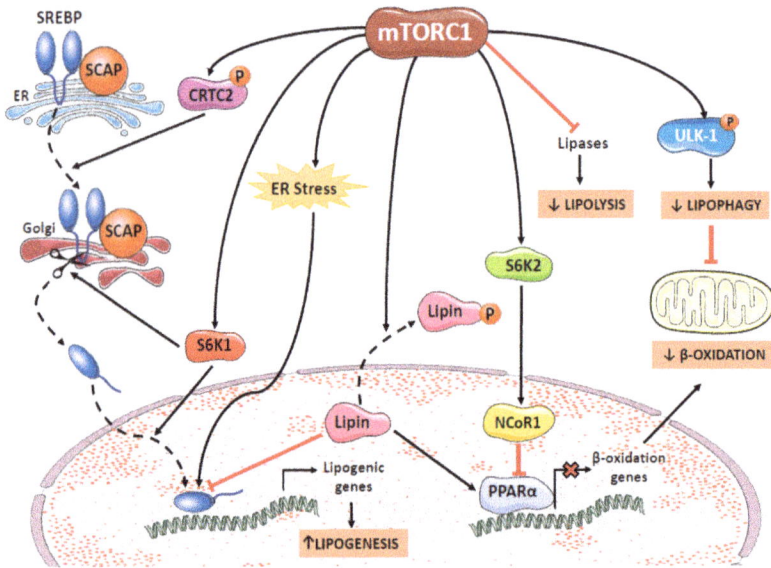

Figure 3. Effects of mTORC1 on lipid metabolism. mTORC1 activates lipogenesis via SREBP1c, partly through S6K1 and also by S6K1-independent mechanisms, such as the phosphorylation of CRTC2 and lipin, which causes its nuclear exclusion, and ER stress induction. In addition, mTORC1 inhibits neutral lipolysis and repress autophagy/lipophagy by phosphorylating ULK-1, which could inhibit fatty acid β-oxidation by lowering substrate availability. mTORC1 may also inhibit PPARα activity by recruiting NCoR1 to the nucleus and by inducing lipin-1 phosphorylation.

mTOR affects lipid metabolism not only by inducing lipogenesis but also by inhibiting lipolysis and lipophagy (Figure 3). Both mTORC1 and mTORC2 can inhibit neutral lipolysis, a process in which cytoplasmic lipases hydrolyse cytoplasmic lipid droplets at a neutral pH [39]. The term lipophagy was coined in 2009 when it was demonstrated that the intracellular lipid content is also regulated by the lysosomal degradation of lipids through autophagy [40]. Since then, lipophagy has been reported to occur in different cell types and be essential for regulating cellular energy metabolism, as it may be activated or inhibited in response to energy requirements [41]. Lipophagy is, in fact, a specialized subtype of autophagy, using the same intracellular machinery and being regulated by the same mechanisms as those associated with autophagy, including mTORC1 [39]. Repression of autophagy by mTORC1 involves the phosphorylation of ULK-1 at Ser-757 [42]. Our studies in female rats revealed that increased phosphorylation of hepatic mTOR after fructose supplementation for two months increased phosphorylated levels of ULK-1 and led to a decrease of autophagic markers, including the LC3B-II/LC3B-I protein ratio [8]. As the inhibition of autophagy promotes hepatic triglyceride accumulation, we hypothesized that this mechanism could be responsible, at least in part, for the hepatic steatosis observed in rats sub-chronically supplemented with liquid fructose.

Finally, the mTOR system may also modulate lipid catabolism by inhibiting fatty acid β-oxidation. This could be a consequence of the inhibition of autophagy by mTORC1, as autophagy causes the breakdown of triglycerides and provides fatty acid substrates for β-oxidation. Activation of mTORC1 and inhibition of autophagy could explain why β-oxidation is inhibited in the livers of female rats after sugar supplementation for two and seven-month, without altering peroxisome proliferator-activated receptor (PPAR)α gene or protein expression [8,9]. Despite a lack of effect on PPARα expression, our results showed that the reduction of β-oxidation by fructose involved lower PPARα activity, as indicated by the reduced nuclear PPARα levels in the livers of fructose-supplemented rats [9]. This could also be related to mTORC1 activation, as mTORC1 has been reported to inhibit PPARα at least by two possible mechanisms, via nuclear receptor corepressor 1 (NCoR1) or lipin-1 [2]. NCoR1 is a transcriptional regulator that binds to several nuclear receptors. The mTORC1 substrate S6K2 has been observed to associate with NCoR1, recruiting it to the nucleus where it represses PPARα transcriptional activity [43]. In hepatic cells lipin-1 acts as a transcriptional activator of β-oxidation genes through PPARα activation. As it was previously mentioned, mTORC1 can induce the phosphorylation and nuclear exclusion of lipin-1, which could lead to the reduction of PPARα activity. There are few studies examining the effects of carbohydrates on lipin-1 in vivo. Vasiljević et al. reported that male rats supplemented with 10% liquid fructose for nine weeks showed increased microsomal levels of lipin-1 in the liver, although the extent of lipin-1 phosphorylation or its concentration in hepatic nuclear fractions were not determined [44]. Furthermore, despite the same treatment increased the nuclear contents of lipin-1 in the hearts of female (but not male) rats, this was not accompanied by increased levels of nuclear PPARα [45]. Moreover, it remains to be established whether this is a specific effect in cardiac cells and whether it is related to mTOR activity.

4. The Effects of mTOR on Carbohydrate Metabolism

mTOR can affect carbohydrate metabolism directly, by controlling hepatic gluconeogenesis, and also indirectly, by regulating pancreatic β-cell mass and activity (Figure 4). Moreover, both mTORC1 and mTORC2 can induce insulin resistance and, thus, dysregulate glucose metabolism.

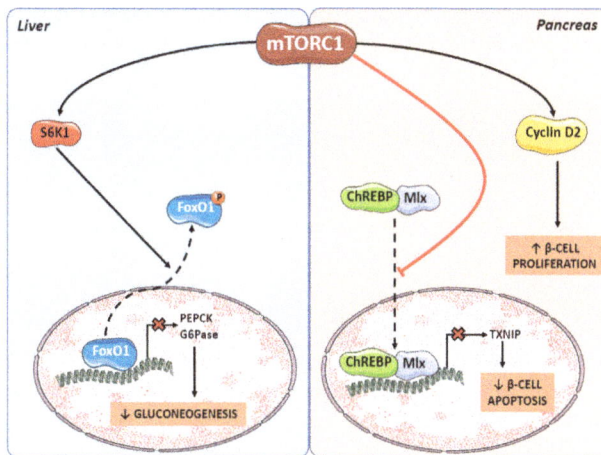

Figure 4. Effects of mTORC1 on carbohydrate metabolism. mTORC1 activation inhibits gluconeogenesis by promoting the phosphorylation and nuclear exclusion of FoxO1 via S6K1, which blocks its transcriptional effect on the main gluconeogenic genes PEPCK and G6Pase. Carbohydrate metabolism may be also indirectly altered by mTORC1 effects on the survival and proliferation of insulin-secreting pancreatic β-cells.

The ability of mTORC1 to control gluconeogesis was demonstrated by experiments in rapamycin-treated rats, which showed that chronic inhibition of the mTORC1-S6K1 pathway increased the hepatic expression of the key gluconeogenic genes encoding phosphoenolpyruvate carboxykinase (PEPCK) and glucose 6-phosphatase (G6Pase) in the liver [46]. The regulation of gluconeogenic gene expression is mediated partly by the transcription factor forkhead box protein O1 (FoxO1). In response to insulin, FoxO1 is phosphorylated by Akt causing its nuclear exclusion and a reduction in PEPCK and G6Pase expression. Interestingly, it has been reported that in rapamycin-treated rats, in which mTORC1 was inhibited, nuclear FoxO1 levels were increased despite hyperinsulinemia, which could account for the increased expression of PEPCK and G6Pase [46]. Although that study did not determine the extent of FoxO1 phosphorylation, Yue et al. [47] showed that the stimulation of mTOR-S6K1 signalling in the mouse hypothalamus increased FoxO1 phosphorylation, whereas treatment with rapamycin (which blocks only mTORC1 when it is administered acutely) reduced FoxO1 phosphorylation. In addition, experiments in liver-specific Rictor knockout mice demonstrated that mTORC2 also controls hepatic gluconeogenesis. Upon refeeding, these mice showed hepatic FoxO1 hypophosphorylation and nuclear localization, together with higher levels of PEPCK and G6Pase mRNA, compared to wild type mice [37]. mTORC2 phosphorylates Akt at Ser-473 and it has been shown that in mTORC2-deficient cells phosphorylation at this position is absent and FoxO1 phosphorylation is specifically reduced [48].

Thus, it seems plausible that both mTORC1 and mTORC2 activation may inhibit gluconeogenesis by promoting FoxO1 phosphorylation via S6K1 and Akt, respectively. Our results in female rats supplemented with simple sugars support this hypothesis. In rats drinking a 10% *w/v* fructose solution for two weeks, mTORC1 activation led to a decrease in PEPCK expression, probably via IRE1 phosphorylation that promoted the splicing of X-box-binding protein (XBP)-1, which is involved in the maintenance of glucose homeostasis [49]. Moreover, chronic glucose and fructose supplementation in rats has been reported to activate mTORC1 (shown by the phosphorylation of peroxisome proliferator-activated receptor gamma coactivator 1-alpha [PGC-1α], a direct target of S6K1 and the absence of Ser-473 Akt phosphorylation), increase FoxO1 phosphorylation and reduce the expression of PEPCK and G6Pase [9]. However, the crosstalk between mTORC1 and mTORC2 is quite complex, as cell culture experiments show that mTORC1-S6K1 signalling induce Rictor phosphorylation, with Akt and FoxO1 phosphorylation increasing when the phosphorylation position of Rictor is mutated [50]. This suggests that mTORC1 signalling could inhibit the mTORC2-Akt pathway, leading to reduced FoxO1 phosphorylation and increased gluconeogenesis.

In addition, mTOR signalling regulates the growth and proliferation of pancreatic β-cells and their ability to secrete insulin, which may also affect glucose homeostasis. Similar to the regulation of gluconeogenesis, both mTOR complexes control β-cell mass and activity, as mice deficient in S6K1 [51] or Rictor [52] exhibit reduced β-cell mass and hypoinsulinemia. The molecular mechanism underlying these effects was recently unravelled [53]. In pancreatic β-cells, mTOR interacts with a complex containing ChREBP and Max-like protein (Mlx), inhibiting its translocation to the nucleus. The ChREBP-Mlx complex regulates the transcription of thioredoxin-interacting protein (TXNIP), which is involved in the apoptosis of β-cells. Thus, the reduced nuclear translocation of ChREBP-Mlx results in reduced TXNIP expression and protects β-cells from apoptosis. Moreover, mTOR not only regulates the number of β-cells but also their specific activity, as mTOR inactivation by the overexpression of a kinase-dead mTOR mutant (which therefore affects both mTORC1 and mTORC2) leads to defective β-cell function without affecting its mass [54].

Carbohydrates, as well as other nutrients, can regulate β-cell proliferation as an adaptive response to the changes in the metabolic environment. It has been recognized for a long time that glucose regulates not only insulin secretion but also the proliferation of β-cells. However, the role of mTOR as a key player in this process has been demonstrated only recently. The proliferative effect of glucose on β-cells involves the activation of an atypical protein kinase C (PKCζ), which activates mTORC1 and subsequently induces cyclin D2 activation [55,56]. Fructose might also have a proliferative effect of on pancreatic β-cells, given the ability of fructose to activate mTORC1. However, excessive fructose consumption might be detrimental, as a high fructose diet (65% fructose in solid form) has been reported to induce pancreatic ER stress and β-cell apoptosis, which are increased when fructose is combined with a high fat diet [57].

5. Concluding Remarks

It is well recognized that overnutrition, together with a sedentary lifestyle, is one of the main drivers of metabolic pathologies such as fatty liver, dyslipidaemia and hyperglycaemia. However, the role of individual nutrients and the mechanisms involved have not been fully elucidated. From our studies in rats supplemented with simple sugars in liquid form (10% w/v) for different periods of time (from two weeks to seven months), we have identified hepatic mTOR, specifically mTORC1, as a key hub that transduces the signals elicited by carbohydrates to activate or inhibit molecular pathways and modulate the metabolism of lipids and carbohydrates. Thus, we have consistently observed that glucose and fructose intake increases mTOR phosphorylation and activates mTORC1. Although the specific underlying mechanism is not fully understood, we have ruled out the involvement of Rheb availability or expression and we have also demonstrated that mTORC1 activation is independent of ER stress. mTORC1 activation by glucose and fructose explains most of the metabolic effects observed in our studies in female rats, including enhanced lipogenesis and reduced gluconeogenesis (Figure 5). Moreover, mTORC1 activation might also inhibit PPARα activity and autophagy which, together with enhanced lipogenesis, contribute to hepatic fat deposition. By these mechanisms sub-chronic administration of fructose (for two months) induced hepatic steatosis in female rats. However, sustained activation of the mTORC1-IRE1 pathway by chronic fructose supplementation could prevent fat deposition in the liver. Moreover, the different extent of mTORC1 activation seems to be responsible for the different effects of fructose and glucose supplementation in rats, as only fructose-supplemented rats displayed significant hyperinsulinemia, which also activates mTORC1. On the other hand, only glucose increases plasma adiponectin levels leading to AMPK activation, which in turn inhibits mTORC1 and therefore has a weaker effect on mTORC1 activation than fructose. The mechanism by which glucose increases adiponectin levels and whether this effect is specific to rodents or may also apply to humans are yet to be established.

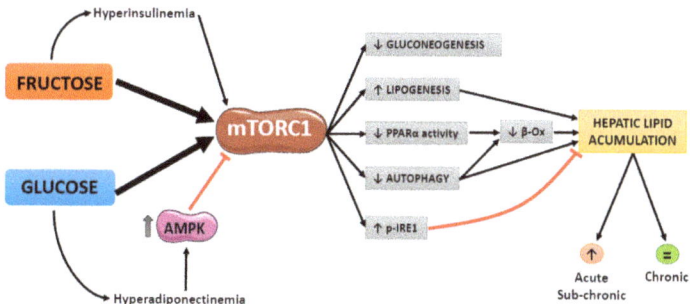

Figure 5. mTORC1 as a key hub transducing the metabolic effects of glucose and fructose in the liver. Fructose activates mTORC1 leading to reduced gluconeogenesis and enhanced lipogenesis which, together with PPARα/β-oxidation activity and autophagy inhibition contribute to hepatic fat deposition observed in our studies after sub-chronic administration of fructose (for two months) in female rats. By contrast, sustained activation of the mTORC1-IRE1 pathway by chronic fructose supplementation could prevent fat deposition in the liver. Fructose-induced hyperinsulinemia, which activates mTORC1 and the increase in plasma adiponectin levels caused by glucose administration, which inhibits mTORC1 via AMPK activation, lead to a different extent of mTORC1 activation by these simple sugars, which seems to be responsible for the different metabolic effects of fructose and glucose supplementation observed in our studies performed in female rats.

Funding: This research was funded by Spanish Ministry of Economy, Industry and Competitiveness (grant numbers SAF2010-15664, SAF2013-42982-R and SAF2017-82369-R), Generalitat de Catalunya (SGR09-00413; SGR13-00066 and 2017 SGR 38) and European Commission FEDER funds. A.M.V. is a predoctoral fellow, BECAL grant program BCAL04-327, from the Government of Paraguay.

Acknowledgments: We thank the University of Barcelona's Language Advisory Service for revising the manuscript.

Conflicts of Interest: The authors declare no conflict of interest.

Abbreviations

4EBP	eIF4E binding protein
AMPK	activating transcription factor 6
ATF6	adenosine monophosphate-activated protein kinase
CRTC2	CREB-regulated transcription coactivator 2
DEPTOR	DEP domain-containing mTOR-interacting protein
ER	endoplasmic reticulum
FoxO1	forkhead box protein O1
G6Pase	glucose 6-phosphatase
IRE1	inositol-requiring enzyme 1
mLST8	mammalian lethal with SEC13 protein 8
Mlx	Max-like protein
mTOR	mechanistic (mammalian) target of rapamycin
mTORC	mTOR complex
NAFLD	non-alcoholic fatty liver disease
NCoR1	nuclear receptor corepressor 1
PDK1	peroxisome proliferator-activated receptor
PEPCK	phosphoenolpyruvate carboxykinase
PERK	phosphoinositide 3-kinase
PGC-1α	phosphoinositide-dependent kinase 1
PI3K	proline-rich Akt substrate of 40 kDa
PPAR	protein kinase RNA-like ER kinase
PRAS40	protein S6 kinases
Raptor	rapamycin-insensitive companion of mTOR
Rheb	Ras-homolog enriched in brain
Rictor	receptor gamma coactivator 1-alpha
S6K1/2	regulatory-associated protein of mTOR
SCAP	SREBP cleavage-activating protein
SREBP	sterol response element-binding protein
TCA	thioredoxin-interacting protein
TSC	tricarboxylic acid
TXNIP	tuberous sclerosis complex
ULK-1	UNC-51-like kinase 1
UPR	unfolded protein response
XBP-1	X-box-binding protein

References

1. Sabatini, D.M. Twenty-five years of mTOR: Uncovering the link from nutrients to growth. *Proc. Natl. Acad. Sci. USA* **2017**, *114*, 11818–11825. [CrossRef] [PubMed]
2. Caron, A.; Richard, D.; Laplante, M. The Roles of mTOR Complexes in Lipid Metabolism. *Annu. Rev. Nutr.* **2015**, *35*, 321–348. [CrossRef] [PubMed]
3. Castellano, B.M.; Thelen, A.M.; Moldavski, O.; McKenna, F.; van der Welle, R.E.; Mydock-McGrane, L.; Jiang, X.; van Eijkeren, R.J.; Davis, O.B.; Louie, S.M.; et al. Lysosomal Cholesterol Activates mTORC1 via an SLC38A9-Niemann Pick C1 Signaling Complex. *Science* **2017**, *355*, 1306–1311. [CrossRef] [PubMed]
4. Saxton, R.A.; Sabatini, D.M. mTOR Signaling in Growth, Metabolism, and Disease. *Cell* **2017**, *168*, 960–976. [CrossRef] [PubMed]

5. Efeyan, A.; Comb, W.C.; Sabatini, D.M. Nutrient-sensing mechanisms and pathways. *Nature* **2015**, *517*, 302–310. [CrossRef] [PubMed]

6. Efeyan, A.; Zoncu, R.; Chang, S.; Gumper, I.; Snitkin, H.; Wolfson, R.L.; Kirak, O.; Sabatini, D.D.; Sabatini, D.M. Regulation of mTORC1 by the Rag GTPases is necessary for neonatal autophagy and survival. *Nature* **2013**, *493*, 679–683. [CrossRef] [PubMed]

7. Soliman, G.A.; Acosta-Jaquez, H.A.; Dunlop, E.A.; Ekim, B.; Maj, N.E.; Tee, A.R.; Fingar, D.C. mTOR Ser-2481 autophosphorylation monitors mTORC-specific catalytic activity and clarifies rapamycin mechanism of action. *J. Biol. Chem.* **2010**, *285*, 7866–7879. [CrossRef] [PubMed]

8. Baena, M.; Sangüesa, G.; Hutter, N.; Sánchez, R.M.; Roglans, N.; Laguna, J.C.; Alegret, M. Fructose supplementation impairs rat liver autophagy through mTORC activation without inducing endoplasmic reticulum stress. *Biochim. Biophys. Acta Mol. Cell Biol. Lipids* **2015**, *1851*, 107–116. [CrossRef] [PubMed]

9. Sangüesa, G.; Montañés, J.C.; Baena, M.; Sánchez, R.M.; Roglans, N.; Alegret, M.; Laguna, J.C. Chronic fructose intake does not induce liver steatosis and inflammation in female Sprague–Dawley rats, but causes hypertriglyceridemia related to decreased VLDL receptor expression. *Eur. J. Nutr.* **2018**. [CrossRef] [PubMed]

10. Rebollo, A.; Roglans, N.; Baena, M.; Padrosa, A.; Sanchez, R.M.; Merlos, M.; Alegret, M.; Laguna, J.C. Liquid fructose down-regulates liver insulin receptor substrate 2 and gluconeogenic enzymes by modifying nutrient sensing factors in rats. *J. Nutr. Biochem.* **2014**, *25*, 250–258. [CrossRef] [PubMed]

11. Acosta-Jaquez, H.A.; Keller, J.A.; Foster, K.G.; Ekim, B.; Soliman, G.A.; Feener, E.P.; Ballif, B.A.; Fingar, D.C. Site-specific mTOR phosphorylation promotes mTORC1-mediated signaling and cell growth. *Mol. Cell. Biol.* **2009**, *29*, 4308–4324. [CrossRef] [PubMed]

12. Lee, M.N.; Ha, S.H.; Kim, J.; Koh, A.; Lee, C.S.; Kim, J.H.; Jeon, H.; Kim, D.-H.; Suh, P.-G.; Ryu, S.H. Glycolytic flux signals to mTOR through glyceraldehyde-3-phosphate dehydrogenase-mediated regulation of Rheb. *Mol. Cell. Biol.* **2009**, *29*, 3991–4001. [CrossRef] [PubMed]

13. Kahn, B.B.; Alquier, T.; Carling, D.; Hardie, D.G. AMP-activated protein kinase: Ancient energy gauge provides clues to modern understanding of metabolism. *Cell Metab.* **2005**, *1*, 15–25. [CrossRef] [PubMed]

14. Zhang, C.S.; Hawley, S.A.; Zong, Y.; Li, M.; Wang, Z.; Gray, A.; Ma, T.; Cui, J.; Feng, J.W.; Zhu, M.; et al. Fructose-1,6-bisphosphate and aldolase mediate glucose sensing by AMPK. *Nature* **2017**, *548*, 112–116. [CrossRef] [PubMed]

15. Inoki, K.; Zhu, T.; Guan, K.-L. TSC2 Mediates Cellular Energy Response to Control Cell Growth and Survival. *Cell* **2003**, *115*, 577–590. [CrossRef]

16. Shimobayashi, M.; Hall, M.N. Making new contacts: The mTOR network in metabolism and signalling crosstalk. *Nat. Rev. Mol. Cell Biol.* **2014**, *15*, 155–162. [CrossRef] [PubMed]

17. Gwinn, D.M.; Shackelford, D.B.; Egan, D.F.; Mihaylova, M.M.; Mery, A.; Vasquez, D.S.; Turk, B.E.; Shaw, R.J. AMPK Phosphorylation of Raptor Mediates a Metabolic Checkpoint. *Mol. Cell* **2008**, *30*, 214–226. [CrossRef] [PubMed]

18. Dibble, C.C.; Manning, B.D. Signal integration by mTORC1 coordinates nutrient input with biosynthetic output. *Nat. Cell Biol.* **2013**, *15*, 555–564. [CrossRef] [PubMed]

19. Alegret, M.; Roglans, N.; Laguna, J.C. Fructose consumption and leptin resistance: What have we learnt from animal studies? In *Leptin: Hormonal Fuctions, Dysfunctions and Clinical Uses*; Nova Science: New York, NY, USA, 2011; pp. 209–230. ISBN 9781611228915.

20. Abdelmalek, M.F.; Lazo, M.; Horska, A.; Bonekamp, S.; Lipkin, E.W.; Balasubramanyam, A.; Bantle, J.P.; Johnson, R.J.; Diehl, A.M.; Clark, J.; et al. ATP Homeostasis in Obese Individuals with Type 2 Diabetes. *Hepatology* **2013**, *56*, 952–960. [CrossRef] [PubMed]

21. Sangüesa, G.; Roglans, N.; Montañés, J.C.; Baena, M.; Velázquez, A.M.; Sánchez, R.M.; Alegret, M.; Laguna, J.C. Chronic Liquid Fructose, but not Glucose, Supplementation Selectively Induces Visceral Adipose Tissue Leptin Resistance and Hypertrophy in Female Sprague-Dawley Rats. *Mol. Nutr. Food Res.* **2018**, *62*, 1800777. [CrossRef] [PubMed]

22. Hu, Y.; Semova, I.; Sun, X.; Kang, H.; Chahar, S.; Hollenberg, A.N.; Masson, D.; Hirschey, M.D.; Miao, J.; Biddinger, S.B. Fructose and glucose can regulate mammalian target of rapamycin complex 1 and lipogenic gene expression via distinct pathways. *J. Biol. Chem.* **2018**, *293*, 2006–2014. [CrossRef] [PubMed]

23. Ruan, H.; Dong, L.Q. Adiponectin signaling and function in insulin target tissues. *J. Mol. Cell Biol.* **2016**, *8*, 101–109. [CrossRef] [PubMed]

24. Walter, P.; Ron, D. The Unfolded Protein Response: From Stress Pathway to Homeostatic Regulation. *Science* **2011**, *334*, 1081–1086. [CrossRef] [PubMed]

25. Moore, C.E.; Omikorede, O.; Gomez, E.; Willars, G.B.; Herbert, T.P. PERK Activation at Low Glucose Concentration Is Mediated by SERCA Pump Inhibition and Confers Preemptive Cytoprotection to Pancreatic β-Cells. *Mol. Endocrinol.* **2011**, *25*, 315–326. [CrossRef] [PubMed]

26. Li, H.; Min, Q.; Ouyang, C.; Lee, J.; He, C.; Zou, M.H.; Xie, Z. AMPK activation prevents excess nutrient-induced hepatic lipid accumulation by inhibiting mTORC1 signaling and endoplasmic reticulum stress response. *Biochim. Biophys. Acta Mol. Basis Dis.* **2014**, *1842*, 1844–1854. [CrossRef] [PubMed]

27. Appenzeller-Herzog, C.; Hall, M.N. Bidirectional crosstalk between endoplasmic reticulum stress and mTOR signaling. *Trends Cell Biol.* **2012**, *22*, 274–282. [CrossRef] [PubMed]

28. Kato, H.; Nakajima, S.; Saito, Y.; Takahashi, S.; Katoh, R.; Kitamura, M. MTORC1 serves ER stress-triggered apoptosis via selective activation of the IRE1-JNK pathway. *Cell Death Differ.* **2012**, *19*, 310–320. [CrossRef] [PubMed]

29. Zhang, K.; Wang, S.; Malhotra, J.; Hassler, J.R.; Back, S.H.; Wang, G.; Chang, L.; Xu, W.; Miao, H.; Leonardi, R.; et al. The unfolded protein response transducer IRE1Î ± prevents ER stress-induced hepatic steatosis. *EMBO J.* **2011**, *30*, 1357–1375. [CrossRef] [PubMed]

30. Yecies, J.L.; Zhang, H.H.; Menon, S.; Liu, S.; Yecies, D.; Lipovsky, A.I.; Gorgun, C.; Kwiatkowski, D.J.; Hotamisligil, G.S.; Lee, C.H.; et al. Akt stimulates hepatic SREBP1c and lipogenesis through parallel mTORC1-dependent and independent pathways. *Cell Metab.* **2011**, *14*, 21–32. [CrossRef] [PubMed]

31. Shimano, H.; Sato, R. SREBP-regulated lipid metabolism: Convergent physiology-divergent pathophysiology. *Nat. Rev. Endocrinol.* **2017**, *13*, 710–730. [CrossRef] [PubMed]

32. Owen, J.L.; Zhang, Y.; Bae, S.-H.; Farooqi, M.S.; Liang, G.; Hammer, R.E.; Goldstein, J.L.; Brown, M.S. Insulin stimulation of SREBP-1c processing in transgenic rat hepatocytes requires p70 S6-kinase. *Proc. Natl. Acad. Sci. USA* **2012**, *109*, 16184–16189. [CrossRef] [PubMed]

33. Li, S.; Ogawa, W.; Emi, A.; Hayashi, K.; Senga, Y.; Nomura, K.; Hara, K.; Yu, D.; Kasuga, M. Role of S6K1 in regulation of SREBP1c expression in the liver. *Biochem. Biophys. Res. Commun.* **2011**, *412*, 197–202. [CrossRef] [PubMed]

34. Lee, G.; Zheng, Y.; Cho, S.; Jang, C.; England, C.; Dempsey, J.M.; Yu, Y.; Liu, X.; He, L.; Cavaliere, P.M.; et al. Post-transcriptional Regulation of De Novo Lipogenesis by mTORC1-S6K1-SRPK2 Signaling. *Cell* **2017**, *171*, 1545–1558. [CrossRef] [PubMed]

35. Han, J.; Li, E.; Chen, L.; Zhang, Y.; Wei, F.; Liu, J.; Deng, H.; Wang, Y. The CREB coactivator CRTC2 controls hepatic lipid metabolism by regulating SREBP1. *Nature* **2015**, *524*, 243–246. [CrossRef] [PubMed]

36. Peterson, T.R.; Sengupta, S.S.; Harris, T.E.; Carmack, A.E.; Kang, S.A.; Balderas, E.; Guertin, D.A.; Madden, K.L.; Carpenter, A.E.; Finck, B.N.; et al. MTOR complex 1 regulates lipin 1 localization to control the srebp pathway. *Cell* **2011**, *146*, 408–420. [CrossRef] [PubMed]

37. Hagiwara, A.; Cornu, M.; Cybulski, N.; Polak, P.; Betz, C.; Trapani, F.; Terracciano, L.; Heim, M.H.; Rüegg, M.A.; Hall, M.N. Hepatic mTORC2 activates glycolysis and lipogenesis through Akt, glucokinase, and SREBP1c. *Cell Metab.* **2012**, *15*, 725–738. [CrossRef] [PubMed]

38. Koo, H.Y.; Miyashita, M.; Simon Cho, B.H.; Nakamura, M.T. Replacing dietary glucose with fructose increases ChREBP activity and SREBP-1 protein in rat liver nucleus. *Biochem. Biophys. Res. Commun.* **2009**, *390*, 285–289. [CrossRef] [PubMed]

39. Zechner, R.; Madeo, F.; Kratky, D. Cytosolic lipolysis and lipophagy: Two sides of the same coin. *Nat. Rev. Mol. Cell Biol.* **2017**, *18*, 671–684. [CrossRef] [PubMed]

40. Singh, R.; Kaushik, S.; Wang, Y.; Xiang, Y.; Novak, I.; Komatsu, M.; Tanaka, K.; Cuervo, A.M.; Czaja, M.J. Autophagy regulates lipid metabolism. *Nature* **2009**, *458*, 1131–1135. [CrossRef] [PubMed]

41. Ward, C.; Martinez-Lopez, N.; Otten, E.G.; Carroll, B.; Maetzel, D.; Singh, R.; Sarkar, S.; Korolchuk, V.I. Autophagy, lipophagy and lysosomal lipid storage disorders. *Biochim. Biophys. Acta Mol. Cell Biol. Lipids* **2016**, *1861*, 269–284. [CrossRef] [PubMed]

42. Russell, R.C.; Yuan, H.-X.; Guan, K.-L. Autophagy regulation by nutrient signaling. *Cell Res.* **2014**, *24*, 42–57. [CrossRef] [PubMed]

43. Kim, K.; Pyo, S.; Um, S.H. S6 kinase 2 deficiency enhances ketone body production and increases peroxisome proliferator-activated receptor alpha activity in the liver. *Hepatology* **2012**, *55*, 1727–1737. [CrossRef] [PubMed]

44. Vasiljević, A.; Veličković, N.; Bursać, B.; Djordjevic, A.; Milutinović, D.V.; Nestorović, N.; Matić, G. Enhanced prereceptor glucocorticoid metabolism and lipogenesis impair insulin signaling in the liver of fructose-fed rats. *J. Nutr. Biochem.* **2013**, *24*, 1790–1797. [CrossRef] [PubMed]

45. Romić, S.; Tepavčević, S.; Žakula, Z.; Milosavljević, T.; Kostić, M.; Petković, M.; Korićanac, G. Gender differences in the expression and cellular localization of lipin 1 in the hearts of fructose-fed rats. *Lipids* **2014**, *49*, 655–663. [CrossRef] [PubMed]

46. Houde, V.P.; Brûlé, S.; Festuccia, W.T.; Blanchard, P.G.; Bellmann, K.; Deshaies, Y.; Marette, A.; Bru, S.; Festuccia, W.T.; Blanchard, P.G.; et al. Chronic rapamycin treatment causes glucose intolerance and hyperlipidemia by upregulating hepatic gluconeogenesis and impairing lipid deposition in adipose tissue. *Diabetes* **2010**, *59*, 1338–1348. [CrossRef] [PubMed]

47. Yue, Y.; Wang, Y.; Li, D.; Song, Z.; Jiao, H.; Lin, H. A central role for the mammalian target of rapamycin in LPS-induced anorexia in mice. *J. Endocrinol.* **2015**, *224*, 37–47. [CrossRef] [PubMed]

48. Oh, W.J.; Jacinto, E. mTOR complex 2 signaling and functions. *Cell Cycle* **2011**, *10*, 2305–2316. [CrossRef] [PubMed]

49. Rebollo, A.; Roglans, N.; Alegret, M.; Laguna, J.C.C. Way back for fructose and liver metabolism: Bench side to molecular insights. *World J. Gastroenterol.* **2012**, *18*, 6552–6559. [CrossRef] [PubMed]

50. Julien, L.-A.; Carriere, A.; Moreau, J.; Roux, P.P. mTORC1-Activated S6K1 Phosphorylates Rictor on Threonine 1135 and Regulates mTORC2 Signaling. *Mol. Cell. Biol.* **2010**, *30*, 908–921. [CrossRef] [PubMed]

51. Pende, M.; Kozma, S.; Jaquet, M.; Oorschot, V.; Burcelin, R.; Le Marchand-Brustel, Y.; Klumperman, J.; Thorens, B.; Thomas, G. Hypoinsulinaemia, glucose intolerance and diminished beta-cell size in S6K1-deficient mice. *Nature* **2000**, *408*, 994–997. [CrossRef] [PubMed]

52. Gu, Y.; Lindner, J.; Kumar, A.; Yuan, W.; Magnuson, M.A. Rictor/mTORC2 is essential for maintaining a balance between β-cell proliferation and cell size. *Diabetes* **2011**, *60*, 827–837. [CrossRef] [PubMed]

53. Chau, G.C.; Im, D.U.; Kang, T.M.; Bae, J.M.; Kim, W.; Pyo, S.; Moon, E.Y.; Um, S.H. mTOR controls ChREBP transcriptional activity and pancreatic β cell survival under diabetic stress. *J. Cell Biol.* **2017**, *216*, 2091–2105. [CrossRef] [PubMed]

54. Alejandro, E.U.; Bozadjieva, N.; Blandino-Rosano, M.; Wasan, M.A.; Elghazi, L.; Vadrevu, S.; Satin, L.; Bernal-Mizrachi, E. Overexpression of kinase-dead mTOR impairs glucose homeostasis by regulating insulin secretion and not β-cell mass. *Diabetes* **2017**, *66*, 2150–2162. [CrossRef] [PubMed]

55. Stamateris, R.E.; Sharma, R.B.; Kong, Y.; Ebrahimpour, P.; Panday, D.; Ranganath, P.; Zou, B.; Levitt, H.; Parambil, N.A.; O'Donnell, C.P.; et al. Glucose Induces mouse β-cell proliferation via IRS2, MTOR, and cyclin D2 but Not the insulin receptor. *Diabetes* **2016**, *65*, 981–995. [CrossRef] [PubMed]

56. Lakshmipathi, J.; Alvarez-Perez, J.C.; Rosselot, C.; Casinelli, G.P.; Stamateris, R.E.; Rausell-Palamos, F.; O'Donnell, C.P.; Vasavada, R.C.; Scott, D.K.; Alonso, L.C.; et al. PKCζ is essential for pancreatic β-cell replication during insulin resistance by regulating mTOR and cyclin-D2. *Diabetes* **2016**, *65*, 1283–1296. [CrossRef] [PubMed]

57. Balakumar, M.; Raji, L.; Prabhu, D.; Sathishkumar, C.; Prabu, P.; Mohan, V.; Balasubramanyam, M. High-fructose diet is as detrimental as high-fat diet in the induction of insulin resistance and diabetes mediated by hepatic/pancreatic endoplasmic reticulum (ER) stress. *Mol. Cell. Biochem.* **2016**, *423*, 93–104. [CrossRef] [PubMed]

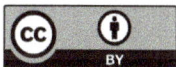

International Journal of
Molecular Sciences

MDPI

Article

Dopamine Receptor Subtypes Differentially Regulate Autophagy

Dongmei Wang [1,2], Xinmiao Ji [1], Juanjuan Liu [1], Zhiyuan Li [1,*] and Xin Zhang [1,3,*]

1   High Magnetic Field Laboratory, Key Laboratory of High Magnetic Field and Ion Beam Physical Biology, Hefei Institutes of Physical Science, Chinese Academy of Sciences, Hefei 230031, China; dongmeiwang@hmfl.ac.cn (D.W.); xinmiaoji@hmfl.ac.cn (X.J.); liujj@hmfl.ac.cn (J.L.)
2   Science Island Branch of Graduate School, University of Science and Technology of China, Hefei 230031, China
3   Institute of Physical Science and Information Technology, Anhui University, Hefei 230601, China
*   Correspondence: lizhiyuan@hmfl.ac.cn (Z.L.); xinzhang@hmfl.ac.cn (X.Z.); Tel.: +86-551-6559-4037 (Z.L.); +86-551-6559-3356 (X.Z.)

Received: 4 April 2018; Accepted: 18 May 2018; Published: 22 May 2018

Abstract: Some dopamine receptor subtypes were reported to participate in autophagy regulation, but their exact functions and mechanisms are still unclear. Here we found that dopamine receptors D2 and D3 (D2-like family) are positive regulators of autophagy, while dopamine receptors D1 and D5 (D1-like family) are negative regulators. Furthermore, dopamine and ammonia, the two reported endogenous ligands of dopamine receptors, both can induce dopamine receptor internalization and degradation. In addition, we found that AKT (protein kinase B)-mTOR (mechanistic target of rapamycin) and AMPK (AMP-activated protein kinase) pathways are involved in DRD3 (dopamine receptor D3) regulated autophagy. Moreover, autophagy machinery perturbation inhibited DRD3 degradation and increased DRD3 oligomer. Therefore, our study investigated the functions and mechanisms of dopamine receptors in autophagy regulation, which not only provides insights into better understanding of some dopamine receptor-related neurodegeneration diseases, but also sheds light on their potential treatment in combination with autophagy or mTOR pathway modulations.

Keywords: dopamine receptor; autophagy; AKT; mTOR; AMPK

1. Introduction

Autophagy is an evolutionarily conserved process that degrades unwanted proteins, cytosol and organelles to maintain cellular and organism homeostasis [1]. Autophagy is executed by autophagy related proteins (ATGs) that are responsible for phagophore formation, nucleation, autophagosome elongation and closure. Among those, ATG8/LC3, the widely used autophagy marker, transforms from cytosolic LC3-I to membrane bound LC3-II when autophagy is induced [2]. Autophagy inhibitors such chloroquine (CQ) and bafilomycin A1 (Baf A1) are frequently used to evaluate the autophagic flux via LC3 turnover assay [3]. Besides ATGs, there are several proteins that can regulate autophagy. For example, AMPK and mTOR, which are essential players of cellular energy balance and organismal growth and homeostasis, could regulate autophagy in response to energy and nutrient availability [4,5]. AMPK consists of α, β, γ subunits and the α-T172 and β-S108 are the main phosphorylation sites for AMPK activity [6,7]. mTOR signaling pathway involves the upstream PI3K-AKT and downstream p70 S6K and 4E-BP1 substrates [8,9], and its dysregulation is associated with numerous human diseases [10–13].

Dopamine receptors (DR), including D1-5 (also called DRD1-5), are originally identified to be the receptors for dopamine, an endogenous neurotransmitter that controls a variety of brain functions, including emotion, cognition and movement [14–16]. As a GPCR (G protein-coupled receptor) member,

Int. J. Mol. Sci. **2018**, *19*, 1540

DR is classified into D1-like (including DRD1 and DRD5) and D2-like (including DRD2, DRD3 and DRD4) families according to their coupled G proteins, Gαs or Gαi [17,18]. Many neurogenic diseases such as Parkinson and Alzheimer's disease were associated with DR dysfunction and relevant agonists or antagonists are used to target DR for therapy or modified to generate effective probes for live imaging [19–23]. Since Zhang et al. reported that compounds with affinity for DRs could modulate autophagy in a screen [24], functions of different DRs agonists and antagonists in autophagy have been examined in cells and animals [25–31]. However, the DR subtype functions in autophagy by themselves were not studied directly.

We previously found that ammonia is an endogenous ligand for DRD3. In addition to its role of inhibiting autophagic flux by modulating intra-vesicular pH, ammonia could also induce autophagy through DRD3 and mTOR [32]. In this paper, we systematically studied the roles of different DR subtypes in autophagy and further investigated the intertwined regulation between DRD3 and autophagy, which seems to be related to AKT-mTOR and AMPK pathways.

2. Results

2.1. Dopamine Receptors D2 and D3 (D2-Like Family) Are Positive Regulators of Autophagy

We previously dissected the mechanism of ammonia-induced autophagy through dopamine receptors D3 (DRD3) and mTOR [32]. To investigate the exact role of DRD3 itself in autophagy, DRD3 knockdown and autophagy inhibitors were combined to examine autophagic flux level changes. When DRD3 was knocked down by DRD3 RNAi, the relative LC3B-II, the autophagosome-bound LC3, was slightly increased (Figure 1A). However, the increased LC3B-II may be the result of increased autophagy induction or decreased autophagic degradation [2]. It has been well accepted that the autophagic flux could be more accurately shown by differences in the relative level of LC3-II between samples in the presence and absence of autophagy inhibitors [2]. In order to examine the autophagic flux in DRD3 knockdown cells, LC3 turnover assay using autophagy inhibitors CQ or Baf A1 was performed [3]. Our results show that the autophagic flux was obviously decreased in the DRD3 RNAi group compared with the negative control group (Figure 1B). Furthermore, the differences were more significant when higher concentration of Baf A1 and prolonged treatment time were used (Figure 1C). These evidences show that DRD3 is a positive regulator of autophagy.

Given that both DRD2 and DRD3 belong to D2-like family of DR, we next examined the role of DRD2 in autophagy regulation. Similarly, LC3 turnover assay also was performed between the negative control and DRD2 RNAi groups as DRD3 RNAi, which indicated that DRD2 knockdown also inhibited autophagic flux shown by the relative differences of LC3B-II (Figure 1D), which implies that DRD2 is a positive regulator of autophagy as well.

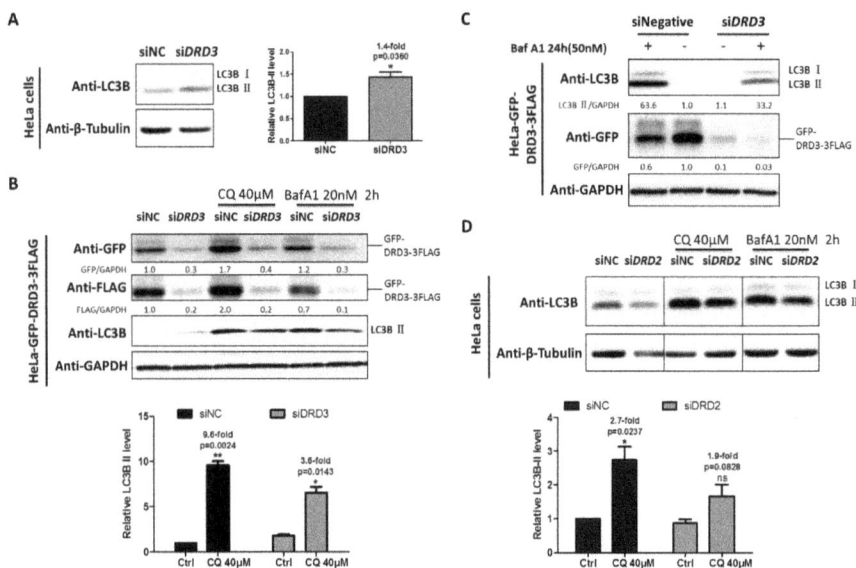

Figure 1. DRD3 and DRD2 knockdown inhibit autophagic flux. (**A**) Dopamine receptor D3 (DRD3) RNAi in HeLa cells was used to test the relative level of LC3B-II. (**B**) DRD3 RNAi was combined with autophagy inhibitors Chloroquine (CQ) (40 μM) or Baf A1 (20 nM) for 2 h to detect the autophagic flux in HeLa cells stably expressing GFP-DRD3-3FLAG. (**C**) DRD3 RNAi was combined with high concentration of Baf A1 (50 nM) for 24 h to examine the autophagic flux in HeLa cells stably expressing GFP-DRD3-3FLAG. (**D**) DRD2 RNAi in HeLa cells was combined with autophagy inhibitors CQ (40 μM) or Baf A1 (20 nM) for 2 h to detect the autophagic flux. Experiments were repeated at least three times and representative Western blots are shown. Densitometric analysis was performed and quantification results were labeled below the corresponding blots. * $p < 0.05$, ** $p < 0.01$.

2.2. Dopamine Receptors D1 and D5 (D1-Like Family) Are Negative Regulators of Autophagy

DRD1 and DRD5 belong to D1-like family, and they are functionally different from the D2-like family members. To investigate the roles of DRD1 and DRD5 in autophagy regulation, HeLa cells stably expressing DRD1 and DRD5 were established using MSCV infection (Figure S1). Furthermore, in order to examine the effect of DRD1 knockdown on autophagic flux, Baf A1 combined with DRD1 RNAi induced higher LC3-II level than the negative control, indicating increased autophagic flux after DRD1 knockdown (Figure 2A). Next we overexpressed DRD1 in HeLa cells and found the DRD1 expression levels were associated with LC3B-II levels (Figure 2B). Moreover, GFP-3FLAG tagged DRD1 was also transiently expressed in 293T cells (Figure 2C), and it was obvious that DRD1 expression decreased LC3B-II in 293T cells as well (Figure 2C), which was consistent with the results in HeLa cells (Figure 2B). Therefore, DRD1 knockdown and overexpression experiments in HeLa and 293T cells all show that DRD1 is a negative regulator of autophagy.

As for the role of DRD5 in autophagy, we also combined overexpression and knockdown experiments. GFP-3FLAG tagged DRD5 was transiently transfected into 293T cells and the LC3-II level was obviously decreased compared to vector control (Figure 2C). We also performed LC3 turnover assay in DRD5 knockdown cells using autophagy inhibitor CQ. It was interesting that DRD5 knockdown could increase the LC3-II level in CQ treated cells, indicating increased autophagic flux. Therefore, DRD5 overexpression and knockdown experiments both show that DRD5 is a negative regulator of autophagy, which is similar to the other D1-like member, DRD1 (Figure 2C,D).

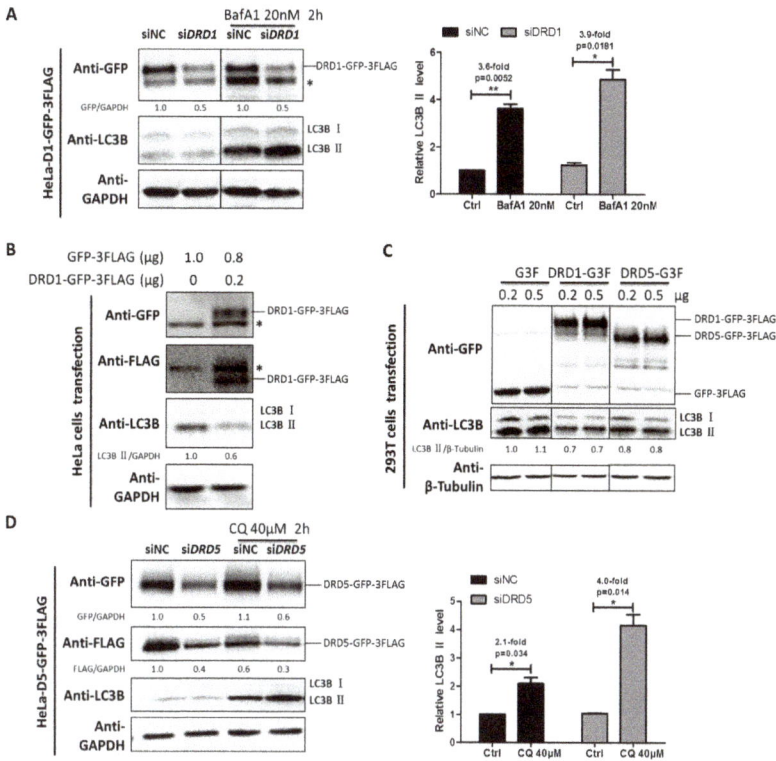

Figure 2. DRD1 and DRD5 knockdown promote autophagic flux. (**A**) DRD1 RNAi was combined with autophagy inhibitor Baf A1 (20 nM) for 2 h to detect the autophagic flux in HeLa cells stably expressing DRD1-GFP-3FLAG. (**B**) Total of 1 μg of MSCV-DRD1-GFP-3FLAG and MSCV-GFP-3FLAG plasmids were transfected into HeLa cells using lipofectamine 2000 for 48 h. (**C**) 0.2 or 0.5 μg MSCV-DRD1/DRD5-GFP-3FLAG or MSCV-GFP-3FLAG plasmid was transfected into 293T cells using lipofectamine 2000 for 48 h. (**D**) DRD5 RNAi was combined with autophagy inhibitors CQ (40 μM) for 2 h to detect the autophagic flux in HeLa cells stably expressing DRD5-GFP-3FLAG. The asterisk (*) indicates the nonspecific band. Experiments were repeated at least three times and representative Western blots are shown. Densitometric analysis was performed and quantification results were labeled below the corresponding blots or in separate panels. * $p < 0.05$, ** $p < 0.01$.

2.3. Both Dopamine and Ammonia Induce Dopamine Receptor Degradation

Dopamine is the well-known endogenous ligand for dopamine receptors. Due to the fact that some ligands could induce the degradation of their receptors [33,34], we therefore studied the effects of dopamine on dopamine receptor degradation. Notably, dopamine induced the D2-like family DRD2 and DRD3 degradation and the GFP fragment accumulation from GFP tagged DRD2 or DRD3 (Figure 3A,B). However, the D1-like family DRD1 and DRD5 were much less affected compared with the D2-like family (Figure 3C,D).

Ammonia, a recently discovered endogenous ligand for DRD3, was shown to induce significant DRD3 degradation and GFP fragment accumulation from GFP tagged DRD3 [32]. Here we examined its effects on the degradation of other dopamine receptors. It is interesting that ammonia induced significant GFP fragment accumulation from GFP tagged DRD2 (Figure 3E), which is similar to DRD3. However, its effect on the D1-like family DRD1 and DRD5 were not as significant as the D2 like family (Figure 3F), which was consistent with the effects of dopamine. Hence, both dopamine and ammonia could induce significant degradation of D2-like family DRs but only moderately affect the D1-like family. In another word, the D2-like family DRs seem to be more sensitive to their endogenous ligand-induced degradation than the D1-like family DRs.

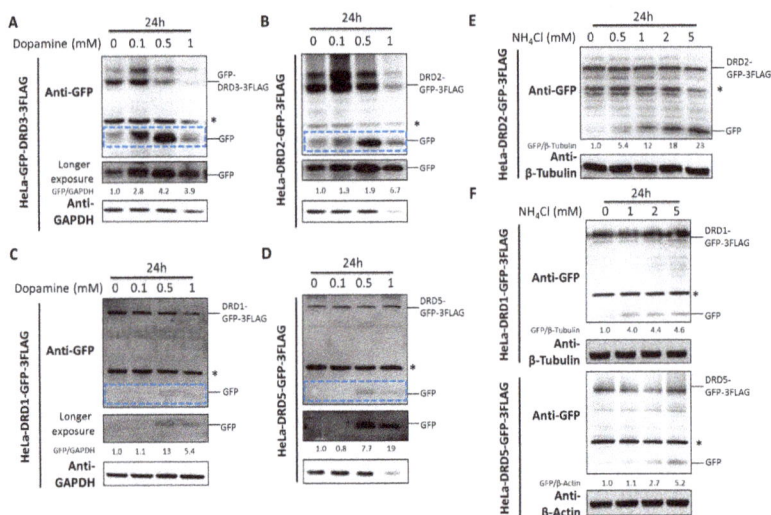

Figure 3. Dopamine and ammonia induce the degradation of D1-like and D2-like dopamine receptors differentially. (**A–D**) HeLa cells stably expressing GFP-3FLAG tagged DRD1, 2, 3 and 5 were treated with different concentrations of dopamine for 24 h. (**E,F**) HeLa cells stably expressing GFP-3FLAG tagged DRD1, 2 and 5 were treated with different concentrations of ammonia for 24 h. The asterisk (*) indicates the nonspecific band. Experiments were repeated at least three times and representative Western blots are shown. Blue dashed frames show the GFP fragment with shorter exposure. Densitometric analysis was performed and quantification results were labeled below the corresponding blots.

2.4. Dopamine and Monoamines Are DRD3 Ligands and Induce DRD3 Internalization and LC3B Increase

Previously, we found that DRD3 is a receptor for ammonia-induced autophagy [32]. Then we pursued structure-activity analysis of DRD3 ligands, where we quantified the induction of autophagy by candidate DRD3 ligands. DRD3's endogenous ligand dopamine contains amine and catechol functional groups, suggesting that DRD3 might bind and sense these moieties. We first tested the effect of dopamine, catechol and ammonium chloride on cells and found that although dopamine and ammonium chloride increased cleaved GFP fragment, catechol did not (Figure 3A and Figure 4A). This indicates that the ligand-receptor recognition may act through the amine or ammonia functionality rather than the hydroxyl. Next, we examined several amine derivatives to find out whether other primary amines can also cause the same effect. Urea was used as a negative control because it is a carbamide, which does not have a free amino group. We found that ethylamine and propylamine both increased the cleaved GFP fragment while urea did not (Figure 4A). To compare their ability to induce GFP-DRD3-3FLAG internalization and modulate autophagy, we examined the localization of GFP-DRD3-3FLAG (Figure 4B). However, since the methanol fix procedure can not differentiate internal antigens from external ones because the methanol permeabilizes the cell membrane, we fixed the cells using formaldehyde and also permeabilized them using 0.1% Triton X-100 to perform immuno-staining. In this way, the membrane part can be better preserved than methanol fix and internalized antigens could be detected simultaneously. As shown in Figure 4C, the signals from cell surface were reduced in dopamine and monoamines treated groups compared with control group, which suggested the internalization of surface GFP-DRD3-3FLAG (Figure 4C). It also indicates similar internalization induced by dopamine and monoamines as in methanol fix (Figure 4B,C). Also, we analyzed LC3B puncta (Figure 4D) in cells that were treated as in Figure 4B. Our results show that propylamine and phenethylamine have the strongest phenotype, while catechol and urea do not increase GFP-DRD3-3FLAG internalization (Figure 4B) or LC3B puncta in cells (Figure 4D). To measure the downstream G protein mediated traditional GPCR signaling pathway, we used cAMP assays to measure the effects of these potential ligands. Consistent with the autophagy results, urea does not affect the cAMP level in CHO-GFP-DRD3-FLAG cells (Figure 4E). However, cAMP assay results of the other ligands do not completely correlate with autophagy induction. For example, catechol also induces cAMP changes similar to dopamine and the ethylamine, while propylamine and phenethylamine-induced cAMP change is much weaker than NH_4Cl (Figure 4E). These indicate that dopamine and monoamines are all DRD3 ligands and they could induce DRD3 internalization and degradation, as well as LC3B increase, which confirms the role of DRD3 in autophagy.

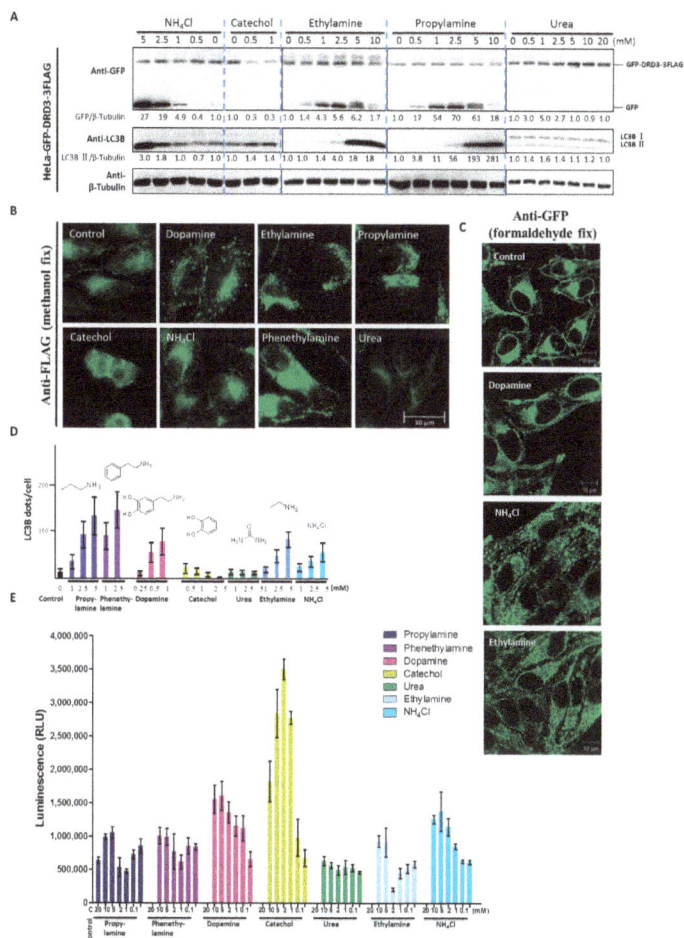

Figure 4. The free amino group is responsible for dopamine and monoamine-induced autophagy and DRD3 internalization. (A) Representative Western blots show GFP fragment and autophagy levels

upon addition of different chemicals. The blue dashed lines are helpful to distinguish different lanes in each group. HeLa cells stably expressing GFP-DRD3-3FLAG were treated with different concentrations of catechol, NH_4Cl, ethylamine, propylamine or urea for 24 h. Densitometric analysis was performed and quantification results were labeled below the corresponding blots. (**B**) GFP-DRD3-3FLAG localizations in cells treated with different chemicals. Immunofluorescence used anti-FLAG antibody to analyze the localization of GFP-DRD3-3FLAG. HeLa cells stably expressing GFP-DRD3-3FLAG were treated with dopamine, catechol, NH_4Cl, ethylamine, propylamine, phenethylamine or urea for 24 h. Cells were fixed with methanol, blocked by AbDil-Tx (containing 0.1% Triton X-100) and then subjected to anti-FLAG antibody staining. Experiments were repeated at least three times and representative results are shown. Scale bar, 10 µm. (**C**) GFP-DRD3-3FLAG localizations in cells treated with dopamine and monoamines. Cells treated as Figure 4B were fixed with 3.7% formaldehyde, blocked by AbDil-Tx (containing 0.1% Triton X-100) and then subjected to anti-GFP antibody staining. Experiments were repeated at least three times and representative results are shown. Scale bar, 10 µm. (**D**) LC3B puncta in cells treated with different chemicals. Quantification results of the LC3B puncta in HeLa cells stably expressing GFP-DRD3-3FLAG treated with different concentrations of ammonia, dopamine, urea, catechol and some monoamines. (**E**) cAMP responses in cells treated with different chemicals. cAMP-Glo experiment was used to measure cAMP level in CHO cells that stably express GFP-DRD3-FLAG upon adding NH_4Cl, dopamine, catechol, urea, ethylamine, propylamine or phenethylamine. Data show mean ± SD from three independent experiments.

2.5. AKT-mTOR and AMPK Are Involved in DRD3-Regulated Autophagy

To find out the downstream signaling pathways for dopamine receptor regulated autophagy, we chose DRD3 and DRD5 as representative D1-/D2-like family receptors for further investigation. Although dopamine agonist such as quinelorane activates PI3K-AKT-mTOR pathway [35,36], little is known for the roles of DR themselves in AKT-mTOR pathway. It was interesting that DRD3 knockdown increased AKT phosphorylation at both Ser-473 and Thr-308 while DRD5 knockdown showed opposite effects (Figure 5A). Furthermore, DRD3 knockdown increased the mTOR substrate phospho-p70-S6K (T389) level while DRD5 knockdown showed opposite effect as well (Figure 5A). These results indicate that the D1 and D2-like family dopamine receptors both can modulate the AKT-mTOR signaling pathway, but in an opposite way.

To further dissect the underlying mechanism for the autophagy regulation function of dopamine receptors, we chose DRD3 for further studies. Although dopamine was reported to regulate AKT-mTOR signaling in human SH-SY5Y neuroblastoma cells [37], the exact role of dopamine on DRD3 is unclear due to the fact that other DRs are also highly expressed in the neuroblastoma cells. Therefore, for their low expression of DRs, HeLa cells were selected for dopamine effects on downstream signaling. HeLa cells stably expressing GFP-DRD3-3FLAG were treated with dopamine or ammonia, the two reported DRD3 ligands, for different time points. Even as short as for 1 h treatment of dopamine could obviously inhibit the mTOR substrate phospho-p70-S6K (T389) phosphorylation. At 8 h, dopamine also induced AKT activation, which is likely due to the negative feedback loop of mTOR signaling excessive inactivation (Figure 5B). Consistently, ammonia also increased AKT phosphorylation (Figure S2) and decreased mTOR substrate phospho-p70-S6K (T389) level [32]. These results confirmed the involvement of AKT-mTOR pathway in dopamine receptor-regulated autophagy.

To further study the relationship between mTOR and dopamine receptors, we established a HeLa cell line stably expressing GFP-3FLAG tagged GIPC1 (GAIP interacting protein, C terminus), the downstream scaffold protein for DRD2 and DRD3. Considering that the basal levels of autophagosome protein LC3B is usually low in untreated cells, we used Baf A1 and ammonia to enrich autophagosomes. Using co-immunoprecipitation (co-IP) experiments, we added extra 0.1% Triton X-100 to the MPER buffer that already contained mild detergent to reduce nonspecific binding. It is obvious that LC3B and mTOR could be pulled out by both GFP-DRD3-FLAG and GIPC1-GFP-3FLAG (Figure 5C). The interaction between mTOR and DRD3 seem to be much weaker than mTOR and GIPC1, which implies that DRD3 may rely on GIPC1 to regulate mTOR.

In addition, we found that AMPK was also affected by DRD3. Specifically, AMPK activity was inhibited by DRD3 knockdown, which is shown by decreased phosphorylation level of AMPK α-T172 and β-S108 (Figure 5D). Interestingly, ammonia-induced AMPK signaling inhibition (Figure 5E) was partially antagonized by DRD3 knockdown, which avoided ammonia-induced excessive AMPK inhibition in DRD3 knockdown cells (Figure 5E, lane 4 and 8). Therefore, our results show that DRD3 knockdown could increase AKT-mTOR activity and decrease AMPK activity. Given that autophagy was regulated by the balance between mTOR and AMPK activity and AKT as the upstream kinase for mTOR [4,5,10], the AKT-mTOR and AMPK pathways might both contribute to the autophagy regulation by DRD3.

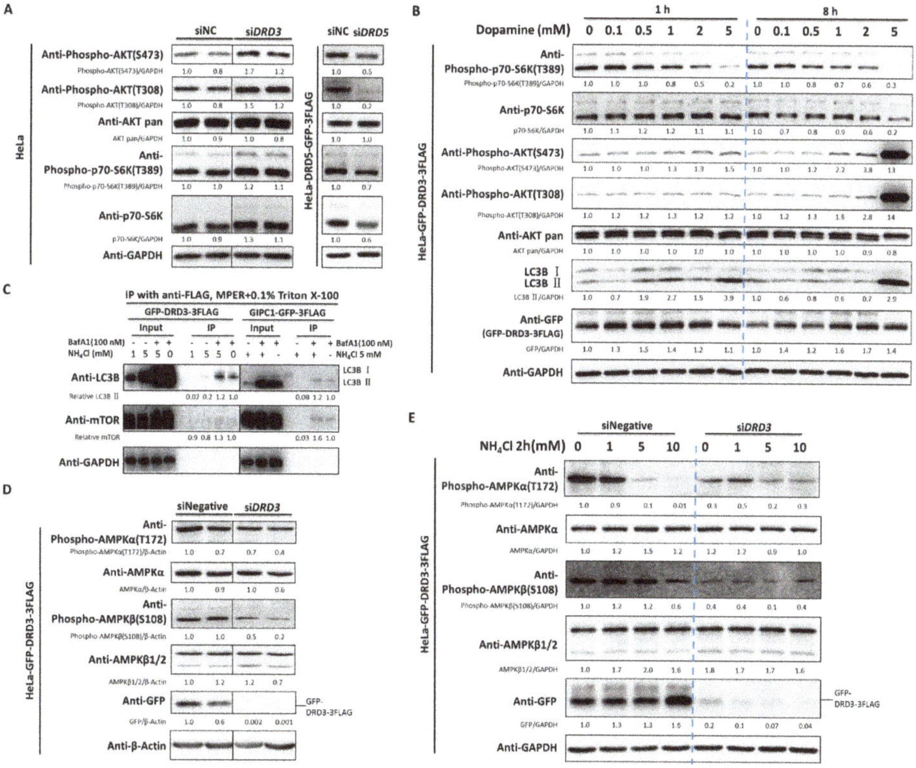

Figure 5. AKT (protein kinase B)-mTOR (mechanistic target of rapamycin) and AMPK (AMP-activated protein kinase) pathways are involved in DRD3-regulated autophagy. (**A**) DRD3 or DRD5 RNAi in HeLa wild type or HeLa cells stably expressing DRD5-GFP-3FLAG. (**B**) HeLa cells stably expressing GFP-DRD3-3FLAG were treated with increasing concentrations of dopamine for 1 h or 8 h. (**C**) Co- Immunoprecipitation using anti-FLAG in HeLa cells stably expressing GFP-DRD3-3FLAG or GIPC1-GFP-3FLAG treated with Baf A1 and/or NH4Cl, in the presence of additional 0.1% Triton X-100 in IP and washing buffers. (**D**) DRD3 RNAi in HeLa cells stably expressing GFP-DRD3-3FLAG decreases AMPK activity shown by AMPKα-T172 and β-S108. (**E**) DRD3 RNAi in HeLa cells stably expressing GFP-DRD3-3FLAG partially antagonizes the effect of ammonia-induced AMPKα-T172 and β-S108 inhibition. The blue dashed lines are used to distinguish different parts of the results for better visualization. Experiments were repeated at least three times and representative Western blots are shown. Densitometric analysis was performed and quantification results were labeled below the corresponding blots.

2.6. Perturbation of Autophagy Machinery Induced DRD3 Degradation Inhibition and Oligomer Increase

The GFP fragment is an intermediate degradation byproduct from GFP-DRD3 because GFP can be degraded in the lysosomes but not the intermediate autophagosomes [38]. At lower concentrations of ammonia, GFP fragment could not be easily detected due to lower GFP-DRD3 degradation rate and robust lysosomal degradation capacity. To further examine the role of autophagy in DRD3 degradation, the autophagy machinery was perturbed to test the DRD3 protein level changes. Knockdown of Beclin-1 or ATG7, two core autophagy components, significantly increased the GFP fragment in lower concentration of ammonia (1 mM, which is not sufficient to induce GFP-DRD3 degradation in control condition), which indicated the role of autophagy in DRD3 degradation (Supplementary Materials Figure S3A,B and Figure 6A). These results indicate that autophagy perturbation could sensitize GFP fragment accumulation, which may be due to the compromised autolysosomal degradation for intermediate GFP induced by lower concentration of ammonia.

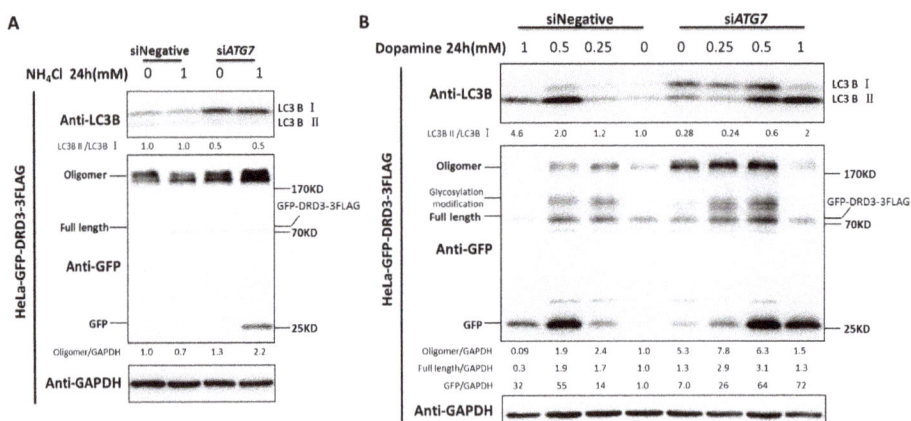

Figure 6. Autophagy inhibition decreases dopamine receptor degradation and increases oligomer formation. (**A**) ATG7 RNAi in HeLa cells stably expressing GFP-DRD3-3FLAG were treated with 1 mM ammonia for 24 h. (**B**) ATG7 RNAi in HeLa cells stably expressing GFP-DRD3-3FLAG were treated with different concentrations of dopamine for 24 h. Experiments were repeated at least three times and representative Western blots are shown. Densitometric analysis was performed and quantification results were labeled below the corresponding blots.

In the meantime, we noticed that the full length of GFP-DRD3 protein level did not increase when autophagy machinery was perturbed (Figure 6A, Figure S3A,B). Given that DRD3 might form oligomers [39], we next examined the oligomer level before and after autophagy machinery perturbance. In fact, the DRD3 oligomer significantly increased after ATG7 knockdown, indicating the conditioned accumulation of DRD3 oligomer by autophagy perturbation (Figure 6A). Therefore, the oligomer-form of DRD3 should also be considered to quantify the total protein amount of DRD3. In addition, since dopamine could induce DRD3 degradation, we further examined the role of autophagy in dopamine-induced DRD3 degradation. The LC3B-I to LC3B-II conversion was also inhibited after ATG7 knockdown, indicating compromised autophagy flux (Figure 6A,B). In the meantime, after 1 mM of dopamine treatment, almost all GFP-DRD3-3FLAG proteins, including the full-length monomer form as well as the oligomer form, were degraded (Figure 6B). However, in ATG7 knockdown cells, there are still some GFP-DRD3-3FLAG monomer and oligomer left, which indicates that the ammonia-induced DRD3 degradation was inhibited by ATG7 knockdown. It was also interesting that ATG7 knockdown could alleviated the cytotoxicity of higher concentrations of dopamine [40], which is likely due to autophagic cell death.

3. Discussion

The different roles of D1-like and D2-like DR subtypes in autophagy regulation may be due to their differentially associated G protein and downstream scaffold proteins. D1-like DR subtypes DRD1 and DRD5 are coupled to Gαs G protein while D2-like DR subtypes DRD2 and DRD3 are coupled to Gαi G protein [17]. Interference of the Gαi with PTX (Pertussis toxin), locking Gαi in the GDP-bound inactive state, could induce autophagy [41]. In addition, D2-like DRD2 and DRD3 are associated with the scaffold protein GIPC and it has been evidenced that GIPC induced autophagy in pancreatic cancer cells [42–44]. We also attempted to clone DRD4 but did not succeed, which is probably due to the high GC content in DRD4 sequence. Moreover, as DRD4 belongs to D2-like family and its gene polymorphism [45] encodes different isoforms, here the complex role of DRD4 variants in autophagy was not discussed. In sum, the differential roles of D1-like and D2-like DRs in autophagy might be due to the different downstream signaling partners.

Some studies show that dopamine receptor agonists or antagonists are involved in autophagy regulation. For example, DRD4 antagonists such as L-741, 742 and PNU 96415E disrupted the autophagy-lysosomal pathway [30]; DRD5 agonists induced autophagy and autophagic cell death [29]; DRD2 antagonists such as raclopride and sertindole induced autophagy [26,31]. Although dopamine receptors agonists or antagonists participated in autophagy regulation, little was known about the exact roles of dopamine receptors themselves in autophagy. Hence, based on our previous report, our study here further confirms that DRs participate in autophagy regulation.

Most GPCRs are internalized by endocytic sorting and degraded by the general lysosome pathway [46,47]. Moreover, brain cannabinoid 1 receptor has been shown to be degraded by autophagy [48]. However, whether DRs are degraded through autophagy pathway is still unknown. Our findings here provide evidences for the autophagic degradation of DRs, which will further strengthen the link between autophagy and GPCRs degradation.

The main finding of our study concerns that expression of DRD2 and DRD3, by itself, without interaction with ligands, induces autophagy, and that the opposite situation occurs in the case of DRD1 and DRD5. Considering the role of autophagy in neurodegenerative diseases [49–51], constitutive expressing DRs in some neurons might be responsible for the formation of misfolded proteins and neuro-degeneration. However, since there are many factors affecting autophagy, other proteins and environmental factors should also be considered for autophagy contribution in some neurodegenerative diseases, such as Parkinson's disease and Huntington's disease when using autophagy as a therapeutic strategy.

There are some evidences showing that DR could form oligomers, such D1-D2, D1-D3 and D2-adenosine A2A receptor [39,52–56]. Here we found that DRD3 preferentially existed as oligomers when autophagy was compromised, which may be a potential indicator for autophagy inhibition in DRD3 associated diseases. However, whether the accumulated DRD3 oligomers have specific function or just aggregate due to degradation inhibition is unknown. In addition, whether and how DRs form oligomers to regulate autophagy also needs to be investigated.

DRs were found as the receptors for dopamine and many neuro-degeneration diseases are associated with their dysfunction. In this paper, we systematically studied the roles of D1-like and D2-like family receptors in autophagy regulation. Our results show that D1-like family receptors DRD1 and DRD5 negatively regulate autophagy, while D2-like family receptors DRD2 and DRD3 positively regulate autophagy. DRD3 generally functions through the downstream cAMP associated signaling cascade to control intracellular events [57]. Here we found that the AKT-mTOR and AMPK pathways might participate in DRD3 regulated autophagy, which will provide some clues for the connection between DR and the intracellular signaling hub. Our findings not only revealed the role of DRD3 in autophagy but also connected DRD3 signaling with the cellular energy and nutrient sensor, mTOR and AMPK, which will broaden the scope of DRD3 study and guide combined therapeutics for DR associated diseases in the future.

4. Materials and Methods

4.1. Cell Culture and Stable Cell Lines Establishment

HeLa and 293T cells were cultured in DMEM (Corning Cellgro, 15-017-CVR, Manassas, VA, USA) supplemented with 10% Fetal Bovine Serum (CLARK Bioscience, Richmond, VA, USA), 2 mM GlutaMAX (Gibco, Carlsbad, CA, USA), 100 units/mL of Penicillin-100 µg/mL of Streptomycin (HyClone, Logan, UT, USA). HeLa-DRD1-GFP-3FLAG, HeLa-DRD2-GFP-3FLAG, HeLa-GFP-DRD3-3FLAG, HeLa-DRD5-GFP-3FLAG, HeLa-GIPC1-GFP-3FLAG cells were maintained in DMEM complete medium with 1 µg/mL puromycin (Selleck, Washington, DC, USA). HeLa-GFP-DRD3-3FLAG cells were established as previously described [32,58]. In addition, HeLa-DRD1/DRD2/DRD5/GIPC1-GFP-3FLAG cells were established similarly. The cDNA for DRD1/DRD2/DRD5/GIPC1 were amplified from HeLa cells and cloned into MSCV vector with GFP-3FLAG in their C-terminus.

4.2. Transient Transfection

HeLa or 293T cells were plated at 30% confluence in 12-well-plate 24 h before experiment. Then cells were transfected for the plasmids of MSCV-GFP-3FLAG, MSCV-DRD1/DRD5-GFP-3FLAG using lipofectamine 2000 (Invitrogen, Waltham, MA, USA) and cultured for another 48 h for Western blots.

4.3. RNAi for Dopamine Receptors, ATG7 and Beclin-1

The RNAi assay was conducted as described before [32]. Briefly, for one well in 12-well-plate, HeLa wild type or the dopamine receptors overexpression cell lines were trypsinized, plated and transfected with 6 µL Hiperfect (Qiagen, Dusseldorf , Germany) and 2.4 µL siRNAs (20 µM) in 100 µL opti-MEM (Gibco, Carlsbad, CA, USA) according to the manufacture's protocol. After 72 h incubation, cells were lysed for Western blots. The sequences of siRNA oligos targeted to human mRNA were as below (5′-3′): Negative or NC: UUCUCCGAACGUGUCACGUTT; *DRD1*: GGACCUUGUCUGUACUCAUTT; *DRD2*: GAAGAAUGGGCAUGCCAAA; *DRD3*: GUACAGCCAGCAUCCUUAA; *DRD5*: GCAGUUCGCUCUAUACCAGTT; *ATG7*: CAACAUCCCUGGUUACAAG; *Beclin-1*: UAAGAUGGGUCUGAAAUUU.

4.4. Western Blots and Co-Immunoprecipitation

Cells were lysed on ice by the M-PER (Thermo Scientific, Waltham, MA, USA) supplemented with protease and phosphatase inhibitors cocktail (Roche, Basel, Switzerland) for 30 min. The whole cell lysate was denatured in the final $1\times$ SDS loading buffer at 95 °C for 5 min. Then the denatured samples were subjected to the SDS-PAGE and subsequent Western blots such as PVDF membrane (Merck, Whitehouse Station, NJ, USA) transfer, primary and HRP-conjugated secondary antibodies incubation. For co-immunoprecipitation, cells were cultured in 10-cm-dish to 95–100% confluence and lysed the same as above. The anti-FLAG M2 monoclonal antibody was incubated with Dynabeads protein G (Invitrogen, Waltham, MA, USA) at room temperature for 45 min on a rotator. The whole cell lysate were centrifuged at $10,000\times g$ for 1 min to get rid of cell debris and the supernatant was mixed with antibody-conjugated Dynabeads protein G at 4 °C for 45 min on a rotator. After washing with ice-cold PBST (PBS with 0.04% Tween-20) three times every 5 min at 4 °C (using the magnet to separate the Dynabeads mixture and the supernatant), the Dynabeads were supplemented with lysis buffer and SDS sample buffer followed by boiling at 95 °C for 5 min. And the supernatant was used as input control. The immunoprecipitates and input were subjected to subsequent SDS-PAGE and Western blots. The chemiluminesence results were obtained using Tanon Fine-do X6 (Shanghai, China) catalyzed by Thermo Scientific (Waltham, MA, USA) or Millipore ECL (Billerica, NJ, USA). Results shown in figures are all representative.

4.5. Immunofluorescence

HeLa cells expressing GFP-DRD3-3FLAG were grown on coverslips and treated with ammonia, dopamine, urea, catechol and some monoamines for 24 h. Cells were washed once with PBS and fixed by -20 °C methanol for 5 min or fixed with 3.7% formaldehyde at room temperature for 15 min and then blocked by AbDil-Tx (TBS-Tx supplemented with 0.1% Triton X-100, 2% BSA and 0.05% sodium azide) at room temperature for 30 min, followed by primary antibodies (FLAG, GFP or LC3B) incubation at 4 °C overnight. The secondary fluorescently conjugated antibodies were incubated at room temperature for 1 h and washed by TBS-Tx (TBS added with 0.1% Triton x-100) and mounted by anti-fade prolong Gold with DAPI (4′,6-Diamidino-2-Phenylindole, Dihydrochloride) (Invitrogen, Waltham, MA, USA). Images were taken using a Leica DMI4000B fluorescent microscope (Leica Camera, Wetzlar, Germany) or Zeiss LSM 710 confocal microscope (Carl Zeiss AG, Oberkochen, Germany). Images shown in figures are all representative results from multiple independent experiments.

4.6. Reagents

The autophagy antibody sampler kit, the antibodies for phospho-S6K (T389/412), S6K, AKT pan, phospho-AKT (Thr-308), phospho-AKT (Ser-473), mTOR, AMPK Antibody sampler kit, the HRP-linked anti-rabbit and anti-mouse IgG antibody were all from Cell signaling technology. The anti-GFP (sc-9996) antibodies were acquired from Santa Cruz. The anti-GAPDH, anti-β-Tubulin and anti-β-Actin antibodies were from Beijing TransGen Biotech (Beijing, China). Dynabeads Protein G was from NOVEX. The secondary antibodies and anti-fade prolong Gold with DAPI were from Molecular Probes. The anti-FLAG M2 monoclonal antibody (F3165), dopamine, chloroquine, NH_4Cl were from Sigma. Ethylamine was from J&K Chemical (Shanghai, China), catechol from Energy Chemical (Shanghai, China), propylamine and phenethylamine from Tokyo Chemical Industry. GlutaMAX supplement was from Gibco. Puromycin dehydrochloride was from Selleck. Bafilomycin A1 was from Cayman. The siRNAs were ordered from GenePharma (Shanghai, China).

4.7. cAMP-Glo Assay

The intracellular cAMP level was monitored by the cAMP-Glo assay (Promega) based on the reciprocal relationship between the cAMP concentration and the bioluminescence value. The decreased luminescence reading reflects higher cAMP level in cells. Briefly, 5000 cells (CHO and CHO-GFP-DRD3-FLAG cells) were plated in white 384-well plate (Corning, Manassas, VA, USA, 3570) 24 h prior to the assay. Cells were washed once with PBS and then were pre-treated with 20 µL compounds of interest in PBS for 25 min before treated with 7.5 µL compounds in the presence of 1 mM IBMX, 200 µM Ro 20-1724 and 10 µM forskolin for 15 min at room temperature. The subsequent steps were performed as the manufacture's protocol indicated. The data were acquired with the Multimode Plate Reader (EnVision, PerkinElmer, Waltham, MA, USA) and analyzed by GraphPad Prism 5 (GraphPad Software, La Jolla, CA, USA).

4.8. Statistical Analysis

ImageJ software (NIH, Bethesda, Maryland, USA) was used for densitometric analysis of Western blots to quantify the relative protein levels. GraphPad Prism 5 was used for Student's t-test. p values < 0.05 were considered as statistically significant.

Supplementary Materials: Supplementary Materials can be found at http://www.mdpi.com/1422-0067/19/5/1540/s1.

Author Contributions: X.Z. initiated and supervised the project. X.Z. and Z.L. designed the experiments. D.W., Z.L., X.J. and J.L. performed the experiments. Z.L. and X.Z. wrote the manuscript. All authors read and approved the final manuscript.

Acknowledgments: We thank Wenchao Wang at High magnetic field laboratory, Chinese Academy of Sciences for a gift of the plasmid GIPC1-GFP-3FLAG in MSCV vector. This work was supported by the National Key Research and Development Program of China (#2016YFA0400900), the Chinese Academy of Sciences "hundred talent program" to Xin Zhang and China Postdoctoral Science Foundation funded project (2016M602045) to Zhiyuan Li.

Conflicts of Interest: The authors declare no conflict of interest.

Abbreviations

4E-BP1	Translation initiation factor 4E-binding protein 1
AKT	Protein kinase B
AMPK	AMP-activated protein kinase
ATG7	Autophagy related protein 7
LC3	Microtubule-associated protein 1 light chain 3
mTOR	Mechanistic/mammalian target of rapamycin
p70-S6K	Ribosomal protein S6 kinase beta-1

References

1. Klionsky, D.J.; Abdelmohsen, K.; Abe, A.; Abedin, M.J.; Abeliovich, H.; Acevedo Arozena, A.; Adachi, H.; Adams, C.M.; Adams, P.D.; Adeli, K.; et al. Guidelines for the use and interpretation of assays for monitoring autophagy. *Autophagy* **2016**, *12*, 1–222. [CrossRef] [PubMed]

2. Mizushima, N.; Yoshimori, T. How to interpret LC3 immunoblotting. *Autophagy* **2007**, *3*, 542–545. [CrossRef] [PubMed]

3. Mizushima, N.; Yoshimori, T.; Levine, B. Methods in mammalian autophagy research. *Cell* **2010**, *140*, 313–326. [CrossRef] [PubMed]

4. Kim, J.; Kundu, M.; Viollet, B.; Guan, K.L. AMPK and mTOR regulate autophagy through direct phosphorylation of Ulk1. *Nat. Cell Biol.* **2011**, *13*, 132–141. [CrossRef] [PubMed]

5. Egan, D.F.; Shackelford, D.B.; Mihaylova, M.M.; Gelino, S.; Kohnz, R.A.; Mair, W.; Vasquez, D.S.; Joshi, A.; Gwinn, D.M.; Taylor, R. Phosphorylation of ULK1 (hATG1) by AMP-activated protein kinase connects energy sensing to mitophagy. *Science* **2011**, *331*, 456–461. [CrossRef] [PubMed]

6. Sanders, M.J.; Ali, Z.S.; Hegarty, B.D.; Heath, R.; Snowden, M.A.; Carling, D. Defining the mechanism of activation of AMP-activated protein kinase by the small molecule A-769662, a member of the thienopyridone family. *J. Biol. Chem.* **2007**, *282*, 32539–32548. [CrossRef] [PubMed]

7. Woods, A.; Vertommen, D.; Neumann, D.; Türk, R.; Bayliss, J.; Schlattner, U.; Wallimann, T.; Carling, D.; Rider, M.H. Identification of phosphorylation sites in AMP-activated protein kinase (AMPK) for upstream AMPK kinases and study of their roles by site-directed mutagenesis. *J. Biol. Chem.* **2003**, *278*, 28434–28442. [CrossRef] [PubMed]

8. Nojima, H.; Tokunaga, C.; Eguchi, S.; Oshiro, N.; Hidayat, S.; Yoshino, K.-I.; Hara, K.; Tanaka, N.; Avruch, J.; Yonezawa, K. The mammalian target of rapamycin (mTOR) partner, raptor, binds the mTOR substrates p70 S6 kinase and 4E-BP1 through their TOR signaling (TOS) motif. *J. Biol. Chem.* **2003**, *278*, 15461–15464. [CrossRef] [PubMed]

9. Freudlsperger, C.; Burnett, J.R.; Friedman, J.A.; Kannabiran, V.R.; Chen, Z.; Van Waes, C. EGFR–PI3K–AKT–mTOR signaling in head and neck squamous cell carcinomas: Attractive targets for molecular-oriented therapy. *Expert Opin. Ther. Targets* **2011**, *15*, 63–74. [CrossRef] [PubMed]

10. Laplante, M.; Sabatini, D.M. mTOR signaling at a glance. *J. Cell Sci.* **2009**, *122*, 3589–3594. [CrossRef] [PubMed]

11. Laplante, M.; Sabatini, D.M. mTOR signaling in growth control and disease. *Cell* **2012**, *149*, 274–293. [CrossRef] [PubMed]

12. Inoki, K.; Corradetti, M.N.; Guan, K.-L. Dysregulation of the TSC-mTOR pathway in human disease. *Nat. Genet.* **2005**, *37*, 19–24. [CrossRef] [PubMed]

13. Johnson, S.C.; Rabinovitch, P.S.; Kaeberlein, M. mTOR is a key modulator of ageing and age-related disease. *Nature* **2013**, *493*, 338–345. [CrossRef] [PubMed]

14. Missale, C.; Nash, S.R.; Robinson, S.W.; Jaber, M.; Caron, M.G. Dopamine receptors: From structure to function. *Physiol. Rev.* **1998**, *78*, 189–225. [CrossRef] [PubMed]

15. Vallone, D.; Picetti, R.; Borrelli, E. Structure and function of dopamine receptors. *Neurosci. Biobehav. Rev.* **2000**, *24*, 125–132. [CrossRef]

16. Liu, C.; Kershberg, L.; Wang, J.; Schneeberger, S.; Kaeser, P.S. Dopamine Secretion Is Mediated by Sparse Active Zone-like Release Sites. *Cell* **2018**, *172*, 706–718. [CrossRef] [PubMed]

17. Beaulieu, J.-M.; Gainetdinov, R.R. The physiology, signaling, and pharmacology of dopamine receptors. *Pharmacol. Rev.* **2011**, *63*, 182–217. [CrossRef] [PubMed]

18. Gainetdinov, R.R.; Premont, R.T.; Bohn, L.M.; Lefkowitz, R.J.; Caron, M.G. Desensitization of G protein–coupled receptors and neuronal functions. *Annu. Rev. Neurosci.* **2004**, *27*, 107–144. [CrossRef] [PubMed]

19. Pavese, N.; Andrews, T.C.; Brooks, D.J.; Ho, A.K.; Rosser, A.E.; Barker, R.A.; Robbins, T.W.; Sahakian, B.J.; Dunnett, S.B.; Piccini, P. Progressive striatal and cortical dopamine receptor dysfunction in Huntington's disease: A PET study. *Brain J. Neurol.* **2003**, *126*, 1127–1135. [CrossRef]

20. Goldman-Rakic, P.S.; Castner, S.A.; Svensson, T.H.; Siever, L.J.; Williams, G.V. Targeting the dopamine D1 receptor in schizophrenia: Insights for cognitive dysfunction. *Psychopharmacology* **2004**, *174*, 3–16. [CrossRef] [PubMed]

21. Johnson, P.M.; Kenny, P.J. Dopamine D2 receptors in addiction-like reward dysfunction and compulsive eating in obese rats. *Nat. Neurosci.* **2010**, *13*, 635–641. [CrossRef] [PubMed]

22. Gerlach, M.; Double, K.; Arzberger, T.; Leblhuber, F.; Tatschner, T.; Riederer, P. Dopamine receptor agonists in current clinical use: Comparative dopamine receptor binding profiles defined in the human striatum. *J. Neural Transm.* **2003**, *110*, 1119–1127. [CrossRef] [PubMed]

23. Vellaisamy, K.; Li, G.; Ko, C.-N.; Zhong, H.-J.; Fatima, S.; Kwan, H.-Y.; Wong, C.-Y.; Kwong, W.-J.; Tan, W.; Leung, C.-H.; et al. Cell imaging of dopamine receptor using agonist labeling iridium(iii) complex. *Chem. Sci.* **2018**, *9*, 1119–1125. [CrossRef] [PubMed]

24. Zhang, L.; Yu, J.; Pan, H.; Hu, P.; Hao, Y.; Cai, W.; Zhu, H.; Yu, A.D.; Xie, X.; Ma, D.; et al. Small molecule regulators of autophagy identified by an image-based high-throughput screen. *Proc. Natl. Acad. Sci. USA* **2007**, *104*, 19023–19028. [CrossRef] [PubMed]

25. Li, C.; Guo, Y.; Xie, W.; Li, X.; Janokovic, J.; Le, W. Neuroprotection of pramipexole in UPS impairment induced animal model of Parkinson's disease. *Neurochem. Res.* **2010**, *35*, 1546–1556. [CrossRef] [PubMed]

26. Yan, H.; Li, W.L.; Xu, J.J.; Zhu, S.Q.; Long, X.; Che, J.P. D2 dopamine receptor antagonist raclopride induces non-canonical autophagy in cardiac myocytes. *J. Cell. Biochem.* **2013**, *114*, 103–110. [CrossRef] [PubMed]

27. Wei, C.; Gao, J.; Li, M.; Li, H.; Wang, Y.; Li, H.; Xu, C. Dopamine D2 receptors contribute to cardioprotection of ischemic post-conditioning via activating autophagy in isolated rat hearts. *Int. J. Cardiol.* **2016**, *203*, 837–839. [CrossRef] [PubMed]

28. Wang, J.D.; Cao, Y.L.; Li, Q.; Yang, Y.P.; Jin, M.; Chen, D.; Wang, F.; Wang, G.H.; Qin, Z.H.; Hu, L.F.; et al. A pivotal role of FOS-mediated BECN1/Beclin 1 upregulation in dopamine D2 and D3 receptor agonist-induced autophagy activation. *Autophagy* **2015**, *11*, 2057–2073. [CrossRef] [PubMed]

29. Leng, Z.G.; Lin, S.J.; Wu, Z.R.; Guo, Y.H.; Cai, L.; Shang, H.B.; Tang, H.; Xue, Y.J.; Lou, M.Q.; Zhao, W. Activation of DRD5 (dopamine receptor D5) inhibits tumor growth by autophagic cell death. *Autophagy* **2017**, *13*, 1404–1419. [CrossRef] [PubMed]

30. Dolma, S.; Selvadurai, H.J.; Lan, X.; Lee, L.; Kushida, M.; Voisin, V.; Whetstone, H.; So, M.; Aviv, T.; Park, N. Inhibition of dopamine receptor D4 impedes autophagic flux, proliferation, and survival of glioblastoma stem cells. *Cancer Cell* **2016**, *29*, 859–873. [CrossRef] [PubMed]

31. Shin, J.H.; Park, S.J.; Kim, E.S.; Jo, Y.K.; Hong, J.; Cho, D.-H. Sertindole, a potent antagonist at dopamine D2 receptors, induces autophagy by increasing reactive oxygen species in SH-SY5Y neuroblastoma cells. *Biol. Pharm. Bull.* **2012**, *35*, 1069–1075. [CrossRef] [PubMed]

32. Li, Z.; Ji, X.; Wang, W.; Liu, J.; Liang, X.; Wu, H.; Liu, J.; Eggert, U.S.; Liu, Q.; Zhang, X. Ammonia induces autophagy through dopamine receptor D3 and MTOR. *PLoS ONE* **2016**, *11*, e0153526. [CrossRef] [PubMed]

33. Strous, G.; Kerkhof, P.V.; Govers, R.; Ciechanover, A.; Schwartz, A. The ubiquitin conjugation system is required for ligand-induced endocytosis and degradation of the growth hormone receptor. *EMBO J.* **1996**, *15*, 3806–3812. [PubMed]

34. Alwan, H.A.; van Zoelen, E.J.; van Leeuwen, J.E. Ligand-induced lysosomal epidermal growth factor receptor (EGFR) degradation is preceded by proteasome-dependent EGFR de-ubiquitination. *J. Biol. Chem.* **2003**, *278*, 35781–35790. [CrossRef] [PubMed]

35. Salles, M.J.; Herve, D.; Rivet, J.M.; Longueville, S.; Millan, M.J.; Girault, J.A.; la Cour, C.M. Transient and rapid activation of Akt/GSK-3beta and mTORC1 signaling by D3 dopamine receptor stimulation in dorsal striatum and nucleus accumbens. *J. Neurochem.* **2013**, *125*, 532–544. [CrossRef] [PubMed]

36. La Cour, C.M.; Salles, M.J.; Pasteau, V.; Millan, M.J. Signaling pathways leading to phosphorylation of Akt and GSK-3beta by activation of cloned human and rat cerebral D(2)and D(3) receptors. *Mol. Pharmacol.* **2011**, *79*, 91–105. [CrossRef] [PubMed]

37. Giménez-Xavier, P.; Francisco, R.; Santidrián, A.F.; Gil, J.; Ambrosio, S. Effects of dopamine on LC3-II activation as a marker of autophagy in a neuroblastoma cell model. *Neurotoxicology* **2009**, *30*, 658–665. [CrossRef] [PubMed]

38. Ni, H.-M.; Bockus, A.; Wozniak, A.L.; Jones, K.; Weinman, S.; Yin, X.-M.; Ding, W.-X. Dissecting the dynamic turnover of GFP-LC3 in the autolysosome. *Autophagy* **2011**, *7*, 188–204. [CrossRef] [PubMed]

39. Nimchinsky, E.A.; Hof, P.R.; Janssen, W.G.; Morrison, J.H.; Schmauss, C. Expression of dopamine D3 receptor dimers and tetramers in brain and in transfected cells. *J. Biol. Chem.* **1997**, *272*, 29229–29237. [CrossRef] [PubMed]

40. Li, Z.; Zhang, X. Autophagic cell death induced by dopamine and monoamines. Unpublished work.

41. Zhang, T.; Dong, K.; Liang, W.; Xu, D.; Xia, H.; Geng, J.; Najafov, A.; Liu, M.; Li, Y.; Han, X. G-protein-coupled receptors regulate autophagy by ZBTB16-mediated ubiquitination and proteasomal degradation of Atg14L. *Elife* **2015**, *4*, e06734. [CrossRef] [PubMed]

42. Bhattacharya, S.; Pal, K.; Sharma, A.K.; Dutta, S.K.; Lau, J.S.; Yan, I.K.; Wang, E.; Elkhanany, A.; Alkharfy, K.M.; Sanyal, A. GAIP interacting protein C-terminus regulates autophagy and exosome biogenesis of pancreatic cancer through metabolic pathways. *PLoS ONE* **2014**, *9*, e114409. [CrossRef] [PubMed]

43. Jeanneteau, F.; Diaz, J.; Sokoloff, P.; Griffon, N. Interactions of GIPC with dopamine D2, D3 but not D4 receptors define a novel mode of regulation of G protein-coupled receptors. *Mol. Biol. Cell* **2004**, *15*, 696–705. [CrossRef] [PubMed]

44. Jeanneteau, F.; Guillin, O.; Diaz, J.; Griffon, N.; Sokoloff, P. GIPC recruits GAIP (RGS19) to attenuate dopamine D2 receptor signaling. *Mol. Biol. Cell* **2004**, *15*, 4926–4937. [CrossRef] [PubMed]

45. Lakatos, K.; Toth, I.; Nemoda, Z.; Ney, K.; Sasvari-Szekely, M.; Gervai, J. Dopamine D4 receptor (DRD4) gene polymorphism is associated with attachment disorganization in infants. *Mol. Psychiatry* **2000**, *5*, 633–637. [CrossRef] [PubMed]

46. Marchese, A.; Paing, M.M.; Temple, B.R.; Trejo, J. G protein-coupled receptor sorting to endosomes and lysosomes. *Annu. Rev. Pharmacol. Toxicol.* **2008**, *48*, 601–629. [CrossRef] [PubMed]

47. Cho, D.; Zheng, M.; Min, C.; Ma, L.; Kurose, H.; Park, J.H.; Kim, K.M. Agonist-induced endocytosis and receptor phosphorylation mediate resensitization of dopamine D(2) receptors. *Mol. Endocrinol.* **2010**, *24*, 574–586. [CrossRef] [PubMed]

48. He, C.; Wei, Y.; Sun, K.; Li, B.; Dong, X.; Zou, Z.; Liu, Y.; Kinch, L.N.; Khan, S.; Sinha, S. Beclin 2 functions in autophagy, degradation of G protein-coupled receptors, and metabolism. *Cell* **2013**, *154*, 1085–1099. [CrossRef] [PubMed]

49. Nah, J.; Yuan, J.; Jung, Y.-K. Autophagy in Neurodegenerative Diseases: From Mechanism to Therapeutic Approach. *Mol. Cells* **2015**, *38*, 381–389. [CrossRef] [PubMed]

50. Nixon, R.A. The role of autophagy in neurodegenerative disease. *Nat. Med.* **2013**, *19*, 983–997. [CrossRef] [PubMed]

51. Menzies, F.M.; Fleming, A.; Caricasole, A.; Bento, C.F.; Andrews, S.P.; Ashkenazi, A.; Füllgrabe, J.; Jackson, A.; Jimenez Sanchez, M.; Karabiyik, C.; et al. Autophagy and Neurodegeneration: Pathogenic Mechanisms and Therapeutic Opportunities. *Neuron* **2017**, *93*, 1015–1034. [CrossRef] [PubMed]

52. Perreault, M.L.; Hasbi, A.; Alijaniaram, M.; Fan, T.; Varghese, G.; Fletcher, P.J.; Seeman, P.; O'Dowd, B.F.; George, S.R. The dopamine D1-D2 receptor heteromer localizes in dynorphin/enkephalin neurons increased high affinity state following amphetamine and in schizophrenia. *J. Biol. Chem.* **2010**, *285*, 36625–36634. [CrossRef] [PubMed]

53. Marcellino, D.; Ferré, S.; Casadó, V.; Cortés, A.; Le Foll, B.; Mazzola, C.; Drago, F.; Saur, O.; Stark, H.; Soriano, A. Identification of dopamine D1–D3 receptor heteromers indications for a role of synergistic D1–D3 receptor interactions in the striatum. *J. Biol. Chem.* **2008**, *283*, 26016–26025. [CrossRef] [PubMed]

Int. J. Mol. Sci. **2018**, *19*, 1540

54. Fuxe, K.; Ferré, S.; Canals, M.; Torvinen, M.; Terasmaa, A.; Marcellino, D.; Goldberg, S.R.; Staines, W.; Jacobsen, K.X.; Lluis, C. Adenosine A2A and dopamine D2 heteromeric receptor complexes and their function. *J. Mol. Neurosci.* **2005**, *26*, 209–220. [CrossRef]

55. Fuxe, K.; Ferré, S.; Genedani, S.; Franco, R.; Agnati, L.F. Adenosine receptor–dopamine receptor interactions in the basal ganglia and their relevance for brain function. *Physiol. Behav.* **2007**, *92*, 210–217. [CrossRef] [PubMed]

56. Guo, W.; Urizar, E.; Kralikova, M.; Mobarec, J.C.; Shi, L.; Filizola, M.; Javitch, J.A. Dopamine D2 receptors form higher order oligomers at physiological expression levels. *EMBO J.* **2008**, *27*, 2293–2304. [CrossRef] [PubMed]

57. Hall, D.A.; Strange, P.G. Comparison of the ability of dopamine receptor agonists to inhibit forskolin-stimulated adenosine 3′ 5′-cyclic monophosphate (cAMP) accumulation via D2L (long isoform) and D3 receptors expressed in Chinese hamster ovary (CHO) cells. *Biochem. Pharmacol.* **1999**, *58*, 285–289. [CrossRef]

58. Zhang, X.; Wang, W.; Bedigian, A.V.; Coughlin, M.L.; Mitchison, T.J.; Eggert, U.S. Dopamine receptor D3 regulates endocytic sorting by a Prazosin-sensitive interaction with the coatomer COPI. *Proc. Natl. Acad. Sci. USA* **2012**, *109*, 12485–12490. [CrossRef] [PubMed]

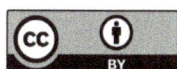

International Journal of
Molecular Sciences

MDPI

Article

Combined Fluid Shear Stress and Melatonin Enhances the ERK/Akt/mTOR Signal in Cilia-Less MC3T3-E1 Preosteoblast Cells

Chi Hyun Kim [1], Eui-Bae Jeung [2] and Yeong-Min Yoo [2,*]

[1] Department of Biomedical Engineering, College of Health Science, Yonsei University, Wonju, Gangwon 26493, Korea; chihyun@yonsei.ac.kr
[2] Laboratory of Veterinary Biochemistry and Molecular Biology, College of Veterinary Medicine, Chungbuk National University, Cheongju, Chungbuk 28644, Korea; ebjeung@chungbuk.ac.kr
* Correspondence: yyeongm@hanmail.net; Tel.: +82-10-2454-5309

Received: 30 August 2018; Accepted: 23 September 2018; Published: 26 September 2018

Abstract: We investigated whether combined fluid shear stress (FSS) and melatonin stimulated signal transduction in cilia-less MC3T3-E1 preosteoblast cells. MC3T3-E1 cells were treated with chloral hydrate or nocodazole, and mechanotransduction sensor primary cilia were removed. p-extracellular signal–regulated kinase (ERK) and p-Akt with/without melatonin increased with nocodazole treatment and decreased with chloral hydrate treatment, whereas p-ERK and p-Akt in FSS with/without melatonin increased in cilia-less groups compared to cilia groups. Furthermore, p-mammalian target of rapamycin (mTOR) with FSS-plus melatonin increased in cilia-less groups compared to only melatonin treatments in cilia groups. Expressions of Bcl-2, Cu/Zn-superoxide dismutase (SOD), and catalase proteins were higher in FSS with/without melatonin with cilia-less groups than only melatonin treatments in cilia groups. Bax protein expression was high in FSS-plus melatonin with chloral hydrate treatment. In chloral hydrate treatment with/without FSS, expressions of Cu/Zn-SOD, Mn-SOD, and catalase proteins were high compared to only-melatonin treatments. In nocodazole treatment, Mn-SOD protein expression without FSS was high, and catalase protein level with FSS was low, compared to only melatonin treatments. These data show that the combination with FSS and melatonin enhances ERK/Akt/mTOR signal in cilia-less MC3T3-E1, and the enhanced signaling in cilia-less MC3T3-E1 osteoblast cells may activate the anabolic effect for the preservation of cell structure and function.

Keywords: fluid shear stress; melatonin; chloral hydrate; nocodazole; MC3T3-E1 cells; primary cilia

1. Introduction

Primary cilium serves as a cellular sensory organelle and mediates mechanosensing or mechanotransduction in tissues including bone, cartilage, endothelium, and kidney [1–5]. The primary cilium has recently been highlighted as an organelle in vertebrate development and human genetic diseases associated with ciliary dysfunction or defects in cilia formation [1]. In bone cells including osteoblasts and osteocytes, the cilia that project from the cell surface and deflect from fluid flow are required for osteogenic and bone-resorptive responses to dynamic fluid flow or fluid shear stress (FSS) [2,6,7]. FSS-induced osteoblasts play an important role in both osteogenesis and osteoclastogenesis. However, its molecular mechanotransduction mechanism is still to be understood [2,6,7]. Malone et al. [2] reported that primary cilia mediate mechanosensing in bone cells by a calcium-independent mechanism, and Kwon et al. [7] showed that primary cilium-dependent mechanosensing is mediated by adenylyl cyclase 6 and cyclic adenosine monophosphate (AMP) without intracellular Ca^{2+} release in bone cells. In a further study, Delaine-Smith et al. [6] investigated how primary cilia respond to FSS and mediate flow-induced calcium deposition in osteoblasts. Saunders et al. described how MC3T3-E1 cells respond to oscillatory fluid flow with an increase in prostaglandin E2 release [8]. Wadhwa et al. demonstrated that FSS induces the transcription of cyclooxygenase-2 through the protein kinase A and protein kinase C signaling pathways [9].

Melatonin functions as a broad-spectrum antioxidant [10–12] and has anti-apoptotic and anti-autophagic effects [13–17]. Moreover, melatonin modulates osteogenic and adipogenic differentiation, in different kinds of mesenchymal stem cells, including dental pulp-derived stem cells and adipose-derived stem cells [18,19]. Recently, Kim and Yoo [20] reported that a combination of FSS and melatonin activates anabolic proteins through the p-ERK in MC3T3-E1 osteoblast cells. Moreover, melatonin has a significant effect on bone formation through the regulation of differentiation in osteoblasts and osteoclasts [21,22], indicating that melatonin may have the potential to regulate anabolic and catabolic responses in bone remodeling. However, the influence of melatonin combined with FSS in cilia-less osteoblasts has not been elucidated. In this study, we investigated whether combined FSS and melatonin stimulated signal transduction in cilia-less MC3T3-E1 osteoblast cells.

2. Results

We investigated whether the combination of FSS and melatonin stimulated signal transduction in cilia-less MC3T3-E1 preosteoblast cells. MC3T3-E1 cells were treated with chloral hydrate (4 mM) for 3 days or nocodazole (10 μg/mL) for 4 h, and then its primary cilia, as sensors of mechanotransduction, were removed (Figure 1). p-ERK and p-Akt with/without melatonin treatment (0.1, 1 mM) were increased with nocodazole treatment and decreased with chloral hydrate treatment (Figure 2), whereas p-ERK and p-Akt in FSS with/without melatonin were increased with cilia-less groups compared to cilia groups (Figure 3).

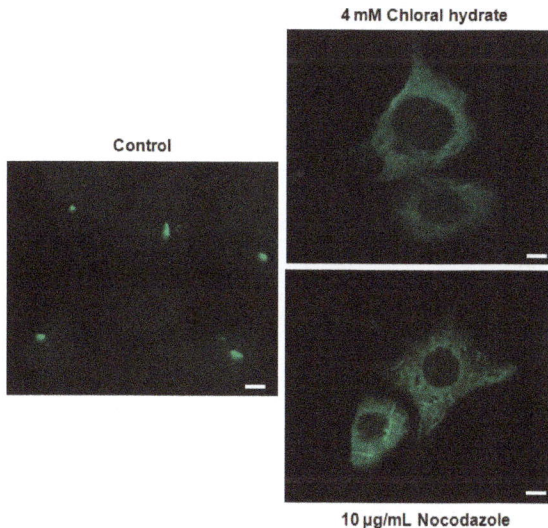

Figure 1. Removal of primary cilia in MC3T3-E1 cells as a sensor of mechanotransduction. MC3T3-E1 cells were treated with chloral hydrate (4 mM) for 3 days or nocodazole (10 μg/mL) for 4 h at 37 °C and 5% CO_2. The cilia in MC3T3-E1 cells were incubated using an anti-vinculin antibody. Scale bar represents 20 μm.

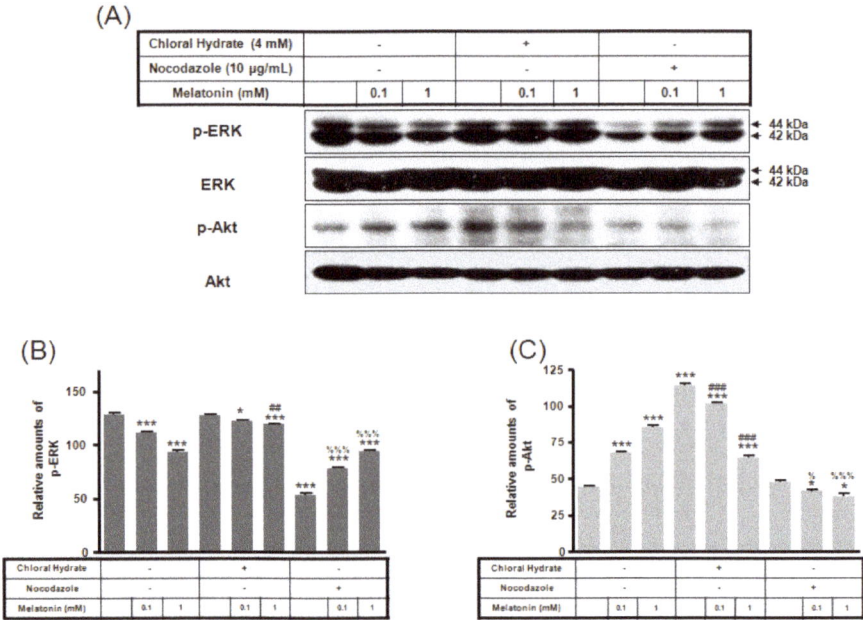

Figure 2. p-ERK and p-Akt expressions in MC3T3-E1 cells with/without melatonin treatment. MC3T3-E1 cells were incubated in α-MEM supplemented with 10% FBS at 37 °C with 5% CO_2. MC3T3-E1 cells in the presence or absence of melatonin (0.1, 1 mM) were treated with chloral hydrate (4 mM) for 3 days or nocodazole (10 µg/mL) for 4 h. p-ERK and p-Akt expressions were identified by Western blots (**A**). p-ERK (**B**) and p-Akt (**C**) expressions were quantified with ImageJ analysis software. * $p < 0.05$, *** $p < 0.001$ vs. FBS alone; ## $p < 0.01$, ### $p < 0.001$ vs. FBS + chloral hydrate; % $p < 0.05$, %%% $p < 0.001$ vs. FBS + nocodazole.

p-mTOR (Ser2481) with/without melatonin treatment was decreased in chloral hydrate treatment, and p-mTORs (Ser2448, Ser2481) were increased in nocodazole treatment (Figure 4). In FSS-plus melatonin treatments, p-mTORs (Ser2448, Ser2481) were significantly increased in cilia-less groups compared to only melatonin treatments in cilia groups (Figure 5). These data indicate that combination with FSS and melatonin enhance ERK/Akt/mTOR signal in cilia-less MC3T3-E1.

Expression of Bcl-2 protein with/without melatonin treatment in chloral hydrate treatment was increased, and Bax protein expression was decreased (Figure 6). In FSS-plus melatonin treatments, expressions of Bcl-2 and Bax proteins in chloral hydrate treatment were significantly increased compared to only melatonin treatments in cilia groups, whereas expression of Bcl-2 protein in nocodazole treatment was significantly increased (Figure 7).

In chloral hydrate treatment with/without FSS, the expressions of Cu/Zn-SOD, Mn-SOD, and catalase proteins were high compared to only melatonin treatments (Figures 8 and 9). In nocodazole treatment, the expression of Mn-SOD protein without FSS was high (Figure 8), and the expression of catalase protein with FSS was low, compared to only melatonin treatment (Figure 9).

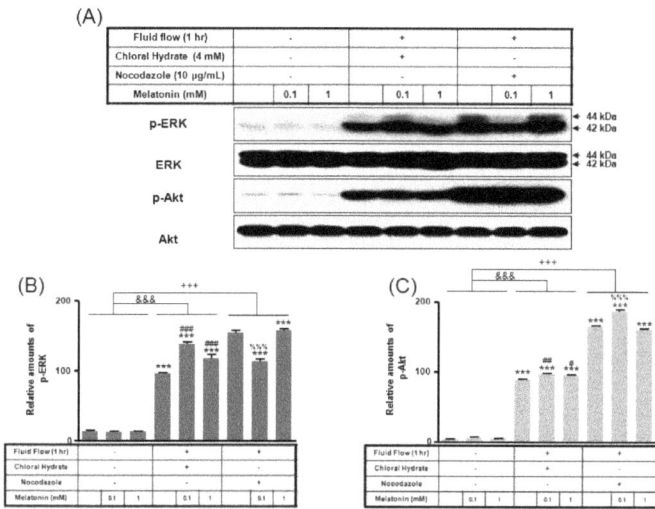

Figure 3. p-ERK and p-Akt expressions in MC3T3-E1 cells with/without fluid shear stress and/or melatonin treatment. MC3T3-E1 cells were incubated in α-MEM supplemented with 10% FBS at 37 °C with 5% CO_2. Fluid flow stress experiments were performed at 1 Hz frequency and ±1 Pa maximum shear stress. MC3T3-E1 cells in the presence or absence of melatonin (0.1, 1 mM) were treated with chloral hydrate (4 mM) for 3 days or nocodazole (10 μg/mL) for 4 h. p-ERK and p-Akt expressions were identified by Western blots (**A**). p-ERK (**B**) and p-Akt (**C**) were quantified with ImageJ analysis software. *** $p < 0.001$ vs. FBS alone; [#] $p < 0.05$, [##] $p < 0.01$, [###] $p < 0.001$ vs. FBS + chloral hydrate; [%%%] $p < 0.001$ vs. FBS + nocodazole; [&&&] $p < 0.001$, no FSS vs. FSS + chloral hydrate; [+++] $p < 0.001$, FSS vs. FSS + chloral hydrate.

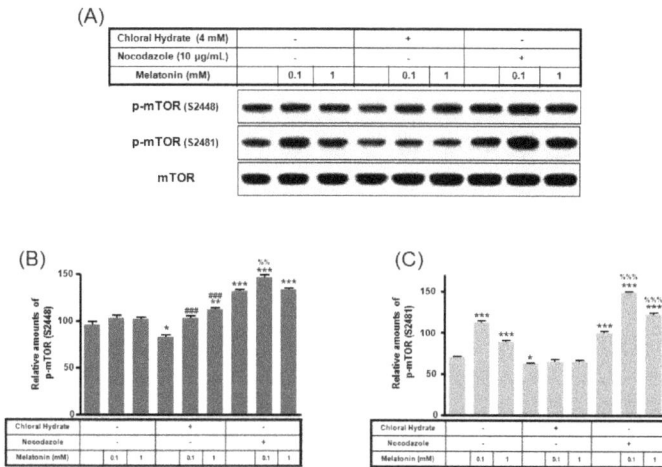

Figure 4. p-mTOR (Ser2448, Ser2481) expressions in MC3T3-E1 cells with/without melatonin treatment. MC3T3-E1 cells were incubated in α-MEM supplemented with 10% FBS at 37 °C with 5% CO_2. MC3T3-E1 cells in the presence or absence of melatonin (0.1, 1 mM) were treated with chloral hydrate (4 mM) for 3 days or nocodazole (10 μg/mL) for 4 h. p-mTOR (Ser2448, Ser2481) expressions were identified by Western blots (**A**). p-mTOR (Ser2448) (**B**) and p-mTOR (Ser2481) (**C**) were quantified with ImageJ analysis software. * $p < 0.05$, ** $p < 0.01$, *** $p < 0.001$ vs. FBS alone; [###] $p < 0.001$ vs. FBS + chloral hydrate; [%%] $p < 0.01$, [%%%] $p < 0.001$ vs. FBS + nocodazole.

(A)

Fluid flow (1 hr)			-		+		+	
Chloral Hydrate (4 mM)			-		+		-	
Nocodazole (10 µg/mL)			-		-		+	
Melatonin (mM)	0.1	1			0.1	1	0.1	1

p-mTOR (S2448)

p-mTOR (S2481)

mTOR

(B)

(C)

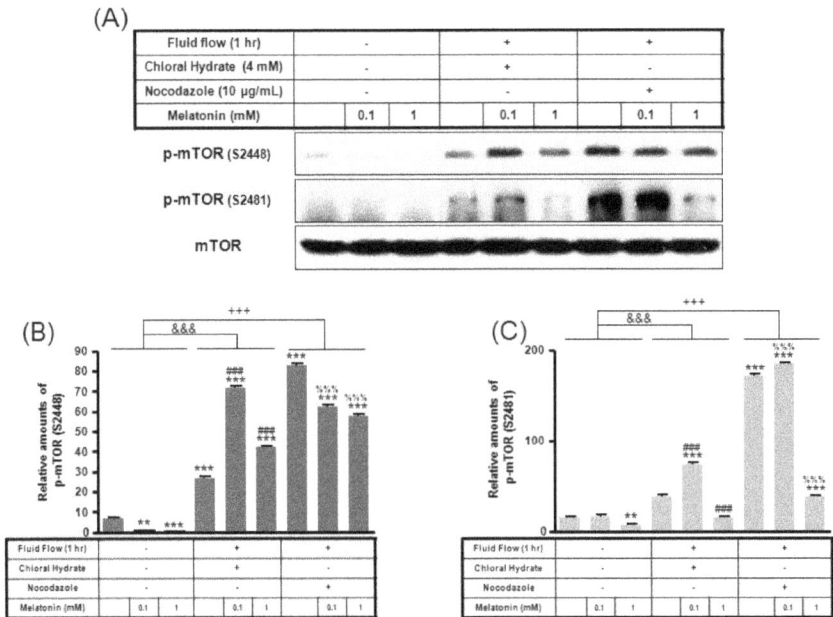

Figure 5. p-mTOR (Ser2448, Ser2481) expressions in MC3T3-E1 cells with/without fluid shear stress (FSS) and/or melatonin treatment. MC3T3-E1 cells were incubated in α-MEM supplemented with 10% FBS at 37 °C with 5% CO_2. Fluid flow stress experiments were performed at 1 Hz frequency and ±1 Pa maximum shear stress. MC3T3-E1 cells in the presence or absence of melatonin (0.1, 1 mM) treated with chloral hydrate (4 mM) for 3 days or nocodazole (10 µg/mL) for 4 h. p-mTOR (Ser2448, Ser2481) expressions were identified by Western blots (**A**). p-mTOR (Ser2448) (**B**) and p-mTOR (Ser2481) (**C**) were quantified with ImageJ analysis software. ** $p < 0.01$, *** $p < 0.001$ vs. FBS alone; ### $p < 0.001$ vs. FBS + chloral hydrate; %%% $p < 0.001$ vs. FBS + nocodazole; &&& $p < 0.001$, no FSS vs. FSS + chloral hydrate; +++ $p < 0.001$, FSS vs. FSS + chloral hydrate.

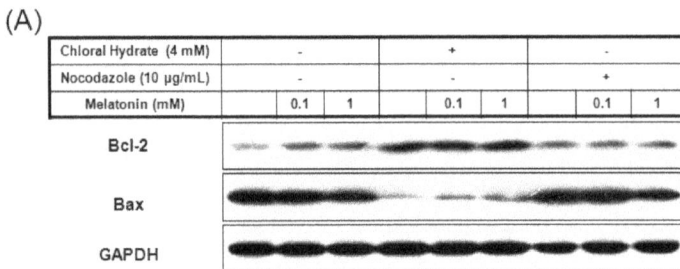

(A)

Chloral Hydrate (4 mM)			-		+		-	
Nocodazole (10 µg/mL)			-		-		+	
Melatonin (mM)	0.1	1			0.1	1	0.1	1

Bcl-2

Bax

GAPDH

Figure 6. *Cont.*

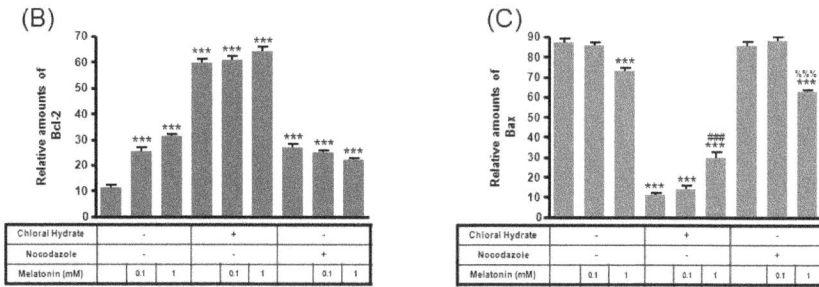

Figure 6. The expressions of Bcl-2 and Bax proteins in MC3T3-E1 cells with/without melatonin treatment. MC3T3-E1 cells were incubated in α-MEM supplemented with 10% FBS at 37 °C with 5% CO_2. MC3T3-E1 cells in the presence or absence of melatonin (0.1, 1 mM) were treated with chloral hydrate (4 mM) for 3 days or nocodazole (10 μg/mL) for 4 h. Bcl-2 and Bax expressions were identified by Western blots (**A**). Bcl-2 (**B**) and Bax (**C**) were quantified with ImageJ analysis software. *** $p < 0.001$ vs. FBS alone; ### $p < 0.001$ vs. FBS + chloral hydrate; %%% $p < 0.001$ vs. FBS + nocodazole.

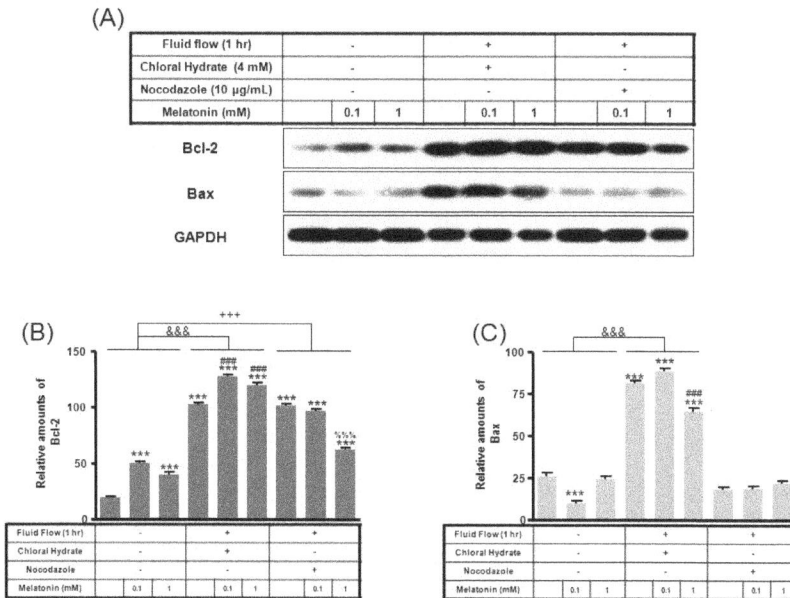

Figure 7. The expressions of Bcl-2 and Bax proteins in MC3T3-E1 cells with/without fluid shear stress and/or melatonin treatment. MC3T3-E1 cells were incubated in α-MEM supplemented with 10% FBS at 37 °C with 5% CO_2. Fluid flow stress experiments were performed at 1 Hz frequency and ±1 Pa maximum shear stress. MC3T3-E1 cells in the presence or absence of melatonin (0.1, 1 mM) treated with chloral hydrate (4 mM) for 3 days or nocodazole (10 μg/mL) for 4 h. Bcl-2 and Bax expressions were identified by Western blots (**A**). Bcl-2 (**B**) and Bax (**C**) were quantified with ImageJ analysis software. *** $p < 0.001$ vs. FBS alone; ### $p < 0.001$ vs. FBS + chloral hydrate; %%% $p < 0.001$ vs. FBS + nocodazole; &&& $p < 0.001$, no FSS vs. FSS + chloral hydrate; +++ $p < 0.001$, FSS vs. FSS + chloral hydrate.

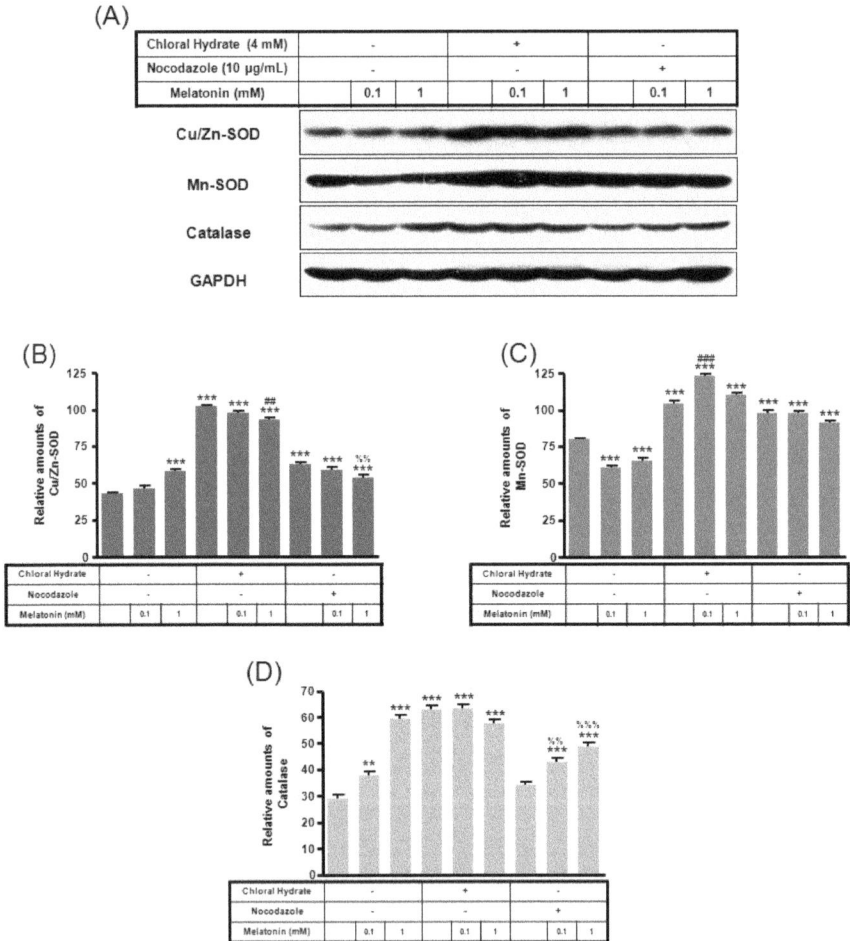

Figure 8. The expressions of Cu/Zn-SOD, Mn-SOD, and catalase proteins in MC3T3-E1 cells with/without melatonin treatment. MC3T3-E1 cells were incubated in α-MEM supplemented with 10% FBS at 37 °C with 5% CO_2. MC3T3-E1 cells in the presence or absence of melatonin (0.1, 1 mM) treated with chloral hydrate (4 mM) for 3 days or nocodazole (10 μg/mL) for 4 h. Cu/Zn-SOD, Mn-SOD, and catalase proteins were identified by Western blots (**A**). Cu/Zn-SOD (**B**), Mn-SOD (**C**), and catalase proteins (**D**) were quantified with ImageJ analysis software. ** $p < 0.01$, *** $p < 0.001$ vs. FBS alone; ## $p < 0.01$, ### $p < 0.001$ vs. FBS +chloral hydrate; %% $p < 0.01$, %%% $p < 0.001$ vs. FBS + nocodazole.

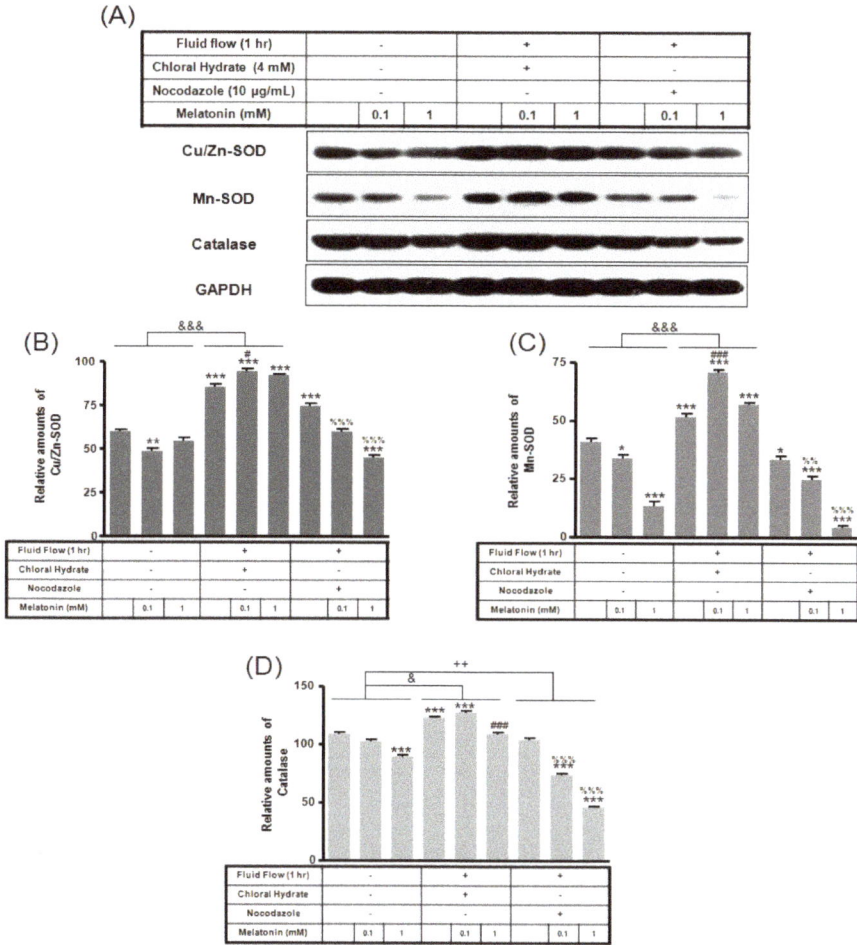

Figure 9. The expressions of Cu/Zn-SOD, Mn-SOD, and catalase proteins in MC3T3-E1 cells with/without fluid shear stress (FSS) and/or melatonin treatment. MC3T3-E1 cells were incubated in α-MEM supplemented with 10% FBS at 37 °C with 5% CO_2. Fluid flow stress experiments were performed at 1 Hz frequency and ±1 Pa maximum shear stress. MC3T3-E1 cells in the presence or absence of melatonin (0.1, 1 mM) treated with chloral hydrate (4 mM) for 3 days or nocodazole (10 µg/mL) for 4 h. Cu/Zn-SOD, Mn-SOD, and catalase proteins were identified by Western blots (**A**). Cu/Zn-SOD (**B**), Mn-SOD (**C**), and catalase proteins (**D**) were quantified with ImageJ analysis software. * $p < 0.05$, ** $p < 0.01$, *** $p < 0.001$ vs. FBS alone; # $p < 0.05$, ### $p < 0.001$ vs. FBS + chloral hydrate; %% $p < 0.01$, %%% $p < 0.001$ vs. FBS + nocodazole; & $p < 0.05$, &&& $p < 0.001$, no FSS vs. FSS + chloral hydrate; ++ $p < 0.01$, FSS vs. FSS + chloral hydrate.

3. Discussion

Our recent study reported that melatonin combined with FSS activates anabolic proteins through p-ERK in MC3T3-E1 preosteoblast cells [20]. This investigation, carried out in MC3T3-E1 osteoblast cells with primary cilia under FSS and melatonin, showed that p-ERK, p-Akt, and p-mTOR (Ser 2481) expressions increased with the addition of 1 mM melatonin compared to 0.1 mM melatonin treatment. The results of the current study show that p-ERK, p-Akt, and p-mTOR in FSS with/without melatonin increased in cilia-less groups compared to cilia groups, suggesting that the enhanced signaling in cilia-less MC3T3-E1 preosteoblast cells may be activated when combined with FSS and melatonin.

In this study, primary cilia were removed with chloral hydrate or nocodazole in MC3T3-E1 cells, demonstrating that the increase of phosphorylation of ERK/Akt/mTOR in cilia-less MC3T3-E1 osteoblast cells under FSS may be activated for the preservation of cell structure and function. Delaine-Smith et al. proved that damage or removal of primary cilia with chloral hydrate inhibited fluid flow-induced mineral/calcium deposition, suggesting that primary cilia were a mechanosensor in bone cells, and highlighting their relevance in clinical treatments of bone disorders caused by dysfunctional responses to loading [6]. Jeon et al. [23] showed that osteoblastic cells with primary cilia by fluid flow stress induced an increase of COX-2 level and PGE2 release via focal adhesions and Akt phosphorylation. Malone et al. [2] suggested that primary cilia, in response to dynamic fluid flow, regulate osteopontin gene expression and MAPK phosphorylation in bone cells via tissue-specific pathways. Praetorius and Spring [24] demonstrated that chloral hydrate did not impair the Ca^{2+} mobilization machinery in MDCK cells, indicating that the primary cilium in MDCK cells functions as a Ca^{2+} sensor. Alenghat et al. [25] reported that nocodazole-treated kidney epithelial cells remove the fluid flow-induced intracellular calcium response, suggesting that disrupting the cytoskeleton in the cytoplasm may influence the function of the primary cilium to maintain its mechanotransduction response. Furthermore, nocodazole impairs tubulin polymerization in human HT-29 colon carcinoma cells, indicating that cellular interactions with the cell cytoskeleton are strongly influenced by fluid flow shear stress [26].

MAPK signaling is activated in osteoblasts that are stimulated with FSS [27–32], and Ca^{2+} change from extracellular Ca^{2+} entry or intracellular Ca^{2+} release is important for ERK activation in osteoblasts [30,33]. However, primary cilium-dependent mechanotransduction in bone cells is mediated by adenylyl cyclase 6 and cyclic AMP without intracellular Ca^{2+} release in bone cells [2,7], whereas another study showed that primary cilia under FSS mediate flow-induced calcium deposition in osteoblasts [6]. Thus, the mechanotransduction pathway on primary cilium dependence and independence may not be unique to bone cells but activates the anabolic effect under FSS [20,34]. For example, bending the primary cilium by suction with a micropipette or by increasing the flow rate of perfusate has been shown to increase extracellular Ca^{2+} in kidney cells, whereas manipulation of the apical membrane does not [35]. Praetorius and Spring also demonstrated that the flow-induced Ca^{2+} response is not inhibited by removal of the primary cilium with 4 mM chloral hydrate treatment [35].

FSS-induced activation of the phosphoinositide-3 kinase (PI3K)/Akt pathway may promote anabolic responses in osteoblasts [20,36,37]. Rangaswami et al. [38] reported that FSS-induced osteoblasts activate Akt/ERK signaling with the anabolic response of bone. Triplett et al. [39] found that FSS may regulate IGF-I-activated p-Akt and p-ERK signaling in osteoblasts. These studies demonstrate that Akt phosphorylation is required for primary, cilia-mediated, FSS-induced upregulation of osteogenic responses. In the present study, p-Akt in FSS with/without melatonin were increased with cilia-less groups compared with cilia groups in MC3T3-E1 cells (Figure 3). Similar to p-ERK increase, FSS in osteoblast activates p-Akt as an important stimulator in the cilium-dependent and cilium-independent mechanotransduction pathways.

Kim and Yoo [20] demonstrated that FSS and melatonin in combination increase the expression of anabolic proteins through the Akt/mTOR in MC3T3-E1 osteoblast cells. Lee et al. [40] provided insights into the mechanisms by which oscillatory shear stress induces osteoblast-like MG63 cells proliferation through the upregulation of PI3K/Akt/mTOR/p70S6K pathways. However, the relevance between the osteoblast-signaling pathway and anabolic proteins expression in response to mechanical stimuli is not currently known. Our present study demonstrated that FSS induces phosphorylation of mTOR in osteoblast cells with/without cilium.

In chloral hydrate treatment with/without FSS, expressions of Bcl-2, Bax, Cu/Zn-SOD, Mn-SOD, and catalase proteins were high compared to only melatonin treatments (Figures 7–9). In nocodazole treatment, expression of Mn-SOD protein without FSS was high (Figure 8), and expression of catalase protein with FSS was low, compared to only melatonin treatments (Figure 9). The effects of FSS increasing antioxidant proteins including Bcl-2, Cu/Zn-SOD, Mn-SOD, and catalase in osteoblast or osteocyte cells are not well known [20,41]. Therefore, it is necessary to study antioxidant proteins under FSS.

In conclusion, we found that combined FSS and melatonin enhance ERK/Akt/mTOR signal in cilia-less MC3T3-E1. The increase of p-ERK/p-Akt/p-mTOR may have resulted from the total influence of combined FSS and melatonin in MC3T3-E1 osteoblast cells with and without cilia, and, especially, the enhanced signaling in cilia-less MC3T3-E1 osteoblast cells may activate the anabolic effect required for the preservation of cell structure and function.

4. Materials and Methods

4.1. Cell Culture

MC3TC-E1 osteoblast cells were purchased from ATCC (Manassas, MD, USA) and cultured in α-minimum essential medium (α-MEM; Gibco BRL, Gaithersburg, MD, USA) with 10% heat-inactivated fetal bovine serum (FBS; Gibco BRL, Gaithersburg, MD, USA) at 37 °C with 5% CO_2.

4.2. Treatment of Chloral Hydrate or Nocodazole and Fluid Flow-Induced Shear Stress

Cells at a density of 1×10^6 cells were placed in glass slides under sterile conditions. Fluid flow stress was produced by a syringe that was driven by an actuator at a frequency of 1 Hz and a maximum shear stress of ±1 Pa. MC3T3-E1 cells in the presence or absence of melatonin (0.1, 1 mM) with the treatment of chloral hydrate (4 mM) for 3 days or nocodazole (10 μg/mL) for 4 h were incubated at 37 °C and 5% CO_2 for 1 h. Control cells were placed in flow chambers for 1 h with no fluid flow.

4.3. Immunofluorescence

Fixed cells were incubated overnight at 4 °C with a vinculin monoclonal antibody (clone 7F9, 1:330, Millipore, San Diego, CA, USA) and incubated with FITC-conjugated goat anti-mouse antibody (1:200, Millipore, San Diego, CA, USA). Fluorescence-labeled cells were visualized by fluorescence microscopy (Carl Zeiss, San Diego, CA, USA).

4.4. Western Blot Analysis

Cells were harvested, washed two times with ice-cold PBS and then resuspended in 20 mM Tris-HCl buffer (pH 7.4) containing 1% NP-40, 0.1 mM phenylmethylsulfonyl fluoride, 5 μg/mL aprotinin, 5 μg/mL pepstatin A, 1 μg/mL chymostatin, 5 mM Na_3VO_4 and 5 mM NaF. The cell lysate was centrifuged at $13,000 \times g$ for 20 min at 4 °C. Protein concentration was determined using the BCA assay (Sigma, St Louis, MO, USA). Proteins were separated by Tris-Glycine SDS-PAGE and then transferred to a polyvinylidene difluoride (PVDF) membrane. The membrane was incubated with antibodies, indicated as follows: p-Akt and Akt (1:1000, Cell Signaling Technology, Beverly, MA, USA); p-ERK and ERK (1:500, Santa Cruz Biotechnology, Santa Cruz, CA, USA); mTOR (1:500, Santa Cruz Biotechnology); Bax and Bcl-2 (1:500, Santa Cruz Biotechnology); catalase, Cu/Zn-SOD, Mn-SOD (1:1000, Cell Signaling Technology), and GAPDH (1:1000, Assay Designs, Ann Arbor, MI, USA). The membrane was exposed to X-ray film; protein bands were scanned and measured using ImageJ analysis software (version 1.37; Wayne Rasband, NIH, Bethesda, MD, USA), and normalized by GAPDH, an internal control.

4.5. Statistical Analysis

Data analysis was performed with Prism software (GraphPad Software Inc., San Diego, CA, USA). Values are presented as means ± SD and considered statistically significant when $p < 0.05$.

Author Contributions: Conceptualization, C.H.K. and Y.-M.Y.; Data curation, E.-B.J.; Formal analysis, C.H.K. and Y.-M.Y.; Funding acquisition, C.H.K.; Supervision, Y.-M.Y.; Validation, Y.-M.Y.; Writing original draft, Y.-M.Y.; Review & editing, C.H.K., E.-B.J. and Y.-M.Y.

Funding: This research was supported by the Basic Science Research Program through the National Research Foundation of Korea (NRF) funded by the Ministry of Education (NRF-2015R1D1A1A01060699).

Conflicts of Interest: The authors declare no conflict of interest.

References

1. Goetz, S.C.; Anderson, K.V. The primary cilium: A signalling centre during vertebrate development. *Nat. Rev. Genet.* **2010**, *11*, 331–344. [CrossRef] [PubMed]

2. Malone, A.M.; Anderson, C.T.; Tummala, P.; Kwon, R.Y.; Johnston, T.R.; Stearns, T.; Jacobs, C.R. Primary cilia mediate mechanosensing in bone cells by a calcium-independent mechanism. *Proc. Natl. Acad. Sci. USA* **2007**, *104*, 13325–13330. [CrossRef] [PubMed]

3. Satir, P.; Pedersen, L.B.; Christensen, S.T. The primary cilium at a glance. *J. Cell Sci.* **2010**, *123*, 499–503. [CrossRef] [PubMed]

4. Egorova, A.D.; Khedoe, P.P.; Goumans, M.J.; Yoder, B.K.; Nauli, S.M.; ten Dijke, P.; Poelmann, R.E.; Hierck, B.P. Lack of primary cilia primes shear-induced endothelial-to-mesenchymal transition. *Circ. Res.* **2011**, *108*, 1093–1101. [CrossRef] [PubMed]

5. Raghavan, V.; Rbaibi, Y.; Pastor-Soler, N.M.; Carattino, M.D.; Weisz, O.A. Shear stress-dependent regulation of apical endocytosis in renal proximal tubule cells mediated by primary cilia. *Proc. Natl. Acad. Sci. USA* **2014**, *111*, 8506–8511. [CrossRef] [PubMed]

6. Delaine-Smith, R.M.; Sittichokechaiwut, A.; Reilly, G.C. Primary cilia respond to fluid shear stress and mediate flow-induced calcium deposition in osteoblasts. *FASEB J.* **2014**, *28*, 430–439. [CrossRef] [PubMed]

7. Kwon, R.Y.; Temiyasathit, S.; Tummala, P.; Quah, C.C.; Jacobs, C.R. Primary cilium-dependent mechanosensing is mediated by adenylyl cyclase 6 and cyclic AMP in bone cells. *FASEB J.* **2010**, *24*, 2859–2868. [CrossRef] [PubMed]

8. Saunders, M.M.; You, J.; Trosko, J.E.; Yamasaki, H.; Li, Z.; Donahue, H.J.; Jacobs, C.R. Gap junctions and fluid flow response in MC3T3-E1 cells. *Am. J. Physiol. Cell Physiol.* **2001**, *281*, C1917–C1925. [CrossRef] [PubMed]

9. Wadhwa, S.; Choudhary, S.; Voznesensky, M.; Epstein, M.; Raisz, L.; Pilbeam, C. Fluid flow induces COX-2 expression in MC3T3-E1 osteoblasts via a PKA signaling pathway. *Biochem. Biophys. Res. Commun.* **2002**, *297*, 46–51. [CrossRef]

10. Jung-Hynes, B.; Reiter, R.J.; Ahmad, N. Sirtuins, melatonin and circadian rhythms: Building a bridge between aging and cancer. *J. Pineal Res.* **2010**, *48*, 9–19. [PubMed]

11. Blask, D.E.; Hill, S.M.; Dauchy, R.T.; Xiang, S.; Yuan, L.; Duplessis, T.; Mao, L.; Dauchy, E.; Sauer, L.A. Circadian regulation of molecular, dietary, and metabolic signaling mechanisms of human breast cancer growth by the nocturnal melatonin signal and the consequences of its disruption by light at night. *J. Pineal Res.* **2011**, *51*, 259–269. [CrossRef] [PubMed]

12. Rodriguez, C.; Mayo, J.C.; Sainz, R.M.; Antolín, I.; Herrera, F.; Martín, V.; Reiter, R.J. Regulation of antioxidant enzymes: A significant role for melatonin. *J. Pineal Res.* **2004**, *36*, 1–9. [CrossRef] [PubMed]

13. Yoo, Y.M.; Yim, S.V.; Kim, S.S.; Jang, H.Y.; Lea, H.Z.; Hwang, G.C.; Kim, J.W.; Kim, S.A.; Lee, H.J.; Kim, C.J.; et al. Melatonin suppresses NO-induced apoptosis via induction of Bcl-2 expression in PGT-β immortalized pineal cells. *J. Pineal Res.* **2002**, *33*, 146–150. [CrossRef] [PubMed]

14. Choi, S.I.; Joo, S.S.; Yoo, Y.M. Melatonin prevents nitric oxide-induced apoptosis by increasing the interaction between 14-3-3beta and p-Bad in SK-N-MC cells. *J. Pineal Res.* **2008**, *44*, 95–100. [PubMed]

15. Joo, S.S.; Yoo, Y.M. Melatonin induces apoptotic death in LNCaP cells via p38 and JNK pathways: Therapeutic implications for prostate cancer. *J. Pineal Res.* **2009**, *47*, 8–14. [CrossRef] [PubMed]

16. Yoo, Y.M.; Jeung, E.B. Melatonin suppresses cyclosporine A-induced autophagy in rat pituitary GH3 cells. *J. Pineal Res.* **2010**, *48*, 204–211. [CrossRef] [PubMed]

17. Kim, C.H.; Kim, K.H.; Yoo, Y.M. Melatonin protects against apoptotic and autophagic cell death in C2C12 murine myoblast cells. *J. Pineal Res.* **2011**, *50*, 241–249. [CrossRef] [PubMed]

18. Basoli, V.; Santaniello, S.; Cruciani, S.; Ginesu, G.C.; Cossu, M.L.; Delitala, A.P.; Serra, P.A.; Ventura, C.; Maioli, M. Melatonin and Vitamin D Interfere with the Adipogenic Fate of Adipose-Derived Stem Cells. *Int. J. Mol. Sci.* **2017**, *18*, 981. [CrossRef] [PubMed]

19. Maioli, M.; Basoli, V.; Santaniello, S.; Cruciani, S.; Delitala, A.P.; Pinna, R.; Milia, E.; Grillari-Voglauer, R.; Fontani, V.; Rinaldi, S.; et al. Osteogenesis from Dental Pulp Derived Stem Cells: A Novel Conditioned Medium Including Melatonin within a Mixture of Hyaluronic, Butyric, and Retinoic Acids. *Stem Cells Int.* **2016**, *2016*, 2056416. [CrossRef] [PubMed]

20. Kim, C.H.; Yoo, Y.M. Fluid shear stress and melatonin in combination activate anabolic proteins in MC3T3-E1 osteoblast cells. *J. Pineal Res.* **2013**, *54*, 453–461. [CrossRef] [PubMed]

21. Sánchez-Barceló, E.J.; Mediavilla, M.D.; Tan, D.X.; Reiter, R.J. Scientific basis for the potential use of melatonin in bone diseases: Osteoporosis and adolescent idiopathic scoliosis. *J. Osteoporos.* **2010**, *2010*, 830231. [CrossRef] [PubMed]

22. Roth, J.A.; Kim, B.G.; Lin, W.L.; Cho, M.I. Melatonin promotes osteoblast differentiation and bone formation. *J. Biol. Chem.* **1999**, *274*, 22041–22047. [CrossRef] [PubMed]

23. Jeon, O.H.; Yoo, Y.M.; Kim, K.H.; Jacobs, C.R.; Kim, C.H. Primary Cilia-Mediated Osteogenic Response to Fluid Flow Occurs via Increases in Focal Adhesion and Akt Signaling Pathway in MC3T3-E1 Osteoblastic Cells. *Cell Mol. Bioeng.* **2011**, *4*, 379–388. [CrossRef]

24. Praetorius, H.A.; Spring, K.R. Bending the MDCK cell primary cilium increases intracellular calcium. *J. Membr. Biol.* **2001**, *184*, 71–79. [CrossRef] [PubMed]

25. Alenghat, F.J.; Nauli, S.M.; Kolb, R.; Zhou, J.; Ingber, D.E. Global cytoskeletal control of mechanotransduction in kidney epithelial cells. *Exp. Cell Res.* **2004**, *301*, 23–30. [CrossRef] [PubMed]

26. Haier, J.; Nicolson, G.L. Role of the cytoskeleton in adhesion stabilization of human colorectal carcinoma cells to extracellular matrix components under dynamic conditions of laminar flow. *Clin. Exp. Metast.* **1999**, *17*, 713–721. [CrossRef]

27. Liu, D.; Genetos, D.C.; Shao, Y.; Geist, D.J.; Li, J.; Ke, H.Z.; Turner, C.H.; Duncan, R.L. Activation of extracellular-signal regulated kinase (ERK1/2) by fluid shear is Ca^{2+}- and ATP-dependent in MC3T3-E1 osteoblasts. *Bone* **2008**, *42*, 644–652. [CrossRef] [PubMed]

28. Jackson, R.A.; Kumarasuriyar, A.; Nurcombe, V.; Cool, S.M. Long-term loading inhibits ERK1/2 phosphorylation and increases FGFR3 expression in MC3T3-E1 osteoblast cells. *J. Cell Physiol.* **2006**, *209*, 894–904. [CrossRef] [PubMed]

29. Gabarin, N.; Gavish, H.; Muhlrad, A.; Chen, Y.C.; Namdar-Attar, M.; Nissenson, R.A.; Chorev, M.; Bab, I. Mitogenic G(i) protein-MAP kinase signaling cascade in MC3T3-E1 osteogenic cells: Activation by C-terminal pentapeptide of osteogenic growth peptide [OGP(10–14)] and attenuation of activation by cAMP. *J. Cell Biochem.* **2001**, *81*, 594–603. [CrossRef] [PubMed]

30. Jessop, H.L.; Rawlinson, S.C.; Pitsillides, A.A.; Lanyon, L.E. Mechanical strain and fluid movement both activate extracellular regulated kinase (ERK) in osteoblast-like cells but via different signaling pathways. *Bone* **2002**, *31*, 186–194. [CrossRef]

31. Alford, A.I.; Jacobs, C.R.; Donahue, H.J. Oscillating fluid flow regulates gap junction communication in osteocytic MLO-Y4 cells by an ERK1/2 MAP kinase-dependent mechanism. *Bone* **2003**, *33*, 64–70. [CrossRef]

32. Jiang, G.L.; White, C.R.; Stevens, H.Y.; Frangos, J.A. Temporal gradients in shear stimulate osteoblastic proliferation via ERK1/2 and retinoblastoma protein. *Am. J. Physiol. Endocrinol. Metab.* **2002**, *283*, E383–E389. [CrossRef] [PubMed]

33. Choudhary, S.; Wadhwa, S.; Raisz, L.G.; Alander, C.; Pilbeam, C.C. Extracellular calcium is a potent inducer of cyclo-oxygenase-2 in murine osteoblasts through an ERK signaling pathway. *J. Bone Miner. Res.* **2003**, *18*, 1813–1824. [CrossRef] [PubMed]

34. You, J.; Reilly, G.C.; Zhen, X.; Yellowley, C.E.; Chen, Q.; Donahue, H.J.; Jacobs, C.R. Osteopontin gene regulation by oscillatory fluid flow via intracellular calcium mobilization and activation of mitogen-activated protein kinase in MC3T3–E1 osteoblasts. *J. Biol. Chem.* **2001**, *276*, 13365–13371. [CrossRef] [PubMed]

35. Praetorius, H.A.; Spring, K.R. Removal of the MDCK cell primary cilium abolishes flow sensing. *J. Membr. Biol.* **2003**, *191*, 69–76. [CrossRef] [PubMed]

36. Norvell, S.M.; Alvarez, M.; Bidwell, J.P.; Pavalko, F.M. Fluid shear stress induces beta-catenin signaling in osteoblasts. *Calcif. Tissue Int.* **2004**, *75*, 396–404. [CrossRef] [PubMed]

37. Pavalko, F.M.; Gerard, R.L.; Ponik, S.M.; Gallagher, P.J.; Jin, Y.; Norvell, S.M. Fluid shear stress inhibits TNF-alpha-induced apoptosis in osteoblasts: A role for fluid shear stress-induced activation of PI3-kinase and inhibition of caspase-3. *J. Cell Physiol.* **2003**, *194*, 194–205. [CrossRef] [PubMed]

38. Rangaswami, H.; Schwappacher, R.; Tran, T.; Chan, G.C.; Zhuang, S.; Boss, G.R.; Pilz, R.B. Protein kinase G and focal adhesion kinase converge on Src/Akt/β-catenin signaling module in osteoblast mechanotransduction. *J. Biol. Chem.* **2012**, *287*, 21509–21519. [CrossRef] [PubMed]

39. Triplett, J.W.; O'Riley, R.; Tekulve, K.; Norvell, S.M.; Pavalko, F.M. Mechanical loading by fluid shear stress enhances IGF-1 receptor signaling in osteoblasts in a PKCzeta-dependent manner. *Mol. Cell Biomech.* **2007**, *4*, 13–25. [PubMed]

40. Lee, D.Y.; Li, Y.S.; Chang, S.F.; Zhou, J.; Ho, H.M.; Chiu, J.J.; Chien, S. Oscillatory flow-induced proliferation of osteoblast-like cells is mediated by alphavbeta3 and beta1 integrins through synergistic interactions of focal adhesion kinase and Shc with phosphatidylinositol 3-kinase and the Akt/mTOR/p70S6K pathway. *J. Biol. Chem.* **2010**, *285*, 30–42. [CrossRef] [PubMed]

41. Bakker, A.; Klein-Nulend, J.; Burger, E. Shear stress inhibits while disuse promotes osteocyte apoptosis. *Biochem. Biophys. Res. Commun.* **2004**, *320*, 1163–1168. [CrossRef] [PubMed]

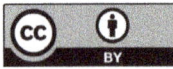